Cancer Immunotherapy
Principles and Practice

Cancer Immunotherapy
Principles and Practice

Second Edition

Editors

Lisa H. Butterfield, PhD
Vice President, Research and Development
Parker Institute for Cancer Immunotherapy;
Adjunct Professor of Microbiology and Immunology
University of California San Francisco
San Francisco, California

Howard L. Kaufman, MD, FACS
Clinical Associate
Division of Surgical Oncology
Massachusetts General Hospital
Harvard Medical School
Boston, Massachusetts

Francesco M. Marincola, MD
President and Chief Scientific Officer
Refuge Biotechnologies
Menlo Park, California

Section Editors
Paolo A. Ascierto, MD
Raj K. Puri, MD, PhD

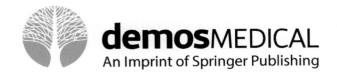

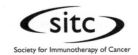

Society for Immunotherapy of Cancer

Springer Publishing Company, LLC
11 West 42nd Street, New York, NY 10036
www.springerpub.com
connect.springerpub.com/

Acquisitions Editor: David D'Addona
Compositor: Exeter Premedia Services Private Ltd.

ISBN: 978-0-8261-3742-5
ebook ISBN: 978-0-8261-3743-2
DOI: 10.1891/9780826137432

22 23 24 25 /7 6 5 4

Medicine is an ever-changing science. Research and clinical experience are continually expanding our knowledge, in particular our understanding of proper treatment and drug therapy. The authors, editors, and publisher have made every effort to ensure that all information in this book is in accordance with the state of knowledge at the time of production of the book. Nevertheless, the authors, editors, and publisher are not responsible for any errors or omissions or for any consequence from application of the information in this book and make no warranty, expressed or implied, with respect to the content of this publication. Every reader should examine carefully the package inserts accompanying each drug and should carefully check whether the dosage schedules therein or the contraindications stated by the manufacturer differ from the statements made in this book. Such examination is particularly important with drugs that are either rarely used or have been newly released on the market.

Library of Congress Control Number: 2021940388

Lisa H. Butterfield: https://orcid.org/0000-0002-3439-9844
Howard L. Kaufman: https://orcid.org/0000-0003-1131-004X
Francesco M. Marincola: https://orcid.org/0000-0001-6423-391X

Contact sales@springerpub.com to receive discount rates on bulk purchases.

Printed in the United States of America by Integrated Books International

Contents

Contributors

Eiman I. Ahmed
Research Specialist
Cancer Research Department
Sidra Medicine
Doha, Qatar

Michelle M. Appenheimer, PhD
Research Associate
Department of Immunology
Roswell Park Cancer Institute
Buffalo, New York

Paolo A. Ascierto, MD
Director
Unit of Melanoma, Cancer Immunotherapy and
    Development Therapeutics
Istituto Nazionale Tumori IRCCS—Fondazione
    "G. Pascale"
Napoli, Italy

Michael B. Atkins, MD
Deputy Director
Georgetown Lombardi Comprehensive Cancer Center;
Scholl Professor and Vice Chair
Department of Medical Oncology
Georgetown University Medical Center
Washington, DC

Deepti Aurora-Garg, PhD
Executive Director, Companion Diagnostics
Merck & Co., Inc
Kenilworth, New Jersey

Isabella Barajon, MD
Department of Biomedical Sciences
Humanitas University
Milan, Italy

Jürgen C. Becker, MD, PhD
Department Head
Translational Skin Cancer Research
German Cancer Consortium (DKTK)
University Medicine Essen
Essen, Germany;
Germany Cancer Research Center (DKFZ)
Heidelberg, Germany

Davide Bedognetti, MD, PhD
Director
Cancer Research Department
Sidra Medicine;
Adjunct Associate Professor
Hamad Bin Khalifa University
Doha, Qatar;
Associate Professor
Department of Internal Medicine and Medical
    Specialties
University of Genoa
Genoa, Italy

Nicky Beelen, MSc
PhD Student
Department of Cell, Developmental and Cancer
    Biology
Oregon Health and Science University
Portland, Oregon

John Bell, PhD
Senior Scientist
Centre for Innovative Cancer Research
Ottawa Hospital, General Campus
Ottawa, Ontario, Canada

Courtney B. Betts, PhD
Research Project Manager
Department of Cell, Developmental and Cancer
    Biology
Oregon Health and Science University
Portland, Oregon

Shailender Bhatia, MD
Associate Professor
Division of Medical Oncology
Department of Medicine
University of Washington
Seattle, Washington

Adrian Bot, MD, PhD
Vice President and Global Head
Department of Translational Medicine
Kite Pharma Inc.
Los Angeles, California

Julie R. Brahmer, MD, MSc
Professor
Department of Oncology;
Director
Thoracic Oncology Program
Johns Hopkins Kimmel Cancer Center
Baltimore, Maryland

Raphael Brandao, MD
Head of Oncology
Moriah Hospital
Sao Paulo, Brazil

Vincenzo Bronte, MD
Professor
Department of Medicine
University Hospital
University of Verona
Verona, Italy

Tullia C. Bruno, PhD
Assistant Professor
Department of Immunology
University of Pittsburgh;
Hillman Fellow for Innovative Cancer Research
Hillman Cancer Center;
Member
Tumor Microenvironment Center;
Member
Cancer Immunology and Immunotherapy
    Program
UPMC Hillman Cancer Center
Pittsburgh, Pennsylvania

Jack D. Bui, MD, PhD
Professor
Department of Pathology
University of California at San Diego
La Jolla, California

Lisa H. Butterfield, PhD
Vice President, Research and Development
Parker Institute for Cancer Immunotherapy;
Adjunct Professor of Microbiology and
    Immunology
University of California San Francisco
San Francisco, California

Lei Cai, MD, PhD
Research Fellow
Department of Surgery
Massachusetts General Hospital
Harvard Medical School
Boston, Massachusetts

William E. Carson III, MD
Professor of Surgery
Vice Chair for Promotion and Tenure
The John B. and Jane T. McCoy Chair in Cancer
    Research;
Associate Director for Clinical Research
OSU Comprehensive Cancer Center
The Ohio State University
Columbus, Ohio

Alessandra Cesano, MD, PhD
Chief Medical Officer
ESSA Pharma
San Francisco, California

Louis F. Chai, MD
Research Fellow
Immuno-Oncology Institute
Roger Williams Medical Center
Providence, Rhode Island

Damien Chaussabel, PhD
Director
Immunology Program;
Principal Investigator
Translational Systems Immunology Laboratory
Sidra Medicine
Doha, Qatar

Nai-Kong V. Cheung, MD, PhD
Enid A. Haupt Endowed Chair
Department of Pediatric Oncology
Memorial Sloan Kettering Cancer Center
New York, New York

Thinle Chodon, MD, PhD
Research Professor
Department of Obstetrics and Gynecology
Biological Sciences Division
The University of Chicago
Chicago, Illinois

Laronna Colbert, MD
Medical Officer
Office of Tissues and Advanced Therapies
Center for Biologics Evaluation and Research
U.S. Food and Drug Administration
Silver Spring, Maryland

Pierre G. Coulie, MD, PhD
Professor
de Duve Institute
University of Louvain
Brussels, Belgium

Lisa M. Coussens, PhD
Hildegard Lamfrom Chair in Basic Sciences
Professor and Chair
Department of Cell, Developmental and Cancer Biology;
Associate Director for Basic Research
Knight Cancer Institute
Oregon Health and Science University
Portland, Oregon

Razvan Cristescu, PhD
Senior Principal Scientist
Merck & Co., Inc
Kenilworth, New Jersey

Bruno Daniele, MD, PhD
Oncology Unit
Ospedale del Mare
Napoli, Italy

Greg M. Delgoffe, PhD
Associate Professor
Department of Immunology
Tumor Microenvironment Center
UPMC Hillman Cancer Center
University of Pittsburgh
Pittsburgh, Pennsylvania

Andrea De Maria, MD
Associate Professor
Department of Health Sciences, Infectious Diseases Unit
University of Genova;
Center for Excellence in Biomedical Research
Laboratory of Molecular Immunology
IRCCS A.O.U. San Martino IST
Genova, Italy

Olivier Demaria, PhD
Research and Development Director
Innate Pharma Research Laboratories
Innate Pharma
Marseille, France

Sandra Demaria, MD
Professor
Department of Radiation Oncology
Department of Pathology and Laboratory Medicine
Sandra and Edward Meyer Cancer Center
Weill Cornell Medical College
New York, New York

Diletta Di Mitri, PhD
Assistant Professor
Department of Biomedical Science
Humanitas University;
Principal Investigator
Tumor Microenvironment Unit
Humanitas Clinical and Research Center IRCCS
Milan, Italy

Alena Donda, PhD
Research Associate
Translational Tumor Immunology Group
Department of Oncology
Faculty of Biology and Medicine
University of Lausanne
Epalinges, Switzerland

Rebekka Duhen, PhD
Cancer Research Scientist
Earle A. Chiles Research Institute
Providence Cancer Center
Portland, Oregon

Jaikumar Duraiswamy, PhD
Biologist
Office of Tissues and Advanced Therapies
Center for Biologics Evaluation and Research
U.S. Food and Drug Administration
Silver Spring, Maryland

Eivind Valen Egeland, PhD
Postdoctoral Researcher
Department of Cell, Developmental and Cancer Biology
Oregon Health and Science University
Portland, Oregon

Colt Egelston, PhD
Assistant Research Professor
Department of Immuno-Oncology
Beckman Research Institute
City of Hope Comprehensive Cancer Center
Duarte, California

Femke Ehlers, MSc
Researcher
Department of Transplantation Immunology
Tissue Typing Laboratory
Maastricht UMC+
Maastricht, Netherlands

Kenneth Emancipator, MD
Executive Medical Director
Early Oncology Development
Merck & Co., Inc
Kenilworth, New Jersey

Leisha A. Emens, MD, PhD
Professor of Medicine
Department of Medicine
UPMC Hillman Cancer Center
University of Pittsburgh
Pittsburgh, Pennsylvania

Sharon S. Evans, PhD
Professor
Department of Immunology
Roswell Park Cancer Institute
Buffalo, New York

Chaohong Fan, MD, PhD
Lead Medical Officer
Oncology Branch
Office of Tissues and Advanced Therapies
Center for Biologics Evaluation and Research
U.S. Food and Drug Administration
Silver Spring, Maryland

Piera Federico, MD, PhD
Oncology Unit
Ospedale del Mare
Napoli, Italy

Robert L. Ferris, MD, PhD
Director
UPMC Hillman Cancer Center;
Hillman Professor of Oncology
Associate Vice-Chancellor for Cancer Research;
Co-Director
Tumor Microenvironment Center;
Professor
Departments of Otolaryngology, Immunology, and
    Radiation Oncology
University of Pittsburgh School of Medicine
Pittsburgh, Pennsylvania

Cristina R. Ferrone, MD
Associate Professor
Department of Surgery
Massachusetts General Hospital
Harvard Medical School
Boston, Massachusetts

Soldano Ferrone, MD, PhD
Professor in Residence
Department of Surgery
Massachusetts General Hospital
Harvard Medical School
Boston, Massachusetts

Thomas Finn, PhD
Microbiologist
Office of Tissues and Advanced Therapies
Center for Biologics Evaluation and Research
U.S. Food and Drug Administration
Silver Spring, Maryland

Alexandra K. Frye, MSc
Research Associate
Earle A. Chiles Research Institute
Providence Cancer Center
Portland, Oregon

David Furman, PhD
Buck AI Platform
Buck Institute for Research on Aging
Novato, California;
Stanford 1000 Immunomes Project
Stanford University School of Medicine
Palo Alto, California;
Austral Institute for Applied Artificial Intelligence
Institute for Research in Translational Medicine (IIMT)
Austral University
Buenos Aires, Argentina

Thomas F. Gajewski, MD, PhD
Professor
Departments of Pathology, Medicine, and the Ben May
    Department of Cancer Research
The University of Chicago Medicine
Chicago, Illinois

Pamela Gallagher, PhD
Scientific Reviewer
Division of Molecular Genetics and Pathology
Office of In Vitro Diagnostics and Radiological Health
Office of Product Evaluation and Quality
Center for Devices and Radiological Health
U.S. Food and Drug Administration
Silver Spring, Maryland

Lorenzo Galluzzi, PhD
Assistant Professor
Department of Radiation Oncology
Sandra and Edward Meyer Cancer Center
Caryl and Israel Englander Institute for Precision Medicine
Weill Cornell Medical College
New York, New York

Paola Ghanem, MD
Postdoctoral Research Fellow
Department of Medical Oncology
Johns Hopkins University
Baltimore, Maryland

Pier Federico Gherardini, PhD
Director
Department of Informatics
Parker Institute for Cancer Immunotherapy
San Francisco, California

Antonio Maria Grimaldi, MD
Vice Director
Unit of Melanoma, Cancer Immunotherapy and
    Development Therapeutics Unit
Istituto Nazionale Tumori IRCCS – Fondazione
    "G. Pascale"
Napoli, Italy

Alexander Guminski, MD
Associate Professor
Department of Medicine
University of Sydney
Sydney, Australia

Weihua Guo, PhD
Postdoctoral Fellow
Department of Immuno-Oncology
Beckman Research Institute
City of Hope Comprehensive Cancer Center
Duarte, California

Dave R. Gupta, MD, MPH
Fellow
Division of Hematology and Oncology
Emory University School of Medicine
Atlanta, Georgia

Omid Hamid, MD
Chief of Research and Immuno-Oncology
Co-Director
Cutaneous Malignancy Program
Cedars-Sinai Cancer
The Angeles Clinic and Research Institute
Cedars-Sinai Affiliate
Los Angeles, California

Farah Hasan, BSc
PhD Candidate and Graduate Research Assistant
Department of Melanoma Medical Oncology
The University of Texas MD Anderson Cancer
   Center
Houston, Texas

Priti S. Hegde, PhD
Chief Scientific Officer
Foundation Medicine, Inc.
Cambridge, Massachusetts

Yingxiang Huang, PhD
Bioinformaticist
Buck Institute for Research on Aging
Novato, California

Syed R. Husain, PhD
Senior Staff Scientist
Office of Tissues and Advanced Therapies
Center for Biologics Evaluation and Research
U.S. Food and Drug Administration
Silver Spring, Maryland

Muhammad Husnain, MD
Assistant Professor
Division of Hematology
Department of Medicine
University of Arizona
Tucson, Arizona

Shyam Kalavar, MPH, CT(ASCP)
Senior Scientific Reviewer
Division of Molecular Genetics and
   Pathology
Office of In Vitro Diagnostics and Radiological
   Health
Office of Product Evaluation and Quality
Center for Devices and Radiological Health
U.S. Food and Drug Administration
Silver Spring, Maryland

Noriyuki Kasahara, MD, PhD
Professor
Department of Neurological Surgery
University of California, San Francisco
San Francisco, California

Jakob Nikolas Kather, MD, MSc
Clinician
Department of Medicine III
University Hospital RWTH Aachen
National Center for Tumor Diseases
Heidelberg, Germany

Steven C. Katz, MD, FACS
Chairman
Immuno-Oncology Institute;
Chief
Immunotherapy Service
Department of Medicine
Roger Williams Medical Center
Providence, Rhode Island;
Associate Professor
Department of Surgery
Boston University School of Medicine
Boston, Massachusetts

Howard L. Kaufman, MD, FACS
Clinical Associate
Division of Surgical Oncology
Massachusetts General Hospital
Harvard Medical School
Boston, Massachusetts

Alper Kearney, PhD
Principal Scientist, Immunology
Astellas Pharma US
South San Francisco, California

Karin M. Knudson, PhD
Staff Researcher and Regulatory Review Fellow
Office of Tissues and Advanced Therapies
Center for Biologics Evaluation and Research
U.S. Food and Drug Administration
Silver Spring, Maryland

Sushil Kumar, PhD
Research Assistant Professor
Department of Cell, Developmental and Cancer
    Biology
Oregon Health and Science University
Portland, Oregon

Theresa M. LaVallee, PhD
Vice President
Translational Medicine and Regulatory Affairs
Parker Institute for Cancer Immunotherapy
San Francisco, California

Peter P. Lee, MD
Bill and Audrey L. Wilder Professor
Department of Immuno-Oncology
Beckman Research Institute
City of Hope Comprehensive Cancer Center
Duarte, California

Robert D. Leone, MD
Instructor
Department of Oncology
Bloomberg-Kimmel Institute for Cancer Immunotherapy
Sidney-Kimmel Comprehensive Cancer Research Center
Johns Hopkins University School of Medicine
Baltimore, Maryland

Ke Liu, MD, PhD
Chief of Oncology
Office of Tissues and Advanced Therapies
Center for Biologics Evaluation and Research
U.S. Food and Drug Administration
Silver Spring, Maryland

Michael T. Lotze, MD
Professor of Surgery, Immunology, and Bioengineering
Senior Advisor
Immune Transplant and Therapy Center
University of Pittsburgh Medical Center
UPMC Hillman Cancer Center
Pittsburgh, Pennsylvania

Jason J. Luke, MD, FACP
Director of the Cancer Immunotherapeutics Center
Division of Hematology/Oncology
University of Pittsburgh
Pittsburgh, Pennsylvania

Thomas A. Mace, PhD
Assistant Professor
Division of Gastroenterology, Hepatology and Nutrition
Department of Internal Medicine
The Ohio State University
Columbus, Ohio

Holden T. Maecker, PhD
Professor
Department of Microbiology and Immunology
Institute for Immunity, Transplantation, and Infection
Stanford University
Palo Alto, California

Luke Maggs, PhD
Research Fellow
Department of Surgery
Massachusetts General Hospital
Harvard Medical School
Boston, Massachusetts

Usha Malhotra, MD
Clinical Director
Merck & Co., Inc
Kenilworth, New Jersey

Alberto Mantovani, MD
Emeritus Distinguished Professor
Department of Biomedical Science
Humanitas University;
Scientific Director
Humanitas Clinical and Research Center IRCCS
Milan, Italy;
The William Harvey Research Institute
Queen Mary University
London, United Kingdom

Kim Margolin, MD
Clinical Professor
Department of Medical Oncology and Therapeutics
    Research
City of Hope Comprehensive Cancer Center
Duarte, California

Francesco M. Marincola, MD
President and Chief Scientific Officer
Refuge Biotechnologies
Menlo Park, California

William H. McBride, PhD, DSc
Emeritus Distinguished Professor
Department of Radiation Oncology
University of California at Los Angeles
Los Angeles, California

Inderjit Mehmi, MD
Department of Medical Oncology
The Angeles Clinic and Research Institute
Cedars-Sinai Affiliate
Los Angeles, California

Theodoros Michelakos, MD
Research Fellow
Department of Surgery
Massachusetts General Hospital
Harvard Medical School
Boston, Massachusetts

Lorenzo Moretta, MD
Director
Immunology Area
Ospedale Pediatrico Bambin Gesù
Rome, Italy

James J. Mulé, PhD
Associate Center Director
Translational Science;
Scientific Director
Cell-Based Therapies
H. Lee Moffitt Cancer Center & Research Institute
Tampa, Florida

David H. Munn, MD
Professor
Department of Pediatrics
Georgia Cancer Center and Medical College of
    Georgia
Augusta University
Augusta, Georgia

Dhaarini Murugan, PhD
Postdoctoral Researcher
Department of Cell, Developmental and Cancer
    Biology
Oregon Health and Science University
Portland, Oregon

Rita Nanda, MD
Associate Professor of Medicine
Department of Medicine
University of Chicago
Chicago, Illinois

Jean Philippe Nesseler, MD
Postdoctoral Fellow
Department of Radiation Oncology
University of California at Los Angeles
Los Angeles, California

Brian Niland, PhD
Biologist
Office of Tissues and Advanced Therapies
Center for Biologics Evaluation and Research
U.S. Food and Drug Administration
Silver Spring, Maryland

Y Nguyen, PhD
Gene Therapy Reviewer
Office of Tissues and Advanced Therapies
Center for Biologics Evaluation and Research
U.S. Food and Drug Administration
Silver Spring, Maryland

Kunle Odunsi, MD, PhD
The Abbvie Foundation Director of the University
    of Chicago Medicine Comprehensive Cancer
    Center;
Dean for Oncology, Biological Sciences Division;
Professor of Obstetrics and Gynecology
The University of Chicago
Chicago, Illinois

Hideho Okada, MD, PhD
Professor
Director
Brain Tumor Immunotherapy Center
Department of Neurological Surgery
University of California, San Francisco
San Francisco, California

Moshe C. Ornstein, MD, MA
Assistant Professor of Medicine
Departments of Hematology and Medical
    Oncology
Cleveland Clinic Taussig Cancer Center
Cleveland, Ohio

Patrick A. Ott, MD, PhD
Clinical Director
Melanoma Center and Center for Immunology;
Associate Professor
Department of Medicine
Dana-Farber Cancer Institute and Harvard Medical
    School
Boston, Massachusetts

Margaret Ottaviano, MD, PhD
Oncology Unit
Ospedale del Mare
Napoli, Italy

Graham Pawelec, PhD, MA
Professor
Department of Immunology
University of Tübingen
Tübingen, Germany;
Consulting Scientist
Health Sciences North Research Institute
Sudbury, Ontario, Canada

Ernesto Perez-Chanona, PhD
Postdoctoral Fellow
Laboratory of Integrative Cancer Immunology
Center for Cancer Research, National Cancer Institute,
    National Institutes of Health
Bethesda, Maryland;
Director of Business Development
CSSI LifeSciences
Glenn Burnie, Maryland

Lina Petersone, PhD
Postdoctoral Research Fellow
Division of Infection and Immunity
Institute of Immunity and Transplantation
University College London
London, United Kingdom

Giulia Petroni, PhD
Postdoctoral Associate
Department of Radiation Oncology
Weill Cornell Medical College
New York, New York

Reena Philip, PhD
Director
Division of Molecular Genetics and Pathology
Office of In Vitro Diagnostics and Radiological Health
Office of Product Evaluation and Quality
Center for Devices and Radiological Health
U.S. Food and Drug Administration
Silver Spring, Maryland

Emilie Picard, PhD
Postdoctoral Fellow
Health Sciences North Research Institute
Sudbury, Ontario, Canada

Gabriella Pietra, PhD
Associate Professor
UOC Immunology
IRCCS Ospedale Policlinico San Martino
Genova, Italy

Violena Pietrobon, PhD
Senior Scientist
Refuge Biotechnologies, Inc.
Menlo Park, California

Larissa Pikor, PhD
Senior Postdoctoral Fellow
Centre for Innovative Cancer Research
Ottawa Hospital
Ottawa, Ontario, Canada

Michael R. Pitter, BA
PhD Student
Department of Pathology
University of Michigan School of Medicine
Ann Arbor, Michigan

Amanda Poissonnier, PhD
Postdoctoral Research Fellow
Department of Cell, Developmental and Cancer Biology
Oregon Health and Science University
Portland, Oregon

Seth M. Pollack, MD
Sarcoma Program Director
The Steven T. Rosen Professor of Cancer Biology;
Associate Professor
Department of Medicine
Northwestern University
Chicago, Illinois

Jonathan D. Powell, MD, PhD
Professor
Department of Oncology
Bloomberg-Kimmel Institute for Cancer Immunotherapy
Sidney-Kimmel Comprehensive Cancer Research
    Center
Johns Hopkins University School of Medicine
Baltimore, Maryland

Raj Puri, MD, PhD
Director
Division of Cellular Gene Therapies
Office of Tissues and Advanced Therapies
Center for Biologics Evaluation and Research
U.S. Food and Drug Administration
Silver Spring, Maryland

Igor Puzanov, MD, MSCI, FACP
Senior Vice President
Clinical Investigation;
Director
Center for Early Phase Clinical Trials
Roswell Park Comprehensive Cancer Center
Buffalo, New York

Lei S. Qi, PhD
Assistant Professor
Department of Bioengineering
Department of Chemical and Systems Biology
ChEM-H Institute
Stanford University
Palo Alto, California

Raju R. Raval, MD, DPhil
Assistant Professor
Department of Radiation Oncology
The Ohio State University
Columbus, Ohio

Stanley R. Riddell, MD
Professor
Program in Immunology
Fred Hutchinson Cancer Research Center;
Professor
Department of Medicine;
Adjunct Professor
Department of Immunology
University of Washington
Seattle, Washington

Darawan Rinchai, PhD
Staff Scientist
Cancer Department
Research Branch
Sidra Medicine
Doha, Qatar

Brian I. Rini, MD
Professor of Medicine
Division of Hematology/Oncology
Vanderbilt University Medical Center
Nashville, Tennessee

Paul F. Robbins, PhD
Associate Scientist
Surgery Branch
National Cancer Institute
National Institutes of Health
Bethesda, Maryland

Jessica Roelands, MSc
PhD Student
Cancer Research Department
Sidra Medicine
Doha, Qatar;
PhD Student
Department of Surgery
Leiden University Medical Center (LUMC)
Leiden, Netherlands

Emanuela Romano, MD, PhD
Director
Department of Oncology
Center for Cancer Immunotherapy
Institut Curie
Paris, France

Pedro Romero, MD
Professor
Translational Tumor Immunology Group
Department of Oncology
Faculty of Biology and Medicine
University of Lausanne
Epalinges, Switzerland

Joseph D. Rosenblatt, MD
Professor
Division of Hematology
Department of Medicine
University of Miami Miller School of Medicine
Miami, Florida

Wendy Rubinstein, MD, PhD
Director, Personalized Medicine
Office of In Vitro Diagnostics and Radiological
    Health
Office of Product Evaluation and Quality
Center for Devices and Radiological Health
U.S. Food and Drug Administration
Silver Spring, Maryland

Ayana T. Ruffin, MS
PhD Candidate
Program in Microbiology and Immunology
Department of Immunology;
Member
Tumor Microenvironment Center
UPMC Hillman Cancer
Pittsburgh, Pennsylvania

Ananthan Sadagopan
Student Researcher
Department of Surgery
Massachusetts General Hospital
Harvard Medical School
Boston, Massachusetts

Robert Saddawi-Konefka, MD, PhD
Resident
Division of Otolaryngology-Head and Neck Surgery
Department of Surgery
UC San Diego School of Medicine
La Jolla, California

Margaux Saillard, MSc
PhD Student
Translational Tumor Immunology Group
Department of Oncology
Faculty of Biology and Medicine
University of Lausanne
Epalinges, Switzerland

Alexander I. Salter, MD, PhD
Postdoctoral Research Fellow
Program in Immunology
Fred Hutchinson Cancer Research Center
Seattle, Washington

Dörthe Schaue, PhD
Associate Professor
Department of Radiation Oncology
University of California at Los Angeles
Los Angeles, California

Nicole C. Schmitt, MD
Associate Professor of Otolaryngology
Co-Director for Translational Research, Head and
    Neck Program
Winship Cancer Institute
Emory University School of Medicine
Atlanta, Georgia

Joseph H. Schwab, MD
Associate Professor
Department of Orthopaedic Surgery
Massachusetts General Hospital
Harvard Medical School
Boston, Massachusetts

Cheryl Selinsky, PhD
Vice President
Research Operations
Parker Institute for Cancer Immunotherapy
San Francisco, California

Mihir M. Shah, MD
Assistant Professor of Surgery
Division of Surgical Oncology
Emory University School of Medicine
Atlanta, Georgia

Ragunath Singaravelu, PhD
Postdoctoral Fellow
Centre for Innovative Cancer Research
Ottawa Hospital, General Campus
Ottawa, Ontario, Canada

Shivani Srivastava, PhD
Assistant Professor
Human Biology Division
Fred Hutchinson Cancer Research Center
Seattle, Washington

Priyanka B. Subrahmanyam, PhD
Research Scientist
Institute for Immunity, Transplantation, and
    Infection
Stanford University
Palo Alto, California

Maya Suzuki, MD
Assistant Professor
Department of Pediatrics
Center for Clinical and Translational
    Research
Kyushu University Hospital
Fukuoka, Japan

Randy F. Sweis, MD
Assistant Professor of Medicine
Section of Hematology/Oncology
Committee on Immunology
Committee on Cancer Biology
University of Chicago
Chicago, Illinois

Zohreh Tatari-Calderone, PhD
Staff Scientist
Immunology Program
Sidra Medicine
Doha, Qatar

Marc Theoret, MD
Deputy Director
Oncology Center of Excellence
U.S. Food and Drug Administration
Silver Spring, Maryland

Victor Tieu, MS
PhD Student
Department of Bioengineering
Stanford University
Palo Alto, California

John M. Timmerman, MD
Professor of Medicine
Division of Hematology and Oncology
David Geffen School of Medicine at UCLA
University of California, Los Angeles
Los Angeles, California

Cornelia L. Trimble, MD
Professor
Departments of Gynecology and Obstetrics,
    Oncology, and Pathology
Johns Hopkins University School of
    Medicine
Baltimore, Maryland

Giorgio Trinchieri, MD
NIH Distinguished Investigator
Chief, Laboratory of Integrative Cancer Immunology
Center for Cancer Research, National Cancer Institute,
 National Institutes of Health
Bethesda, Maryland

Selma Ugurel, MD
Professor of Medicine
Department of Dermatology
University Medicine Essen
Essen, Germany

Nicolas van Baren, MD, PhD
Senior Scientist
de Duve Institute
University of Louvain
Brussels, Belgium

Ramjay S. Vatsan, PhD, CQA
Team Leader, Gene Therapy Branch
Division of Cellular and Gene Therapies
Office of Tissues and Advanced Therapies
Center for Biologics Evaluation and Research
U.S. Food and Drug Administration
Silver Spring, Maryland

Ilio Vitale, PhD
Group Leader
Italian Institute for Genomic Medicine (IIGM)
Torino, Italy;
Candiolo Cancer Institute, FPO - IRCCS
Candiolo, Italy

Massimo Vitale, PhD
Team Leader
UOC Immunology
IRCCS Ospedale Policlinico San Martino
Genova, Italy

Eric Vivier, DVM, PhD
Innate Pharma Research Laboratories
Innate Pharma;
Aix Marseille University
CNRS, INSERM, CIML;
Assistance Publique des Hôpitaux de Marseille
Immunology
Hôpital de la Timone
Marseille Immunopole
Marseille, France

Lucy S. K. Walker, BSc, PhD
Professor of Immune Regulation
Division of Infection and Immunity
Institute of Immunity and Transplantation
University College London
London, United Kingdom

Ena Wang, MD
Executive Director
Translational Oncology
Allogene Therapeutics
South San Francisco, California

Lei Wang, PhD
Associate Professor
Department of Immuno-Oncology
City of Hope Comprehensive Cancer Center
Duarte, California

Sarah Warren, PhD
Senior Director
Translational Science
NanoString Technologies
Seattle, Washington

Andrew D. Weinberg, PhD
Adjunct Professor
Departments of Molecular Microbiology and Immunology
School of Medicine
Oregon Health and Science University;
Member and Judith A. Hartman Endowed Chair
Laboratory of Basic Immunology
Earle A. Chiles Research Institute
Providence Cancer Center
Portland, Oregon

Mathias Wenes, PhD
Postdoctoral Fellow
Translational Tumor Immunology Group
Department of Oncology
Faculty of Biology and Medicine
University of Lausanne
Epalinges, Switzerland

Allen Wensky, PhD
Biologist
Office of Tissues and Advanced Therapies
Center for Biologics Evaluation and Research
U.S. Food and Drug Administration
Silver Spring, Maryland

Theresa L. Whiteside, PhD
Professor
Departments of Pathology, Immunology, and
 Otolaryngology
University of Pittsburgh Cancer Institute
Hillman Cancer Center
Pittsburgh, Pennsylvania

Jon M. Wigginton, MD
Chief Medical Officer
Cullinan Oncology
Cambridge, Massachusetts

Jacklyn Woods, PhD
Laboratory Manager
Department of Cell, Developmental and Cancer Biology
Oregon Health and Science University
Portland, Oregon

Teppei Yamada, MD, PhD
Research Fellow
Department of Surgery
Massachusetts General Hospital
Harvard Medical School
Boston, Massachusetts

Cassian Yee, MD
Professor
Department of Melanoma Medical Oncology
Department of Immunology
The University of Texas MD Anderson Cancer Center
Houston, Texas

Patricia A. Young, MD
Assistant Clinical Professor
Division of Hematology & Oncology
David Geffen School of Medicine at UCLA
University of California, Los Angeles
Los Angeles, California

Hua Yu, PhD
Billy and Audrey L. Wilder Professor in Tumor
    Immunotherapy
Associate Chair and Professor
Department of Immuno-Oncology;
Co-Leader
Cancer Immunotherapeutics Program
City of Hope Comprehensive Cancer Center
Duarte, California

Jianda Yuan, MD, PhD
Senior Medical Director
Division of Translational Oncology
Department of Early Oncology Development
Merck & Co., Inc
Kenilworth, New Jersey

Bryan S. Yung, MS
Graduate Student
Department of Pharmacology
University of California San Diego
La Jolla, California

Yu Zhang, MD
Research Assistant Professor
Division of Hematology
Department of Medicine
University of Miami Miller School of Medicine
Miami, Florida

Weiping Zou, MD, PhD
Charles B. de Nancrede Professor
Professor of Pathology, Immunology, Biology,
    and Surgery
University of Michigan School of Medicine
Ann Arbor, Michigan

Preface

Much has happened in immuno-oncology since the launch, in June of 2017, of the first edition of *Cancer Immunotherapy, Principles and Practice*. The field has been propelled by a surging tailwind incited by the awarding of the 2018 Nobel Prize in Physiology or Medicine to James P. Allison and Tasuku Honjo *"for their discovery of cancer therapy by inhibition of negative immune regulation"* and by innumerable approvals by the U.S. Food and Drug Administration of products related to immune modulation, adoptive cellular transfer, oncolytic viruses, and other therapeutics affecting the immune status of the host and/or of the tumor microenvironment. Several combinations and respective permutations have been tested in clinical trials. Advances have been made in the understanding of determinants of immune responsiveness and toxicity. Basic concepts have been explored in experimental models and through clinical observation such as the role of immunogenic cell death and mutational burden as alternative, yet nonexclusive, biomarkers of cancer immunogenicity. The roles of low-dose fractionated radiotherapy, chemotherapeutics, and pathway inhibitors have been tested in the clinic for their ability to induce antitumor immunity and as potential adjuvants to immunotherapy. Appreciation of the role of germline contributions to immune responsiveness and treatment-related toxicity has improved. A clearer categorization has been delineated about circumstantial influences that may affect a patient's ability to respond to immunotherapy such as environmental, behavioral, and anamnestic factors, as well as concurrent morbidities; among them, the role of nutrition and of the variability of the gut microbiota as modulators of patients' immune status. The importance of product *"fitness"* for adoptive cell therapy is increasingly appreciated as a determinant of clinical effectiveness and long-term benefit. This recognition, in turn, stimulates interest in the production of better cellular products not only by improving cell culture processes but also through the application of gene editing technologies and DNA targeting for gene expression modulation and cellular reprogramming without permanent structural alteration of the genome. On the analytical side, novel methods have improved the resolution of correlative studies including single-cell sequencing, high-parameter cellular and tissue profiling, multiplex/multidimensional platforms, high content bioinformatics, and artificial intelligence platforms.

These achievements constitute a fertile ground for continuous developments that pave the way to future innovation.

This plethora of developments has attracted to the field an ever increasing number of participants from industry and academia, spanning basic to applied sciences. Investments in biotechnology are converging from other areas of cancer research to test small molecules and chemotherapy agents that may cause immunogenic death of cancer cells, adding to their primary oncolytic purpose the attractive possibility of opening a therapeutic window for immunotherapy by temporarily converting immune-deserted tumors into immune-active cancer microenvironments. These are just a few examples of the expansion of an ecosystem attracting other scientific disciplines to explore their complementarity and impact on immune-based treatments of cancer, based on the premise that immune-mediated rejection of cancer leads to long-term benefit superior to results achieved with other anticancer modalities.

In these last few years, the involvement of clinicians in immunotherapy has rapidly expanded while skepticism is waning. A new generation of oncologists has emerged equipped with deeper understanding of experimental and clinical immunology, which better prepares them to deal with the unique pharmacodynamics of immunotherapy agents and the management of their toxicity in patients. Growing interest is reflected by the exponential growth in the number of participants to the Society for Immunotherapy of Cancer (SITC) Annual Meeting and the breadth of its activities rooted in the fertile ground of basic science and rapidly stretching toward application in clinical settings. Industry, investors, quality experts, payors, and other stakeholders interested in the financial repercussions of the expanding cancer ecosystem increasingly appreciate the potential impact of immuno-oncology on improving cancer patient outcomes. Increasing participation by a larger group of scientific, clinical, mathematical, and policy professionals in SITC activities fertilizes the quality of the Annual Meeting by including considerations that go beyond the realms of science and clinical practice into the benefit of a healthy financial future associated with longer patient survival that can sustain and prioritize immuno-oncology research.

Challenges remain and will keep us all busy. There are practical challenges, such as access to costly therapies in both experimental and clinical settings. In particular, the cost of adoptive cell therapies bearing genetically modified products such as chimeric antigen receptors or synthetic T cell receptors remains a challenge. New closed culture systems and improved products may streamline production, including the development of off-the-shelf allogeneic products that can be applied to broader patient populations. From the clinical development point of view, the costs of carrying candidate therapeutics from conception to licensing remain daunting. Still, no fully representative preclinical model has been defined to accurately predict the clinical effectiveness of candidate therapeutics; therefore, continued innovation is needed there as well. The accuracy of evidence-based tools that can guide patient selection during study design and feed the development of precision-guided therapeutics remains limited in spite of continuous technical advancements. More patient-derived biospecimen data needs to be accrued to develop useful surrogate biomarkers with compelling predictive and prognostic value. Attention to better understanding the causes of immune-related toxicities and strategies for preventing or treating these are also a high priority for the field.

In accord with the rapid development of the field, regulatory and payer agencies are still struggling to keep pace and ensure that rapid approval of promising drugs is rapidly translated to the clinic and ensure sufficient patient access. Finally, the ultimate beneficiaries of these efforts, the patients and their families, though increasingly empowered through open access information, need educational support to make truly informed decisions.

Conceptual challenges remain the salient ones: How can we match the mechanisms of action of a product with an individual patient's cancer immune biology? How can the benefit of immuno-oncology approaches expand to immune-resistant or non-immunogenic tumors? Adoptive cell therapy may offer the solution; however, besides its practical complexity, it still shows limited benefit in the context of solid tumors. The reasons for the difference in effectiveness remain manifold, spanning lack of trafficking to tumor sites, limited penetration into tumor nests, tumor heterogeneity, and subjection to overbearing immune suppression. The biology of immune exclusion (defined as accumulation of T cells around the periphery of tumor nests) remains paradoxical. In this case, trafficking may not represent a primary limitation as it could be assumed that the presence of endogenous T cells corroborates the existence of sufficient chemoattraction. Then, what can be done to overcome the mechanical and/or functional barriers that limit T cell penetration within tumor cells and, therefore, their effectiveness? More needs to be done to investigate this intriguing biology.

The SITC has expanded efforts to respond to the exponential growth of educational needs by offering primers at the Annual Meeting, itinerant courses to healthcare providers domestically and internationally, topical meetings and task forces addressing salient questions related to the field, specifying guidelines for patient toxicity management, policy and quality benchmark development, and informing on other themes as they emerge through the SITC portal. Partnering with other professional societies, nonprofits, and groups supporting patients and the field has broadened SITC's impact. In this context, SITC leadership decided to update, refine, and broaden the legacy established by the first edition of this textbook by providing a second edition that targets primarily young basic and clinical investigators but is informative to as many other constituencies as possible. The new edition updates chapters of the first edition while introducing new ones to cover emerging concepts.

It made sense that the original editors, supported by the SITC staff, assured continuity to the effort. As in the first edition, we included as contributors as many thought leaders as possible and we cannot thank them enough for their enthusiastic response. Chapters for textbooks can be painstakingly overbearing, but all contributors managed to complete their part to bring together cutting-edge insights that every translational investigator and practicing clinician needs to know about tumor immunology and immunotherapy. The textbook is still divided into five sections: Basic Principles of Tumor Immunology, Cancer Immunotherapy Targets and Classes, Immune Function in Cancer Patients, Disease-Specific Treatments and Outcomes, and Regulatory Aspects of the Biological Therapy of Cancer. We tried to cover through these sections the continuum from basic principles to practical and clinically relevant information to allow critical understanding of the development and testing of novel therapeutics, companion diagnostics, and useful biomarkers, and inform about the regulatory processes that support the safe and efficient delivery of immunotherapy to patients with cancer.

In addition, the chapter on the history of immunotherapy was not only preserved but updated to honor and recognize those who pioneered and championed the field along its ups and downs and provide the reader with a better appreciation of its evolution.

As mentioned in the first edition, we want to emphasize that the book is not meant to cover all aspects of tumor immunology, particularly those in rapid evolution. Indeed, the field is a compound science that includes two overlapping disciplines, immunology and cancer biology, that in turn include several aspects of human and experimental genetics, cell biology, molecular biology, systems biology, computational biology, epidemiology, and bioinformatics. Plenty of textbooks cover basic concepts relevant to the two areas and their related subdisciplines. In this textbook, we endeavored to focus on converging concepts and peculiarities relevant to the cross-talk between the host's immune reaction and neoplastic tissues.

Furthermore, we were concerned about producing a contemporary textbook reflecting as close as possible the current status of the field. However, considering the rapid evolution of cancer immunotherapy, particularly in the clinic, it is impossible to claim complete success: the number of successful clinical trials and corresponding regulatory licensing are still growing at an accelerated pace. Similarly, correlative studies are producing a wealth of new information that accumulates beyond the scope of the textbook. Thus, this book focuses predominantly on educating and guiding the neophyte through a critical interpretation of upcoming results and the development of solid foundations for the understanding of salient concepts related to efficacy and toxicity in experimental and clinical settings within the context of alternative treatments and potential combinations.

Because some areas are likely to progress more rapidly than others, we are planning to complement the information included here with additional updates presented as reviews in the SITC official journal—the *Journal for ImmunoTherapy of Cancer*—which in turn has experienced tremendous growth during the last few years. In addition, SITC has developed several initiatives and task forces tackling fundamental issues, whose outcomes can be easily followed through the SITC website (www .sitcancer.org).

We hope that the readers, especially those new to this exciting field, will enjoy this book and find in it useful information to complement the other SITC activities, and that they will be inspired to become active members of the rapidly expanding tumor immunology community.

Lisa H. Butterfield, PhD
Howard L. Kaufman, MD
Francesco M. Marincola, MD

About the Society for Immunotherapy of Cancer

Immunotherapy has become a cornerstone of modern cancer treatment, offering hopes of extended survival and disease control for many patients with malignancies that once carried universally dismal prognoses. Now considered by many to be a fourth pillar alongside the traditional triumvirate of surgery, chemotherapy, and radiation, the ascendancy of immunotherapy has by no means followed a straightforward trajectory. Indeed, in the very early days of the discipline, the very notion of immunological control of cancers was considered by many to be "witchcraft." Only thanks to the tireless efforts of innumerable practicing oncologists, basic and translational scientists, and clinical trial participants all along the bench-to-bedside pipeline has cancer immunotherapy become the standard of care—gaining many regulatory approvals, recognition by the Nobel Prize, and, most importantly, improving patients' lives. Throughout the years, the Society for Immunotherapy of Cancer (SITC) has supported these advances by pursuing its core mission to improve cancer patient outcomes by advancing the science, development, and application of cancer immunology and immunotherapy.

The SITC was established in 1984 by 40 founding members as the Society for Biological Therapy. Since then, SITC's membership base has grown to more than 4,600 people, representing greater than 35 medical specialties in 63 countries around the world. Although the society's name has evolved throughout the decades, the core values of interaction/integration, innovation, translation, and leadership in the field have remained a through line for SITC's aim to one day make the word "cure" a reality for cancer patients everywhere.

Founded with strong dedication to translational research—from bench to bedside and back—SITC has long been a unique nexus for diverse perspectives aligned toward a common purpose. Bringing together academicians, as well as industry and regulatory bodies, SITC became a leading force for advancing the science and application of cancer immunotherapy. Throughout the decades, the society has evolved and grown while always remaining dedicated to improving patient outcomes. That mission drives the society to foster connections between all aspects of the cancer immunology and immunotherapy community. As the field saw more and more successes, FDA approvals for immunotherapy accelerated, and immunological control of cancer became mainstream, the SITC community has expanded even further, now including many stakeholder groups such as community oncologists, oncology pharmacists, nurses, emergency department physicians, and patients and patient advocacy representatives.

Education has always been a cornerstone of the society's activities, both for the purpose of scientific exchange between its members, as well as introducing immunotherapy to a wider world of healthcare providers, researchers, and trainees who may be new or peripheral to the field. In addition to convening high-caliber scientific symposia, workshops, and conferences, the society provides ongoing education and outreach activities, including professional development courses for young investigators, collaborative endeavors with global oncology and immunotherapy societies, and ongoing educational opportunities. Additionally, the society's official journal, *Journal for ImmunoTherapy of Cancer*, is now ranked among the top oncology and immunology journals. Open access and peer-reviewed since its launch to ensure that top-tier research is freely available around the globe, the journal offers a venue for all of the immunotherapy community members to share their findings and access the latest research in the field. The journal publishes papers ranging from basic tumor immunology to clinical trial reports and clinical practice guidelines, and its individual sections are edited by leading experts from around the world in the numerous disciplines that encompass the immunotherapy field.

The SITC strives to advance the science and application of immunotherapy by advocating for research funding and support, setting standards, and identifying priorities for the future of immunotherapy. In addition, collaborations with like-minded domestic and international organizations, government and regulatory agencies, scientific associations, and patient advocacy groups allow the society to further enhance its impact. Through activities such as scientific publications, guidelines, and policy initiatives, the SITC serves as a beacon for the field, always imbued with the ultimate goal to improve outcomes for cancer patients everywhere.

This textbook, now in its second edition, was developed by the society to serve as a comprehensive reference that presents the history of the field, basic science, and current clinical application. The authors hope that this resource will help cultivate the next generation of leaders in tumor immunology and cancer immunotherapy, so that tomorrow's innovators will keep challenging the thinking and bring the field even further forward. It is an exciting time for cancer immunotherapy—advances in technology continue to add nuanced understanding to even the most fundamental principles of our field—and the SITC remains dedicated to advancing the discipline for many years to come.

Acknowledgments

As with any scientific endeavor, the writing of this textbook was a true labor of love and a collaborative effort, supported throughout the process in ways large and small by a great number of names. First and foremost, the editors extend their sincere recognition to patients and patients' families, whose brave participation in clinical trials has enabled so many of the lifesaving advances that are now standard of care. The editors also offer their deepest gratitude to the past pioneers in immuno-oncology who paved the way for the current renaissance in our field, as well as the volunteer leaders of the SITC, who nurtured this textbook through its inception, first edition, and this current update.

The editors thank the SITC for supporting the project. In particular, the authors wish a heartfelt thanks and their profound appreciation to Tara Withington, CAE, Executive Director Emeritus of SITC, whose pioneering vision and leadership throughout the years helped grow the society into the world-leading organization that it is today. Additionally, the editors thank the section editors for their tireless efforts in developing the high-quality scientific content found within these pages as well as the SITC staff, Matthew Erickson and Angela Kilbert, for their support throughout the writing process. Finally, the editors are grateful to the publisher, Demos Medical Publishing, and its staff, specifically David D'Addona and Jaclyn Shultz, for their assistance in the book development.

Abbreviation List

4-1BBL	4-1BB ligand
A2A	adenosine 2A receptor
AA	accelerated approval
AACR	American Association for Cancer Research
Ab	antibody
Ab3′	anti-carbohydrate GD2 antibody
ABZI	amidobenzimidazole
ACT	adoptive cell transfer
ADCC	antibody-dependent cellular cytotoxicity
ADCP	antibody-dependent cell-mediated phagocytosis
AE	adverse event
AFP	α fetoprotein
AHR	aryl hydrocarbon receptor
aKG	a-ketoglutarate
ALC	lymphocyte count
ALL	acute lymphoblastic leukemia
ALNs	axillary lymph nodes
ALT	alanine transaminase
AML	acute myeloid leukemia
AMP	adenosine phosphate
AMPK	adenosine phosphate-activated protein kinase
APC	antigen-presenting cell
ANXA1	annexin A1
AP-1	activator protein 1
AP2	adaptor protein complex
API	active pharmaceutical ingredient
APM	antigen processing machinery
ARG1	arginase-1
ASCO	American Society of Clinical Oncology
AST	aspartate transaminase
ATP	adenosine triphosphate
AVA	adventitious viral agents
B2M	β-2-microglobulin
B-ALL	B-cell acute lymphoblastic leukemia
BBB	blood–brain barrier
BCAP31	B cell receptor-associated protein 31
BCCs	basal cell carcinomas
BCDM	B cell-deficient mice
BCG	Bacillus Calmette–Guérin
BCL	B lymphocyte chemoattractant
BCMA	B cell maturation antigen

BCR	B cell receptor
BCT	blood collection tube
BiTEs	bi-specific T cell engagers
BLA	biological license application
BLADE	Boolean logic and arithmetic through DNA excision
BMS	Bristol Myers Squibb
B_{reg}	regulatory B
BTD	breakthrough therapy designation
BTK	bruton tyrosine kinase
bTMB	blood tumor mutation burden
BUF	buffer
C	cysteine
C/T	cancer/testis
C5aR	complement 5a receptor
CAFs	cancer-associated fibroblasts
CAIX	carbonic anhydrase IX
CALR	calreticulin
cAMP	cyclic adenosine monophosphate
CAR	chimeric antigen receptor
CASP2	caspase 2
CASP3	caspase 3
CASP8	caspase 8
CBM	CARMA1-BCL10-MALT1
CBTRUS	Central Brain Tumor Registry of the United States
CCL	CC chemokine ligand
CCR	CC chemokine receptor
CD	cluster of differentiation
CD	cytosine deaminase
CD200R	CD200 receptor
CDC	complement-dependent cytotoxicity
cDC	conventional DC
CDN	cyclic dinucleotide
cDNA	complementary DNA
CEA	carcinoembryonic antigen
CEACAM1	carcinoembryonic antigen cell adhesion molecule 1
CED	convention-enhanced delivery
cfDNA	cell-free DNA
CFRs	Code of Federal Regulations
CGAS	GMP-AMP synthase
cGMP	current good manufacturing practice
CGP	comprehensive genomic panels

CHI	checkpoint inhibitors	Cy/Flu	cyclophosphamide and fludarabine
CHL	classic Hodgkin's lymphoma	CyTOF	cytometry by time-of-flight
CHOMP	circuits of hacked orthogonal modular proteases	DAMP	damage-associated molecular pattern
CIK	cytokine-induced killer	DAMPs/PAMPs	danger- or pathogen-associated molecular patterns
CLIA	Clinical Laboratory Improvement Amendments	DART	dual-affinity re-targeting
CLL	chronic lymphocytic leukemia	DC	dendritic cell
CLND6	claudin 6	DCIS	ductal carcinoma in situ
CLTX	chlorotoxin	DDA	dimethyldioctadecylammonium
CMC	chemistry, manufacturing, and control	DDR	DNA damage response
		DFS	disease-free survival
CMC	complement-mediated cytotoxicity	DHFR	dihydrofolate reductase
CMV	cytomegalovirus	DIPG	diffuse intrinsic pontine glioma
CNS	central nervous system	DLBCL	diffuse large B cell lymphoma
CNS	conserved noncoding sequence	DLT	dose-limiting toxicitie
COA	certificate of analysis	DMG	diffuse midline glioma
COG	Children's Oncology Group	dMMR	deficient mismatch repair
CPI	checkpoint inhibitor	DOPE	dioleoylphosphatidylethanolamine
CPP	critical process parameter	DR3	death receptor 3
CPS	combined positive score	Ds	double-stranded
CPT	cell preparation tube	DSP	digital spatial
CQA	critical quality attributes	DST	desmosomal protein dystonin
CR	complete response	EAE	experimental autoimmune encephalomyelitis
CRC	colorectal carcinoma		
CREB	cAMP response element-binding	EBV	Epstein-Barr virus
CRF	case report form	ECM	extracellular matrix
CRI	cancer-related inflammation	ECOG	Eastern Cooperative Oncology Group
CRISPR	clustered regularly interspaced short palindromic repeats		
		eCTD	electronic common technical document
cRIT	compartmental radioimmunotherapy	EDTA	(ethane-1,2-diyldinitrilo) tetraacetic acid
CRP	C-reactive protein		
CRPC	castration-resistant prostate cancer	EFS	event-free survival
CRS	cytokine release syndrome	EGF	epidermal growth factor
CRT	calreticulin	EGFR	epidermal growth factor receptor
CSC	cancer stem cell	EGFRt	truncated epidermal growth factor receptor
CSF	cerebral spinal fluid		
CSF	colony-stimulating factor	EGFRvIII	epidermal growth factor receptor variant III
CSF1R	colony-stimulating factor 1 receptor		
CT	cancer testis	EIF2AK3	eukaryotic translation initiation factor 2 α kinase 3
CTA	cancer-testis antigen		
CTAG1B	cancer/testis antigen 1B	EIF2S1	eukaryotic translation initiation factor 2 subunit α
CTC	circulating tumor cells		
ctDNA	circulating tumor DNA	ELISA	enzyme-linked immunosorbent assay
CTGF	connective tissue growth factor		
CTL	cytotoxic T lymphocyte	EMT	epithelial-mesenchymal transition
CTLA4	cytotoxic T lymphocyte-associated protein 4	EMT6-B	EMT-6 tumor-educated B cells
		ENTPD1	diphosphohydrolase 1
CTX	cyclophosphamide	EOC	epithelial ovarian cancer
CX3CL	C-X3-C-motif chemokine ligand	EOP	end of production
CXCL	C-X-C chemokine ligand	EOPC	end of production cells
CXCL1	C-X-C motif chemokine ligand 1	EORTC	European Organization for Research and Treatment of Cancer
CXCL10	C-X-C motif chemokine ligand 10		
CXCL8	C-X-C motif chemokine ligand 8	ER	endoplasmic reticulum

ERBB2IP	Erbb2-interacting protein
ESCC	esophageal squamous cell carcinoma
ESMO	European Society for Medical Oncology
ETBF	enterotoxigenic B. fragilis
ETC	endogenous T-cell
Ezh2	enhancer of zeste homolog 2
FABP	fatty acid-binding protein
FACS	fluorescence activated cell sorting
FAK	focal adhesion kinase
FAO	fatty acid oxidation
FAS	fatty acid synthase
FBS	fetal bovine serum
FcgRIIb	Fc-g receptor IIb
FcR	Fc receptor
FDA	U.S. Food and Drug Administration
FFPE	formalin-fixed paraffin-embedded
FGF	fibroblast growth factor
FITC	fluorescein isothiocynate
FKBP	FK506-binding protein
FL	follicular lymphoma
FACS	fluorescence activated cell sorting
FOXC1	factor forkhead box C1
Foxp3	forkhead box protein 3
FRB	FKBP-rapamycin binding
FRC	fibroblastic reticular cell
FRET	fluorescence resonance energy transfer
FTD	fast track designation
GALT	gut-associated lymphoid tissue
GALV	gibbon ape leukemia virus
GAPVAC	glioma-actively personalized vaccine
GBM	glioblastoma
G-CSF	granulocyte colony-stimulating factor
GD2	disialoganglioside
GEJ	gastric/gastroesophageal junction
GEP	gene expression profile
GES	gene expression signature
GI	gastrointestinal
GIST	gastrointestinal stromal tumors
GITR	glucocorticoid-induced tumor necrosis factor receptor-related gene
GLA	glucopyranosyl lipid adjuvant
GM-CSF	granulocyte-macrophage colony-stimulating factor
GMP	granulocyte–monocyte progenitor
gp100	glycoprotein 100
GPCR	G-protein–coupled receptor
GSK	GlaxoSmithKline
GSK-3β	glycogen synthase kinase-3β
GVHD	graft-versus-host disease

GWAS	genome-wide association study
HA-1	histocompatibility antigen HA-1
HAMA	human anti-mouse antibody
HAVCR2	hepatitis A virus cellular receptor 2
HBP	hexosamine biosynthetic pathway
HBV	hepatitis B virus
HCC	hepatocellular carcinoma
HCV	hepatitis C virus
HDAC	histone deacetylase
HDACi	histone deacetylase inhibitor
hDCT	human dopachrome tautomerase
HER2	human epidermal growth factor receptor 2
hERV	human endogenous retroviruse
HEV	high endothelial venule
HGD	high-grade dysplasia
HGF	hepatocyte growth factor
HGSC	high-grade serous cancer
HIF-1	hypoxia-inducible factor 1
HIF-1α	hypoxia-inducible factor 1α
HIF	hypoxia-inducible factor
HLA	human leukocyte antigen
HLN	healthy lymph node
HMGB1	high mobility group box 1
HNSCC	head and neck squamous cell carcinoma
HPV	human papilloma virus
HR+	hormone receptor-positive
HRE	hypoxia response elements
HSC	hematopoietic stem cell
HSCs	hepatic stellate cells
HSCT	hematopoietic stem cell transplant
HSP90AA1	Hsp90 α-family class A member 1
HSPA1A	heat shock protein family A (Hsp70) member 1A
HSPA4	heat shock protein family A member 4
HSV	herpes simplex virus
HSV-1	herpes simplex virus type 1
HSV-TK	herpes simplex virus thymidine kinase
HVEM	herpes virus entry mediator
IAP	inhibitor of apoptosis protein
IBD	inflammatory bowel disease
ICAM	intercellular adhesion molecule
ICANS	immune effector cell-associated neurotoxicity syndrome
iCAR	inhibitory chimeric antigen receptor
iCasp9	inducible caspase 9
ICB	immune checkpoint blockade
ICC	investigator's choice chemotherapy
ICD	immunogenic cell death
ICD-O-3	International Classification of Disease Oncology
ICI	immune checkpoint inhibitor

ICOS	inducible T cell co-stimulator	KLH	keyhole limpet hemacyanin
ICR	immunologic constant of rejection	L1CAM	neural cell adhesion molecule L1
IC	immune cell	LAG	lymphocyte activation gene
IDH	isocitrate dehydrogenase	LAG-3	lymphocyte activation gene 3
IDO	indoleamine 2,3 dioxygenase	LAK	lymphokine-activated killer
IFN α	interferon-α	LAMP1	lysosomal-associated membrane protein 1
IFN	interferon		
IFNβ	interferon-β	LC-MS/MS	liquid chromatography/mass spectrometry
IFNγ	interferon-γ		
IFP	immunomodulatory fusion protein	LCMV	lymphocytic choriomeningitis virus
Ig	immunoglobulin	LDA	leukocyte-dependent antibody
IgE	immunoglobulin E	LDH	lactate dehydrogenase
IgG	immunoglobulin G	LFA	lymphocyte function-associated antigen
IgM	immunoglobulin M		
IgV	immunoglobulin variable	LLC	Lewis lung cancer
IHC	immunohistochemistry	LM	leptomeningeal
IKKα	IκB kinase α	LMP	latent membrane protein
IL	interleukin	LMS	leiomyosarcoma
IL-10	interleukin 10	LNP	lipid nanoparticle
IL13Rα2	interleukin 13 receptor subunit alpha 2	LOA	letter of authorization
		LOS	loss of function
IL-2	interleukin 2	LPT	local peripheral treatment
IL-2R	interleukin 2 receptor	LRP1	LDL receptor-related protein 1
ILA	induced lymphocyte activation	LSEC	liver sinusoidal endothelial cell
ILC	innate lymphoid cells	LSECtin	liver sinusoidal endothelial cell lectin
IMC	imaging mass cytometry		
iMCs	immature myeloid cells	LTFU	long-term follow-up
IND	investigational new drug	LT-α	lymphotoxin-α
iNOS	inducible nitric oxide synthase	mAb	monoclonal antibody
IO	immuno-oncology	MAGE	melanoma-associated antigen
IPEX	immune dysregulation, poly-endocrinopathy, enteropathy, and X-linked syndrome	MAGE-A	melanoma-associated antigen A
		MAGE-A3	melanoma-associated antigen A3
		MAIT	mucosal-associated invariant T
iPSCs	induced pluripotent stem cells	MAMP	microbe-associated molecular pattern
irAE	immune-related adverse event		
iRANO	immunotherapy response assessment for neuro-oncology	MAPK	mitogen-activated protein kinase
		MART-1	melanoma antigen recognized by T cells 1
IRES	internal ribosome entry site		
irRC	immune-related response criteria	MAS	macrophage antivtion syndrome
ISG	interferon-stimulated gene	MCA	methylcholanthrene
ITD	immune-mediated tissue-specific destruction	M-CSF	macrophage colony-stimulating factor
ITF	invasive tumor front	MDSC	myeloid-derived suppressor cell
ITIM	immunoreceptor tyrosine-based inhibitory motif	MESA	modular extracellular sensor architecture
iTME	immune tumor microenvironment	MHC	major histocompatibility complex
ITSM	immunoreceptor tyrosine-based switch motif	MIANA	minimal information about neoantigen assays
IUO	investigational use only	MIATA	minimal information about T cell assays
IVD	in vitro diagnostic device		
JAK	Janus kinase	MIBG	metaiodobenzylguanidine
KC	keratinocyte chemoattractant	MIBI	multiplexed ion beam imaging
KIM-1	kidney injury molecule-1	MLANA	melan-A
KIR	killer cell immunoglobulin–like receptor	MLKL	mixed-lineage kinase domain-like pseudokinase

MLTC	lymphocyte-tumor cell cultures	NY-ESO-1	cancer/testis antigen 1
MM	metastatic melanoma	ODE	ordinary differential equation
MMP9	matrix metallopeptidase 9	OPN	osteopontin
MMR	mismatch repair	ORR	objective response rate
MnSOD	manganese superoxide dismutase	ORR	overall response rate
moAbs	monoclonal antibodies	OS	overall survival
MPT	mitochondrial permeability transition	OTU	operational taxonomic unit
		OV	oncolytic virus
MRCL	myxoid/round cell liposarcoma	OXPHOS	oxidative phosphorylation
MRD	minimal residual disease	PAMP	pathogen associated molecular pattern
MRI	magnetic resonance imaging		
mRNA	messenger RNA	PANX1	pannexin 1
MS	mass spectrometry	PARP	poly-(ADP-ribose) polymerase
MSI	microsatellite instability	PB	peripheral blood
MSN	mesoporous silica NP	PBMC	peripheral blood mononuclear cell
MSS	microsatellite stable	PCAWG	Pan-Cancer Analysis of Whole Genomes
MTD	maximum tolerated dose		
mTOR	mammalian target of rapamycin	PCD	programmed cell death
mTORC1	mammalian target of rapamycin complex 1	PCNA	proliferating nuclear cell antigen
		PCR	polymerase chain reaction
MTPI	modified toxicity probability interval	PD	progressive disease
		PD-1	programmed cell death 1
MUC1	Mucin 1	PDA	pancreatic ductal adenocarcinoma
MUC16	Mucin 16	PDAC	pancreatic ductal adenocarcinoma
MVB	master viral bank	PD-1	programmed cell death 1
MVGTs	microbial vectors used for gene therapy	pDC	plasmacytoid DC
		PDGF	platelet-derived growth factor
NAS	nucleic acid sensing	PDIA3	protein disulfide isomerase family A member 3
NCCN	National Comprehensive Cancer Network		
		PD-L1	programmed cell death ligand 1
NCI	National Cancer Institute	PDT	photodynamic therapy
NCR	natural cytotoxicity receptor	PET	positron emission tomography
NDV	Newcastle disease virus	PFS	progression-free survival
NET	neutrophil extracellular trap	PGE2	prostaglandin E2
NFAT	nuclear factor of activated T cells	PHA	phytohemagglutinin
NF-κB	nuclear factor κB	PI3K	phoshoinositide 3-kinase
NGS	next-generation sequencing	PICI	Parker Institute of Cancer Immunotherapy
NHEJ	nonhomologous end joining		
NHL	non-Hodgkin lymphoma	PKB	protein kinase B
NICD	Notch intracellular domain	PKC	protein kinase C
NIR-PIT	near-infrared photoimmunotherapy	PMA	premarket approval application
NK	natural killer	PMEL	premelanosome protein
NKCEs	natural killer cell engagers	pMHC	peptide-major histocompatibility complex
NKG2D	NKG2-D type II integral membrane protein		
		PMN	polymorphonuclear leukocyte
NKT	natural killer T cell	pMO	patrolling monocyte
NLR	neutrophil-to-lymphocyte ratio	PNAd	peripheral node addressin
NLR	nucleotide-binding oligomerization domain-like receptor	PPA2	protein phosphatase 2
		PPAR	peroxisome proliferator-activate receptor
NO	nitric oxide		
NPCR	National Program of Cancer Registry	PR	partial response
		PRAME	preferentially expressed antigen in melanoma
NSCLC	non-small cell lung cancer		
NT5E	5'-nucleotidase ecto	PRC2	polycomb repressive complex 2
nUPLC-MS/MS	high-resolution mass spectrometry	PRIT	pretargeted RIT

PRR	pattern recognition receptor	sCD25	soluble CD25
PS	phosphatidylserine	SCFA	short-chain fatty acid
PSA	prostate specific antigen	scFv	single-chain variable fragment
PTEN	phosphatase and tensin homolog	SCID	severe combined immunodeficient
PTM	post-translational modification	SCLC	small-cell lung cancer
pT_{reg}	peripherally induced regulatory T cell	SD	stable disease
		SEER	Surveillance Epidemiology and End Result Program
PVR	poliovirus receptor	SERD	selective ER destroyer
QiP	quality in pathology	SGOC	serine glycine one-carbon pathway
RA	retinoic acid	siRNA	small interfering RNA
RA	rheumatoid arthritis	SIRPα	signal-regulatory protein α
RAE1	retinoic acid early transcript 1	SLE	systemic lupus erythematosus
RANO	response assessment in neuro-oncology	SLN	sentinel lymph node
		SLP	asynthetic long peptide
RASER	rewiring of aberrant signaling to effector release	SNAP25	synaptosomal-associated protein 25
RB	retinoblastoma	SNV	single-nucleotide variants
RBD	receptor-binding domain	SOC	standard of care
RCC	renal cell carcinoma	SPA	special protocol assessment
RCD	regulated cell death	SRS	stereotactic radiosurgery
RCV	replication competent viruses	SS	synovial sarcoma
RECIST	response evaluation criteria in solid tumors	STAT	signal transducers and activators of transcription
RET	rearranged during transfection	STING	stimulator of interferon genes
RFA	radiofrequency ablation	STS	soft tissue sarcomas
RFS	recurrence-free survival	SUPRA	split universal programmable
RFS	relapse-free survival	synNotch	synthetic Notch
RGMb	repulsive guidance molecule B	TAA	tumor-associated antigen
RIG-I	retinoic acid-inducible gene-1	TACE	transarterial chemoembolization
RIT	radioimmunotherapy	TAF	tumor-associated fibroblast
RLR	RIG-I-like receptor	TAM	tumor associated macrophage
RMAT	regenerative medicine advanced therapy	TAN	tumor-associated neutrophil
		TAP1	transporter 1, ATP-binding cassette subfamily B member
RNA	ribonucleic acid	TAP2	transporter 2, ATP-binding cassette subfamily B member
RNAi	RNA interference		
RNAP	RNA polymerase		
RNAseq	RNA sequencing	TA	tumor antigen
RNS	reactive nitrogen species	TCA	tricarboxylic acid
ROR1	receptor tyrosine kinase–like orphan receptor-1	TCGA	The Cancer Genome Atlas
		T_{conv}	conventional T
ROS	reactive oxygen species	TCR	T cell receptor
RP-HPLC	reversed-phase high-performance liquid chromatography	TCR-Seq	T cell receptor high throughput sequencing
rRNA	ribosomal ribonucleic acid	TCs	tumor cells
RRV	retroviral replicating vectors	TDB	trehalose 6,6′-dibehenate
RTK	receptor tyrosine kinase	TdLNs	tumor-draining lymph nodes
RUO	research use only	Teff	effector cell
S1P	sphingosine 1-phosphate	TET	ten-eleven translocation
SADA	self-assembling disassembly antibody	T_{EX}	exhausted T cells
		TEX	tumor-derived exosomes
SB	Sleeping Beauty	Tfam	transcription factor A
SBRT	stereotactic body radiation therapy	Tfh	follicular T helper cells
SCC	squamous cell carcinoma	TGF	transforming growth factor
SCCHN	squamous cell carcinoma of the head and neck	TGF-β	transforming growth factor beta
		TGF-β1	transforming growth factor beta 1

TGS	third-generation sequencing	TSA	tumor-specific antigens
Th1 and 2	types 1 and 2 of helper cells	TSCC	tongue squamous cell carcinoma
Th1	T helper cell 1	T_{scm}	T memory stem cells
Th17	T helper 17	TSLP	thymic stromal lymphopoietin
Th2	T helper cells	TSLPR	thymic stromal lymphopoietin receptor
TI	thymus independent		
TIDC	tumor-infiltrating dendritic cell	tT_{reg}	thymic T regulatory cell
TIGIT	T cell immunoreceptor with immunoglobulin and ITIM domain	TVEC	talimogene laherparepvec
		UC	urothelial cancer
TIL	tumor infiltrating lymphocyte	UCB	umbilical cord blood
TIM	T cell immunoglobulin and mucin domain	UHPLC/MS	ultrahigh performance liquid chromatography/mass spectrometry
TIS	tumor inflammation signature		
TKI	tyrosine kinase inhibitors	uPA	urokinase/plasminogen activator
TLR	Toll-like receptor	UPS	undifferentiated pleomorphic sarcoma
TLS	tertiary lymphoid structures		
TMB	tumor mutation burden	VAMP1	vesicle-associated membrane protein 1
TMB-H	tumor mutational burden-high		
TME	tumor microenvironment	VCN	vector copy number
TNBC	triple-negative breast cancer	VEGF	vascular endothelial growth factor
TNF	tumor necrosis factor	VEGFR	vascular endothelial growth factor receptor
TNFR	tumor necrosis factor receptor		
TNFRSF	tumor necrosis factor receptor superfamily	VLP	virus-like particle
		VRE	vancomycin-resistance enterococci
TNFα	tumor necrosis factor alpha	VSV	vesicular stomatitis virus
TPS	tumor proportion score	WES	whole exome sequencing
TRAC	T cell receptor alpha constant	WGS	whole genome sequencing
T_{reg}	regulatory T	WHO	World Health Organization
TRIF	TIR-domain-containing adapter molecule 1	WMS	whole metagenomic sequencing
		WT-1	Wilms tumor antigen 1
TRMN	tumor-rejection mediating neoepitope	WVB	working viral bank
		ZFN	zinc-finger nuclease

History of Cancer Immunotherapy

Michael T. Lotze and Michael B. Atkins

KEY POINTS

- The first cancer immunotherapies used nonspecific immunostimulants including oncolytic viruses with the then-unknown mechanisms of action that rarely limited tumor growth but provided impetus for creation of the Biologic Response Modifiers Program (BRMP) of the National Cancer Institute (NCI; prior to the 1980s).

- The second generation of immunotherapies utilized well-characterized recombinant cytokines including interleukin-2 (IL-2) and interferon alpha (IFNα). These agents were associated with substantial toxicity when utilized at effective doses but demonstrated objective responses in up to 25% of patients with less than 10% complete responses (prior to the 1990s). Most of the complete responses were durable for >10 years. Other cytokines, including IFNγ, IL-4, IL-7, IL-10, IL-12, IL-15, IL-18, IL-25, and so on, failed to provide substantive benefit, although anecdotal responses were observed. These two cytokines were the first effective immunotherapies.

- The third generation of immunotherapies utilized humanized and human monoclonal antibodies (mAbs) to cell surface receptor proteins present on tumor cells (human epidermal growth factor receptor 2 [HER2]/Neu, epidermal growth factor receptor [EGFR], etc.) and were integrated into cancer care (prior to the 2000s).

- Vaccination strategies using the available peptide, whole tumor, recombinant proteins, dendritic cells (DCs), and adjuvants were only modestly successful (heteroclitic glycoprotein [gp]100 vaccine with IL-2, anti-idiotype vaccines following effective chemotherapy, and long peptides for human papillomavirus [HPV] E6, E7 in precancerous lesions; prior to the 2000s).

- The modern era of immunotherapy launched with the extraordinary efficacy (and toxicities) of mAbs to immune checkpoints in patients with lung cancer, melanoma, renal cancer, bladder cancer, Hodgkin's disease, Merkel cell tumor, head and neck cancer, and over a dozen other malignances (2005–present).

- Current application of cellular therapies including chimeric antigen receptor (CAR) T cells and expanded tumor-infiltrating lymphocytes (TIL) engage the highly evolved communication network of immunity within the host, recognizing that T cells are the "drug," and represents early emergent therapies that have been or shortly (2020) will be realized after substantial steadfast cellular engineering (1990s–present).

- The modern treatment of patients with cancer has increasingly integrated immunotherapy with conventional surgical and radiation oncologic, chemotherapeutic, anti-angiogenic, vascular normalizing, and molecularly targeted therapy strategies (2018–present).

- Efforts are underway to develop biomarkers that identify how individual cancers evade the immune response and to provide precise therapies or combinations, where available, that disable these mechanisms as personalized therapies (the future).

The organism possesses certain contrivances by means of which the immunity reaction, so easily produced by all kinds of cells, is prevented from acting against the organism's own elements and so giving rise to auto toxins . . . so that one might be justified in speaking of a "horror autotoxicus" of the organism. These contrivances are naturally of the highest importance for the existence of the individual.

—P. Ehrlich and J. Morgenroth, Studies on Haemolysins: Fifth Communication, *Berliner klin. Wochenschrift* (1901), No. 10.

INTRODUCTION

Indeed, we live in an era where the "contrivances" have been identified and serve as a basis for the modern immunotherapy of cancer, utilizing checkpoint inhibitor antibodies to CTLA4 and PD1/PDL1 (Exhibit 1.1). The relationship between cancer regression and infection dates back even further to the 18th century, and perhaps earlier. Recognition of the relationship between erysipelas due to *Streptococcus pyogenes* and remission of tumors was first credited to W. Busch in 1866, and F. Fehleisen confirmed these results in 1882. In subsequent clinical work by Coley, the injection of toxins derived from bacteria (from *Serratia marcescens* and *Streptococcus*, Coley's toxin) into cancer patients to induce systemic inflammation led to tumor regression in rare patients, many of them with what were called sarcomas and possibly melanomas (also known as melanosarcomas in the past). The ability to capitalize on this observation was hindered by its rarity and the lack of understanding of the underlying biologic and immunologic processes. As a consequence, the field of cancer immunotherapy lay largely dormant for decades. Similarly, although viruses could be recovered from tumors, their first use as oncolytic agents, initiated in murine studies performed at Sloan Kettering by Alice Moore over 70 years ago, awaited modern virology and recombinant DNA technologies to evolve.[1,2] More modern applications, positing a role for oncolytic viruses to promote an expansion and recruitment of T cells, useful for ex vivo expansion emerged.[3]

In the 1950s, the notion emerged that factors derived from dead and dying (often irradiated) tumor cells could promote the growth of a small inoculum of tumors that would not otherwise grow in the mouse.[4-7] Although not understood at the time, the current appreciation of the role of damage associated molecular pattern (DAMP) molecules can be traced to these early studies.[8-10]

In the 1960s and 1970s, the reemergence of interest in cancer immunotherapy was focused on the intratumoral and systemic administration of bacterial products or extracts, such as bacillus Calmette–Guérin (BCG) and *Corynebacterium parvum* (*C. parvum*), to nonspecifically enhance overall immune function. Although the activity of these intratumoral injections was well documented, further development was hindered by limited insight into the concepts of unique or shared tumor antigens, the nature of antigen presentation and T cell recognition, the biology of dendritic cells (DCs), and the factors involved in stimulating, expanding, and maintaining an immune response.[11-18] Likewise, the critical alterations in cancer cells with either primary genomic instability (pediatric tumors, glioma, sarcomas) or secondary genomic instability (most adult tumors) subsequent to chronic inflammation were not fully recognized. Indeed, we now recognize that the *pas de deux* between the tumor and

the immune response has been carried out for more than 75–10 years before the tumor is recognized clinically. Individual loss of major histocompatibility complex (MHC) molecules, immune editing of particular oncogene mutations (e.g., p53), and immune infiltrate characterized by tumor-infiltrating lymphocytes (TILs) and tumor-infiltrating dendritic cells (TIDCs) are evidence of this ongoing dialogue. Indeed, the T cell response to tumor arises to recognize individual neoepitopes within the tumor, something abundantly apparent now,[19] but shrouded in the past by lack of a deep understanding of either tumor immunology or cancer biology.

In the 1970s and 1980s, lymphocyte CD4 and CD8 subsets were identified and cytokines such as the interferons (IFNs)[20] and interleukin-2 (IL-2)[21] that induced activation and proliferation of T cells and natural killer (NK) cells when administered to patients were explored. Furthermore, the advent of recombinant DNA technology enabled these cytokines to be produced in quantities sufficient to deliver pharmacologic doses to patients with cancer.[22] Studies with high doses of recombinant IL-2[23] produced durable responses in a small subset of patients with either metastatic melanoma or renal cell carcinoma (RCC). Administration of recombinant IFNα prevented tumor recurrence in a subset of patients with high-risk melanoma,[24] prompting U.S. Food and Drug Administration (FDA) approval of these agents—the first immunotherapeutics.

These nonspecific immune activators were associated with significant toxicities and in many patients induced the activation of countervailing immunosuppressive properties, greatly limiting their therapeutic index and overall applicability. Efforts to expand on this early success, through the development of combination regimens, investigation of other cytokines (IL-1, IL-3, IL-4, IL-10, IL-12, IL-18, IL-21, etc.), and application in other tumor types, were largely unsuccessful. Nonetheless, the initial studies with cytokines served as "proof of principle" that the immune system, if properly activated, could produce durable cancer control or "cure" in select individuals with specific tumor types, thus leading to sustained interest in the immunotherapy field.

The first evaluation of T cells as opposed to antibodies or cytokines was performed by Fefer, Cheever, and Greenberg[25] in the friend virus-induced leukemia (FBL3) murine lymphoma model. Subsequent studies in the Greenberg laboratory demonstrated that a second signal, normally provided by CD28 crosslinking by DCs, could be similarly provided by ablation of the E3 ligase, CBL-B.[26] In 1980, lymphokine-activated killer (LAK) cells were administered alone as the first cell therapy for cancer in patients, but without efficacy.[21,23,27-30] In late 1987, the results of adoptive transfer of LAK cells with IL-2 in 157 patients with advanced melanoma were first presented.[31] LAK activity mediated by IL-2-activated

NK cells and T cells was shown to have potent in vitro activity against non-cultured fresh tumor; however, combinations of IL-2 and LAK were found to have at best only modest advantage over IL-2 alone in prospective randomized studies, with about 10% deep complete responses.[32]

Identification of tumor antigens and insights into the biology of antigen presentation also yielded a large number of diverse and novel cancer vaccine trials. Sadly, most of the trials in patients with advanced disease produced low levels of objective responses, and most trials in the adjuvant setting eventually showed no meaningful benefit.[33] Studies with TIL confirmed that immune cells, if isolated from the tumor microenvironment and expanded in IL-2, could recognize tumor-specific antigens and mediate important antitumor effects. When administered to patients with melanoma following lymphodepleting chemotherapy, TIL combined with high-dose (HD) IL-2 could induce tumor regressions in many patients whose disease was refractory to HD IL-2 alone and served as the basis for the first gene therapy trials.[34–36] The investigation of TIL therapy prompted substantial evolution in the understanding of the requirements for the optimal application of this approach, including (a) use of tumor fragments to allow egress of TIL, (b) specialized culture flasks to allow more effective gas exchange, (c) application of nonmyeloablative chemotherapy to enhance homeostatic proliferation of the adoptively transferred cells with concomitant ablation of the residual immunosuppressive cells, (d) more rapid expansion of cells early in culture (young TIL), and (e) identification and selection of neoepitope reactive T cells.[37] In the setting of melanoma and anecdotally other tumors, objective response rates increased to as much as 56%.[38] Higher dose IL-2 regimens in melanoma also, by meta-analysis, appeared to enhance responses.[39] Together, these insights suggested that effective immunotherapy was frequently being limited by regulatory mechanisms for controlling immune activation and a potent immunosuppressive tumor microenvironment.

Subsequent research identified a raft of immunosuppressive factors, including cells, cytokines, and proteins (checkpoints), within the tumor microenvironment that dampened an ongoing or induced immune response (presumably limiting the "horror autotoxicus" noted previously). Many of these factors, particularly the immune checkpoints, were presented on the cell surface and therefore were targetable with specific monoclonal antibodies (mAbs). Remarkably, targeting of these checkpoints, particularly the programmed death 1 (PD-1)/programmed death ligand-1 (PD-L1) checkpoint, led to unleashing of the tumor-directed immune response in the tumor microenvironment and producing tumor regressions in a variety of tumor types with manageable toxicity.[40–44] These observations provided both an explanation for the previously limited effects of immunotherapy and a path on which to move forward. This chapter describes in more detail the history of immunotherapy (Exhibit 1.1), which laid the foundation for the current clinical promise of this approach and sets the stage for the more in-depth discussions throughout this textbook.

EXHIBIT 1.1 TIMELINE OF MODERN IMMUNOTHERAPY DEVELOPMENT

1940	• First viral oncolysis by Alice Moore at Sloan Kettering
1950	• Parke Davis takes Coley's toxins out of the formulary
1960	• Autologous and allogeneic melanoma cancer vaccines (subsequently disproved)
1970	• Intratumoral bacillus Calmette–Guérin
1980	• Lymphokine activated killer cells
1990	• Interferon alpha, Interleukin 2
2000	• Tumor infiltrating lymphocytes (TIL); gene marking
	• Chimeric Antigen Receptor T Cells (CART)
	• FDA approved the first cancer vaccine, sipuleucel-T (DC)
2010	• Immune checkpoints (CTLA4, PD1, PDL1)
	• Oncolytic herpes/GM-CSF approved
2022	• Predicted TIL approval for clinical use by FDA

FDA, U.S. Food and Drug Administration.

EARLY DAYS OF IMMUNOTHERAPY

Bacterial Toxins

If one were to trace the genesis of immunotherapy, the most appropriate place in the United States to begin might be in 1891, with William B. Coley.[45] Dr. Coley was a bone sarcoma surgeon at the Bone Tumor Service of Memorial Hospital in New York City. In 1890, Dr. Coley lost a young patient to Ewing's sarcoma and had sought to discover a more therapeutic course of action. He learned of a patient seen at New York Hospital 7 years prior with a non-operable neck tumor who had apparent resolution of his tumor following the development of erysipelas. Dr. Coley personally sought out this patient, a German immigrant in Lower Manhattan by the name of Stein. Years later, the patient still showed no signs of cancer recurrence. A remarkably similar story launched the career of Steven Rosenberg, who had a patient with an inoperable gastric cancer at the Roxbury Veterans Administration Hospital who many years later was found to have had a spontaneous regression confirmed during a cholecystectomy.[46] The first report of a relationship between erysipelas due to *S. pyogenes* infection and remission of tumors was credited to the German physician W. Busch in 1866. Other physicians such as Diedier, Paget, Bush, and Burns had noted a similar relationship between infection and tumor regression[47] based in part on Ehrlich's early side chain theory as a mechanism for immune recognition. Armed with these examples, Coley began to experiment with bacterial mixtures and devised what was to be labeled Coley's toxin, a preparation of chopped meat bouillon inoculated with *Streptococci* and *Serratia*, incubated for several weeks and then thermally sterilized.[47] He injected his first patient with this mixture in 1891 and observed shrinkage in the tumor soon thereafter. Spurred on by this initial success, Coley continued his injections and by 1895 had treated 84 patients with some additional successes.[47]

Despite this apparent promise, there was considerable suspicion in the scientific community about these observations for a variety of reasons: (a) Dr. Coley had poorly controlled and poorly documented patient follow-up[45] and (b) his toxins varied in preparation, effectiveness, and route of administration. As a consequence, he met with fierce resistance from many, including the head of Memorial Hospital, the famed pathologist Dr. James Ewing, who espoused the application of radiation therapy as a more effective therapy. Interestingly, some even questioned if Coley's patients had actually had a diagnosis of cancer to begin with. Nevertheless, Coley's toxin made its way into production in 1899 and was widely used and marketed for more than 30 years. Gradually, this toxin became less accepted as a useful treatment and

in 1952 its production was finally halted. Ten years later, the FDA denied recognition of Coley's toxin as a proven drug, rendering its use illegal.

Though Coley's toxin never regained its prior standing, his work was carried on by his children. His son, an orthopedic surgeon, continued to advocate use of the toxin as adjuvant therapy for patients with resected cancers. His daughter, Helen Nauts, a cancer researcher, tabulated hundreds of cases showing near-complete tumor regression and garnered enough support to found the Cancer Research Institute, which remains in existence today. Even a one-time rival, Dr. Codman, conducted a controlled study in 1962 showing dramatic response in 20 of 92 cancer patients.[48,49] Coley, for all the scientific community's disbelief, was on to something and consequently has come to be considered by many the honorary "Father of Cancer Immunotherapy."

Ehrlich's Magic Bullet

Paul Ehrlich was a Jewish internist practicing in Berlin in the late 19th century.[47] Early on he made contributions to the fields of histology characterizing granulocytes and mast cells. In 1885, Ehrlich began publishing his thoughts on the nature of cellular receptors.[50] He argued that the uptake of oxygen and other molecules required specific receptors and that harmful compounds took advantage by binding to these receptors. In 1897, three years after Hermann Emil Fischer postulated his "lock and key" model for enzymes, Ehrlich proposed his "side chain theory."[51] This stated that cells expressed side chains on their surface and that these side chains had the ability to recognize and bind specific molecules, which he called "antigens." Side chain binding of antigens promoted the creation of additional side chains that were released into the extracellular fluid to counter the antigen.[51] In 1900, Ehrlich renamed his receptive side chains "receptors."[51] Ehrlich began exploring the creation of chemicals that could target these receptors and how these chemicals could be made less toxic. He envisioned a Zauberkugel, a "magic bullet" chemical that would bind only with its target and therefore have no toxic effects. Ehrlich's "magic bullet" concept was primarily focused on infectious etiologies in his time. His laboratory was able to synthesize the antisyphilis agent, Salvarsan, the first "synthetic chemotherapy."[51] Salvarsan and its derivatives were the preferential treatment of syphilis until the arrival of penicillin in the early 1940s.[51] Years later, his idea of a chemical, able to specifically bind cellular structures, would have profound ramifications in targeted oncologic treatment and presaged the discovery of antibodies that could specifically block receptor–ligand interactions.

MONOCLONAL ANTIBODIES

The ability of the immune system to recognize foreign compounds and living organisms, and to produce proteins (antibodies) that react with them, is one of the crucial means by which the body defends itself against disease. Although each antibody targets a specific antigenic target, in a typical immune response to an illness, many different types of antibodies are produced in response to the variety of antigenic targets presented to the immune system. In addition, the so-called "Network Theory," advanced by Niels Jerne suggested that in response to the unique antibody 1 (the idiotype), an antibody 2 (the anti-idiotype) emerged that recognized the unique targeting antibody 1, and an antibody 3 (the anti-anti-idiotype) to Ab2, and so on.[52,53] The complexity of the immune response with NK, NKT, alpha beta T cells, and gamma delta T cells was only dimly perceived then and this notion of interacting networks among and between adaptive immune type should be reexamined. The ability to administer large numbers of antibodies targeting a single antigen presented on a particular cell was seen as a potentially valuable approach to cancer treatment—the realization of the "magic bullet" proposed by Ehrlich.

The use of polyclonal antisera was limited by the inability to reproducibly obtain high-titer antisera to tumors. Nonetheless, in the early 1960s, these techniques were able to identify several cancer-specific antigens, including carcinoembryonic antigen, alpha-fetoprotein, and even p53.[54-56] Cell surface antigens expressed by human cancers also included altered glycosylation of molecules such as Muc1[57] and a variety of targets that are overexpressed, mutant, or variably expressed compared with other tissues.

A transformative technology was the development of mAbs championed by George Köhler and Cesar Milstein.[58] This was accomplished by fusing myeloma cells with antibody-secreting mouse spleen cells that had been immunized against specific antigens. This technique, called *somatic cell hybridization*, produced a series of fused cells called *hybridomas*, each of which was immortal and secreted a limitless supply of a single mAb. This pioneering research by Köhler and Milstein led to their sharing the 1984 Nobel Prize in Physiology or Medicine with Niels Jerne and launched the era of antibody therapy. Interestingly, they promoted use of mAbs to help mankind and it was Croce and Koprowski[59] who demonstrated their therapeutic use, leading to several modern biotech companies developing these strategies for clinical use (Centocor, Amgen, Immunex, and Genentech).

Early efforts used murine mAbs[60] that could bind and image tumor, but were limited in their effectiveness by their immunogenicity. Subsequent work was able to create mAbs that were either chimeric or fully human, enabling them to be administered to patients without triggering an anti-antibody immune response that caused both toxicity and their prompt elimination. Subsequent efforts focused on targeting individual tumor molecules were able to surmount the considerable obstacles in target and construct selection and highlight potentially supportive and limiting roles of the immune system, ultimately transforming mAbs into agents for human cancer therapy.

mAbs have proven to be powerful additions to the therapeutic armamentarium for a wide range of human diseases, including many types of cancer. The class of antibody most frequently used clinically is immunoglobin G (IgG). IgG is further divided into subclasses, each with unique and sometimes overlapping properties, including the ability not only to target and interfere with cell signaling but also to induce cell death through properties of their Fc domains,[61] enabling antibody-dependent cellular toxicity (ADCC).[62,63]

The initial focus of antibody-mediated cancer therapy was to target cell surface proteins that are aberrantly expressed on tumor cells. Trastuzumab, pertuzumab, and cetuximab, mAbs that target the receptors of the epidermal growth factor family, have been FDA approved for the treatment of subsets of patients with breast or colon cancer. By directly binding to these membrane-bound receptors, these antibodies inhibit the receptors' activity, resulting in dampened function of the downstream signaling cascades.

The company IDEC was initially charged with developing anti-idiotypic antibodies to tumor-specific antibody molecules expressed on the cell surface.[64] This was only possible in about a quarter of the patients with lymphoma, and Nabil Hanna reasoned that perhaps an antibody to all B cells might be useful, leading to the development and approval by the FDA of rituximab for certain B cell non-Hodgkin lymphomas, the first mAb therapy approved for treating cancer patients. A growing body of work has demonstrated that both the variable and constant regions mediate the effects of rituximab by inducing complement-dependent cytotoxicity (CDC) and ADCC.[65]

This information has led to the development of novel anti-CD20 antibodies selected for their superiority in inducing CDC and ADCC based on their physical properties that may alter binding with Fc receptors on immune effector cells.[66] Other clinically useful direct targets of mAbs in cancer therapy include vascular endothelial growth factor (VEGF; bevacizumab) and receptor activator of nuclear factor kappa-B ligand (RANK-L; denosumab); however, efforts to target other proteins such as SMADc and the insulin-like growth factor receptor have been unsuccessful.

A variety of toxin-conjugated antibodies and so-called bytes using antibodies to CD3 crosslinked to antibodies to other molecules such as CD19 have also obtained recent FDA approval. However, the remarkable success of the checkpoint inhibitor antibodies targeting cytotoxic T lymphocyte–associated protein 4 (CTLA-4), PD-1, and PD-L1 over the past decade have made antibodies the most versatile and effective of anticancer agents. These checkpoint inhibitor antibodies function by essentially taking the physiologic brakes off of T cells, immune cells with innate cytolytic properties, enabling restoration of effective antitumor tumor activity. Checkpoint inhibitor antibodies have revitalized interest in immunotherapy and are proving to be the backbone for the lion's share of immunotherapy research.

Bacillus Calmette–Guérin and *Corynebacterium parvum*

The next advance in immunotherapy came during the 1970s from an unlikely source. The scourge of the 19th century, tuberculosis, would prove a bellwether for immunotherapy. In 1929, Raymond Pearl first reported an inverse association between cancer and tuberculosis in autopsy patients.[67] Subsequently, in 1935, Holgren reported successful treatment of some gastric cancer patients with BCG.[67] Years later, Rosenthal noted that the reticuloendothelial system could be activated by BCG.[68] Armed with this information, Old et al. in the 1960s showed that BCG had activity against experimental tumors in mouse models.[69] Then, in 1974, Morton treated 151 patients with melanoma by direct intratumoral injection of BCG, and noted that a fourth of those patients remained free of disease for 1–6 years.[70] According to Morton's initial report, 91% of melanoma nodules injected had complete regression and 70% of uninjected melanoma nodules had regression.[70] These observations led Morton and colleagues to include BCG as a vaccine adjuvant administered to patients with resected stage III and IV melanoma, an approach that continued to be investigated into the early 21st century before it was ultimately shown to be inferior to BCG alone in phase III trials.[70] These results, while ending the study of canvaxin, an allogeneic irradiated melanoma vaccine (see subsequently), left open the possibility that BCG injection, by itself, may produce beneficial effects.

Another area where BCG immunotherapy was actively investigated was in the treatment of non-muscle-invasive bladder cancer. Coe and Feldman[71] first described a delayed hypersensitivity reaction in the bladder following injection of live BCG in 1966.[67] Then, in 1976, Morales[72] reported on a clinical trial of nine patients with recurrent superficial bladder cancer given six weekly treatments of intravesical BCG. He observed a 12-fold reduction in bladder tumor recurrence compared with historical controls. A follow-up controlled study by Lamm et al.[73] confirmed reduction in tumor recurrence with intravesical administration, leading to its FDA approval for treatment of carcinoma in situ of the bladder in 1989,[72] perhaps the longest period between the development of a drug (1920s) and its approval. This approval was expanded to include Ta or T1 papillary tumors of the bladder in 1998. Intravesical BCG continues to be used for the treatment of patients with recurrent superficial bladder cancer and although its precise mechanism of action is not fully understood, BCG continues to be a component of combination immunotherapy regimens for this disease.

Alongside BCG, *C. parvum* injection also generated interest as a potential cancer immunotherapy. Currie showed that intradermal *C. parvum* following cyclophosphamide produced complete and lasting regression in murine models.[74] The time from chemotherapy to immunotherapy was noted to be critical, with a 12-day interval curing 70% of the mice.[74] More recently Zitvogel and colleagues have demonstrated that so-called immunogenic chemotherapy is dependent on HMGB1 and ATP release (as DAMPs) and calreticulin exposure.

Despite this early data, a clinical trial in patients with melanoma comparing surgical excision with and without adjuvant *C. parvum* injections showed no survival difference at 3 years.[75] However, a subset analysis of patients with melanomas greater than 3 mm in thickness showed a 73% 3-year[75] disease-free survival rate in the *C. parvum* group versus 33% in the operation alone control group,[75] suggesting a possible value of this approach in patients with higher-risk melanomas. This observation was never pursued in a subsequent trial and therefore remains to be validated.

CYTOKINES AND NONSPECIFIC IMMUNE ACTIVATORS

Cytokines, literally "cell movers," are secreted proteins that have pleiotropic effects, including regulation of innate immunity, adaptive immunity, and hematopoiesis. Distinct cytokines often have overlapping effects providing a level of redundancy to the immune system; indeed, the characteristics of cytokines include redundancy, pleiotropism, synergy, and antagonism. The first cytokines identified for cancer treatment were the IFNs. The name *interferon* was adopted based on the ability of these agents to "interfere" with viral infection of cells. Subsequently, many characterized cytokines were referred to as interleukins because they were principally produced by and acted on leukocytes, primarily released following folding and posttranslational modification in the Golgi, and subsequent clipping of a leader sequence. They are joined by the tumor necrosis factor (TNF) family of cytokines, the transforming growth factor-beta

(TGF-β) family of cytokines, and the so-called leaderless cytokines high mobility group Box 1 (HMGB1), the fibroblast growth factors (FGFs), and the extended IL-1 family (IL-1α and β, IL-18, IL-33, and IL-37 and IL-38).

Cytokines play a critical role in the recognition, persistence, and elimination of malignancies by the immune system. Mice that are deficient in IFNγ, the type I or type II IFN receptors, or elements of their downstream signal transduction intermediates have a higher frequency of tumors compared to control mice.[76,77] Thus, cytokines play a critical role in immune surveillance, further promoting consideration of their use as cancer immunotherapeutics. The development of recombinant DNA technology allowed production of cytokines in sufficient quantities to enable their utility as antitumor agents to be tested in the clinic.

Interferon

IFNα, initially referred to as leukocyte IFN, is comprised of a group of at least 12 distinct proteins[78] encoded by 13 distinct genes. These are IFNα1, IFNα2, IFNα4, IFNα5, IFNα6, IFNα7, IFNα8, IFNα10, IFNα13, IFNα14, IFNα16, IFNα17, and IFNα21. Only single copies of the other type I IFNs, IFN-beta (IFNβ), IFN-epsilon, IFN-kappa, and IFN-omega genes are found, with the human IFNα gene family sharing 70% to 80% amino acid homology, and 35% with IFNβ. Recombinant IFNα2a, IFNα2b, and IFNα2c differ by one to two amino acids and are the forms of IFNα that have been tested clinically.[78] In the United States, IFNα2a is sold under the trade name Roferon (Roche) and IFNα2b is available as Intron A (Merck). IFNα2c is available in Europe as Berofor (Bender). These compounds have never been compared in a randomized fashion; however, their spectrum of activity is likely to be quite similar. Soon after their development, these agents were tested in virtually every cancer type and showed reproducible efficacy in a few diverse settings. The antitumor effects were sufficient to support FDA approval for IFN in patients with hairy cell leukemia (HCL), chronic myelogenous leukemia (CML), RCC (in combination with bevacizumab), and as adjuvant therapy for patients with resected high-risk melanoma.[79] Subsequently, IFNαs, conjugated to polymer polyethylene glycol (PEG)–IFN, to increase the half-life and allow for longer dosing intervals and long exposure times, have been introduced.[80] Pegylated IFNα2a (Pegasys, Roche) and pegylated IFNα2b (PEG-Intron, Merck) are the two forms of PEG–IFN that are available in the United States.[81,82] These agents are widely used in combination with ribavirin in the treatment of hepatitis C and have gained approval as adjuvant treatment for patients with stage III melanoma,[83] now largely supplanted by checkpoint inhibitors.[84–88]

IFNs have a pleiotropic mechanism of action. In HCL, CML, and RCC, IFN's mechanism of action appears to be more antiproliferative or antiangiogenic rather than immune based, as continued administration appeared to be necessary to maintain benefit. Although IFNs were initially viewed as breakthrough therapies in these three diseases, their use was soon superseded by agents that more directly inhibit relevant tumor cell pathways in each malignancy (e.g., pentostatin, imatinib, and the VEGF pathway inhibitors).

In contrast, IFNs exhibited more typical immune effects in patients with melanoma. Responses to single-agent IFNs in patients with metastatic melanoma were observed in approximately 15% of patients, with those with low metastatic tumor burden responding best, perhaps presaging its clinical activity in the adjuvant setting.[89] A maximally tolerated dose regimen of IFNα2B involving a 4-week intravenous induction followed by a year of subsequent maintenance was developed by Kirkwood et al. and tested in the adjuvant setting in a series of Eastern Cooperative Oncology Group coordinated trials.[90] A similar set of trials was carried out in Europe, largely involving lower or intermediate doses of IFNα2A.[91–93] In the aggregate, these studies showed an approximately 1-year delay in median relapse-free survival, a 20% relative reduction in relapse, and an 11% relative reduction in death in patients with high-risk melanoma.[94] This high dose (HD) IFN regimen showed the most robust impact on overall survival, leading to its FDA approval in the United States in 1996. This survival benefit, though small, was associated with autoimmune phenomena such as vitiligo, thyroid dysfunction, and increased titers of autoantibodies,[95] suggesting a T cell–mediated immune mechanism of action and establishing these factors as hallmarks of effective immunotherapy, at least in patients with melanoma. It is unclear whether a survival advantage or similar immune effects occur with lower or intermediate-dose IFN or PEG–IFN in patients with advanced melanoma, suggesting that the HD bolus induction period might be essential to activating the critical components of the immune system.

The toxicities of IFN therapy can be broken down into five major categories: constitutional, neuropsychiatric, gastrointestinal, hematologic, and autoimmune. Constitutional symptoms are the most common, with more than 80% of patients in the HD IFN trials reporting fever and fatigue.[96] Additionally, more than half report headache and myalgias.[96] The majority of these symptoms can be controlled with nonsteroidal anti-inflammatory drugs (NSAIDs); however, severe fatigue often requires a treatment hiatus with a subsequent dose reduction for amelioration. This considerable toxicity for HD IFN, together with its marginal survival benefit, has increasingly limited its use even in the adjuvant setting and highlighted the need for more effective adjuvant treatments for patients with high-risk melanoma.

High-Dose IL-2

In 1976, Morgan, Ruscetti and Gallo demonstrated the existence of a growth factor present in the conditioned medium of lectin-stimulated human peripheral blood mononuclear cells that could indefinitely sustain the ex vivo proliferation of human T cells.[97] Interestingly, this factor capable of expanding T cells was discarded because it did not expand leukemic cells, as the Gallo lab was seeking. A visiting Israeli scientist, Isaac Witz, was surprised that they could grow T cells and encouraged them to report their findings. This initial report was followed in short order by the isolation, biochemical characterization, and, ultimately, the cloning of what was then termed T cell growth factor (TCGF).[98] Subsequently designated IL-2, this factor was shown to be a 15 kDa polypeptide made up of 153 amino acids, the first 20 of which form a signal sequence that undergoes proteolytic cleavage during secretion (as a member of the "leadered" group of cytokines). The molecule has cysteine residues at positions 58, 105, and 125, the first two of which form an intramolecular disulfide bridge. The third cysteine is not essential for biological activity and can be replaced with alternative amino acids to minimize polymerization and increase shelf life—an approach taken in the development of the recombinant human IL-2, aldesleukin (Proleukin) initially developed by Cetus, then Chiron, then Novartis, then Prometheus/Nestle and now distributed by Clinigen. Several other IL-2 analogues are now in testing efforts designed to limit support of regulatory T cells (T_{reg} cells).[99]

In addition to its proliferative effects, IL-2 induces a capillary leak syndrome allowing tissue entry of immune cells as well as the synthesis of an array of secondary cytokines, including HMGB1, IL-1β, IFNγ, TNF, IL-5, IL-6, and lymphotoxin.[100] Several of these secondary cytokines are detectable in the circulation of patients with cancer receiving IL-2 immunotherapy (see subsequently) and thought by many investigators to contribute to the side effects of IL-2.[101] The biological effect of IL-2 arguably most pertinent to its use as an antitumor agent may be its ability to enhance the cytolytic activity of antigen-specific cytotoxic T cells (CTLs) and NK cells,[102] promoting the increase in perforin and granzyme B.

Based on these in vitro studies, IL-2 underwent extensive evaluation as an antitumor agent in a variety of murine tumor models. In these models, IL-2—used either alone, in combination with other cytokines, or in conjunction with the adoptive transfer of various ex vivo–activated lymphoid cells—eradicated a wide range of local and metastatic tumors. Early studies demonstrated that IL-2 used alone could reduce or eliminate pulmonary metastases from methylcholanthrene-induced sarcoma and melanoma cell lines and that this antitumor effect was strictly dependent on the dose of IL-2 administered.[103] In some animal models, tumor eradication by IL-2 administration resulted in immunization against the tumor. In other studies, in which mice were immunized with DCs pulsed with tumor lysates, the concurrent systemic administration of IL-2 enhanced the efficacy of the vaccine.[104] In several studies, the effects of IL-2 could be enhanced by the concurrent administration of LAK cells generated by culturing splenocytes ex vivo in media containing IL-2.[105] Mice bearing hepatic micrometastases from poorly immunogenic mouse colon adenocarcinoma-105 (MCA-105) or MCA-102 sarcomas or MC-38 adenocarcinoma cells, for example, were highly responsive to treatment with the combination of IL-2 and LAK cells, but unresponsive to LAK cells alone and only partially responsive to IL-2. In pulmonary metastases models, NK cells could be eliminated at day (D) 7 following tumor injection without impact on tumor response, but this elimination of NK cells at D3 partially abrogated the effects of IL-2 therapy. Furthermore, when TIL were isolated, activated with IL-2, and tested in vitro for cytolytic activity against autologous tumor cells, they were shown to be 50- to 100-fold more potent than IL-2-activated splenocytes (LAK cells).[106]

Taken all together, this preclinical work laid the foundation for clinical studies with IL-2. Although initial studies with purified IL-2 showed limited efficacy, studies with recombinant human IL-2 (aldesleukin) enabled dose escalation to maximally tolerated doses, which when combined with LAK cells produced groundbreaking antitumor efficacy. In initial studies performed by Rosenberg, Lotze, and colleagues at the National Cancer Institute (NCI) Surgery Branch (NCI SB), tumor responses were observed in more than 30% of patients with advanced melanoma and kidney cancer.[103] This remarkable result generated substantial enthusiasm for the promise of immunotherapy, leading to the formation of the NCI Biologic Response Modifiers Program (BRMP), the creation of the NCI-sponsored Extramural IL-2 LAK Working Group, which subsequently became the Cytokine Working Group (CWG), and the formation of the Society for Biologic Therapy (SBT), which subsequently became the Society for Immunotherapy of Cancer (SITC). The Extramural IL-2/LAK Working Group validated the initial results of the NCI SB with IL-2 and LAK and subsequently showed, in conjunction with the NCI SB investigators, that in contrast to mouse models, LAK cells added no significant clinical benefit. A compilation of phase II studies with HD IL-2 alone showed that it produced responses in approximately 25% of patients with advanced melanoma or RCC, with complete responses being extremely durable.[70,75,107,108] In fact, long-term follow-up of responders on these initial studies established that patients still responding after 30 months rarely experienced disease progression, suggesting that they were likely "cured." These early studies led to the FDA approval of HD IL-2 for patients with metastatic RCC in 1992 and advanced melanoma in 1998.

HD IL-2, like IFN, is a nonspecific immune activator, and therefore its administration was associated with significant side effects.[109,110] This toxicity was related to the release of secondary cytokines from activated immune cells that produced a cytokine release associated with fever, rigors, capillary leak syndrome, hypotension, and multiorgan dysfunction. This has been called a systemic autophagic syndrome,[111,112] as it is associated with reversible organ dysfunction rather than true parenchymal damage. Though this toxicity was quickly reversed by withholding treatment and, therefore, was manageable, it limited the use of HD IL-2 to patients with intact organ function treated at select centers skilled in the management of these side effects and prevented its broad application in malignancies besides melanoma and RCC. Currently, it is presumed that HDs are needed to exceed the capacity of T_{reg} cells to consume the IL-2 and limit its access to T effector cells, at least in the setting of patients with melanoma.

Attempts throughout the 1990s to develop a cytokine-based regimen with a better therapeutic index, through use of lower doses of IL-2, combinations of IL-2 with IFN, chemotherapy or peptide vaccines, efforts to dissociate the antitumor effects of HD IL-2 from its toxicity, or the study of more T cell selective cytokines such as IL-4, -6, -12, -18, and -21, were all largely unsuccessful.[113–118]

Consequently, efforts in the early 21st century turned to trying to identify those patients most likely to respond, in order to limit the needless exposure to IL-2 toxicities of patients not destined to benefit. Studies in patients with melanoma suggested that those most likely to benefit had a normal lactic dehydrogenase (LDH; perhaps indicating the absence of tumor necrosis)[119] and an inflamed tumor microenvironment (perhaps indicating preexisting tumor-specific T cells). Further preliminary data suggested that in many patients, IL-2 tended to activate suppressor cells rather than effector cells[120] and that some genetically determined immune regulatory component, as evidenced by the frequent association of IL-2 response with autoimmune conditions such as vitiligo and thyroid dysfunction, was necessary to achieve benefit.[121,122]

As in mouse models, TIL when isolated and expanded in vitro with IL-2 were shown to recognize melanoma cells. Re-administration of these TIL following lymphodepleting chemotherapy (presumably to eliminate immunosuppressive factors in the tumor microenvironment) produced antitumor responses even in patients whose disease had progressed following HD IL-2.[123] TIL/IL-2 therapy was labor intensive and required inpatient therapy, and thus was not readily translatable to most academic medical centers until commercial efforts were developed and refined. Thus, addressable barriers for effective cancer immunotherapy helped identify the critical role for reactivated tumor-specific T cells in the process.

Taken together, aggregate findings suggested that the immune system, when properly activated in the right host and tumor, could produce durable responses, and that immune cells within the tumor microenvironment recognize the tumor, although their tumor lytic activity was being thwarted by suppressive factors. These critical observations both kept the immunotherapy field alive and prompted the search for targetable immunosuppressive factors within the tumor microenvironment as a way of enhancing or unleashing antitumor immunity.

Recognizing the critical role of cytotoxic T cells in antitumor immunity has restored interest in trying to create cytokines that could preferentially stimulate cytotoxic T cell growth and proliferation without simultaneously activating T_{reg} cells. For IL-2 these efforts have focused on modifying its biologic activity by limiting its ability to bind to the alpha chain component of the high affinity IL-2 receptor. This has been accomplished through a variety of approaches including coupling IL-2 to the IL-2Rα chain, adding pegylation in order to block its binding to the IL-2Rα chain, or modifying the protein to limit its ability to interact with the IL-2Ra.[99,124,125] Similar pegylation strategies have also tested with IL-10.[126] In addition, other cytokines such as IL-7 and IL-15 have been investigated that in preclinical models might be more cytotoxic T cell selective. Finally, efforts are underway to try to target cytokines such as IL-2 or IL-12 directly to the tumor microenvironment, thereby reducing the systemic toxicity associated with high dose systemic administration.[127–130] Whether any of these approaches will result in similar efficacy as seen with HD-IL-2 at doses that enable safe outpatient administration remains to be determined.

VACCINES

Prophylactic vaccines have changed the natural history of many infectious diseases and hopefully will have a dramatic impact on SARS CoV-2, the cause of the 2020 pandemic.[131–133] Consequently, the development of vaccines that could stimulate the immune system to recognize and destroy cancer cells has been a major focus of immunotherapy research for decades. Many vaccine approaches have been tried, and several have shown promise in early phase trials compared to historical controls. However, with a few notable exceptions, randomized controlled phase III trials have failed to confirm the benefit of these vaccines relative to standard therapies, observation, or placebo. Nonetheless, examination of these approaches in the light of our recent understanding of tumor immunology provides insight into the likely limitations of previous vaccine approaches that can inform current and future cancer vaccine development.

Early approaches focused on whole tumor cell vaccines using autologous tumor cells. Although this approach had the advantage of exposing the immune system to all tumor-associated antigens, it meant that each vaccine had to be individually made, increasing the cost and time needed to prepare these samples.[134] Autologous whole tumor cell vaccines have universally failed to show benefit in phase III trials, including studies with GVAX (a granulocyte macrophage colony-stimulating factor [GM-CSF]-transduced autologous tumor cell vaccine) given alone or in combination with other agents.[135,136]

To overcome these limitations inherent in autologous vaccination strategies, researchers have explored vaccines that induced immunity to shared antigens that are common on specific tumor lineages. These shared antigens included tissue differentiation antigens (e.g., cancer testes antigens) that were re-expressed on dedifferentiated cancer cells from tumors of the same tissue of origin and less commonly on differentiated normal tissues as well as overexpressed or aberrantly expressed antigens. The latter include proteins such as HER2/neu and the epidermal growth factor receptor (EGFR), which are overexpressed in breast cancers and many epithelial cancers, and MUC-1, a heavily glycosylated protein that is expressed on the luminal surface of normal glandular cells, but is aberrantly expressed on the surface of many types of adenocarcinomas and thus conceivably not subject to immune tolerance. These latter antigens came to be known collectively as *cancer antigens*. Approaches to vaccinating against shared antigens included the use of mixtures of allogeneic tumor cells together with an immune adjuvant, or the direct vaccination against putative cancer antigens administered as whole proteins. Allogeneic tumor cell vaccines that showed some benefit in phase II trials, but not in phase III trials, include Canvaxin (a allogeneic whole-cell vaccine combining melanoma lines with BCG), Melacine (a similar polyvalent melanoma vaccine), as well as belagenpumatucel-l (an allogeneic tumor vaccine modified to limit secretion of TGF-β2).[134,137,138] As noted previously, Canvaxin showed exciting results compared with historical controls in patients with resected stage IV melanoma, with as many as 40% of patients remaining alive at 5 years. However, in randomized phase III trials comparing Canvaxin to BCG alone in patients with resected stage III or stage IV melanoma, the BCG alone control arm was found to produce superior survival.[70] Taken together, these studies illustrate some of the pitfalls of using historical controls to assess the efficacy of adjuvant therapies, including, but not limited to, stage migration over time related to improved imaging techniques and patient selection, particularly the requirement for patients to be disease free on post-resection imaging. They also raised the possibility that certain vaccinations, in the absence of co-stimulation, might induce immune suppression or immune tolerance, rather than enhanced antitumor effects.

With the discovery of DCs and their ability to present processed proteins or peptides on MHC molecules to specific T cell populations,[139] vaccination approaches shifted to the use of specific peptides (usually human leukocyte antigen [HLA]-0201 restricted) either alone or pulsed onto HLA-restricted autologous DCs or the direct injection of tumor DNA or RNA into DCs, enabling them to process and present either the shared antigens or all of the tumor antigens. Further, these 9 to 15 amino acid peptides were sometimes mutated to produce a substitution of an amino acid in order to enhance their antigenicity. Although vaccination strategies using these approaches have largely been equally disappointing, a couple of approaches have produced more promising results.

In 1996, Murphy published a phase I clinical trial showing that autologous DCs pulsed with prostate-specific membrane antigen resulted in cellular immune response and decreased prostate-specific antigen (PSA) in patients with advanced prostate cancer.[140] Building on this approach, the sipileucel-T vaccine strategy was developed, which involved the use of an autologous antigen-presenting cell cultured with prostatic acid phosphatase linked to GM-CSF. A phase III placebo-controlled trial in patients with advanced prostate cancer treated with sipileucel-T showed a 4.5-month improvement in overall survival (but without apparent objective tumor responses).[141] Subsequent trials confirmed this overall survival benefit,[142] leading to the FDA approval (the first for a cell therapy) of sipileucel-T for men with castration-resistant prostate cancer.[143] Despite this reproducible survival benefit, the absence of efficacy surrogates such as clinical response, PSA decline, or laboratory correlates, together with the expense of producing an individualized autologous product, have limited the use of this agent and hindered its further development.

A phase II trial conducted at the NCI SB involving HD IL-2 and a mutated heteroclitic gp-100 peptide vaccine in HLA A2+ patients with advanced melanoma showed an overall response rate of 42%, significantly higher than what would have been expected with HD IL-2 alone.[144] This result led to a multicenter randomized phase III trial of HD IL-2 with or without the gp100 peptide vaccine in a similar patient population, which showed an improved response rate (22.1% vs 9.7%), improved progression-free survival (PFS), and a trend toward improved overall survival (17.6 vs 12.8 months, $p = .01$) for the vaccine-containing arm.[145] Although this result suggested that the immune response could be enhanced through specific peptide vaccination, the lower-than-anticipated response rate in the IL-2 alone arm and the failure of this same peptide to enhance the efficacy of checkpoint inhibitors such as ipilimumab[146] or nivolumab[147] has called into question the validity or at least the generalizability of this observation. Further, although many studies with peptide vaccines were successful at inducing high levels of antigen-specific T cells, this immune activation rarely correlated with clinical benefit, suggesting that either the vaccine-specific T cells did not recognize these antigens in the context of the tumor, did not travel to the tumor, or were stymied once they reached the tumor microenvironment.

Recently, it has become apparent that the immune system typically recognizes neoantigens/neoepitopes rather than shared antigens on tumors, and that tumors, survive by using a variety of means of evading the resultant immune response generated against these neoantigens. Taken together, this suggested that for vaccines to be effective, they must involve the autologous tumor cells and likely be combined with factors that sustain any induced response. This has led to strategies involving fusions of autologous tumor cells with DCs,[148] direct tumor injection of substances that enhance tumor neoantigen expression (e.g., genetically engineered oncolytic viruses),[149,150] genes coding for Toll-like receptor agonists and IFN-gamma inducers (e.g., stimulator of interferon genes[51,151]), or more recently neoantigen vaccines.[152] It is noteworthy that a phase III trial (Oncovex Pivotal Trial in Melanoma [OPTiM]) involving intralesional administration of talimogene laherparepvec, T-VEC, a genetically engineered oncolytic herpes simplex virus expressing GM-CSF, to patients with metastatic melanoma, showed improved response rates and median overall survival compared to GM-CSF injections alone, resulting in its FDA approval in 2015.[153] Furthermore, studies combining T-VEC with checkpoint inhibitors, either ipilimumab[154] or pembrolizumab,[155] in patients with melanoma showed apparent improvements in antitumor efficacy relative to the single agents, suggesting a possible way forward for tumor vaccine therapy. Phase III trials comparing oncolytic viral vaccines or TLR agonists together with immune checkpoint inhibitors versus the immune checkpoint inhibitor alone have been launched with results eagerly awaited.

OVERCOMING IMMUNOSUPPRESSIVE FACTORS

Because of the largely disappointing data with vaccines and cytokines (for all except a few diseases), increased attention was given during the 1990s to the concept that effective immunotherapy was limited by regulatory mechanisms for controlling immune activation and an immunosuppressive tumor microenvironment. Several factors were implicated, including inhibitory ligand–receptor interactions, which limited T cell activation and function (CTLA-4); immunosuppressive cytokines (e.g., TGF-β, IL-4, IL-6, and IL-10); immunosuppressive

cells (e.g., T_{reg} cells, myeloid-derived suppressor cells [MDSCs]); and cell signaling disruption (via class 1 antigen loss, down modulation of T cell receptor [TCR] zeta chain expression and indoleamine 2,3-dioxygenase [IDO] secretion). Together or separately, these factors constrained immune-activating signals, contributed to tumor-induced immune suppression, and likely inhibited the antitumor immune response. In retrospect, and in view of the many known mechanisms for counteracting the stimulatory effects of cytokines and vaccines and for suppressing immune responses in the tumor microenvironment, it seems surprising that a subset of patients with advanced disease could respond so well to IL-2.

Two clinical approaches that entered the clinic in the early part of the 21st century heralded the new era of cancer immunotherapy: immune checkpoint inhibitors and cumulative advances in adoptive cellular therapy.

Immune Checkpoint Inhibitors

The first breakthrough came from preclinical and clinical studies, which demonstrated the substantial antitumor effects of blocking inhibitory ligand–receptor interactions that served as physiologic brakes on the immune system. The principal "immune checkpoints" discovered and targeted for clinical development were CTLA-4 and the PDL1-PDL1 pathway. Their discovery by James Allison and Tasuku Hanjo led to their jointly receiving the 2018 Nobel Prize in Physiology or Medicine. Lieping Chen,[156–158] Gordon Freeman,[40,159–162] and Arlene Sharpe[160,162] also played seminal roles in developing this area.

Administration of antagonist antibodies to CTLA-4 (ipilimumab or tremelimumab) to patients with advanced melanoma led to tumor responses in 10% to 20% of patients.[147,163] Ipilimumab prolonged median survival of patients with metastatic melanoma in randomized phase III trials,[147] and like HD IL-2, the responses were sufficiently durable to produce a tail (20–24% alive at 3 or more years)[164] on the overall survival curve[165] despite treatment generally stopping after 12 weeks. This result led to the FDA approval, in 2011, of ipilimumab for the treatment of patients with advanced melanoma.

Observations made in clinical studies of anti-CTLA-4 generated new paradigms for safe management of patients and interpretation of clinical results from immunotherapy trials. Administration of CTLA-4 antibodies was associated with reactivated T cell immunity against many normal tissues, leading to a raft of immune-related adverse events beyond the thyroid dysfunction and vitiligo observed in patients receiving IL-2 or HD IFN.[146] These include dermatitis, colitis, hepatitis, and hypophysitis. Algorithms were developed for successful management of these adverse events with corticosteroids and other immune modulatory agents which—interestingly, in contrast to their use in the context of cytokine therapy—did not appear to interfere with the anti-tumor immune response once it was established.[166] Unconventional tumor response patterns were also observed, including initial progression of disease, so-called pseudo-progression, followed by clear-cut tumor regression, which in many cases persisted following treatment cessation. In addition, in a subset of patients who responded to anti-CTLA-4 and subsequently developed disease progression, a second "re-induction" course of anti-CTLA-4 could produce additional anti-tumor activity.[167] These observations contributed to the finding that the survival benefit from ipilimumab greatly exceeded what would have been anticipated based on its response rate or median PFS and suggested that landmark survival or "treatment free survival" might be better indicators of ipilimumab efficacy.

Efforts were subsequently focused on the discovery and targeting of other immune checkpoints that might be relevant to cancers in addition to melanoma. The discovery that PD-L1 on tumor cells served to suppress the function of PD-1 expressing activated CTLs in the tumor microenvironment provided a target that could be inhibited in a more selective way than CTLA-4. Targeting the PD-1–PD-L1 interaction provided a means of unleashing the suppressed T cell response in situ.[159–162] Remarkably, as described in various sections of this book, antagonist antibodies against this single immune inhibitory pathway demonstrated unprecedented and clinically relevant anticancer activity in a subset of patients across at least 20 different types of malignancy.[168,169] From late 2014 until the end of 2020, the anti-PD-1 agents nivolumab, pembrolizumab, and cemiplimab and the anti-PD-L1 agents atezolizumab, durvalumab, and avelumab have received FDA approval for the treatment of patients with advanced melanoma and high risk melanoma, metastatic and stage III non-small cell lung cancer, advanced kidney cancer, advanced urothelial cancer, head and neck cancer, hepatocellular cancer, gastric and esophageal cancer, Merkel cell cancer, squamous cell cancer of the skin, and Hodgkin disease.[85,170–173] In addition, anti-PD1 therapy became the first treatment approach to be approved based on a tissue agnostic biomarker of tumor mutational load.[174–176] Because PD-1 pathway blockers, as noted previously for ipilimumab, have their most profound impact on overall survival, virtually all randomized phase III trials conducted to date comparing PD-1 pathway blockers have shown superior survival related to standard therapies. Furthermore, in contrast to CTLA-4 antibody therapy, the toxicities associated with anti-PD-1 blockade appear to be fairly minor, with less than 15% of patients typically experiencing any type of grade 3 immune-related toxicities.[177] The tolerability of these agents has made it possible to consider combinations of anti-PD-1/PD-L1 with practically any type of therapy and their study in the adjuvant setting.

More than any other development in this field, the broad clinical activity of anti-PD-1 and anti-PD-L1 antibodies energized the pharmaceutical and biotech industry to initiate or expand preclinical and clinical research programs for cancer immunotherapy agents. As a result, several new immune modulatory agents advanced into the clinic, and a large number of combination trials were initiated, most based on blockade of the PD-1/PD-L1 pathway. The first combination to be tested involved nivolumab with ipilimumab. In phase I studies involving patients with melanoma, the combination produced rapid and deep tumor responses in more than 50% of patients,[178] and phase II and III trials suggested that the combination was superior in terms of tumor response and median PFS to either single agent.[179,180] Similar enhanced efficacy was suggested for the combination in patients with non-small cell lung cancer, kidney cancer, bladder cancer, and ovarian cancer[181–185] leading to the FDA approval of this combination in several of these disease settings. Thus, combination immunotherapy appears to be superior to anti-PD-1 alone, thereby opening the floodgates for the study of various combinations in a multitude of diseases and settings.

The last several years have produced an explosion of trials, which have established benefits of PD1 pathway blockers in combination with standard treatments relative to the standard treatment alone resulting in additional FDA approvals. Such studies have included combinations of PD-1/PD-L1 blockers with cytotoxic chemotherapy in non-small cell and small cell lung cancer;[186,187] breast cancer;[188] anti-angiogenic agents in kidney, liver and endometrial cancer;[189–193] and molecularly targeted therapy in patients with melanoma.[194] Most of these approvals have been based on an improvement in response rate and median PFS for the combination. How these combinations would compare to an anti-PD-1/PD-L1-based pure immunotherapy regimen as initial treatment, especially when using more typical immunotherapy endpoints such as durable response, landmark PFS, or OS rates and treatment-free survival, remains to be established.

In addition to these mixed combination regimens, considerable effort has gone into creating pure immunotherapy combinations that might overcome the additional immunosuppressive factors within the tumor microenvironment and/or enhance the immunogenicity of the tumor itself, in some cases turning a T cell depleted or "cold" tumor microenvironment into a T cell replete or "hot" microenvironment. Among the multitude of combinations being pursued are studies involving tumor antigen or neoantigen vaccines, cytokines, agonist antibodies, inhibitors of other immune checkpoints, and inhibitor MDSCs, T_{reg} cells, or other immunosuppressive factors such as IDO or adenosine within the tumor microenvironment.[195] Of note, initial data from phase 2 studies with anti-PD-1 and the IDO inhibitor epacadostat appeared extremely promising, yet the phase III trial of pembrolizumab plus epacadostat proved no better than pembrolizumab alone in the treatment of patients with advanced melanoma.[196,197] This disappointing result has prompted a call for more definitive preclinical and early clinical data including either single agent efficacy and/or efficacy of the combination in patients with resistance to PD-1 pathway blockade, before committing resources to large scale randomized phase 3 trials.

Furthermore, the availability of multiple treatment approaches and potential clinical trial options for patients with various diseases has stimulated efforts to identify predictive biomarkers of immunotherapy responsiveness and resistance and thereby aid in both rational combination therapy development and treatment selection.

Adoptive Cellular Therapy

An alternative approach to overcoming the suppressive tumor microenvironment involved the administration of genetically modified autologous T cells targeting specific cancer-related antigens.[198,199] This could be done in the form of TIL in which TCRs for a shared tumor antigen (e.g., NY ESO1) or a tumor-specific neoantigen were inserted before being expanded in vitro in IL-2 and re-administered in large numbers following lympho-depleting chemotherapy. The function of these genetically modified T cells or tumor infiltrating lymphocytes could be enhanced by coadministration of IL-2,[39] the co-transduction of stimulatory cytokines such as IL-12, or sustained through the coadministration of PD-1 pathway blockers. These approaches have produced dramatic responses in a few patients with a variety of individual tumor types,[200,201] suggesting that this might be a key to treating patients with solid tumors in which the immunosuppressive factors in the tumor microenvironment could not be identified and/or blocked. Recently, multiple successful trials of TIL have been reported from several academic sites for patients with melanoma[116,202-205] and from commercial groups preparing for registration in melanoma and cervical cancer.

An alternative to modified T cell therapy is the adoptive cell transfer with T cells modified to express chimeric antigen receptors (CARs). CARs are receptors combining tumor-specific binding domains (single-chain variable fragment from a mAb) fused with T cell intracellular signaling domains.[206] In 1989, Zelig Eshhar generated a chimeric TCR from a T cell constant domain fused to a 2,4,6-trinitrophenyl (TNP) antibody variable domain. He transfected these into a CTL hybridoma and observed functioning of this TCR. He also observed that the transfected cells expanded through IL-2 production and were cytolytic against TNP-bearing cells of various strains and species.[207] This indicated that these T cells killed target-bearing cells in an HLA unrestricted fashion. Initial studies in mouse models showed promise, but the first clinical trials showed no reduction of tumor burden, likely due to lack of exogenous co-stimulation.[206] Second-generational CARs were developed that included co-stimulatory molecules such as CD28, 4-1BB, OX40, CD27, and ICOS[206] within the chimeric transgene.

These second-generation CAR T cells have been created targeting a variety of tumor-related shared antigens such as CD19, CD22, and mesothelin, and studied in clinical trials. The most success has been seen with CD19 CAR T cells targeting CD19 expressing hematological malignancies. In 2010, Kochenderfer and Rosenberg treated a patient who had heavily pretreated advanced follicular lymphoma with autologous CAR T cells engineered to target CD19.[208] The patient experienced a partial remission lasting 32 weeks with absent B cells and low immunoglobulins following treatment.[208] In 2015, Porter and June reported on a series of 14 patients with relapsed or refractory chronic lymphocytic leukemia who were treated with autologous T cells transfected with the anti-CD19 lentivirus.[209] They observed an overall response rate of 57%, with four complete and persistent remissions.[209] Perhaps the most promising results, though, were observed in patients with acute lymphoblastic leukemia (ALL). Maude et al observed complete remission in 90% of patients, primarily children with ALL, treated with the anti-CD19 CAR T cells.[210] Similar phase 1 studies at other institutions have confirmed this antitumor activity with overall response rates of 88%.[211] CAR T cells have also been tested in patients with chemotherapy-refractory multiple myeloma targeting CD138, with four of the five patients having stable disease for longer than 3 months.[212] Recent studies demonstrating CART cells responding to BCMA as a target antigen have also been reported.[213,214] Subsequent studies in the United States and China have shown substantial antitumor response.

Treatment of patients with solid tumors using CAR T cells has been less fruitful. One study using Epstein Barr-specific T cells, engineered to express neuroblastoma disialoganglioside GD2, showed complete remission in 3 of 11 patients with neuroblastoma.[215] Another phase I/II study used anti-HER2 CAR T cells on HER2-positive sarcoma.[216] Of the 19 patients treated this way, four had stable disease from 3 to 14 months.[216] Recently similar studies have been reported targeting the tumor-associated antigen IL-13 receptor alpha 2 (IL-13Rα2) chain.[217]

It has been hypothesized that many individual factors could be contributing to the decreased efficacy of CAR T cells in solid compared to hematologic malignancies. First, T cells must travel to the tumor site, and this can be impaired if there are mismatches in chemokine or adhesion mechanisms.[218] The notion that vascular normalization rather than anti-angiogenesis should be pursued has been championed by Rakesh Jain, with recent suggestions that such strategies can facilitate tumor perfusion leading to enhanced antitumor immune responses.[219–224] There is a also a concern that to enhance specificity and avoid off-tumor/on-target toxicity, CAR T cells must be directed against tumor-specific antigens.[225] To date, most studies have focused on "self" antigens rather than tumor neo-antigens.[225] Once the T cells infiltrate the tumor, they must overcome oxidative stress, nutritional depletion, acidic pH, and hypoxia of the tumor environment.[218] Soluble factors and suppressive cytokines secreted by tumor cells may also inhibit the T cells.[218] Additionally, the tumor microenvironment may contain immunosuppressive immune cells such as regulatory T cells and MDSCs, as well as tumor-associated macrophages, mast cells, plasmacytoid DCs, and neutrophils.[218] T cell activation-induced surface molecules, such as PD-1, might be expressed and negatively regulate the antitumor response.[218] Given the nearly limitless possibilities for engineering the T cells *ex vivo*, a number of these potential obstacles will likely be addressed through additional modifications of the T cell product prior to therapy.

CONCLUSION

It has been a long and storied road to our current understanding of tumor immunology. Initial observations by Busch, Coley, and others that bacterial preparations could induce tumor regression were noted, but then fell out of favor for decades. Ehrlich's idea of a magic bullet for cellular receptors eventually led to the concept of employing mAbs to target specific surface proteins on tumor cells and eventually immune cells. The first substantial clinical benefits of immune inducing agents were seen with the local administration of BCG in the treatment of patients with skin metastases from melanoma or superficial bladder cancer. These results spurred interest in identifying approaches to activate anticancer immunity in a more systemic fashion.

Investigations with early immunotherapies, such as HD IL-2 performed within the NCI SB and the CWG,[225,226] established that activated T cells could produce durable clinical responses and cures in a subset of patients with metastatic melanoma or kidney cancer. Subsequent research, also spearheaded by the NCI SB, determined that many tumors contained immune cells that, when reactivated and expanded *ex vivo* and re-administered following lympho-depleting chemotherapy, could eradicate melanoma in up to 56% of patients not responsive to HD IL-2. These seminal observations sustained interest in cancer immunotherapy through a long period of frustration spanning a quarter of a century between 1985 and 2010 and spawned efforts to reactivate TIL *in situ*. These efforts were rewarded by the discovery and targeting of immune checkpoints, such as PD-1 and its ligand (PD-L1), and thereby unleash of effective antitumor immunity. Antibodies against the PD-1/

PD-L1 pathway have produced antitumor responses—with little toxicity—not only in patients with advanced melanoma and kidney cancer, but also in at least 20 other tumor types, revolutionizing both immunotherapy and the broader field of cancer therapy.

Combining CTLA-4 and anti-PD-1 antibodies produced antitumor activity superior to anti-PD-1 monotherapy in melanoma, establishing proof of principle that these immunosuppressive mechanisms were not redundant, paving the way for further exploration of this approach and other combination strategies including combinations with both conventional cancer therapies and novel immunotherapies. The existence and power of these immunoregulatory checkpoints served to highlight why early efforts with immunotherapies were largely ineffective, while at the same time providing a means to potentially improve their efficacy. Further, the demonstrated power of unleashed antitumor immunity has fueled efforts to generate or expand TIL in less inflamed or non-PD-1 pathway-protected tumors or, failing that, to manufacture *ex vivo* antitumor immune cells that can be adoptively transferred into patients to aggressively attack tumor-associated antigens.

We now know that cancer is both a disease of the cancer cell AND the host response. Thus, the future of cancer immunotherapy looks incredibly bright. Future progress will require integration of both cancer biology and tumor immunologic principles. The current and proposed investigations with cancer immunotherapy promise to forever change not only the way we treat many (if not most) cancers, transforming the field of oncology in ways that now seem obvious but required years of painstaking work, insights into fundamental immunology, and the emergence of technologies capable of revealing the complexity and diversity latent in the adaptive immune response.

KEY REFERENCES

Only key references appear in the print edition. The full reference list appears in the digital product on Springer Publishing Connect: connect.springerpub.com/content/book/978-0-8261-3743-2/chapter/ch01

   4. Revesz L. Effect of tumour cells killed by x-rays upon the growth of admixed viable cells. *Nature*. 1956;178(4547):1391–1392. doi:10.1038/1781391a0
  25. Cheever MA, Greenberg PD, Fefer A, Gillis S. Augmentation of the anti-tumor therapeutic efficacy of long-term cultured T lymphocytes by in vivo administration of purified interleukin 2. *J Exp Med*. 1982;155(4):968–980. doi:10.1084/jem.155.4.968
  56. Köhler G, Milstein C. Continuous cultures of fused cells secreting antibody of predefined specificity. *Nature*. 1975;256(5517):495–497. doi:10.1038/256495a0
 180. Wolchok JD, Chiarion-Sileni V, Gonzalez R, et al. Overall survival with combined nivolumab and ipilimumab in advanced melanoma. *N Engl J Med*. 2017;377(14):1345–1356. doi:10.1056/NEJMoa1709684
 184. Hellmann MD, Rizvi NA, Goldman JW, et al. Nivolumab plus ipilimumab as first-line treatment for advanced non-small-cell lung cancer (CheckMate 012): results of an open-label,

phase 1, multicohort study. *Lancet Oncol.* 2017;18(1):31–41. doi:10.1016/S1470-2045(16)30624-6

201. Tran E, Turcotte S, Gros A, et al. Cancer immunotherapy based on mutation-specific CD4+ T cells in a patient with epithelial cancer. *Science.* 2014;344(6184):641–645. doi:10.1126/science.1251102

208. Kochenderfer JN, Wilson WH, Janik JE, et al. Eradication of B-lineage cells and regression of lymphoma in a patient treated with autologous T cells genetically engineered to recognize CD19. *Blood.* 2010;116(20):4099–4102. doi:10.1182/blood-2010-04-281931

Basic Principles of Tumor Immunology

Francesco M. Marincola

Introduction to Basic Sciences: The Caduceus of Cancer-Immune Responsiveness and Cancer Biology

Francesco M. Marincola and Michael T. Lotze

KEY POINTS

- Cancer is a disorder of genes driven by the development of genomic instability. In children, primary genomic instability arises during embryogenesis prior to the functional maturation of the immune system. Almost all adult tumors arise in the setting of chronic inflammation and the associated stress, resulting in secondary genomic instability. Although almost all tumors have reparative proliferation as a consequence of untoward and excessive cell death, the release of damage-associated molecular pattern molecules (DAMPs) promotes a wound healing phenotype. Programmed cell death (apoptosis, necroptosis, ferroptosis) and programmed cell survival (autophagy) are coordinated in stressed cells with the resultant outcome dependent on other cell-intrinsic and -extrinsic factors. Fundamentally, cancers emerge with heightened autophagy and limited ability to undergo programmed cell death. The immune response to tumors initiates with recruitment of innate immune effectors in response to release of DAMPs and an elicited adaptive immune response. The major sources of antigenic moieties in cancer are primarily the neo-epitopes arising from mutated genes/frameshifts in non-driver mutations, and secondarily against so-called oncofetal or tumor-testis antigens reexpressed during tumor development.

- Immunotherapy against cancer exploits this natural and broadly conserved immunological behavior. This is better defined as immune-mediated tissue-specific destruction (ITD). ITD is responsible not only for rejection of neoplastic tissues but also for flares of autoimmunity, destruction of pathogen-containing cells during acute infections, rejection of allogeneic transplants, and graft versus host disease. The occurrence

of cancer rejection is consistently associated with the activation of a transcriptional signature that is identical to that observed in other facets of ITD and defined, therefore, as the immunologic constant of rejection (ICR). Tumor rejection is the extreme manifestation of a continuum of immune surveillance against cancer as the ICR signature is associated also with a favorable predictive and prognostic implication. Tumors that naturally express ICR genes are more likely to respond to immunotherapy and are associated with better survival. Tumor rejection is a multifactorial phenomenon in which three categories of determinants play a fundamental role: genetic background of the host and post genetic adaptations, somatic evolution of the neoplastic cells, and environmental factors such as microbiome and comorbidities. Notably, the genetic background of the host affects the genetic makeup of cancer cell biology and overlaps with it as cancer cells carry the same functional variants of the host's genome.

- Escape from immune detection can be related to failure of T cell entry into tumors. T cells traffic across "normal" endothelia expressing activation markers follow chemokine gradients from specialized dendritic cells within the tumor. So-called cold tumors arise due to altered pathways in tumors including enhanced Wnt/Beta catenin signaling and PTEN loss. An altered tissue biology including hypoxia, variant nutrient availability, and enhanced K+ release by dead and dying cells as well as other DAMPs causes "lymphoplegia" with limited functionality of recruited cells within the tumor microenvironment. In addition, loss of antigen expression stealth cancer cells from recognition by T cells.

- Contrasting biology with autoimmunity. Contrary to other forms of ITD, cancer rejection is characterized by genomic instability of the target tissue adding complexity to the understanding of its mechanisms. As a corollary, studying other forms of ITD, such as autoimmunity, can provide insights about non-neoplastic determinants of tissue rejection related to the genetic background of the host, its post-genetic adaptations, environmental influences, and comorbidities.

- Anticancer immunotherapy. Immuno-oncology (IO) focuses on fundamental reductionist biology as well as a systems biology approach. Interference with cellular sociology, particularly the interaction between cancer and normal cells as well as stromal and immune cells that counter-regulate each other's functional status, is a means to circumvent advanced cancer (for example, targeting FAP or CD39 on stromal cells). Other anticancer treatments that target intracellular mechanisms are now being evaluated for their direct or indirect immunologic effects (for example, the use of CBL-B inhibitors to enhance T cell survival and IL-2 production). Most current cancer immunotherapies are aimed at extracellular targets while other approaches such as chemotherapy and targeted therapies are aimed against intracellular targets. Both immunologic and cancer biologic approaches will need to be combined to enhance the effectiveness of anticancer therapy, and this is the major challenge for the next generation of therapeutics.

Asclepius derived his name from healing soothingly and from deferring the withering that comes with death. For this reason, therefore, they give him a serpent as an attribute, indicating that those who avail themselves of medical science undergo a process similar to the serpent in that they, as it were, grow young again after illnesses and slough off old age; also because the serpent is a sign of attention, much of which is required in medical treatments. The staff also seems to be a symbol of some similar thing. For by means of this it is set before our minds that unless we are supported by such inventions as these, in so far as falling continually into sickness is concerned, stumbling along we would fall even sooner than necessary.
—Lucius Annaeus Cornutus, 66 AD, Theologiae Graecae Compendium

MODERN IMMUNOTHERAPY OF CANCER

Surprisingly, the use of the Asclepius (and subsequently the Caduceus) symbol represents how a destructive animal, the snake, could be used to demonstrate healing. The snake exuviates, shedding its skin to enable escape from death, with the Asclepius presenting the physician's role of avoiding death for life, modeled by the god of healing.[1] Indeed, the destruction wrested by cancer initially, and subsequently by iatrogenic insults inflected by the use of cytotoxic strategies is now giving way to a deeper understanding of immune mechanisms, serving to promote healing and control cancer. The last three decades introduced immunotherapy as a new modality of cancer treatment, emergent with proven benefits over standard therapy with the availability of cytokine therapies such as *interleukin* (*IL*)-2 and interferons, cellular therapies with *tumor-infiltrating lymphocytes* (*TIL*)[2] and *chimeric antigen receptor* (*CAR*) T cells,[3,4] and most recently the use of antibodies targeting immunosuppressive molecules. These more recent agents have clearly improved survival and reduced toxicity. Peculiar to immunotherapy are the long-term effects observable in responding patients, who are often permanently cured with long tails of the survival curve. Thus, several immunotherapies received U.S. Food and Drug Administration approval resulting in health improvement but also supporting a multi-billion-dollar industry. Foremost among immunotherapies stand "checkpoint inhibitors." However, only a limited proportion of patients benefit. Identifying the anlage of cancer immune resistance and correcting it will extend curative treatments to the majority of patients while optimizing the cost-effectiveness of clinical trial design through an evidence-based prioritization of actionable targets and/or their combinations.

MOST MALIGNANT TUMORS IN ADULTS ARE EPITHELIAL

Epithelial tumors (in order of deaths in the United States annually: lung, colon, breast, pancreas, and prostate) arise in the setting where three fundamental processes are balanced: the critical need to maintain internal or external barriers with the environment; allow selective transport of nutrients, waste, or metabolites across a permeable set of cells; and husbandry of the immune sentinels sensitive to breaching of these barriers. Cancer arises in the setting where these three principles of balance and counter-regulation are distorted by perpetual stress, first external in the form of pathogens or tissue damage/injury and then internalized by the emergent barrier-promoting epithelial tumors. Although T cells responsive to epithelial tumors can now be identified,[5–7] their ability to mediate important antitumor effects when adoptively transferred have been limited. Clearly, there is additional biology waiting to be discerned. For example, the CD2/CD58(LFA-3) interaction, although identified early in the panoply of cluster determining/cluster of differentiation molecules in the last century, has still to be considered in its evolutionary biology or importance in T cell responses to tumor.[8,9]

DAMAGE-ASSOCIATED MOLECULAR PATTERN MOLECULES INCLUDING HMGB1 PROMOTE THE TUMOR MICROENVIRONMENT AND LOCAL AND SYSTEMIC AUTOPHAGY

The universal response to stress in cells is the enhancement of autophagy whether this be genomic stress, ER stress, nutrient stress, hypoxia, or viral or opportunistic bacterial infections.[10–13] When cells are stressed, they release HMGB1[12,14] and other intracellular proteins such as histones.[15] Furthermore, autophagy can limit immune responses, in part by degrading major histocompatibility molecules,[16] necessary for conventional αβ T cell recognition as well as consuming deposited granzymes.[17,18] Thus, within the tumor is a wound-healing response that never fully resolves as a consequence of emergent genomic instability and the reparative response with proliferation. The consequences of this phenomenon are the release of "reducing" equivalents from the cells following necrosis with the obligate need to oxidize these components and diminish their biologic activity.[19] One of the oxidant means to promote cell death is a more recently recognized form of cell death, ferroptosis,[20,21] which is opposed by the System Xc for import of molecular cysteine. The cycles of micro-thrombosis and resultant micro-necrosis in tissues promote rounds of emergent tissue instability. This is driven in part by HMGB1 release from platelets[22,23] regulated in part by the inflammasome and the Bruton's tyrosine kinase. Release of HMGB1 and other DAMPs stimulates the release of chemokines, promoting recruitment of innate immune cells and initiation of what the late Charles Janeway called Signal 0 in the immune response.[24] Other factors in the tumor microenvironment include the release of the lymphoplegia-inducing cation K+,[25] the relative ability of T cells to sense high or low oxygen,[26] nutrient availability,[27] and a variety of other host factors[28] that will be discussed in detail in Chapter 10, which is dedicated to T cell differentiation and function in the tumor microenvironment. One of the hallmarks of cancer is avoiding apoptotic death; interestingly, much of what we had thought was necrotic death now appears to be a form of regulated cell death known as necroptosis, driving the development of the innate and subsequent adaptive immune response to cancer.[29–32] Similarly, exuberant autophagy in tumor cells can limit expression of MHC class I molecules and thereby obviate an adaptive immune response.[33,34] Interestingly, transcriptional signatures related to autophagy have been shown to bear a prognostic connotation in the context, for instance, of prostate and lung cancers.[35,36]

INNATE IMMUNITY INITIATES THE IMMUNE RESPONSE AGAINST CANCER

The innate immune cells in the tumor including the embryologically deposited tissue macrophages and natural killer (NK) cells and those recruited over activated endothelium allow initiation and recruitment of the subsequent adaptive immune response.[37,38] The endogenous innate immune activation mediated by exogenous DAMPs such as HMGB1, endogenous STING signaling,[39] and subsequent stress ligands expressed on tumor cells interacting with receptors such as NKG2D on NK and T cells allows the induction of autophagy, release of IFN-γ, and upregulation of class I and II molecules, enabling interrogation by the emergent T cell response. The *receptor for advanced glycation end products (RAGE)* is an MHC class III encoded molecule that serves as a DAMP receptor and the only identified cell surface DNA receptor; it promotes activation of the inflammasome[40] and response to neutrophil extracellular traps.[10] Although there has been substantial interest in exploiting these innate immune effectors in the tumor microenvironment, it is clear that one needs an effective T cell adaptive immune response to mediate the important deep responses possible with immunotherapy. Understanding how innate immune cells and effector mechanisms initiate and sustain or counter-regulate the adaptive immune response is a critical and poorly understood aspect of modern tumor immunology.

T CELLS ARE CENTRAL TO THE IMMUNE RESPONSE TO CANCER

Probably one of the most exciting and convincing demonstrations of the critical role of T cells in molding the natural history of cancer[41] is not only the emergence of tumors in the setting of primary and secondary immune deficiencies, but also the ability of the adoptive transfer of ex vivo expanded tumor infiltrating lymphocytes in mediating antitumor effects.[2] T cells recognize viral epitopes[42] and neoepitopes derived from mutant so-called passenger mutations[5,43–45] as well as driver mutations such as KRAS.[46,47] These can be recognized and can mediate important antitumor effects when adoptively transferred. Such neoepitope-recognizing cells can be identified in the tumor tissue[45] as well as in the blood.[48] Attempts to target solid tumors with chimeric antigen receptor T cells has been stalled by the difficulty of identifying suitable unique targets on the tumor cell surface that can be recognized by antibodies.[49,50]

ACQUIRED RESISTANCE TO T CELLS INVOLVES TUMOR INTRINSIC AND EMERGENT CHANGES IN THE TUMOR MICROENVIRONMENT

During the period of Darwinian interaction of the tumor and the associated host immune response, specific changes associated within the tumor can limit the recruitment of T cells. These so-called cold tumors[28,37,51,52] are dictated by lack of recruitment of critical dendritic cell subpopulations (CD103+, CD141+), expression of PI3K,[53] PTEN loss,[54] or overexpression of Wnt/βcatenin pathway molecules.[28] In addition, secondary to the genetic instability intrinsic to cancer cells, often tumors lose antigen processing and presenting mechanisms and, therefore, become unrecognizable to T cells.

IMMUNOTHERAPY AGAINST CANCER EXPLOITS A NATURAL AND BROADLY CONSERVED IMMUNOLOGICAL BEHAVIOR

Direct study of cancer tissues performed by obtaining serial biopsies of the same lesions before and during immunotherapy identified a specific transcriptional signature associated exclusively to the phase of therapy in which a cancer is rejected by host cells.[55] The signature comprises activation of *interferon (IFN)*-g associated genes including *signal transducer and activation of transcription factor-1 (STAT-1), interferon regulatory factor-1 (IRF-1)*, and *human leukocyte antigen (HLA)* molecules, immune effector genes such as perforin and granzyme, and chemokine receptors CXCR3 and CCR5 and their ligand chemokines. Various studies performed in humans or experimental models serially followed the kinetics of tumor rejection in response to various forms of immunotherapy and demonstrated that the activation of the immune-rejection signature is a conserved, broad behavior that extends also to other forms of *immune-mediated tissue-specific destruction (ITD)* such as rejection of allografts,[56–58] graft-versus-host disease,[59,60] and several autoimmune disorders.[61] This observation leads to the realization that tumor rejection is a facet of a conserved immunologic phenomenon associated with the activation of a common transcriptional signature that we named the Immunologic Constant of Rejection.[62] Thus, understanding immune-mediated tumor rejection can benefit from the study of other auto-destructive phenomena mediated by the immune system, and basic immunological principles that apply to other immune pathologies may be just as relevant in the field of immune oncology. For this reason, the following chapters, although predominantly focused on the interactions between cancer and immune cells and their products, have been prepared by immunologists with broad expertise in the basic mechanisms of immune recognition. It should be emphasized that immune-mediated cancer destruction differs dramatically from other forms of ITD because of the genetic instability of the target organ, which is specific to neoplastic tissues and in some cases viral genomic instability. Therefore, the study of other immune pathologies may simplify the understanding of the role that nonneoplastic factors such as the genetic background of the host or environmental exposure may play on immune rejection.[63–69]

TUMOR REJECTION IS THE EXTREME MANIFESTATION OF A CONTINUUM OF IMMUNE SURVEILLANCE

A transcriptional signature largely overlapping to the ICR signature has been described in association with the infiltration of CD8 expressing T cell in intratumoral and peritumoral areas. This signature bears a favorable prognostic connotation in a multivariate analysis where other canonical prognostic indicators were taken into consideration.[70,71] Such signatures were originally described in colon cancer patients[70–72] and subsequently documented as an independent prognostic biomarker for most other cancer types.[73] Recently, a multinational consortium including a large number of institutions led by the Society for Immunotherapy of Cancer (SITC) validated the robustness of this prognostic marker.[74] At the same time, various investigators observed that the same transcripts included in the ICR, when expressed in pretreatment biopsies, predict responsiveness to immunotherapy including responsiveness to checkpoint inhibitors.[75–77] Thus, it is likely that immune responsiveness of cancer spans a continuum of immune surveillance that goes from proclivity to respond to immunotherapy, to maintenance of a favorable natural course of disease throughout different stages of evolution independent of treatment.[78] Upon enhanced activation, the same processes lead to its ultimate outcome, the rejection of the neoplastic tissue.[79] Individual stages of cancer progression may be related to quantitative aspects of the ICR signature activation.[79,80] Possibly, at the lowest level of activation, the ICR signature does not affect the natural behavior of the tumor until a perturbation is applied through immune stimulation that further activates a naturally occurring but lingering immune recognition, turning it into a full blown acute rejection (predictive signatures). At a higher level of activation, the immune system can slow the progression of tumors independent of treatment (prognostic signature). Only when the activation is optimized is treatment regression observed. The recognition of this signature may, therefore, serve as a tool to stratify patients likely to respond to therapy or to monitor its outcome as a surrogate marker of response as will be discussed extensively in the subsequent sections of this textbook. Obviously, the question remaining revolves around the reason(s) why only a fraction of patients present with a tumor expressing the ICR signature.[63,64]

TUMOR REJECTION IS MULTIFACTORIAL; IN PARTICULAR, CANCER REJECTION IS CHARACTERIZED BY GENETIC INSTABILITY OF THE TARGET TISSUE, ADDING COMPLEXITY TO THE UNDERSTANDING OF ITS MECHANISMS

Cancer immune responsiveness is a multifactorial phenomenon dependent upon several elements; each of them necessary, but not sufficient. Experimental and clinical evidence suggests that there are four categories of factors determining immune responsiveness: (a) genetic background of the host, (b) somatic makeup of individual cancers, (c) hidden environmental factors such as the microbiome and comorbidities,[81] and (d) the diversity within the aggregate rearranged T and B cell receptors, collectively the "adaptome."[82] However, the weight born by each category is not conclusively determined due to limited access to accurate biometrical information and often-insufficient computational infrastructure to support congregated multivariate, high-density data analysis. For instance, querying germline and cancer whole genome sequencing repositories is a challenge that only a few institutions can face. Additionally, integration of data derived from individual experimental and clinical sources and adding temporal dimensions is exponentially challenging. Lessons learned by autoimmunity suggest that the genetic background of the host and its post-genetic adaptations are strong determinants in the proclivity to activate ITD phenomena.[83–87] These include epigenetic factors such as micro-RNA induction of an immune suppressive tumor microenvironment.[88] However, the weight that the genetic background of the host plays in immune responsiveness has not been conclusively studied in humans although several observations suggest that it may be important not only as a determinant of immune responsiveness but also of treatment-related autoimmune toxicity.[64,89,90] It has also become apparent, at least in experimental models, that environmental factors such as the gut microbiota can affect responsiveness of distant tumors to various forms of therapy including immunotherapy.[91,92] Finally, to add complexity to the problem, the neoplastic tissue offers a specific challenge determined by its genetic instability exemplified in particular by tumor micro-satellite instability, which may in turn determine immune responsiveness.[93] It appears that the high-mutational load associated with DNA repair defects, DNA damage, and associated likelihood to develop neoantigens is an important factor in determining immune responsiveness.[94–98] In addition, the genetic instability of neoplastic cells increases the chance for selection under immune pressure of cells capable to escape immune recognition as well as exemplified by loss of HLA molecules[99] or loss of antigen processing elements.[100] Moreover, genetic instability affects a large number of oncogenic processes that in turn mold a highly unstable cancer biology prone to immunogenic cell death.[63,64,67,68,101]

A panoply of factors affects the emergence and function of suitable T cells including the presence of negative suppressor of cytokine signaling family members including CISH,[102] the critical role of maintaining mitochondrial mass[27,103,104] in T cells, and somewhat surprisingly the ability of an established immune response in

T cells to affect the ability of naïve T cells to emerge.[105,106] It was recently reported that enhanced glycolysis activity in breast cancer is associated with pro-tumor immunity mediated through the IL-17 signaling pathway.[107] Diversity within the TCR repertoire has increasingly been identified as being critical for enhancing an immune response to cancer in a variety of settings.[106,108–112] These complex determinants of immune responsiveness and immune escape will be discussed extensively in the following chapters including mechanisms to enhance the former and circumvent the latter.

INITIATING AN IMMUNE RESPONSE: THE OUTSTANDING QUESTION

The activation of the ICR signature is a powerful prognostic and predictive biomarker of immune responsiveness in several cancer histologies undergoing different types of immunotherapy.[67,70,71,74–77,101,113–117] Thus, molecular taxonomies defined by the ICR represent surrogate biomarkers of favorable outcome for explorative studies applied to large data sets including those for which no outcome information is available. This strategy may provide "off-the-shelf" insights about the mechanism determining the favorable phenotype allowing educated assumptions for trial design. For instance, current drug development in cancer immunotherapy focuses on testing additional checkpoint inhibitors as single agents or in combination. As the number of candidate products grows, companies need to rank the sequence of testing to mitigate the extraordinary cost of clinical trials and prioritize patients' accrual into trials with highest likelihood of success. It is becoming apparently clear that the biology of checkpoint interactions with their ligands is most often redundant and affects the same immune landscapes, predominantly immunogenic tumors.[63,67,118] Thus, these therapeutics when given in combination are likely to offer benefit only in a limited number of circumstances where compensatory immune resistance limits the effectiveness of monotherapy targeting only one mechanism of immune regulation at the time.[63,64,118] Thus, the assumption that novel generations of checkpoint inhibitors may apply to tumors that do not respond to the current ones is not substantiated. Known checkpoint inhibitors are co-expressed with the ICR genes in the immune favorable phenotype as a compensatory mechanism against active anticancer immunity.[63] There is no evidence that these mechanisms are activated in immunologically "silent" cancers. Thus, the preclinical categorization of expression of novel checkpoint mechanisms in tumors unlikely to respond to immunotherapy is a good example of how the ICR assumption can be used to prioritize clinical trial selection for proof of principle testing of novel therapeutics.

INTEGRATING CANCER BIOLOGY AND TUMOR IMMUNOLOGY

We now need to take the rich armamentarium of targeted agents that affect tumor biology and discern whether they might be useful for direct use in combination with immunotherapies or to alter immune cells. We know that chemotherapy treatment itself can induce PD-L1 expression[119] and that the subsequent induction of autophagy associated with resistance to chemotherapy can be in part overcome with pharmacologic mediators.[120] Furthermore, chemotherapy treatment can enhance sensitivity to innate immune effectors.[121] A rich area of investigation will assess how small molecules can affect T cell function.[122] Integrating cancer biology and tumor immunology will be critical for the future development and cross-talk between these two fields.

BACK TO CANCER BIOLOGY

Immunotherapy shifted the development of anticancer drugs to systems biology, focusing on the relationship among neoplastic and environmental cells rather than the intrinsic biology of cancer traditionally targeted by therapeutics that selectively kill uncontrollably dividing cells. Thus, most current immunotherapy targets primarily extra-cellular interactions while chemotherapy and pathway inhibitors target intracellular mechanisms. The basic assumption supporting immunotherapy is that at the dawn of cancer, neoplastic cells are recognized and destroyed by immune surveillance.[123] Through an evolutionary process, some of the progeny become less recognizable and a conglomerate of cancer tissue develops.[124] As the cancer forms into new tissue, it requires a structure that can sustain its growth and provide nutrients. At this stage, cancer cells exploit mechanisms used by normal cells in response to injury by producing factors that attract cells capable of initiating tissue repair including angiogenesis.[125,126] Vascular normalization, conversely, is designed to not kill the tumor by limiting blood supply but rather to promote the ability of immune cells to gain access to the tumor to mediate immunologic control.[127–130] This process, however, is promiscuous since it also attracts immune cells that in wounded tissues are meant to protect against foreign pathogens. In cancer the immune cells may be recognized as foreign molecules produced by mutated cancer cells that did not go through thymic scrutiny. Regulatory cells that limit the extent of the immune response counterbalance this immune recognition. The balance between effector and regulatory cells is mediated through cell-to-cell interactions by checkpoint mechanisms. In growing tumors, the balance is skewed in favor of tolerance mechanisms. Immunotherapy, when successful, alters this balance by blocking these checkpoints and tumors are rejected. However, it is possible that immune resistant cancers adopt completely different mechanisms to assure a supportive microenvironment devoid of immune reactivity. In such cases, checkpoint inhibitor therapy will never work and billions of dollars will be wasted testing products in the wrong patient populations.

It is possible that immune resistant cancers evolved to survive in the host by selectively secreting factors that support tissue regeneration but not immune surveillance, spontaneously fine-tuning the mechanisms of wound repair. If this hypothesis is correct, only a better understanding of the intrinsic cancer cell biology determining this "clean" behavior will identify corrective measures targeting intracellular pathways and turning immune silent tumors into immunologically active ones. Data to explore this question are already available in open access repositories and an in silico analysis of germline, somatic, and phenotypic information can already kick start the solution of the problem. More will need to be done to validate the causality of findings by testing concepts identified by this strategy in pre-clinical models.

COMPLEX PROBLEMS DO NOT NECESSARILY DEMAND COMPLEX SOLUTIONS

When the biology of a complex problem is understood, its solutions may turn out to be simpler than anticipated.[131] Step-by-step the plethora of hypotheses put forward to explain cancer immune responsiveness is converging into a theory of everything,[63,67,118,132] thanks to modern inductive approaches based on high-throughput discovery corroborated by experimental validation.[133] Current consensus is that the immune biology of solid tumors can be demarcated into three fundamental landscapes: immune-active, immune-deserted, and immune-excluded.[63,66,134] These immune phenotypes occur at about equal frequency across solid cancers,[135,136] and with their diverse biology, they present distinct opportunities for intervention. Recently, we proposed a strategy to integrate compelling data from various paradigms into a *"Theory of Everything."* Founded upon this unified theory, we proposed the creation of a task force led by SITC aimed at systematically addressing salient questions relevant to cancer immune responsiveness and immune evasion[64] that encompass all aspects of genetics, tumor cell biology, immunology, and environmental sciences pertinent to the understanding of this multifaceted problem. We believe that future investigations should concentrate on this integrative approach to dissect the fundamental determinants of each phenotype and several chapters of the new edition will attempt to exemplify this principle.

CONCLUSION

In conclusion, cancer immunotherapy is rapidly evolving and is perhaps one of the most active areas of investigation at the present time. The current success demonstrated by recent therapies, particularly with checkpoint inhibitors on one side and with adoptive transfer of cells recognizing surface molecules expressed by cancer cells, is strong evidence that cancer is susceptible to immune mechanisms. A deeper understanding of the cell biology determining cancer phenotypes and orchestrating immune responsiveness will likely allow tumor eradication and/or control.

KEY REFERENCES

Only key references appear in the print edition. The full reference list appears in the digital product on Springer Publishing Connect: connect.springerpub.com/content/book/978-0-8261-3743-2/part/part01/chapter/ch02

14. Huang J, Xie Y, Sun X, et al. DAMPs, ageing, and cancer: the 'DAMP Hypothesis'. *Ageing Res Rev*. 2015;24(Pt A):3–16. doi:10.1016/j.arr.2014.10.004

28. Spranger S, Bao R, Gajewski TF. Melanoma-intrinsic beta-catenin signalling prevents anti-tumour immunity. *Nature*. 2015;523(7559):231–235. doi:10.1038/nature14404

62. Wang E, Worschech A, Marincola FM. The immunologic constant of rejection. *Trends Immunol*. 2008;29(6):256–262. doi:10.1016/j.it.2008.03.002

68. Galluzzi L, Vitale I, Warren S, et al. Consensus guidelines for the definition, detection and interpretation of immunogenic cell death. *J Immunother Cancer*. 2020;8(1):e000337corr1. doi:10.1136/jitc-2019-000337corr1

70. Galon J, Costes A, Sanchez-Cabo F, et al. Type, density, and location of immune cells within human colorectal tumors predict clinical outcome. *Science*. 2006;313(5795):1960–1964. doi:10.1126/science.1129139

115. Wang E, Miller LD, Ohnmacht GA, et al. Prospective molecular profiling of melanoma metastases suggests classifiers of immune responsiveness. *Cancer Res*. 2002;62(13):3581–3586. https://cancerres.aacrjournals.org/content/62/13/3581

136. Kather JN, Suarez-Carmona M, Charoentong P, et al. Topography of cancer-associated immune cells in human solid tumors. *Elife*. 2018;7:e36967. doi:10.7554/eLife.36967

3

Genomic Determinants of Cancer Immune Response and Resistance

Alessandra Cesano

KEY POINTS

- Traditionally, the search for factors influencing the outcome of cancer therapy has been highly tumor-centric, resulting in a now well characterized, yet still incomplete, view of the complex molecular and cellular dynamics relevant to cancer progression and to treatment response.

- More recently, evidence that oncoproteins can support more than cellular transformation and growth has been accumulating, and it is now well accepted that there is a complex interplay between genomic/epigenomic alterations and tumor immune response that can impair induction or execution of local antitumor immune response, ultimately impacting disease prognosis and therapeutic responses.

- To this regard the Cancer Genome Atlas (TCGA)-Pan Cancer Atlas (www.cell.com/pb-assets/consortium/pancanceratlas/pancani3/index.html) is an invaluable achievement that has advanced oncogenes understanding and increased the appreciation of the interconnectedness by which oncogenic signaling pathways can produce profound systemic effects and altered immune function, ultimately supporting cancer growth.

- Understanding the main genomic factors implicated in the tumor-immune response (or lack thereof) has important practical implications for the development and clinical application of both predictive biomarker and immunotherapeutic approaches.

INTRODUCTION

Long before the advent of modern genomic technologies, associations between certain cancer histologic sub-types and differences in response to therapeutics were described

and leveraged for disease management in the clinic. More recently, with the advent of high-density data generation such as next generation sequencing, the field has gained tremendous insight into the molecular underpinnings of these clinicopathologic observations and distinct genomic aberrations have been shown to frequently define specific cancer sub-types and to confer notable differences in therapeutic sensibility of major clinical relevance.[1,2]

From an immunological point of view, in the immunocompetent host, tumors develop along a continuum of immunogenic potential manifested by phenotypes with different levels and distribution of T cell infiltration.[3,4] Specifically, three main immune phenotypes have been described:[4] (a) the inflamed phenotype, a.k.a. "hot," (b) the immune-excluded phenotype, and (c) the immune-desert phenotype (the last two currently considered to be immunologically "cold" tumors). T cell infiltrated tumors are characterized by type I IFN activation, CD8+ T cells functionally oriented toward a Th1 phenotype, the presence of T cell-attracting chemokines, competent antigen presentation, and cytotoxic effector molecules.[5] Immune-excluded tumors refer to tumors with an immune suppressed tumor microenvironment (TME) represented by T cell embedded in the stromal TME with high TGF-β signaling, myeloid inflammation, and high expression of cytokines such as IL-8 and IL-6 and VEGF (the latter associated with angiogenesis).[6] Lastly, immune desert tumors represent a tumor virtually devoid of immune infiltration or antigen presentation molecules. These tumors are characterized by remarkable genetic stability and highly proliferative capacity.[5,6] Importantly, these different immune phenotypes have clinical relevance since in the context of checkpoint inhibition, the non-inflamed phenotypes have been associated with inferior clinical outcomes.[7] Furthermore, the tumor immune phenotypes occur independently of individual cancer ontogenesis although the prevalence of each one varies in tumors with different cells of origin.[6]

The majority of the data supporting the molecular classification of such immune phenotypes have been generated by clustering samples according to the level of inflammation present in the TME (i.e., T cell inflamed

25

versus non-T cell inflamed) using gene expression profiling and then integrating genetic/genomic information obtained by DNA sequencing.[7] In this regard, the Cancer Genome Atlas (TCGA)-Pan Cancer Atlas (www.cell.com/pb-assets/consortium/pancanceratlas/pancani3/index.html) has been a foundational achievement that has advanced the understanding of oncogenes and increased the appreciation of the interconnectedness by which oncogenic signaling pathways can produce profound systemic effects and alter the immune function to support cancer growth.[8–10]

Several of these factors, particularly the overall somatic tumor mutation burden (TMB), have shown potential utility in the prediction of response to immunotherapy.[11,12] However, qualitatively genomic characterization of tumors (i.e., characterization of the immune effects of specific mutations versus just counting the tumor mutation load) is emerging as being equally informative from a biomarker and therapeutic point of view.[13]

This chapter provides an overview of the genomic factors implicated in the cancer response to immune surveillance and describes the implications of these findings for the development of both patient selection biomarkers and immunotherapeutic approaches.

Generally speaking, tumor-specific influences on the immune response can be schematically classified into two groups (Figure 3.1):[13]

1. Factors that affect the "visibility" of the tumor by the host immune system
2. Factors that affect the "susceptibility" of the tumor to an effective immune response

TUMOR IMMUNE "VISIBILITY"

In addition to the influence on oncogenic signaling and proliferative potential, genomic mutations may have profound impact on antitumor immunity and can contribute to the "visibility" of the tumor by the immune system.[13] This is largely shaped by the antigenic characteristics of the tumors but may be affected by other influences of these oncogenic alterations on the tumor cells themselves as well as on the TME. An important practical corollary of these observations is that therapeutic targeting of oncogenically activated signaling pathways may also affect the antitumor immune response in a therapeutically relevant way.

Tumor Mutation Burden (TMB)

Generally speaking, tumor immune visibility is dependent on the presence or absence of molecular moieties that can be recognized as "non-self" by components of the host immune system (i.e., antigens).[13,14] These antigens have different levels of tumor cell specificity, that is, differentiation/lineage-specific antigens aberrantly expressed, absent, or only found during ontogenesis (a.k.a., cancer associated antigens)[14] or tumor-cell specific neoantigens derived from the protein product of somatically mutated tumor genes; the latter are felt to predominantly mediate an effective antitumor immune response because neoantigen-reactive T cells escape central deletion during T cell ontogenesis.[15]

The mutational landscape varies across tumor types[16] and is shaped by factors influencing carcinogenesis, which can be exogenous (such as UV irradiation

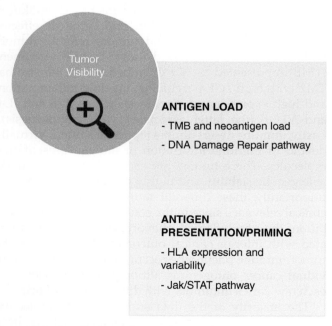

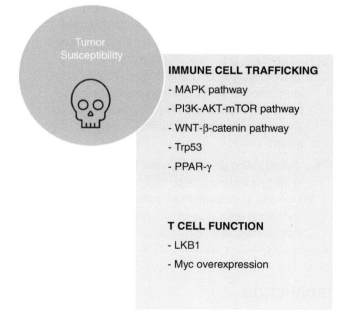

Figure 3.1 Genetic determinants of cancer immune response/resistance.

HLA, human leukocyte antigen; TMB, tumor mutation burden.

and cigarette smoking) or endogenous (such as DNA-Damage-Repair [DDR] gene defects) (e.g., BRCA or Mis-Match-Repair [MMR] gene alterations).[17] Interestingly, response to checkpoint inhibitors (CPI) is positively associated with TMB in individual tumor types.[18,19] In fact, TMB and neoantigen load were among the earliest biomarkers of clinical response to CPI identified. Snyder et al.[11] first showed that higher TMB was associated with response to the CTLA-4 inhibitor ipilumimab in melanoma. This observation was subsequently validated in the context of PD-1/PD-L1 blockade.[12] Further supporting the relationship between TMB with clinical responses to CPI, tumors carrying MMR gene alterations demonstrate an increased sensitivity to checkpoint blockade likely due to an increase in TMB and neo-antigen load (i.e., microsatellite instability high [MSI-H] tumors).[17] Indeed, demonstration of MSI-H or MRR deficiency upon biomarker testing forms the basis for the first tumor agnostic drug approval made by the U.S. Food and Drug Administration (FDA) for anti-PD-1 therapy in 2017.[20] The practical limitation of measuring TMB as predictive biomarker in the context of CPI has been currently mitigated by robust estimation of overall mutational load using data obtained from targeted next generation sequencing technologies now accessible to the clinic. On June 16, 2020, the FDA granted accelerated approval to pembrolizumab (KEYTRUDA, Merck & Co., Inc.) for the treatment of adult and pediatric patients with unresectable or metastatic tumor mutational burden-high (TMB-H) [≥10 mutations/megabase (mut/Mb)] solid tumors, as determined by an FDA-approved test (i.e., FoundationOne CDx test, Foundation Medicine Inc.), who progressed following prior treatment and who have no alternative treatment options.[21] In addition, cancer gene panel mutational profiling by liquid biopsy represents a promising alternative mutational-burden-related methodology for predicting immunotherapy response, as reported in an analysis of non-small cell lung cancer (NSCLC) patients enrolled in clinical trials of the anti-PD-L1 agent atezolizumab.[22]

Although the connection between TMB and neoantigen load provides a biologic explanation underlying CPI response in TMB-H tumors, TMB alone does not reliably predict response in all patients.[19] Identification of additional genomic factors that influence response is imperative to better understand and predict patient outcomes and refine therapeutic strategies.

Furthermore, it is now well understood that genomic instability is not the only source of cancer antigens in tumors. Diseases like clear cell carcinoma, a subset of prostate and ovarian cancers, have a high prevalence of human endogenous retroviruses (hERVs).[23-25] hERVs integrated in the human genome are largely silenced in normal cells but can become dysregulated and re-expressed in cancer, and they can serve as a tumor antigen

signal. In addition to hERVs, viruses such as Epstein-Barr, hepatitis B, hepatitis C, human papillomavirus, and Merkel cell polyomavirus may also provide a strong source of immunogenic antigens in certain tumor types such as HNC, HCC, cervical, Merkel cell carcinoma, and gastric cancers thus provide increased immune "visibility" to those tumors.[26]

Antigen Presentation Machinery

The dynamic of immune activation in response to the tumor cell mutational repertoire is modulated by additional factors that affect the expression, processing, and intrinsic immunogenicity of putative antigens.

The presentation of antigens by human leukocyte antigen (HLA) molecules to T cell receptors, typically defined as "signal 1," is at the basis for T cell-mediated antitumor immune responses. Engagement of "signal 1" is essential for naïve T cell activation and, therefore, the successful application of most immunotherapeutic modalities, including CPI, personalized cancer vaccines, and antigen-directed T cell therapies.[27]

The complex process involved in cleaving a peptide, loading into a MHC molecule, transporting to the cell surface, and ensuring its stability is essential to induce the antigenic T cell response required for tumor clearance.[28] However, several steps can "go wrong" along the way in this multi-step process as described next.

It is well established that tumor cells can evolve to escape immune recognition by reducing antigen-presenting HLA proteins on their surface (HLA loss), thus creating a mechanism that can propagate resistance.[29] Several mechanisms of HLA loss have been described, both at a genetic ("hard loss") and epigenetic ("soft loss") level.[29,30] They can directly affect the HLA class I complex and its transcriptional regulation (e.g., IFN signaling pathway) or indirectly target genes that are part of the antigen presentation machinery (APM).

In a recent study from the TRACERx consortium using 258 tumor regions from 88 prospectively acquired tumors, 56% of lung adenocarcinomas and 78% of lung squamous cell carcinomas showed evidence for genetic disruption of the antigen presentation process, either through HLA loss of heterozygosity (HLA LOH) or APM mutations.[31]

Beta-2 microglobulin (B2M) is an essential component of major histocompatibility complex (MHC) and is required for cell surface expression of MHC class I and antigen presentation. In a small study of melanoma patients treated with CPI, complete loss of both copies of the B2M gene was only observed in non-responders, whereas the absence of tumor-specific expression, frameshift mutations, and LOH of the B2M gene were observed in ~30% of patients with progressive disease and were found more frequently in non-responders than in responders.[32]

Adding another layer of complexity, the MHC-II complex (encoded by HLA-DP, HLA-DM, HLA-DO, HLA-DQ, and HLA-DR) is canonically expressed by professional APCs to present antigens to CD4+ cells. In the absence of tumor MHC-I expression, MHC-II expression functions as a complementary means of activating T helper cells. This synergistic relationship highlights the importance of assessing pre-treatment expression levels for both MHC complexes.[33]

While evidence of HLA loss has been documented in a variety of tumor types[34] albeit mostly in small cohorts, a systematic evaluation of the combined frequency and relative contributions of "hard" and "soft" HLA loss across tumor types is warranted. Only by capturing all mechanisms of HLA loss we can accurately estimate their impact on outcomes in different treatment settings, and devise strategies to overcome resistance, circumvent it, or even prevent an early tumor from evolving an HLA loss phenotype.

TUMOR IMMUNE "SUSCEPTIBILITY"

A tumor's visibility to the immune system does not automatically imply its clearance as numerous distinct factors can also influence its susceptibility to immune attack.[28]

Therefore, although immune visibility is necessary to the establishment of an inflamed TME, it is not sufficient to guarantee tumor clearance.

JAK/STAT Signaling Pathway

The JAK/STAT family of signaling pathways has long been known to play important roles in several immunological functions with established links between JAK/STAT germline mutations and immune-related diseases.[35] The particular implications of the JAK/STAT pathway in immunotherapy are related to its role in IFN-γ downstream signaling. IFN-γ signaling defects have been repeatedly implicated in cancer immunotherapy failure, including copy number losses of IFN-g pathway genes (principally IFNGR1/2, IRF1, and JAK2) in patients failing to respond to anti-CTLA-4 therapy.[36] Loss of function mutations in JAK1/2 have also been described in patients with melanoma with either primary[37] or secondary resistance to anti-PD-1 drugs.[38] Manguso et al.[39] demonstrated via in vivo CRISPR knock out screen that tumors lacking elements of the JAK/STAT pathway failed to upregulate MHC I molecules and were likely to evade immune surveillance. In addition, because IFN-γ signaling results in the upregulation of PD-L1,[40] PD-1/PD-L1 inhibitors are most efficacious when the JAK/STAT pathways are intact or even potentiated. In fact, amplification of chromosomal region 9p24.1, which includes the genes PD-L1, PD-L2, and JAK2, was found to be a biomarker for high PD-1 response rates in Hodgkin lymphoma:[41] expression of PD-L1 is augmented in this case not only directly, via amplification of PD-L1 itself, but also indirectly through a more active JAK/STAT pathway. A study of four melanoma patients who experienced relapses following PD-1 blockade bolstered these findings, as two of the four resistant tumors harbored JAK1 or JAK2 inactivating mutations.[37]

Therefore, as described in the previous section, variation in HLA gene expression and levels of the MHC class I and II complexes can shape the antitumor response by modulating the "visibility" of tumor antigens by the adaptive immune system. Simultaneously, variations in the JAK/STAT pathway modulate IFN-γ and PD-L1 expression levels and consequently T cell cytotoxicity. Any alterations disrupting the complex interaction of these pathways can enable tumor immune escape. Therefore, the JAK/STAT pathway and HLA variability should be analyzed jointly when considering their effect on CPI response.

Canonical Oncogenic Pathways

Confirming the intricate relationship between immune response and tumor progression, alterations in several canonical oncogenes (activated by gain of function alterations) and tumor suppressor genes (inactivated by loss of function alterations) have also been recently associated with response to CPI particularly in the "cold" tumor immune-phenotypes.[42] The co-evolution of tumors and their TME was further elucidated in a recent publication in which TCGA analysis immunologically landscaped 10 canonical cancer pathways.[43] A noteworthy aspect of this analysis explored the mutual exclusivity and co-occurrence of these pathways, with co-occurrent patterns indicating potential oncogenic synergies that can promote resistance to therapy and potentially immune evasion.[43]

The majority of these altered genes function in the MAPK-ERK, PI3K-AKT-mTOR, and WINT/β-catenin pathways, all of which are firmly established as oncogenic signaling pathways with longstanding evidence for relevance in tumor formation and progression.[44] As several of these genes are targets of known inhibitors, any significant associations between these genes and CPI response may be leveraged to select combination therapies of CPI with such inhibitors.

WNT/β-Catenin Pathway

The first tumor-intrinsic oncogene pathway mediating immune exclusion identified was the WNT/β-catenin pathway in metastatic melanoma.[45]

Analyses of human melanoma samples revealed that upregulation of WNT/β-catenin pathway signaling was associated with lack of T cells in both primary tumors and distant metastases.[46] Further analyses in a genetically engineered mouse model of conditional BRaf^V600E and inducible β-catenin revealed a causal relationship between activation of β-catenin signaling, lower T cell infiltration, and lack of response to checkpoint inhibition.[46,47] Possible mechanisms involve low chemokine production (e.g., CCL4, CXCL9, CXCL10) and reduced prevalence of BATF3+ dendritic cells in the TME resulting in diminished T cell infiltration and trafficking.[46,47] A similar analysis of human urothelial bladder cancers in TCGA database revealed that non-T cell inflamed bladder tumors were associated with increased WNT/β-catenin pathway activation.[48] Thus, pharmacological inhibition of WNT/β-catenin signaling may be a strategy to restore T cell entry in at least some non-T cell inflamed tumors and facilitate response to checkpoint inhibitors. The prevalence of this mechanism of immune evasion across cancer types is not yet conclusively defined.

MAPK-ERK Pathway

The MAPK-ERK pathway is involved in a number of diverse cellular processes such as proliferation, differentiation, motility, survival, and its oncogenic role has been well documented.[49] An emerging body of evidence has also identified a role of the MAPK pathway in regulating the immune response in the TME. In mouse models across various cancer histology, inhibition of the pathway using MAPK/ERK inhibitors resulted in enhanced T cell infiltration, IFN-γ production, and MHC class I expression, suggesting that combinations of MAPK inhibitors with CPI may improve outcomes in these patients.[50-52] Interestingly, the MAPK pathway is also essential for T cell activation and function,[53] suggesting that MAPK inhibitors can, on the other side, negatively affect conventional T cell response.

Co-mutation with MAPK pathway genes is also associated with specific immune profiles and response to CPI in a cancer type-dependent context. KRAS, a MAPK pathway gene, is one of the most frequent oncogenic drivers in lung adenocarcinoma, and its co-mutation with STK11 or TP53 (both loss of function alterations) defines genomic subtypes with distinct mutational load and immune profiles.[54,55]

PI3K-AKT-mTOR Pathway

The PI3K-AKT-mTOR pathway is a key signal transduction system comprising several oncogenes and is involved in essential cellular processes such as survival, proliferation, and differentiation.[56] Loss of the tumor suppressor phosphatase and tensin homolog (PTEN) gene, a negative regulator of the pathway, results in a constitutively activated pathway and aberrant tumor growth.[57] Recent studies have shown that, in metastatic melanoma, loss of PTEN correlates with decreased intratumoral T cell infiltration and reduced responsiveness to PD-1 therapy.[58] Mechanistically, loss of PTEN results in increased activation of the PI3K-AKT pathway which in turn results in increased production of immunosuppressive

cytokines such as VEGF, CCL2, and regulatory T cells (T_{reg} cells) recruitment, while rendering the TME less permeable to $CD8^+$ T cells.[59] These observations provide a rationale for developing a therapeutic approach using specific PI3K inhibitors in combination with CPI for tumors with PTEN deletion. It is well established that PTEN loss, inactivation, and attenuation is a common genetic feature in multiple cancers, with PTEN LOH found in more than a quarter of glioblastomas, prostate cancers, breast cancers, and melanomas.[59] Of note, genetic alterations in PTEN and the WNT/β-catenin pathways appear to be mostly non-overlapping, thus suggesting that these may represent distinct mechanisms of immune evasion.[59]

Other Oncogenic Pathways

Emerging data have suggested the potential for additional oncogenic pathways to affect antitumor immunity, some of which are briefly summarized next.

The serine/threonine liver kinase B (LKB1 aka STK11) is a suppressor gene mutated in a diverse range of cancers where it is associated with worse prognosis.[60,61] Loss of LKB1 may mediate immune evasion through the recruitment of inhibitory cell populations to the tumor microenvironment by increased expression of CCL2 by tumor cells and increased pro-tumorigenic macrophage density in the TME.[62] These findings suggest that targeting aberrant cytokine/chemokine signaling or immunosuppressive cell populations might be a promising therapy strategy against LKB1-deficient tumors.

The transcription factor MYC regulates cell proliferation, differentiation, and survival and is overexpressed in many cancers.[63,64] The MYC oncogene regulates tumor cell expression of two immune checkpoints involved in cancer cell immune evasion, PD-L1, and CD47,[65] the latter of which is an antiphagocytic protein that inhibits the ingestion of tumor cells by macrophages and DC, ultimately impairing the ability of APC to prime effector T cells.

Utilizing a mouse lung cancer model of conditional $KRAS^{G12D}$ and inducible Myc, Kortlever et al.[66] provide an example of oncogenic cooperation between *KRas* and *Myc* to produce highly proliferative tumors with an inflamed, angiogenic, and immunosuppressed stroma. Particularly noteworthy in this study is the ability of Myc overexpression to rapidly clear the tumor environment of innate and adaptive immune lymphocytes, namely T, B, and natural killer (NK) cells. Several additional reports provide evidence that gain of functional Myc activity, through amplification or constitutive expression, can influence antitumor immunity and response to immunotherapy.[67-69]

Inactivating mutations of the tumor suppressor gene Trp53 (p53) have been associated with reduced immune infiltration[70] both in experimental models and clinically[71] in breast cancer. These effects seem to be related to a wide range of changes in chemokine production associated with dysregulation of the p53 pathway; the broader applicability of these findings to other tumor types need to be investigated.

In an immune competent model of breast cancer, Hanna et al.[72] demonstrated that dysregulation of the hedgehog pathway can also have a profound impact on the composition and functionality of the tumor-infiltrating cells including M1 and M2 macrophages, MDSCs, T_{reg} cells, dendritic cells, and T cells including CD8 cells and Th1 and Th2 cells. Their work suggests that these effects are (at least partly) manifested through altered gene expression profiles and kinase activity. Complementary work in an engineered mouse model of gastric cancer suggests that hedgehog signaling may alter the TME through additional mechanisms including upregulation of PD-L1 expression.[72]

Studies of T cell excluded bladder cancers have identified the PPARγ and FGFR3 as possible drivers of the non-T cell inflamed phenotype. Mechanistically, activation of the PPARγ pathway in vitro leads to a reduction in IL-6, IL-8, CCL2, CCL5, TNF, and CXCL10.[73]

Besides "hard coded" genetic modifications, epigenetic mechanisms can also play a role in differential tumor cell gene expression and thus immune infiltration. One example of such a mechanism is the regulation of chemokine gene expression in human ovarian cancers.[74] The gene loci for the chemokine CXCL9 and CXCL10 were found to be epigenetically silenced in ovarian cancer, resulting in deficient T cell recruitment in the TME. It is conceivable that expression of additional immunologically relevant genes might be similarly affected by epigenetic mechanisms which remain to be investigated. If such a regulation is present, it would suggest that histone deacetylase inhibitors and/or DNA methyltransferase inhibitors have the potential to augment adaptive immunity within the TME and expand effectiveness of cancer immunotherapies.

Finally, activation of oncogenes or loss of tumor suppressor genes not only exert an intrinsic influence on the biology and behavior of cancer cells but also appear to indirectly interfere with the induction and effector function of antitumor immune responses. For instance, rapidly proliferating tumors alter the metabolic conditions in the TME to create a hostile environment for the function and proliferation of T cells.[75,76] T cells depend on similar glycolytic pathways as tumor cells for survival and function. Increased hypoxia, lactic acid production, presence of an acidic TME, and lipogenesis all together alter the immune metabolism of T cells affecting TCR engagement, T cell effector function, differentiation, and proliferation.[76]

CONCLUSION

Our future conceptualization of what matters for good outcomes in cancer immunotherapies requires an integrated understanding of what contributes to cancer formation and immune evasion in the first place.

Intrinsic cancer cell biology can directly orchestrate the immune environment of tumors. These pathways have been implicated in determining the immune landscape and consequently the response to cancer immunotherapy. This in turn can be related to distinct mutational and/or epigenetic patterns responsible for disruption of these pathways creating an integrated model to explain cancer immune response/resistance from the genetic code all the way to transcriptional, translational, and post-translational modulation.

Though the diverse pathways described in this chapter operate at first glance in different domains, they play a convergent role in affecting immune response through modulation of either tumor visibility or tumor immune susceptibility. The interconnectedness of these apparently disparate biological processes demonstrates the need for a holistic approach to patient stratification. Alterations in the pathways and mechanisms described previously have the potential to join traditional biomarkers such as TMB and PD-L1 expression as a way to stratify patients to maximize the efficacy of CPI or other immunotherapies and to inform the development and clinical implementations of novel biomarkers and immunotherapeutic approaches.

KEY REFERENCES

Only key references appear in the print edition. The full reference list appears in the digital product on Springer Publishing Connect: connect.springerpub.com/content/book/978-0-8261-3743-2/part/part01/chapter/ch03

4. Hegde PS, Karanikas V, Evers S. The where, the when, and the how of immune monitoring for cancer immunotherapies in the era of checkpoint inhibition. *Clin Cancer Res.* 2016;22(8):1865–1874. doi:10.1158/1078-0432.CCR-15-1507

5. Galon J, Angell HK, Bedognetti D, et al. The continuum of cancer immunosurveillance: prognostic, predictive, and mechanistic signatures. *Immunity.* 2013;39(1):11–26. doi:10.1016/j.immuni.2013.07.008

7. Trujillo JA, Sweis RF, Bao R, et al. T cell-inflamed versus non-T cell-inflamed tumors: a conceptual framework for cancer immunotherapy drug development and combination therapy selection. *Cancer Immunol Res.* 2018;6(9):990–1000. doi:10.1158/2326-6066.CIR-18-0277

13. Andrews MC, Reuben A, Gopalakrishnan V, et al. Concepts collide: genomic, immune, and microbial influences on the tumor microenvironment and response to cancer therapy. *Front Immunol.* 2018;9:946. doi:10.3389/fimmu.2018.00946

28. Chen DS, Mellman I. Oncology meets immunology: the cancer-immunity cycle. *Immunity.* 2013;39(1):1–10. doi:10.1016/j.immuni.2013.07.012

42. Spranger S, Gajewski TF. Impact of oncogenic pathways on evasion of antitumour immune responses. *Nat Rev Cancer.* 2018;18(3):139–147. doi:10.1038/nrc.2017.117

44. Hanahan D, Weinberg RA. Hallmarks of cancer: the next generation. *Cell.* 2011;144(5):646–674. doi:10.1016/j.cell.2011.02.013

4

Human Tumor Antigens Recognized by T Lymphocytes

Nicolas van Baren and Pierre G. Coulie

KEY POINTS

- Human tumors bear antigens that can be recognized by autologous CD4 or CD8 T cells. These antitumor T cells can be found in the blood or in the tumors of some patients before any anticancer treatment.

- Tumor antigens can be of high tumoral specificity. They consist of antigenic peptides derived from proteins encoded by genes that are mutated in the tumor cells; epigenetically activated in tumor and germinal cells (the latter of which do not carry human leukocyte antigen [HLA] molecules), such as the *MAGE* genes; or those of viral origin.

- The other tumor antigens are of low tumoral specificity, such as the melanocytic differentiation antigens or those encoded by genes that are overexpressed in tumor cells as compared to normal cells.

- While almost all antigens mentioned earlier are derived from intracellular proteins, antigens recognized by antibodies, and therefore also by chimeric antigen receptor (CAR) T cells, are surface antigens. Very few of these antigens display a high tumoral specificity.

- Tumoral specificity is the major concern when using antigens in cancer immunotherapy. In most common tumors, the number of tumor-specific antigens is low.

- Predicting the full spectrum of antigens displayed on the cells of a given tumor remains almost impossible. Even though DNA sequencing allows us to list candidate mutated antigens exhaustively, only a small proportion (estimated at less than 10%) is processed and present at the cell surface. There are no reliable tools yet to predict which ones.

INTRODUCTION

Most current efforts in cancer immunotherapy aim to induce tumor-specific T cell responses in cancer patients, in order to obtain tumor rejections or to prevent recurrence. Antitumor effects have been observed after direct administration of tumor-specific T cells to human patients, after immunization with antigens recognized by such T cells, and after nonantigen-specific stimulation of T cells through the blockade of inhibitory pathways. In addition, it appears that antitumor T cells also exert a clinically meaningful antitumor effect either spontaneously, or following radiotherapy, on some types of chemotherapy or administration of monoclonal antibodies against the tumor cells or their microenvironment. The recognition of tumor-specific antigens by T lymphocytes holds a pivotal role in these processes.

TUMOR ANTIGEN DISCOVERY PROCESS

The molecular identification of human tumor antigens recognized by T cells has followed three main approaches. In the first approach, the starting material is a population of tumor-specific T cells, preferably a T cell clone. They can be derived through autologous mixed lymphocyte-tumor cell cultures (MLTC), in which T lymphocytes from the patient's blood or tumor are restimulated in vitro with the autologous tumor cells. Thus, from the beginning of the identification work, one knows that the examined antigen is naturally processed in the tumor cells and expressed at their surface at a level high enough for T cell recognition. The antigenic peptide itself can be identified with a genetic approach, by cloning its encoding gene with the transfection of a DNA or complementary DNA (cDNA) library prepared from the autologous tumor line.[1] This historical approach has been used extensively for melanomas, from which cell lines can readily be derived with a success rate close to 50% for metastatic tumors. However, for other cancers, the establishment of a tumor cell line is, even with current technology, a daunting if not impossible task. MLTCs reveal T cells that are restimulated by the autologous tumor cells. In most cases, they do not provide the co-stimulatory signals required for T cell priming. Thus, antitumor T cells obtained from MLTCs have been primed in vivo and derive from the self-tolerant T cell repertoire. It is therefore not surprising that, with the exception of melanocytic differentiation antigens, most tumor antigens identified with the MLTC/genetic approach prove to be of high tumoral specificity. Having derived antitumor T cells with the recognized tumor line or tissue at hand, another approach to identify the antigen consists in the immunoaffinity purification of detergent-solubilized human leukocyte antigen (HLA)–peptide complexes from the tumor cells, followed by acid elution of the antigenic peptides and their purification and identification with liquid chromatography-coupled tandem mass spectrometry.[2,3] The resulting "HLA-ligandome" consists mostly of nonantigenic normal self-peptides and also the tumor-specific antigenic peptides. During the purification steps, the various fractions can be tested for T cell recognition by adding them to cells bearing the appropriate presenting HLA molecule. In the third approach, often referred to as "reverse immunology,"[1] one does not start from antitumor T cells, but from the sequence of a gene of particular interest. It can be a mutated oncogene, a gene that is selectively expressed or overexpressed in tumors, or, in the serological analysis of expression of cDNA libraries (SEREX) methodology, a gene encoding a protein against which cancer patients have mounted an antibody response.[4] The work then consists in finding a candidate antigenic peptide encoded by this gene; predict and possibly verify its binding to HLA molecules; use it to prime or restimulate T cells in vitro to derive HLA/peptide-specific T cells; and, last but not least, verify that these T cells recognize also the cells that naturally express the HLA and gene of interest. There is a fairly high dropout rate using this procedure, mainly at its final step. To identify antigenic peptides that are candidate tumor antigens, the reverse immunology approach benefits today from progress in DNA sequencing and bioinformatics. The former allows us to identify in exome and RNA sequencing data those mutations that are present in genes expressed in a tumor. The latter provides algorithms that predict to some extent the processing and very well the binding affinities of mutated peptides to a wide array of HLA class I or class II alleles.[5] These methods can provide a large number of candidate tumor antigens, only a fraction of which are actually processed in the tumor cells and presented at their surface for T cell recognition. Fed by the growing list of identified antigenic peptides and their presenting HLA molecules, machine learning algorithms are starting to provide shorter and more accurate lists of candidate antigens.[6,7]

CLASSES OF HUMAN TUMOR ANTIGENS RECOGNIZED BY T CELLS

Antigens of High Tumoral Specificity

Tumor antigens of three classes, according to the genetic mechanism that drives their expression, are absent from the surface of normal cells. Therefore, the T cells that recognize these antigens can have a strict tumoral specificity, a crucial concept in immunotherapy. These antigens are encoded by genes that are mutated in the tumor cells, by cancer-germline genes, or by viral genes.

Antigens Encoded by Mutated Genes

We refer to tumor antigens encoded by mutated genes as "mutated" antigens, a clear though formally incorrect designation as it is the gene that is mutated. They are often designated as neoantigens or neoepitopes, because they newly appear with the development of a tumor. However, new antigens can also be encoded by viral genes, by cancer-germline genes, or by tumor-specific posttranslational modifications of peptides. The first mutated tumor-specific antigens were identified on the murine mastocytoma cell line P815[8] and a few years later on human malignant melanomas.[9,10] Gene mutations produce new antigenic peptides through several mechanisms. Of these, by far the most common is the change of one amino acid that results from a single-nucleotide variation in the encoding gene. The new amino acid can produce an antigenic peptide by either of two mechanisms (Figure 4.1). Its side chain can be noncovalently bound into one of the pockets present in the floor of the peptide-binding groove of one of the six HLA class I molecules present in the tumor cells, thus anchoring the peptide in the HLA molecule. Antigenic peptides presented by HLA class I molecules have two allele-specific anchoring residues, usually at positions 2 or 3 and at the C-terminus (usually position 9). The wild-type peptide is not antigenic because it cannot be anchored in, and therefore presented by, any of the HLA class I molecules of the tumor cells. Web-based software tools such as the pioneer SYFPEITHI[11] or the neural network–based NetMHCpan-4.0[12] predict which sequences of a polypeptide or protein can bind to the given HLA class I or class II molecules, with a computed binding affinity. The other mechanism of antigenicity of a new amino acid is the creation of a new epitope, that is, the part of the antigenic peptide that is recognized by the T cell receptor (TCR). Here, wild-type and mutated peptides contain the same residues that anchor them into HLA molecules and are therefore presented to T cells. During the establishment of natural tolerance, the naïve T cells that recognize the wild-type peptide are deleted or inactivated. Other naïve T cells recognize the new antigenic peptide on the tumor cells. Their TCR usually contacts

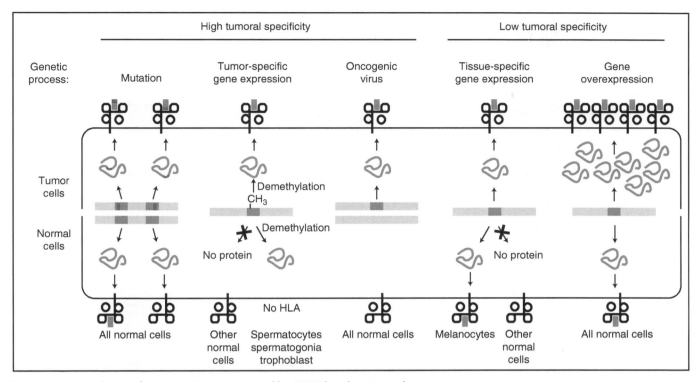

Figure 4.1 Main classes of tumor antigens recognized by CD8 T lymphocytes on human tumors.

HLA, human leukocyte antigen.

the side chain of the mutated amino acid, but the latter can also modify the shape of the presented peptide at other positions, with TCR recognition at a distance from the position of the mutated residue. Thus, the new epitope is not necessarily the new amino acid encoded by the mutated gene. Other mechanisms whereby gene mutations can produce new antigenic peptides include indels with either the addition or removal of one or several amino acids, the extension of the coding sequence beyond the normal stop codon, chimeric coding sequences straddling the junctions of chromosome translocations, or the change of the open reading frame of the coding sequence (Figure 4.2). The latter mechanism is particularly active in mismatch repair-deficient (MMR-d) tumors. In these tumors, which comprise a subset of mainly colorectal, gastric, and endometrial carcinomas, inactivation of a DNA repair enzyme such as MLH1, MSH2, or MSH6 in the tumor cells leads to the accumulation of altered microsatellites (repeats of single nucleotides or very short nucleotide sequences) that are present in the coding sequence of many genes. The resulting frameshifted proteins produce many aberrant peptides. Consistently, MMR-d tumors express a wide range of mutated antigens, are frequently infiltrated by T cells, and carry a relatively better prognosis.[13]

Mutated Antigens in Cancer Immunotherapy

Mutated antigens have several advantages in cancer immunotherapy; first and foremost, tumor specificity. T cells that recognize mutated antigenic peptides do not recognize normal cells and are thus truly tumor specific. A second advantage is that some mutated antigens are encoded by cancer driver genes, decreasing the possibility of immune escape of the tumor cells following a loss, or a loss of expression, of the mutated allele. Oncogenes that have been shown to encode mutated antigens recognized by T cells present in cancer patients include *CDK4*,[10] *NRAS*,[14] *KRAS*,[15] and *BRAF*[16] with nonsynonymous single nucleotide variants (SNV); *CASP8* with a mutated stop codon and a longer open reading frame;[17] and several fusion genes, all listed in Vigneron et al.[18] However, as expected from the observation that the majority of mutations present in tumor cells do not appear to participate in tumor development, most mutated antigens are encoded by passenger mutations. A third advantage of mutated antigens is their great diversity in some tumors. Their number is expected to increase with the mutation rate: it is higher in lung carcinomas and melanomas associated with mutations induced by tobacco carcinogens and ultraviolet radiation, respectively, or in tMMR-d tumors (see the previous text). Patients with

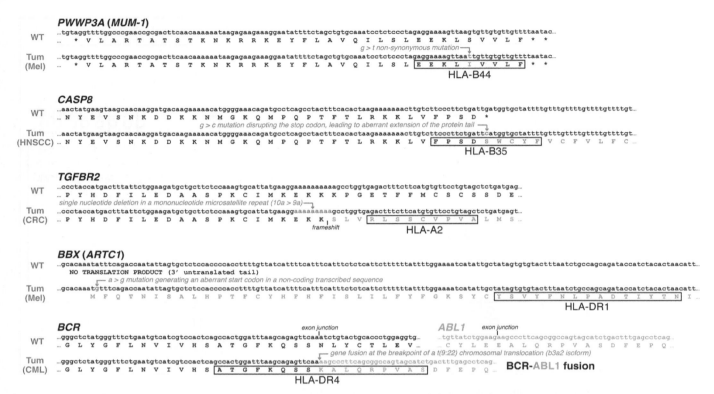

Figure 4.2 Different molecular mechanisms leading to mutated peptides recognized by antitumoral T lymphocytes. Each mechanism is illustrated by one example selected from the Cancer Antigenic Peptide Database (caped.icp.ucl.ac.be/Peptide/list).[18] The cDNA sequence of the target gene is shown in small letters and its translation product in capital letters, with a star indicating a stop codon. The genetic alteration in the tumor cells is indicated and described in red. The resulting amino acid changes are displayed in green. The T cell-recognized peptide is boxed, with its HLA presenting molecule below. Of note, other genetic alterations leading to mutated peptides, such as insertion or deletion of one or a few in-frame codons, or changes in splice acceptor sites, are very likely to exist, but are not reported here because of insufficient published documentation.

CML, chronic myeloid leukemia; CRC, colorectal carcinoma (MMR-d subtype); HNSCC, head and neck squamous cell carcinoma; Mel, melanoma; Tum, tumoral sequence; WT, wild-type sequence.

these tumors are more likely to respond clinically to immunostimulatory antibodies targeting the cytotoxic T lymphocyte–associated antigen 4 (CTLA-4) or programmed death 1 (PD-1) pathways.[19-22] Interestingly, frameshifting indel mutations, which can generate more than one antigenic peptide, appear to have a greater impact than missense mutations in eliciting clinical response.[23,24] A disadvantage of mutated antigens is that most of them are unique to individual tumors, preventing their use in generic vaccines. Nevertheless, the identification of mutated antigens for each individual tumor has become possible. Exome sequencing of the tumor and of normal cells, coupled with RNA-Seq of the tumor, identifies the nonsynonymous mutations in genes that are expressed in the tumor. Then peptides of eight to 11 amino acids, containing the mutated residue at any position, can be tested in silico for their binding to each of the six HLA class I alleles of the patient (HLA typing also can be obtained from the sequencing data), with algorithms

such as Net-MHC. It generates a list of candidate-mutated antigenic peptides, with their predicted binding affinities to HLA class I molecules. We are still missing reliable methods to predict which of these peptides are actually processed in the tumor cells: many of them will either not be produced—usually the C-terminus of the antigenic peptide depends on the cleavage of a precursor polypeptide by one of the three proteases of the proteasome or immunoproteasome—or will be destroyed by proteases or peptidases present in the cytosol or endoplasmic reticulum, or will undergo posttranslational modifications. Thus, for now, DNA sequencing and bioinformatics provide only a list of candidate peptides that contains those that are actually presented to T cells by surface HLA molecules of the tumor cells.

As mentioned earlier, there is a method that provides an unbiased view of the antigenic peptides that are presented by surface HLA molecules: start from lysed cells, immunoprecipitate HLA molecules, elute the antigenic peptides, and identify them with mass spectrometry. The resulting collection of peptides is called the HLA ligandome. Combining high-throughput DNA sequencing and HLA ligandomics allows us to identify for every patient the mutated antigenic peptides that are displayed at the surface of tumor cells. Vaccination of cancer patients with such antigenic peptides has started, with the demonstration of T cell responses against the vaccine antigens.[25] There are of course limitations to this methodological approach, one of them being the number of required cells, 10^8 to 10^9 for a detection of less abundant peptides.

Antigens Encoded by Cancer-Germline Genes

Cancer-germline genes were discovered by Boon et al. when a tumor-specific cytotoxic T lymphocyte (CTL) clone from a melanoma patient was found to recognize an antigenic peptide encoded by a new gene, *MAGEA1*.[26,27] *MAGEA1* is part of a family of 25 genes organized in three clusters, *MAGEA*, *MAGEB*, and *MAGEC*, all located on the X chromosome.[28] Other families of cancer-germline genes located on the X chromosome include *CTAG* with genes *CTAG1B* (NY-ESO-1) and *CTAG2* (*LAGE-1*),[29] *GAGE*,[30] and *SSX*.[31] Several of them were identified by screening tumor cDNA expression libraries with antitumor immunoglobulin G (IgG) present in the serum of tumor-bearing patients, a method called SEREX, developed by Pfreundschuh et al.[32] Subsequently, cDNA subtraction procedures or database mining have led to the identification of additional cancer-germline genes.

The hallmark of the cancer-germline genes is their pattern of expression (Figure 4.1). They are silent in normal somatic tissues, except in male and female germline cells and in trophoblastic cells (Figure 4.3),[33,34] but they are expressed in a substantial fraction of a large range of tumors (Table 4.1).

The expression of cancer-germline genes in normal tissues was tested initially with semiquantitative real-time quantitative reverse transcription polymerase chain reaction (RT-PCR) amplifications and subsequently with RT-qPCR. Today, mining large collections of RNA-Seq data allows us to detect very low levels of expression that have thus far gone unnoticed. The sensitivity will increase even more with RNA-Seq data of enriched populations of cells that are rare in a given tissue, and with single cell RNA-Seq. Therefore, it is impossible to exclude that some cancer-germline genes are expressed at a very low level in many cells of a given tissue or at a high level in a minority of cells. The latter possibility can be suspected if rare cells are clearly stained by antibodies to the relevant protein. In 2013, Morgan et al. reported that two cancer patients experienced fatal brain toxicity following the adoptive transfer of T cells transduced with a TCR recognizing a MAGEA3 peptide presented by HLA-A2 molecules.[35] It turned out that this TCR also recognized a MAGEA12 peptide that differs from the MAGEA3 peptide by a single amino acid, and that gene *MAGEA12* was expressed at very low levels in the brain.[35] The low level of *MAGEA12* expression in various parts of the brain can now be readily detected in some publicly available RNA-Seq data. To date, the expression of the other *MAGEA*, *MAGEB*, and *MAGEC* genes in normal tissues remains limited to germline and trophoblastic cells. Cancer-germline genes are expressed in tumors and more frequently in melanomas or bladder, head and neck, and lung carcinomas (Table 4.1). Expression is rare or absent in tumor types such as leukemia, glioblastoma, or renal cell carcinoma. Cancer-germline genes are frequently coactivated, and positive tumors tend to express several of them. The mechanism of activation involves the demethylation of the promoter of these genes, as suggested by the initial observation that treating a nonexpressing melanoma line with the DNA methylation inhibitor 5-aza-2'-deoxycytidine activated gene *MAGEA1*,[36] and was confirmed by showing that the *MAGEA1* promoter was methylated in normal somatic tissues but demethylated in germ cells and in the tumor cells that expressed the gene.[37] Demethylation

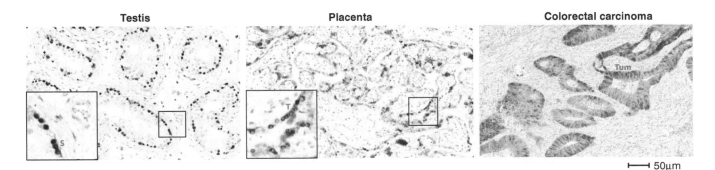

Figure 4.3 Tissue expression profile of a MAGE protein. The indicated formalin-fixed, paraffin-embedded tissues were stained with an anti-MAGEA9 monoclonal antibody (positive cells appear in brown). MAGEA9 is detected in spermatogonia (S), trophoblast (T), and tumor cells (Tum), but not in the other cell types present in these tissues.

Table 4.1 Proportions of Tumors Expressing Cancer-Germline Genes

HISTOLOGICAL TYPE	MAGE							MAGE		BAGE		GAGE			LAGE1	LAGE2 NYESO1	
	A1	A2	A3	A4	A6	A12	n	A10	n	1	n	1, 2, 8	3–7	n	1	1,2	n
Cutaneous melanoma																	
Primary lesions	25	52	55	18	59	34	83	24	17	12	41	29	41	79	33	17	6
Metastases	46	70	74	28	72	62	243	47	236	31	145	41	50	211	19	20	80
Squamous cell lung carcinoma	44	42	48	59	53	28	93	41	32	9	53	40	43	77	33	31	39
Lung adenocarcinoma	43	47	45	37	49	37	49	44	16	17	29	34	39	44	49	38	39
Head and neck squamous cell carcinoma	29	36	48	54	55	26	89	30	23	6	89	25	28	89	35	24	17
Esophageal squamous cell carcinoma	53	53	63	74	68	26	19	43	14	6	17	47	47	17	20	10	10
Bladder carcinoma																	
Superficial (<T2)	14	11	16	23	19	10	70	20	69	3	35	3	3	35			
Infiltrating (≥T2)	32	43	57	45	57	34	53	38	53	26	34	25	35	40	47	47	15
Prostate carcinoma	18	18	18	0	23	5	22	10	10	0	20	15		20	27	27	11
Breast carcinoma	19	9	13	6	15	13	136	4	28	12	68	10		154	23	23	13
Colorectal carcinoma	0	13	17	11	22	11	46	0	23	0	42	0		42	0	0	9
Renal cell carcinoma	5	0	0	2	0	5	44	0	24	0	36	0		34	0	0	8
Sarcoma	10	19	19	29	14	10	21	0	13	0	13	31		16	19	37	16
Leukemia	0	0	0	1	0	0	112	0	25	0	18	0	0	45	0	0	13
Myeloma (stages I-II)	0	0	0	0	0	0	11	0	11	0	11	0	9	11	9	0	11
Myeloma (stage III)	41	26	41	22	37	26	27	11	27	26	27	48	56	27	70	33	27

Expression was measured by RT-PCR using total RNA and primers specific for each gene. The proportion (%) of tumors expressing each gene is shown.

n, number of tumor samples tested; RT-PCR, reverse transcription polymerase chain reaction.

and activation of cancer-germline genes in tumors correlates with global genome hypomethylation.[38] A study conducted on microdissected samples of ovarian tumors confirmed that intratumor heterogeneity of cancer-germline gene expression correlated with promoter and global DNA methylation status.[39] DNA hypomethylation is more frequent in advanced tumors, in line with the observation that cancer-germline genes are more frequently expressed in advanced tumors such as metastatic versus primary melanomas[40] or infiltrating versus superficial bladder carcinomas (Table 4.1).[40,41]

The expression of cancer-germline genes in germ cells and in trophoblastic cells does not lead to the presence at the surface of these cells of antigens that can be recognized by T cells, because in the healthy state these cells are devoid of HLA molecules. Therefore, it is misleading to refer to the antigens that are encoded by cancer-germline genes as "cancer-testis antigens," as it suggests that testicular autoimmunity is a concern when using these antigens in immunotherapy. We favor the terms "cancer-germline" for the genes and "MAGE-type" for the antigens.

MAGE-Type Antigens in Cancer Immunotherapy

The main advantage of MAGE-type antigens is that they are shared between patients, with obvious opportunities for the development of vaccines or adoptive transfer of specific T cells. However, candidate patients have to be tested for the expression of the relevant genes in their tumor, which leads to the problem of the level of gene or protein expression that suffices for T cell recognition. The very same problem is present when analyzing gene expression data, for example, *MAGEA3* expression in a given type of tumors, to define predictive or prognostic biomarkers. Cancer patients have been vaccinated with MAGE-type antigenic peptides or proteins, or with recombinant viruses containing cancer-germline gene sequences, without signs of autoimmunity.[42–46] Adoptive transfer of T cells recognizing MAGE-type antigens, either naturally or after TCR transduction, has been followed by tumor regression without severe side effects.[35,47–50] However, strong toxicities were encountered when the transferred T cells carried modified TCRs that had not been filtered by the mechanisms of natural tolerance.[35,51] Therapeutic vaccination with protein MAGEA3 and adjuvant AS15 was not efficacious in patients with non-small-cell lung cancer or melanoma.[42,52] Anti-MAGEA3 B cells and CD4 T cells were stimulated by the vaccine, as indicated by anti-MAGEA3 IgG responses. There were little, if any, CD8 responses. Whether anti-MAGE vaccination modalities that induce strong CD8 T cell responses, such as recombinant viruses,[53] possibly combined with PD-1 blockade, reach clinical efficacy remains a key issue 20 years after MAGE discovery through the anti-MAGEA1 CD8 T cell clone of a melanoma patient.[26]

Viral Antigens and Their Use in Cancer Immunotherapy

Approximately 20% of cancers are linked to infectious agents.[54] The study of mouse tumors induced with oncogenic viruses showed in the 1960s that tumor rejections could be observed after recognition of viral antigens.[55] In the 1980s, Townsend et al. demonstrated how viruses were a source of antigenic peptides presented to CTLs by MHC class I molecules.[56,57] Therefore, immunization against viral antigens through vaccination or adoptive cell transfer is explored for cancer immunotherapy. For the antigens encoded by the E6 and E7 oncoproteins of human papillomavirus (HPV)-16, clinical responses have been observed in patients with vulvar intraepithelial neoplasia vaccinated with adjuvanted long peptides.[58,59] Even though mutated antigens can be more immunogenic than HPV antigens,[60] prolonged survival was observed in patients with advanced cervical cancer treated with an HPV vaccine during chemotherapy, which reduces numbers of immunosuppressive myeloid cells.[61] Anti-HPV immunizations could also be applied to the head and neck cancer patients with an HPV⁺ tumor.[62] Adoptive transfer of Epstein-Barr virus-specific T cells has met some clinical success.[63] About 80% of Merkel-cell carcinomas, rare and aggressive skin cancers, are associated with the oncogenic Merkel-cell polyoma virus.[64] The polyoma virus–negative tumors are ultraviolet (UV) induced and characterized by a high mutational load.[65] Interestingly, both types of Merkel-cell carcinomas respond to blocking anti-PD-1 or anti-PD-L1 antibodies.[66,67] It is very likely that CTLs recognizing either viral or mutated antigenic peptides contribute to these clinical responses.

Antigens of Low Tumoral Specificity

Tissue Differentiation Antigens

Differentiation antigens were discovered in melanomas with the surprising observation that patients had CTLs that recognized both tumor cells and normal melanocytes.[68] The target antigens were shown to be derived from melanocyte-specific proteins such as tyrosinase (TYR), Melan-A/MART-1 (MLANA), and Pmel17/gp100 (PMEL).[18] Tolerance to melanocytic antigens is thus incomplete, which was unexpected. The melanocytic antigen MLANA deserves a comment. Two-thirds of HLA-A2 patients with advanced metastatic melanoma have, in their metastases, detectable levels of CD8 T cells recognizing $MLANA_{26-35}$ peptide EAAGIGILTV presented by HLA-A2 molecules.[69] The frequency of blood CD8 T cells that recognize this antigen in healthy HLA-A2 individuals is approximately 8×10^{-4}.[70,71] This frequency of naïve anti-MLANA T cells is very high, in contrast with the frequencies of circulating CD8 T cells against other HLA–peptide combinations, which have been estimated at 4 to 40×10^{-7}, thus two or three orders of magnitude lower.[72,73] The main reason for this high frequency was found to be a high thymic output, which suggested that negative selection of the anti-$MLANA_{26-35}$ T cells was incomplete.[70] Recently, the MLANA polypeptide present in medullary thymic epithelial cells, which drive negative selection, was found to be misinitiated and truncated, lacking the sequence encoding peptide EAAGIGILTV.[74] These results explain why the corresponding anti-$MLANA_{26-35}$ T cells escape from central tolerance. The $MLANA_{26-35}$ peptide was often used in vaccines and the resulting frequencies of memory T cells could reach several percent of the blood CD8⁺ T cells.[75] However, the processing of peptide $MLANA_{26-35}$ in melanoma cells appears to be inefficient, with several components of the antigen processing machinery that either do not produce or destroy the peptide.[76] Nonmelanoma cancer patients do not appear to have spontaneous T cell responses against tissue differentiation antigens of their tumor, suggesting that melanomas have a unique immunogenicity profile. The mechanisms of natural tolerance should prevent strong T cell responses to tissue differentiation antigens, and melanocytes are thus far the only clear exception. Inducing such T cell responses, by vaccination if that proves possible, or by adoptive T cell transfer, should be considered with great caution.

Differentiation Antigens in Cancer Immunotherapy

Melanocyte differentiation antigens have been used to actively or passively immunize patients with metastatic melanoma. On the side of active immunization, advanced melanoma patients treated with high-dose interleukin-2 (IL-2) and a PMEL peptide had a higher tumor response rate and longer progression-free survival than those receiving IL-2 alone.[77] Clinical responses were observed in metastatic melanoma patients after vaccination with dendritic cells loaded with PMEL and TYR peptides.[78] While the adoptive transfer of bulk, ex vivo amplified TILs, which very often contain CD8 T cells recognizing melanocyte antigens, has been followed by complete tumor responses in ±20% of metastatic melanoma patients,[79] a recent work indicates that this proportion drops to ±4% when all the transferred T cells recognize these differentiation antigens.[80] Possible explanations for these disappointing results are the heterogeneity of melanocyte antigens in melanomas, and a poor affinity of the T cells as a result of tolerance even if incomplete. As expected, strong T cell responses to melanocyte differentiation antigens can lead to ocular and systemic autoimmunity.[81–83] Prostatic differentiation antigens can be safely used against prostate cancer cells after prostatectomy. Antigenic peptides have been described that are derived from prostate-specific antigen or prostatic acid phosphatase, which are absent from other tissues.[84,85] Patients with minimally symptomatic castration-resistant prostate cancer appear to experience a clinical benefit from vaccination with sipuleucel-T, which is composed of autologous monocytes pulsed with a fusion protein incorporating prostatic acid phosphatase and granulocyte macrophage colony-stimulating factor (GM-CSF).[86,87] An ongoing phase III trial is investigating vaccination with recombinant poxviruses encoding prostate-specific antigen and the co-stimulatory molecules B7-1, ICAM-1, and LFA-3 in patients with metastatic castration-resistant prostate cancer (PSA-TRICOM).[88] No signs of serious autoimmunity were reported with these two vaccines.

Overexpressed Antigens

Productive T cell recognition requires a minimal number of HLA–peptide complexes displayed at the surface of the stimulatory or target cell. This minimal number varies according to the functional states of T cell and antigen-presenting cell, but can be as low as one.[89] This threshold provides a theoretical opportunity for tumor specificity of T cells recognizing peptides derived from proteins that are overexpressed in tumor cells as compared to normal cells. This overexpression is not tested easily. Quantification of gene expression is readily done, but the results are affected by the proportions of tumor cells in the sample. At the protein level, the difficulty is to quantify histochemical staining, which is not an easy task. Considering that, in addition, antigen recognition by T cells can be exquisitely sensitive, and much more so than the recognition by most antibodies, it is almost impossible to predict whether a given "overexpressed" antigen, or T cells recognizing it, can be used safely. It is only through repeated clinical experiments that one can be reassured about the safety of these antigens and prudence suggests us to consider only antigens with a very high difference of expression between tumoral and normal cells or tissues.

Overexpressed Antigens in Cancer Immunotherapy

The oncogene encoding the growth factor receptor ERBB2 (or human epidermal growth receptor [HER]-2/neu) is overexpressed in many epithelial tumors, including ovarian and breast carcinomas, as a result of gene amplification and increased transcription. More than a dozen ERBB2 antigenic peptides presented by HLA class I molecules have been defined[18,90] and several of them were used in vaccines[91] without harmful side effects.

The gene encoding transcription factor Wilms tumor protein 1 (WT1) is expressed at 10-fold to 1,000-fold higher levels in leukemic cells, in which it contributes to the malignant phenotype, than in normal CD34+ cells.[92,93] Tumor regressions following WT1 vaccination have been reported, without signs of autoimmunity.[94–96] Patients with leukemia received an allogeneic hematopoietic cell transplant followed by an infusion of donor-derived CTL clones directed against a WT1 peptide presented by HLA-A2. A decrease in the number of leukemic cells was observed without evidence of on-target toxicity.[97] Anti-WT1 TCR gene therapy also was shown to be safe and clinically efficient.[98]

Several other peptides or proteins are considered for cancer immunotherapy based on their higher expression in tumors than in normal tissues. The apoptosis inhibitor protein survivin is overexpressed in many tumors. T cells from an HLA-A2 donor were transduced with a transgenic HLA-A2-restricted anti-survivin TCR. They underwent apoptosis as a result of fratricide due to survivin expression in activated T lymphocytes,[99] indicating the inability of this TCR to differentiate between the lower and higher levels of the survivin antigenic peptide on normal and tumoral cells, respectively. Interestingly, this anti-survivin TCR was derived from an allogenic non-HLA-A2 donor. Recently, an anti-survivin TCR isolated from an HLA-A2 donor proved capable of targeting tumor cells overexpressing survivin but not the activated T cells that expressed lower levels of the anti-apoptotic protein.[100] Structurally, the selective tumor specificity was associated with more TCR contacts with the survivin peptide. This result indicates that thymic selection can filter out TCRs that recognize an antigen present at a low level in normal cells while sparing some TCRs that recognize the same antigen present at high levels in tumor cells. It suggests that survivin as well as other overexpressed tumor antigens may be safe targets if one uses carefully selected TCRs. Gene *PRAME* was found to be expressed at higher levels in almost all melanomas and in many other tumors, including a sizeable proportion of leukemias, than in most normal tissues.[101,102] However, *PRAME* is also expressed in some normal tissues such as testis, endometrium, adrenals, or ovary.[101] The distribution of *PRAME*-positive cells in these tissues is unknown and it is possible that a few normal cells express *PRAME* at levels comparable to those observed in tumors. *PRAME* was shown to be expressed in medullary thymic epithelial cells,[103] which might lead to central tolerance. Rare anti-*PRAME* T cells have been derived from cancer patients and from normal individuals.[101,104,105] *PRAME* expression in normal tissues raises a cautionary flag and it remains unclear whether PRAME antigens are safe cancer targets. The carcinoembryonic antigen (CEA) family results from the expression of a set of highly related glycoproteins (CEACAM1-21) involved in cell adhesion.[106,107] It is present especially in colon, breast, and ovarian carcinomas and in fetal gastrointestinal tissue. However, its expression is also observed in normal adult colonic mucosa, lung, and lactating breast tissue. It is considered to be overexpressed in colon carcinomas. CEA can be shed from cells and its detection in serum is a tumor marker. Patients with metastatic colon cancer received T cells transduced with a TCR-recognizing peptide CEA$_{691-699}$ presented by HLA-A2. Tumor regression as well as severe transient colitis were observed.[108]

OTHER TYPES OF TUMOR ANTIGENS

Many CD4 or CD8 tumor-specific T cells derived from cancer patients were found to recognize antigenic peptides that could not have been predicted on the basis of the five mechanisms discussed earlier. Several peptides were derived from abnormal gene products such as intronic or reverse strand transcripts,[9,109] from polypeptides translated from alternate open reading frames,[110-112] or contained a posttranslational modification that was essential for T cell recognition, such as phosphorylation[113,114] or asparagine deamidation following deglycosylation.[115-117] The most unexpected posttranslational modification observed in antigenic peptides presented

by HLA class I molecules was the splicing in the final peptide of noncontiguous sequences of the source protein.[117-120] Peptide splicing, even sometimes in the reverse order, was shown to occur in the proteasome.[119] Spliced antigenic peptides are difficult to identify with T cells, and it is not yet quite straightforward with bioinformatical analyses of peptides eluted from HLA class I molecules.[121] Their proportion in the HLA ligandome is still a matter of debate but 1% to 5% is the most probable range.[122,123] HLA-ligandome experiments have shown that some antigenic peptides could be eluted from HLA molecules of tumor cells but not or much less so from those of normal cells.[124-126] These differences in ligand density were not accounted for by differences in mRNA copy numbers.[126] The reasons for these discrepancies are not clear, and differences of antigen processing between tumoral and normal cells could be part of the explanation. As nicely shown by the group of T. van Hall, one such difference is present in TAP-deficient tumor cells.[127]

TUMOR ANTIGENS RECOGNIZED BY ANTIBODIES OR CHIMERIC ANTIGEN RECEPTORS

We mention some of these antigens in this chapter because they can now be targeted by T cells through chimeric antigen receptor (CAR) or bispecific T cell engager (BiTE) antibodies. Cancer patients produce antibodies that recognize antigens that are displayed on the surface of their tumor cells or that are released from dead tumor cells. Antibodies to the latter antigens cannot directly target tumor cells and their relevance for anticancer immunity is unclear. Antibodies to the former antigens include several tumor-targeting monoclonal antibodies that are among the most successful anticancer drugs. Tumor antigens thus far targeted by such antibodies are not strictly tumor specific, but are overexpressed on tumor cells as compared to normal cells, or are differentiation antigens. The growth factor receptor encoded by the HER-2/neu oncogene is overexpressed in 10% to 30% of breast tumors[128] and in a fraction of bladder, esophageal, gallbladder, stomach, and uterine carcinomas.[129] The anti-HER-2/neu monoclonal antibody trastuzumab is an effective anticancer therapy, improving survival among patients with ERBB2-amplified breast carcinomas.[130] This clinical activity has been attributed to inhibition of intracellular signaling by HER-2, as the antibody targets tumors that are addicted to HER-2 activation. However, there is increasing evidence in preclinical models and in patients that the therapeutic effect of trastuzumab depends also on innate immunity through Fc receptor (FcR)-mediated cytotoxicity by natural killer (NK) cells and on adaptive immunity through T cells.[131] HER-2 is not tumor specific, and cardiac dysfunction, with congestive heart failure in patients treated with trastuzumab alone, that is, without anthracycline-containing chemotherapy, was noted in several studies. Toxicity was much more severe when a patient received T cells engineered to directly recognize HER-2: T cells transduced with a CAR based on trastuzumab caused lethal toxicity in a patient who received 10^{10} CAR T cells after myeloablative conditioning.[132] The carbonic anhydrase IX (CAIX/G250 antigen) is a surface antigen considered to be overexpressed in more than 90% of renal clear cell carcinomas. It is also present on some normal cells including bile duct epithelial cells. Encoded by a hypoxia-inducible gene, its overexpression is linked to von Hippel–Lindau (VHL) dysregulation, a tumor suppressor protein involved in HIF1α degradation. Liver toxicity was observed in renal cancer patients after adoptive transfer of T cells transduced with a single-chain antibody based on the anti-CAIX monoclonal antibody G250.[133]

Several cell surface markers are differentiation antigens. Many of them have been described on hematopoietic cells. CAR T cells targeting the B cell antigen CD19 have yielded impressive results in patients with acute lymphoblastic leukemia at the cost of B cell aplasia, an on-target off-tumor toxicity that is manageable with intravenous administration of immunoglobulins.[134-136] Time will tell whether other surface differentiation antigens can be targeted by CAR T cells or by BiTE antibodies with an acceptable toxicity profile. Potential targets include the prostate-specific membrane antigen (PSMA) encoded by the folate hydrolase 1 (FOLH1) gene, and tumor-associated carbohydrate antigens. The latter are present on several glycoproteins and especially Mucin 1. In tumors, deregulated O-glycosylation leads to truncated mono- and disaccharides known as pan-carcinoma antigens Tn and SialylTn.[137] Gangliosides, carbohydrate moieties linked to a lipid molecule (ceramide) anchored in the plasma membrane, are another example.

CONCLUSION

Somewhat unforeseeable as it was, using the currently most successful cancer immunotherapy drugs does not require us to have prior knowledge of which antigens are present in a given tumor. The immunostimulatory antibodies like those that target the CTLA-4 and PD-1 pathways appear to restimulate antitumor T cells previously primed during spontaneous antitumor T cell responses in the patient and, probably, to prime new antitumor T cells. The whole gamut of the available tumor antigens is expectedly targetable by all these antitumor T cells. It is anticipated that the clinical efficacy of these immunostimulatory antibodies, and of others that are under clinical development, will augment through their combination with drugs that mitigate the tumoral immunosuppressive environment and with active or passive immunization against tumor antigens. It is obvious that when known tumor antigens are to be used in immunotherapy they should be tumor specific to avoid T cell–mediated damage to healthy tissues and that multiple antigens or "driver" antigens decrease the probability of selecting antigen-loss tumor cell variants. The case in point is mutated antigens corresponding to oncogenic gene products. However, these ideal tumor antigens are scarce and the choice of antigens remains a difficult task. In practice, it is simplified by the observation of antigen spreading. Active immunization against one tumor antigen, even poorly immunogenic, may lead to T cell responses against other tumor antigens.[25,138,139] It has been observed also after adoptive transfer of antitumor T cells.[47,140] The mechanisms behind antigen spreading are not clearly understood. They probably involve antigen release following tumor cell destruction, as well as intratumoral secretion by activated T cells of cytokines that decrease local immunosuppression or attract T cells and other immune cells. Through their cytokine and chemokine secretion, antitumor CD4 T cells are possibly as efficient as cytolytic CD8 T cells in inducing this antigen-spreading effect. Two conditions prevent antigen spreading in cancer immunotherapy: a paucity of tumor antigens, either primary or secondary to selection by successful tumor immune attacks, and a strongly immunosuppressive microenvironment in the tumor. There is little we can do about the former, except maybe for using immunotherapy at earlier disease stages, but we can still work on the latter by deciphering and inhibiting the main mechanisms of immunosuppression.

KEY REFERENCES

Only key references appear in the print edition. The full reference list appears in the digital product on Springer Publishing Connect: connect.springerpub.com/content/book/978-0-8261-3743-2/part/part01/chapter/ch04

9. Coulie PG, Lehmann F, Lethé B, et al. A mutated intron sequence codes for an antigenic peptide recognized by cytolytic T lymphocytes on a human melanoma. *Proc Natl Acad Sci USA*. 1995;92(17):7976–7980. doi:10.1073/pnas.92.17.7976
10. Wölfel T, Hauer M, Schneider J, et al. A p16INK4a-insensitive CDK4 mutant targeted by cytolytic T lymphocytes in a human melanoma. *Science*. 1995;269(5228):1281–1284. doi:10.1126/science.7652577
22. Van Allen EM, Miao D, Schilling B, et al. Genomic correlates of response to CTLA-4 blockade in metastatic melanoma. *Science*. 2015;350(6257):207–211. doi:10.1126/science.aad0095
24. Mandal R, Samstein RM, Lee KW, et al. Genetic diversity of tumors with mismatch repair deficiency influences anti-PD-1 immunotherapy response. *Science*. 2019;364(6439):485–491. doi:10.1126/science.aau0447
25. Carreno BM, Magrini V, Becker-Hapak M, et al. Cancer immunotherapy: a dendritic cell vaccine increases the breadth and diversity of melanoma neoantigen-specific T cells. *Science*. 2015;348(6236):803–808. doi:10.1126/science.aaa3828
26. van der Bruggen P, Traversari C, Chomez P, et al. A gene encoding an antigen recognized by cytolytic T lymphocytes on a human melanoma. *Science*. 1991;254(5038):1643–1647. doi:10.1126/science.1840703

5

Structural and Functional Defects in HLA Class I Antigen Processing Machinery in Cancer Cells: Molecular Mechanisms and Clinical Relevance

Lei Cai, Theodoros Michelakos, Teppei Yamada, Luke Maggs, Ananthan Sadagopan, Joseph H. Schwab, Cristina R. Ferrone, and Soldano Ferrone

KEY POINTS

- A fully functional human leukocyte antigen (HLA) class I antigen processing machinery (APM) is required for the synthesis and expression on cancer cell membrane of HLA class I antigen-tumor antigen (TA) peptide trimolecular complexes. These complexes mediate the interactions of cancer cells with cognate T cells. Abnormalities in HLA class I APM component expression and/or function result in defective and/or lack of TA peptide presentation by HLA class I antigens to cognate cytotoxic T cells, providing cancer cells with a mechanism to escape from recognition and destruction by the host's immune system.

- HLA class I APM component expression in cancers has been analyzed mostly utilizing immunohistochemical staining methods. Formalin-fixed paraffin-embedded tissue sections are the substrate of choice. HLA class I APM component-specific monoclonal antibodies (mAbs) are used as probes. Immunohistochemical methods are advantageous compared to Western blotting and DNA- or RNA-based methods, because they provide information about the expression at the protein level of the molecule of interest, its cellular distribution, the degree of heterogeneity in its expression in a malignant lesion, and the spatial relationship among cells present in a tumor section.

- Many types of defects in HLA class I APM component expression have been identified. They range from total HLA class I loss/downregulation to selective loss/downregulation of one HLA class I APM component. Epigenetic mechanisms underlie the majority of HLA class I APM component defects, with no specific mechanism operating in any given cancer type. The only known exception is represented by the defects caused by BRAF mutations, which are restricted to the cancer types bearing these mutations. In the majority of cases, HLA class I APM component defects may be corrected by rationally designed strategies which counteract the underlying epigenetic mechanisms.

- A review of 237 papers revealed that the frequency of expression defects ranges from 36% to 80% for HLA class I heavy chain, from 17% to 73% for β2m, and from 0% to 100% for APM components. A higher frequency of defects was found in the gene products of the HLA-A locus than in those of the HLA-B/C loci. In many cancer types, HLA class I APM component downregulation has been found to be associated with cancer aggressiveness and poor prognosis.

- A fully functional HLA class I APM appears to be required for the therapeutic efficacy of checkpoint-specific mAb-based immunotherapy of malignant diseases. HLA class I APM component expression defects may play a role in the resistance to checkpoint-specific mAb-based immunotherapy. Whether HLA class I APM component defects represent useful biomarkers to select and monitor patients treated with this type of immunotherapy remains to be assessed.

INTRODUCTION

The impressive clinical responses observed in a proportion of patients with many cancer types treated with immune checkpoint-specific monoclonal antibodies (mAbs)[1-3] have provided convincing evidence that in humans—like in mice—the immune system can recognize and eliminate malignant cells. Therefore, it plays an important role in the pathogenesis and clinical course of malignant diseases. These impressive results have convinced even the most skeptical clinical and experimental oncologists that immunotherapy is an effective therapy for the treatment of many types of malignant diseases. It is somehow surprising that this additional clinical evidence was needed to convince oncologists about the value of immunotherapy for the treatment of malignant diseases. Overwhelming evidence has shown that immunotherapy with mAbs which recognize molecules expressed on malignant cells is very effective in the treatment of many types of solid and hematological cancers.[4,5] As a result, mAbs with this specificity have been for many years integral components of the armamentarium routinely used for the treatment of many types of solid and hematological malignancies.

The mechanism underlying the antitumor activity of immune checkpoint-specific mAb-based immunotherapy is represented by the unleashing of T cells, which recognize and destroy cancer cells. The interactions between cancer cells and cognate T cells are mediated by a trimolecular complex which results from the selective binding of a tumor antigen (TA) peptide to the HLA class I allele heavy chain-β2 microglobulin (β2m) complex. The peptide included in the trimolecular complex is in most, if not all, cases a mutated peptide, which was formerly referred to as a "unique" TA.[6] The synthesis of the HLA class I antigen-TA peptide trimolecular complex and its transport to the cancer cell membrane requires a fully functional HLA class I antigen processing machinery (APM). Abnormalities in the expression and/or function of HLA class I APM components result in defective and/or lack of HLA class I antigen-TA peptide complex expression providing cancer cells with an escape mechanism from recognition and destruction by the host's immune system. Therefore, HLA class I APM appears to play a crucial role in the outcome of immune checkpoint-specific mAb-based immunotherapy of malignant diseases. Nevertheless, limited attention has been paid to the expression and function of HLA class I APM components in cancers of patients treated with immune checkpoint-specific mAb-based immunotherapy, although (a) abnormalities in HLA class I APM component expression have been described in all the cancer types analyzed, (b) these abnormalities have clinical significance as they are associated with the clinical course of many malignancies, (c) HLA class I loss in cancers because of the selective pressure imposed by TA-specific immune response induced or enhanced by cancer vaccines may be associated with loss of clinical response,[7,8] and (d) acquired resistance to immune checkpoint-specific mAb-based immunotherapy has been described in patients with metastases which do not express HLA class I because of β2m loss.[9-11]

Therefore, in this chapter we will (a) describe the structure and function of HLA class I APM, as well as the methodology presently available to analyze the expression of its components in cancer tissues, (b) review the information in the literature about the frequency of HLA class I APM component defects in malignant diseases, (c) discuss the clinical significance of these defects, (d) review the information in the literature about the molecular mechanisms underlying these defects and discuss the potential use of this information to design rational strategies to correct these defects, and (e) discuss the potential impact of HLA class I APM component defects on the outcome of immune checkpoint-specific mAb-based immunotherapy and their potential use as biomarkers to select patients to be treated with this modality.

HLA CLASS I APM STRUCTURE AND FUNCTION

Recognition of cancer cells by cognate T cells is mediated by HLA class I antigen-TA peptide complexes. Their synthesis and expression require a fully functional HLA class I APM which generates 8 to 12 amino-acid long peptides from TA, loads them on HLA class I antigens, and transports them to the cell membrane for presentation to cognate T cells (Figure 5.1). Specifically, mostly, although not exclusively, endogenous proteins are degraded by proteasome isoforms and their active subunits to peptides with the correct length and sequence for HLA class I binding. The proteasome is a multimeric protein complex formed by the 20S catalytic core, which has two outer rings of 7 α-subunits (α1–α7),[12] two inner rings of 7 β-subunits (β1–β7),[13,14] and two regulatory 19S (or PA700) particles on both ends of the core (Figure 5.2). Importantly, when the three β-subunits—β1, β2, and β5—are replaced by the interferon-γ (IFNγ) inducible subunits—low molecular weight protein-2 (LMP2, also called β1i), 7 (LMP7, β5i), and 10 (LMP10, β2i), respectively—the immunoproteasome[15,16] is formed at the catalytic core. Proteasome and immunoproteasome differ in their enzymatic activity and in their ability to generate major histocompatibility complex (MHC) class I restricted peptides.[17,18] Once these immunogenic peptides are generated, they are shuttled by the heterodimeric transporter associated with antigen processing (TAP) complex, which is formed by two non-covalently linked subunits, named TAP1 and TAP2, into the lumen of the endoplasmic reticulum (ER). The TAP complex forms a pore on the ER membrane allowing the peptides to enter the ER lumen.[19-21] There, the newly synthesized HLA class I heavy chain is stabilized by calnexin, and then associates with β2m.[22] Subsequently, the HLA class I dimer binds to

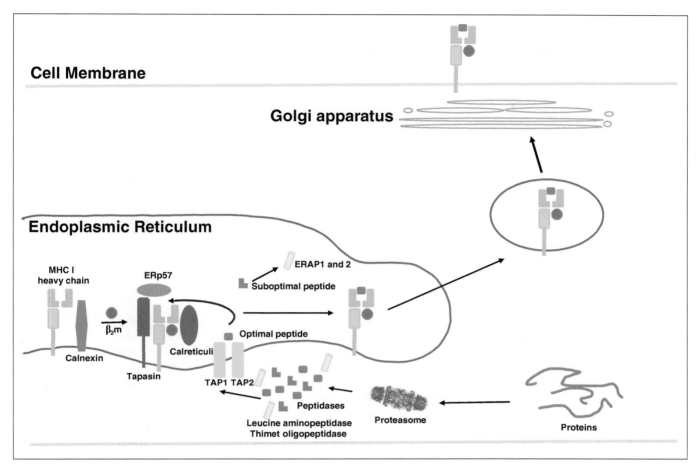

Figure 5.1 Structure of HLA class I APM.

APM, antigen-processing machinery; ERAP, endoplasmic reticulum aminopeptidase; ERp57, endoplasmic reticulum resident protein 57; HLA, human leukocyte antigen; MHC, major histocompatibility complex; TAP, transporter associated with antigen processing; β2m, β2 microglobulin.

the chaperone molecules calreticulin, endoplasmic reticulum resident protein 57 (ERp57), and tapasin, generating the peptide loading complex which is loaded with peptides.[23–27] The resulting trimeric complex—HLA class I heavy chain, β2m, and peptide—transverses the Golgi apparatus, shuttles to the cell membrane, and fuses with it. As a result, the HLA class I peptide complex is exposed extracellularly and can be recognized by the cognate T cell receptor (TCR) expressed on CD8+ T cells. A well-controlled, orderly, stepwise progression of this pathway is required in order for the immunogenic peptide to reach the cell membrane loaded onto HLA class I molecules and interact with cognate CD8+ T cells.

METHODOLOGY TO DETECT HLA CLASS I APM COMPONENT EXPRESSION IN TUMOR TISSUES

Historical Perspective

Immunohistochemical staining of tumor tissue sections with mAbs is the most widely used technique to measure HLA class I APM component expression in cancer tissues. This technique has the advantage to provide information about the expression at the protein level of the molecule of interest, its cellular distribution, the degree of heterogeneity in its expression within a malignant lesion, and the spatial relationship among cells present in a tumor section. The probes used in the early studies included allo-antisera and few xeno-antisera. Allo-antisera recognize HLA class I alleles. In contrast, xeno-antisera for the most part contain either a major antibody population specific for a framework epitope (i.e., an epitope shared by the gene products of the HLA class I loci) or multiple antibody populations specific for distinct epitopes expressed on overlapping subpopulations of the gene products HLA-A, -B, and -C loci. In the latter case, the staining pattern resembles that obtained with an antiserum recognizing a framework epitope. Staining of tissue sections with allo- and xeno-antisera in IHC reactions suffered from the high background caused most likely by the contaminating antibodies present in the polyclonal allo- and xeno-antisera

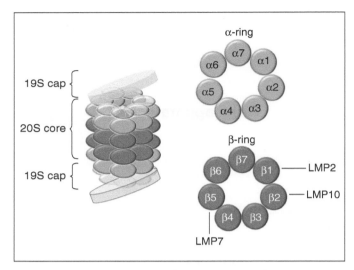

Figure 5.2 Proteasome and immunoproteasome structure.

in addition to the availability in limited amounts of the HLA class I allele-specific allo-antisera. These limitations represented a major obstacle to studies aiming to characterize HLA class I expression in normal and pathological tissues. This scenario dramatically changed in the 1980s when HLA class I-specific mAbs were developed. Because of their high degree of specificity, their availability in large amounts in a standardized form, and the lack of contaminating antibodies in the preparations used for staining, mAbs eliminated the limitations imposed by conventional allo- and xeno-antisera on the analysis of HLA class I expression in tissues. As a result, a large number of studies were performed and published. A search in PubMed showed that after 1980, the number of published studies per year has been steadily increasing until it plateaued in 2005. The results of these studies have convincingly shown that defects in HLA class I expression are the rule and not the exception in all cancer types. An unexpected result of these studies was the restricted HLA class I distribution in normal tissues. Contrary to what was believed, HLA class I antigens are not expressed on the surface of all types of nucleated cells as they are not detectable in hypophysis, thyroid, and seminiferous tubule cells, nor in hepatocytes and adipocytes.[28]

HLA class I APM component-specific mAbs became available only in the 2000s.[29–31] These reagents have been used to analyze HLA class I APM component expression in surgically removed tumors. As one would expect, the cancer types and the number of samples analyzed for each cancer type are markedly lower than those analyzed for HLA class I expression. Like HLA class I, APM components have been found to be downregulated in all the cancer types tested, although with differences among the APM components and among the cancer types analyzed.

One might ask whether mAbs that recognize HLA class I-peptide trimolecular complexes have been developed[32]

and used to measure their expression on cell lines and in normal and malignant tissues. A number of mAbs with this claimed specificity have been described in the literature.[33] Their specificity has not been corroborated by independent laboratories in most, if not all, cases.[34] In addition, these reagents do not detect HLA class I-TA peptide trimolecular complexes in surgically removed cancer tumors, most likely because the expression level of these complexes is below the sensitivity of the IHC method used.

Substrates Used to Detect HLA Class I APM Component Expression in Tumors

In early studies, frozen cancer tissues have been used as substrates, since the epitopes recognized by most, if not all, the available antibodies, whether monoclonal or polyclonal, are lost most likely because of the heating required for several steps of the fixation-embedding procedure. However, frozen tissues have not become popular in clinical practice because of the many limitations associated with their use for other common diagnostic purposes. First, frozen tissues do not maintain their structural and cellular details; therefore, the staining patterns are at times difficult to interpret. Second, they are not easy to handle, as they require special equipment and freezers for their preparation and storage, which increase the handling costs. These limitations have stimulated investigators, especially those with interest in analyzing HLA class I APM component expression in solid tumors, to develop antibodies which recognize epitopes of these molecules retained in formalin-fixed paraffin-embedded (FFPE) tissues. In most cases, reagents with these characteristics have been developed utilizing denatured molecules as immunogens. A list of HLA class I-specific mAbs that stain FFPE sections is presented in Table 5.1. The availability of mAbs with

Table 5.1 List of Antibodies That Stain Formalin—Fixed Paraffin—Embedded Tissues

TARGET	ANTIBODIES
HLA-A,B,C	EMR8-5
	Mouse anti-human HLA class I antibody (MBL)
	EP1395Y, #ab70328 (Abcam)
	Mouse anti-human HLA-ABC antibody (DAKO)
	Anti-HLA-ABC antibody (Santa Cruz)
HLA-A	HCA2
HLA-B	Anti-HLA-B antibody (Santa Cruz)
HLA-BC	HC10
β2m	L368
	Mouse anti-human β2m antibody (Santa Cruz)
	NAMB-1
	Rabbit polyclonal anti-β2m antibody (Polysciences)
	Rabbit polyclonal anti-β2m antibody (A0072, DAKO)
	Rabbit polyclonal anti-β2m antibody (A072, Glostrup)
	Rabbit polyclonal anti-β2m antibody (Novacastra)
	Rabbit polyclonal anti-β2m antibody (Biotechnology)
	EMR-B6
	BBM.1 (Santa Cruz)
	D8P1H (Cell Signaling)
LMP2	Mouse anti-human LMP2 antibody (Millipore)
	Rabbit anti-LMP2 antibody (Mamhead)
	SY-1
	LMP2 antibody (Abcam)
LMP7	Mouse anti-human LMP7 antibody (Abcam)
	HB-2
	Rabbit anti-LMP7 antibodies (Mamhead)
	SY-3
LMP10	TO-6
	TO-7
TAP1	Rabbit anti-human TAP1 antibody (Santa Cruz)
	NOB-1
	AK1.7
	TO-1
TAP2	Rabbit anti-human TAP2 antibody (Abcam)
	NOB-2
	TAP2 antibody (Santa Cruz Biotechnology)
	SY-2
	TAP2-specific mAb (BD Biosciences Pharmingen)
	Monoclonal mouse IgG antibody against TAP2 (MBL International)
	Mouse anti-TAP2 mAb 429.4
Calnexin	TO-5
	Calnexin antibody (Shanghai Jingtian, Biotechnology)
	MAB3126
	CSA-630
Calreticulin	Goat anti-calreticulin antibody (ab39818, Abcam)
	Anti-calreticulin (FMC75, Abcam)
	Anti-calreticulin (Biotechnology)
	Anti-calreticulin (006-661, #z9700, Upstate)
	TO-11
	SPA-600
ERp57	TO-2
	Anti-ERp57 antibody (Santa Cruz)
	PDIA3 (ab154191, Abcam)
Tapasin	TO-3
	Anti-tapasin antibody (Abcam)
	NBP1-86968 (Novus Biologicals)
	Anti-tapasin antibody (14373, Santa Cruz)

β2m, β2 microglobulin; HLA, human leukocyte antigen; LMP, low-molecular-weight protein; mAb, monoclonal antibody; TAP, transporter associated with antigen processing.

this reactivity pattern has allowed the use of FFPE tissue sections as substrates in immunohistochemical reactions. They have the advantage to maintain cellular and structural details and to facilitate the analysis of the spatial relationship among cells present in a tumor section. Furthermore, they provide the opportunity to use collections of archived tumors in retrospective studies, since most of the tumor samples are stored as FFPE tissues. However, FFPE tissue sections have their own limitations. Most important among them is the dissociation of the HLA class I complex during the fixation procedure most likely because of the heating required in several steps of the procedure. The dissociation of β2m from HLA class I heavy chain, the two HLA class I antigen subunits, results in the loss of the expression of the conformational epitopes which define HLA class I alleles. Therefore, FFPE tumor tissue sections cannot be utilized to assess HLA class I allele expression in tumor samples. Analysis of these substrates provides only information about the expression of the isolated subunits of HLA class I antigens.

In contrast, assessment of the expression of HLA class I alleles encoded in a cancer cell requires the use of frozen tissue sections. In these substrates, the two subunits of HLA class I antigens are associated and the complex expresses the polymorphic epitopes which define HLA class I alleles. However, their identification in tissues is hampered by the limitation that only a small number of the many mAbs which recognize HLA class I alleles function properly in IHC with frozen tissues. The replacement of antibody-based HLA typing techniques with DNA-based molecular typing has had a negative impact on the development of mAbs specific for HLA class I alleles.

Scoring of HLA Class I APM Component Expression in Cancers

Stained tissue sections can be scored by determining the percentage of stained cancer cells. To reduce the variability among laboratories in evaluating HLA class I APM component expression, in 1996, the HLA and Cancer component of the 12th International Histocompatibility Workshop proposed a classification system to assess the expression of these molecules in cancers.[35] According to this classification system, lesions are scored as negative, heterogeneous, and positive, when the percentage of stained cancer cells in the entire lesion is less than 25%, between 25% and 75% inclusive, and more than 75%, respectively. More recently, the H-score[36,37] has been introduced to quantify HLA class I APM component expression. This score is calculated by the formula $H\text{-}score = \sum Pi(I)$, where I is the intensity (range, 0–3) and Pi is the percentage of stained cancer cells varying from 0% to 100%. This scoring method is a popular semiquantitative system, and is recommended by leading organizations such as the Society of Clinical Oncology and the College of American Pathologists for scoring the expression of many markers such as hormone receptors in breast cancer.[38] However, surprisingly, this scoring method has been used only to a limited extent to evaluate HLA class I expression in tissues.[39,40] Therefore, the available information is not sufficient to compare the H-score with other scoring methods which have been widely used for many years. Nevertheless, the H-scoring system is attractive since it can be analyzed as a continuous variable and it takes into account both the staining intensity and the percentage of stained cells. However, it has some limitations. Specifically, the intensity threshold is subjective, leading to operator-dependent variation in the results. Furthermore, the staining intensity is dependent on the concentration of the mAb and the overall IHC technique used, thus decreasing the reproducibility of the results. Therefore, the H-score should be evaluated by multiple laboratories in a workshop, an approach which has already had a major positive impact on the progress of the HLA field.

It should be noted that IHC assays provide very useful and clinically relevant information. However, they do not provide information about the function of HLA class I APM. In this regard, lack of expression of one or more components is more informative than their detection, since the latter does not prove that the expressed molecules are functional.

Molecular Methods to Evaluate HLA Class I APM Component Expression in Cancers

Western blotting has been used to measure HLA class I APM component expression at the protein level in cancers. This assay has the advantage that a positive result most likely reflects the expression of the tested molecule in the sample analyzed and not the cross reactivity of the antibody used with an unrelated molecule. However, this assay provides no information about the distribution of the molecule tested in the cancer cell population analyzed. Furthermore, unless the tested malignant cell population is separated from non-malignant cells, the molecule isolated from the non-malignant cells contaminating the cancer cell population may "confound" the results in terms of its expression level in malignant cells. Finally, Western blot cannot detect HLA class I alleles, since the corresponding epitopes are lost when HLA class I subunits are dissociated during the electrophoresis step. Similar limitations apply to RNA- and DNA-based techniques which have been proposed to assess HLA class I APM component expression, although they can identify the polymorphism of HLA class I heavy chains.

HLA CLASS I APM COMPONENT DEFECTS IN CANCER

Defect Types

A review of the literature which has described HLA class I APM component expression in a large number of surgically removed cancers and of cell lines in short- and long-term culture has shown that the association between malignant transformation of cells and defects in HLA class I APM component expression is the rule more than the exception. Many defect types have been identified. Defects in β2m-HLA class I heavy chain-peptide complex expression will be distinguished from those affecting the other components of HLA class I APM. The defects in HLA class I trimolecular complex expression include:

1. **Total lack of HLA class I trimolecular complex expression.** This phenotype is generally caused by lack of β2m expression because of structural defects. These defects are not corrected by cytokines known to modulate HLA class I expression, such as IFNγ. This phenotype causes resistance to recognition and lysis by cognate T cells. Contrary to the general belief, this phenotype does not trigger lysis by natural killer (NK) cells, unless target cells express NK cell-activating ligands;

2. **HLA class I trimolecular complex downregulation.** This phenotype can be caused by (a) defects in the loading of peptides on β2m–HLA class I heavy chain complexes which result in instability of the β2m–HLA class I heavy chain dimer; (b) epigenetic downregulation of β2m; and (c) epigenetic downregulation of HLA class I heavy chain. These defects are generally correctable by targeting the underlying mechanisms. This phenotype causes resistance to recognition and lysis by cognate T cells, when the expression levels of the targeted HLA class I trimolecular complex is below that required to mediate interactions between target cells and cognate T cells. It may cause increased susceptibility to recognition and lysis by NK cells, when the level of HLA class I alleles reacting with KIR is not sufficient to inhibit the activity of NK cells and target cells express NK cell activating ligands;

3. **Downregulation or loss of one haplotype (i.e., HLA class I alleles encoded by the genes present in one of the chromosomes #6 [of paternal or maternal origin] which carry the MHC region).**[41] This phenotype is generally caused by loss of one of the chromosomes #6 or the region of the chromosomes #6 which carries the MHC region. This phenotype may cause abnormalities in the recognition and lysis of target cells by T cells that use the defective HLA class I allele as the restricting element. On the other hand, it is not likely to affect the recognition and lysis of target cells by NK cells;

4. **Downregulation or loss of the gene products of HLA-A, -B, or -C loci.** This phenotype is generally caused by abnormalities in the mechanisms that regulate the expression of these antigens. The expression of downregulated HLA class I can usually be restored by correcting the dysregulatory mechanism(s). It may cause abnormalities in the recognition and lysis of target cells by T cells, which target the defective HLA class I trimolecular complex. In addition, downregulation or loss of the gene products of HLA-B or -C loci may enhance recognition and lysis of target cells by NK cells; and

5. **Selective downregulation or loss of one HLA class I allele.** Downregulation may be caused by epigenetic mechanism(s) (Figure 5.3), while loss may be caused by mutations that inhibit the transcription or translation of the gene encoding the defective HLA class I allele. Correction of the latter defect requires transfection of abnormal cells with a wild-type gene encoding the defective allele. In contrast, the former defect may be corrected with a strategy that counteracts the mechanisms causing the HLA class I allele downregulation. This phenotype affects the recognition and lysis of target cells by T cells, which use the defective HLA class I allele as a restricting element, but is not expected to affect the interactions of target cells with NK cells.

It should be noted that although in the majority of cancers HLA class I abnormalities are in the form of downregulation or loss, there are also examples of abnormal upregulation. They include the appearance of HLA class I on cancers derived from normal cells that display no or barely detectable HLA class I expression. Examples of this abnormality include cancers derived from hypophysis, thyroid, hepatocytes, seminiferous tubules, and adipocytes.[28]

APM Component Downregulation and Loss

Defects in APM components include (a) downregulation of one or more APM component(s). This constitutes the majority of defects. This phenotype may be caused by epigenetic mechanism(s) and may be corrected by a strategy(ies) that counteract(s) it(them). This phenotype may have a negative impact on the generation of TA peptide(s), their transport to the endoplasmic reticulum, their loading on β2m-HLA class I heavy chain dimers, and/or transport of β2m-HLA class I heavy chain-peptide complexes to the membrane of cancer cells. As a result, this phenotype may have a negative impact on the recognition and lysis of target cells by cognate T cells. In addition, it may enhance the recognition and lysis by NK cells of target cells, provided that the downregulated HLA class I alleles include those which interact with KIRs and NK cell-activating ligands that are expressed on target cells.

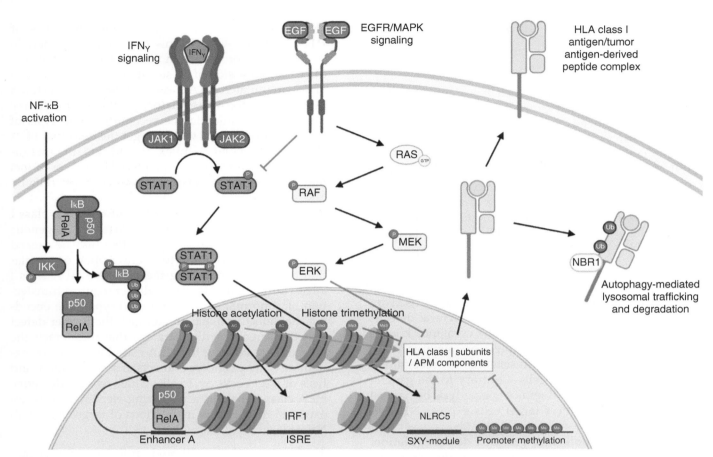

Figure 5.3 Epigenetic regulation of HLA class I APM component expression in cancer cells. Canonical NF-κB activation results in degradation of IκB and liberation of free NF-κB (p50/RelA dimer). Nuclear binding of NF-κB to promoter regions of HLA class I APM components, most notably the conserved cis-acting regulatory element enhancer A, promotes HLA class I APM component transcription. STAT1 activation by IFNγ results in IRF1 binding to ISRE and NLRC5-mediated transactivation of transcription factors on the SXY-module. These effects enhance HLA class I APM component expression. However, EGFR activation suppresses STAT1 signaling, downregulating HLA class I APM component expression. Likewise, MAPK activation (by KRAS, BRAF, etc.) is also implicated in HLA class I APM component downregulation, though the mechanism is unknown. Histone acetylation upregulates HLA class I APM component expression by increasing chromatin accessibility to transcription factors, while histone trimethylation has the opposite effect. Similarly, methylation of the promoter regions of HLA class I APM components represses their transcription, downregulating their expression. Lastly, the autophagy receptor NBR1 can mediate lysosomal trafficking and degradation of the assembled HLA class I–TA peptide complex.

APM, antigen processing machinery; EGFR, epidermal growth factor receptor; HLA, human leukocyte antigen; IFN, interferon; MAPK, mitogen-activated protein kinase; ISRE, interferon-sensitive response element; TA, tumor antigen.

The molecular mechanisms underlying HLA class I APM component downregulation are discussed in detail in the section "Molecular Mechanisms Underlying Defects in HLA Class I APM Components in Cancers"; (b) loss of one or more APM component(s). This phenotype may be caused by structural mutation(s) in both alleles of the gene(s) encoding the defective component(s). As described for β2m, the loss of HLA class I APM components is caused by two events. This phenotype may have a negative impact on the generation of peptide(s) from TAs, their transport to the endoplasmic reticulum, their loading on β2m-HLA class I heavy chain dimers, and/or transport of β2m-HLA class I heavy chain-peptide complexes to the membrane of cancer cells. As a result, this phenotype may have a negative impact on the recognition and lysis of target cells by cognate T cells. In addition, it may enhance the recognition and lysis of target cells by NK cells, provided that HLA class I alleles that interact with KIR are downregulated and NK cell-activating ligands are expressed on target cells; (c) upregulation of one or more APM components. Examples of this type of abnormality include high expression of the proteasome subunit delta in bladder cancer and of the chaperone molecules calnexin in lung adenocarcinoma[42] and colorectal cancer,[43] and calreticulin in pancreatic cancer.[44,45] The mechanisms underlying these abnormalities are not known. Similarly, it is not known whether these abnormalities have an impact on interactions of cancer cells with cognate T cells and/or with NK cells. However, these phenotypic changes appear to have clinical relevance, since they may be associated with the clinical course of the disease. For instance, delta upregulation has been reported to be associated with shorter survival in patients with bladder cancer. Assuming that this association is neither a fortuitous event nor a technical artifact, but reflects a cause-effect relationship and an immunologic mechanism, one might hypothesize that the negative impact of delta upregulation on patients' survival is caused by defects in patients' immune response against their own cancers because of unbalanced production of peptides from TAs. Furthermore, high calnexin expression in lung and colon cancer has been shown to be associated with poor disease-free and overall survival. This association has been suggested to reflect the involvement of calnexin in the unfolded protein response (UPR) and its role in cancer cell growth, invasion, and migration.[42] Lastly, high calreticulin expression has been found to be an independent predictor of poor survival in pancreatic cancer. This finding can be explained by the involvement of calreticulin in the activation of the MAP/ERK pathway.[44] As discussed later, this pathway has been shown to downregulate HLA class I expression and to promote cancer cell proliferation; and (d) changes in cellular distribution of one or more components. This type of change has been described for the immunoproteasome subunit LMP10 in oral cancer and appears to have clinical significance, since a low nuclear LMP10 expression has been reported to be associated with a favorable clinical outcome in HPV-positive cancers, whereas its moderate/high cytoplasmic expression appeared to be correlated with a good clinical outcome in HPV-negative cancers.[46] Furthermore, as a result of the UPR, calreticulin may migrate to the cell membrane where it acts as an "eat me" signal.[45,47] The mechanism(s) underlying these changes as well as their impact on interactions of target cells with cognate T cells and/or NK cells are not known.

Frequency of Defects in HLA Class I APM Component Expression

A review of the literature describing defects in HLA class I APM component expression in malignant tumors has been performed. This review has been limited to studies that have utilized mAbs recognizing epitopes shared by the gene products of HLA-A, -B, and -C loci, the gene products of HLA-A locus, and the gene products of HLA-B and -C loci, and APM components. Papers that describe loss of haplotypes or of HLA class I alleles have not been included, since the number of studies describing cancers

with these defects in the literature is small and not sufficient to draw definitive conclusions. Therefore, the frequency of HLA class I APM component defects reported for each of the cancer types analyzed is likely to be an underestimate of the defects present in them, also because previous results[48] suggest that selective HLA class I allele losses are not detected by staining cancer tissue sections with mAbs which recognize framework or locus-specific epitopes. Furthermore, studies in cancers originating from cells that normally do not express HLA class I molecules (ex. hypophysis, thyroid, hepatocytes, seminiferous tubules, and adipocytes) have been excluded. Lastly, studies performed by staining FFPE tissues with the mAb W6/32 have not been included, since this mAb does not stain FFPE tissues, as indicated by the manufacturer's instructions.[49,50] Therefore, the staining patterns described in the literature are likely to be a technical artifact.

Altogether, 237 papers[40,44,45,51–268] have been reviewed; of those, 190 have analyzed HLA class I heavy chain antigen expression in 19 cancer types, 91 β2m expression in 18 cancer types, and 54 APM component expression in 17 cancer types. With the exception of intrahepatic cholangiocarcinoma and pancreatic ductal adenocarcinoma, at least 127 samples of each cancer type have been analyzed for HLA class I heavy chain expression, at least 67 for β2m expression, and at least 10 for APM component expression. The total number of cancer samples analyzed for HLA class I heavy chain expression is 23,954, that for β2m expression is 8,248, and that for APM component expression is 3,446. The most studied APM component is TAP1 (36 studies, 2,487 cases) and the least studied one is LMP10 (5 studies, 250 cases). The total frequency of HLA class I heavy chain defects ranges between 36% in urinary bladder cancer and 80% in penile cancer. The total frequency of β2m expression defects ranges from 17% in bone and soft tissue cancer and 73% in ocular melanoma (Figure 5.4). The total percentage of APM component defects ranges between 0% and 100%. The total percentage of immunoproteasome subunit LMP2, LMP7, and LMP10 defects ranges between 0% (cervical cancer, LMP10) and 100% (brain cancers, LMP7). The total frequency of defects for the two TAP subunits, TAP1 and TAP2, ranges between 13% (breast cancer, TAP2) and 97% (prostate cancer, TAP1). Lastly, the total percentage of defects for the chaperone molecules calnexin, calreticulin, ERp57, and tapasin ranges between 0% (brain cancers, ERp57) and 100% (brain cancers, calreticulin; renal cancer, tapasin; Table 5.2).

The difference in the frequency of defects is likely to reflect both biological and methodological-variables. The latter include the following:

1. **Substrate utilized in the IHC reaction.** Among the reviewed studies, 138 used FFPE tissues, and 46 frozen tissues. The frequency of defects found testing

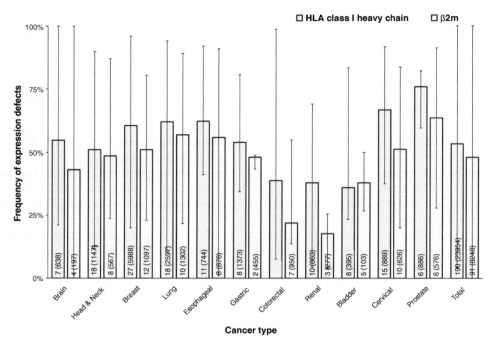

Figure 5.4 Frequency of HLA class I heavy chain and β2m expression defects in cancer types. Only cancer types in which HLA class I heavy chain expression was analyzed in more than 300 cases have been included in the graph. The number of included studies (number of cases) for each cancer type is presented within each bar. Error bars represent the highest and lowest expression defect frequency reported.

HLA, human leukocyte antigen; β2m, β2 microglobulin.

Table 5.2 Lowest and Highest Frequency of Expression Defects of Each HLA Class I APM Component

HLA CLASS I APM COMPONENT	LOWEST FREQUENCY		HIGHEST FREQUENCY	
	(%)	TUMOR SITE	(%)	TUMOR SITE
HLA-A/B/C	35.8	Kidney	80.3	Penis
β2m	16.7	Bone/soft tissue	72.7	Eye (melanoma)
LMP2	18.7	Colon/rectum	94.4	Prostate
LMP7	14.4	Colon/rectum	100	Brain
LMP10	0	Cervix	90.9	Eye (melanoma)
TAP1	24.1	Breast	96.6	Prostate
TAP2	13.2	Breast	87.8	Brain
Calnexin	1.2	Colon/rectum	90.9	Eye (melanoma)
Calreticulin	3.3	Skin (melanoma)	100	Brain
ERp57	0	Brain	87.2	Stomach
Tapasin	7.1	Skin (melanoma)	100	Kidney

Note: The tumors in which the minimum and maximum values have been reported are shown. Minimum and maximum values represent the average frequency of defects for each tumor (not individual studies).

APM, antigen processing machinery; β2m, β2 microglobulin; HLA, human leukocyte antigen; LMP, low-molecular-weight protein; TAP, transporter associated with antigen processing.

FFPE tumors was significantly higher ($p < .001$) than that found testing frozen tumors (54% of the 20,272 FFPE tumor samples analyzed, as compared to 45% of the 2,237 frozen tumors analyzed);

2. **Characteristics of the mAbs used as probes.** Some studies have utilized mAbs which recognize an epitope restricted to the gene products of HLA-A locus such as mAb HCA2[51,59,60,63,67,72,93,98,100,103,123,124,129,131,145,146,150,153,162,170,181,182,201,230,257,268–270] or of HLA-B and -C loci such as mAb HC10,[40,52,55,59,60,63,69,71,72,75,91,93,98,100,103–107,109,123,124,129,132–134,140,141,143,145–147,150,153,155,156,158–160,162,166,170,174–177,181,182,201,229,237,240,268–271] whereas other studies focus on mAbs which recognize an epitope shared by the gene products of HLA-A, HLA-B, and HLA-C loci such as mAb EMR8-5[54,76,77,82–86,95,97,108,118,126,128,154,163,167,169,179,183,190,233–236,238,241,242,245,247,250,252,254,256,258,260–262,265,272] and other studies focus on mAbs which recognize an epitope shared by classical and non-classical HLA class I antigens such as mAb W6/32.[80,81,102,120,122,127,135,142,144,149,151,249,251,263,267,273–275] Needless to say, the studies utilizing only the mAb HC10 provide incomplete information since they do not detect the defects present in the gene products of the HLA-A locus which are more frequent than those present in the gene products of the HLA-B and -C loci, as will be discussed later.

Although a clear difference was not found in the frequency of HLA class I expression defects detected with mAbs recognizing framework epitopes and those recognizing locus-specific epitopes, a significant difference ($p < .001$) was found in the frequency of defects detected with mAbs recognizing the gene products of the HLA-A locus and of those detected with mAbs recognizing the gene products of the HLA-B/-C loci. Specifically, the mAb HCA2, which recognizes an epitope selectively expressed by the gene products of the HLA-A locus,[269,270] detected defects in 53% of the 3,143 cancer samples analyzed, while the mAb HC10, which recognizes an epitope selectively expressed by the gene products of the HLA-B and -C loci,[269–271] detected defects in 44% of the 3,210 cancer samples tested. This difference was found in all the cancer types in which both mAbs were tested. Although the role of the characteristics of the mAbs tested cannot be excluded, this difference probably reflects the differential susceptibility of the gene products of the HLA class I loci to genetic mutations and/or epigenetic changes.

3. **Sensitivity of the IHC assay.** This variable is influenced by the antigen retrieval method and by the criteria utilized to score the stained slides.

The biological variables include (a) characteristics of the cancer types included in the study. The frequency of HLA class I APM component defects increases with disease progression in some cancer types. For instance, in cancers of the oral mucosa, the frequency of HLA class I expression defects is higher in the malignant compared to the premalignant lesions;[276] (b) frequency of mutations and patient's immune response to his cancer. Development of tumors with HLA class I APM component defects reflects the outgrowth of cancer cells which have acquired the ability to avoid the host's immune system attack since they have developed escape mechanism(s). This mechanism raises the possibility that the mutation load may play a role in the frequency of HLA class I APM component defects, since a high cancer mutation load is likely to induce a strong immune response. The latter will in turn exert a strong selective pressure on a cancer cell population, which will facilitate the outgrowth of cancer cells carrying escape mechanisms.[277] This possibility is supported by the higher frequency of HLA class I APM component defects found in microsatellite instable (MSI) colon cancer than in microsatellite stable (MSS) colon cancer (e.g., 60%–61% in MSI vs 17%–30% in MSS cancers).[63,98]

4. **Length of interval between the time of malignant transformation of cells and diagnosis.** A long interval provides more chances for cancer cells to develop mutations that may affect HLA class I APM components and to host's immune system to develop an immune response to his cancer. The combination of mutations with immune response is likely to facilitate the outgrowth of cancer cells with HLA class I APM defects. As a matter of fact, the frequency of HLA class I APM component defects is high in malignancies like breast and prostate cancer which have a slow clinical course; and

5. **Epigenetic downregulation of HLA class I APM component expression in cancer cells.** In recent years there has been increasing evidence that the HLA class I APM component and TA expression can be modulated by the activation of many signaling pathways and by changes in the expression of proteins involved in chromatin/DNA modification.

Primary and Metastatic Tumors

A few studies have analyzed the frequency of HLA class I APM component defects in metastatic tumors and compared it to that in autologous or allogeneic primary tumors. Cordon-Cardo et al. were the first to report that the frequency of HLA class I expression defects in metastases from many cancer types was higher than that described in primary cancers of different histotype, since HLA class I antigens were not detected in 75% of the metastases analyzed.[58] HLA class I expression defects were suggested to provide metastatic cells with an escape from immune surveillance. In subsequent studies these analyses have been extended to other APM components.

With few exceptions these studies were performed with metastases to lymph nodes. HLA class I antigens, LMP2, LMP7, TAP1, TAP2, calnexin, and/or tapasin were reported to be downregulated in metastases as compared to primary tumors in melanoma, head and neck squamous cell carcinoma, breast cancer, and/or ovarian cancer.[55,66,91,92,107,148,151] Surprisingly, comparison of the phenotype of brain metastases with that of autologous breast primary cancers detected no significant difference.[113] The latter results, however, have to be interpreted with caution, since only 15 cancer samples were analyzed.

MOLECULAR MECHANISMS UNDERLYING DEFECTS IN HLA CLASS I APM COMPONENTS IN MALIGNANT CANCERS

Multiple molecular mechanisms underlie HLA class I APM component loss or downregulation in malignant cells. They can be divided into two major groups: (a) selective or total loss of HLA class I APM component expression: these abnormalities are caused by structural mutations in the genes which encode HLA class I APM components and (b) selective or total HLA class I APM component downregulation: these abnormalities are caused by epigenetic mechanisms or structural mutations in genes which regulate HLA class I APM component expression.

Selective or Total Loss of HLA Class I APM Component Expression Caused by Structural Mutations

HLA Class I Heavy Chain

Mutations have been identified in the genes encoding HLA class I heavy chains in most, if not all, the cancer types analyzed. The frequency of mutations is higher in the genes encoding HLA-B heavy chains than in those encoding HLA-A and HLA-C heavy chains. However, no marked difference has been found in the frequency of mutations among the gene products of each of the HLA-A, -B, and -C loci. The cancer types analyzed do not appear to differ in the frequency of mutations present in HLA class I heavy chains. Furthermore, no hotspot has been identified in HLA class I heavy chain sequences. Lastly, the mutations found in HLA class I heavy chain encoding genes range from large deletions to single base deletions.[278–282] They inhibit either transcription or translation of the mutated gene.

β2m

In the late 1980s, a number of studies investigated the mechanisms underlying total HLA class I loss, which could not be restored by IFNγ. These studies were facilitated by the development of colon cancer and melanoma cell lines with defective HLA class I expression. Lack of HLA class I expression that could not be restored by IFNγ was shown to be caused by lack of expression of functional β2m, which is required for the transport of HLA class I heavy chains to the cell membrane and the expression of epitopes which define HLA class I alleles. A number of abnormalities were identified. As observed with HLA class I heavy chain, they range from loss of large fragments of β2m gene to single nucleotide deletions. These mutations in most cases inhibit the translation of mRNA, but do not affect the transcription of β2m encoding gene.[283] This information is important also from a practical viewpoint, since RNA-based assays may give misleading results about β2m expression in cancer biopsies.[284-286] Although the mutations are distributed randomly in β2m genes, a mutation hotspot has been suggested to be located in the CT repeat region in exon 1 of the β2m gene.[283] The available evidence suggests that the mutation type in the β2m gene may be influenced by T cell immunotherapy.[287] In this regard, the internal dinucleotide "CT" deletion has been found in three of five melanoma cell lines established from patients receiving T cell–based immunotherapy,[287] but only in one (Me1386)[288] out of five melanoma cell lines established from patients not treated with this immunotherapy type.[282,289] The relationship between outgrowth of cancer cells harboring certain genomic instability types and type/extent of T cell-mediated immune selective pressure is supported by the different frequency of β2m gene mutations identified in different colon carcinoma types.[284-286] The β2m gene CT deletion has been found in microsatellite instable (MSI)[290] colon carcinomas but not in chromosomal instability (CIN)-positive[290] colon carcinomas. MSI cancers are infiltrated by a large number of activated cytotoxic CD8+ T cells, and this infiltration is associated with a longer survival.[291–294]

Mutations in the two co-dominant β2m encoding genes have not been described. A more frequent mechanism is represented by inactivation of one gene because of a mutation and by loss of the chromosome #15 or of the region which carries the wild-type β2m gene.[295] Therefore, loss of β2m expression results from two events: the available evidence[296–298] is compatible with the possibility that the loss of a wild-type β2m gene is chronologically the first event and mutation in the other β2m allele is the second one. The data generated by the TCGA Research Network (http://cancergenome.nih.gov/) suggest that the frequency of β2m mutations varies among cancer types; it ranges from a minimum of 1% in lung, esophageal, bladder, and ovarian cancer, to a maximum of 6% in gastric and colorectal cancer. However, these values have to be interpreted with caution, since a recent analysis of PDXs established from lung cancer reported a higher frequency of β2m mutations.[137]

APM Components

The frequency of mutations found in APM components in the cancer types analyzed is markedly lower than that found in β2m and in HLA class I heavy chains in all the malignancies analyzed. Like β2m, APM components are encoded by two co-dominant genes. Therefore, as described for β2m, APM component loss requires two events which in the few characterized cases have resulted to be different from those identified for β2m. Loss of TAP1 in a squamous cell lung cancer cell line[299] and of tapasin in a melanoma cell line[287] have been shown to be caused by a cancer-unrelated germline mutation in combination with a cancer-related repression of the other allele. In contrast, no germ-line mutations have been identified so far in β2m encoding genes; all the mutations that cause β2m loss are cancer-related. As discussed elsewhere,[300] it is not known at present whether this difference reflects a lower genetic stability of the β2m locus and/or the involvement of APM in crucial alternative functions in malignant cells.

Selective or Total HLA Class I APM Component Downregulation Caused by Dysregulatory Mechanisms

Comparison of the frequency of mutations identified in HLA-A heavy chains, HLA-B heavy chains, HLA-C heavy chains, β2m, and APM components with that of the abnormalities identified in the corresponding proteins in all the cancers analyzed has shown that the latter have a significantly higher frequency in all the cancer types analyzed. The difference between the combined frequency of defects at the protein level and the maximum frequency of mutations is at least 39% (14% vs. 53%), 42% (6% vs. 48%), and 39% (6% vs. 45%) for HLA class I heavy chains, β2m, and HLA class I APM components, respectively.

These differences suggest that at least 3/4 of the defects found in HLA class I APM components at the protein level are likely to be caused by epigenetic mechanisms. This finding has several implications in terms of our understanding of the pathogenetic mechanisms underlying HLA class I APM abnormalities in cancer cells and in terms of therapeutic strategies to correct them. Several epigenetic mechanisms have been found to affect HLA class I APM component expression by cancer cells and their ability to generate peptides from TAs, process them, and present them to cognate T cells. There is no general mechanism underlying HLA class I APM component defects in all cancer types; in addition, no specific mechanism has been identified for any specific cancer type. The following mechanisms have been identified in a number of cancer types.

MAPK Signaling Pathway

In several cancer types including head and neck cancer and melanoma, mitogen-activated protein kinase (MAPK) pathway activation downregulates HLA class I APM component expression.[301] Their level may be restored by inhibiting MAPK activation as described in head and neck cancer cells treated with the EGFR-specific mAb cetuximab[302] and in BRAF mutant melanoma cells treated with a BRAF inhibitor.[303] Treatment with a BRAF inhibitor and adoptive immunotherapy with T cells transduced with a TA-specific T cell receptor inhibited the growth of human BRAF mutant melanoma cells grafted in immunodeficient mice.[303] In the case of EGFR inhibition, HLA class I APM component upregulation was shown to be mediated by STAT1 activation/upregulation via several distinct mechanisms.[302] These changes in HLA class I APM component expression level have functional significance, since they are associated with an increased susceptibility of cancer cells to recognition and elimination by cognate T cells. The clinical relevance of these results is suggested by the association of HLA class I APM component upregulation in head and neck cancers with clinical responses in patients treated with the EGFR-specific mAb cetuximab.[304] Immunological events are likely to play a role in this association because tumors of patients who respond to therapy are infiltrated by lymphocytes.

IFN Pathway

Cytokine activation of the IFN pathway, primarily IFNγ, is known to induce HLA class I upregulation on cancer cells through stimulation of HLA class I APM gene transcriptional regulators (STAT1, IRF1, NLRC5). Modulation of this pathway, which is found in several cancer types, is associated with changes in HLA class I expression level.[9,305] IFNγ treatment can restore HLA class I APM component expression on cancer cells[306,307] and therefore increase T cell-mediated lysis.[308] However, defects in the IFNγ signal transduction pathway, such as JAK1 or JAK2 mutations, confer resistance to IFNγ-mediated HLA class I APM component upregulation.[309–311] Melanoma cells with JAK2 deletion also possessed reduced basal HLA class I APM component expression.[311] Similarly, HLA-A expression was downregulated on melanoma cells in tumors from patients with STAT1 mutations.[312]

NF-κB Pathway

Similarly to the IFN pathway, the NF-κB pathway regulates HLA class I expression by malignant cells in some cancer types.[313,314] Therefore, restoration or upregulation of NF-κB signaling in cancer cells may enhance their susceptibility to the antitumor activity of cognate T cells through increased HLA class I expression as well as improve the efficacy of checkpoint inhibition therapy.[315]

Methylation

Hypermethylation of the HLA-A, -B, and -C heavy chains; β2m; and APM component encoding gene promoter regions may cause HLA class I APM component downregulation or loss.[130,316,317] This mechanism has been found to underlie defects in HLA class I APM component expression in melanoma,[318] nasopharyngeal cancer,[319] and esophageal squamous cell carcinoma[130] cell lines. In some cases, these defects have been identified also in the cancers from which the cell lines have originated. The expression level of the downregulated molecules can be restored by treating cells with demethylating agents such as azacitidine and decitabine. This phenotypic change has functional relevance, since it is associated with an increased susceptibility of target cells to recognition by cognate T cells in vitro.[318,320] One additional finding is noteworthy because of its relevance to the use of demethylating agents in the area of immunotherapy of malignant diseases. Demethylating agents have been shown in a mouse model of mammary carcinoma and mesothelioma to markedly enhance the efficacy of immunotherapy with immunological checkpoint-specific mAbs.[321,322] This result provides a strong rationale for combining demethylating agents with T cell-based immunotherapies for the treatment of patients bearing tumors with HLA class I APM defects caused by hypermethylation.

Histone Acetylation and Methylation

The histone acetylation level modulates chromatin accessibility to transcription factors leading to regulation of gene expression. Defective histone acetylation underlies the HLA class I APM component downregulation frequently found in Merkel cell carcinoma cells, as their expression can be restored both in vitro and in vivo with histone deacetylase (HDAC) inhibitors.[323] At pharmacological doses the latter compounds can also enhance the in vitro susceptibility of human breast and prostate cancer cell lines to recognition by cognate T cells by upregulating many HLA class I APM component expressions.[324] The mechanism suggested for this effect is a cellular survival response to ER stress mediated through the UPR. Irrespective of the mechanism, the described data argue for the combination of HDAC inhibitors with T cell-based immunotherapy such as that with checkpoint inhibitors, in order to enhance its efficacy. Other mechanisms such as trimethylation of histone H3 at lysine 27 (H3K27me3) have been reported to contribute to HLA-B downregulation in CML, embryonal carcinoma, and neuroblastoma cell lines in vitro and MHC class I transactivator NLRC5 downregulation in the CML cell line. This histone modification could be reversed through inhibition

of the enhancer of zeste homolog 2 (EZH2), the key enzymatic component of the polycomb repressive complex 2 (PRC2) which promotes trimethylation of histone H3 at lysine 27. The generated H3K27me3 inhibits transcription. In fact, EZH2 inhibition upregulated several HLA class I APM components in small cell lung cancer cells and reversed their in vitro resistance to T cell-mediated killing.[325]

Autophagy

Autophagy was recently reported to be involved in the regulation of HLA class I antigen-TA peptide complex expression on PDAC cells, which demonstrate high autophagic flux. The ubiquitinated HLA class I trimolecular complex is bound by the autophagy receptor NBR1, and these complexes traffic to the lysosome for degradation. In vitro treatment of PDAC cells with chloroquine, which inhibits autophagy, upregulated HLA class I subunit expression, but did not affect HLA class I APM component expression.[326] The in vivo relevance of these data is indicated by the increased therapeutic efficacy of dual immune checkpoint blockade against PDAC and increased CD8+ T cell infiltration in tumors in mice treated with chloroquine.[326] The clinical relevance of these results is indicated by the increased tumor lymphocyte infiltration and decreased autophagy in PDAC patients treated with chloroquine in combination with gemcitabine/nab-paclitaxel as compared to those treated with chemotherapy alone.[327] This is compatible with the possibility that inhibition of autophagy with chloroquine upregulates HLA class I APM component expression.

CLINICAL SIGNIFICANCE OF HLA CLASS I APM COMPONENT DEFECTS IN CANCER CELLS

Several lines of evidence suggest that HLA class I APM component defects may play a role in the pathogenesis and clinical course of malignant diseases. Analysis of normal colon mucosa in subjects with familial adenomatous polyposis who are prone to the development of multiple adenomas has detected defects in HLA class I expression.[328] These abnormalities do not appear to be restricted to the colon since they have been found also in normal cervical and vulvar tissues and in pre-neoplastic lesions.[206,329,330] Because of the crucial role played by HLA class I antigens in the recognition of cancer cells by cognate T cells, these abnormalities have been suggested to provide normal and premalignant cells with an escape mechanism from immune surveillance.

In many cancer types, HLA class I APM component downregulation is associated with clinicopathologic characteristics of the disease. Specifically, HLA class I APM component downregulation or loss is associated with larger tumor size (ex. intrahepatic cholangiocarcinoma[150]),

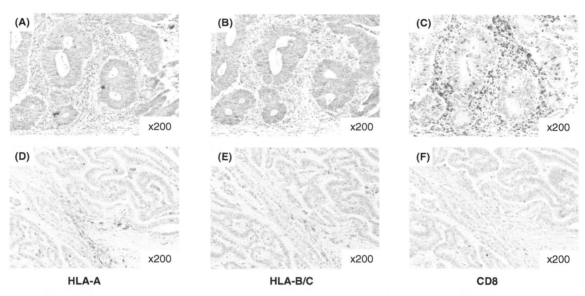

Figure 5.5 **Correlation of HLA class I antigen expression with CD8⁺ T cell infiltration in formalin-fixed, paraffin-embedded colorectal cancer lesions stained with HLA class I antigen-specific and CD8-specific mAbs.** Tumor tissue sections were IHC stained with mouse HLA-A-specific mAb HCA2, HLA-B/C-specific mAb HC10, and CD8-specific mAb. The positive expression of HLA-A (A) and HLA-B/C (B) with high CD8⁺ T cell infiltration (C) was compared with low/negative expression of HLA-A (D) and HLA-B/C (E) with low CD8⁺ T cell infiltration (F). Magnification is indicated.

HLA, human leukocyte antigen; IHC, immunohistochemical; mAbs, monoclonal antibodies.

higher grade (ex. breast[40,175] and lung cancer[144]), and higher stage (ex. melanoma[91]). Furthermore, higher HLA class I APM component expression is correlated with an increased number of tumor infiltrating lymphocytes, which are predominantly found peri-tumorally (Figure 5.5).[97,112,166] In many cancer types, an association has been found between high HLA class I APM component expression in primary tumors and favorable prognosis in terms of frequency of metastatic disease, as well as disease-specific, disease-free, and overall survival.[44,55,56,66,80,81,84,86,91,94,110,126,132,134,136,146,153,158,161–163,177,183] This association, which in some cases involves also CD8⁺ T cell infiltration and the PD-1/PD-L1 axis, argues in favor of the role of HLA class I antigens in the recognition of cancer cells by cognate T cells. It is noteworthy that, in some tumors, HLA class I APM component loss from cancer cells is associated with disease recurrence in patients who had initially responded clinically to T cell-based immunotherapy.[331–334] This finding is likely to reflect the outgrowth of cancer cell subpopulations which escape the selective pressure imposed by the induced or enhanced T cell immunity, because of defects in the HLA class I antigen-TA peptide trimolecular complex expression. As previously mentioned, these complexes mediate the interaction between target cells and cognate T cells. The frequency of this scenario is likely to increase with the growing use of checkpoint inhibitor-based immunotherapy.

In some cases,[318,335] multiple genetic and epigenetic defects which are often caused by different mechanisms have been found in tumors and the derived cell line(s). At least two examples of coexisting defects in HLA class I APM components have been identified in melanoma cell lines. In one, structural mutations caused HLA-A2 and TAP1 loss (Figure 5.6A).[335] In another cell line, HLA-A3 downregulation caused by hypermethylation of its promoter was associated with tapasin loss caused by a germ line mutation of one gene copy along with a somatic loss of the other gene copy (Figure 5.6B).[318] Those phenotypes may reflect the development of multiple escape mechanisms by cancer cells that are subjected to selective pressure exerted by cognate T cells with different fine specificity. These findings highlight the plasticity of the cancer cell population, which has the ability to adapt to the hostile tumor microenvironment, as well as that of the immune system, which allows T cells to adjust to changes in the phenotypic and functional properties of the targeted cancer cell population.

The extent to which HLA class I expression plays a role in the clinical course of malignant diseases is influenced by the interference of confounding factors, such as high PD-L1 expression. Indeed, a study of HLA class I and PD-L1 expression in intrahepatic cholangiocarcinoma (ICC) has shown that HLA class I expression by ICC cells was associated with favorable clinical course

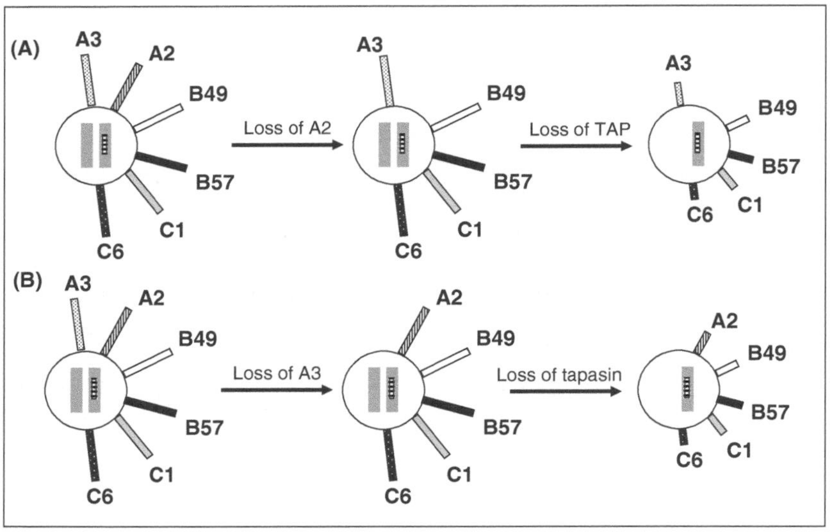

Figure 5.6 Role of the plasticity of cancer cells and patients' immune system in the development of multiple HLA class I APM defects in a cancer cell population subjected to immune selective pressure. A. Outgrowth of HLA-A2 negative melanoma cells from an HLA-A2 positive melanoma cell population subjected to selective pressure exerted by TA-specific, HLA-A2-restricted T cells, followed by loss of TAP and subsequent downregulation of HLA class I molecule expression. B. Loss of HLA-A3 caused by hypermethylation of its promoter was associated with tapasin loss caused by a germline mutation of one gene copy along with a somatic loss of the other gene copy.

APM, antigen-processing machinery; HLA, human leukocyte antigen; TA, tumor antigen; TAP, transporter associated with antigen processing.

of the disease only if PD-L1 was not, or was barely, detectable.[150] Similarly, high HLA class I expression was associated with short recurrence-free and overall survival when PD-L1 was highly expressed in esophageal squamous cell carcinoma.[85] Caution has to be exercised in interpreting these results because each study has been performed only in one center and the results have not been confirmed independently. Furthermore, the number of patients investigated is relatively small.

An unexpected finding described in the literature is the shorter survival of patients with low HLA class I expression level in their tumors, as compared to those with lack of or high HLA class I expression level. This association has been described in patients with breast, colorectal, penile, and cervical cancer.[67,74,176,201] This bimodal association has been suggested to reflect the antitumor activity of NK cells and cognate T cells with cancer cells which lack or express high HLA class I levels, respectively. On the other hand, the short survival of patients with low HLA class I expression in their tumors reflects the resistance of cancer cells to both cognate T cells and NK cells. The cytotoxic activity of NK cells is inhibited by interactions of cancer cell HLA class I antigen with NK cell KIRs; cognate T cells do not recognize cancer cells because of the defective presentation of TA peptides by downregulated HLA class I antigens.

POTENTIAL ROLE OF HLA CLASS I APM COMPONENT DEFECTS IN RESISTANCE TO TREATMENT WITH CHECKPOINT INHIBITOR-BASED IMMUNOTHERAPY

There is general agreement that the impressive clinical responses described in patients with various cancer types treated with immune checkpoint inhibitors-based immunotherapy are mediated by the antitumor activity of unleashed cognate T cells. The target of this immune response has been suggested to be in most cases a HLA class I antigen-TA peptide trimolecular complex.[336] Crucial to its synthesis and expression on cancer cell membrane is the role of the HLA class I APM, which has to generate the peptides from the mutated protein(s), load them on β2m-HLA class I heavy chain dimers, and transport the resulting trimers to the cancer cell membrane. Clinical evidence has convincingly shown that not all cancer types and only a proportion of patients with a given cancer type respond to immune checkpoint inhibitor-based immunotherapy.[1–3] Furthermore, in a percentage of patients, which varies among the cancer types studied, the clinical responses have a limited duration. These clinical findings have stimulated interest in identifying biomarkers that are predictors of clinical responses and/or are useful to monitor the clinical course of the disease. A number of potential biomarkers have been proposed. They include PD-L1 expression level, PD-L2 expression level, relative eosinophil count, relative lymphocyte count, tumor T cell infiltrate, gene expression profile, mutational load, mismatch repair status, TCR clonality, myeloid-derived suppressor cell infiltrate, T regulatory cell infiltrate, and ICOS[+] CD4[+] T cell infiltrate.[337–350] Only assays to measure PD-L1 expression have been FDA approved. None of the assays appears to have become the standard to select and monitor patients.

To the best of our knowledge, there are limited studies on the role of HLA class I APM component defects in response to checkpoint inhibitor therapy. The scant information in this area is surprising given the role of HLA class I APM in the interactions between cancer cells and unleashed cognate T cells, the frequent presence of HLA class I APM component defects in cancers, and the clinical relevance of these defects. However, there is an increasing number of reports showing that the level of HLA class I APM expression is associated with the response to checkpoint inhibition.[351,352] On the other hand, the loss of HLA class I expression caused by a β2m mutation is associated with poor response to checkpoint inhibition therapy. For instance, β2m loss by cancer cells because of structural mutations has been reported to be associated with resistance to checkpoint inhibition in a patient with melanoma who had a relapse while being treated with an anti-PD-1 mAb,[9] in a colorectal cancer patient refractory to anti-PD-1 therapy,[10] and in metastatic melanoma patients unresponsive to either anti-PD-1 or anti-CTLA-4 therapy.[11] Moreover, in an analysis of the TCGA human skin cutaneous melanoma cohort, HLA class I downregulation[351] and HLA class I APM component downregulation[352] were associated with resistance to anti-CTLA-4 therapy. Similarly, β2m loss has been shown to confer resistance to anti-PD-1 therapy in mice bearing tumors derived from lung cancer[353] or melanoma cell lines.[354] Interestingly, the role of HLA class I expression in response to checkpoint inhibition appears to be influenced also by the anatomic site of the metastasis where the HLA class I downregulation is documented.[355]

In cases where epigenetic HLA class I APM component downregulation is involved, strategies to reverse this downregulation have been generally effective in enhancing efficacy of immune checkpoint blockade. The anti-CTLA4 mAb ipilimumab in combination with the DNA methyltransferase inhibitor guadecitabine, which upregulates HLA class I heavy chain expression, induced complete or partial clinical responses in 26% (5/19) of patients with unresectable melanoma.[356] Likewise, in mice, irinotecan upregulated MHC class I expression in breast cancer in vivo, and synergized with an anti-PD-L1 mAb resulting in better control of tumor growth than monotherapy.[357] Similarly, the EZH2 inhibitor GSK126 upregulated MHC class I expression in a murine oral squamous cell cancer (OSCC) cell line in

vitro and in tumor-bearing mice, and restored sensitivity of anti-PD-1 mAb of OSCC tumors resistant to this therapy.[358] Lastly, autophagy inhibition with chloroquine, which was shown to increase MHC class I expression, sensitized PDAC cells to dual immune checkpoint blockade in mice and increased CD8[+] T cell infiltration in treated cancers.[326]

It must be noted, however, that there are exceptions to the role of HLA class I expression in response to checkpoint inhibition-based therapy. For instance, a high response rate to checkpoint inhibitors has been described in lymphoma, although this cancer type harbors HLA class I defects in high frequency.[359] Furthermore, in a group of melanoma patients, HLA class II, not I, expression level has been associated with response to PD-1/PD-L1 blockade.[360] Additionally, HLA class I downregulation in melanoma patients failed to predict resistance to anti-PD-1 therapy.[351] Similarly, in a patient with Merkel cell carcinoma refractory to anti-PD-1 therapy, the combination of the HDAC inhibitor panobinostat and an anti-PD-L1 mAb stabilized the disease for only 3 months, in spite of HLA-A, β2m, TAP1, TAP2, LMP2, and LMP7 upregulation and increased CD8[+] T cell infiltration density.[361] Likewise, in mice, in an OSCC tumor treated with the combination of an anti-PD-1 mAb and GSK126 (EZH2 inhibitor), despite MHC class I upregulation, there was no control of tumor growth.[358] Lastly, both β2m-knockout and Ifngr1-knockout urothelial tumors (which do not express MHC class I antigens) were still responsive to anti-PD-1 and/or anti-CTLA-4 therapy in mice.[362]

CONCLUSION

Testing of a large number of surgically removed tumors mainly with immunohistochemical assays has convincingly shown that abnormalities in HLA class I expression are present in all the cancer types analyzed, although with different frequency. The information in the literature about APM component expression in cancer is less extensive. Nevertheless, there is convincing evidence that the expression of these molecules is frequently defective in most, if not all, cancer types analyzed. As observed for HLA class I subunits, there are differences in the frequency of defects among the APM components and among the cancer types tested. The HLA class I abnormalities we have described have clinical relevance, since they are associated with the histopathological characteristics of tumors and/or with clinical characteristics such as disease-free survival and overall survival. The abnormalities in HLA class I APM component expression we have described are caused by genetic and epigenetic mechanisms, the latter being much more frequent than the former ones. The latter finding implies that HLA class I APM defects may be corrected by rationally designed and clinically relevant strategies. As briefly discussed in this chapter, at least in animal model systems, growing evidence is compatible with the possibility that strategies which restore HLA class I APM component expression and function in malignant cells may enhance the therapeutic efficacy of T cell-based immunotherapy. Given that an increasing number of mechanisms has been implicated in HLA class I APM downregulation, strategies aiming to restore HLA class I expression will need to be guided by identification of the underlying molecular mechanism in each individual tumor. If additional experimental evidence corroborates this conclusion, then characterization of HLA class I APM component expression and function in the targeted cancer should be included among the tests to evaluate patients to be treated with T cell-based immunotherapy. This information will contribute to the rational design of effective combinatorial strategies

KEY REFERENCES

Only key references appear in the print edition. The full reference list appears in the digital product on Springer Publishing Connect: connect.springerpub.com/content/book/978-0-8261-3743-2/part/part01/chapter/ch05

12. Kloetzel PM. The proteasome and MHC class I antigen processing. *Biochim Biophys Acta.* 2004;1695(1–3):225–233. doi:10.1016/j.bbamcr.2004.10.004

24. Ortmann B, Androlewicz MJ, Cresswell P. MHC class I/beta 2-microglobulin complexes associate with TAP transporters before peptide binding. *Nature.* 1994;368(6474):864–867. doi:10.1038/368864a0

28. Natali PG, Bigotti A, Nicotra MR, et al. Distribution of human class I (HLA-A,B,C) histocompatibility antigens in normal and malignant tissues of nonlymphoid origin. *Cancer Res.* 1984;44(10):4679–4687. https://cancerres.aacrjournals.org/content/44/10/4679

30. Wang X, Campoli M, Cho HS, et al. A method to generate antigen-specific mAb capable of staining formalin-fixed, paraffin-embedded tissue sections. *J Immunol Methods.* 2005;299(1–2):139–151. doi:10.1016/j.jim.2005.02.006

277. Chang CC, Ferrone S. Immune selective pressure and HLA class I antigen defects in malignant lesions. *Cancer Immunol Immunother.* 2007;56(2):227–236. doi:10.1007/s00262-006-0183-1

278. Brady CS, Bartholomew JS, Burt DJ, et al. Multiple mechanisms underlie HLA dysregulation in cervical cancer. *Tissue Antigens.* 2000;55(5):401–411. doi:10.1034/j.1399-0039.2000.550502.x

351. Rodig SJ, Gusenleitner D, Jackson DG, et al. MHC proteins confer differential sensitivity to CTLA-4 and PD-1 blockade in untreated metastatic melanoma. *Sci Transl Med.* 2018;10(450):eaar3342. doi:10.1126/scitranslmed.aar3342

6

Systems Biology of T Cells

David Furman and Yingxiang Huang

KEY POINTS

- Systems biology is defined as the quantification of the molecular elements of a biological system and integration of that information to study biological systems using computational and statistical methods, from which hypotheses could be made for further investigation.

- Tumor–immunity interactions and the functional dynamics of the tumor microenvironment are complex and multiscale, which highlights the requirement of systems biology-based approaches, for the purpose of characterizing the tumor microenvironment and developing strategies for cancer therapy.

- Systems biology approaches provide numerous applications to the field of cancer biology, including identification of potential biomarkers and therapeutic targets, elucidation of the biological pathways associated with the disease pathology, assessment of drug efficacy, identification of patients' subpopulation based on their response to the treatment, and prediction of drug toxicity.

- Systems biology has two branches: (a) knowledge discovery or data mining and network analysis and (b) simulation-based analysis.

- Knowledge discovery or data mining and network analysis integrate different data types into networks and biological pathways revealing hidden patterns from large sets of experimental data and form hypotheses based on that.

- Simulation-based analysis tests a hypothesis theoretically using mathematical models, and provides explanations for observed behaviors to make experimentally testable predictions for further exploration.

INTRODUCTION

The emergence of molecular biology has provided remarkable progress in understanding the components and the function of biological systems. We have in-depth knowledge of the basic molecular level mechanisms of a biological system, such as replication, transcription, translation, and so forth. The complete DNA sequence information is available for humans and many other organisms as well. A large number of gene sets and their transcriptional products have been identified, and advanced technologies are available to obtain extensive gene expression profiles and study them at the messenger RNA (mRNA) and protein levels. Although the identification of individual biological components and their function is crucial, it is important to understand how these biological components interact with each other and function as a whole system.

Systems biology is an emerging field in biology and aims at understanding the biological process as a whole system instead of its isolated parts, by considering as many of its components as possible, and examining their properties and molecular interaction networks. It uses the application of experimental, computational, and theoretical modeling techniques and studies biological systems in most aspects, from the molecular level, through the cellular, and to the behavioral levels. Broadly, "systems biology" is defined as the quantification of the molecular elements of a biological system and integration of that information to study the biological systems using computational and statistical methods, from which hypotheses could be made for further investigation.[1]

In the past five decades, several attempts have been made to understand biology at the system level, but most of these focused mainly on the physiological level of a given biological system because of the paucity of molecular data and lack of advanced computational and biological technologies.[2] The remarkable technological breakthroughs in the past 10 years, particularly in genome sequencing, high-throughput proteomics, and metabolomics technologies, enable us to collect comprehensive data sets and have renewed the global interest in systems biology approaches. Since then, systems biology has been applied in different areas of life science research, including oncology and immunology. Regulatory agencies, including the U.S. Food and Drug Administration (FDA), encourage the use of the systems biology approaches as they may help to improve drug discovery, safety, and efficacy.[3]

Decades of scientific studies evidence the involvement of the immune system in cancer pathology and clinical outcome. Cells and molecules of the immune system are fundamental components of the tumor environment, and they can recognize and eliminate the malignant cells by eliciting an immune response against tumor-specific antigens.[4,5] Encouraging observations from cancer immunology studies led to the development of cancer immunotherapy, which is an emerging therapeutic option for the treatment of cancer. Cancer immunotherapy enhances host immunity to recognize and eliminate malignant cells either by stimulating a specific component of the immune system or counteracting immune suppressive signals in the tumor microenvironment. There have been successes in developing immunotherapies utilizing immune checkpoint inhibitors, antitumor antibodies, adoptive T cell therapy, natural killer (NK) cell therapy, and dendritic cell therapy, which led to the development of multiple FDA-approved immunotherapies, including sipuleucel-T and ipilimumab.[6]

However, tumor cells often resist immune-mediated cell death and induce an immunosuppressive microenvironment that favors the growth of immunosuppressive cell populations, such as regulatory T cells (T_{reg} cells), thereby escaping from detection and destruction by the host immune response.[7] Tumor–immunity interaction and the functional dynamics of the tumor microenvironment are complex; therefore, it highlights the requirement of systems biology-based approaches for the purpose of characterizing the tumor microenvironment and developing strategies for cancer therapy. Systems biology approaches provide numerous applications to the field of cancer biology including screening and identification of potential biomarkers for the prognosis and diagnosis of diseases; elucidation of the biological pathways associated with the disease pathology and clinical outcome; identification of the therapeutic targets and understanding their mode of action; assessment of drug efficacy; identification of patients' subpopulation based on their response to the treatment; and prediction of the drug toxicity. Overall, systems biology garners huge attention and has been applied extensively in cancer research in recent times. In this chapter, we will first introduce the available systems biology data resources and the various "omics" technologies employed to collect large sets of data.

We then describe the application of systems biology in cancer immunology with a focus on T cells and immunotherapy.

RESOURCES AND TOOLS USED TO GENERATE DATA FOR SYSTEMS BIOLOGY APPROACHES

The remarkable advancements in omics technologies enable us to collect a large set of data required for systems biology-based approaches. In the past few years, large-scale projects have generated a tremendous amount of omics data from molecular analysis of patient tumor samples, which have been made available to the scientific community. In this section, we have provided a list of various public domains where the different sources and types of data are available (Table 6.1A and 6.1B), and then described the different omics technologies commonly used to examine the biology of tumors and the immune system in a system-wide fashion.

Omics Technologies

Cytometry by Time-of-Flight

Cytometry by time-of-flight (CyTOF), otherwise called mass cytometry, is a new technology for multiparameter single-cell analysis, which combines technologies of mass spectrometry (MS) and flow cytometry. CyTOF has the ability to resolve more than 40 metal probes with no or minimal signal overlap as it uses heavy metal ions as antibody labels, and signals are detected as separate spectra lines in mass spectroscopy. This enables collection of a large amount of data that reveal unprecedented depth in the phenotypic and functional characterization of cells in biological samples, including cell hematopoiesis,[8,9] cellular responses to drugs,[8,10] T cells specific for viral antigens,[11–13] circulating and tumor-infiltrating T_{reg} cells in different tumor samples,[14–17] and more recently to address changes in immune cells associated with aging and chronic inflammatory conditions.[18–20]

Next-Generation Sequencing

Next-generation sequencing enables the collection of gene and transcript expression profiles, as well as detection of alternative splicing, single nucleotide variants, mutations in tumor cells, and amplifications in the whole genome and transcriptome. It employs a methodology that includes template preparation, sequencing and imaging, and data analysis. The methodology starts with the construction of a DNA or a complementary DNA (cDNA) library from which new DNA fragments are synthesized. Then the sequencing occurs through a cycle of washing and flooding the fragments in a sequential order; as nucleotides incorporate into the growing DNA

Table 6.1 (A) Public Database for Cancer Genomic Data and (B) Public Database for Immunology Data

NAME OF RESOURCE	URL	DESCRIPTION
(A)		
The Cancer Genome Atlas	cancergenome.nih.gov	Database on copy number, gene, and microRNA expression, epigenetic data from >11,000 patients with 33 types of cancer
International Cancer Genome Consortium	icgc.org	Comprehensive catalogs of genomic abnormalities, including somatic mutations, abnormal expression of genes, epigenetic modifications in tumors from 50 different cancer types and/or subtypes
NCBIdbGaP	www.ncbi.nlm.nih.gov/gap	Stores and distributes the data from studies that investigate the interaction of genotype and phenotype
COSMIC	cancer.sanger.ac.uk/cosmic	Provides mutation range and frequency statistics based on the choice of gene and/or cancer phenotype
Oncomine	www.oncomine.org/resource/login.html	Cancer microarray database with a web-based data-mining platform
Gene Expression Ominibus	www.ncbi.nlm.nih.gov/geo	Microarray, next-generation sequencing, and other forms of high-throughput functional genomics data repository
ArrayExpress	www.ebi.ac.uk/arrayexpress	Archive of functional genomics data of many human cancer cell lines
Tumorscape	portals.broadinstitute.org/tumorscape/pages/portalHome.jsf	Provides copy number alterations across multiple cancer types
cBioPortal for Cancer Genomics	www.cbioportal.org	Provides visualization, analysis, and download of large-scale cancer genomics data sets covering 147 cancer studies
CellMiner	discover.nci.nih.gov/cellminer	A database and online query tool to facilitate the integration of molecular and pharmacological data sets on NCI-60 cell lines
European Genome-Phenome Archive	www.ebi.ac.uk/ega/	A database containing many sequencing and genotyping experiments of which over >50% are cancer related
Genomics of Drug Sensitivity in Cancer	www.cancerrxgene.org	Largest database of drug sensitivity and drug response in cancer cells
NONCODE	www.noncode.org	Database dedicated to non-coding RNA, which has important implications in cancer
(B)		
Immuno Polymorphism Database	www.ebi.ac.uk/ipd	Database and tools to study polymorphisms in genes of the immune system
IMGT/HLA	www.ebi.ac.uk/ipd/imgt/hla	Provides a specialist database for sequences of human major histocompatibility complex
IMGT/mAb-DB	www.imgt.org/mAb-DB	Resources on monoclonal antibodies with diagnostic or therapeutic indications, fusion proteins for immune applications, composite proteins for clinical applications, and relative proteins of the immune system with clinical indications
Cancer Testis Database	www.cta.lncc.br	Collection of information on cancer-testis antigen genes, their gene products, and immune responses

(continued)

Table 6.1 (A) Public Database for Cancer Genomic Data and (B) Public Database for Immunology Data (*continued*)

NAME OF RESOURCE	URL	DESCRIPTION
Peptide Database	www.cancerresearch.org/scientists/ events-and-resources/peptide-database	Human tumor antigens recognized by CD4+ or CD8+ T cells
The Cancer Immunome Atlas	tcia.at/about	A database containing intratumoral immune landscapes and the cancer antigenomes
ImmPort	www.immport.org/shared/home	Data repository available for free immunological data archiving, dissemination, analyses, and reuse
ImmGen	www.immgen.org/Databrowser19/ DatabrowserPage.html	Gene-expression database for all characterized immune cells in the mouse for construction of gene regulatory network in immune cells

SNP, single nucleotide polymorphism.

strand, they are digitally recorded as a sequence. Next-generation sequencing has numerous applications in cancer immunology and, in particular, it enables a very broad approach to T cell receptor (TCR) repertoire analysis,[21–24] which provides us with insights as to which TCR sequences are important for the response to different tumor antigens.

Soluble Protein Multiplexing Analysis

xMAP Luminex and the MesoScale Discovery (MSD) platforms are the most popular technologies in multiplexing the analysis of soluble proteins such as cytokines and chemokines. In the xMAP technology, microsphere beads are color-coded into 500 distinct sets. Each bead set can be coated with a reagent specific for a particular assay, allowing the capture and detection of specific analytes from a sample. A light source then excites the internal dyes that identify each microsphere particle with many readings made on each bead set, which validates the results. This technology shares common components with general flow cytometry instruments such as lasers, fluidics, and optics. Using this process, the xMAP technology allows multiplexing of up to 500 unique bioassays within a single sample. On the other hand, the MSD platform is similar to a multiplexed enzyme-linked immunosorbent assay (ELISA). Individual spots on a microtiter plate are coated with capture reagents for the analytes of interest, which are then detected with enzyme-linked detector antibodies. An electrochemiluminescent substrate is then used to create a light signal that is quantitated by the instrument. The advantages of this detection system include high sensitivity and a wide dynamic range, as well as minimal interference from the matrix factors.

A vast number of studies have addressed the changes in cytokine profiles under multiple clinical conditions.

For instance, these technologies have been used to evaluate the association between cytokine profiles and the risk of lung cancer,[25] to measure systemic inflammation in colon cancer,[26] to examine tumor-induced inflammatory states in the progression of breast cancer,[27] as well as evaluate many other tumor types.

Mass Spectrometry

MS is often used to measure metabolites in biological materials. In MS experiments, samples are subjected to methanol extraction and split into aliquots for analysis by ultrahigh performance liquid chromatography/MS (UHPLC/MS) in the positive, negative, or polar ion mode and by gas chromatography/MS (GC/MS). Metabolites are identified by automated comparison of ion features to a reference library of chemical standards followed by visual inspection for quality control. There are two approaches in metabolomics: targeted metabolomics and untargeted metabolomics or metabolic profiling. In targeted metabolomics, defined sets of structurally known and biochemically annotated metabolites are quantified, and it is based on a previous understanding of biochemical pathways. In contrast, untargeted metabolomics is the comprehensive analysis of all the measurable analytes in a sample including chemical unknowns. Many have recognized untargeted metabolomics as having an unprecedented value in bringing clarity to complex "omics" data. The reason for this is that metabolites are a proxy to the phenotype and the metabolome is the very end product of the genetic setup of an organism, as well as the sum of all influences it is exposed to, such as nutrition, environmental factors, or treatment. Untargeted metabolomics includes analysis of large arrays of metabolites, thereby extracting biochemical information that reflects functional endpoints of biological events.

Another application of MS includes the development of technologies to analyze the human leukocyte antigen (HLA) ligandome.[28–33] Briefly, HLA complex molecules are isolated from a patient's cancer tissue samples or primary cell line by immunoaffinity purification methodology using pan-HLA class monoclonal antibodies or allele-specific antibodies. The purified HLA peptides are loaded on high-pressure reverse-phase liquid-chromatography coupled to MS and the resulting spectra are matched to spectra of theoretical peptides derived from a reference customized database. The identified peptides are then validated using T cell-based assays.

APPLICATION OF SYSTEMS BIOLOGY APPROACHES IN CANCER BIOLOGY

In general, systems biology has two branches: (a) knowledge discovery or data mining and network analysis, which reveals the pattern from a large set of experimental data and forms hypotheses, and (b) simulation-based analysis, which tests hypotheses theoretically using mathematical models and provides predictions for further exploration. In the following sections, we discuss how these two branches of systems biology aid cancer immunology (Figure 6.1).

Application of Systems Biology in Data Mining, Network, and Pathway Analysis

Genomics, transcriptomics, proteomics, and metabolic high-throughput technologies available today enable the measurement of tens of thousands of molecular targets per sample simultaneously. In the longitudinal studies of aging at Stanford University,[34–44] the investigators profiled peripheral blood in hundreds of healthy individuals of different ages (20–96 years) using multiple technological platforms, including mass and flow cytometry, xMAP system, transcriptomics, and metabolomics. In such studies of influenza vaccine responses, individuals were recruited and whole blood was collected three times per year (before and 7 and 28 days

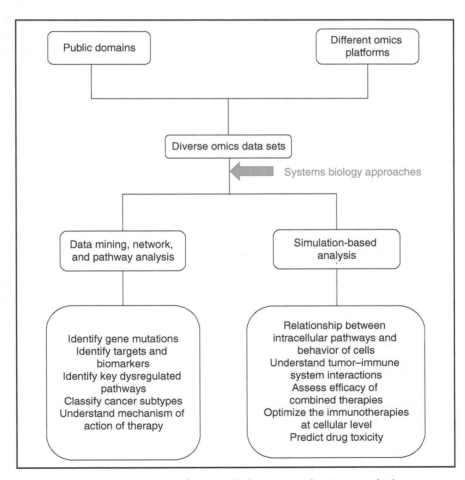

Figure 6.1 Application of systems biology approaches in cancer biology.

after vaccination). The Stanford longitudinal cohort was initiated in the year 2007 and a large number of participants have been screened and followed for more than 8 years, enabling temporal characterization of the changes observed in healthy populations and creating a snapshot reference of healthy immune systems.

Whole genome and whole exome sequence data, mutations, rearrangements, copy number variation, and expression data at mRNA, micro-RNA, protein, and metabolite levels are being generated from various tumor entities using various high-throughput technologies and these are readily publicly available. The real value of these different data sets in the field of cancer biology could be realized only if these heterogeneous data are integrated and interpreted in a meaningful way. A study that investigated the stage-specific alterations of the genome, transcriptome, and proteome during colorectal carcinogenesis found that changes were mostly observed in gene expression and less so in protein abundance when comparing tumor tissues with control tissues.[45,46] Furthermore, the integration of omics data with clinical parameters is critical for most of the clinical studies. Overall, these observations highlight the necessity of integrating data across a multitude of omics platforms, a task that requires infrastructure and tools of bioinformatics, such as the GLMNET, an extremely efficient R package that fits a number of generalized linear models[36] for the integration of diverse data types.

Computational systems biology tools offer excellent aid to integrate different data types into networks and to reveal the information in the complex data. For example, gene co-expression networks can be constructed with similar global expression profiles and used to identify key transcriptional regulators.[38,47–50] The key transcriptional factors, for instance, STAT3 and CEBP, were identified as major regulators of mesenchymal transformation in glioblastoma using gene network approaches.[51] Palomero et al. employed an integrative systems biology approach to investigate the transcriptional programs activated by NOTCH1, which plays an important role in T cell development and pathogenesis of human T cell lymphoblastic leukemia and found that c-MYC is a critical mediator.[52,53]

Another important application of systems biology is its capability of analyzing high-throughput data from the perspective of biological pathways. Analysis of molecular expression profiles with the help of computational tools can lead to the identification of altered pathways in cancer patients. This pathway-based analysis is useful to identify genes associated with the diseases and to separate them from those changes that may occur by random chances or are reactive to causative perturbations to genes or pathways. This approach is also useful to identify the common biological pathways affected by cancer.

For example, a set of different cancer patients might have deleted different components that are involved in the same pathway. Gene or protein expression analysis alone does not help us classify those patients, as they do not share a defect in a common gene or protein. However, by projecting the gene mutation data into a biological pathway analysis, the etiology of the disease in those patients can be interpreted easily (Figure 6.2). Recently, many computational tools have been developed to integrate and visualize the data in order to identify the functionally important cancer genome alterations and pathways altered (Table 6.2). Here we describe the application of data mining and network analysis in detail to discover tumor antigens and characterize tumor-infiltrating T lymphocytes.

Identification of Tumor-Associated T Cell Antigens

Tumor-associated T cell antigens are well-known candidates for the development of cancer-specific vaccines and are used for the ex vivo expansion of patient-derived tumor-specific T cells before adoptive T cell therapy and preparation of specific TCR or chimeric antigen receptor transduced T cells. The identification of tumor antigens includes the steps described in the following paragraphs. But first, the selection of the tumor-associated antigen is a critical process, and there are a few fundamental requirements for the antigen to be a potential tumor antigen target. These requirements include aberrant expression in tumor cells while no or limited expression occurs in normal tissue, immunogenicity, and a role in tumor development. Here, we explain how computation tools can help us identify potential tumor-associated antigens/peptides.

First, tumor proteins can be identified by comparing the sequence data obtained from tumor tissue and matched normal tissues. There are numerous computational tools available for variant detection, annotations, and interpretation (Figure 6.3).[54] Furthermore, the most biologically relevant alterations among all somatic mutations are selected by either identifying the functional impact of genetic variants using publicly available annotation databases such as Ensembl, RefSeq (for genes and transcripts), NONCODE, Body map (for non-coding RNA), Pfam, and Interpro (proteins), or assessing the recurrence and frequency of particular mutations or pathway and network analysis.

Once tumor-specific proteins are identified, they have to be tested for immunogenicity, and relevant major histocompatibility complex (MHC) peptides should be predicted. There are computational algorithms and technologies available for this purpose (Table 6.3). Most of these epitope mapping algorithms work on the fact that epitopes link together into the binding groove of MHC class I and II molecules through the interaction between

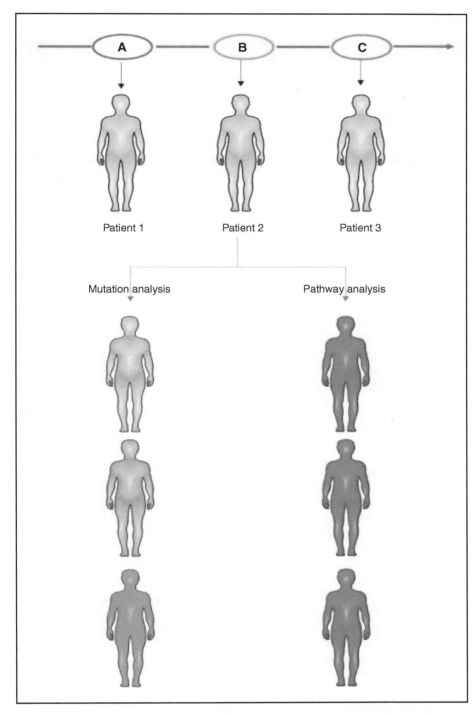

Figure 6.2 **Application of pathways analysis in identifying the etiology of disease in cancer patients.** A pathway-based analysis is useful to identify the common biological pathways affected by cancer. As shown in the figure, three different cancer patients, patient 1, patient 2, and patient 3, have different mutations such as A, B, and C, respectively, which involve the same pathway. By projecting the gene mutation data into a biological pathways analysis, the common altered pathway in those patients can be easily interpreted when compared to healthy individuals with unaltered sequences.

R groups present in their side chains and pockets located on the floor of the MHC.[55,56] More recently, MS-based approaches have been used to discover naturally processed class I and class II tumor-associated peptides. Walter et al. used an integrative approach, called the Tubingen approach,[57] for the identification of potential

Table 6.2 Computational Tools Available for Data Integration and Visualization

NAME OF TOOL	URL	DESCRIPTION
Cytoscape	www.cytoscape.org	An open-source platform for visualizing complex networks and integrating the networks with other data types
Pathway Commons	www.pathwaycommons.org	Pathway Commons is a portal to access biological pathway information collected from public pathway databases
NetWalker	netwalkersuite.org	Application for functional analyses of large-scale genomics data sets within the context of molecular networks
LINCS (Library of Integrated Network-Based Cellular Signatures)	www.lincsproject.org	Creates a network-based understanding of biology, cataloging changes in gene expression, and other cellular processes in response to perturbations
COPASI	www.copasi.org	Software for simulation and analysis of biochemical networks and their dynamics
Virtual Cell (Vcell)	www.nrcam.uchc.edu	Virtual Cell is a computational environment for modeling and simulation of cell biology
Reactome Sky Painter	www.reactome.org	A tool to calculate the statistical significance of affected pathways and visualize pathways
PathwayExplorer	genome.tugraz.at/pathwayexplorer/pathwayexplorer_description.shtml	Web-based tool to visualize data on publicly available biological pathways
VisANT	visant.bu.edu	Visualization and analysis tool for biological networks and pathways

therapeutic vaccine candidates for renal cancer (Figure 6.4).[57] The Tubingen approach uses tumor gene expression profiling, HLA peptide repertoire analysis by MS, in vitro human T cell assays, and computational tools for epitope prediction and data mining.[57–59]

The peptide repertoire available for MHC binding is a limiting step in determining T cell epitope immunogenicity.[60] Therefore, there are efforts to profile the entirety of HLA-associated peptides that cytotoxic T cells scan for. In the form of the Human Immuno-Peptidome Project,[61] the project aims to annotate, store, and share MS-produced HLA-associated peptides from around the world as well as connect data sets in existing popular sites such as IEDB. Referred to as immunopeptidomics or HLA ligandome, the profiling of HLA-associated peptides from human tissues using current updated MS technologies allows for the new ways to identify nonself tumor-specific mutant neo-antigens and peptide-specific cancer immunotherapies.[30,62,63] Accompanying the massive data sets generated are new tools to analyze the data and generate reproducible results. For example, MHCquant automatically processes immunopeptidomics data and generates annotated epitopes.[64] It is a pipeline that compiled existing standard methods, whereas database search using COMET is used to identify peptides and proteins.[65] In

addition to annotating epitopes, other platforms such as MAPDP provide downstream tools for peptide-binding affinity prediction, HLA genotyping, and the generation of personalized proteome databases.[66] As the known repertoire of HLA-associated peptides grows with the new MS technology and organization of immunopeptidomics databases and tools, adequate epitope data sets becomes available for training and benchmarking T cell epitope predictions,[67,68] allowing for more accurate prediction and personalized immunotherapy.

Cellular Characterization of Immune Infiltrates in Tumors

The investigation of the cellular composition of lymphocyte infiltrates in tumors provides us with knowledge on the interaction between the tumor and immune system, which leads to the identification of predictive markers and the development of novel therapeutic strategies. To characterize the lymphocyte population, imaging and cellular phenotyping by flow cytometry are the most widely used techniques. However, because of their inherent limitations, computational genomic tools are being used to obtain a comprehensive picture of tumor lymphocyte infiltrates. The gene expression profile for

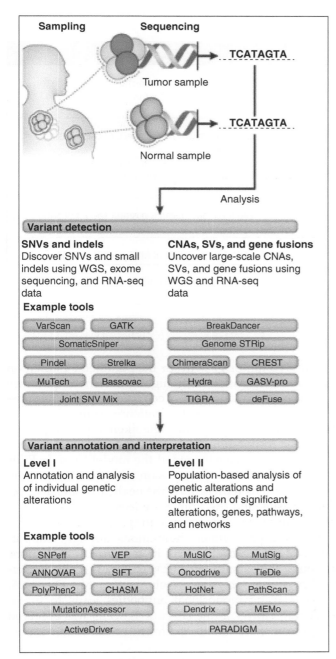

Figure 6.3 Computational tools available for variant detection, annotation, and interpretation. Tumor and healthy tissue samples are sequenced using high-throughput technologies. After alignment, small alterations (single nucleotide variations [SNVs], insertions and deletions [Indels]), and large alterations (copy number aberrations [CAN], structural variants [SV], and gene fusion) are identified, annotated, and analyzed either individually (level I) or collectively (level II) using a range of computational tools.

WGS, whole genome sequencing.

Source: Reproduced with permission from Ding L, Wendl MC, McMichael JF, Raphael BJ. Expanding the computational toolbox for mining cancer genomes. *Nat Rev Genet.* 2014;15(8):556–570. doi:10.1038/nrg3767

the individual cell population, which is interpreted by computational methods including gene set enrichment analysis and deconvolution methods, provides information on the composition of tumor-infiltrating lymphocytes (Figure 6.5).[42]

Gene set enrichment analysis evaluates microarrays or RNA sequence data at the level of gene sets, which are assembled based on prior biological knowledge. ImmuneSigDB and TCGA are the major resources for the collection of gene sets. The goal of gene set enrichment analysis is to rank the genes either by comparing their expression between two biological states or assessing a degree of differential expression of a gene in a particular gene set. Deconvolution methods infer specific cell proportion in an unknown cell mixture using reference expression matrix and computer algorithms. Computational approaches like CIBERSORT and ImmuneCellAI have been introduced for inferring the leukocyte subpopulation from bulk tumors.[69,70] It uses a signature expression matrix for 22 leukocyte subpopulations. Similar to the gene expression profile, deconvolution methods also infer cell lineage–specific DNA methylation patterns to detect and quantify the lymphocyte subpopulation. Although the availability of reference data for cell lineage–specific DNA methylation patterns from the purified lymphocyte cell population is limited, these methods hold potential for determining the composition of tumor infiltrates from bulk tumor tissue.[71,72]

APPLICATION OF SIMULATION-BASED ANALYSIS

An important feature of systems biology is the concept of modeling the dynamics of biochemical networks. A number of complex processes that take place in tumor–immune system interactions in a nonlinear way are amenable to mathematical modeling, which helps to suggest explanations for observed behaviors and to make experimentally testable predictions. The most common methods in simulating the interaction between the tumor and immune system are differential equations and rule-based models. We have provided a few simulation models that are developed to describe the tumor–immune system interactions and the role of T cells in developing immunotherapy for cancer.

Application of Simulation Models in Understanding Basics of Tumor–Immune System Interactions

An effective antitumor immune response is predominantly mediated by cytotoxic T cells and NK cells. Numerous mathematical models have been developed to describe the interaction between cytotoxic lymphocytes and a growing tumor. Those models enabled the

Table 6.3 Computational Algorithms for T Cell Epitope Prediction

WEBSERVER	URL	DESCRIPTION
NetMHCcons 1.1	www.cbs.dtu.dk/services/NetMHCcons	Works based on artificial neural network. Prediction can be made for peptide of any length. Consensus method for predicting MHC class I epitopes
PickPocket 1.1	www.cbs.dtu.dk/services/PickPocket	Predict peptide binding to any known MHC molecules using position-specific weight matrices
EpiJen	www.ddg-pharmfac.net/epijen/EpiJen/EpiJen.htm	Predicts MHC class I epitopes based on proteasome cleavage, TAB binding, and MHC binding
RANKPEP	imed.med.ucm.es/Tools/rankpep.html	Predicts MHC class I and II epitopes using a position-specific scoring matrix
EpiTOP	www.pharmfac.net/EpiTOP	Proteochemometric model for prediction of MHC class II epitopes
IEDB T cell epitope prediction tools	tools.immuneepitope.org/main/tcell	Set of tools includes MHC class I and II binding predictions, as well as peptide processing predictions

MHC, major histocompatibility complex.

identification of biologically significant parameters based on the numerical estimates, interpretation, and prediction of a number of phenomena that occur in the tumor environment.

Kuznetsov et al. developed an ordinary differential equation (ODE)-based generic model, which mimics the interaction between cytotoxic T lymphocytes and growing cells in a tumor and explains the possible influence of cytotoxic T lymphocytes on the phenomena of "sneaking through" of the tumor and formation of the tumor "dormant" state.[73] A discretized version of Kuznetsov et al.'s model takes it a step further where the nuance of the complex dynamic behavior of cancer growth is simulated.[74] Such behavior follows a growth pattern of periodic regression followed by re-expansion of the tumor. A mathematical model developed by Matzavinos et al., based on partial differential equation (PDE), described the spatiotemporal dynamics pattern of growth of a solid tumor in the presence of cytotoxic T lymphocytes.[75] They focused on the analysis of the spatiotemporal dynamics of tumor cells, immune cells, tumor–immune cell complexes, and chemokines in an immunogenic tumor and suggested that cytotoxic T lymphocytes could play an important role in the control of tumor dormancy. This model might be used to assess the time interval between the primary treatment and the recurrence of an immunogenic tumor.[75] Another mathematical model, developed by de Pillis et al. based on differential equations, described the dynamics of tumor–immune system interaction with a focus on the role of NK cells and CD8 T cells in tumor surveillance.[76] Using published data on CD8+ T-tumor and NK-tumor lysis by chromium release assays

and in vivo tumor growth for the parameter estimation and model validation, they highlighted the importance of focus on increasing CD8+ T cell activity and direct positive correlation between the patient-specific efficacy of the CD8+ T cell response and the likelihood of a patient favorably responding to immunotherapy treatments.[76] Further studies have extended the model from de Pillis et al. to model tumor progression with three interacting cell populations representing the healthy tissue, the neoplastic tissue, and the immune effector cells, as well as the cells' dynamics in response to chemotherapy.[77]

Recent experimental observations strongly support the involvement of T_{reg} cells in the growth of tumors. Although the expansion of CD4+CD25+ T_{reg} cells accelerates the tumor progression, elimination of CD4+CD25+ T_{reg} cells using monoclonal antibodies leads to tumor rejection.[78] However, the effect of T_{reg} cells was observed only in some, but not all, the forms of tumors. This phenomenon was explained by Leon et al. using a mathematical model in which they predicted that (a) there is an existence of two alternative dynamic modes of tumor growth, named as growth without T_{reg} cells and growth with T_{reg} cells, and (b) the existence of which type of mode depends on the dynamical properties of the tumor.[79] If the tumors have a high intrinsic growth rate, low immunogenicity, and ability to resist destruction, it induces expansion of only the effector cells, but not T_{reg} cells. The expansion of effector cells, however, does not control the growth of the tumor because of its larger size and fast growing kinetics. If the tumors have a low growth rate, relatively high immunogenicity, and more sensitivity for the destruction by T cells, the tumor induces a balanced

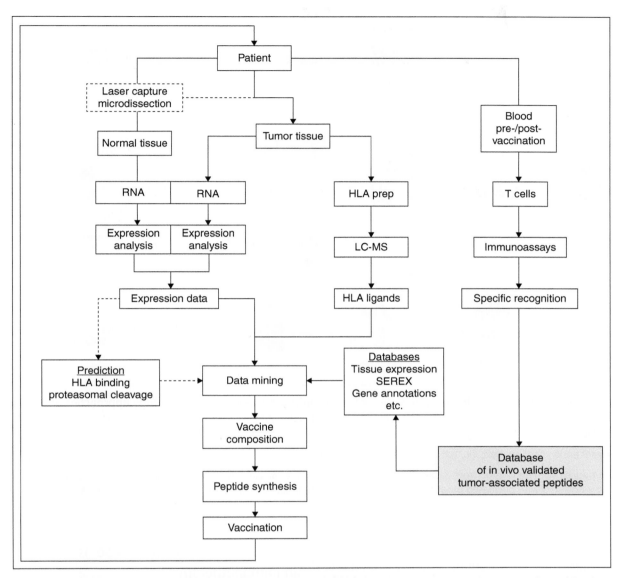

Figure 6.4 **Tubingen approach for the identification of tumor-associated antigens.** An integrative approach used for the identification of tumor-associated antigens. This approach combines tumor gene expression profiling, HLA peptide repertoire analysis by mass spectrometry, in vitro human T cell assays, and computational tools for epitope prediction and data mining.

HLA, human leukocyte antigen; LC-MS, liquid chromatography/mass spectrometry; SEREX, serological analysis of expression cDNA libraries.

Source: Reproduced with permission from Singh-Jasuja H, Emmerich NPN, Rammensee H-G. The Tubingen approach: identification, selection, and validation of tumor-associated HLA peptides for cancer therapy. *Cancer Immunol Immunother.* 2004;53(3):187–195. doi:10.1007/s00262-003-0480-x

expansion of both regulatory and effector T cells.[79] Such findings have been used to model the response of T_{reg} cells in cytokine-induced killer chemotherapy of pancreatic cancer. By mitigating the action of T_{reg} cells, a combination of cytokine-induced killer immunotherapy and immuno-suppressive chemotherapy can increase survival.[80]

Webb et al. developed a model to describe the importance of the Fas/FasL system in tumor–immune system interaction.[81] This model showed that the constitutive expression of Fas ligand by tumor cells is one of the potential mechanisms of immune evasion as it is able to interact and induce apoptosis in T cells that bear the Fas receptor. This model also predicted that enzymatic cleavage of Fas ligand into soluble Fas ligand by matrix metalloproteinase (MMP) can act as an inhibitor to the Fas ligand-induced cell death. This model has

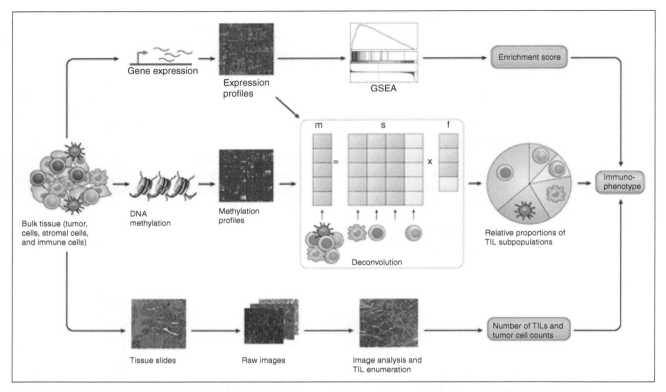

Figure 6.5 Characterization of cellular composition of tumor infiltrates using systems biology approaches. The composition of tumor-infiltrating lymphocytes in the tumor tissue is estimated from different entities using individual or a combination of computational tools (i.e., GSEA, deconvolution, and/or image analysis).

GSEA, gene set enrichment analysis; TIL, tumor-infiltrating lymphocytes.

Source: Reproduced with permission from Sasaki S, Sullivan M, Narvaez CF, et al. Limited efficacy of inactivated influenza vaccine in elderly individuals is associated with decreased production of vaccine-specific antibodies. *J Clin Invest.* 2011;121(8):3109–3119. doi:10.1172/jci57834

two clinical implications: (a) cancer therapies, which use broad-spectrum MMP inhibitors as potential therapeutic agents based on the concept that elevated MMP levels in the tumor are associated with invasion and angiogenesis. The predicted adverse effect of MMP inactivation on conversion from FasL to soluble FasL could counterbalance the therapeutic effects and (b) numerous attempts that aim to activate T lymphocytes via antigenic peptide presentation and co-stimulation may be impacted as Fas/FasL interactions are shared by these approaches.[81] What was missing from the model proposed by Webb et al. was taking into account how the tumor escapes from one or both arms of the adaptive and innate immune systems.[82] Mahasa et al. proposed a more nuanced model by including NK cells and the activated CD8+ cytotoxic T lymphocytes into their differential equations and showing that tumor cells evolve and survive from both cytotoxic arms of the immune system, which could be mitigated by introducing NK cell-based immunotherapy.

Application of Simulation Models in Immunotherapy

Adoptive immunotherapy with tailored T cells (e.g., TCR engineered, CAR T cells, tumor-infiltrating lymphocytes [TILs]) has been proven to be effective against certain types of tumors. However, there are still many questions that remain unanswered, including what would be the optimal number of tumor-specific T cells to be administered; or what schedule would be most effective, and how to improve the efficacy of the immunotherapy, despite experimental data indicating that in some cases the larger the number of TILs, the more efficacious the therapy.[83] Mathematical modeling provides an analytical framework to answer these questions.

Kronik et al. constructed a mathematical model to aid in the design of more efficacious glioblastoma adoptive immunotherapy.[84] This model could retrieve published clinical trial results of efficacious alloreactive CTL immunotherapy for glioblastoma and predicted the reason for the failure of cellular adoptive immunotherapy as the administered dose was 20-fold lower than that required for therapeutic efficacy. This analysis also suggested that glioblastoma could be eradicated with a higher dose of alloreactive T cells.[84] A different tumor–immune dynamics model developed by Kronik et al. provided information such as the minimally required T cell dose and T cell functionality depending on the growth and size of a tumor for a clinical study.[85] Kogan et al. suggested that their mathematical model was able to estimate the optimal levels and time of T cell infusion on a per-patient basis to theoretically reduce tumor load or to even eliminate the tumor.[86]

Many mathematical models investigated the effects of cytokines on improving tumor adoptive cell therapy. Two mathematical models developed by Kirschner and Panetta[87] and Wilson and Levy[88] indicate that interleukin-2 (IL-2) and transforming growth factor-β (TGF-β) can augment the effect of cancer immunotherapy, respectively. The model developed by Kim et al. shows the combination of immunotherapy and imatinib treatment to optimally sustain the antileukemia T cell response.[89] It was also shown that during treatment, the cancer cell population generally falls below detection, evading the immune system. Careful timing of administration of treatment is needed to maintain a strong immune response throughout. To this end, models have been shown to use population dynamics and treatment responses to identify better drug administration regimes.[90,91]

CONCLUSION

The rapid technological developments of omics platforms speed up the discovery of relevant genes, proteins, and other molecules and their interaction in the development of cancer and disease symptoms. Considering the nonlinear nature of the biochemical processes and different time scale of the cellular processes, the generation of large sets of data makes the global picture more complex and difficult to interpret. We argue that it is not possible to understand the dynamic and multicellular nature of the immune system–cancer relations simply from the molecular and cell biology data without computational tools and approaches. Systems biology approaches are able to integrate diverse experimental data sets and build network models that mimic the cancer system. In this way, it is possible to obtain better insights into complex molecular mechanisms in tumor development and immunotherapies, and identify potential biomarkers and therapeutic targets that can be translated into practical clinical use.

KEY REFERENCES

Only key references appear in the print edition. The full reference list appears in the digital product on Springer Publishing Connect: connect.springerpub.com/content/book/978-0-8261-3743-2/part/part01/chapter/ch06

35. Furman D. Sexual dimorphism in immunity: improving our understanding of vaccine immune responses in men. *Expert Rev Vaccines.* 2015;14:461–471. doi:10.1586/14760584.2015.966694

54. Ding L, Wendl MC, McMichael JF, Raphael BJ. Expanding the computational toolbox for mining cancer genomes. *Nat Rev Genet.* 2014;15(8):556–570. doi:10.1038/nrg3767

61. Caron E, Aebersold R, Banaei-Esfahani A, et al. A case for a human immuno-peptidome project consortium. *Immunity.* 2017;47:203–208. doi:10.1016/j.immuni.2017.07.010

69. Hackl H, Charoentong P, Finotello F, Trajanoski Z. Computational genomics tools for dissecting tumour-immune cell interactions. *Nat Rev Genet.* 2016;17:441–458. doi:10.1038/nrg.2016.67

74. Moghtadaei M, Hashemi Golpayegani MR, Malekzadeh R. Periodic and chaotic dynamics in a map-based model of tumor-immune interaction. *J Theor Biol.* 2013;334:130–140. doi:10.1016/j.jtbi.2013.05.031

80. He D-H, Xu J-X. A mathematical model of pancreatic cancer with two kinds of treatments. *J Biol Syst.* 2017;25:83–104. doi:10.1142/S021833901750005X

7

Activation of CD4$^+$ T Lymphocytes

Lina Petersone and Lucy S. K. Walker

KEY POINTS

- CD4$^+$ T cells control both cell-mediated and humoral immunity.

- Secondary lymphoid organs bring together naïve T cells and cells presenting protein antigens.

- T cell activation is mediated by antigen, co-stimulation, and cytokines.

- The best defined co-stimulatory receptor on T cells is CD28, which is bound by B7-1 (CD80) and B7-2 (CD86).

- CD4$^+$ T cells can differentiate into different subsets with distinct migration patterns and cytokine production.

INTRODUCTION

CD4$^+$ T lymphocytes control both cell-mediated and humoral immune responses to protein antigens and are, therefore, justifiably called the "conductors of the immunological orchestra." Not surprisingly, elucidating the biology of these cells is a key to understanding protective immunity and immunological diseases and developing therapies for autoimmune diseases and cancer. It is for these reasons that in the past two decades there has been great interest in studying CD4$^+$ T cells and remarkable advances in our understanding of this cell population. This chapter reviews the activation of CD4$^+$ T cells, and the next chapter discusses how the responses of these cells are regulated.

THE IN VIVO ANATOMY OF T CELL ACTIVATION

All immune responses, including the responses of T cells, are initiated and develop in the secondary (peripheral) lymphoid organs—the lymph nodes, spleen, and mucosa—and the skin-associated lymphoid tissues (Figure 7.1).[1] Naïve T cells constantly recirculate through these organs. Antigens enter through epithelia (the common routes of entry of microbes) or are produced in tissues (e.g., in tumors and organ transplants). The protein antigens of these microbes, tumors, and grafts are captured by dendritic cells that are present in all tissues and are transported to secondary lymphoid organs, mainly under the influence of the chemokines CCL19 and CCL20, which are produced in the lymphoid organs. These chemokines are recognized by the receptor CCR7, which is expressed on activated dendritic cells and naïve T cells, and serves to bring together in the same anatomic region dendritic cells carrying their antigenic cargo and naïve T cells capable of recognizing the antigen. In the lymphoid organs, the naïve T cells are in rapid motion, scanning the surfaces of dendritic cells for antigens that the T cells can see. If the T cell antigen receptor (TCR) of a T cell encounters its cognate antigen, then that T cell is rapidly arrested on the surface of the dendritic cell and forms a tight synapse with the dendritic cell. This allows the antigen to deliver activating signals to the T cell; the nature of these and associated signals is described in more detail later. Naïve T cells also express high levels of the receptor for a phospholipid, sphingosine 1-phosphate (S1P), which is present at higher concentrations in the lymph and the blood than in the lymphoid organs. This receptor, called S1PR1, directs the exit of cells out of the lymphoid organs into the circulation. When a T cell recognizes an antigen, it transiently downregulates S1PR1 and is thus retained in the lymphoid organ for long enough to complete its activation program. Once the T cell has gone through its activation sequence, it re-expresses S1PR1 and exits the lymphoid organ to search for the source of the antigen (microbe or tumor) and mediate its protective function.

Although it is possible that some immune responses can be initiated at peripheral sites, such as the site of a tumor, it seems unlikely that this is a major location for the initial activation of naïve cells, for several reasons. Most naïve T cells do not traffic through nonlymphoid peripheral tissues, and these tissues are not organized structurally in a way that would support the migratory events and cell–cell interactions needed for the development of immune responses. It is, therefore, likely that immune responses to tumors develop in draining lymph nodes and other secondary lymphoid organs, much like responses to microbes and transplants. Once effector cells are produced, they do migrate to peripheral tissues

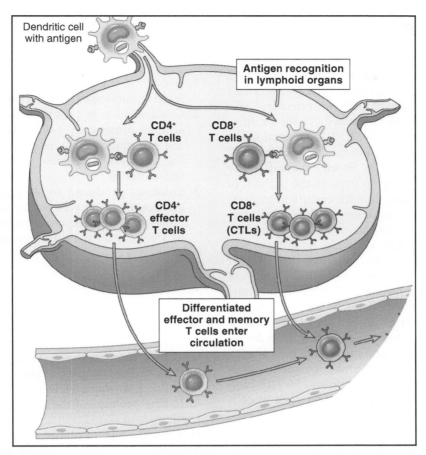

Figure 7.1 The induction of T cell responses. Dendritic cells capture protein antigens, transport the antigens to lymph nodes, and display peptides (attached to MHC molecules) to naïve CD4⁺ and CD8⁺ T cells. The T cells are activated to proliferate and differentiate into effector and memory cells, which exit the node, enter blood vessels, and migrate to sites of antigen entry.

MHC, major histocompatibility complex.

Source: Adapted with permission from Kumar V, Abbas AK, Aster JC. *Basic Pathology*. 9th ed. Elsevier; 2012.

and are activated to perform their functions in these tissues, as described later.

Protein antigens that are captured by the dendritic cells are processed in these cells to generate peptides that bind to major histocompatibility complex (MHC) molecules, and the peptide–MHCs are displayed on the surface.[2] The TCRs of CD4⁺ T cells recognize peptides presented by class II MHC molecules (human leukocyte antigen [HLA]-DR, –DQ, and –DP in humans). As *HLA* genes are highly polymorphic, different individuals express different allelic forms of HLA molecules, and these molecules present different sets of peptides. As a result, the peptide recognition specificity of T cells varies in individuals who inherit different HLAs. In other words, even the same microbe or tumor might generate different peptides that are displayed by the HLA molecules of different individuals. This feature of T cell antigen recognition makes it challenging to define the fine specificities of T cells in humans. Various approaches can be used to quantify antigen-specific T cells in healthy individuals or patients. For example, multimers of HLA molecules loaded with peptides can be used to bind to cells expressing the relevant TCR.[3] Alternatively, a mixed population of cells may be stimulated with the relevant antigen and the responsive cells detected by their production of cytokine or their upregulation of activation markers. However, these assays are technically difficult, have to be individualized for each person, and have not yet become a standard practice in clinical immunology. As a result, there is little information on the numbers of antigen-specific T cells in humans, especially in disease situations. This limitation has been a major problem in understanding the pathogenesis of autoimmune diseases, the success or failure of antitumor immunity, and the way to develop effective vaccines.

SEQUENCE OF T CELL ACTIVATION

The process of T cell activation moves through a stereotypic sequence of steps, each associated with functional and phenotypic alterations (Figure 7.2).[1] Within 2 to 3 hours of receiving activation signals, which are described later, CD4[+] T cells secrete the cytokine interleukin-2 (IL-2). IL-2 functions as a growth factor to drive the proliferation of antigen-activated T cells (IL-2 also functions to control immune responses by maintaining regulatory T cells, as discussed in Chapter 8). Shortly thereafter, the antigen-activated T cells begin to express the α chain of the IL-2 receptor (CD25), and thus the complete trimeric IL-2 receptor, and become responsive to the growth factor. IL-2, acting in concert with other activating signals, drives the T cells to enter the cell cycle. As antigen recognition is required for the production of IL-2 and for the expression of CD25, the antigen-specific T cells are the ones that proliferate preferentially in an immune response. The result is an expansion of the antigen-specific clones of T cells. It is estimated that CD4[+] T cells expand 100- to 1,000-fold from the starting population of naïve cells, and CD8[+] cells expand as much as 10,000- to 100,000-fold. Thus, the small number of naïve T cells specific for an antigen (estimated to be 1 in 10^5–10^6 lymphocytes) is converted into a much larger pool of cells specific for the same antigen.

Some of the progeny of the expanded antigen-specific clones differentiate into effector and memory cells, which are described in more detail subsequently. A distinct population of CD4[+] T cells functions to control harmful immune responses. These regulatory T cells (T_{reg} cells) are discussed in Chapter 8.

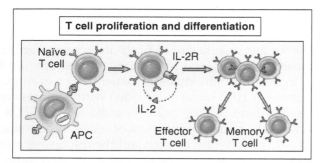

Figure 7.2 Steps in the activation of T cells. Naïve T cells recognize MHC-associated peptide antigens displayed by APCs. The T cells secrete the cytokine IL-2 and express high-affinity receptors for IL-2, and this growth factor stimulates the proliferation of T cells. Some of the progeny of the proliferated cells differentiate into effector and memory cells.

APC, antigen-presenting cell; IL-2, interleukin-2; MHC, major histocompatibility complex.

Source: Adapted with permission from Kumar V, Abbas AK, Aster JC. *Basic Pathology.* 9th ed. Elsevier; 2012.

SIGNALS FOR T CELL ACTIVATION

Three types of external signals function cooperatively to activate naïve as well as memory T cells.

1. *Antigen* is the necessary first signal and its requirement ensures specificity in the subsequent response.
2. *Co-stimulation* is provided by a set of molecules on antigen-presenting cells (APCs) that ensure that the immune system responds to potentially harmful invaders but does not react against harmless self-antigens.
3. *Cytokines* produced by APCs and other cells in the environment, as well as by the T cells themselves, "fine-tune" the response by stimulating proliferation of T cells and their differentiation into different types of effector cells.

Antigen Recognition By T Cells

As discussed at the beginning of this chapter, the TCRs of T cells have evolved to recognize peptides displayed on MHC molecules. The coreceptor (CD4 or CD8) simultaneously recognizes the MHC molecules and recruits kinases to the complex in order to initiate biochemical signaling pathways. Molecules associated with the TCR, including proteins of the CD3 complex and the ζ chain, participate in signal transduction.[4] These signaling molecules form a cluster of membrane proteins on each T cell that binds to ligands on APCs and brings the cells into close apposition, forming a structure called an immune synapse. The intracellular consequences of signal transduction by the TCR complex and coreceptors is the assembly of enzymes and substrates on adaptor proteins that ultimately activate transcription factors that initiate T cell responses.

In addition to the specific recognition and signaling components of the TCR–coreceptor complex, T cells express adhesion molecules, such as integrins, that bind to their ligands on APCs and stabilize the interaction. In addition, as discussed in the following section, T cells express receptors for co-stimulators and cytokines that serve critical roles in the responses of the cells.

Co-Stimulation

The two-signal hypothesis of lymphocyte activation stated that the first signal is provided by antigens and the second signal is provided by microbes or by innate immune responses to microbes. The requirement for "signal 2" is the reason why the immune system responds best when it needs to, that is, when it is faced with a pathogen. This hypothesis has been broadened to include not only microbes but also damaged and necrotic cells as the inducers of second signals. In T cells, the second signal is referred to as *co-stimulation*. The co-stimulators that provide this signal are expressed on APCs, mainly in response to microbes and products of dead cells, and the receptors that detect and respond to co-stimulators are expressed on T cells.

The CD28-B7 Families

The best-defined co-stimulators for T cells are the B7 molecules, B7-1 (CD80) and B7-2 (CD86), which are recognized by CD28 on T cells. CD28 was discovered as an activating receptor by a search for antibodies that cooperated with anti-TCR antibodies to elicit maximal responses of human T cells *in vitro*. The ligands for CD28 were then shown to be the B7 molecules. Further analysis of CD28 homologs has revealed at least three other receptors that are structurally similar, and the ligands for these receptors are homologous to the B7 proteins (Figure 7.3).[5]

Some fascinating conclusions have emerged from the studies of these receptors and ligands. First, some members of the CD28 family deliver activating signals and are appropriately called co-stimulators, but other members of the family that shut off immune responses are thus inhibitors. These inhibitory receptors include cytotoxic T-lymphocyte–associated antigen 4 (CTLA-4;

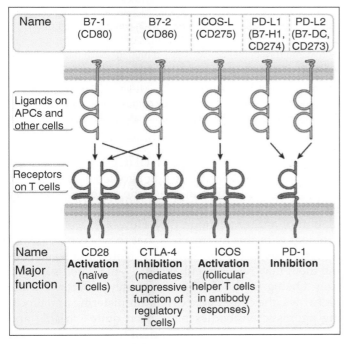

Name	B7-1 (CD80)	B7-2 (CD86)	ICOS-L (CD275)	PD-L1 (B7-H1, CD274)	PD-L2 (B7-DC, CD273)
Ligands on APCs and other cells					

Name	CD28	CTLA-4	ICOS	PD-1
Major function	**Activation** (naïve T cells)	**Inhibition** (mediates suppressive function of regulatory T cells)	**Activation** (follicular helper T cells in antibody responses)	**Inhibition**

Figure 7.3 Members of the B7-CD28 families of co-stimulators and co-inhibitors. Several ligands homologous to B7 are expressed on APCs and engage receptors expressed on T cells. Different pathways stimulate or inhibit T cell responses.

APC, antigen-presenting cell; CTLA-4, cytotoxic T-lymphocyte–associated antigen 4; ICOS, inducible T cell co-stimulator; PD-1, programmed death 1.

Source: Adapted with permission from Abbas AK, Lichtman AH, Pillai S. *Basic Immunology*. 5th ed. Elsevier; 2016.

CD152) and programmed death 1 (PD-1; CD279). They play important roles in regulating immune responses to self-antigen and foreign antigens, and they are being exploited for the immunotherapy of cancer. We discuss the functions of the inhibitory receptors in Chapter 8. Remarkably, both the best-defined activating receptor CD28 and the best-defined inhibitory receptor CTLA-4 recognize B7 molecules. How the recognition of the same ligands by two different receptors can lead to dramatically different functional outcomes is a fascinating question that we will address when we discuss the inhibitory receptors (Chapter 8). The second important conclusion about the CD28 family is that even the activating receptors in the family serve largely distinct functions. CD28 is essential for activating naïve T cells and thus for initiating primary immune responses to protein antigens, whereas inducible T cell co-stimulator (ICOS) is more important for the development and function of T follicular helper (Tfh) cells and thus for antibody responses in germinal centers.

Important questions about the CD28-B7 families of receptors and ligands remain unanswered. Are B7-1 and B7-2 functionally redundant or do they serve distinct roles? The bulk of the available data suggests that they can, indeed, exhibit redundancy, but there are differences in their kinetics of expression and binding affinity to CD28 and CTLA-4, raising the possibility that they could have distinct functions in physiological settings. Furthermore, interactions between PD-L1 and B7-1 but not B7-2 expressed *in cis* (on the same cell) have been described. It has been shown that these interactions prevent PD-L1 binding to its receptor PD-1 and reduce B7-1 binding to CTLA-4 but not CD28, which raises further questions about the interplay between CD28-B7 family members in immune regulation (Figure 7.4).[6]

Another question that remains to be answered is whether the B7 molecules signal back into APCs. The conventional view is that the B7 molecules engage CD28 and CD28 signals to the T cells. The possibility of reverse signaling by B7, leading to changes in APCs, has been raised by some experimental studies, but the nature of these reverse signals has not been established, despite extensive investigation,[7] and their importance remains a matter of speculation. What biochemical signals are induced in T cells by CD28? There is evidence that CD28 enhances TCR-mediated signals and may also initiate signals of its own, but the relative contribution of these classes of signals to the T cell response is not well understood.[8] The cytoplasmic tail of CD28 contains several highly conserved tyrosine-based motifs as well as proline-rich sequences that permit the recruitment of intracellular proteins containing SH2 or SH3 domains. Ligation of CD28 increases the sensitivity of T cells to TCR engagement, allowing them to respond to lower doses of antigen, and also augments IL-2 production and

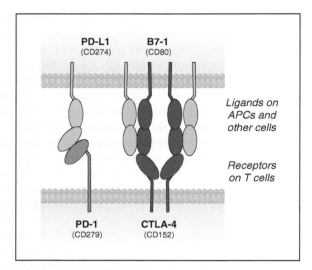

Figure 7.4 **PD-L1 and B7-1 (CD80) interact *in cis* (on the same cell).** B7-1 can form heterodimers with PD-L1, which affects B7-1 binding to CTLA-4 and blocks the PD-L1–PD-1 binding site. Thus, B7-1–PD-L1 interactions affect both the CTLA-4 and PD-1 pathways.

APC, antigen-presenting cell; CTLA-4, cytotoxic T-lymphocyte associated antigen 4; PD-1, programmed death 1.

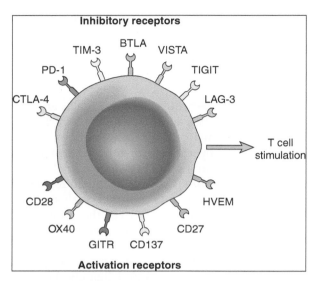

Figure 7.5 **Activating and inhibitory receptors of T cells.** T lymphocytes express a large number of receptors that are known to stimulate or inhibit the activation of these cells. The relative engagement of these receptors determines the net outcome of T cell activation.

BTLA, B and T cell attenuator; CTLA-4, cytotoxic T-lymphocyte–associated antigen 4; GITR, glucocorticoid-induced TNFR-related gene; HVEM, herpes virus entry mediator; LAG-3, lymphocyte activation gene; PD-1, programmed death 1; TIGIT, T cell immunoreceptor with Ig and ITIM domains; TIM, T cell immunoglobulin mucin; VISTA, V-domain Ig suppressor of T cell activation.

Source: Adapted with permission from Mellman I, Coukos G, Dranoff G. Cancer immunotherapy comes of age. *Nature.* 2011;480(7378):480–489. doi:10.1038/nature10673

promotes T cell survival. Furthermore, CD28 engagement appears to play a role in the remodeling of the actin cytoskeleton during T cell activation,[9] controlling access of TCR signaling molecules to their substrates, perhaps explaining why TCR- and CD28-mediated signaling events have proved so hard to disentangle.

It is generally accepted that microbial products are the most potent inducers of co-stimulators in APCs, but the role of co-stimulation in antitumor immune responses and the way co-stimulators are induced in the absence of an infection are still not answered with any certainty. One hypothesis is that as tumors outstrip their blood supply, tumor cells become necrotic and release products that activate the APCs and induce the expression of co-stimulators. Therapies that increase tumor cell death, such as chemotherapy and radiation, may increase the expression of co-stimulators and thus promote antitumor immunity, which cooperates with the toxic therapies to enhance tumor rejection. These are reasonable hypotheses, but there is actually little evidence to support them, especially in humans.

Other Co-Stimulators and Inhibitors

Since the discovery of the CD28-B7 families, many more co-stimulatory receptors and ligands have been described (Figure 7.5).[10] Many of these receptors are members of the tumor necrosis factor (TNF)-receptor superfamily, and their ligands are homologous to the cytokine TNF. Gene knockouts and experiments with blocking and stimulating antibodies in mice have shown that several of these receptors co-stimulate T cells; these include OX40

(CD134), 4-1BB (CD137), and GITR (CD357). This has led to considerable interest in using agonistic antibodies to provide co-stimulation at the same time as inhibitory receptors are blocked, in order to provide maximal stimulation of antitumor immunity. However, one potential problem with this approach is that these co-stimulatory receptors are also expressed on T_{reg} cells, and so activating them may result in enhanced T_{reg}-mediated suppression. Owing to the dual and opposing effects of these pathways, the consequences of administering and blocking agonistic antibodies have been quite variable and unpredictable and often dependent on the experimental system and context.

Inhibitory receptors unrelated to CTLA-4 and PD-1 have also been described. Three of the best known are TIM-3, LAG-3, and TIGIT.[11] They belong to different protein families, and all have been shown to inhibit T cell activation. In preclinical models, blocking each of these has shown enhanced antitumor immunity, and the first clinical trials with blocking antibodies have yielded promising results, especially when used in combination with PD-1 blockade.[12,13]

Cytokines

The major cytokine involved in early T cell responses is IL-2, discussed earlier in this chapter. Other cytokines are involved in the differentiation and functions of effector and memory T cells and are discussed briefly subsequently.

EFFECTOR AND MEMORY CD4⁺ T CELLS

The end result of T cell activation is the differentiation of naïve cells into antigen-specific effector and memory cells. Effector cells are the cells responsible for the ultimate *effect* of the immune response, which is to eliminate microbes and other sources of antigens (tumors and transplants). They are short-lived, and the majority of them die after the antigen is eliminated. Memory cells are functionally quiescent but are capable of surviving for long periods, and they respond rapidly and effectively on repeat encounters with the specific antigen, thus displaying *memory* for prior antigen exposure. Naïve, effector,

and memory cells can be distinguished by phenotypic and functional characteristics (Figure 7.6).[14] It is still not clear what mechanisms determine whether a particular T cell that has responded to antigen and co-stimulation becomes an effector or a memory cell. These distinct outcomes are associated with the expression of different transcription factors and probably epigenetic alterations, but whether the choice of these pathways is stochastic or driven by specific signals remains to be established.

Subsets of Effector CD4+ T Cells

One of the most informative discoveries in immunology was the identification of subpopulations of CD4⁺ T cells that make different cytokines and serve distinct functions. The first two of these to be discovered were called Th1 and Th2 (types 1 and 2 helper) cells, and the third was named Th17 because its defining cytokine is IL-17. These subsets differ in their cytokine products, functions, and roles in disease (Figure 7.7).[1,15] They

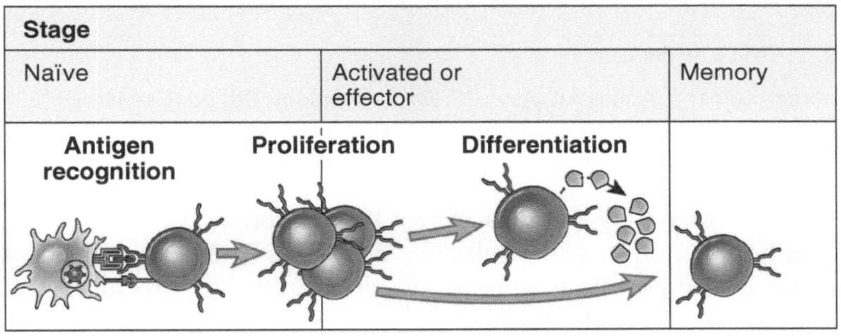

Stage		
Naïve	Activated or effector	Memory

	Naïve	Activated or effector	Memory
Migration	Preferentially to secondary lymphoid organs	Preferentially to inflamed tissues	Preferentially to inflamed tissues, mucosal tissues
Frequency of cells responsive to particular antigen	Very low	High	Low
Effector functions	None	Cytokine secretion; cytotoxic activity	None
Cell cycling	No	Yes	+/−
Surface protein expression			
IL-2R (CD25)	Low	High	Low
I-Selectin (CD62L)	High	Low	Variable
IL-7R (CD127)	Moderately high	Low	High
Adhesion molecules: integrins, CD44	Low	High	High
Chemokine receptor CCR7	High	Low	Variable
Major CD45 isoform (humans only)	CD45RA	CD45RO	CD45RO; variable
Morphology	Small; scant cytoplasm	Large; more cytoplasm	Small

Figure 7.6 Characteristics of naïve, effector, and memory T cells. Following antigen recognition, naïve T cells can differentiate into short-lived effector cells or long-lived memory cells. Some of the important features of these cells are summarized.

IL, interleukin.

Source: Adapted with permission from Abbas AK, Lichtman AH, Pillai S. *Cellular and Molecular Immunology.* 8th ed. Elsevier; 2015.

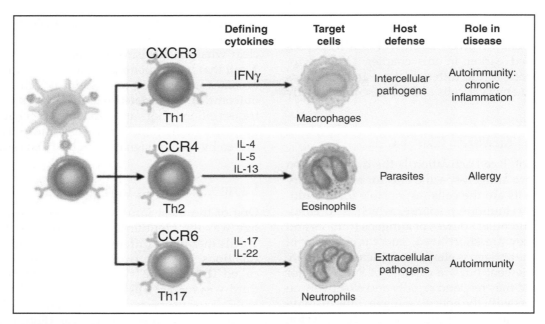

Figure 7.7 Subsets of CD4⁺ effector T cells. CD4⁺ T cells can differentiate into subpopulations called Th1, Th2, and Th17 that secrete distinct sets of cytokines, act on different targets, provide defense against different types of infectious pathogens, and play a role in various inflammatory diseases.

IFNγ, interferon-γ; IL-2, interleukin-2; Th1, T helper cells 1.

Source: Adapted with permission from Kumar V, Abbas AK, Aster JC. *Basic Pathology*. 9th ed. Elsevier; 2012.

also differ in the transcription factors they express. A fourth subset consists of T follicular helper (Tfh) cells; these cells position themselves in the germinal centers of lymphoid organs and help B cells to make high-affinity antibodies. Numerous other "subsets" have been described based on cytokine production and transcription factor expression, including Th9 and Th22 cells; whether these are stable subpopulations is not established. In fact, the stability or plasticity of all these subsets is a topic of continuing debate. It is generally believed that with repeated or prolonged stimulation, each subset becomes progressively and stably committed to one path and becomes increasingly resistant to conversion.

The major subsets of CD4⁺ T cells can all develop from the same starting naïve cell. Which differentiation path the T cell follows is largely determined by the cytokines to which it is exposed at the time of activation. In response to intracellular microbes, such as mycobacteria, dendritic cells and macrophages produce IL-12 and natural killer (NK) cells produce interferon-γ (IFNγ), and these two cytokines work together to drive T cells toward the Th1 pathway. Th1 cells produce IFNγ, which is the most potent macrophage-activating cytokine known, and it activates macrophages to kill intracellular bacteria such as mycobacteria. Th2 cells are induced in response to helminths and other antigens. The cytokines that drive

Th2 responses are poorly defined and may include IL-10 and IL-4. Th2 cells make IL-4, which induces immunoglobulin E (IgE) production; IL-5, which activates eosinophils; and IL-13, which has diverse actions. This subset is especially important for allergic reactions and probably for defense against helminths. Fungi and some bacteria activate dendritic cells to produce IL-1, IL-6, and IL-23, which together promote the development of naïve T cells into Th17 cells. Th17 cells secrete IL-17 and other cytokines that recruit neutrophils, which destroy extracellular bacteria and fungi. Most chronic inflammatory diseases (other than allergies) are associated with the activation of Th1 and/or Th17 cells.

The subsets of T cells show distinct migration patterns, based largely on the expression of chemokine receptors and adhesion molecules. Th1 cells express the chemokine receptor CXCR3, which recruits them to the sites of infection. Th2 cells express CCR4 (and CCR3), which directs them to epithelial tissues, and Th17 cells express CCR6, which is also involved in the migration to inflammatory sites.

Role of CD4⁺ T Cell Subsets in Tumor Immunity

T cell subset cells also play different roles in immunity to tumors.[16,17] The abundance of Th1 cells in a tumor infiltrate is associated with a better prognosis,[18,19]

presumably because Th1-activated macrophages are effective at destroying tumor cells. In contrast, the abundance of Th2 cells frequently indicates worse outcomes, perhaps because Th2 cytokines inhibit the development of Th1 cells. In addition, Th2-associated inflammation is believed to promote tumor growth and angiogenesis. Few evidence exists for other CD4 T cell subsets; however, in the setting of colorectal carcinoma, Th17 and Th22 cells appear to be associated with poor outcomes, while in contrast a high density of Tfh cells at the center of the tumor is associated with good clinical outcomes.[20,21]

Cytokines made by different subsets of T cells trigger distinct pathways of macrophage activation that have different impacts on tumor growth.[22] IFNγ made by Th1 cells induces what is called classical macrophage activation, in which the macrophages acquire the ability to destroy phagocytosed microbes and tumor cells. In contrast, Th2 cytokines induce a different type of macrophage response, called alternative activation, and these macrophages promote tissue repair, angiogenesis, and scarring. It has been postulated that classically activated macrophages serve to eliminate tumors, whereas alternatively activated macrophages promote tumor development and growth. These ideas highlight the observation that inflammation can be pro-tumorigenic and may explain the association between cancer and infections with hepatitis B and C viruses and the bacterium *Helicobacter pylori*.[19,23]

Memory CD4+ T Cells

Memory cells may arise from effector cells that have not died at the end of an immune response, or memory cell development may be a distinct pathway from that of effector cells. Although this basic question is not fully resolved, it is known that memory cells express anti-apoptotic proteins that keep them alive and they cycle slowly, thus self-renewing, a property characteristic of stem cells. In CD4+ memory cells, survival and low-level proliferation are driven by the cytokine IL-7, which is produced by stromal cells in many tissues. Memory cells also respond more rapidly to antigen challenge than naïve cells, probably because many of the genes that encode key effector molecules are fixed in an "open" configuration in memory cells and become transcriptionally active very quickly after stimulation by the antigen. Generating abundant memory cells is, of course, an important goal of vaccination for infections and tumors.

Memory cells are heterogeneous in terms of migration and function. The two major subsets of memory T cells are called *central* and *effector*. Central memory cells migrate preferentially to secondary lymphoid organs and are not potent effectors but can proliferate rapidly on antigen challenge to generate a large pool of effector cells. Effector memory cells tend to migrate to peripheral tissues such as the gut, airways, and skin and are capable of rapid effector functions on antigen challenge. Thus, the central memory pool provides the reserve for large secondary responses, and the effector memory pool performs the key defensive functions.

The capacity for immunological memory is a hallmark of the adaptive immune response and is thought to play a key role in establishing effective antitumor immunity. Consistent with this idea, patients with primary tumors that exhibit a high infiltration of memory CD4+ T cells are less likely to experience tumor recurrence.[24] In colorectal cancer, the density of tumor-infiltrating cells expressing the memory T cell marker CD45RO has been shown to be significantly associated with longer cancer-specific and overall survival.[25] Thus, the generation of a memory T cell response and the positioning of memory T cells within the tumor mass appear to be important for successful antitumor immunity.

CONCLUSION

This chapter has summarized the basic biology of CD4+ T cells and pointed out the possible involvement of these cells in defense against tumors. The next, companion, chapter focuses on the regulation of T cell activation, and the way regulatory pathways are being exploited for improved therapy of tumors.

ACKNOWLEDGMENTS

The contribution of Professor Abul K. Abbas to this chapter in the previous edition is greatly appreciated.

KEY REFERENCES

Only key references appear in the print edition. The full reference list appears in the digital product on Springer Publishing Connect: connect.springerpub.com/content/book/978-0-8261-3743-2/part/part01/chapter/ch07

1. Kumar V, Abbas AK, Aster JC. *Basic Pathology*. 9th ed. Elsevier; 2012.
4. Smith-Garvin JE, Koretzky GA, Jordan MS. T cell activation. *Annu Rev Immunol*. 2009;27:591–619. doi:10.1146/annurev.immunol.021908.132706
5. Abbas AK, Lichtman AH, Pillai S. *Basic Immunology*. 5th ed. Elsevier; 2016.
6. Sugiura D, Maruhashi T, Okazaki IM, et al. Restriction of PD-1 function by cis-PD-L1/CD80 interactions is required for optimal T cell responses. *Science*. 2019;364(6440):558–566. doi:10.1126/science.aav7062
10. Mellman I, Coukos G, Dranoff G. Cancer immunotherapy comes of age. *Nature*. 2011;480(7378):480–489. doi:10.1038/nature10673
14. Abbas AK, Lichtman AH, Pillai S. *Cellular and Molecular Immunology*. 8th ed. Elsevier; 2015.
24. Fridman WH, Pagès F, Sautès-Fridman C, Galon J. The immune contexture in human tumours: impact on clinical outcome. *Nat Rev Cancer*. 2012;12(4):298–306. doi:10.1038/nrc3245

Regulation of Cell-Mediated Immunity: The Biology of Checkpoints and Regulatory T Cells

Lucy S. K. Walker and Lina Petersone

KEY POINTS

- We balance immune defense against microbial pathogens and cancers with the need for tolerance toward self-antigens and harmless antigens.

- Failure of self-tolerance is the basis of autoimmunity.

- Cancers can co-opt tolerance pathways to avoid immune-mediated rejection.

- Central tolerance acts on developing lymphocytes and peripheral tolerance acts on mature lymphocytes.

- Peripheral T cell tolerance can be mediated by anergy, regulatory T cells (T_{reg} cells), or deletion.

- Cytotoxic T-lymphocyte–associated antigen 4 (CTLA-4) and programmed death 1 (PD-1) are the key pathways for peripheral T cell regulation.

- Blockade of CTLA-4 and PD-1 promotes antitumor immunity but can simultaneously promote autoimmunity.

INTRODUCTION

The healthy immune system exists in a state of equilibrium in which the need to be activated to defend the host against microbial pathogens is constantly balanced by the need to prevent or control reactions against self and other harmless antigens, such as commensal microbes (Figure 8.1). In order to maintain this equilibrium, the system has evolved to develop numerous mechanisms whose primary function is to inhibit responses against harmless antigens. Some chronic infections and many cancers have acquired the ability to exploit these same mechanisms to prevent immune reactions against themselves; in fact, the ability to evade host immune defense is one of the hallmarks of cancer.[1] To understand how cancers have learned to evade host responses and the

way oncologists can exploit the immune system to treat cancer, we first need to understand the basic biology of immune regulation. In this chapter, we review some of the major mechanisms that suppress cell-mediated immune responses.

It is useful to start our discussion by defining terms that are commonly used in this context. "Regulation" is a broad term that refers to all mechanisms that prevent, inhibit, or terminate immune responses to self-antigens and foreign antigens. "Tolerance" is defined as the inability of the immune system to respond to an antigen as a result of exposure to that antigen. Its major importance lies in tolerance to self-antigens, as discussed later. Tolerogenic antigens fail to elicit productive immune responses and to generate effector and memory cells; instead, they shut down immune responses. "Exhaustion" refers to a phenomenon in which immune cells do make an initial effector response, but this response is terminated prematurely, before the source of antigen can be eliminated. It is the result of prolonged or repeated exposure to an antigen. It was first described in chronic viral infection, but the same phenomenon may occur with tumor. Many of the mechanisms of tolerance may also be responsible for inducing exhaustion in an immune response.

Most regulatory mechanisms have been studied in the context of tolerance to self-antigens, and that is mainly how we discuss these mechanisms. Throughout, we refer to the relevance of these mechanisms to tumor immunity.

IMMUNOLOGICAL TOLERANCE: BASIC PRINCIPLES

Tolerance is an actively induced phenomenon of antigen-specific unresponsiveness. Its induction requires specific recognition of antigen and failure to elicit an effective immune response. The significance of tolerance is that all individuals are tolerant of their own (self) antigens, and failure of self-tolerance is the underlying cause of autoimmunity. However, the importance of tolerance goes well beyond self-tolerance and autoimmunity.

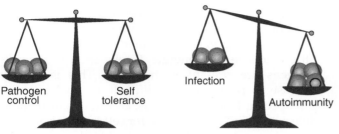

Figure 8.1 The balance of lymphocyte activation and control. Lymphocytes are poised to respond to foreign (e.g., microbial) antigens to provide host defense against pathogens, but lymphocytes also have to be controlled by the mechanisms of tolerance and regulation to prevent reactions against self and other harmless antigens (e.g., commensal microbes and environmental antigens).

Many microbes and cancers invoke the mechanisms of tolerance to avoid immune attack. These mechanisms can be exploited therapeutically, inducing tolerance to treat autoimmune and allergic diseases and graft rejection or blocking tolerance to promote immune responses against tumors and perhaps some microbes. All these strategies are now approved for patients or are in clinical trials, so the phenomenon of tolerance occupies a central place in basic and translational immunology.

Immunologists have classified self-tolerance into two groups based on the immunological compartment where it occurs (Figure 8.2).[2] "Central tolerance" is unresponsiveness induced in the central (generative) lymphoid organs, which are the thymus for T cells and the bone marrow for B cells.[3] Mature lymphocytes are generated

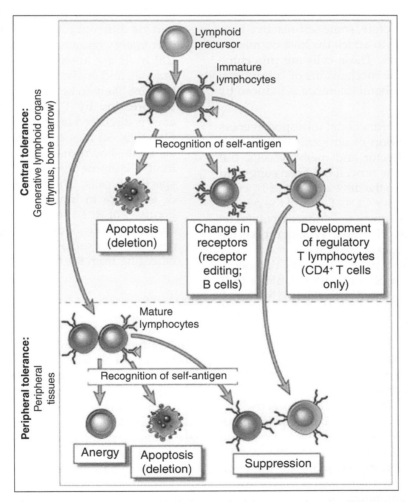

Figure 8.2 Mechanisms of central and peripheral tolerance. Central tolerance is induced in the generative lymphoid organs when immature lymphocytes recognize antigens (typically self-antigens) with high affinity and die, change their receptors, or develop into regulatory cells. Peripheral tolerance is induced in peripheral organs when mature lymphocytes recognize antigens in the absence of full activating signals and are inhibited, suppressed by regulatory cells, or killed.

Source: Reproduced with permission from Abbas AK, Lichtman AH, Pillai S. *Cellular and Molecular Immunology*. 8th ed. Elsevier; 2015.

from hemopoietic precursors in these organs. As many self-antigens are also present in these organs, lymphocytes with specific receptors for these antigens encounter them before the lymphocytes are fully mature. Antigen recognition by immature lymphocytes leads not to the activation (as it does in mature cells) but to the death of many of the cells. This phenomenon is called "negative selection." As a result, many potentially dangerous self-reactive lymphocytes are deleted from the pool of lymphocytes that mature and enter peripheral tissues. Immature B cells are able to express new antigen receptors (a process called "receptor editing"). Also, some CD4+ T cells are not killed, but they develop into regulatory T cells (T_{reg} cells), described later. The net result of these processes is that the lymphocytes that reach functional maturity are purged of potentially dangerous self-reactive cells.

Central tolerance is, however, imperfect. Not all self-antigens are present in the thymus and bone marrow, and not all self-reactive immature cells in these organs are eliminated. Therefore, some self-reactive lymphocytes with the potential to attack the host do mature and enter peripheral tissues. These cells are prevented from causing damage by the mechanisms of "peripheral tolerance."[4] In T cells, peripheral tolerance is induced by three main mechanisms:

- **Anergy.** Anergy refers to functional unresponsiveness induced by the recognition of antigen. Anergic cells cannot develop into effector and memory cells, but they may survive for some time. It has been suggested that anergy is a prelude to the development of T_{reg} cells; in other words, self-reactive CD4+ T cells in the peripheral tissues first become functionally inactive (anergic) and then differentiate into T_{reg} cells.[5] Whether this is the usual fate of anergic T cells is unknown.

  There are two known mechanisms of anergy (Figure 8.3).[6] First, anergic cells show a block in T cell receptor (TCR)-mediated signaling. This block may result from the activation of ubiquitin ligases that tag TCR-associated signaling proteins for proteasomal degradation, thus reducing the intracellular pool of signaling intermediates. Second, anergy is induced when there is a greater engagement of inhibitory receptors such as cytotoxic T-lymphocyte–associated antigen 4 (CTLA-4) relative to activating receptors such as CD28. This may be because tolerogenic antigens are presented by antigen-presenting cells (APCs) that express low levels of co-stimulators; in this setting, the inhibitory receptors are preferentially engaged. Exhausted T cells also show increased expression of many inhibitory receptors, and the defective responses associated with T cell exhaustion are in large part because of the actions of these inhibitory receptors. The role of inhibitory receptors in maintaining T cell unresponsiveness is discussed in detail later.

Most of the evidence for anergy as a mechanism of tolerance has come from experimental models, often using genetically modified mice. There is little evidence that anergic T cells specific for self-antigens are present in humans.[7] This is mainly because it is technically difficult to analyze antigen-specific T cells in humans, and so it is difficult to detect anergic T cells specific for self-antigens or other tolerizing antigens. However, with the increasing interest in immune responses specific for tumor antigens, it is likely that many studies examining the characteristics of these cells will appear. An obvious and important question is the contribution of anergy to the failure of antitumor immunity. Data from mouse models suggest that tumor-specific CD4 T cells may be driven toward anergy or T_{reg} cell induction rather than effector fates in tumor-draining lymph nodes.[8] In patients with autoimmunity, or allergy, autoantigens or allergens may be administered in different forms and via different routes with the goal of inducing specific anergy or activation of T_{reg} cells. Numerous clinical trials are attempting to induce tolerance in this manner, and analyses of the T cells in treated individuals are likely to be informative.

- **Suppression by T_{reg} cells.** This mechanism of tolerance is discussed later.
- **Deletion.** Studies conducted mostly in mouse models have shown that some tolerogenic antigens may inhibit immune responses by inducing apoptosis of specific T cells. The importance of this mechanism of tolerance in humans is largely unknown, partly because of the problems inherent in quantifying antigen-specific T cells and partly because, as the T cells die, they are often rapidly replaced by new cells emerging from the thymus.

IMMUNE CHECKPOINTS MAINTAINED BY INHIBITORY RECEPTORS

The concept that the outcome of antigen recognition is controlled by a balance between the engagement of activating and inhibitory receptors was most convincingly first demonstrated in natural killer (NK) cells. Subsequently, the same principle has been shown to be relevant to T and B lymphocytes, and it is also probably true for other cells in the immune system, such as dendritic cells. In Chapter 7, we introduced this idea for T cells, which is the focus of our discussion. The stops in T cell activation that are induced and maintained by these inhibitory receptors have been called "checkpoints." We also introduced the two best understood T cell inhibitory receptors, CTLA-4 (CD152) and programmed death 1 (PD-1; CD279), both members of the CD28 family. Subsequently, we consider the functions and mechanisms of action of each of these receptors and then their implications for cancer immunotherapy.

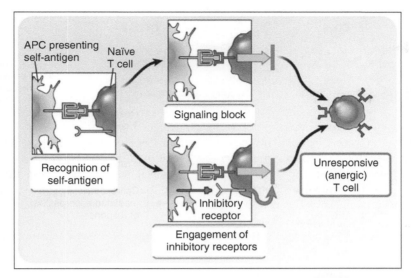

Figure 8.3 Mechanisms of T cell anergy. T cells that recognize antigens in the absence of co-stimulation or other signals become unresponsive, by shutting down activating signals from the antigen receptor complex or by engaging inhibitory receptors (the so-called coinhibitors).

APC, antigen-presenting cell.

Source: Reproduced with permission from Abbas AK, Lichtman AH, Pillai S. *Basic Immunology*. 5th ed. Elsevier; 2016.

Cytotoxic T-Lymphocyte–Associated Antigen 4 (CD152)

CTLA-4 was discovered in a complementary DNA (cDNA) library generated from cytotoxic T lymphocytes, but it is expressed mainly on T$_{reg}$ cells and activated conventional (responding) T cells. It is structurally homologous to the co-stimulatory receptor CD28 and, as for CD28, its ligands are B7-1 (CD80) and B7-2 (CD86). Distinct from CD28, it exhibits a predominantly intracellular location, and only a small fraction of the total CTLA-4 pool is present on the cell surface at any one time. This is a result of continual endocytosis of CTLA-4 molecules because of a conserved motif in their cytoplasmic domain that associates with the clathrin adaptor protein complex, AP2.

The first insights into the biology of CTLA-4 came from *in vitro* experiments demonstrating that it counteracted the stimulatory actions of CD28 and inhibited the activation of CD4$^+$ T cells (Figure 8.4). This was soon followed by the creation of gene knockout mice, which developed fatal systemic inflammatory disease, thus establishing the essential role of CTLA-4 as a controller of immune activation. The inflammatory disease is likely because of autoimmunity directed against multiple self-antigens, although it is not known which antigens are targeted by the autoimmune attack when CTLA-4 is eliminated. More recent observations have confirmed this essential role of CTLA-4 in humans as well: cancer patients treated with antibodies that block CTLA-4 and

individuals with loss-of-function mutations in the *CTLA4* gene also develop multisystem inflammatory lesions.

Mechanisms of Action of CTLA-4

CTLA-4 inhibits T cell responses through its expression on both conventional and T$_{reg}$ cells (Figure 8.5). Conventional T cells that are activated by antigen and co-stimulation

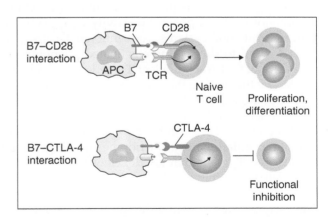

Figure 8.4 The opposite consequences of CD28 and CTLA-4 engagement. Engagement of the co-stimulatory receptor CD28 by B7 ligands at the time of T cell antigen recognition results in enhanced T cell responses, but the engagement of CTLA-4 inhibits T cell responses.

APC, antigen-presenting cell; CTLA-4, cytotoxic T-lymphocyte–associated antigen 4; TCR, T cell receptor.

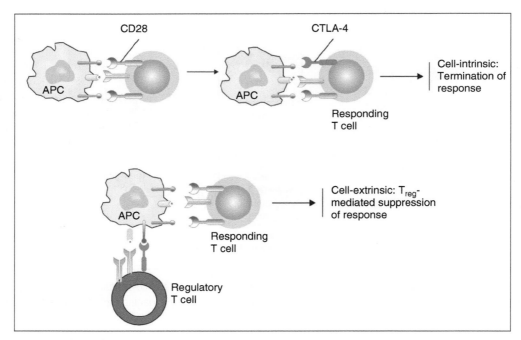

Figure 8.5 CTLA-4 functions on both conventional cells and T$_{reg}$ cells. CTLA-4 is expressed on responding T cells following activation and terminates further activation of these cells. CTLA-4 expressed on T$_{reg}$ cells inhibits the activation of responding T cells, when both cells are recognizing antigen displayed by the same APC (cell-extrinsic action of CTLA-4).

APC, antigen-presenting cell; CTLA-4, cytotoxic T-lymphocyte–associated antigen 4; T$_{reg}$, regulatory T.

begin to express CTLA-4 and can use it to terminate their own response. This likely involves CTLA-4 outcompeting CD28 for access to their shared ligands. T$_{reg}$ cells constitutively express CTLA-4 and can use it to block the activation of conventional (responding) T cells. Although both pathways have been demonstrated experimentally, the emerging consensus is that CTLA-4 mainly functions as a mediator of the suppressive activity of T$_{reg}$ cells. In fact, in experimental systems, conventional T cells lacking CTLA-4 fail to show a hyperactivated phenotype in the presence of CTLA-4-sufficient T$_{reg}$ cells. This was first suggested by the finding that in mixed bone marrow chimeras, comprising CTLA-4$^{-/-}$ and CTLA-4$^{+/+}$ cells, the CTLA-4-deficient cells were controlled by the normal T cells. Deletion of CTLA-4 in Foxp3^{+} cells largely mimics the systemic inflammatory phenotype of the germline knockout, and T$_{reg}$ cells that are deficient in CTLA-4 frequently fail to exhibit regulatory function in adoptive transfer experiments.

The early studies to define the mechanisms of action of CTLA-4 were interpreted to show that it delivers inhibitory signals to T cells. Although this would explain the inhibitory activity of CTLA-4 in conventional T cells, it does not explain the cell-extrinsic mechanism of action. In addition, the cytoplasmic domain of CTLA-4 does not contain a well-defined immunoreceptor tyrosine-based inhibitory motif (ITIM). More recent studies have shown

that CTLA-4 works primarily as a competitive inhibitor of CD28. CTLA-4 tightly binds to B7 molecules on the surface of APCs and removes these molecules by a process of trans-endocytosis, thus making them unavailable for the activating receptor CD28 (Figure 8.6). As CTLA-4 has a 20- to 50-fold higher affinity for B7 ligands than does CD28, it readily outcompetes CD28, especially when B7 levels on APCs are low (as when the APCs are presenting self-antigens or tumor antigens, compared to antigens from microbes, which tend to induce more B7). CTLA-4 can work as a competitive inhibitor of CD28 signaling, regardless of whether it is expressed on responding T cells or adjacent T$_{reg}$ cells, as long as the T$_{reg}$ cells are in contact with the same APCs as are the responding cells (see Figure 8.5). This mechanism of action is unique among immune receptors, because this is a rare situation in which an activating receptor (CD28) and an inhibitory receptor (CTLA-4) share the same B7 ligands, thus setting up the potential for competition. The action of CTLA-4 as a competitive inhibitor also explains why patients with heterozygous mutations[9,10] (affecting only one of the two alleles of the gene) show the disease phenotype—losing half the functional CTLA-4 molecules from a cell is likely enough to impair its role as a competitor of CD28.

The available evidence suggests that CTLA-4 mainly inhibits the activation of naïve CD4^{+} T cells during the initiation of immune responses in secondary lymphoid

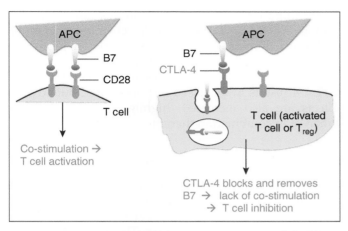

Figure 8.6 The role of CTLA-4 as a competitive inhibitor of CD28. In the absence of CTLA-4 (left panel), CD28 on T cells engages B7 molecules (CD80, CD86) on APC and stimulates T cell responses. When CTLA-4 is present (right panel), it binds to B7 with higher affinity than CD28 does and also removes B7 molecules from APCs by trans-endocytosis, thus reducing the availability of co-stimulators and inhibiting T cell activation.

APC, antigen-presenting cell; CTLA-4, cytotoxic T-lymphocyte–associated antigen 4; T_{reg}, regulatory T.

organs. This involves the control of co-stimulatory ligand (B7) expression on dendritic cells (DC), with migratory DC subsets being especially targeted.[11] Since migratory DC transport tumor antigens to the tumor-draining lymph node, anti-CTLA-4 antibodies may interrupt the regulation of B7 expression on these cells. CTLA-4 may also inhibit the activation of CD8[+] T cells, either directly or by limiting T cell help for the development of CTLs. As it controls the early, co-stimulation-dependent steps in T cell responses, mutation or blockade of the receptor leads to severe dysregulation of all cell-mediated immune responses. This is different from PD-1, described in the following section, which probably functions mainly to control the effector phase of CD8[+] T cell responses (Table 8.1). Patients with mutations in the *CTLA4* gene also develop a systemic immune dysregulation syndrome involving a progressive loss of B cells and a consequent antibody deficiency, suggesting that CTLA-4 directly or indirectly influences antibody production.

Programmed Death 1

PD-1 was discovered as an inhibitor of immune responses and is thus called because it was thought to be involved in programmed death (apoptosis) of T cells. Subsequent studies showed that it is related structurally to CD28 and CTLA-4. Gene knockout mice develop autoimmune diseases, but the diseases are less severe, more variable, and show later onset than the diseases seen in CTLA-4-knockout mice. In the bone marrow of chimeric mice that contain a mixture of PD-1–deficient cells and normal cells, the mutant and not the normal T cells are hyperactivated, demonstrating that the function of PD-1 is cell-intrinsic. This simple experiment reveals a fundamental difference between the PD-1 and the CTLA-4 pathways, as therapeutic inhibition of PD-1 would be predicted to affect only the PD-1–expressing cells, whereas inhibition of CTLA-4 would affect CTLA-4–negative cells too as a result of its cell-extrinsic mechanism of action.

Great interest in PD-1 was spurred by the finding that, in a mouse model of chronic viral infection, CD8[+] CTLs are induced, but these effector cells become nonfunctional (exhausted), allowing the virus to establish latent infection. Exhausted T cells express high levels of PD-1 (as well as other inhibitory receptors), and their function can be rescued by blocking PD-1. A similar role for PD-1 has been demonstrated in chronic viral infections in humans, such as HIV and hepatitis C. In addition to exhausted PD-1[+] cells, PD-1[+] CD8[+] T cells with stem cell-like properties have been recently described in mouse and human tumors. In response to checkpoint immunotherapy, these cells can differentiate into CD8[+] effector cells and promote tumor control.[12]

PD-1 is also expressed on B cells, particularly peritoneal cavity B-1 cells and germinal center B cells and is thought to have an inhibitory function in these cells as well.

PD-1 binds to two ligands, PD-L1 (CD274) and PD-L2 (CD273), which are expressed on a wide variety of cell types, including APCs, parenchymal cells, and tumor cells.[13] The current model for the mechanism of action of PD-1 is that it delivers inhibitory signals, perhaps dependent on tyrosine phosphatases, which inhibit TCR-mediated signals. Unlike CTLA-4, the cytoplasmic domain of PD-1 contains both an ITIM and an immunoreceptor tyrosine-based switch motif (ITSM). The precise nature of the "off-signals" generated by PD-1 is not defined but may involve recruitment of the tyrosine phosphatase SHP-2 to the PD-1 ITSM motif and subsequent inactivation of effector molecules such as Zap70 in T cells and Syk in B cells. However, repeated or persistent antigen stimulation induces high levels of PD-1 on the antigen-activated T cells. This receptor functions as a cell-intrinsic terminator of lymphocyte activation in situations of chronic antigen exposure. Thus, PD-1 is a feedback inhibition mechanism that limits prolonged or excessive immune activation and the attendant tissue damage. As tumors are persistent and can provide a chronic source of antigen, they too can engage this pathway and thus evade immune responses. Unlike CTLA-4, there is little evidence that PD-1 is involved in the suppressive action of T_{reg} cells.

The mechanisms of action and functions of PD-1 are different from those of CTLA-4, although there may be some overlap (Table 8.1). Some of these differences

Table 8.1 Actions of CTLA-4 and PD-1

ACTIVITY	CTLA-4	PD-1
Major site of action	Secondary lymphoid organs	Peripheral tissues
Stage of immune response that is inhibited	Induction	Effector phase
Cell type that is inhibited	CD4$^+$ > CD8$^+$	CD8$^+$ > CD4$^+$
Main signals inhibited	CD28 co-stimulation (by blocking and removing B7 from APCs)	Chronic antigen receptor stimulation
Role in T$_{reg}$-mediated suppression of immune responses	Yes	Probably no
Role in defective response of "exhausted" T cells	Maybe, but not critical	Yes
Inflammatory reactions following blocking antibody therapy	Severe	Milder

CTLA-4, cytotoxic T-lymphocyte–associated antigen 4; PD-1, programmed death 1; T$_{reg}$, regulatory T.

account for the less severe inflammatory reactions seen after the PD-1 blockade compared to the CTLA-4 blockade. As described in Chapter 7, recent studies have demonstrated interactions between PD-L1 and B7-1 (CD80) that impair their binding to PD-1 and CTLA-4. Understanding these interactions in different settings will be essential for predicting functional outcomes of co-blockade with anti-CTLA-4 and anti-PD-L1.[14]

Other Inhibitory Receptors

In Chapter 7, we mentioned several other inhibitory receptors belonging to various protein families (see Figure 7.3, Chapter 7). The physiological roles and mechanisms of action of these receptors are still active fields of study, and attempts to target them for cancer immunotherapy are in early clinical trials. A key goal is to define whether particular inhibitory receptors target common or distinct pathways, in order to shed light on which therapeutic approaches might be most suitable for use in combination. In this respect, it has been shown that PD-1 and lymphocyte-activation gene 3 (LAG-3) act synergistically to inhibit autoimmunity in mice.[15] In cancer, early clinical trials separately studying blockade treatments of

T cell immunoglobulin and mucin-domain containing protein-3 (TIM-3), LAG-3, and T cell immunoglobulin and ITIM domain (TIGIT) have all shown promising clinical potential when combined with co-blockade of PD-1.[16,17] Combining antibodies that target PD-1 and CTLA-4 results in increased response rates, but adverse effects are also increased, highlighting the challenge inherent in combination therapies.

Checkpoint Blockade for Cancer Immunotherapy

The discovery of CTLA-4 as an inhibitor of T cell responses prompted some investigators to ask if tumors engage this control pathway and whether blocking it stimulates antitumor immunity. The first such experiment, done with a transplantable melanoma in mice, showed dramatic tumor rejection induced by blocking CTLA-4 with a specific antibody. This led to clinical trials of anti-CTLA-4 antibody in patients with melanoma, and the birth of *checkpoint blockade* as an effective cancer immunotherapy.[18] Predictably, blocking CTLA-4 also resulted in inflammatory disease in treated patients, and this adverse effect, which was sometimes severe, limited the use of this therapy.[19] Subsequent studies in preclinical models and in patients showed that blocking PD-1 or its major ligand, PD-L1, also resulted in regression of melanomas and other tumors, with generally less adverse inflammatory reactions. Checkpoint blockade is now an accepted form of immunotherapy for many cancers.

The success of checkpoint blockade has established a new paradigm in immunology. Previous attempts to induce immune responses have been dominated by stimulation approaches, which were based on the early successes of vaccination, the classical immune-stimulation strategy. Checkpoint blockade demonstrates that it is possible to stimulate responses by "removing the brakes." In fact, eliminating regulation may be more successful in cancer than vaccination alone, because a hallmark of cancer is its ability to inhibit immune responses. In addition, cancer is a situation in which vaccines usually have to be therapeutic, not only prophylactic, so by the time the vaccine is administered the tumor has already established mechanisms that prevent effective immune responses. More recent immunotherapy protocols are using combinations of checkpoint blockade and vaccination, an approach that has a strong biological rationale.

A fundamental question that emerges is: Why do T cells responding to cancers engage these inhibitory receptors and thus prevent immune responses? Although there is not a definite answer to this question, there are some plausible hypotheses. It may be that cancers activate innate immunity weakly (compared to microbes), and therefore the level of B7 co-stimulators expressed on APCs is relatively low. This is the situation when the high-affinity receptor CTLA-4 is preferentially engaged, resulting in a block in the response. The possibility with PD-1 is more straightforward: Tumors may evolve to express PD-L1 and this directly engages PD-1 expressed on chronically activated T cells, thus shutting off the response of the T cells. Whether other factors in the tumor environment contribute to the engagement of these inhibitory receptors is a topic of active investigation.

REGULATORY T CELLS

The second major and well-defined mechanism of peripheral tolerance involves T_{reg} cells. The idea that some lymphocytes suppress other lymphocytes is an old one and gave rise to the field of "suppressor T cells" more than 40 years ago. Problems in purifying and characterizing these cells and their biologically active products led to growing skepticism about the importance, and even existence, of suppressor cells. The idea was resurrected in the 1990s with much better definitions using more advanced technology. The cells that were shown to inhibit immune responses were called "T_{reg} cells" (Figure 8.7).[2,19] Their importance was definitively established by the discovery of genetic mutations in mice and humans that interfered with the development and functions of these cells and resulted in severe autoimmune diseases. T_{reg} cells are now recognized as a central component of immune regulation, with roles in preventing autoimmunity and antitumor immunity, as

well as preventing rejection of the fetus and elimination of harmless commensal microbes.

The T_{reg} cells that inhibit immune responses are CD4$^+$, express high levels of the interleukin 2 receptor (IL-2R) α chain (CD25), and stably express the transcription factor Foxp3. Many other phenotypic markers as well as epigenetic modifications have been described in these cells. In addition, other populations of "T_{reg} cells" that suppress immune responses have been described, but the only ones that are known to prevent autoimmunity in mice and humans are the Foxp3$^+$ CD4$^+$ cells. Mutations of the *Foxp3* gene are the cause of the severe autoimmune disease IPEX (for immune dysregulation, polyendocrinopathy, enteropathy, and X-linked syndrome) in humans and the disease called scurfy in mice. Knockout of the *Foxp3* gene replicates these diseases, is associated with a loss of Foxp3$^+$ T cells, and can be rescued by the transfer of normal Foxp3$^+$ T cells. Thus, this cell population satisfies "Koch's postulates" for cells that prevent autoimmunity.

Most T_{reg} cells specific for self-antigens arise in the thymus as a consequence of the recognition of self-antigens in this organ; they are called thymic T_{reg} cells (and were previously known as "natural" T_{reg} cells because they are present throughout life). As mentioned earlier, many self-reactive immature T cells that recognize self-antigens in the thymus are deleted. The process through which some escape this fate and instead develop into

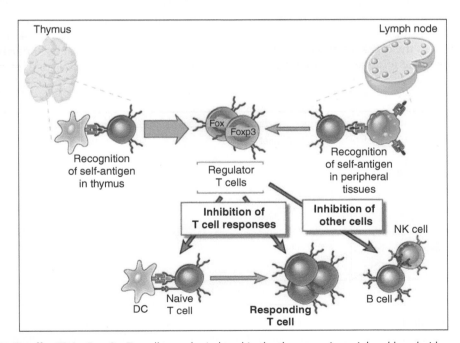

Figure 8.7 Regulatory T cells. CD4+ Foxp3+ T_{reg} cells may be induced in the thymus or in peripheral lymphoid organs. T_{reg} cells suppress immune responses by inhibiting the activation and functions of different lymphocyte populations.

DC, dendritic cell; NK, natural killer cell; T_{reg}, regulatory T.

Source: Reproduced with permission from Abbas AK, Lichtman AH, Pillai S. *Cellular and Molecular Immunology.* 8th ed. Elsevier; 2015.

T_{reg} cells is not clearly understood, but it is likely to be related to the sensitivity of the TCR to antigens and the availability of the factors that control the size of the T_{reg} cell niche.[20] T_{reg} cells can also be generated in the periphery; these are called peripheral T_{reg} cells (and previously, adaptive or induced T_{reg} cells). Peripheral T_{reg} cells may be induced by self-antigens that are not present in the thymus and by antigens that are only encountered in the periphery, such as paternal antigens in the fetus, antigens of commensal microbes, and tumor antigens, especially those produced by mutated genes that are not normally present.

Populations of T_{reg} cells may be distinguished by activation status and site of residence, as well as phenotypic markers and transcription factor expression. Resting, activated, and memory T_{reg} cells have been described in various models in mice and humans. T_{reg} cells may reside mainly in secondary lymphoid organs and in peripheral, nonlymphoid tissues and may migrate between these compartments. They have distinctive transcriptional signatures according to their tissue environment. T_{reg} cells within tumors may share transcriptional features with tissue-specific T_{reg} cells in the same location; for example, tumor-resident T_{reg} cells in melanoma share common features with skin T_{reg} cells.[21]

Role of IL-2 in T_{reg} Maintenance

In Chapter 7, we described IL-2 as an autocrine growth factor that is required for the proliferation of antigen-stimulated T cells early in an immune response. As a result of this well-known function of the cytokine, it was predicted that knockout of the *IL-2* gene in mice would result in an immunodeficiency. It came as a surprise when, in fact, knockout of the gene encoding IL-2 or the α or β chain of the IL-2R led not to immune deficiency but to lympho proliferation and various manifestations of autoimmunity. This unexpected result was explained by the demonstration that Foxp3+ T_{reg} cells require the growth factor IL-2 for their survival and functional competence. In the absence of this cytokine or its receptor, T_{reg} cells are not maintained, and the result is uncontrolled lymphocyte activation and autoimmunity.[22] As T_{reg} cells do not themselves make IL-2, they likely get this growth factor from conventional T cells responding to self-antigens and other antigens (Figure 8.8).[23] It is now believed that these conventional responding T cells make small amounts of IL-2, which first and preferentially act on T_{reg} cells in the environment, and the T_{reg} cells are activated to impose control on the immune response. The implications of this function of IL-2 for the development of new therapies are discussed later.

Mechanisms of Action of T_{reg} Cells

Although dozens of mechanisms of action of T_{reg} cells have been reported,[24] only some are well supported by data from experimental models and humans. The following are the best-defined mechanisms.

- **CTLA-4-mediated suppression of immune responses.** One of the canonical features of Foxp3+ T_{reg} cells is the stable expression of CTLA-4. As we discussed earlier, CTLA-4 on T_{reg} cells may remove B7 from APCs and thus shut off immune responses (see Figures 8.5 and 8.6). The ability of anti-CTLA-4 antibody to promote T cell responses may be at least partly related to blocking of the receptor on T_{reg} cells or even depletion of the cells.

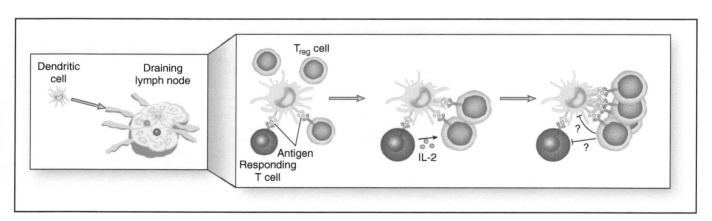

Figure 8.8 The role of IL-2 in the function of T_{reg} cells. When effector cells and T_{reg} cells recognize antigen displayed by an APC, the effector cell produces IL-2, which acts on the T_{reg} cells, stimulates their proliferation and suppressive activity, and thus limits the responses of the effector cells.

APC, antigen-presenting cell; IL-2, interleukin-2; T_{reg}, regulatory T.

Source: Adapted with permission from Carrizosa E, Mempel TR. Immunology: in the right place at the right time. *Nature*. 2015;528(7581):205–206. doi:10.1038/nature16312

- **Secretion of immunosuppressive cytokines.** Some T_{reg} cells produce inhibitory cytokines such as IL-10 and transforming growth factor-β (TGF-β), which inhibit immune responses. T_{reg} cells that are induced by culture with these cytokines and secrete the cytokines have been called "Tr1 cells"; these may or may not express Foxp3. IL-10 may be especially important for regulating immune responses in mucosal tissues, particularly the gut, because deletion of the IL-10 gene selectively in Foxp3$^+$ cells causes colitis but not other manifestations of autoimmunity.
- **Consumption of IL-2.** As T_{reg} cells express high levels of IL-2R, they absorb this growth factor from the environment of immune activation. The resultant depletion of IL-2 may lead to defective T cell proliferation.

These mechanisms of suppression are not mutually exclusive. The same T_{reg} cells may use more than one of these mechanisms. There may also be subsets of T_{reg} cells that rely mainly on one or the other mechanism to mediate their suppressive effects.

Role of T_{reg} Cells in Antitumor Immune Responses

Numerous experimental models have demonstrated that depletion of T_{reg} cells enhances antitumor immunity. However, there is no direct evidence that tumors activate T_{reg} cells specific for tumor antigens at different stages of their growth. Meta-analyses of the reported immune infiltrates in tumors have revealed an extremely variable picture in which high numbers of T_{reg} cells appear to predict either better or worse patient outcomes depending on the tumor type.[25] Nevertheless, depleting T_{reg} cells or blocking their suppressive functions is likely to promote antitumor immune responses and eradication of the tumors.

Therapeutic Approaches for Manipulating T_{reg} Cells

Many attempts to deplete T_{reg} cells or inhibit their actions are ongoing in preclinical tumor models. The approaches include targeting surface markers of T_{reg} cells, such as CD25 and GITR, with depleting antibodies. The limitation of such approaches is that no marker is unique to T_{reg} cells, and most of these surface proteins are transiently or stably expressed on activated and effector T cells as well. Other approaches include agents that inhibit the suppressive cytokines produced by T_{reg} cells, including IL-10 and TGF-β. The risk of all such treatments is that they unleash the immune system and lead to exaggerated responses against self-antigens and other harmless antigens, thus triggering inflammatory reactions.

There is also a great interest in the converse strategy of increasing T_{reg} cell numbers or functions to treat autoimmune diseases. One such approach is to administer low doses of IL-2, or use mutants of IL-2 that bind preferentially to CD25, thus activating T_{reg} cells. Thus, our new understanding of immune regulation has prompted us to move from using IL-2 to promote immune activation in cancer to using it to promote immune suppression in autoimmunity. Cell therapy with *ex vivo*-activated T_{reg} cells is also being tried in patients.

CONCLUSION

Understanding immune regulation is one of the dominant themes of modern immunology. Elegant experimental models have provided many insights into the complex pathways that regulate immune responses, and many of these insights are being translated to the understanding and treatment of diseases. Perhaps the most impressive accomplishment in this field has been the development of therapies that aim to promote or reduce regulation for autoimmune disease or cancer. Much remains to be learned about the induction and maintenance of antigen-specific tolerance in humans, and the way these mechanisms are disturbed during various disease states. Answering these questions requires the development of new technologies for studying antigen-specific lymphocytes in patients and examining effector and regulatory populations in tissues. Clinical successes and the need for more fundamental information undoubtedly drive the development of these technologies. It is not too optimistic to believe that knowledge about immune regulation will continue to grow rapidly and will lead to a better understanding of diseases as well as to even more new therapeutic advances.

ACKNOWLEDGMENTS

The contribution of Professor Abul K. Abbas to this chapter in the previous edition is greatly appreciated.

KEY REFERENCES

Only key references appear in the print edition. The full reference list appears in the digital product on Springer Publishing Connect: connect.springerpub.com/content/book/978-0-8261-3743-2/part/part01/chapter/ch08

2. Abbas AK, Lichtman AH, Pillai S. Cellular and Molecular Immunology. 8th ed. Elsevier; 2015.
4. Walker LSK, Abbas AK. The enemy within: keeping self-reactive T cells at bay in the periphery. *Nat Rev Immunol.* 2002;2(1):11–19. doi:10.1038/nri701
6. Abbas AK, Lichtman AH, Pillai S. *Basic Immunology.* 5th ed. Elsevier; 2016.
9. Kuehn HS, Ouyang W, Lo B, et al. Immune dysregulation in human subjects with heterozygous germline mutations in CTLA4. *Science.* 2014;345(6204):1623–1627. doi:10.1126/science.1255904
10. Schubert D, Bode C, Kenefeck R, et al. Autosomal dominant immune dysregulation syndrome in humans with CTLA4 mutations. *Nat Med.* 2014;20(12):1410–1416. doi:10.1038/nm.3746
18. Allison JP. Checkpoints. *Cell.* 2015;162(6):1202–1205. doi:10.1016/j.cell.2015.08.047
23. Carrizosa E, Mempel TR. Immunology: in the right place at the right time. *Nature.* 2015;528(7581):205–206. doi:10.1038/nature16312

9

B Cells in Solid Tumors: Their Role in Tumor Pathogenesis and Antitumor Immunity

Muhammad Husnain, Yu Zhang, and Joseph D. Rosenblatt

KEY POINTS

- B cells may promote the development of progression of cancer, attenuate antitumor immune response, or, alternatively, mediate antitumor effects by killing tumor cells directly, through antibody production or by enhancing adaptive antitumor responses.

- Various mechanisms are involved in regulatory B (B_{reg}) cell suppression of immunity: promoting regulatory T cell (T_{reg} cell) activation and expansion; secretion of suppressive cytokines (e.g., interleukin [IL]-10, IL-35, transforming growth factor beta [TGF-β]), and inhibitory molecules expressed on the cell surface (e.g., programmed cell death-ligand 1 [PDL-1]) leading to inhibition of T and/or natural killer (NK) cell cytotoxic activity.

- Evidence for B cell suppression of antitumor immunity has been seen in multiple murine models and in a variety of human solid tumor settings, including hepatocellular carcinoma, melanoma, and ovarian, breast, pancreatic, and lung cancers.

- Tumor-infiltrating B cells, which are often contained within "tertiary lymphoid structures," may also mediate antitumor response in a variety of tumors, including melanoma, non-small cell lung cancer (NSCLC), and cervical, breast, renal cell, and oropharyngeal cancer.

INTRODUCTION

The role of B cells in the formation and production of antibodies is well known. B cells are phenotypically and functionally heterogeneous and may play a variety of roles in the adaptive immune system; they may serve as antigen-presenting cells, as regulators of CD4+ T cell differentiation, or may produce cytokines that regulate CD4+, CD8+ T cell, and natural killer (NK) cell activity.

Increasing evidence suggests an important role for B cells in the modulation of immune response to tumors.[1–13] Depending upon the tumor setting, B cells may promote the development or progression of cancer, attenuate antitumor immune response, or, alternatively, mediate antitumor effects by killing tumor cells directly, through antibody production, or by enhancing adaptive antitumor immune responses. Improved understanding of the role played by B cells in modulating antitumor response and shaping the tumor microenvironment may provide new avenues for therapeutic intervention through selective depletion of B_{reg} subpopulations. In this review, we will focus on the role of B cells in modulating tumor immunity, and discuss mechanisms of B cell regulatory and effector function that affect tumorigenesis, tumor growth and metastatic spread, and antitumor immune response.

B CELL SUPPRESSION OF ANTITUMOR IMMUNITY: EARLY EVIDENCE

While a role of regulatory T cells (T_{reg} cells) in the suppression of antitumor immunity has been well documented, accumulating evidence points to a potential suppressive role for B cells as well. B cells with suppressive phenotype are called regulatory B (B_{reg}) cells. B cells have been demonstrated to play a significant role in modulating immune responses in a variety of autoimmune disorders, including autoimmune encephalomyelitis,[14] systemic lupus erythematosus,[15–17] type 1 diabetes mellitus,[18] and multiple sclerosis.[19]

Early observations regarding a possible role of B lymphocytes in modulating antitumor immunity were reported by Brodt et al. in studies of syngeneic methylcholanthrene-induced tumors in C57BL/6 mice, which demonstrated that treatment of tumor-bearing mice with anti-mouse immunoglobulin M (IgM) serum, leading to B cell depletion, reduced tumor growth and metastasis.[5] Following this, Moach et al.[6] in a murine skin cancer model and Qin et al.[7] in mammary adenocarcinoma mice (TS/A) demonstrated augmented antitumor immunity in B cell-deficient mice (BCDM). Qin also noted that enhanced cytotoxic T lymphocyte (CTL)-mediated antitumor immunity and suppressed the growth of TS/A tumors in BCDM, which was reversed following adoptive transfer of B cells.

Using three different tumor cell lines (Rous sarcoma virus-induced CSA1M fibrosarcoma, radiation-induced OV-HM ovarian carcinoma, and methylcholanthrene-induced BAMC-1 fibrosarcoma), Wijesuriya et al. showed that the elimination of B cells from the splenic population of tumor-bearing mice resulted in enhanced interferon (IFN)-γ production by tumor-specific T cells in response to tumor.[20] The suppressive effects of B cells appeared to depend upon the ability of CD40+ B cells to downregulate IL-12 production by antigen-presenting cells.[20] Shah et al. demonstrated that other solid tumors, such as the MC38 murine colon carcinoma and the EL-4 thymoma, were rejected immunologically in BCDM, while the adoptive transfer of B cells into BCDM reversed tumor resistance.[8] However, the adoptive transfer of CD40⁻⁻ B cells into BCDM also restored growth of MC38 colon carcinoma in vivo, suggesting that factors in addition to CD40 signaling were involved in dampening of the antitumor responses in vivo.[8] In both the MC38 colon and EL-4 thymoma models, tumor rejection in BCDM was associated with enhanced antitumor Th$_1$ cytokine and cytolytic responses, which were reversed upon adoptive B cell reconstitution of BCDM.[8]

MECHANISMS OF B CELL SUPPRESSION OF ANTITUMOR IMMUNITY

A variety of different mechanisms have been implicated in the suppression of antitumor immunity. Inoue et al.[3] and Tao et al.[21] studied EL4 engineered to express the Friend murine leukemia virus gag antigen (EL4-gag), D5 mouse melanoma, and MCA304 sarcoma mouse models. They demonstrated that B$_{reg}$ function depended upon IL-10 production by B cells, and that decreasing IL-10 production by B cells led to enhanced antitumor immune responses.[3,21] In contrast, Zhang et al. showed that although in the EMT-6 murine breast cancer model tumor growth was dependent on the presence of B cells, and mediated by B$_{reg}$ conversion of CD4+ T cells to FoxP3+ T$_{reg}$ cells, tumor growth did not depend upon direct IL-10 secretion by B cells.[22] EMT-6 mammary tumor-infiltrating B (TIL-B) cells expressed increased levels of the checkpoint inhibitory ligand programmed cell death-ligand 1 (PDL-1), membrane-bound latency associated peptide/transforming growth factor beta (LAP/TGF-β), CD80, and CD86 relative to non-infiltrating splenic B cells.[23] Tumor-educated B cells, co-cultured with EMT-6 cells, suppressed CD4+ and CD8+ T cell proliferation, Th1 cytokine secretion, and NK-cell proliferation (Figure 9.1).[22,23,24] Although a subset of LAP/TGF-β, expressing B cells could be induced to produce IL-10 following stimulation with lipopolysaccharide (LPS),

demonstrating that an IL-10-producing population was contained within the TIL-B cells, EMT-6 tumor growth could nevertheless be "rescued" through adoptive transfer of IL-10⁻/⁻–deficient B cells. Adoptive transfer of B cells restored tumor growth and decreased cytolytic T cell activity, reduced tumor infiltration by CD8+ T cells and NK cells, and reduced production of cytolytic T cells.

B CELL EFFECTS ON TUMOR ANGIOGENESIS

In addition to immune-suppressive effects, B cells appeared to augment angiogenesis in several murine models. Yang et al. studied the B16 melanoma and Lewis Lung Cancer (LLC) mouse models and showed that B cells augmented tumor angiogenesis in a manner that was dependent on activation of signaling by STAT3. STAT3 was persistently activated in TIL-B cells. When B16 mouse melanoma cells or LLC mouse lung tumor cells were implanted into *Rag1*⁻/⁻ mice, in the presence or absence of either STAT3+/+ or STAT3⁻/⁻ B cells, the presence of STAT3 +/+ B cells in the tumor microenvironment increased tumor angiogenesis and accelerated growth of both B16 melanoma and LLC lung tumors, while the addition of STAT3⁻/⁻ B cells showed reduced angiogenesis and tumor growth.[25] B cells isolated from tumor tissues and the tumor-draining lymph nodes showed increased expression of proangiogenic genes, such as *S1PR1, MMP9, HIF1α, and vascular endothelial growth factor (VEGF;* Figure 9.2).[25]

Zhang et al. demonstrated that CD5+ B cells promoted tumor growth in a B16 melanoma mouse model as compared to CD5⁻ B cells. These CD5+ B cells could bind to IL-6 in the absence of IL-6Rα and lead to activation of STAT3 via gp30 and its downstream kinase JAK2.[26] CD5+ B cells demonstrated activation of STAT3 in several different human tumor tissues, including prostate, ovarian, and lung cancer tissues. These studies pointed to a novel role of STAT3-activated B cells in promoting tumor progression through effects on angiogenesis as well as antitumor immunity.

B CELL EFFECTS ON METASTASES

In addition to the effects on immunity and angiogenesis, B cells have been directly implicated in the promotion of metastases. Olkhanud et al. showed that tumor-induced B$_{reg}$ cells in a 4T1 murine mammary cancer model constitutively expressed STAT3 and promoted lung metastasis through TGF-β–mediated conversion of CD4+ T cells to FoxP3 T$_{reg}$ cells.[9] The 4T1 tumors did not metastasize into the lungs In the absence of tumor-induced B$_{reg}$ cells, due to reduced conversion of T cells into T$_{reg}$ cells. Phenotypically, these tumor-induced B$_{reg}$ cells were CD19+CD25ʰⁱCD69ʰⁱ. These tumor-induced B$_{reg}$ cells expressed high levels of B7-H1, CD80, and CD86, as well as intermediate levels of IgM and low levels of CD62L.[9]

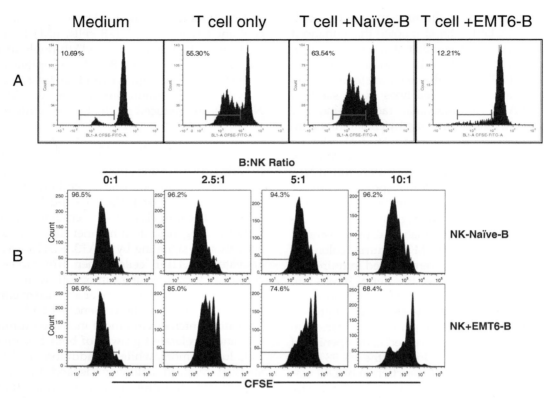

Figure 9.1 Tumor-educated B cells suppress T and NK cell proliferation. Naïve B cells were co-cultured with mitomycin C-treated EMT-6 breast cancer cells for 2 days (1:1 ratio) to yield EMT-6 tumor-educated B cells (EMT6-B). Murine CD19+ B cells were positively selected as naïve B cells. **(A)** Tumor-conditioned B cells suppress T cell proliferation in vitro. CFSE-labeled purified T cells were stimulated with plate-bound anti-CD3/CD28 antibodies. Purified naïve B cells or EMT6-B were added to the co-culture at a B:T cell ratio of 10:1. About 3 days later, cells were harvested and surface stained for CD3+ T cells. Live CD3+ T cell proliferation was assessed based on CFSE expression. The percentage of proliferating CD3 cells is indicated for each co-culture condition. **(B)** Tumor-educated B cells suppress NK cell proliferation in vitro. NK cells were isolated from naïve BALB/c mice and labeled with CFSE. CFSE-labeled NK cells were co-cultured with EMT6-B or naïve B cells at the indicated B:NK ratio and stimulated with mIL-15 for 4 days. NK cell proliferation was evaluated by flow cytometry for CFSE. The percentage of proliferating cells is indicated for each group.

CFSE, carboxyfluorescein succinimidyl ester dye; NK, natural killer.

Guan et al. studied 134 patients with breast cancer and showed that CD19+CD24+CD38+ B cells were found in a higher percentage in breast tissue and the peripheral blood of patients with invasive breast cancer compared to patients with benign tumors or healthy individuals.[27] These B cells secreted IL-10 and when co-cultured with T cells from patients with invasive breast cancer induced formation of PDL-1–dependent CD4+FoxP3+ T cells.[27] Ishigami et al. studied the role of tumor-infiltrating lymphocytes (TILs) in patients with breast cancer and showed that tumor-infiltrating IL-10+CD25– B$_{regs}$ were associated with a significantly increased rate of metastasis and played a role in the induction of T$_{reg}$ cells.[28] Whether reduction in tumor-infiltrating B$_{reg}$ could augment response to checkpoint inhibitors such as nivolumab in patients with breast cancer remains an open question.

More recently, Yan et al. studying the 4T1 breast cancer model also proposed a highly novel role for pathogenic antibodies in the promotion of metastases. These investigators demonstrated that tumor-induced B cells promoted lymph node metastasis through the production of pathogenic immunoglobulins against heat shock protein family A member 4 (HSPA4). HSPA4 is a member of the HSP70 family of tumor antigens. Immunoglobulin against HSPA4 antigen seemed to promote tumor cell chemotaxis to the lymph node matrix via a CXCR4–SDF-1α interaction. CXCR4 expression and SDF-1α secretion were significantly upregulated when tumors were treated with pathogenic immunoglobulin as compared to normal immunoglobulin leading to metastatic spread to lymph nodes. Pathogenic immunoglobulin bound to membrane glycosylated HSPA4 to activate the CXCR4/SDF-1α axis and led to breast cancer lymph node metastasis. Pathogenic immunoglobulin was able to enhance phosphorylation of IkBα and p65, which are markers of NF-kβ activation. B^{null} mice (Igμ heavy-chain

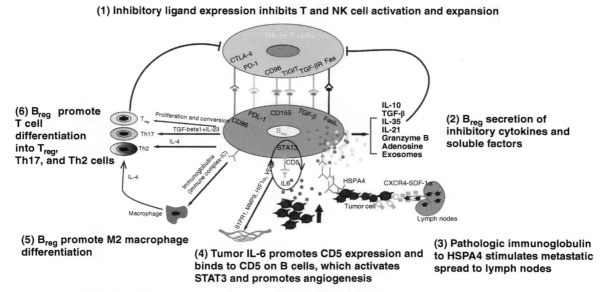

Figure 9.2 **Protumorigenic B_{reg} effects on antitumor immune response, angiogenesis, and metastatic potential. (1)** B_{reg} may express membrane ligands such as TGF-β or PDL-1, which bind to inhibitory and checkpoint receptors expressed on NK or T cells to reduce NK or T cell cytokine release, proliferation, or cytotoxic function and suppress antitumor immune response. **(2)** B_{reg} secrete cytokines such as IL-10, IL-21, or soluble factors such as adenosine that inhibit immune effector function. **(3)** B cell may secrete pathogenic antibodies directed against tumor antigens such as HSPA4 in breast cancer cells, which in turn stimulate tumor cell expression of chemokine receptors such as CXCR4. Locally secreted SDF-1α chemokine attracts CXCR4+ tumor cells leading to metastasis to lymph nodes and bone marrow. **(4)** CD5 on the B cell surface can bind to tumor-secreted IL-6, leading to phosphorylation of STAT3, which promotes expression of proangiogenic factors, such as VEGF, that stimulate tumor angiogenesis. **(5)** B cell-secreted immunoglobulins form immune complexes that promote tumor-associated macrophage differentiation (TAM, or M2) leading to CD4+ T cell differentiation into Th2, and suppression of antitumor Th1 response. **(6)** B_{reg} cells can promote T_{reg} cell proliferation and convert conventional CD4+ T cells into inducible T_{reg} cells, as well as stimulate Th2 or Th17 differentiation. Details in text.

B_{reg}, regulatory B cell; CFSE, carboxyfluorescein succinimidyl ester dye; HSPA4, heat shock protein family A member 4; IL, interleukin; NK, natural killer; PDL-1, programmed cell death-ligand 1; TGF-β, transforming growth factor beta; T_{reg}, regulatory T.

knockout) showed significantly reduced pathogenic immunoglobulin and lymph node metastasis.[29] High levels of serum HSPA4 immunoglobulin antibodies were reported in patients with breast cancer and appear to correlate with poor prognosis.[29] This mechanism, if confirmed independently, may have identified an important new role for paraneoplastic antibody production by B cells in breast cancer pathogenesis and suggests new approaches for predicting metastatic spread and possibly for prevention of metastases.

B CELLS IN PROSTATE, PANCREATIC, GASTROINTESTINAL, AND HEPATOCELLULAR CANCERS AND OTHER SOLID TUMORS

Ammirante et al. in a murine prostate cancer model showed that castrate resistance was promoted by B cells in prostate cancer cells. Using a prostate cancer mouse model, they showed that androgen-deprived prostate cancer is infiltrated by B cells that produce cytokines that activate IkB kinase α (IKKα), a catalytic subunit of NF-kβ. Depletion of B cells prevented IKKα activation

and delayed growth of castrate-resistant prostate cancer. IKKα induces phosphorylation and nuclear translocation of E2F1 and its recruitment to the *Bmil* promoter, leading to progression of castrate-resistant prostate cancer.[2,30] Shalapour et al. further reported that these tumors were more responsive to oxaliplatin in BCDM but acquired oxaliplatin resistance following adoptive transfer of B cells. The immunosuppressive B cells expressed IgA, IL-10, and PDL-1, and elimination of B cells facilitated CTL-dependent eradication of tumors,[10] suggesting a role for B cells in modulating immune response following cytotoxic chemotherapy.

Lee et al. using Kras (G12D) pancreatic ductal adenocarcinoma (PDAC) mouse model, as well as human tumors, demonstrated that HIF1α deletion accelerated tumor growth and was accompanied by significant increase in influx of a so called "B1b" B cell subtype. B1b cells are a subset of mature B cells and have a CD19+CD43+IgM^{hi}CD5- phenotype. B cell depletion with an anti-CD20 antibody in HIF1α-deficient mice inhibited tumor progression and suppressed pancreatic tumorigenesis.[31] Using the same Kras (G12D) PDAC mouse model Pylayeva-Gupta et al. showed that these B cells were CD1d(hi)CD5[+] and that a protumorigenic effect was mediated by IL-35.[32] The growth of orthotopic pancreatic cancer was significantly reduced in BCDM but was rescued following adoptive transfer of CD1d[hi]CD5[+] B cells.[32] The protumorigenic effect of B cells was mediated in part by IL-35-induced tumor cell proliferation. IL-35 secreted by CD1d[hi]CD5[+] B cells led to further expansion of IL-35[+]B$_{reg}$ cells. IL-35 has also been reported to be upregulated in sera of patients with pancreatic cancer.[33] IL-35-induced B$_{reg}$ cells were shown to inhibit T$_H$17 and T$_H$1 T cell generation and promote the expansion of T$_{reg}$ cells leading to the growth of tumor.[34]

Das et al. showed that a key component of B cell receptor (BCR) signaling, Bruton's tyrosine kinase (BTK), played a potential role in regulation of CD1d[hi]CD5[+] B$_{reg}$ cells. Treatment with BTK inhibitor tirabrutinib-inhibited CD1d[hi]CD5[+] B$_{reg}$ differentiation and production of IL-10 and IL-35 increased stromal CD8[+]INF-γ[+] cytotoxic T cells and reduced tumor cell proliferation in mice bearing orthotopically implanted Kras G12D-pancreatic cancer.[35] In a PDAC mouse model, Gunderson et al. showed that tumor growth was dependent on a cross talk between B cells and FcR-γ[+] tumor-associated macrophages. Treatment of PDAC-bearing mice with a BTK inhibitor resulted in reprogramming of macrophages toward a T$_H$1 phenotype (induced expression of T$_H$1 cytokines, IL-12, TNF-α, IL-6, and IL-1-β) that enhanced CD8[+] T cell cytotoxicity and suppressed tumor growth.[36] This led to a phase III clinical trial of the BTK inhibitor ibrutinib versus placebo, in combination with nab-paclitaxel and gemcitabine, in the first line treatment of patients with metastatic pancreatic adenocarcinoma (ClinicalTrials.gov: NCT02436668). However, the human study failed to show a statistically significant improvement in progression-free or overall survival.[36,37]

Shi et al. studied the role of B$_{regs}$ in 60 healthy volunteers and 60 patients with esophageal cancer.[38] They demonstrated that the percentages of CD19[+]CD5[+]FoxP3[+], IL-10, and TGF-β-producing B$_{regs}$ were significantly higher in the peripheral blood of patients with esophageal cancer compared to healthy adults and declined after surgery, suggesting that B cells might be playing a role in tumor progression.[38] In other studies, Mao et al. showed that exosomes from patients with esophageal squamous cell carcinoma (ESCC) increased expression of IL-10 and the PD-1 checkpoint on B$_{reg}$ cells.[39] Genes related to the Toll-like receptor (TLR) 4 and mitogen-activated protein kinase (MAPK) signaling pathways were differentially expressed in B$_{reg}$ cells, and the authors postulated that ESCC-derived exosomes activated TLR4 and MAPK signaling pathways, leading to PD-1 expression and IL-10 secretion in B cells.[39] Similarly, Lundgren et al. analyzed tissue microarrays from 154 cases of epithelial ovarian cancer and showed that CD20[+]CD138[+] and immunoglobulin κ C-expressing B cells were associated with significantly higher tumor grade, showing that B$_{reg}$ cell infiltration in epithelial ovarian cancer had a significant impact on tumor progression.[40]

B$_{reg}$ cells may also play a significant role in the development of lung cancer. Peripheral blood mononuclear cells from patients with lung cancer had higher frequencies of CD19[+]CD24[hi]CD27[+] B$_{reg}$ as compared to control healthy donors. Co-culture of peripheral blood mononuclear cells with LPS-stimulated cancer cells significantly increased the proportion of CD19[+]CD24[hi]CD27[+] and CD19[+]IL-10[+] B cells and increased the number of T$_{reg}$ cells, suggesting that B$_{reg}$ cells promote tumor growth by inhibiting CD4[+] T cell proliferation while promoting T$_{reg}$ expansion.[41] Seo et al. showed that in patients with non-small cell lung cancers (NSCLCs), both tumor-associated macrophages and B$_{reg}$ cells were immunosuppressive and showed decreased cytolytic activity of CD8 T cells in the presence of B cells and macrophages.[42]

Human hepatocellular carcinoma (HCC) is another human tumor with accumulating evidence for B cell modulation of immunity. Wang et al. showed that CD19[+]CD5[+]CD1d[hi] B$_{regs}$ correlated positively with the presence of CD4[+]CD25[+]CD127[low] T$_{reg}$ cells and advanced stage of primary hepatic carcinoma.[43] Shao et al. showed that in patients with HCC, increased intrahepatic B cells at tumor margins were associated with tumor invasion, advanced tumor stage, and tumor recurrence. They showed that human B$_{regs}$ promoted HCC growth in SCID mice independent of T$_{reg}$ cells. Human B$_{regs}$ appear to promote growth and invasiveness of HCC in vitro through CD40/CD154 signaling.[44]

Xiao et al. identified a unique subset of TIL-B cells that expressed higher levels of PD-1 and constituted 10% of all B cells in advanced stage HCC. These PD-1[hi] B cells were CD5[(hi)]CD24[(±)]CD27[(hi/+)]CD38[(dim)]. The authors postulated that PD-1[hi] B cells play a significant role in suppressing tumor-specific T cell immunity and promote cancer growth via IL-10 secretion following engagement of PD-1 by HCC tumor-expressed PDL-1.[45] Ye et al. reported significantly higher TIM-1[+] CD5[high]CD24[-]CD27±CD38[+] B$_{reg}$ cell infiltration in HCC compared with normal tissue. B cells activated by tumor-derived exosomes via TLR 2/4 and MAPK expressed TIM-1 and were capable of suppressing CD8[+] T cells.[46] TIM-1[+] B cells co-cultured with CD8[+] T cells suppressed CD8[+] T cell proliferation and decreased CD8 production of TNF-α and INF-γ.[46]

Wu et al. showed that levels of circulating PDL-1[+] B cells were elevated in patients with melanoma and correlated with tumor stage, with highest levels seen in stage IV with bone metastasis. PDL-1+ B$_{regs}$ were phenotypically IgM[+]IgD[+]CD20[+]CD27[-] and could act as T cell suppressors. When CD4[+] or CD8[+] T cells were incubated with these PDL-1[+] B cells from patients with metastatic melanoma, it showed significantly reduced expression of INF-γ compared to incubation with B cells from healthy donors. Higher levels of expression of PDL-1 on B cells correlated with greater reductions in INF-γ expression.[46,47]

Wang et al. reported that PD-1[+] B$_{reg}$ cells were significantly upregulated in patients with differentiated thyroid tumors. PD-1[+] B$_{regs}$ expressed PDL-1, suppressed the proliferation of CD4[+] and CD8[+] T cells, and blockade of PDL-1 increased proliferation and viability of T cells in vitro.[48]

Zhou et al. reported that CD19[+]IL-10[+] B$_{regs}$ were significantly increased in the microenvironment of tongue squamous cell carcinoma (TSCC), and predicted poor overall survival. In vitro experiments showed that B$_{regs}$ increased significantly after co-culture with TSCC cell lines and converted CD4[+] T cells into CD4[+]Foxp3[+] T$_{reg}$ cells.[49]

A diagram summarizing several mechanisms implicated in B$_{reg}$ suppression of antitumor immunity and enhancement of tumor growth and metastasis is presented in Figure 9.2.

SUMMARY

Accumulating evidence indicates that B$_{reg}$ cells may play a significant role in the suppression of innate and adaptive immune response, through inhibition of CD4[+], CD8[+] T cell and NK expansion and activation, and through the promotion of T$_{reg}$ cell expansion and suppressive function. These B$_{reg}$ cells exert their suppressive function and promote tumor growth through the elaboration of cytokines such as IL-10, TGF-β, and IL-35, expression of Granzyme B and/or Fas-L, and presentation of checkpoint ligands such as PDL-1. Induction of a B$_{reg}$ phenotype may be stimulated by tumor exosomes, cytokines, or through direct interaction with tumor cells expressing negative regulatory molecules such as PDL-1. Increased understanding of mechanisms of suppression and better phenotypic characterization of B$_{regs}$ may lead to novel approaches that will enhance the effects of immunotherapy and facilitate immune tumor rejection.

B CELLS MAY MEDIATE ANTITUMOR EFFECTS: THE ROLE OF TERTIARY LYMPHOID STRUCTURES

While the previously cited studies in both murine and human settings implicate B$_{reg}$ activity in the suppression of antitumor immunity, many other studies suggest that, depending upon the context, B cells may actually facilitate tumor rejection. Solid tumors in humans often contain significant B cell populations, suggesting a role for these cells in shaping the tumor microenvironment.[50,51]

The presence of TIL-B cells have been reported to confer a positive prognosis in several tumors. Schmidt et al. showed that TIL-B cells correlated with positive prognosis patients with breast cancer.[50] Erdag et al. showed that increased proportions of TIL-B cells correlated with increased survival in metastatic melanoma.[51] Nedergaard et al. showed that peritumoral CD20[+] B cells were significantly lower in patients with cervical squamous cell carcinoma in whom disease relapsed, as compared to patients without relapse, suggesting TIL-B cells conferred a protective effect.[52] Al-Shibli et al. studied the prognostic role of epithelial and stromal lymphocyte infiltration in NSCLC. They showed that increasing epithelial CD8[+], stromal CD8[+], epithelial CD20[+], stromal CD20[+,] and stromal CD4[+] lymphocyte infiltration correlated with improved disease-specific survival in patients with NSCLC, suggesting that infiltrating B effector cells played a role in antitumor immune response.[53] Berntsson et al. studied the role of CD20[+]CD138[+] and immunoglobulin κ[+]B cells in tissue microarrays with tumors from 557 cases of colorectal cancer and demonstrated that a higher density of CD20[+] cells correlated with an improved overall survival and lower T-stage. CD138 and IGKC expression on B cells also correlated with an improved overall survival (OS).[54]

In patients with infection, inflammation, or autoimmune diseases, ectopic lymphoid structures called tertiary lymphoid structures (TLSs) may form within the tissues. TLS seems to play a significant role in infection and inflammation. Recently, there has been increasing evidence for a beneficial role for TLS in tumor immunity.[55] The presence of TLS has been linked to improved immunotherapy responses and is associated with improved overall survival in patients with soft tissue sarcoma, melanoma, and renal cell carcinoma, respectively.[56–58]

Hladikova et al. showed higher expression of B cell-related genes and higher concentration of CD20[+] B cells in human papillomavirus (HPV)-associated oropharyngeal squamous cell carcinoma. CD20[+] TIL-B cells formed non-organized aggregates within oropharyngeal squamous cell carcinoma tumor tissue. High density of TIL-B cells was associated with local CXCL9 chemokine production and increased levels of CD8[+] T cell infiltration and were predictive of improved prognosis in these patients.[59]

B cells could theoretically augment antitumor immune response by antigen presentation, antibody production, and/or through the local production of cytokines. Hansen et al. showed that in medullary carcinoma of breast, improved clinical outcome was associated with the presence of increased lymphoplasmacytic infiltrate in tumor stroma. They showed that a humoral antibody response against actin was antigen-driven, affinity-maturated, and appeared to be stimulated by an increased rate of apoptosis within the tumor.[60,61] Human lung cancer tissue xenotransplanted into SCID mice showed that human immunoglobulin production from TIL-B cells was observed in xenotransplanted mice and the levels of immunoglobulin were significantly higher in mice in whom tumor regressed, compared to mice in whom tumor progressed, suggesting that immunoglobulin produced by TIL-B cells played a role in reducing tumor growth.[62] In another report, B cell depletion with an anti-CD20 antibody in the B16 melanoma model resulted in increased tumor growth and lung metastasis and also impaired induction of INF-γ secreting CD4[+] and CD8[+] T cells in tumor-draining lymph nodes in response to challenge with B16 melanoma cells.[63] These and other results also suggest that widely used anti-CD20 antibodies may not be an optimal method of depleting immunosuppressive B_{reg} cells in solid tumors and might actually impair antitumor immunity.

Luther et al. showed that B lymphocyte chemoattractant (BCL) expression in pancreatic islets led to the development of TLSs.[64] Lymphotoxin-α is also thought to play a role in the formation of lymphoid-like structures in the tumor microenvironment containing aggregates of T cells, antigen-presenting cells, and B cells.[65] In patients with lung cancer, TLS with high density of follicular B cells correlated with long-term survival both in patients with early stage lung cancer and in patients with advanced lung cancer.[66] Mechanisms leading to TLS formation and a beneficial B cell-mediated response, as opposed to induction of immunosuppressive B_{regs} and reduction in antitumor immunity, remain poorly understood and are an important target for further study in both murine and human settings.

CONCLUSION

B cells have a wide variety of phenotypes and may play a regulatory role in suppression of antitumor immunity or alternatively may have an effector phenotype and augment antitumor immunity. A variety of phenotypic markers have been associated with B_{reg} cells in human and murine tumors, and the phenotype may vary between different malignancies. B_{reg} suppression of immunity is associated with activation or expansion of T_{reg} cells and inhibition of T and/or NK cell cytotoxic activity. Antitumor activity has been associated with production of antitumor antibodies, a direct protective effect through tumor-infiltrating B lymphocytes or through the

formation of tertiary lymphoid structures. The emerging biology suggests that interventions directed at depletion of B_{reg} may be possible to augment antitumor immunity. However, depletion of B_{reg} cells with anti-CD20 antibodies or through blocking B cell function by blocking BTK receptors on B cells has not demonstrated significant benefit. Alternative strategies such as targeting CD38, CD19, IL-10, inhibitory ligands, or downstream cytokines may prove more useful. More precise characterization of B_{reg} and B effector phenotype, downstream signaling mechanisms, and gene expression profiles of B_{reg} may facilitate selective targeting of B_{reg} in an effort to augment antitumor immunity. These strategies could be used to increase the efficacy of immunotherapies such as anti-PD-1–directed checkpoint blockade, bispecific T cell engagers, chimeric antigen receptor T cells (CAR T) cells, and other antitumor immunotherapies.

KEY REFERENCES

Only key references appear in the print edition. The full reference list appears in the digital product on Springer Publishing Connect: connect.springerpub.com/content/book/978-0-8261-3743-2/part/part01/chapter/ch09

4. Zhang Y, Gallastegui N, Rosenblatt JD. Regulatory B cells in anti-tumor immunity. *Int Immunol*. 2015;27(10):521–530. doi:10.1093/intimm/dxv034
7. Qin Z, Richter G, Schüler T, Ibe S, et al. B cells inhibit induction of T cell-dependent tumor immunity. *Nat Med*. 1998;4(5):627–630. doi:10.1038/nm0598-627
10. Shalapour S, Font-Burgada J, di Caro G, et al. Immunosuppressive plasma cells impede T-cell-dependent immunogenic chemotherapy. *Nature*. 2015;521(7550):94–98. doi:10.1038/nature14395
23. Zhang Y, Morgan R, Chen C, et al. Mammary-tumor-educated B cells acquire LAP/TGF-β and PD-L1 expression and suppress anti-tumor immune responses. *Int Immunol*. 2016;28(9):423–433. doi:10.1093/intimm/dxw007
45. Xiao X, Lao XM, Chen MM, et al. PD-1[hi] identifies a novel regulatory B-cell population in human hepatoma that promotes disease progression. *Cancer Discov*. 2016;6(5):546–559. doi:10.1158/2159-8290.CD-15-1408
55. Engelhard VH, Rodriguez AB, Mauldin IS, et al. Immune cell infiltration and tertiary lymphoid structures as determinants of antitumor immunity. *J Immunol*. 2018;200(2):432–442. doi:10.4049/jimmunol.1701269
57. Cabrita R, Lauss M, Sanna A, et al. Tertiary lymphoid structures improve immunotherapy and survival in melanoma. *Nature*. 2020;577(7791):561–565. doi:10.1038/s41586-019-1914-8

10

Functional Status of T Cells: Stemness Versus Terminal Differentiation

Alessandra Cesano, Alper Kearney, and Francesco M. Marincola

KEY POINTS

- Cytotoxic T cells come in different levels of differentiation—*T memory stem cells* (T_{scm}) are T lymphocytes endowed with stem cell-like properties, such as self-renewal aptitude, and the multipotent capacity to reconstitute the entire spectrum of memory and effector T cell subsets.[1,2] Human T_{scm} represents a small fraction (~2%–3%) of circulating T lymphocytes sitting astride naïve T cells (T_0) and *central memory T cells* (T_{CM}). They present with a peculiar functional, metabolic, and differentiation profile that enhances their antitumor properties predominantly by assuring their long-term memory functions.

- "Exhaustion" is a most frequently referred-to term that outlines the status of T cell dysfunction—Other terms are used to define T cell dysfunction, including the irreversible concept of "senescence." In the original definition, exhausted T cells (T_{EX}) are described as cells with languishing response to chronic (tonic) and/or repeated antigen stimulation by viruses and tumor cells. In extreme cases, chronic stimulation leads to irreversible exhaustion and "clonal deletion." Tumor-infiltrating lymphocytes (TILs) are a good example of dysfunctional T cells, and it is likely that most cancers are populated with T_{EX} because a continuous stimulus is delivered in the absence of sufficient co-stimulation in an immunosuppressive tumor microenvironment (TME).

- T_{scm} display a specific genetic, epigenetic, and transcriptional profile—Transcriptional and epigenetic regulation of T cell stemness depends on several signaling pathways that also operate in embryonic and adult stem cells. Moreover, the epigenetic progression of T cell differentiation suggests that chromatin accessibility is regulated in a gradual manner supporting the progressive model of T cell evolution. Similar processes are associated with control of stemness resulting in the open chromatin states in chromosomal regions controlling functionality responsible for nimble response to antigen. In addition, epigenetic control of T cell differentiation is dependent upon the reciprocal expression of several small noncoding microRNAs.

- The metabolic milieu dramatically affects T cell function and differentiation in the TME—Following the original expansion, most T cells undergo programmed apoptotic cell death during the contraction phase. However, a number of cells return to a quiescent anamnestic state capable of mounting a rapid response to subsequent antigen encounters. These evolutionary stages are demarcated by specific metabolic transitions that mirror functional needs. In addition, T cells need to adapt to circumstantial factors related to the heterogeneity of the TME by sustaining effector functions, while proliferating and overcoming unfavorable environmental signals. In this process, the T cells must balance the metabolic demands of energy maintenance, cell survival, and persistence with those of rapid proliferation and inflammatory function that adopt different strategies.

- Clinical considerations suggest that better fitness of T cells will increase their antitumor effectiveness—The longevity, self-renewal potential, and the capacity for immune reconstitution make T_{scm} ideal candidates for adoptive cell therapy since success is highly dependent upon T cell engraftment, peak of expansion, and persistence. Thus, the understanding that intrinsic T cell characteristics, as well as extrinsic factors, can affect T cell differentiation, metabolism, and function, and ultimately clinical outcomes in the setting of adoptive cell transfer (ACT), has spurred a series of therapeutic strategies targeting either the T cell product and/or the TME in order to improve the therapeutic effectiveness of ACT.

INTRODUCTION

T memory stem cells (T_{scm}) are T lymphocytes endowed with stem cell-like properties, such as self-renewal aptitude and the multipotent capacity to reconstitute the entire spectrum of memory and effector T cell subsets.[1,2] Human T_{scm} represent a small fraction (~2%–3%) of circulating T lymphocytes sitting astride naïve T cell (T_0) expressing cluster of differentiation (CD)45RA, CC chemokine receptor (CCR)-7, CD62L, CD28, CD27, and the interleukin (IL)-7Rα and central memory T cell (T_{CM}) expressing CD95, C-X-C chemokine receptor (CXCR)-3, IL-2Rβ, CD58, CD11a, and lymphocyte function-associated antigen 1/CD11A (LFA 1/CD11A).[3,4] The latter differentiate them from CCR7- and CD62L- effector memory T cells (TEM) and their CD45RA+ terminally differentiated ($T_{EMRA/EFF}$) offspring.[5,6] With the exception of $T_{EMRA/EFF}$ cells, a major demarcating step in T cell differentiation is the switch upon T cell activation from CD45RA to the CD45RO isoform, which stands as the prototypical marker for antigen-experienced T cells (Figure 10.1). Expression of CCR7 and CD62L allows antigen-experienced T cells to patrol central lymphoid organs.

T cell activation and differentiation are accompanied by dramatic shifts in cellular metabolic programs, which fulfill their bioenergetic, biosynthetic, and redox demands.[7–11] Specifically, quiescent naïve T cells and memory T cells rely on fatty acid oxidation (FAO) and oxidative phosphorylation (OXPHOS) to maintain their basic energy level, cellular function, and viability,[12,13] while activated T cells predominantly engage in aerobic glycolysis, the pentose phosphate pathway, and glutaminolysis to drive proliferation and subsequent effector functions.[14–17] This metabolic transition is dependent upon the induction of the transcription factor Myc.[12]

Thus, according to Lanzavecchia's progressive differentiation model, T_{scm} represent minimally differentiated T cells that maintain the proliferative properties of naïve and central memory cells.[18] Their characterization and relevance in health and disease have been amply discussed elsewhere, while this chapter focuses on their relevance as determinants of anticancer immune responsiveness and as components of adoptive cell transfer (ACT).[19]

In practice, stemness is often used in reference to a condition of T cell *"fitness"* positively associated with the effectiveness of ACT in the treatment of cancer. Several other terms have been introduced that refer to favorable or detrimental T cell qualities, such as polyfunctionality,[20] hyporesponsiveness, dysfunction, exhaustion, senescence, and degrees of sequential differentiation that determine their fate according to environmental signals.[21–23]

It is becoming increasingly appreciated that T cell differentiation and function are affected not only by the intensity and frequency of cognate T cell stimulation and co-stimulatory signaling but also by other metabolic

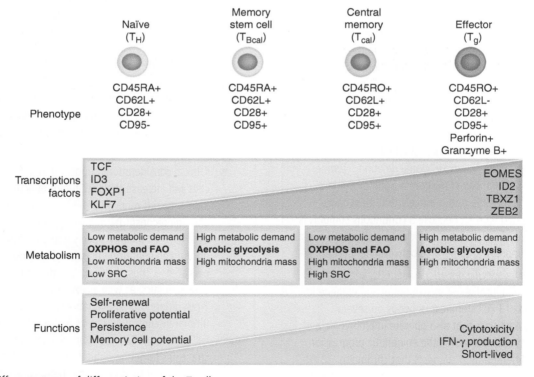

Figure 10.1 Different stages of differentiation of the T cell compartment.

FAO, fatty acid oxidation; IFN-γ, interferon-γ; OXPHOS, oxidative phosphorylation; SRC, spare (reserve) respiratory capacity.

factors that affect T cell function within the tumor micro-environment (TME). However, it should be emphasized that intrinsic functional characteristics of T cells determine their likelihood of success, and they can be observed ex vivo before administration.[3] These intrinsic properties likely affect T cells' ability to proliferate and traffic to the tumor site independent of circumstantial variables encountered upon arriving in the TME that further shape their destiny.[24] In addition, a stem cell memory-like phenotype can be reversed in vitro from differentiated T cells by adopting reprogramming techniques used in regenerative medicine, suggesting a certain degree of plasticity that may modulate ACT effectiveness during manufacturing as well as after delivery into patients.[25-36]

Unpublished observations in the late 1990s by Wang E pointed at an essential requirement for the effectiveness of ACT products: studying by whole genome transcriptional profiling approximately 200 retention samples saved at the time of administration of tumor-infiltrating lymphocytes (TILs) to patients with metastatic melanoma. Wang observed that effector T cell differentiation consistently excluded effectiveness. The observation was then so counterintuitive that it was never published, awaiting for an independent cohort validation. However, this seminal observation led to the collaborative characterization of stem cell-like T cells in experimental settings.[3] Subsequently, several preclinical studies demonstrated a negative correlation between the level of differentiation of T cells and their anticancer potential.[30,37] Now, T_{scm} is a well-established concept in clinical settings. In fact, multiple clinical studies reported an association between the administration of phenotypically and functionally T_{scm}-like (e.g., polyfunctionality in cytokine production) chimeric antigen receptor (CAR) engineered T cells and in vivo persistence, which results, in turn, in favorable outcomes.[20,38] Conversely, therapeutic failures have been associated with attenuated CAR T cell expansion and rapid attrition of CAR T effector cells.[39]

SEMANTICS

While experimentally the concept of T_{scm} is well accepted, it remains unclear to what extent it describes dynamic aspects of T cell function in distinct in vitro or in vivo conditions or it abides by a strictly sequential path of differentiation with limited potential for reversibility. Particularly in humans, it is unclear whether T cell persistence and distribution in the peripheral circulation, trafficking to tumor site, infiltration, and survival in the TME follow rigid blueprints rather than flexible plasticity.[40] For example, can T_{scm} become exhausted? And if they do, is this a reversible condition while exhaustion of other T cell subsets may reach a point of no-return associated with incremental epigenetic rearrangements?[41] Consequently, is environmental adaptation through

metabolic plasticity strictly linked to the status of differentiation of T cells or, at least, partially, does it reflect momentary adaptations of a given T cell subset within a bidirectional spectrum?[40,42] For instance, activated T cells display a glucose-sensitive metabolic checkpoint controlled by the energy sensor AMP-activated protein kinase (AMPK) that regulates mRNA translation and glutamine-dependent mitochondrial metabolism to maintain T cell viability.[42] However, it is unclear whether this metabolic checkpoint affects the status of differentiation along the spectrum from T_{scm} to T_{EM}.

This lack of clarity is reflected by the different appellations offered to describe functional statuses of T cells and associated markers, as well stated by Schietinger and Greenberg:[43] *"with the identification of phenotypic traits shared in different settings of T cell dysfunction, distinctions between such states have become blurred, resulting in confused use in the literature of the words exhaustion, tolerance, anergy, and ignorance"* (Table 10.1).[43]

CHARACTERISTICS OF T CELL EXHAUSTION (T_{EX})

"Exhaustion" is a most frequently referred-to term that outlines a status of T cell dysfunction,[23,43-52] occasionally associated with the irreversible concept of "senescence,"[53] the latter generally reserved for CD8+ T cells.[48] In the original definition, exhausted T cells (T_{EX}) are described as cells with languishing response to chronic (tonic) and/or repeated antigen stimulation by viruses and tumor cells.[23] In extreme cases, chronic stimulation leads to irreversible exhaustion and "clonal deletion" of pathogen-specific T cells;[54] whether the same occurs in the case of cancer remains to be determined.[55] Moreover, contrary to chronic viral infections, TILs may suffer a dysfunctional state for additional reasons beyond tonic antigen stimulation due to the immunosuppressive TME. It is implied that most growing cancers are populated with T_{EX} because, similarly to chronic infection, a continuous stimulus is delivered in the absence of sufficient co-stimulation in an immunosuppressive TME. Indeed, frequently TILs exhibit a T_{EX} phenotype with impairment of cytokine production and expression of most inhibitory receptors, including programmed cell death protein-1 (PD-1), lymphocyte activation gene (LAG)-3, CD160, CD244/2B4, T cell immunoglobulin, and mucin-domain containing-3/hepatitis A virus cellular receptor 2 (TIM-3/HAVCR2), and cytotoxic T lymphocyte-associated protein 4 (CLTA-4).[56-62]

Interestingly, Sade-Feldman et al. reported a specific subtype of T_{EX} expressing both CD39 (an enzyme in the adenosine pathway) and TIM-3 that is characterized by significant reduction in the expression of tumor necrosis factor (TNF)-α and interferon (IFN)-γ though maintaining IL-2 producing capacity. The dual inhibition of TIM-3 and CD39 reconstituted their antitumor effectiveness in experimental mouse models.[62] This is consistent with

Table 10.1 Connotations of CD8$^+$ T Cell Status and Function

BY	ATTRIBUTION	ABBREVIATION	DEFINITION
Status			
Potency	Totipotent	N.A.[†]	Stem cells that can form all cell types in the body plus embryonic cells
	Pluripotent	N.A.[†]	Stem cells that can give rise to all of the cell types that make up the body
	Multipotent	N.A.[†]	Stem cells that can develop into more than one cell type but are more limited than pluripotent cells within a specific organ/tissue development
CD8 T cell differentiation	Naïve	T_0	A naïve T cell has not yet encountered the respective cognate antigen
	Stem cell-like*	T_{SMC}	Memory T lymphocytes endowed with the stem cell-like ability to self-renewal and the multipotent capacity to reconstitute the entire spectrum of T cell subsets
	Central memory	T_{CM}	Antigen-experienced T cells that lack tissue homing properties but display lymph node-homing receptors and maintain self-renewal capacity
	Effector memory	T_{EM}	Antigen-experienced T cells that lack lymph node-homing receptors and display reduced self-renewal capacity but maintain effector functions
	Terminally differentiated	$T_{EMRA/EFF}$	CD45RA$^+$ subtype of T_{EM} maintaining effector functions only
Function			
	Dysfunctional	N.A.[†]	General term referring to dissonance between expected and observed function sub-categorized according to following nomenclature
	Exhausted	T_{EX}	Hyporesponsive after chronic stimulation (originally used for viral infections but applied also to cancer)
	Senescent (natural)	N.A.[†]	Irreversible, permanent cell-cycle arrest associated with telomere shortening (Hayflick limit)
	Senescent (premature)	N.A.[†]	A potentially reversible telomere-independent process induced by cellular stress
	Quiescent	N.A.[†]	In reversible cell-cycle arrest
	Anergic (in vitro)	N.A.[†]	Dysfunctional due to antigen stimulation in absence of co-stimulatory signals
	Anergic (in vivo)	N.A.[†]	Also referred to as "adaptive tolerance." Due to suboptimal in vivo stimulation due to lack of co-stimulatory inflammatory signals
	Ignorant	N.A.[†]	Peripheral potentially self-reactive T cells non-responsive due to physical separation (immune privilege, immune exclusion) from antigen-bearing targets or insufficient antigen density. Antigen-inexperienced close to naïve T cells with potential to become functional
	Self-tolerance (central)	N.A.[†]	Deletion of self-reactive T cell by thymic selection
	Self-tolerance (peripheral)	N.A.[†]	Antigen-experienced T cells rendered tolerant by peripheral deletion, suppressive mechanism(s), or self-induced apoptotic death

*For a comprehensive view of memory T cell subtypes and their functional status, refer to Martin et al.,[5] Willinger et al.,[6] and Schietinger and Greenberg.[43]

[†]N.A. Abbreviation not applicable or used in this chapter.

other experimental observations, in which checkpoint inhibitors were combined with inhibition of CD73 (also involved in the adenosine pathway) to enhance anticancer effectiveness.[63]

T_{EX} are characterized by reduced proliferative capacity. However, T_{EX} are not a homogeneous and static population but include T cells at different stages of the exhaustion process as well as progenitors of exhausted T cells.[64] A progenitor stem cell-like subpopulation, described as PD-1[+] TCF1[+] CXCR5[+] TIM-3[-], gives rise to terminally differentiated exhausted cells that are PD-1[+] TCF1[-] CXCR5[-] TIM-3[+].[65-67] In between the progenitor and terminally differentiated exhausted cells, there exists an intermediate or "pre-exhausted" population, which has been credited for efficacy of PD-1 blockade in reinvigorating T cells in chronic viral infection and in cancer.[64,66,68]

The T cell exhaustion process is associated with gradual loss of cytokine production, manifesting with reduced expression of IL-2, progressing to reduced TNF-α, and, ultimately, IFN-γ, the last coupled with reduced degranulation.[44,69] In parallel, the exhaustion process is also associated with a gradual increase in expression of inhibitory surface receptors, including PD-1, LAG-3, CD160, CD244/2B4, TIM-3, B- and T cell attenuator (BTLA), and CLTA-4.[70]

Concurrent expression of inhibitory receptors on T_{EX} has been suggested to stem from a centrally controlled, coordinate transcriptional regulation of co-inhibitory gene modules induced by master transcription factors, such as PR domain zinc finger protein 1 (PRDM1/Blimp-1) and c-MAF in an IL-27-dependent way[26] or T-box transcription factor-21 (TBX21/T-bet) and Eomesodermin/T-box brain protein 2 (Eomes/TBR2)[71] (Table 10.2). Even though T-bet is up in T_{EX} compared to T_0, it is still lower than in T_{EM} or $T_{EMRA/EFF}$. Thus, T-bet expression is principally associated with stemness and proliferation rather than exhaustion, which Eomes is known for. In addition, the expression of other transcription factors has been associated with the exhausted phenotype, including TNF receptor-associated factor 1 (TRAF1)[72] and the T cell receptor-induced factors basic leucine zipper transcription factor (BATF),[73] and interferon regulatory factor (IRF) 4.[74] Characteristically, Eomes[hi]-PD-1[hi] T_{EX} cells display strongly suppressed proliferative capacity but still exhibit strong cytotoxic activity in spite of the coordinated expression of most co-inhibitory receptors.[75] It is notable that combined blockade of PD-1 and TIM-3[76] or PD-1 and LAG-3[70] can prevent exhaustion in chronic viral infection models at the T_{EM} but not at the $T_{EMRA/EFF}$ stage.[66,68]

IKAROS family transcription factors IKAROS (IKZF1), HELIOS (IKZF2), and AIOLOS (IKZF3), which are involved in lymphoid differentiation, are also implicated in T cell exhaustion. In chronic viral infection, while TCF1 downregulation was associated with CD8 T cell exhaustion, HELIOS and KLF4 upregulation were associated with CD4 T cell exhaustion.[77] More recently, treatment with the immunomodulatory drug lenalidomide, which selectively degrades IKAROS and AIOLOS,[78] decreased exhaustion in CAR T cells in in vitro chronic antigen stimulation assays.[79] However, the mechanism and extent of the contribution that IKAROS family transcription factors make to CD4 and CD8 T cell exhaustion remains to be determined.

The mechanism leading to exhaustion is intimately related to chronic antigen stimulation, the activation of the nuclear factor of activated T cells (NFAT) transcription factor, along with distinct transcriptional programs NFAT participates in. Acute TCR stimulation leads to upregulation of NFAT and AP-1 transcription factors; however, chronic stimulation leads to upregulation of NFAT without sufficient AP-1. During productive activation of a T cell, NFAT:AP-1 complexes bind promoters of activation-related target genes and initiate a transcriptional program that results in upregulation of effector cytokines, such as IL-2 and IL-4, and other T cell activation genes.[80] However, NFAT, in the absence of its partner AP-1, binds promoters of a different set of genes that result in induction of anergy and exhaustion.[81-83] Partnerless NFAT is the master regulator of a broad selection of exhaustion-related genes, including transcription factors thymocyte selection-associated high mobility group box protein (TOX), IRF4, HELIOS, nuclear receptor subfamily 4 group A member (NR4A) 2, and NR4A3, as well as inhibitory receptors PD-1, TIM-3, and LAG-3.[82,84] In fact, a mutant NFAT engineered to not interact with AP-1 strongly induces exhaustion,[82] while overexpression of AP-1 transcription factor c-JUN prevents exhaustion.[85] Ultimately, the balance between NFAT and AP-1 transcription factors governs the fate of stimulated T cell between productive activation and exhaustion.[86] Once NFAT initiates the exhaustion transcriptional program, downstream transcription factors NR4A1, NR4A2, and NR4A3, in cooperation with TOX1 and TOX2 and in part by antagonizing AP-1, drive the T cell into a hyporesponsive state.[87-89] Exhausted CD8 T cells in both viral infection and cancer models had elevated levels of NR4A and TOX transcription factors, as well as enrichment of binding motifs for NR4A within accessible chromatin.[87,88] Conversely, NR4A triple knock-out CAR T cells display enrichment of DNA motifs for nuclear factor-kappa b (NF-κB) and AP-1, transcription factors involved in T cell activation, and achieve superior tumor control in vivo.[87] Similarly, TOX double knock-out CAR T cells also yield superior tumor control in vivo.[88] Both NR4A triple knock-out and TOX double knock-out CAR T cells show increased cytokine expression, decreased inhibitory receptor expression, and enrichment of binding motifs for NF-κB and AP-1 transcription factors. Overall, NFAT and its downstream effectors NR4A and TOX exert a comprehensive control of transcriptional programs that result in CD8 T cell exhaustion.

Table 10.2 Transcriptional Regulators of Memory CD8⁺ T Cell Status and Function

TRANSCRIPTION FACTOR	ABBREVIATION	IMPLICATION	MECHANISM OF ACTION
T cell factor 1/7	TCF1/TCF7	Stemness	The human *TCF7* gene encodes the TCF1 protein activating Wnt/β-catenin signaling. TCF1 protein expression occurs in CD39^{low}, TIM-3^{low} TIL. In mice, its expression is regulated by **c-Myb.**
Zinc finger E-box binding homeobox 2	ZEB2	Differentiation	In mice, its expression is regulated by **c-Myb**. Promotes T cell differentiation.
Inhibitor of DNA-binding 3	ID3	Stemness	Master regulator of T cell memory differentiation induced by TGF-β
	LEF1	Stemness	Wnt/β-catenin signaling transducer
Forkhead box P1	FOXP1	Stemness	
Signal transducer of activation and transcription 3	STAT-3		Activated by IL-21; suppresses T cell differentiation. This can also be mediated by IL-6, IL-10, and TGF-β through the SMAD pathway. STAT-3 activates in turn KLFs.
Kruppel-like factors	KLF		Promote cell quiescence and lymphoid organ homing.
T-box transcription factor-21	TBX21/T-bet	Stemness	Maintenance of cytokine production and proliferation and progenitor function
TNF receptor-associated factor 1	TRAF1	Stemness	Increased T cell survival and effector function *in vivo*
Let family, miRNA 26a/b, 29 a/b, 30a-5P, 142-5P,		Stemness	
miRNA-155	miRNA-155	Stemness	
miRNA 21, 146		Differentiation	
Mammalian target of rapamycin	mTOR	Differentiation	Restraint of mTOR-mediated protein translation by rapamycin can enhance self-renewal and limit differentiation.
miRNA-29	miRNA-29	Differentiation	Suppresses function of Eomes, TBX21, and IFN-γ.
c-Jun	c-Jun	Prevention of exhaustion	Heterodimer component together with c-Fos of the AP-1 complex that prevents exhaustion upon tonic stimulation and terminal differentiation driving expression of IL-2.
Cytokine-inducible SH2-containing protein	CISH	Exhaustion	Member of the SOCS family. Induced by IL-2, IL-3, and antigen-dependent TCR. signaling induced proteasomal degradation of PLC-g1, promoting expansion and cytokine polyfunctionality.
Src homology 2 (SH2) domain-containing inositol polyphosphate 5-phosphatase 1	SHIP-1	Exhaustion (Terminal diff.)	In mice, the expression is suppressed by miR-155. SHIP-1 suppressed Phf19, which promotes terminal differentiation of T cells.
PR domain zinc finger protein 1	PRMD1/ BLIMP-1	Exhaustion	Regulation of co-inhibitory receptor module (PD-1, TIM-3, LAG-3, and TIGIT)
c-MAF	c-MAF	Exhaustion	Regulation of co-inhibitory receptor module (PD-1, TIM-3, LAG-3, and TIGIT)
Eomesodermin/T-box brain protein 2	Eomes/TRB2	Exhaustion	Suppression of cytokine production and proliferation and maintenance of cytotoxic function.
Basic leucine zipper factor	BATF	Exhaustion	TCR-induced AP-1 transcription factor that induces expression of immune regulatory genes, such as PD-1, reducing proliferation and cytokine production. Expression associated with CD39^{hi}, TIM-3^{hi} TIL.
Interferon regulatory factor 4	IRF4	Exhaustion	TCR-induced AP-1 transcription factor driving checkpoint expression

IL, interleukin; PD-1, programmed cell death protein-1; TGF-β, transforming growth factor beta; TIL, tumor-infiltrating lymphocyte.

To a certain degree, exhaustion is neither an irreversible status of terminal differentiation nor a totally unresponsive T cell state, but rather reversible adaptive hyporesponsiveness to environmental conditions. The reversible state may apply to the population rather than the cellular level. Currently, there is not enough data to conclude that individual cells at the true exhaustion stage can be rescued. More likely, PD-1 blockade does not reinvigorate $T_{EMRA/EFF}$ exhausted cells but allows progenitors to give rise to a less exhausted population that can mount an antitumor immune response. It is likely that $T_{EMRA/EFF}$ exhausted cells are irreversibly stuck in a state of exhaustion/hyporesponsiveness to antigen. The ultimate transition toward the acquisition of a terminally differentiated exhausted state by $T_{EMRA/EFF}$ is a progressive process epigenetically imprinted and independent of circumstantial factors. However, according to some investigators, T_{EX} also embody a degree of differentiation ultimately dependent upon epigenetic modifications.[90,91] For instance, terminally differentiated T_{EX} do not express the T cell factor 1 (TCF1; protein product of the TCF7 gene),[92] while the self-renewing TCF1 expressing T cells from which they derive display T_{scm} properties.[62] This difference can be ascribed to intrinsic histone deacetylase activity of the TCF1 protein.[92] Moreover, the TOX transcriptional regulator has been implicated in the modulation of exhaustion through epigenetic reprogramming, which questions the potential to reverse exhaustion;[23] this phenomenon is referred to as premature senescence. Indeed, T cell senescence is dependent upon two distinct cellular mechanisms: replicative senescence and premature senescence.[53] The former represents an age-related natural progression related to repeated cell divisions leading to shortening of the telomere ends, also referred to as the Hayflick limit.[93,94] The latter is a telomere-independent process induced by cellular stress.[95] Senescence and exhaustion may be particularly pertinent to ACT when T cells administered to cancer patients face the challenges of repeated divisions in the context of potential stress signals associated with an unfavorable TME.[53] For a more comprehensive discussion of the different statuses of dysfunction of T cells that also include tolerance to self-antigens, ignorance due to suboptimal stimulation, and anergy induced by stimulation in the absence of co-stimulation in vitro or in vivo (adaptive tolerance), we refer the reader to a review by Schietinger A. and Greenberg P.D.[43]

In practical terms, T_{EX} span from T_{EM} to more terminally differentiated effector cells that lack proliferative potential and cytokine production capacity while still able to exert some cytotoxic properties.[49,52] T_{EX} express multiple inhibitory receptors as summarized extensively by Catakovic et al.[52] Interference with their respective ligands by immune checkpoint blockade has been shown to at least in part recover T_{EX} function, suggesting partial reversibility of the dysfunctional status at the population level.[49-51] This recovery has been attributed to new effector cells that arise from PD-1$^+$ TCF1$^+$ progenitors rather than invigoration of terminally differentiated exhausted cells.[66,68,96]

An intrinsic signaling pathway implicated in T cell dysfunction and premature exhaustion/senescence is mediated by the suppressor of cytokine signaling (SOCS) gene family, of which one member, cytokine-inducible SH-containing protein (CISH), plays a central role. CISH is activated upon T cell stimulation by IL-2 in vitro[97] and in vivo,[98] as well as in response to TCR signaling.[31] Although SOCS family members act by blocking STAT5 activation, after TCR stimulation CISH also targets directly the TCR intermediate phospholipase C-γ 1 (PLC-γ1) for proteasomal degradation, resulting in reduced T cell proliferation and production of cytokines.[31] Genetic deletion of this gene in CD8$^+$ T cells restores expansion, functional avidity, cytokine polyfunctionality, and durable regression of established tumors.

Overexpression of c-Jun, a component of the heterodimer AP-1 complex, prevents CAR T cells exhaustion and diminishes terminal differentiation, resulting in enhanced, IL-2-dependent expansion, increased functional capacity, and improved antitumor efficacy.[85] In an exhaustion assay delivering tonic signaling, CAR T cells demonstrated higher expression of exhaustion markers such as PD-1, TIM-3, LAG-3, and CD39, and suffered an almost complete suppression of IL-2 production (but not IFN-γ). Moreover, these cells lost expression of CD62L while becoming CD45RA positive (marker of $T_{EMRA/EFF}$ cells), and were characterized by increased expression of effector genes and decreased expression of LEF1, TCF7, ILO7R, and KFL2. These changes were associated with increased chromatin accessibility to exhaustion-associated genes while that to memory-associated genes such as IL-7R was reduced. All these changes were prevented by the engineered overexpression of c-Jun that compensated for a relative deficiency of c-Jun/c-Fos AP-1 heterodimers typical of CAR T_{EX}. Interestingly, c-Jun overexpression increased the frequency of T_{scm} and T_{CM} cells based on the expression of the canonical differentiation markers CD62L and CD45RA underlying the principle that exhaustion may be, conceptually, at least in practical terms, a reciprocal facet of T cell stemness, while terminal differentiation is the canonical reciprocal of stemness. Exhaustion is more like a corruption of the entire gamut of T cell differentiation, all the way from T_{scm} to $T_{EMRA/EFF}$ PD-1$^+$ TCF1$^+$ progenitors are like exhausted T_{scm}, while PD-1$^+$ TCF1$^-$ exhausted cells are like functional status of terminally differentiated $T_{EMRA/EFF}$.

CHARACTERISTICS OF T MEMORY STEM CELLS (T_{SCM})

Multiple lines of evidence indicate that T_{scm} possess stem cell-like attributes not shared by other antigen-experienced T cells such as stronger regenerative potential and multipotent capabilities to reconstitute the full diversity of memory and effector T cell subsets upon serial transplantation.[3]

In the previous section, we described different levels of T cell dysfunction that may or may not be related to their level of differentiation, underlying the notion that in some cases dysfunction may be reversed while in others it may be irreversible, leading ultimately to clonal deletion. With this background, we now explore specific characteristics of T_{scm} that may prevent or mitigate T cell degeneration into a dysfunctional state. This will include observations beyond the defining cell surface hallmarks, since T_{scm} are characterized by peculiar and broader transcriptional, epigenetic, and metabolic properties (Figure 10.1).

Capacity for immune reconstitution as a hallmark of stemness was originally dependent upon clonogenic animal observations.[99,100] In humans, in the context of hematopoietic stem cell transplantation using cell derived from haploidentical donors, it was subsequently observed that T_{scm} differentiate directly from naïve precursors in vivo[101,102] and can reconstitute the entire repertoire of memory T cell subsets.[101] Similar observations were made with the adoptive transfer of genetically modified virus-specific T cells.[103] Adoptive transfer of genetically engineered T cells, incorporating a transgene that allows their distinction from endogenous T cells, demonstrated that T_{scm} can maintain their precursor potential for decades compared with more differentiated T cell subsets. These observations were made in the context of gene therapy to treat immune deficiencies,[104] as well as adoptive transfer of CAR T cells for the treatment of neoplastic disorders.[105] Thus, the potential for differentiation of T cells is restricted during the maturation process to T_{scm} that stand at the apex of Lanzavecchia's progressive model.[18]

Functionally, T_{scm}, similarly to T_{CM}, bear increased capacity for IL-2 secretion and reduced capacity of IFN-γ production compared to T_{EM}, while TNF-α remains comparable.[106] Differently from T_{CM}, T_{scm} express CD95 and IL-2Rβ, display a diluted content of TCR excision circles, possess a higher capability to rapidly release cytokines upon activation, and proliferate more efficiently in response to IL-15.[3] In addition, both T_{scm} and T_{CM} can activate telomerase to maintain replicative potential.[107]

Transcriptional and epigenetic regulation of T cell stemness depends on several signaling pathways that also operate in embryonic and adult stem cells, including Wnt-β-catenin, TGF-β receptor signaling/SMAD, STAT-3, and forkhead box O (FOXO).[2,108] STAT-3 regulates stemness by inducing Kruppel-like factors (KLF), which promote cell quiescence and expression of lymphoid organ-homing signals.[109,110] Moreover, transcriptional profiling denotes a progressive transition from T_{scm}

to T_{EM} coupled to a gradual decrease in the activation of the Wnt-β-catenin signaling transducers TCF1 and lymphoid enhancer-binding factor 1 (LEF1), members of the KLF family, Forkhead box P1 (FOXP1), and the inhibitor of DNA-binding 3 (ID3), all highly active in T_{scm} (Table 10.2). Conversely, ID2, Eomes, PRDM1/BLIMP-1, and zinc finger E-box binding homeobox 2 (ZEB2) follow the opposite pattern to promote differentiation and have been implicated in T cell exhaustion. Some of these transcription factors have complicated/pleiotropic roles. For instance, Eomes and T-bet usually have opposite effects. Eomes plays a role in memory, especially T_{CM}, differentiation, which is close in terms of functionality and markers to T_{scm}. Yet, T_{EX} are Eomes[high]. T-bet plays a role in effector T cells. It also represses PD-1, yet T_{EX} are T-bet[low]. More recently, Gautam et al.[111] observed in a syngeneic mouse model that the transcription factor c-Myb regulates CD8[+] T cell stemness, promoting antitumor immunity. In the mouse model, c-Myb regulated contemporarily two putative regulators of stemness by activating TCF1 to enhance T cell memory and repressing ZEB2 that promotes T cell differentiation.

In addition, epigenetic control of T cell differentiation is dependent upon the reciprocal expression of several small noncoding microRNAs (mRNAs).[112,113] For instance, in mouse models, miR-155 prevents T cell senescence and functional exhaustion through epigenetic silencing of drivers of terminal differentiation by downregulation of the expression of the AKT inhibitor Src homology 2 (SH2) domain-containing inositol polyphosphate 5-phosphatase 1 (SHIP1). The latter releases the activation of Polycomb repressor complex 2, promoting the expression of the associated factor PHF19.[114]

A significant role in T cell stemness/differentiation is played by STAT-3 and SMAD signaling, which can be triggered by Th17-type polarizing cytokines, such as IL-6, IL-21, and TGF-β. This observation suggests commonalities between CD8 memory cells and Th17 polarized T cells related to the maintenance of a stem cell-like phenotype.[115–117] In addition, TGF-β has been shown to suppress the expression of BLIMP-1 while activating ID3, which, in turn, promotes accumulation of T_{scm}/T_{CM} cells in ex vivo stimulated human T cells expanded for ACT.[118] However, TGF-β has also been shown to induce an iT$_{reg}$-like phenotype and accelerate exhaustion upon repeated antigen challenge in mesothelin/28Z CAR T cells.[119] Fittingly, knocking out TGF-β receptor 2 (TGFBR2) in CAR T cells has led to enhanced expansion and efficacy in vivo. All in all, the pleiotropic role TGF-β plays in T cell stemness, exhaustion, and persistence is not a settled matter.

The TCF1 transcription factor is centrally involved in T cell stemness, and its expression by CD8 T cells in the TME is positively correlated with response to checkpoint blockade therapy.[62] Moreover, reduction in open chromatin at the TCF1-related genomic regions has been associated with nonreprogrammable dysfunction of PD-1^{hi} T cells.[41,62] The expression of TCF1 in melanoma patients is associated with a CD39$^-$ TIM-3$^-$ population of T$_{scm}$-like T cells. On the contrary, T$_{EX}$-like CD39$^+$ TIM-3$^+$ T cells display high expression of BATF,[120] due to its participation in these pathways. Since TCF1 participates in Wnt-β-catenin signaling, which is critical to preserving T cell stemness,[120] it is increasingly recognized as a major modulator of the T$_{scm}$ phenotype.

At the transcriptional level, T$_{scm}$ are closest to T$_{CM}$, including the predominant role played by the Wnt/β-catenin signaling pathway essential for T$_{CM}$ formation and long-term-survival.[3,120–123] The mammalian target of rapamycin (mTOR) signaling pathway is also a major modulator for both T$_{CM}$ and T$_{scm}$ development, promoting their differentiation toward a T$_{EM}$ stage while inhibition by rapamycin stimulates the generation of T$_{CM}$.[124,125] Moreover, AKT, a serine/threonine-specific protein kinase in the PI3K-Akt pathway, augments mTOR signaling and controls CD8$^+$ T cell differentiation, and its blockade increases T$_{CM}$ numbers sparing T$_{EMRA/EFF}$ cells from exhaustion and apoptosis.[126]

The epigenetic progression of T cell differentiation suggests that chromatin accessibility is regulated in a gradual manner supporting the progressive model of T cell evolution,[18] according to which T$_{scm}$ represent the least differentiated among antigen-experienced T cells.[28] Indeed, naïve, T$_{CM}$, and T$_{EM}$ phenotypes are associated with specific epigenetic and chromatin states affecting DNA methylation, histone modification, reorganization of nucleosomes, and expression of regulatory noncoding RNAs.[127,128] Similar processes are associated with control of stemness,[129] resulting in the open chromatin states in chromosomal regions controlling functionality responsible for nimble response to antigen. As T cells differentiate away from T$_{scm}$ and lose stemness, they also transition from a plastic epigenetic state to an imprinted state that is resistant to reprogramming.[41] In this model, PD-1 expression by TILs correlated with a shift from a reversible to a fixed state that paralleled progressive chromatin changes.

Emerging evidence suggests that the metabolic program is highly regulated following T cell activation to support cellular growth in size, clonal expansion, lineage polarization, acquisition of effector functions, and differentiation.[40] Indeed, cell metabolism is a critical factor in determining the activity and fate of T lymphocytes,[130] including the development of regulatory T cells (T$_{reg}$ cells).[131] As mentioned before, development of T$_{EM}$ and T$_{scm}$ is dependent upon FAO, increased mitochondrial size, low mitochondrial membrane potential, *spare* (reserve) respiratory capacity (SRC) (amount of extra ATP that can be produced by OXPHOS in response to sudden increases in energy demand),[34,121,124,132,133] and low glycolytic metabolism.[34,35,134] Interestingly, these metabolic characteristics can be induced experimentally through conditioning of T cells in vitro in the presence of IL-7, IL-21,[135,136] and the β-catenin stabilizing glycogen synthase-3β inhibitor TWS119.[121] Conversely, aerobic glycolysis promotes the formation of short-lived T$_{EM}$ and terminally differentiated T$_{EMRA/EFF}$.[34,35,134] (Figure 10.1).

CELLULAR METABOLISM AND HYPOXIA

Upon antigen stimulation, and in proper co-stimulatory conditions, T cells rapidly transition from a quiescent to an active state characterized by increase in cell size, enhanced metabolism, and proliferation requiring an outburst of energy production. Gradually, and dependent upon environmental factors, T cells differentiate into a heterogeneous population with variable phenotypic and functional characteristics, among which, paramount for CD8 T cells, is the performance of effector functions (Table 10.1). Following the original expansion, most T cells undergo programmed apoptotic cell death during the contraction phase. However, a number of cells return to a quiescent anamnestic state capable of mounting a rapid response to subsequent antigen encounters. These evolutionary stages are demarcated by specific metabolic transitions that mirror functional needs (Figure 10.1). Therefore, while naïve T cells rely on OXPHOS, the response of antigen-exposed T cells to meet progressively higher energetic demands is a gradual metabolic shift from OXPHOS and FAO by T$_{scm}$ and T$_{CM}$[133,137,138] to enhanced energy production by T$_{EM}$ and T$_{EMRA/EFF}$, which include pentose phosphate pathway activation, aerobic glycolysis, and glutaminolysis to support ATP generation and provide biosynthetic intermediates.[40,139,140] T cells, more than any other tissue-resident cell, are equipped to be deployed in different organs during stressful circumstances like acute or chronic infections where extensive tissue damage and regeneration concomitantly occur. Thus, adaptability and metabolic plasticity are a central feature of T cell biology that allows metabolic homeostasis in harsh and rapidly evolving environments. As well discussed by Slack et al.,[40] plasticity includes (a) adaptability to regional and functional differences throughout the body, (b) differentiation into specialized lineages to adapt to condition-specific demands, and (c) energetic reprogramming to sustain distinct functions while competing in a metabolically hyperactive microenvironment for substrates, among which glucose and glutamine, together with oxygen availability, play a paramount role. These physiologic processes can be disrupted by several factors that limit the availability of substrates for the different metabolic strategies adapted by the cells. This applies particularly to the metabolic derangement of the TME due to competition with the high energy consumption of constantly replicating cancer cells and the stromal responses that lead to heightened consumption of glucose and essential amino acids, such as glutamine, tryptophan, cysteine, glycine, and arginine.[10] This is, in turn, compounded by mostly hypoxic conditions that simultaneously induce the production of immunosuppressive byproducts, such as lactate, adenosine, and kynurenine.[141–144] T cells required to function in a wide range of nutrient-deficient environments, such as infectious, inflammatory, and tumor sites, must therefore utilize alternative sources of nutrients including autophagy-dependent processing of intracellular substrates or scavenging of extracellular molecules to recycle into bioenergetics resources.[40]

When all else fails, metabolic and functional disruption of T cells occurs as a hallmark of neoplasia, often determining the outcome of anticancer immunotherapy.[35,130,145] Intrinsically, increased mitochondrial metabolism and generation of reactive oxygen species (ROS) in response to T cell activation leads in one way to sustenance of effector function and proliferation at the cost of compromised self-renewal capacity of T_{scm} and T_{CM}.[9] T cell differentiation and their functional activity have been shown to be metabolically linked,[10,146] suggesting that targeting intrinsic metabolic properties of T cells associated with enhanced antitumor efficacy by reprogramming metabolic pathways may increase the efficacy of T cell-based therapies, as later described. In addition, T cells need to adapt to circumstantial factors related to the heterogeneity of the TME by sustaining effector functions while proliferating and overcoming unfavorable environmental signals. In this process, the T cells must balance the metabolic demands of energy maintenance, cell survival, and persistence with those of rapid proliferation and inflammatory function that adopt different strategies.[10] In particular, T_{scm} and T_{EM} depend on increased FAO and SRC,[130,132] while extensive glycolysis leads to the development of $T_{EMRA/EFF}$[134] and oxidative metabolism to quiescence and loss of effector function.[147] Thus, long-term survival is predominantly dependent on quiescence status and fatty acid metabolism, while proliferative and effector functions require higher energy expenditure sustained by a switch from OXPHOS to aerobic glycolysis (Figure 10.1). It remains unclear why T cells adopt a less efficient metabolism in an already oxygen-replete environment.[148,149] Moreover, T cells with high mitochondrial membrane potential (Dψm) and high production of ROS suffer reduced anticancer effectiveness in spite of increased in vitro functionality and increased expression of effector genes, while high SRC promotes persistence of T_{scm}.[34] Conversely, suppression of glucose metabolism (for instance, via pharmacologic inhibition of Akt) limits T cell differentiation and results in enhanced antitumor activity.[29,134]

Nutrient competition in the commensal TME community may also interfere with T cell differentiation and function as an extrinsic factor (Figure 10.2). Glucose deprivation caused by the Warburg effect or hypoxia-driven glycolytic metabolism suppresses T

cell function.[150] Maintenance of T cell metabolic fitness may increase their effectiveness in vivo upon transfer by sustaining a T_{scm} phenotype with reduced glycolysis requirement and enhanced FAO utilization through the enhancement of STAT-3 activity[136] and Wnt/β-catenin signaling.[120] In summary, high metabolic activity of T cells is associated with proliferation and enhanced effector functions but leads toward short-term survival and terminal differentiation and consequent poor antitumor activity, while low metabolic activity is associated with T_{scm} phenotype, longer persistence, and plasticity. This, in turn, fosters progression into a T_{EM} and ultimately a $T_{EMRA/EFF}$ phenotype upon engagement with tumor cells after successful trafficking and expansion in the TME at a later stage to exert a full effector activity (Figure 10.2).

Because of the profound effects that intrinsic or environmental alterations in metabolism may have on T cell differentiation and function, it is important to focus on TME factors that may affect metabolism. Among them, hypoxia plays a paramount role,[151] which, in turn, leads to several aspects of cancer biology, including stemness, dormancy, and intercellular communication in the TME. For instance, chronic hypoxia is a major driver of cancer stemness due to hypoxia-inducible factor (HIF), α-dependent activation of stemness factors, and epithelial-mesenchymal transformation (EMT)-inducing factors. In addition, HIF-α can activate TGF-β and Wnt signaling that, besides promoting cancer cell survival, have powerful effects on T cell differentiation and function.[152–154] Cancer cells, even in physioxic conditions, utilize preferentially a glycolytic metabolism referred to as "aerobic glycolysis" or Warburg effect, possibly in adaptation to disruption of normal tissue physiology.[155] In hypoxic conditions, glycolytic metabolism is promoted further by HIF-α-induced expression of glycolysis programs.[156] The direct and indirect role that hypoxic conditions play on T cell differentiation and function are manifold and occasionally contradictory. For instance, Gropper et al. reported that culture of CD8 T cells under hypoxic conditions enhances the levels of granzyme B and their cytolytic function by speeding their maturation process.[157] Thus, the direct effect of hypoxia on T cells appears to foster a transformation from T_{scm}/T_{CM} to T_{EM}/T_{EMRA}. In addition, hypoxia induces increased expression of TIM-3 and LAG-3, which parallels the phenotype of TILs found in tumor deposits in vivo underlying the notion that T cells generated under hypoxic conditions in vitro closely resemble TILs. These data are concordant with the concept that OXPHOS promotes stemness, while glycolytic metabolism induces effector function as previously discussed and may be related to the hypoxic conditions encountered by T cells in the TME.

Another important alteration germane to the TME is dysregulated potassium levels.[146] Overabundance of this electrolyte suppresses T cell function by limiting nutrient

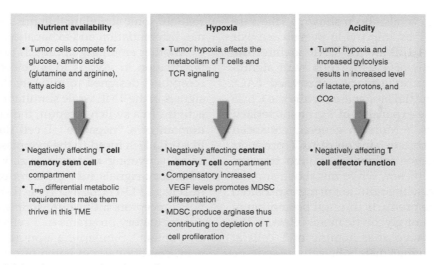

Figure 10.2 Nutrient availability, hypoxia, and acidity in the TME.

MDSC, myeloid-derived suppressor cell; TCR, T cell receptor; TME, tumor microenvironment; T_{reg}, regulatory T cells; VEGF, vascular endothelial growth factor.

uptake, promoting autophagy, and reducing histone deacetylation at effector and exhaustion loci. This, in turn, promotes stemness with improved persistence and maintenance of multipotency.

CLINICAL IMPLICATIONS

The previous considerations bear important implications for cancer immunotherapy and, in particular, for ACT approaches. Specifically, the understanding that intrinsic T cell characteristics, as well as extrinsic factors, can affect T cell differentiation, metabolism, function, and ultimately clinical outcomes in the setting of ACT has spurred a series of therapeutic strategies targeting either the "T cell product" and/or the TME in order to improve the therapeutic effectiveness of ACT.

The longevity, self-renewal potential, and the capacity for immune reconstitution make T_{scm} ideal for ACT approaches. In fact, success of ACT is highly dependent upon T cell engraftment, peak of expansion, and persistence.[37,158–167] Moreover, the administration of cells with higher fractions of T_{scm}-like CD62L[+], CD28[+], and CD27[+] T cells has been shown to correlate with objective tumor responses suggesting that less-differentiated T cells are therapeutically superior.[30,37,105,166,168–171] Yet, in spite of these recurrent observations, unselected T cells are still used in most clinical trials. This is partly due to the small number of circulating T_{scm}[3] as a limiting step for the generation of starting material in clinical-grade manufacturing of ACT products. However, based on emerging clinical data showing that the initial differentiation status of a patient's apheresed T cells may significantly impact the efficacy and persistence of the infused product, different approaches are being investigated aimed at modulating the T cell

product differentiation during the in vitro manufacturing and/or using synthetic biology tools.[38] For instance, it is possible to preferentially expand T_{scm}-like cellular products by different strategies that include particular cytokine milieus such as the presence of IL-7 and IL-15; the former stimulating the development of T_{scm} and the latter sustaining their expansion.[37,172,173] As an alternate to IL-15, IL-21 has also been considered due to its higher effectiveness in slowing T cell differentiation and, therefore, maintenance of the T_{scm} pool[135,174] by specifically activating STAT-3 that promotes the expression of the Wnt/β-catenin-related factor TCF1 and LEF1.[135,136] In particular, IL-21 has the unique capability among the common γ-chain cytokines to activate STAT-3, which is a key-suppressor of T cell differentiation.[108] T_{scm} express IL-6Rα that can also promote their stemness through activation of STAT-3.[175] Moreover, IL-23, which is known to induce proliferation of memory and Th17 cells, can promote a STAT-3-mediated transcriptional program resulting in superior expansion and resistance to exhaustion.[176] In addition to cytokines and based on the current understanding of the connections between T cell differentiation and T cell metabolism, limiting glycolysis during ex vivo expansion by using AKT inhibitors (favoring T cell memory)[89] or inducing mitochondrial fusion pharmacologically (using DRP1 inhibitor Mdivi-1),[177] thus favoring OXPHOS and T cell memory phenotype, are also under evaluation.

An alternative to using ex vivo manufacturing cytokine cocktails or small molecules to affect T cell differentiation is to adopt synthetic biology approaches to hard wire the production of such cytokines directly into the T cells. For instance, CAR T cells that constitutively secrete cytokines, termed "armored" CARs,[178] have been created to enhance proliferation and function.

Metabolic patterns have also been shown to increase the effectiveness of ACT by improving persistence. For instance, inclusion of 4-1BB in the CAR architecture promotes the outgrowth of $T_{SCM/CM}$ cells with significantly enhanced respiratory capacity, increased FAO, and enhanced mitochondrial biogenesis, while the CD28 domain leans toward the expansion of T_{EM} characterized by enhanced glycolysis.[179] More in general, enhanced metabolism during ex vivo expansion of ACT products decreases their persistence following in vivo transfer, reducing their overall efficacy, while metabolic supplementation (for instance, with arginine during expansion) can yield more effective products through promotion of oxidative and reduction of glycolytic metabolism.[180] The opposite may occur in vivo after homing of T cells at the tumor site, where higher metabolic activity may be necessary for antitumor effector functions,[134] which may be particularly relevant in the case of restricted glucose availability due to the Warburg effect.[150] This is corroborated by the observation by Gropper et al.[157] that CD8 T cells cultured in hypoxic conditions display a higher level of effector functions. In contrast, others have shown that hypoxia and anaerobic glycosylation in the TME promotes expansion of T_{reg} cells, which hamper T cell effectiveness.[181]

The substantial difference observed in clinical persistence between the CD28 containing CAR constructs such as CD19/28Z and the 4-1BB-containing ones such as CD19/BBZ CAR T cell products has been a topic of intense study. Recent findings indicate that in 28Z CAR T cells, recruitment of LCK kinase to the protein complex around CAR leads to constitutive basal phosphorylation of CD3Z and consequently enhanced CAR signaling upon encountering antigen, while in BBZ CAR T cells recruitment of SHP-1 phosphatase leads to blunting of CAR signaling.[182,183] In addition, 28Z CAR, through its YMNM motif, interacts with GRB2 and contributes to a stronger Ca^{+2} flux and PLCγ1 activation.[184] Strong T cell activation by 28Z CAR, due to constitutively phosphorylated CD3Z and GRB2 interaction, leads to accumulation of partnerless NFAT, where abundance of NFAT homodimers, which induce exhaustion, exceeds abundance of NFAT:AP-1 complexes, which are required for productive T cell activation. Therefore, the reason for very limited persistence of 28Z CAR T cells in clinic may lie in NFAT-mediated exhaustion.

The site of transgene integration during the engineering of T cell products has also been shown to have significant impact on CAR T cell function. A study with a CD19/28Z CAR used CRISPR to insert the CAR gene under the control of the TCR promoter (i.e., at the TRAC locus), while simultaneously knocking out the TCR via insertion of the CAR gene.[185] The results indicate enhanced proliferation, more memory T cells, and much less exhaustion, which was hypothesized to be due to reduced tonic signaling that pushes T cells toward terminal differentiation and exhaustion.

Another emerging approach to manipulate T cell differentiation in vivo is to engineer T cells with "switch receptors" designed to mitigate the effects of inhibitory signals in the TME while simultaneously enhancing T cell activity. In a switch receptor, the ligand-binding external domain of a "negative" T cell function regulator (e.g., PD-1, IL-4) is fused to the cytoplasmic signaling domain of an activating molecule (e.g., CD28 or IL-7) to turn inhibitory signals into inducers of T cell metabolic fitness (e.g., PD-1/CD28 or IL-4/IL-7).[186,187] Other synthetic notch receptors induce transcriptional activation of various regulatory programs in T cells in response to antigen encounter.[188] Similarly, a non-gene editing, nonpermanent, conditional regulation of cellular programs adopts an antigen encounter-dependent nuclease-deactivated CRISPR-associated interference system.[189] By introducing several single guide RNAs, it is possible to conditionally prevent in synchrony the activation of multiple genes that have suppressive effects on the CAR T cells. This strategy is safer than standard gene editing because it is fully reversible and does not cause permanent changes in DNA structure/sequence. At the same time, this approach bypasses severe toxicities due to the systemic administration of immune-modulatory products.

Finally, T cells can be reprogrammed toward an induced pluripotent stem cells (iPSCs) cell-like status by enforced expression of the Yamanaka factors OCT4, SOX2, KLF4, and MYC. These T cell-derived iPS cells retain the original T cell receptor rearrangements and cognate recognition of antigen.[190–192] Thus, it may be possible in the future to apply this principle to the generation of large numbers of multipotent T_{scm} from later stages of differentiation, including $T_{EMRA/EFF}$ cells.[192] On the same line, Adorno et al.[193] have shown that USP16 modulates Wnt signaling in mammalian cells, affecting their expansion and self-renewal potential. Usp16 downregulation increases stem cell self-renewal and decreases senescence in multiple tissues, including T cells, and the modulation of its function may delay exhaustion and senescence to maintain the T_{scm} pool.

In summary, a plethora of approaches is emerging from a deeper understanding of the T cell biology relevant to successful eradication of cancer. Although stemness is not the only factor limiting the multifactorial determinism of cancer immune responsiveness,[19] it is likely to play a major role for both hematological malignancies and for solid tumors.

CONCLUSION

One of the major hurdles in cancer therapy is lack of homing, engagement, and activation of T cells in an immunosuppressive environment.[194] Although these hurdles are multifactorial, it is becoming increasingly evident that a more robust T cell endowed with functional plasticity is a major factor in inducing and maintaining effective anti-tumor immune responses. This chapter outlines some basic principles that are evolving in time but emphasize the need to address T cell function as a dynamic component of anticancer immunotherapy.

KEY REFERENCES

Only key references appear in the print edition. The full reference list appears in the digital product on Springer Publishing Connect: connect.springerpub.com/content/book/978-0-8261-3743-2/part/part01/chapter/ch10

1. Gattinoni L, Speiser DE, Lichterfeld M, Bonini C. T memory stem cells in health and disease. *Nat Med.* 2017;23(1):18–27. doi:10.1038/nm.4241

10. O'Neill LA, Kishton RJ, Rathmell J. A guide to immunometabolism for immunologists. *Nat Rev Immunol.* 2016;16(9):553–565. doi:10.1038/nri.2016.70

19. Bedognetti D, Ceccarelli M, Galluzzi L, et al. Toward a comprehensive view of cancer immune responsiveness: a synopsis from the SITC workshop. *J Immunother Cancer.* 2019;7(1):131. doi:10.1186/s40425-019-0602-4

35. Sukumar M, Kishton RJ, Restifo NP. Metabolic reprograming of anti-tumor immunity. *Curr Opin Immunol.* 2017;46:14–22. doi:10.1016/j.coi.2017.03.011

36. Henning AN, Roychoudhuri R, Restifo NP. Epigenetic control of CD8(+) T cell differentiation. *Nat Rev Immunol.* 2018;18(5):340–356. doi:10.1038/nri.2017.146

47. Wang JC, Xu Y, Huang ZM, Lu XJ. T cell exhaustion in cancer: Mechanisms and clinical implications. *J Cell Biochem.* 2018;119(6):4279–4286. doi:10.1002/jcb.26645

194. Wang E, Cesano A, Butterfield LH, Marincola F. Improving the therapeutic index in adoptive cell therapy: key factors that impact efficacy. *J Immunother Cancer.* 2020;8(2):e001619. doi:10.1136/jitc-2020-001619

11

The Innate Immune System: Macrophages and Neutrophils

Alberto Mantovani, Isabella Barajon, and Diletta Di Mitri

KEY POINTS

- Tumor-associated macrophages (TAMs) and tumor-associated neutrophils (TANs) sustain cancer-related inflammation (CRI).

- Cancer-mediated signals confer to TAMs and TANs, a tumor-supporting role.

- High-dimensional technologies unveiled a prominent heterogeneity in the composition and functional state of tumor-infiltrating myeloid cells.

- Frequency and transcriptional features of TAMs and TANs have been associated with a poor prognosis in many tumor types.

- Myeloid targeting showed efficacy in several tumor models.

INTRODUCTION

The tumor microenvironment (TME) is composed of a variety of immune cells that sustain cancer-related inflammation (CRI)[1,2] and are fundamental players in the initiation and progression of tumors. The formation of an inflammatory niche can precede tumor initiation and can be mediated by chronic inflammatory conditions.[3] In other circumstances, the recruitment of immune components to the tumor bed is a consequence of neoplastic development and follows intrinsic cancer-related events, such as genetic modifications that cause tumorigenesis and alter the tumor secretome.[4] Myeloid cells are key components of the tumor immune infiltrate, and tumor-associated macrophages (TAMs) and tumor-associated neutrophils (TANs) are essential mediators of CRI.[1,2,5-8] In tumors, TAMs and TANs have been described to foster tumor cell proliferation and invasiveness to enhance angiogenesis, and to promote immunotolerance.[6,9,10] Importantly, both TAMs and TANs can mediate resistance to standard of care therapies and immunotherapies in certain contexts.[11-13] Here, we review the state of the art about tumor-infiltrating myeloid cells. We focus on the transcriptional landscape of myeloid cells in tumors and we recapitulate the role of TAMs and TANs in tumor initiation and progression and in response to therapies.

MYELOID CELLS IN CANCER

Tumor-Associated Macrophages

Macrophages are a crucial component of the innate immune response and play a fundamental role in development, tissue homeostasis and repair and during infections. Macrophages are plastic cells that modify their phenotype in response to external activating stimuli. As a consequence, in tissues, macrophages can cover a large spectrum of polarization states that differ in cytokine profile, metabolism, and antigen presentation properties.[14-16] Importantly, macrophages represent one of the most abundant immune subsets in the TME. In cancer, macrophages can employ both protumoral and antitumoral functions. Substantial evidence shows that cancer-mediated signals and stimuli deriving by immune infiltrating subsets confer to TAMs, a tumor-supporting role, both in situ and at the metastatic site.[7,17] For instance, in pancreatic carcinoma and breast carcinoma, interleukin-4 (IL-4) and IL-13 play a major role as orchestrators of TAMs function.[18,19] Among other cytokines secreted by tumor cells, colony-stimulating factor 1 (CSF-1) and transforming growth factor beta (TGF-β) have been shown to promote the protumoral polarization of TAMs.[8] In addition, upon exposure to lactic acid, derived by aerobic glycolytic activity of tumor cells, TAMs acquire tumor-promoting functions, driven by hypoxia-inducible factor-1α (HIF-1α).[20]

TAMs are mainly derived from monocytic precursors that are recruited to the tumor bed and once there differentiate. The recruitment of monocytes is thus a key determinant of macrophage abundance in tumors and is mediated by a variety of secreted factors released by cancer cells or other components of the TME.[21] Crucial inducers of monocyte recruitment are chemochines, such as CCL2, CCL5, and CXCL1, and a variety of myeloid modulators, such as CSF-1R and TGF-β.[7,22,23] Importantly, most of these factors also modulate the differentiation of monocyte to macrophages and in a second step, the functional state of TAMs. For instance, inhibition of CSF-1R in tumors results in both macrophage depletion and functional reprogramming, depending on the tumor type and the pharmacological approach utilized.[24–26] Recently, retinoic acid (RA) has been reported to mediate the differentiation of tumor-infiltrating monocytes to macrophages in a model of sarcoma. The inhibition of RA signaling in the TME restored T cell–mediated antitumor immunity.[27]

Tumor-Associated Neutrophils

Neutrophils account for about 60% of all leukocytes in the peripheral blood in homeostatic conditions. They are key players of the innate immune system and play a central role in the acute phase of immune response.[28–31] Mostly known as phagocytes and orchestrators of other immune subsets against infections, neutrophils are now recognized as a prominent component of the TME. Production of cytokines by tumor cells results in alteration of hemopoiesis and consequent neutrophilia in the peripheral blood, which correlates with prognosis in most tumor types.[32–34]

The tumor-associated secretome is responsible for the recruitment of TANs to the tumor bed. Granulocyte colony-stimulating factor (G-CSF) can be considered the main promoter of neutrophil mobilization from the bone marrow and has a crucial role in their recruitment to cancer. Furthermore, CXC chemokines (e.g., CXCL1, CXCL2, CXCL5, CXCL6, and CXCL8/IL-8) are highly expressed by tumor cells and by the component of the TME and mediate the accumulation of TANs in cancer by interacting with the CXCR1 and CXCR2 receptors expressed on their surface. Tumor-derived oxysterols and complement components have also been shown to mediate neutrophil recruitment in mouse tumors.[35–40]

The release of secreted factors by tumor cells, stroma, and infiltrating immune components of the TME affects the polarization of TANs and confers the protumorigenic functions. For instance, in primary carcinogenesis and transplantable lung tumors, TGF-β has been reported to induce the polarization of infiltrating neutrophils to a tumor-supporting functional state (N2 neutrophils) that is featured by the release of arginase-1 (ARG1), CCL17, and CXCL14.[41] On the other hand, in early non-small cell lung cancer (NSCLC), interferon beta (IFNβ), in combination with IFNγ and granulocyte-macrophage colony-stimulating factor (GM-CSF), was shown to induce the expression of major histocompatibility complex class II (MHCII) on neutrophils, which is associated with antigen-presenting capabilities and antitumoral properties.[42,43]

HIGH-DIMENSIONAL SINGLE-CELL PROFILING OF TUMOR-INFILTRATING MYELOID CELLS

With the advent of new molecular technologies based on high-dimensional single-cell profiling, such as single-cell RNA sequencing (scRNAseq) and mass cytometry by time-of-flight (CyTOF), many progresses have been made in the analysis of the TME. The immune landscape of hepatocellular carcinoma was recently dissected, and a similar approach was also applied to melanoma, non-small cell lung cancer (NSCLC), kidney cancer, and breast cancer.[44–46] These reports gave insights in the composition of the immune infiltrate in cancer and discovered new players, previously unidentified cell-to-cell interactions, and novel mechanisms of immune regulation. Recently, scRNA-based technologies have disclosed the complexity of cancer-infiltrating myeloid cells, including TAMs and TANs, in diverse cancer types.[47–49] For instance, combination of two scRNAseq strategies based on either full-length or 3′ scRNA-seq technologies unveiled a prominent heterogeneity in the composition and functional state of myeloid cells infiltrating liver cancer. This approach identified a subset of TAMs in which the protumoral and proinflammatory polarization states coexist. This subset correlates with poor prognosis in liver cancer patients.[46] Moreover, scRNAseq in CRC tumors from patients and mouse models unveiled the infiltration of two TAMs subsets showing a transcriptional dichotomy, which differed for their activation and angiogenic potential. Treatment with anti-CSF-1R depleted only a portion of TAMs and resulted in the emergency of a resistant cluster that deserves further investigation.[50]

Recent studies based on single-cell approaches have also characterized neutrophils. These reports gave new insights in the differentiation steps that neutrophils undergo during development and identified diverse subsets of neutrophils that display distinct functional properties.[51,52] Moreover, scRNAseq applied to infiltrating immune populations in NSCLC patients and tumor-bearing mice affected by lung cancer identified a multiplicity of neutrophil subsets that cover a continuum of functional states. Notably, infiltrating neutrophils showed conserved modules of gene expression within mouse and human lung cancer samples.[49]

MYELOID CELLS IN TUMOR INITIATION AND PROGRESSION

Tumor-Associated Macrophages and Cancer

Under the influence of the TME, macrophages assume protumorigenic capabilities. TAMs sustain tumor growth and progression, promote invasion and metastasis, and mediate immune evasion.[53,54] Consistent with these findings, the abundance of TAMs at the tumor bed have been associated with a poor prognosis in many tumor types. Remodeling and destruction of the extra-cellular matrix mediated by TAMs have been reported to promote cancer invasiveness. Indeed, in tumors, TAMs produce enzymes and proteases, which include cathepsins, matrix metalloproteases, and serine proteases,[55] that are associated with metastasis formation.[56,57] In addition, urokinase/plasminogen activator (uPA) produced by macrophages correlates with metastatic dissemination in a breast cancer model.[58] Release of matrix metalloproteases by TAMs has been reported in tumors and contributes to matrix remodeling and enhanced tumor cell invasion.[59,60]

In several cancer models, TAMs have been reported to mediate metastatic dissemination. The abundance of infiltrating macrophages, regulated by CSF-1, correlates with the metastatic potential of breast cancer.[61] On the same line, blockade of CSF-1R impairs tumor invasion mediated by microglia in a model of glioblastoma.[62] In mammary tumors, TAMs facilitate cancer invasion by a synergistic interaction with tumor cells, based on epidermal growth factor (EGF) and CSF-1.[63] Furthermore, macrophage-derived osteopontin (OPN) has been described to promote cell invasion in a model of human hepatoma.[64] An additional mechanism that impacts tumor dissemination is the promotion of angiogenesis and lymphangiogenesis by TAMs. In tumors, macrophages release proangiogenic growth factors and chemokines that facilitate vessel formation, thus fueling cancer cells and inducing tumor cell migration to distant sites.[65–69]

In a recent report, macrophages infiltrating colorectal carcinoma (CRC) liver metastasis were investigated.[70] TAMs were classified based on morphology into small and large using an artificial intelligence algorithm. Infiltration with large macrophages, but not with total macrophages, was strongly associated with poor prognosis and survival in CRC metastasis. Macrophage morphology was correlated with transcriptional profiles at bulk and single-cell levels. The transcriptional profiles included lipid metabolism, complement, and mediators of inflammation.

Tumor-Associated Neutrophils and Cancer

Upon the conditioning of the TME, TANs acquire protumorigenic properties, which include induction of cancer cell proliferation, promotion of angiogenesis, support of metastatic dissemination, and suppression of innate and adaptive immunity.[32]

In tumors, neutrophils secrete a variety of cytokines and growth factors that promote tumor cell proliferation and metastasis formation. On this regard, EGF, hepatocyte growth factor (HGF), and platelet-derived growth factor (PDGF) have been reported to impact cancer growth.[71,72] In a mouse model of breast carcinogenesis, the

macrophage-$\gamma\delta$ T cells axis is responsible for the recruitment of immunosuppressive neutrophils that, in turn, regulate the formation of lung metastases.[73] Moreover, neutrophils have been reported to support metastasis formation by preparing the metastatic niche. In lung and liver premetastatic sites, neutrophils produce factors that mediate the extravasation of cancer cells and facilitate their implantation and subsequent growth.[74,75] Notably, neutrophils have also been described to interact with circulating tumor cells in the blood and to carry cancer to the metastatic sites.[76,77]

An additional mechanism exerted by TANs to facilitate tumor progression and extravasation is the promotion of angiogenesis. In human cancer, neutrophils have been shown to directly modulate tumor angiogenesis through the release of secreted factors that include vascular endothelial growth factor (VEGF), Bv8, CXCL8, and matrix metallopeptidase 9 (MMP-9).[72,78] In a model of pancreatic cancer, TANs have been reported to be the major source of MMP-9. In this context, the release of MMP-9 by neutrophils causes an angiogenic switch in dysplastic islets.[79] Beside a direct impact on tumor migration, the release of MMP-9 by TANs also mediates the release and activation of VEGF, which in turn results in the promotion of angiogenesis.[80] Notably, experiments in tumor-bearing CCR2-deficient mice, which display a significant reduction of macrophage infiltration to the tumor, detected an elevated MMP9 expression by neutrophils, indicating that TANs and TAMs may exert a complementary proangiogenetic activity in cancer.[81]

PROGNOSTIC SIGNIFICANCE OF MYELOID CELLS IN CANCER

The abundance of TAMs at the tumor bed have been associated with a poor prognosis in many tumor types. A meta-analysis performed on epithelial tumors and melanoma recently reported the association of CD68 expression—a pan marker for human macrophages—and overall survival (OS) across most cancers analyzed. Notably, the localization of TAMs and the expression of polarization markers, such as CD204, CD206, and CD163, influenced the grade of correlation with OS.[82] These evidences are consistent with previous findings that associated macrophage number and worse prognosis in diverse tumor types, comprising gastric cancer, urogenital cancer, head and neck cancers, and so forth.[83] For instance, CD206+ M2-TAMs correlate with OS, tumor stage, and vascular invasion in hepatocellular carcinoma.[84] Interestingly, an additional study showed that CD169+ macrophages correlate with good OS in this tumor type, thus further supporting the hypothesis that TAMs subpopulations that differ in functional state may have an opposing predictive value.[85] In breast cancer, the distribution of CD68+ and CD163+ TAMs was found to be associated with tumor proliferation and the presence of lymph node metastasis, while the abundance of TAMs correlate with OS in nonmetastatic breast tumors.[86] Also in classic Hodgkin's lymphoma (CHL), TAM infiltration was associated with poor survival.[87,88] Interestingly, in contrast with other cancer types, CRCs showed an inverse association between TAMs and OS.[83]

As previously mentioned, TAMs have been described to influence response to therapy in certain cancers. In pancreatic adenocarcinoma, the abundance of infiltrating macrophages are associated with response to chemotherapy and have been proposed as prognostic markers that may guide therapy decision-making.[89] Furthermore, TAMs number is predictive of good clinical outcome in follicular lymphoma (FL) patients treated with rituximab and chemotherapy.[90] On the contrary, the abundance of TAMs were associated with poor response to neoadjuvant chemotherapy in esophageal cancer and were shown to correlate with poor prognosis in FL treated with multiagent chemotherapy.[91,92]

As for neutrophils, high TANs infiltration is associated with adverse prognosis in most cancers.[93,94] A high neutrophil-to-lymphocyte ratio (NLR) in blood became a prognostic marker of poor clinical outcome in diverse cancer types, such as melanoma, breast, prostate, and gastric cancer.[95] Nevertheless, the prognostic relevance of NLR is controversial in certain cancers (lung cancer, breast cancer, and CRC)[33] and its relevance in the clinic remains to be proven.[34] A large study on 39 tumors, which estimated immune cells abundance by using the CIBERSORT, indicated infiltrating neutrophils were the most significant adverse prognostic factor.[96] Accordingly, in NSCLC, an elevated neutrophil count was statistically significantly associated with poor OS and short progression-free survival in a cohort of chemo-naïve patients.[97] Nevertheless, in certain human tumors, high levels of TANs were associated with a better clinical outcome. In CRC, the infiltration of CD66b+ neutrophils was found to be significantly associated with increased survival, and combined infiltration of neutrophils and CD8+ cells resulted in a favorable clinical outcome when compared with the presence of CD8+ cells alone.[98,99] Moreover, in undifferentiated pleomorphic sarcoma (UPS), gene expression analysis on human data sets showed that neutrophil infiltration is associated with an antitumoral T cell response and correlates with a better clinical outcome.[100]

SUPPRESSION OF ADAPTIVE IMMUNITY BY MYELOID CELLS

Most tumors are surrounded by an immunosuppressive microenvironment. TAMs and TANs suppress the adaptive immune response by mean of a diversity of mechanisms. For instance, L-arginine metabolism plays a central role in TAMs- and TANs-mediated immunosuppression. Both macrophages and neutrophils release ARG1, which drives arginine depletion at the tumor bed, with consequent inhibition of CD8 T cell growth and activation.[21,101–104] Notably, the mechanisms that induce T cell suppression may vary depending on tumor type. For instance, ARG1 neutralization was not effective in a model of ovarian cancer. Here, the expression of B7-H4 by TAMs was the prominent negative regulator of tumor-associated T cell immunity (Figure 11.1).[105]

Recently, PI3Kγ has been reported to play a role in the establishment of an immunosuppressive microenvironment in breast cancer. In this context, PI3Kγ inhibition results in a transcriptional switch of infiltrating TAMs from an immunosuppressive to an immune-stimulating phenotype. Consistent with this, pharmacological approaches combining PI3K inhibition and immunotherapy resulted in a synergistic effect in tumor-bearing mice, with a reduction in tumor growth and extension of survival.[9] Finally, class IIa histone deacetylase (HDAC) inhibitors tested in breast cancer are able to alter TAMs polarization toward a proinflammatory state that promotes a functional CD8-mediated antitumor immune response that depends on the IFNγ axis.[106]

An additional mechanism of suppression exerted by TAMs and TANs is represented by the expression of surface molecules, such as programmed cell death ligand 1 (PD-L1), PD-L2, and V-domain Ig suppressor of T cell activation (VISTA), that engage immune checkpoint receptors on T cells (Figure 11.1).[107–109]

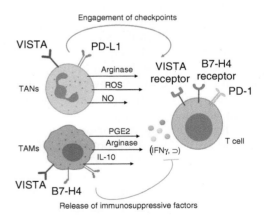

Figure 11.1 Suppression of adaptive immunity by myeloid cells. TAMs and TANs suppress the adaptive immune response by mean of a diversity of mechanisms. The release of immunosuppressive factors and the engagement of checkpoint receptors drive the inhibition of T cell activation.

IFNγ, interferon gamma; IL-10, interleukin 10; NO, nitric oxide; PD-1, programmed cell death protein 1; PD-L1, programmed cell death ligand 1; PGE2, prostaglandin E2; ROS, reactive oxygen species; TAMs, tumor-associated macrophages; TANs, tumor-associated neutrophils; VISTA, V-domain Ig suppressor of T cell activation.

MYELOID CELLS AND IMMUNOTHERAPIES

In recent years, checkpoint blockade inhibitors entered in the clinic for the treatment of most cancer types. Their efficacy is based on the disruption of the interaction between cytotoxic T-lymphocyte-associated protein 4 (CTLA-4) and programmed cell death protein 1 (PD-1) with the respective ligands, which results in removal of T cell tolerance and restoration of T cell–mediated antitumor immunity.[110,111] Myeloid components, such as macrophages and neutrophils, are main factors in the immunosuppression mediated by immune checkpoint in cancer.[112] As a consequence, the investigation of myeloid cell dynamics in cancer may be utilized to predict response to immunotherapies.[15,113]

PD-L1 was found to be expressed in immune-infiltrating subsets, including macrophages, across several human tumors, and its expression in the TME correlates with response to anti-PD-L1 therapy.[112] In hepatocellular carcinoma, the expression of PD-L1 on peritumoral monocytes was reported to increase with disease progression and to correlate with reduced survival. The expression of PD-L1 on monocytes was sustained by an autocrine pathway dependent on TNF-α and interleukin-10 (IL-10).[114] These results were further confirmed in glioblastoma and in models of melanoma and breast cancer.[115] In tumor-bearing mice, PD-L1 engagement was also shown to promote a protumorigenic state in TAMs, which was reverted upon PD-L1 inhibition in vivo.[115] Interestingly, beside the expression of PD-L1, TAMs have been reported to expose on their surface of the molecule PD-1, both in primary human cancers and mouse models. In this context, the abrogation of PD-1/PD-L1 interaction, by mean of a neutralizing antibody, resulted in increased phagocytic activity of TAMs versus the tumor cells.[116]

Combinatorial approaches targeting checkpoint blockades and TAMs may improve the efficacy of currently available immunotherapies and are under preclinical and clinical investigation.[117,118] For instance, combined treatment of tumor-bearing mice with anti-PD-1 and anti-CTLA-4 antibodies and inhibition of the CSF-1R (by mean of the PLX397 antagonist) showed a striking synergistic effect in pancreatic cancer models and completely blocked tumor initiation and progression.[119] TAMs-mediated ADCP that follows therapeutic antibody treatment has been recently reported to promote immunosuppression in the TME of breast cancer in patients and mouse models. Following phagocytosis of tumor DNA, macrophage upregulate PD-L1 and contribute to immunosuppression. In this context, combinatorial approaches combining anti-Her2 therapeutic antibody and immune checkpoint blockade restored T cell and NK cell–mediated cytotoxicity and increased therapeutic efficacy.[120] In addition, combination of ARG1 inhibitors and immune checkpoint blockade showed synergistic effects in colon and breast cancer models.[121]

Less is known about the role of PD-1/PD-L1 and CTLA-4 pathways in TANs. PD-L1 expression on neutrophils has been described to be mediated by proinflammatory stimuli and has a prognostic significance in hepatocellular carcinoma and gastric carcinoma.[107,122–124] PD-1 expression was detected on granulocyte–monocyte progenitors (GMPs) in a model of melanoma. Genetic disruption of PD-1 on myeloid cells resulted in tumor inhibition in this context.[125] On this line, combinatorial immunotherapies targeting TANs have also been tested. In castration-resistant prostate cancer (CRPC), multikinase inhibitors targeting granulocytic cells awaken the antitumor activity of immune checkpoint blockades that did not show efficacy when administered alone.[126]

CONCLUSION

Macrophages and neutrophils are key components of the TME. Depending on the environmental stimuli, tumor type, and progression stage, infiltrating myeloid cells may exert both tumor-promoting and antitumoral functions. The advent of high-dimensional single-cell–based techniques gave new insights in the comprehension of the mechanisms that regulate the behavior of infiltrating macrophages and neutrophils in cancer. Furthermore, preclinical and clinical trials that investigated the efficacy of myeloid targeting in tumor models and patients pave the way for the development of new immune-based combinatorial approaches in cancer. In the next future, it will be crucial to exploit the knowledge that these efforts provided to further explore the possibility to target myeloid components for cancer therapy.

KEY REFERENCES

Only key references appear in the print edition. The full reference list appears in the digital product on Springer Publishing Connect: connect.springerpub.com/content/book/978-0-8261-3743-2/part/part01/chapter/ch11

2. Mantovani A, Allavena P, Sica A, Balkwill F. Cancer-related inflammation. *Nature*. 2008;454(7203):436–444. doi:10.1038/nature07205

6. Coussens LM, Zitvogel L, Palucka AK. Neutralizing tumor-promoting chronic inflammation: a magic bullet? *Science*. 2013;339(6117):286–291. doi:10.1126/science.1232227

15. Mantovani A, Marchesi F, et al. Tumour-associated macrophages as treatment targets in oncology. *Nat Rev Clin Oncol*. 2017;14(7):399–416. doi:10.1038/nrclinonc.2016.217

32. Coffelt SB, Wellenstein MD, de Visser KE. Neutrophils in cancer: neutral no more. *Nat Rev Cancer*. 2016;16(7):431–446. doi:10.1038/nrc.2016.52

34. Jaillons PA, di Mitrid S, Bonecchi R, Mantovani A. Neutrophil diversity and plasticity in tumour progression and therapy. *Nat Rev Cancer*. 2020;20:485–503. doi:10.1038/s41568-020-0281-y

35. Gabrilovich DI, Ostrand-Rosenberg S, Bronte V. Coordinated regulation of myeloid cells by tumours. *Nat Rev Immunol*. 2012;12(4):253–268. doi:10.1038/nri3175

96. Gentles AJ, Newman AM, Liu CL, et al. The prognostic landscape of genes and infiltrating immune cells across human cancers. *Nat Med*. 2015;21(8):938–945. doi:10.1038/nm.3909

12

Natural Killer Cell Effector Mechanisms Against Solid Tumors and Leukemias and Their Exploitation in Immunotherapy

Andrea De Maria, Lorenzo Moretta, Gabriella Pietra, and Massimo Vitale

KEY POINTS

- In the past, natural killer (NK) cells have been indistinctly considered as potent antitumor effector cells. Most recent advances revealed the complexity of this cell population showing that antitumor NK effector functions can be modulated along the cell life span and differently distributed among defined NK subsets and body compartments.

- Cells residing in the tumor microenvironment, as well as tumor cells themselves, release a variety of immunosuppressive factors that inhibit NK cell function and/or their capability to migrate into the tumor lesions.

- The development of NK cell immunotherapeutic strategies is driven by outstanding characteristics of these cells, including the absence of antigen-specificity, preformed perforin storage, shorter in vivo survival compared to T cells, and "preferential" targeting of cancer stem cells.

- NK cell immunotherapy in hematologic malignancies so far has scored superior results compared to solid malignancies. The case of haploidentical bone marrow transplantation and killer Ig-like receptors (KIR)-mismatch represents a milestone in this area.

- Strategies aiming at ex vivo NK cell activation and in vivo NK cell redirecting or de-inhibition are being actively pursued to target hematologic malignancies and cancer stem cells in solid tumors. Several tools for NK cell immunotherapy already entered clinical testing and in some cases are in clinical practice.

NATURAL KILLER CELL EFFECTOR MECHANISMS AND THEIR DISTRIBUTION AMONG DISTINCT NATURAL KILLER CELL SUBSETS AND BODY COMPARTMENTS

Natural Killer Cell Effector Mechanisms

Natural killer (NK) cells are thought to represent one of the major host effector cells to control the insurgence, evolution, and spread of tumors.[1–8] To do that, NK cells are endowed with powerful weapons directed not only against different infections driven by viruses or intracellular bacteria but also against tumor cells. These ammunitions are represented by cytokines such as TNF-α and IFN-γ,[9–12] members of the tumor necrosis factor/tumor necrosis factor receptor (TNF/TNFR) family such as TNF-related apoptosis inducing ligand (TRAIL) and FAS-L[9] expressed on the cell surface, and a number of preformed cytolytic granules stored in the cytosol.[13–15] TNF-α and IFN-γ can induce or amplify cell death of different tumor cell lines. Consistent with these data, IFN-γ has also recently been shown to play an essential role in targeting tumors in vivo. TRAIL and FAS-L can be expressed at the NK cell surface, empowering NK cells to induce apoptosis of TRAIL-R+ or FAS+ tumor cells.[16,17] The cytolytic granules are secretory lysosomes containing effector molecules such as serine proteases, mainly granzymes A and B, and the highly cationic molecule granulysin, which is capable of damaging bacterial and mitochondrial membranes.[13–15] In addition, granules also contain accessory molecules, including the pore-forming perforins and the proteoglycan serglycin, which play a critical role in granule maturation and safe storage of perforins and granzyme B.[13,18] By the engagement of defined activating NK receptors and specific adhesion molecules, NK cells can recognize tumor cells and interact with them forming the "activating immunological synapse," where they polarize the granules and release their content in the synaptic cleft.[19–21] Once released outside the cell, the granule components act cooperatively. Perforins form pores at the target cell surface to facilitate the entry of effector molecules. Inside the target cell, granzymes induce different pro-apoptotic pathways through caspase activation and mitochondrial depolarization, while granulysin causes mitochondrial damage.[13–15,22,23]

At variance with death receptor- or cytokine-mediated cell death induction, granule-dependent cytolysis is potent and rapid, and needs to be tightly controlled by a large array of activating or inhibitory surface NK cell receptors. In humans, these receptors include a complex group of clonally distributed HLA-I-specific inhibitory receptors (KIRs and NKG2A)[24–27] and several activating receptors (including NKG2D, DNAM-1, and the natural cytotoxicity receptors [NCRs]: NKp46, NKp30, NKp44; Table 12.1).[63,69–74] In addition, NK cells express the activating counterparts of HLA-I specific receptors (i.e., activating KIRs and NKG2C; Table 12.1).[75–77] Currently, the specificity of these latter receptors for HLA-I molecules has been formally defined only for KIRDS1, KIR2DS4, and NKG2C, and their role in addressing NK cytotoxicity has not yet been clearly defined.[36–38,43] However, several lines of evidence indicate that they could be involved in the recognition of virally infected cells.[41,78–81] The type and the quantity of receptors involved in NK-target cell interaction dictate the nature (activating vs. inhibitory) of the immunological synapse and the consequent granule release. Many tumor cell lines often express the ligands for different activating receptors and show reduced expression of HLA-I molecules, thus representing potential NK-sensitive targets in vivo (see Table 12.1). For a long time, this idea fueled research to exploit NK cells in cancer immunotherapy. However, only in recent years has their possible use in the clinics become feasible for certain hematologic malignancies, while it is still uncertain for solid tumors. One of the reasons for the long-standing frustrating results is that only recently the real phenotypic and functional heterogeneity of NK cells and their distribution within the body compartments was unveiled.

Phenotypic and Functional Heterogeneity of Natural Killer Cells

Natural Killer Cell Subsets

Besides tumor cell killing, NK cells exert additional functions, including the release of chemokines and cytokines (CCL3, CCL5, and GM-CSF, in addition to IFN-γ, TNF-α)[1,82] and regulatory interactions with dendritic cells (DC), macrophages, monocytes, granulocytes, and T cells.[1,83–86] Moreover, NK cells can variably potentiate their functions in response to different cytokines, including IL-2, IL-15, IL-12, IL-18, and IFNs α/β,[1,87] or to several Pathogen Associated Molecular Patterns (PAMPs; by mean of NK-expressed TLR2, 3, 7, 9).[28]

NK cells circulate in the blood, where they represent approximately 10% to 15% of lymphocytes, and can migrate, and perhaps recirculate, in peripheral tissues and secondary lymphoid organs.[88,89] In this way, they can patrol the body and also encounter, in specific sites, different immune cell types, giving rise to regulatory events. Cytotoxicity and cytokine production are different among specific NK cell subsets in peripheral blood (PB) and lymph nodes (L.N.). These subsets represent NK cells in sequential stages of differentiation. "Terminally differentiated" PB CD56^{dim}CD16^{bright} NK cells expressing CD57 and KIR molecules display high cytotoxic potential and were believed to have limited ability to secrete IFN-γ. The latter concept has been, however, revised recently following the observation that this NK cell subset promptly releases high quantities of IFN-γ upon NCR triggering although for a limited time (<8–12hrs).[90] The CD56^{dim}CD16^{bright}CD57-KIR-NKG2A$^+$ PB NK cells exert both functions at intermediate levels. Finally, less differentiated CD56^{bright}CD16^{dim}CD57-KIR-NKG2A^{++} NK cells, which preferentially locate in L.N., and are poorly represented in PB, express low perforin levels, are poorly cytotoxic but release large amounts of IFN-γ upon cytokine stimulation.[87,91–93]

Plasticity of Natural Killer Cell Effector Functions and Acquisition of Memory-Like Phenotype

It has been proposed that the acquisition of full cytotoxic capabilities can occur only when NK cells have been exposed to autologous MHC-I molecules and have engaged their KIRs and/or NKG2A receptors during their development.[94] The finding that mature NK cells could also reduce or increase their cytolytic potential upon respective cross transfer into MCH-I-/- or wild type mice,[95,96] and that anergic/unlicensed NK cells could acquire full competence during viral infection, suggested that NK cells could actually plastically adapt to milieu perturbations independent of their maturation stage.[97] A further level of complexity is determined by the finding that NK cells could develop "memory-like" properties[98,99] in response to certain viral infections (namely CMV). This phenomenon has been initially described in mice, where CMV infection could induce a population of CMV-specific long-lived LY49H+ NK cells displaying more efficient effector properties after re-challenge with the virus.[100] This cell population could be identified in the liver, spleen, lungs, kidney, and PB.[98] In humans, it has been shown that CMV infection can induce the expansion of NK cells expressing the activating receptor NKG2C.[79,101] The studies conducted in patients receiving haploidentical hematopoietic stem cell (HSC) transplantation for the therapy of high-risk leukemias have recently provided new insights. Indeed, CMV infection or reactivation induced the rapid maturation

Table 12.1 Major Receptor-Ligand Pairs Involved in the Regulation of Natural Killer Cytolytic Activity

NK RECEPTOR	EFFECT ON CYTOLYSIS	LIGAND(S)	LIGAND EXPRESSION ON NONTRANSFORMED CELLS	LIGAND(S) EXPRESSION ON TUMOR CELLS	REF.
KIR2DL1	Inhibitory	HLA-I allotypic determinants (C2 epitope)[a]	Almost all cell types	Potentially down-regulated[b]	28–32
KIR2DL2/3	Inhibitory	HLA-I allotypic determinants (C1/C2 epitopes)[a]	Almost all cell types	Potentially down-regulated[b]	28–32
KIR2DL4	Inhibitory	Nonclassical HLA-I (HLA-G)	Decidua, thymus, cornea, endothelial, and erythroid precursors	Up-regulated in different tumors (melanoma, lungs)	32–34
KIR2DL5	Inhibitory	?	?	?	28,30,35
KIR3DL1	Inhibitory	HLA-I allotypic determinants (Bw4 epitope)[a]	Almost all cell types	Potentially down-regulated[b]	28–32
KIR3DL2	Inhibitory	HLA-I allotypic determinants (alleles HLA-A3/A11)	Almost all cell types	Potentially down-regulated[b]	28–32
KIR2DS1	Activating	HLA-I allotypic determinants (C2 epitope)[a]	Almost all cell types	Potentially down-regulated[b]	28–32,36,37
KIR2DS2	Activating	?	?	?	28–32
KIR2DS4	Activating	HLA-I allotypic determinants (certain HLA-C alleles HLA-A11)	Almost all cell types	Potentially down-regulated[b]	28–32,38,39
		?	?	HLA-I[neg] melanoma cell lines[c]	
KIR2DS5	Activating	?	?	?	28–32,39,40
		?	HIV-infected HLA-Bw4(Ile80)+ cells	?	28–32,41,42
KIR3DS1	Activating	Nonclassical HLA-I (HLA-F)	?	?	
NKG2A:CD94 heterodimer	Inhibitory	Nonclassical HLA-I (HLA-E)	Almost all cell types	Potentially down-regulated[b]	26,28–32,43
NKG2C:CD94 heterodimer	Activating	Nonclassical HLA-I (HLA-E)	Almost all cell types	Potentially down-regulated[b]	28–32,43

(continued)

Table 12.1 Major Receptor-Ligand Pairs Involved in the Regulation of Natural Killer Cytolytic Activity (*continued*)

NK RECEPTOR	EFFECT ON CYTOLYSIS	LIGAND(S)	LIGAND EXPRESSION ON NONTRANSFORMED CELLS	LIGAND(S) EXPRESSION ON TUMOR CELLS	REF.
LIR1/ILT2 /LILRB1	Inhibitory	Certain HLA-A,B,C, alleles	Almost all cell types	Potentially down-regulated[b]	44
		Nonclassical HLA-I (HLA-G)	Decidua, thymus, cornea, endothelial, and erythroid precursors	Up-regulated in different tumors (melanoma, lungs)	
		UL18 viral HLA homologue	CMV-infected cells	?	
IRp60	Inhibitory	PS[d]	Plasma membrane lipidic bilayer inner leaflet: live cells outer leaflet: apoptotic cells	Plasma membrane lipidic bilayer outer leaflet: tumor cells	45,46
NKp30	Activating	BAT3[e]/BAG6[f]	Intracellular or in exosomes released by DC upon stress/activation stimuli	Up-regulated in tumor cells: Raji (Burkitt lymphoma), 293T (human embryonic kidney transformed cells)	47–50
		B7-H6	Monocytes and neutrophils upon stimulation with TLR ligands or proinflammatory cytokines	Highly expressed in Carcinomas Leukemias LymphomasMelanomas	51,52
		HSPG[g]	All cells	Up-regulated/modified in different tumor cell lines: HeLa (cervical cancer), PC3 (prostate cancer), 1106 (melanoma), PANC-1 (pancreatic ductal carcinoma	53
NKp46	Activating	?	Pancreatic b-cells, Liver stellate cells	Highly expressed on a variety of tumor cell lines[h]	47,54
		HSPG[g]	All cells	Up-regulated/modified in different tumor cell lines: HeLa (cervical cancer) PC3 (prostate cancer) 1106 (melanoma) PANC-1 (pancreatic ductal carcinoma)	53
		Influenza virus HA Sendai virus HN	Infected cells	?	55
		CFP[i] (properdin)	Soluble factor	?	56

(*continued*)

Receptor	Type	Ligand	Expression	Tumor/Cells	Ref
NKp44	Activating	21spe-MLL5[h] isoform	Not expressed	Tumor cells of hematopoietic and nonhematopoietic origin: erythroleukemia, B-lymphoma, T cell leukemia, Melanoma, Kidney, bladder, and cervical carcinomas	57
		HSPG[g]	All cells	Up-regulated/modified in different tumor cell lines: HeLa (cervical cancer), PC3 (prostate cancer), 1106 (melanoma), PANC-1 (pancreatic ductal carcinoma)	53
		NID1[m]	Component of the Basement Membrane	Different tumor cell lines: SH-SY-5Y (neuroblastoma), A172 (glioblastoma), C-32 (melanoma), A2774 (ovarian carcinoma), JEG-3 (placental choriocarcin), A549 (lung carcinoma)	58
		PDGF-DD[n]	Soluble factor	Different tumor cells including glioma cell lines	59
		HLA-DP (subset of molecules)	Up-regulated during inflammation	?	60
		Influenza virus HA, Sendai virus HN	Infected cells	?	55
NKG2D	Activating	MICA-B, ULBP1-6	Induced by stress signals (DNA damage, heat shock)	Up-regulated in tumors of epithelial and non-epithelial origin	61,62
DNAM-1	Activating	CD112/Nectin2, CD155/PVR[l]	At low levels on monocytes, DC and activated CD4+ T cells. Expressed within cell junctions	Upregulated or expressed outside cell junctions in different tumor cells: Melanoma, Neuroblastoma, Lung, cervical, colon, ovarian, kidney carcinoma, Glioblastoma, T cell leukemia, Myeloid leukemia	63,50
2B4	Activating	CD48	Lymphocytes, monocytes, endothelial cells	Lymphomas, multiple myelomas	64,65

(continued)

Table 12.1 Major Receptor-Ligand Pairs Involved in the Regulation of Natural Killer Cytolytic Activity (*continued*)

NK RECEPTOR	EFFECT ON CYTOLYSIS	LIGAND(S)	LIGAND EXPRESSION ON NONTRANSFORMED CELLS	LIGAND(S) EXPRESSION ON TUMOR CELLS	REF.
NKp80/KLRF1	Activating	AICL[m]	Myeloid cells (up-regulated by TLR engagement)	Up-regulated on different tumor cells of hematopoietic and nonhematopoietic origin: U937 (histiocytic lymphoma); THP1 (acute monocytic leukemia) K562 (myelogenous leukemia); HeLaS3; and ME180 (carcinomas)	66,67,68

[a] HLA-I alleles bearing the indicated epitopes: C1 = HLA C alleles bearing Lys80, C2 = HLA C (and some HLA B) alleles bearing Asn80, HLA Bw4 = HLA B (and some HLA A) alleles bearing Ile80 or Thr80.

[b] A general HLA-I down-regulation or specific HLA-I loci deletion or protein expression decrease has been frequently observed in tumor cells.

[c] The expression of the ligand has been suggested by its reactivity with human recombinant KIR2DS4-Fc chimera and/or by mAb-mediated blocking of the receptor in functional assays.

[d] PS = PhosphatidylSerine.

[e] BAT3: HLA-B-associated transcript 3.

[f] BAG6: BCL-2-associated athanogene 6.

[g] HSPG: heparan sulfate proteoglycans (NKp46, NKp44, and NKp30 may recognize epitopes that are specifically expressed on tumor cells).

[h] The expression of the ligand has been suggested by its reactivity with human recombinant NKp46-Fc chimera and/or by mAb-mediated blocking of the receptor in functional assays.

[i] CFP: Complement factor P.

[j] 21spe- MLL5: Mixed-lineage leukemia-5 containing 21spe exon.

[m] NID1: Nidogen-1.

[n] PDGF: Platelet-derived growth factor - dimeric isoform DD.

[o] PVR = Poliovirus receptor.

[p] AICL: Activation-induced C-type lectin.

and expansion of NKG2C+ cells in HSCT recipients. This cell population persisted for months after clearance of the infection. Remarkably, these cells appeared to be terminally differentiated as they expressed the KIR⁺CD57⁺ phenotype and displayed potent cytolytic activity against tumor cells.[79,102,103] Another study on NKG2C-/- patients provided evidence that CMV infection could induce the expansion of activating KIR⁺ cells.[81] In summary, available data indicate that the induction of memory cells involves specific NK subsets expressing clonally distributed activating receptors possibly recognizing specific viruses. So far, no specific NK subset has been identified or characterized by clonally distributed receptors recognizing tumor-expressed antigens. Indeed, the activating receptors involved in tumor cell recognition are roughly expressed on the whole NK cell population. Therefore, in the case of tumors, the expansion of specific memory cells may not occur or, anyway, it may be hardly tracked unless new "memory" markers could be identified on NK cells. In this context, important progress in the characterization of NK cells in cancer patients and within the tumor tissues is provided by new tools for high dimensional analyses of single cells, which enable the simultaneous evaluation of a broad number of markers involved in tumor cell recognition, signaling, metabolism, or transcription regulation. These new tools, such as polychromatic flow cytometry, mass cytometry, and single-cell RNA sequencing (RNAseq), have been recently used to accurately define different NK cell subsets and functional characteristics, including maturational stages, memory or adaptive features, or education/licensing status.[104–106] In a recent study, it has also been shown that mitochondrial autophagy promotes the generation of NK cell memory in CMV-infected mice;[107] while another study described mitochondrial morphologic changes during the acquisition of a memory phenotype on T cells.[108] Thus, the study of mitochondrial dynamics could provide new hints not only to track memory acquisition by NK cells but also to investigate new ways to exploit this phenomenon for immunotherapy. Remarkably, NK cells endowed with memory-like properties (i.e., responding promptly to inflammatory cytokines or tumor cell interaction) have been successfully induced in vitro by using different strategies, and their efficacy in tumor control are under investigation at the preclinical and clinical level.[109–111]

Distribution and Features of Natural Killer Cells in Peripheral Tissues

The potential of NK-based therapies, especially in solid tumors, is dependent upon their distribution and nature in peripheral tissues. This aspect of NK cell biology still represents a rapidly evolving area of research as, for many years, the lack of specific markers or appropriate reagents, and the difficulty in obtaining biological materials, has hampered the study of noncirculating NK cells. Growing information on NK cell subset characterization in both mice and humans, and the development of improved cell isolation techniques and in situ imaging, made possible recent advances. Various studies conducted in humans under either healthy or pathological conditions indicate that NK cells are quite widely distributed in peripheral tissues.[88,112,113] NK cells have been described in secondary lymphoid tissues (SLT), spleen, liver, lungs, uterus, intestinal mucosa, kidney, breast, skin, adipose tissues, and joints.[88,89,113–119]

In SLT, NK cells represent a small fraction of the local lymphocyte population, while in other tissues, such as liver, kidney, uterus, and lungs, their frequency among lymphocytes is higher, ranging from 10% to 20% in lungs to over 50% in the uterus.[88,89,114,115] At variance with SLT, in many tissues, including lungs, kidney, breast, and liver, a considerable fraction of NK cells express the CD56^dim phenotype. These cells have also been demonstrated to express NCR and KIR (lungs and liver),[120,121] and high perforin levels (colon, liver, kidney, and lungs).[114] These findings suggest that CD56^dim cells residing in tissues are competent when needed, as they are terminally differentiated cytotoxic cells (i.e., express KIRs and perforin) and express activating receptors (e.g., NCR), whose triggering induces killing of NK targets. Nevertheless, CD56^bright cells are largely represented in many tissues, reaching percentages that are much higher than those observed in PBNK cells. For example, approximately 50% of liver NK cells are represented by CD56^bright cytokine-producing cells. Intrahepatic CD56^bright NK cells express low levels of perforins but can exert effector functions using TRAIL, which is induced in these cells upon IFN-α stimulation.[122] In the uterus, particularly in decidual tissue during the first trimester of pregnancy, the majority of NK cells express CD56 at high levels (i.e., CD56^bright). However, these cells frequently express KIRs and are characterized by unique functional properties. CD56^bright decidual NK cells are poorly cytotoxic; rather, they contribute to the maintenance of pregnancy through different mechanisms. They produce cytokines and chemokines that are involved in angiogenesis and tissue building/remodeling (such as CXCL8, VEGF, CXCL12, and CXCL10).[119,123] Furthermore, they favor proliferation of regulatory T (T_{reg}) cells, a cell population that is thought to play a crucial role in supporting the maternal-fetal tolerance.[124]

An important question regarding peripheral tissue NK cells regards their origin, that is, whether they derived from NK cells that recirculate between PB and tissues, or are stably resident in a given tissue. It has been recently proposed that the surface molecules CD69, CD103, and CD49a could represent putative markers of tissue-resident lymphocytes in mice and humans.[115] Analysis of available data in the literature has shown that about a half of NK cells in the liver and SLT and the large majority of lung NK cells are CD69⁻CD103⁻CD49a⁻, which reflects a circulating NK cell phenotype. According to this analysis, CD56^dim cells essentially represented tissue-circulating NK cells, while tissue-resident NK cells included virtually all CD56^bright and a fraction of CD56^dim cells present in the analyzed tissues. The picture is changing as recent evidence suggests that the phenotype of lung-resident NK cells includes the co-expression of CD103, CD69, and CD49a.[125] These observations suggest that "terminally differentiated" PB NK cells transiently circulate or are recruited in different tissues. This notion is further supported by well-established data indicating that the CD56^dim CD16^+ cells express CXCR1, ChemR23, and CX₃CR1 and respond to CXCL8 and CX₃CL1,[87,126] a group of chemokine-receptors and chemokines driving lymphocytes through endothelium toward inflamed tissues. The origin of tissue-resident NK cells has not yet been completely clarified. Some of them may derive from circulating mature NK cells establishing residency in the tissues upon environmental stimuli; other cells (conceivably those expressing the CD56^bright phenotype) might have been generated from precursors that are already present in the tissues or which may be derived from the circulation.

The characterization of tissue-resident NK cells opens an additional question regarding their unequivocal identification among other innate lymphoid cells (ILC).[127,128] Three major groups of ILC have been characterized on the basis of the type of released cytokines and/or expressed transcription factors. Group 1 ILCs include conventional CD56^dim and CD56^bright NK cells (Tbet^+EOMES^+) and IFN-γ-producing ILC1s (Tbet^+). Group 2 ILCs (RORα^+GATA3^+) produce IL-4, IL-5, and IL-13. Group 3 ILCs comprise lymphoid tissue-inducer cells (RORγt^+), producing IL-17 and IL-22; NCR^+ ILC3s (RORγt^+), producing IL-22; and NCR⁻ ILC3s (RORγt^+), producing IL-17 and IL-22. Apparently, none of the non-NK ILCs are endowed with cytotoxic capability, although some of them express NKp44 or NKp46, which are among the most important activating NK-receptor molecules, whose triggering induces NK-mediated cytotoxicity. In addition, the CD127 ILC marker can also be expressed by certain CD56^bright cells. Therefore, it should be considered that the definition of the NK cell population in tissues based on single markers, even if highly specific (such as NKp46), may have overestimated the size of conventional NK cells, at least in those tissues (such as tonsils or intestinal mucosa) in which the presence of NCR^+ ILC has been documented.

As final considerations, it should be recalled that the composition of NK cell populations and the mechanisms that regulate their homeostasis in the tissues could be heavily modified by alterations of the local microenvironment occurring during the generation and the progression of the tumor lesion and by the concurrent recruitment of specialized NK cells derived from novel CD34^+ cell precursors with marked tissue-homing characteristics.[129]

EXPLOITATION OF NATURAL KILLER CELL EFFECTOR MECHANISMS AGAINST HEMATOLOGIC MALIGNANCIES

Natural Killer Cells Kill Malignant Tumor Cells of Hematologic Origin

Since the first discovery of NK cells, considerable efforts have been devoted to assess the extent of their antitumor activity, trying to define the number and type of NK-susceptible cell targets. In humans, the erythroleukemia cell line K562 represented one of the first described NK targets.[130] Subsequently, NK cells have been shown to kill in vitro a number of established or primary cell lines from different hematologic malignancies, including T and B leukemias, myelogenous leukemias, lymphomas, and multiple myelomas.[66,131–134] Blocking experiments using specific mAbs demonstrated that most activating NK receptors, including the NCRs, NKG2D, and DNAM-1, could be involved in the recognition and killing of transformed cells from various hematologic malignancies.[131] Thanks to the progressive identification of the NK-R ligands (whose list is presently still incomplete!); it has been possible to show that, indeed, activating NK-R ligands can be highly, and/or ectopically, expressed on many tumor cells including hematologic malignancies (Table 12.1). As previously mentioned, the engagement of activating NK receptors by their ligands is crucial to the formation of the activating synapse and the killing of the target through the release of cytolytic granules. The fact that cytolytic granules could represent the major effector mechanism in the elimination of tumor cells is further suggested by a recent study by Chia et al. showing an extraordinarily high incidence of hematologic malignancies in patients carrying defects in the perforin gene.[135]

The importance of the NK cell antitumor effector activity in tumor surveillance is corroborated by many studies showing that NK cells are frequently suppressed/altered in hematologic malignancies. For years, tumor-mediated suppressive effects and the incomplete knowledge of NK cell biology frustrated attempts to successfully employ these cells for therapy, until the breakthrough of the haploidentical HSCT (see the text that follows).

Suppression of Natural Killer Cells in Hematologic Malignancies

It is well established that leukemia cells, primarily the leukemic stem cells (LSC), may be particularly resistant to different chemotherapeutic drugs.[136–139] In particular, one of the consequences of the acquisition of drug-resistant phenotype by leukemic cells is the emergence of cross-resistance against immune effector cells. Leukemia-elusion from recognition by the immune system can be achieved through several mechanisms.[140] Different reports revealed that the patient autologous PB NK cells often show phenotypic and functional defects at diagnosis. Activating receptors, such as DNAM-1, NKp30, and NKp46, display low-expression levels on patient NK cell surfaces[141–143] paralleled by an increased expression of CD94/NKG2A inhibitory receptor.[144] Along with the phenotypic defects, cytolytic activity and TNF-α and/or IFN-γ production are also impaired.[142–144] These defects are associated with poor clinical outcomes. Interestingly, the NK cell phenotype and function can be restored ex vivo in patients undergoing successful therapy, thus achieving complete remission. This observation underlies the role of acute myeloid leukemia (AML) blasts in inhibition of NK cell function.[145] Such perturbation in PB NK cell physiology can also be observed in myelodysplastic syndromes (MDS), in which PB NK cells show severe defects, including down-regulation of activating receptors,[146] reduced cytotoxic potential,[146,147] and reduced cytokine-induced proliferation in vitro.[147] Several mechanisms are involved in the suppression of NK cell function in hematological malignancies, including alterations in the expression of some activating receptors through cell-to-cell contacts, production of immunosuppressive soluble factors by leukemic cells, and defects in the normal lymphopoiesis.

Reduction in activating receptor expression by autologous NK cells may be the result of a continuous exposure to the cognate ligands expressed by AML blasts, leading to an exhaustion of the NK cell cytotoxic activity.[148,149] Other receptors such as CD96 and CD200 (OX2), expressed by NK cells and by some AML, respectively, have been recently identified as suppressors of patient's NK cell cytotoxic and cytokine production during the antitumor response.[150,151] In addition to cell-to-cell contact-based inhibition, various soluble molecules, including soluble ligands of activating NK receptors, soluble factors, such as TGF-β or IL-10, ROS, and tryptophan catabolites, can inhibit NK cell functions. In AML patients' serum, the presence of soluble NKG2D-L (including MICA, MICB, and ULBP2) is associated with a down-regulation of the surface NKG2D expression, leading to an impairment in NKG2D-mediated NK cell activity.[152] Soluble ligands can also be detected in the serum bound to tumor-derived exosomes.[153,154] Exosomes from leukemia/lymphoma cells can express NKG2D-L, leading to an inhibition of the NK cell activation.[153] However, while soluble BAG6 (an NKp30 ligand) released by lymphocytic leukemia cells works as an inhibitory ligand of NKp30,[154] exosome-bound BAG6 activates NK cells in chronic lymphocytic leukemia (CLL).

Soluble inhibitory factors, such as IL-10 and TGF-β, may also play a significant inhibitory role in PMID 17134371. In this context, sera derived from AML patients have been shown to contain microvesicles bearing TGF-β on their surface, resulting in impairment of NK cell function.[155] Besides immunosuppressive molecules, products of the leukemic cell metabolism can also be released by AML blasts. For example, in leukemic blasts, enhanced tryptophan catabolism leads to an immunosuppressive environment. Thus, overexpression of the IDO enzyme catalyzes tryptophan degradation by producing l-kynurenine, which can directly affect NK cell function.[156] Furthermore, some AML types, characterized by specific mutation patterns (including activating RAS mutations or PLT3/ITD mutation),[157,158] produce high levels of ROS that, in turn, can induce NK-cell defects in the expression of activating receptors, such as NKp46 and NKG2D.[159]

A central issue is whether leukemia cells may influence the survival of normal stem cells and their differentiation into immune cells with potential anti-leukemia activity. Increasing evidence supports the notion that in AML, BM environment influences healthy hematopoiesis by affecting BM cell populations. Normal CD34$^+$CD38$^+$progenitors were found reduced in BM of AML patients, likely resulting from impediment to differentiation of the HSC-progenitor progression.[160] Consequently, NK cell differentiation in the BM seems to be affected by AML. Malignant cells may contribute to generate an aberrant BM niche.[161] Recent work by Vasold et al. suggests a role for aberrant BM mesenchymal stromal cells (α-SMA$^+$ mesenchymal stem cells) and hypoxia in the reduction of NK cell cytotoxic activity against autologous AML blasts.[162] Recently, we have shown that IL-1β-releasing AML blasts could inhibit the recovery of CD34$^+$-derived CD161$^+$CD56$^+$ cells, resulting in a reduced generation of ILC3 and NK cells.[163] In the context of hematopoietic stem cell transplant (HSCT), it is possible that IL-1β released by residual AML blasts may alter the BM microenvironment and suppress the proliferation of NK cell precursors. Since in patients receiving haplo-HSCT NK, cells play a fundamental role in clearing residual leukemia blasts after the conditioning regimen, it is possible that AML-mediated suppression could play a dominant suppressive role. Altogether, these observations indicate that AML blasts modify the BM environment, including stromal cells, precursor cells, and mature immune cell populations.

Natural Killer Cell–Based Therapeutic Approaches

Most attention in tumor immunotherapy has concentrated on the augmentation of adaptive immunity; in particular, adoptive T cell transfer, including the generation of chimeric antigen receptor (CAR)-carrying T cells and on checkpoint inhibition by targeting inhibitory receptors expressed on tumor-specific T cells.

There is ample evidence, however, as discussed earlier, that NK cells are deeply affected by the tumor and its microenvironment and that changes in their functional repertoire result in reduced activity, thus contributing to increased invasion and metastasis.

The evidence of NK cell–impaired function suggests a potential for its reversal as a novel anti-cancer immunotherapy. In fact, the relevance of addressing NK cells as an immunotherapeutic tool is provided by a number of studies showing their essential role in immune surveillance against cancer cells. Indeed, defects in the development of NK cells or their function result in recurrent severe viral infections and increased risk of developing cancer.[164] In particular, higher risk of developing cancer is observed in individuals with reduced NK cell cytotoxic activity.[165]

Thus, restoration of NK cell function is an attractive option that is actively being pursued. Importantly, this strategy has already provided satisfactory results in the area of bone marrow transplantation for AML and multiple myeloma (MM).

Several aspects of NK cell biology and function considerably differ from T cells. These differences may be considered as assets in the exploitation of NK cells, alone or in combination with other strategies. Among these, the absence of antigen-specificity, preformed perforin storage, shorter in vivo survival, and "preferential" targeting of cancer stem cells are the outstanding characteristics that drive the development of NK cell immunotherapeutic strategies.

In general, NK cell–targeting therapies may act in vivo in the tumor microenvironment or use adoptive transfer of ex vivo prepared NK cells.

In the first case, the administration of substances that are acting directly on NK cells in the tumor microenvironment or that may engage in activating NK cell receptors or inhibitory NK cell receptors should be considered to overcome the immunosuppressive effect of the tumor/tumor microenvironment. An approach is represented by the in vivo administration of cytokines that induce NK cell expansion and activation. The list of cytokines includes Il-2, -12, -15, -18, -21, and type I interferons. The in vivo administration of these cytokines to sustain NK cell activity has been evaluated in patients with cancer, demonstrating minimal or no clinical effects. Repeated injections of rhIL-2 are generally well tolerated, but no clinical advantage of IL-2 therapy has been recorded.[166] This lack of effect is caused in part by the activation of T_{reg} cells that express the high-affinity IL-2 receptor (CD25) and may inhibit NK cell function, and by T_{reg}-NK cell competition for IL-2. Diphtheria-toxin-IL-2 fusion protein pre-treatment to deplete T_{reg} cells improved complete remission and disease-free survival in patients with AML undergoing haploidentical NK cell infusion.[167] No convincing clinical advantage has been recorded so far with the administration of IL-12 or IL-18. There is some promise with the use of IL-21 in the immunotherapy of metastatic tumors,[168] when co-administered with tumor-targeting mAbs.[169] Its effects, however, are pleiotropic, are not limited to NK cells, and extend also, among others, to T cells, NKT cells, and monocytes/macrophages.[170,171] IL-21 administration is being developed in the immunotherapy of HIV, showing some promise in the SIV model of macaque infection.[170,172,173] There is still caution in the clinical development of IL-21 as a therapeutic agent, due to its involvement in allergy/autoimmune conditions, including systemic lupus, inflammatory bowel disease, and rheumatoid arthritis.[170,174,175] The administration of IL-15 as an NK cell–targeting immunotherapeutic tool has the advantage of selectively sustaining NK cell activation and expansion (and not T_{reg} cell expansion)[176] and allowing achievement of antitumor effect in selected studies, where allogeneic NK cells are adoptively transferred after IL-15 activation.[177] An additional prospect is the use of molecules that inhibit inhibitory or immunosuppressive signaling (TGF-ß, PI3K)[178,179] in the tumor microenvironment. An ongoing clinical trial (NCT02304419) is investigating the effectiveness of one of the molecules: galunisertib, a TGF-ß receptor kinase I inhibitor.[179] In conclusion, the administration of cytokines to activate NK cells for cancer immunotherapy will focus in the future on combinations with adoptively transferred NK cells, as exemplified by ongoing studies combining adoptive transfer of NK cells and IL-15 for the treatment of solid and hematological cancers (NCT01385423 and NCT01875601), the transfer of genetically modified NK cells expressing IL-15 to increase antitumor activity,[180] or the administration of IL-15 super-agonists (IL-15SA/IL-15RαSu-Fc; ALT-80) to boost antitumor activity of NK cells and CD8+CTL.[181]

A second approach to NK cell targeting in vivo has recently emerged from the observations that some cytotoxic drugs display NK cell–modulating activity beyond their original activity against cancer cells. Histone deacetylase inhibitors (valproate, trichostatin A, vorinostat, romidepsin, chidamide), demethylating agents (azacytidine, decitabine), proteasome inhibitors (bortezomib), immunomodulatory drugs (thalidomide, lenalidomide, pomalidomide), and tyrosine kinase inhibitors (TKI; imatinib, dasatinib, sorafenib) can contribute to antitumor cytotoxicity by increasing NK cell activity directly, through increased antibody-dependent cell cytotoxicity, or via increased expression of NK-activating ligands in tumor cells (e.g., MIC-A/B, ULBP).[182] Within the same agents, some have NK cell–stimulating effects while others may reduce NK cell activity. For example, the majority of TKI abolish NK cell function with the exception of imatinib, which activates NK cells through DC stimulation.[178]

A third strategy is represented by the administration of mAbs or soluble ligands that trigger activating receptors on the surface of host NK cells. Monoclonal antibodies specific for antigens expressed by cancer cells have a dual mechanism of action mediated by the two portions of the antibody. Fab fragments bind receptors on the surface of cancer cells, thus inducing apoptosis or influencing tumor growth, while the Fc portion recruits effector cells that recognize bound antibodies on the cancer cell surface, including monocytes, neutrophils, and NK cells. In this context, recognition of bound Fc by NK cells via CD16 induces antibody-dependent cellular cytotoxicity (ADCC), which plays a pivotal function in the antitumor effect. Tumor targeting that exploits NK cell triggering via CD16 includes treatment with trastuzumab (mAb to ErbB2 (HER2)), cetuximab (mAb to epidermal growth factor receptor), or rituximab (mAb to the B cell–specific surface antigen CD20). Indeed, single nucleotide polymorphisms in the genes encoding the Fc correlate with clinical responses to tumor-targeting mAbs.[183,184] Accordingly, combination of cytokines that enhance NK cell activity together with the administration of anti-tumor mAbs results in increased NK cell activity and increased rate of clinical response.[185,186] Focus has been dedicated to improve these mAbs activities by molecular engineering to obtain higher Fc affinity for CD16, and to reduce CD16 shedding by disintegrin and metalloprotease inhibitors following NK cell activation.[187,188] Recent work shows that ADAM 17 and other small molecule inhibitors of metalloproteinase may have an independent antitumor mechanism of action in addition to limiting CD16 shedding from NK cell surface.[189,190]

In addition to mAbs, bispecific or trispecific NK cell engaging constructs represent an alternative strategy to target NK cells and tumor cells and efficiently induce ADCC in vivo. Strategies considering the administration of bispecific antibodies were devised years ago and lost some appeal after noting that drug-resistant cancer cell populations emerged. Renewed interest has been recently stimulated by trispecific antibodies that incorporate CD133, CD16 Fv domains with IL-15,[191] and by targeting other activating receptors on NK cells.

A novel target for NK cell triggering in vivo is represented by CD137 (4-1BB, TNFSFR9 product). Its triggering as a co-stimulating molecule increases the anti-lymphoma activity of the effect of rituximab (anti-CD20)[192] or the efficacy of cetuximab (anti-EGFR).[193] In a recent trial in patients with head and neck cancer, the anti-CD137 agonist urelumab increased cetuximab-activated NK cell survival, DC maturation, and tumor antigen cross-presentation. In addition, upregulation of CD127 by intra-tumoral NK cells correlated with FcgRIII polymorphism.[194]

Finally, a fourth possibility for NK-based immunotherapy is represented by reverting NK cell inhibition in the tumor microenvironment using checkpoint blockade with agents masking inhibitory receptors expressed on NK cells.

Checkpoint inhibitors are currently being successfully used to release T cell activity in vivo. Administration of anti-PD1 and anti-CTLA4 alone or in combination has successfully entered clinical practice in the immunotherapy of solid tumors, including melanoma, colorectal cancer, renal cancer, and lymphoma.[195–197] It has been demonstrated recently that NK cells may express PD-1.[198] In vivo administration of anti-PD1 may thus not only disrupt T cell but also NK cell checkpoint blockade. In addition, in the case of anti-PD-L1 mAbs, NK cell–mediated ADCC may contribute to the effects observed on tumor control, in addition to the checkpoint release of T cell activity. Additional strategies to release NK cell activity are represented by the use of mAbs blocking KIRs on NK cells.[199,200] While a trial in multiple myeloma failed to show effects for the mAb when used alone in AML,[201] a recombinant version of the anti-KIR mAb, lirilumab (IPH2102), is currently being evaluated in combination with anti-CD20 or lenalidomide in solid and hematological cancers.[202,203] The disruption of the NKG2A-HLA-E interaction represents an additional option for NK cell targeting. A blocking mAb to NKG2A (IPH2201; monalizumab) is currently being evaluated alone or in combination for the treatment (ibrutinib, cetuximab, durvalumab) of solid cancers. It has been shown to be quite effective in association with cetuximab in patients with recurrent or metastatic HNSCC.[204] Monalizumab is currently under investigation in association with anti-PD-1 durvalumab in metastatic solid tumors, in non-small cell lung cancer (NSCLC; advanced solid tumors, NCT02671435, and NSCLC, NCT03833440), and as maintenance therapy after allo-SCT (hematologic malignancies, NCT02921685).

Another family of inhibitory receptors is represented by TACTILE CD96 and TIGIT, which unlike KIRs and NKG2A are not HLA-specific. These molecules are expressed by NK cells, bind nectin (CD112) and PVR (CD155), and counteract the activating effect of DNAM-1[205] with preferential inhibition of cytotoxicity (TIGIT) or IFN-γ production (TACTILE).[205] mAbs that block CD96 are effective in reducing metastasis in mice and act in synergy with mAbs that inhibit PD-1 and CTLA-4 and may need to be co-administered for maximal NK cell checkpoint blockade.[150,206]

TIM-3 is another checkpoint-inhibiting molecule that is currently being investigated for its potential to inhibit T cell activity in exhausted cells.[207] TIM-3 is also expressed by NK cells with inducible phenotype and binds Galectin 9, and its targeting reverses exhaustion in NK cells in melanoma patients.[208] TIM-3-targeting needs further development before entering clinical application.

An alternate strategy to the in vivo stimulation of functionally impaired NK cells is represented by adoptive transfer in the autologous or allogeneic setting of NK cells activated ex vivo. In addition, increasing efforts are focusing on the genetic modification of NK cells to induce chimeric antigen receptors.

A common approach to adoptive transfer of NK cells in patients with cancer is the collection of unmodified NK cells, their expansion in vitro, and in vivo reinfusion. Recent protocols have improved the ability to expand NK cells for adoptive transfer in vivo.[209] This approach has limited application in acute leukemias and has shown limited efficacy in determining clinical responses in metastatic and nonmetastatic solid tumors since re-infused NK cells remain in the circulation and have limited tumor-homing ability.[210]

On the contrary, the transfer of allogeneic NK cells in KIR-mismatched donors has shown remarkable results in patients undergoing hematopoietic stem cell transplantation for AML.[211] On the basis of the expression of inhibitory or activating KIR in NK cells and of the HLA class I alleles expressed on target cells (e.g., leukemia blasts), it is now possible to identify different groups of alloreactive NK cells[212] and suitably use the matches to exploit NK cell versus leukemia activity while avoiding GvHD[213] in pediatric and adult patients with AML.[214]

Engineering and redirecting NK cells against specific tumor antigens is another option that is being investigated. This can exploit chimeric antigen receptor (CAR) technology devised for CAR T cell immunotherapy.[215] So far, the CAR-NK technology is largely in the preclinical phase of development, although some trials are already underway. Compared to CAR T immunotherapy, CAR-NK adoptive transfer offers distinct benefits including the advantage of exploiting KIR-HLA mismatches; a shorter half-life, thus limiting the extent of adverse effects; and maintenance of antitumor effectiveness in spite of down-modulation of HLA class I molecules that are necessary for CAR T cell antigen recognition.[216] There are some hindrances to the widespread use of CAR-NK cell immunotherapy due to the relative difficulty of expanding large numbers of NK cells, their sensitivity to cryo-preservation, and relative resistance to infection/transfection.[217] For these reasons, an active area of scientific clinical interest is oriented to NK-92, a transformed cell line constituted by activated NK cells,[218] which are irradiated before infusion.[219] NK-92 cells may be engineered to express recombinant tumor-targeting receptors against both hematologic and solid tumors.[219,220]

The Breakthrough of Haploidentical HSCT

In the absence of an HLA-matched donor, alternative donors/sources of HSCs, such as unrelated umbilical cord blood and HLA-haploidentical relatives, are being increasingly used.[221] Family members identical for one HLA haplotype and fully mismatched for the other (i.e., haploidentical) can serve as HSC donor. Donor T cell depletion has been shown to reduce acute and chronic GvHD, albeit at the cost of slower T cell recovery.[222] Optimization and increase in number of donor CD34+ cell proved to be effective in avoiding transplant failure and ensuring engraftment in a wide range of diseases in addition to high-risk leukemias.[223]

A turning point in T cell–depleted haplo-HSCT came from the observation that donor NK cell allo-reactivity due to KIR-HLA mismatch sharply reduces the risk of graft rejection and of leukemia relapse protecting recipients from GvHD.[211] Altogether, studies confirming the benefit of KIR-mismatched NK cells in T cell–depleted haplo-HSCT represented a true revolution.[224,225] The administration of KIR-mismatched NK cells provides a GVL effect of donor NK cells against leukemic recipient cells, thus preventing relapse and protecting, together with T cell depletion, the generation of allo-specific T cells initiating GvHD.[213]

Phenotypic identification of the alloreactive NK-cell subset and evaluation of the NK cytolytic activity against leukemic cells represent important criteria in donor selection. Multicolor flow cytometric analysis, using appropriate combinations of monoclonal antibodies (mAbs), allows the identification and definition of the size of the alloreactive NK-cell population.[212] Genotypic analysis can be combined with flow-cytometry to explore donor-recipient KIR mismatches to suitably select haplo-HSCT donors.[226] Interestingly, alloreactive NK cells can be detected for long periods of time (up to 4 years) after transplantation. In some patients, the magnitude of the alloreactive NK-cell population may be even larger in the recipient than in the donor, suggesting that they had been selected/expanded preferentially in vivo.[211,212,225]

Other Natural Killer Cell–Based Immunotherapeutic Strategies Against Hematological Malignancies

Following the demonstration of the anti-leukemia effect of alloreactive NK cells infused in haplo-HSCT, a setting of adoptive transfer of allogeneic NK cells after chemotherapy without HSCT proved to induce remission in nine of 15 AML patients.[227] The same approach resulted in a 100% 2-year event-free survival in 10 pediatric patients with AML.[228] Chemotherapy consisting of cyclophosphamide and fludarabine followed by donor-recipient inhibitory KIR-HLA-mismatched NK cells is well tolerated by patients, results in successful engraftment, and is a promising novel therapy for reducing the risk of relapse in patients with myeloid malignancies treated with conventional chemotherapy.

Another NK cell–targeting treatment is represented by the combination of the immunomodulatory compounds lenalidomide and pomalidomide[229] for a review on the mode of action) in combination with rituximab (anti-CD20) in relapsed/refractory B-cell lymphomas and chronic lymphocytic leukemia.[230,231] Besides increasing ADCC,[232] lenalidomide also increases tumor cell expression of NK cell receptor ligands. Its administration is negatively affected by long-term steroid treatment.[233,234]

In other hematologic malignancies, the administration of mAbs specific for antigens expressed by neoplastic cells has proven advantageous as in the case of rituximab (anti-CD20) for lymphomas. The effect is mediated by the Fab portion of the mAb that induces apoptosis in lymphoma cells. The FcγR portion has proven to mediate NK cell–dependent ADCC as part of its action and polymorphisms of the FcγR influence response to treatment.[183] Accordingly, improvements in the affinity of Fc portions of therapeutic mAbs improves the NK cell immunotherapeutic targeting and range of malignancies where these drugs may be employed.[235] These effects may also work for nonhematological tumors treated with antitumor mAbs.

Bortezomib, an inhibitor of 26S proteasome, decreases MHC class I molecule expression on cancer cells[236] and induces expression of NK cell receptor ligands and may be used for the treatment of multiple myeloma with the administration of adoptively transferred NK cells.[237] Also lenalidomide, a drug successfully used in MM, increases NK cell ligand expression, augments actin remodeling, and lowers the threshold for NK cell activation.[238]

Inhibitors of KIR signaling on NK cells have been developed to clinical grade in order to release NK cell function. In MM, KIR-inhibiting mAb (IPH2101), which is safe and well tolerated in AML and MM,[199] showed no clinical efficacy in patients with smoldering MM,[201] but holds promise in combination with lenalidomide or rituximab.[202,239]

EXPLOITATION OF NATURAL KILLER CELL EFFECTOR MECHANISMS AGAINST SOLID TUMORS

Natural Killer Cells Kill Malignant Cells From Solid Tumors

As in the case of hematologic malignancies, transformed cells derived from many solid tumors variably express ligand(s) for one or more of the major activating NK receptors (Table 12.1). Thus, the engagement of the NCRs, DNAM-1, and NKG2D, and the release of the cytolytic granules represent a crucial NK effector mechanism for the killing of solid tumor-derived cells. It should be noted that additional TRAIL-mediated mechanisms of tumor cell killing might be active in the liver. As previously mentioned, a considerable fraction of total liver NK cells can express TRAIL upon IFN-α stimulation and play a role in the control HCV infection.[122] However, analysis of NK cells extracted from liver perfusates at the time of living donor liver transplantation showed that large majority liver of NK cells expressed TRAIL upon exposure to IL-2 and displayed strong cytotoxicity against a hepatocellular carcinoma cell line.[17]

The use of CAR-expressing NK cells (CAR-NK) is also being pursued in solid tumors.

In spite of the many studies characterizing the antitumor activity of NK cells both in vitro and in animal models, the exploitation of these cells for the cure of solid tumors has proven very hard to realize so far. These difficulties are essentially related to the negative effects that the local tumor microenvironment can exert directly on the NK cell effector mechanisms and/or on the process of tumor infiltration.

Tumor Microenvironment and the Evasion From the Natural Killer Cell Attack

Natural Killer Cell Migration to the Tumor Site

Major factors that control NK cell migration into inflamed tissues, parenchyma, or secondary lymphoid organs (SLO) are adhesion molecules, chemokine receptors, and chemokine gradients. Owing to the expression of a large array of chemokine receptors, NK cells can respond to a number of soluble chemotactic factors, such as CCL5 (RANTES), CCL7, and CCL8 (macrophage chemotactic protein, MCP-2,–3), CCL3 (MIP-1alpha), CXCL8 (IL-8), CXCL9 (MIG), CXCL12 (SDF-1), CCL2 (MCP-1), CX3CL1 (fractalkine), CXCL10 (IP-10), CCL21 (SLC), and CCL19 (ELC). The two major blood NK cell subsets (i.e., CD56bright and CD56dim NK cells) are characterized by different expressions of adhesion molecules and chemokine receptors and, therefore, they show different migration capabilities. CD56dim NK cells express CXCR1 (IL-8 receptor), CX3CR1 (fractalkine receptor), CXCR2, and low levels of CXCR3. By contrast, CD56bright NK cells express L-selectin (a pivotal molecule for the interaction with lymph node high endothelial venules), CCR7 (CCL19 and CCL21 receptor), CCR5 (CCL5, CCL3, CCL4 [formerly rantes, MIP1a, MIP1b] receptor), and CXCR3 (CXCL9 and CXCL10 [formerly MIG and IP10] receptor). These differences in chemokine receptor expression are accountable for the preferential migration of CD56bright cells and CD56dim NK cells into SLO and inflamed tissues, respectively. However, so far it is not known whether CD56bright and CD56dim NK cell subsets are differentially recruited to the tumor because of their diverse chemokine receptor repertoire.[87,240]

NK cell infiltrates have been detected in various solid tumors. Remarkably, it has been reported that the presence of high NK cell infiltration is associated with a more favorable outcome, at least in some tumors, including colorectal carcinoma, squamous cell lung, breast, and gastric cancer.[241] Thus, strategies that would increase infiltration of NK cells into tumors would be a likely approach to enhance antitumor efficacy. To date, only little is known about chemokines or other factors governing accumulation of NK cells in tumors and tumor metastases. These factors are largely dependent on the tumor type and tumor microenvironment. Deregulated NK cell migration to the tumor microenvironment has been suggested by studies that found that low numbers of NK cells are associated with tumors in colorectal cancer.[242]

It is possible that NK cell recruitment in solid tumor tissue might be regulated by CXCR3 and CX3CR1 chemokine receptors. Experimental cancer models have shown that gene therapy CX3CL1/fractalkine and CCL2 can stimulate tumor rejection by enhancing infiltration and activation of NK cells.[243,244] In addition, a recent report indicates that when exposed to IL-15 and glucocorticoids, NK cells express a high level of CXCR3, thus increasing their potential to infiltrate CXCL10+ melanoma tumors. Hence, in humans, CD56bright could be preferentially recruited to the tumor site[114,245] due to their high surface expression of CXCR3. Also, CD56dim NK cells have been detected in human lung tumors, colorectal cancer, and melanoma LN metastases.[242,246,247] In the latter case, the enrichment of CD56dim NK cells might reflect a preferential recruitment of these cells by IL-8 producing tumor tissue.[247]

Recent evidence obtained in CRC suggests that in spite of the presence in CRC tissue of high concentrations of attracting chemokines for both CD56bright and CD56dim NK cell subsets, NK cells are not in contact with tumor cells but rather locate within the parenchyma surrounding tumors.[242] This relative lack of physical contact between NK cells and neoplastic cells is further supported by other studies in melanoma and gastrointestinal stromal tumors (GIST).[248,249] These observations suggest that chemokines alone seem to be insufficient to mediate the recruitment of NK cells in the tumor nest. Thus, besides chemokines, other factors could enhance the recruitment of NK cells. In particular, Pachynski et al. showed that at least in a melanoma model, chemerin, an important chemoattractant, enhances infiltration of innate immune cells expressing the chemerin receptor CMKLR1 (i.e., NK cells, T cells, and DCs) into tumors.[250] Our group has recently demonstrated that NK cells, upon interaction with melanoma cells, can release a form of high mobility group box-1 (HMGB1) protein endowed with chemotactic properties for activated NK cells.[251]

Moreover, NK cells can recruit to the tumor site DC able to effectively prime T cell–mediated immunity. In human cancers, intratumoral CCL5, XCL1, and XCL2 transcripts closely correlate with gene signatures of both NK cells and conventional type 1 DC (cDC1) and are associated with increased overall patient survival in several cancer types.[252] In addition, these innate cells, through secretion of FLT3L, control the abundance of intratumoral stimulatory DC and their frequency that directly correlates with survival in patients with melanoma receiving anti–PD-1 therapy.[253]

Knowledge of factors enhancing NK cell accumulation in tumors might help design more effective NK cell–based immunotherapies against cancer. For this reason, it is important to identify and exploit factors regulating NK cell accumulation in tumors to improve the success of antitumor therapies.

Natural Killer Cells in the Tumor Lesions

In humans, NK cells have been documented to infiltrate solid tumors where they usually comprise only a minor population. Immunohistochemical staining detected NK cells in tumor biopsies of different histotypes, including lung, gastric, colorectal, and H&N cancers. These early studies suggested that NK cells might be effective during antitumor responses since the presence of high numbers of tumor-infiltrating NK cells correlated with good prognosis of cancer patients. A caveat of these studies was that NK cell infiltration of tumor tissues had been determined by the analysis of CD56 and/or CD57 expression, two markers not sufficiently restricted to NK cells. CD57 and CD56 can be expressed by some CD8+ T cell subsets in certain tumor types such as melanomas, while CD57 defines only a subset of highly differentiated/mature CD56dim NK cells. In most of the recently performed studies, NK cells have been detected by the use of CD56 and/or NKp46 surface markers. However, non-NK ILCs can express these markers and some studies might have misclassified ILCs as NK cells.

Staining for NKp46 (a marker that is expressed by all NK cells and some ILCs) revealed that certain solid malignancies, including RCC and GIST, are infiltrated by a significant number of NK cells. By contrast, other studies reported that in solid tumors NK cells are scarce. Besides their actual numbers and relative frequency, a key limiting factor to assess intratumoral capacity of NK effector cells is the measurement of their functional capabilities. Several reports have shown that NK cells present at the tumor site are enriched in CD56bright subset and/or display a functional impairment. Tumor-infiltrating NK cells from cancer patients often display reduced expression of the main activating receptors, resulting in reduced antitumor activity. In breast cancer, NK-TILs are enriched in CD56bright cells that expressed activating molecules (NKp44, CD25, and CD69) like mature activated NK cells but exhibit low levels of NKp30, NKG2D, DNAM-1, and CD16 and poor cytotoxic potential.[245] Similarly in peritoneal effusions, NK cells (PE-NK) from ovarian cancer patients are mainly CD56bright cells.[254] On the other hand, in early-stage NSCLCs NK-TILs are mostly CD56dim, show reduced expression of activating receptors (NKp30, NKp80, CD16, and DNAM-1), and decreased degranulation and cytokine release.[246] In RCC, infiltrating NK cells express high levels of CD94/NKG2A inhibitory receptor contributing to decreased NK cell activity, while in GIST patients, NK cells display a CD56[bright] CD16-KIR- phenotype and are found to express predominantly the immunosuppressive NKp30c isoform.[255] Finally, a recent report indicates that the HCC microenvironment induces the accumulation in the liver of CD11b-CD27- NK cell subsets endowed with poor cytotoxic capacity and potential to produce IFN-γ.[256] In addition, tumor-infiltrating NK cells are usually not in direct contact with neoplastic cells, but they are rather located within the stroma.

Natural Killer Cell Suppression: Influence of the Tumor Microenvironment on Natural Killer Cell Function

Despite strong NK cytolytic activity against tumors observed in vitro, tumor-infiltrated NK cells often display a suppressed phenotype. Indeed, tumor-residing cells or tumor cells themselves, as well as various microenvironmental immune suppressive factors present at the tumor site, can hinder NK cell function.

Different cell types present in the tumor microenvironment can be polarized toward a type 2 response and/or produce suppressive factors (such as IL-10 and TGF-β). Within the tumor tissue, tumor-associated macrophages (TAMs) and other myeloid cells constitute a major component of the immune infiltrate.[257] These cells of myeloid origin may affect NK cell function, as reported in two studies analyzing myeloid-derived suppressor cells (MDSC) or TAM isolated from patients with hepatocellular carcinoma (HCC). The immune-suppression is mediated by different mechanisms such as production of IL-10, TGF-β, reactive oxygen species (ROS), or depletion of intracellular L-arginine.

Another immune-suppressive cell population present at the tumor site is represented by T_{reg} cells. Their accumulation in tumors correlates with impaired immune function and poor prognosis. Along this line, T_{reg} cell expansion and low NK cell activity has been detected in GIST and HCC patients. T_{reg} cells isolated from patients with GIST inhibit NK cells through membrane-bound TGF-β.[258] In addition, T_{reg} cells express the high-affinity IL-2 receptor alpha (CD25, IL-2ra) and consequently they could also interfere with NK cell activation by competing for IL-2 availability released by activated CD4+ T cells.

Among the tumor-associated stromal cells, activated fibroblasts, often termed tumor-associated fibroblasts (TAF), are considered to play a role in mediating suppressive activity toward NK cells in the tumor microenvironment. TAF derived from melanoma, HCC, and colorectal carcinomas were shown to inhibit NK cell activity through cell-to-cell contact and through secretion PGE2, which could abrogate IL-2-induced up-regulation of NKp44, DNAM-1, and NKp30 activating receptors.[249,259,260]

Tumor cells themselves can directly contribute to NK immune suppression by a variety of inhibitory mechanisms. Our group showed that melanoma-derived IDO and/or PGE2 could inhibit the surface expression of NKp30, NKp44, and NKG2D on NK cells that are required for target cell recognition and killing.[261]

Other soluble factors such as TGF-β, IL-4, macrophage migration inhibitory factor (MIF), MUC-16, and adenosine.[262] can interfere with NK cell function. In particular, TGF-β has been shown to down-regulate the expression of NKG2D and NKp30 activating receptor,[263] while IL-4 affects the ability of NK cells to release cytokines.[264] Ovarian tumor cells can release/express both MIF and MUC-16 glycoprotein, are able to down-regulate NKG2D, and interfere with the formation of the immunological synapses between NK and tumor cells, respectively.[265] Another potential escape mechanism described in tumors of different hystotypes involves shedding, through proteolytic cleavage, of a soluble form of MICA that, in turn, induces down-regulation of NKG2D receptor, leading to the inhibition of NK cell function.[266,267] In addition, similarly to the NKG2D ligand MICA, soluble forms of BAT3/BAG6 and B7H6 (both ligands of NKp30) have been recently described.[154,167] Although shedding of ligands recognized by activating receptors represents a strategy employed by tumor cells to escape from NK cell recognition (possibly by inducing NK cell desensitization), a recent report showed that, in mice, a shed form of MULT1 (a high-affinity NKG2D ligand) stimulated tumor rejection and increased surface expression of NKG2D.[268] A reduction of NK cell cytotoxic activity by tumor cells can also be mediated by inhibitory signals induced by the engagement of NKp44 receptor with its ligand termed "proliferating nuclear cell antigen (PCNA)," a molecule overexpressed in different tumor types.[269] Phosphatidylserine (PS) expressed on apoptotic tumor cells represents an additional mechanism to dampen NK cell cytotoxicity since PS is recognized by the IRp60 (CD300a) inhibitory NK receptor.[45]

In order to gain further insight about the functional states of human NK cells in solid tumor, a recent study analyzed the transcriptome of TI-NK cells isolated from human melanoma metastases compared with circulating NK cells.[270] Single-cell RNA-seq analysis of TI-NK cells has identified different NK cell subsets with specialized gene expression programs. Some NK cell subsets are found to express high levels of XCL1 and XCL2 chemokine genes that are critical for cross-presenting XCR1[+] DCs recruitment into tumors,[252] whereas other subsets show a higher perforin and granzyme B expression.

This analysis also reveals that TI-NK cells express higher levels of the KRCL1 gene encoding NKG2A inhibitory receptor in comparison to circulating NK cells.[270]

Importantly, the physical status of the tumor microenvironment may also affect NK cell function, thus preventing their ability to eliminate tumor cells. It is now well known that hypoxia (a condition that often characterizes tumor tissues) can both favor the selection of tumor cells with increased invasive and metastatic potential and alter the phenotypic and functional features of tumor-infiltrating immune cells. Along this line, we have recently described that, under hypoxia, NK cells cultured in the presence of activating cytokines (including IL-2, IL-15, IL-12, and IL-21) display a low surface expression of major activating NK receptors and an impaired capability of killing infected or tumor target cells. However, remarkably, the triggering function of the Fc g receptor CD16 is not significantly altered by hypoxia, thus allowing NK cells to maintain their capability of mediating ADCC. These data give hints for a more extensive exploitation of antibody-based immunotherapies.[271]

Finally, tumor cells may also affect the ability of NK cells to enter a solid tumor site. In this context, it has recently been shown that neuroblastoma-derived TGF-β could skew the NK cell chemokine-receptor repertoire.[272]

Natural Killer Cell Evasion Through Tumor-Cell Immune-Editing

Tumor cells may develop different strategies to evade the NK-cell-mediated attack. For example, NK cells have also been reported to play a role in cancer-immune editing process. Several lines of evidence, obtained in animal models, demonstrated that, particularly during the elimination and escape phases, NK cells could shape tumor cell phenotype, thus reducing tumor immunogenicity.[273]

Subsequently, several pieces of evidence suggest that in humans NK cells could also edit malignant cells and reduce their antigenicity. For example, as a consequence of chronic interactions with NK cells, tumor cells can display an altered expression of ligands for either inhibitory or activating receptors. In particular, our group has recently reported that NK cells could favor the selection of tumor cells that are poorly recognized by the NK cells themselves. Thus, upon interaction with NK cells, melanoma cells up-regulate the surface expression of both classical and nonclassical HLA class I molecules (such as HLA-E), thus becoming resistant to NK cell–mediated killing. In this experimental setting, NK cell–derived IFN-γ plays a major role in the up-regulation of HLA class I expression on tumor cells.[274] Another mechanism by which tumor cells may evade NK cell–mediated recognition is the modulation of NKG2D ligands at their surface.[275]

Possible Natural Killer-Based Therapies Against Solid Tumors

The exploitation of NK cells against solid tumors is lagging behind their use for the immunotherapy of hematological malignancies. Lack of animal models and limits in the capability to expand human NK cells in vitro contribute to the delay. However, poor localization into the tumor and the absence of proliferation when they reach the tumor represent the major hindrance. Despite these difficulties, several approaches exploiting NK cell immunotherapy are currently in the clinical or preclinical phase, and might soon show promising results.

Tumor-targeting immunotherapy using mAbs specific for antigens expressed on cancer cells greatly benefits from the contribution of NK cells, which bind the mAb Fc and exert ADCC activity. mAbs specific for the EGFR, such as cetuximab and panitumumab, are used in the treatment of metastatic colon cancer. Cetuximab enhances CD126-dependent NK cell cytotoxicity on EGFR⁺ cell lines.[276] In a dose-finding phase I study in patients with advanced colorectal or head and neck cancer, the administration of cetuximab combined with daily lenalidomide showed dose-dependent increases of NK cell ADCC with increasing doses of lenalidomide and evidence of antitumor activity for the combination therapy.[277]

Migration and presence of NK cells in tumor tissue have been reported to occur at low frequency. Recent evidence shows that the presence of NK cell infiltrates in primary tumors, when assessed by isolation or by transcriptional signature analysis, predicts accurately lack of tumor recurrence.[278] Accordingly, strategies to improve migration of NK cells into tumor tissue represent a major effort for new strategies of solid tumor treatment with the help of NK cell immunotherapy. Migration of NK cells into tissues is regulated by CXCR3. Induction of the expression of CXCR3 ligands (CXCL9-11) by transfected tumor cells could increase adoptively transferred NK cell migration in a melanoma xenograft model.[279] Strategies inducing local production of CXCL9-11 in tumor tissue may represent a future approach.

In addition to the reduced migration of NK cells into solid tumor tissue, various factors within the tumor microenvironment may contribute to reduce NK cell function, as previously indicated. For this reason, an area where NK cell immunotherapy may have future prospects of success is in the treatment of minimal residual disease, or in the selective clearing of cancer stem cells (CSC). CSC represents a defined subset of cancer cells with exclusive ability to generate the growth and spread of a tumor, giving rise to a more differentiated cell progeny. They may represent variable fractions of tumor cells (2%–20%),[280,281] and may be identified by the expression of surface antigens that are absent in other tumor cells. In particular, when compared to tumor cell progenies, they may display reduced expression of MHC class I molecules and increased expression of ligands recognized by NK cell–activating receptors in colorectal carcinoma, melanoma, and glioblastoma. Accordingly, they are more susceptible to NK cell–mediated lysis.[282–285] For these reasons, strategies exploiting the NK cell immunotherapeutic potential should target CSC, possibly with the use of adoptive transfer of activated NK cells. Within this frame, an approach that is being considered is the administration of IL-15-stimulated NK cells after haplo-HCT in pediatric patients with solid tumors.[177] The procedure is feasible and safe; however, the usefulness of the approach is questionable in heavily pretreated patients. For the treatment of solid tumors, the timing of NK cell immunotherapy when combined with chemotherapy (which may affect host NK cell function) as well as the most relevant target, that is, CSC population, should be carefully considered to design the most useful strategy to deliver NK-based therapy.

CONCLUSION

Over recent years, major advances in the area of NK cell biology have allowed researchers to achieve considerable insight on how the tumor and tumoral milieu negatively affect NK cell phenotype and functional characteristics. The growth of our knowledge in this area allowed researchers to identify treatment strategies and tools supporting NK cell immunotherapy.

After years of toddler and teenage experiences, NK cell immunotherapy is coming of age and will represent a consistent part of the immunotherapy against malignancy. Additional work will be needed to achieve full maturity exploring and applying the whole set of tools to target stem cancer cells, to prevent and limit recurrent/metastatic disease, and to achieve routine access to NK cell manipulation for reinfusion or adoptive transfer.

KEY REFERENCES

Only key references appear in the print edition. The full reference list appears in the digital product on Springer Publishing Connect: connect.springerpub.com/content/book/978-0-8261-3743-2/part/part01/chapter/ch12

1. Vivier E, Raulet DH, Moretta A, et al. Innate or adaptive immunity? The example of natural killer cells. *Science.* 2011;331(6013):44–49. doi:10.1126/science.1198687

6. Vitale M, Cantoni C, della Chiesa M, et al. An historical overview: the discovery of how NK cells can kill enemies, recruit defense troops, and more. *Front Immunol.* 2019;10:1415. doi:10.3389/fimmu.2019.01415

8. Chiossone L, Dumas PY, Vienne M, Vivier E. Natural killer cells and other innate lymphoid cells in cancer. *Nat Rev Immunol.* 2018;18(11):671–688. doi:10.1038/s41577-018-0061-z

24. Moretta A, Vitale M, Bottino C, et al. P58 molecules as putative receptors for major histocompatibility complex (MHC) class I molecules in human natural killer (NK) cells. Anti-p58 antibodies reconstitute lysis of MHC class I-protected cells in NK clones displaying different specificities. *J Exp Med.* 1993;178(2):597–604. doi:10.1084/jem.178.2.597

27. Pende D, Falco M, Vitale M, et al. Killer Ig-like receptors (KIRs): their role in NK cell modulation and developments leading to their clinical exploitation. *Front Immunol.* 2019;10:1179. doi:10.3389/fimmu.2019.01179

47. Moretta A, Bottino C, Vitale M, et al. Activating receptors and coreceptors involved in human natural killer cell-mediated cytolysis. *Annu Rev Immunol.* 2001;19:197–223. doi:10.1146/annurev.immunol.19.1.197

78. Gumá M, Budt M, Sáez A, et al. Expansion of CD94/NKG2C+ NK cells in response to human cytomegalovirus-infected fibroblasts. *Blood.* 2006;107(9):3624–3631. doi:10.1182/blood-2005-09-3682

82. Fauriat C, Long EO, Ljunggren HG, Bryceson YT. Regulation of human NK-cell cytokine and chemokine production by target cell recognition. *Blood.* 2010;115(11):2167–2176. doi:10.1182/blood-2009-08-238469

90. de Maria A, Bozzano F, Cantoni C, Moretta L. Revisiting human natural killer cell subset function revealed cytolytic CD56(dim)CD16+ NK cells as rapid producers of abundant IFN-gamma on activation. *Proc Natl Acad Sci USA.* 2011;108(2):728–732. doi:10.1073/pnas.1012356108

98. Cerwenka A, Lanier LL. Natural killer cell memory in infection, inflammation and cancer. *Nat Rev Immunol.* 2016;16(2):112–123. doi:10.1038/nri.2015.9

111. Romee R, Rosario M, Berrien-Elliott MM, et al. Cytokine-induced memory-like natural killer cells exhibit enhanced responses against myeloid leukemia. *Sci Transl Med.* 2016;8(357):357ra123. doi:10.1126/scitranslmed.aaf2341

114. Carrega P, Bonaccorsi I, Di Carlo E, et al. CD56(bright)perforin(low) noncytotoxic human NK cells are abundant in both healthy and neoplastic solid tissues and recirculate to secondary lymphoid organs via afferent lymph. *J Immunol.* 2014;192:3805–3815. doi:10.4049/jimmunol.1301889

125. Marquardt N, Kekäläinen E, Chen P, et al. Unique transcriptional and protein-expression signature in human lung tissue-resident NK cells. *Nat Commun.* 2019;10(1):3841. doi:10.1038/s41467-019-11632-9

204. André P, Denis C, Soulas C, et al. Anti-NKG2A mAb is a checkpoint inhibitor that promotes anti-tumor immunity by unleashing both T and NK cells. *Cell.* 2018;175(7):1731–1743. doi:10.1016/j.cell.2018.10.014

270. de Andrade LF, Lu Y, Luoma A, et al. Discovery of specialized NK cell populations infiltrating human melanoma metastases. *JCI Insight.* 2019;4(23)e133103. doi:10.1172/jci.insight.133103

13

Immunogenic Cell Death and Cancer

Ilio Vitale, Sarah Warren, and Lorenzo Galluzzi*

KEY POINTS

- Mammalian cells succumbing to stress can elicit an adaptive immune response against dead cell-associated antigens.

- Successful adaptive immunity downstream of immunogenic cell death (ICD) involves an antigenic component, an adjuvant component, and a microenvironmental component.

- None of these components is ultimately intrinsic to dying cells as each of them depends (at least in part) on the immunological configuration of the host.

- Multiple anticancer agents, including specific chemotherapeutics, targeted molecules, and radiation therapy, can elicit *bona fide* ICD.

- Combining clinically relevant ICD inducers with immune checkpoint blockers holds promise for the treatment of cold tumors.

INTRODUCTION

Regulated cell death (RCD) is a form of cellular demise that relies on dedicated molecular machinery.[1] RCD can occur physiologically, in the context of (post-)embryonic development and adult tissue turnover, as well as pathophysiologically, as a consequence of failing adaptation to intracellular or extracellular stress.[1–3] That said, stress-induced RCD also constitutes a mechanism of adaptation, de facto allowing the organisms to eliminate cells damaged beyond recovery and hence unable to mediate their functions and therefore potentially dangerous.[4,5] Notably, the molecular machineries involved in purely physiological variants of RCD, commonly referred to

as programmed cell death (PCD), and in stress-induced RCD exhibit considerable overlap.[6,7]

For a long time, RCD has been viewed as an immunologically silent or even tolerogenic entity, as opposed to accidental necrosis, a nonregulated form of cell death with potent proinflammatory (but generally poor immunogenic) consequences.[8–10] This notion is largely derived from the fact that PCD, which occurs several million instances per day in an adult body, cannot be systematically linked to the activation of an immune response. However, over the past two decades, a number of stress-driven RCD modalities with immunogenic potential have been characterized, including specific variants of apoptosis and regulated necrosis, such as mitochondrial permeability transition (MPT)-driven necrosis, necroptosis, and ferroptosis.[1,11–17] In particular, preclinical and clinical findings demonstrated that, under select conditions, stress-driven RCD can elicit adaptive immune responses specifically targeting dead cell-associated antigens. Such functionally unique forms of RCD are commonly known as immunogenic cell death (ICD). In line with notion, the Nomenclature Committee for Cell Death has recently proposed to define ICD as "a form of RCD that is sufficient to activate an adaptive immune response in immunocompetent syngeneic hosts."[1] Thus, cells succumbing to ICD are capable of priming adaptive immunity in a specific host, ultimately driving the activation of cytotoxic T lymphocytes (CTLs) and the establishment of long-term immunological memory against dead cell-associated antigens.[18–20]

In preclinical studies, multiple perturbators of intracellular homeostasis have been demonstrated to exert "on-target" immunostimulatory effects by inducing ICD. These agents include a variety of infectious pathogens that colonize cells (i.e., viruses and intracellular bacteria); conventional chemotherapeutic, such as anthracyclines, oxaliplatin, and taxanes; targeted anticancer agents like the epidermal growth factor receptor (EGFR)-targeting drug cetuximab; radiation therapy; and various forms of photodynamic therapy.[20–22] In this setting, the

*Authors' Disclosure: IV has no conflicts of interest to disclose. SW is an employee and stockholder at NanoString Technologies. LG has received consulting fees from OmniSEQ, Astra Zeneca, Inzen, and the Luke Heller TECPR2 Foundation, and he is member of the Scientific Advisory Committee of Boehringer Ingelheim, The Longevity Labs, Onxeo, and OmniSEQ.

activation of robust adaptive immune responses downstream of ICD depends not only on the physicochemical nature, dose, and schedule of the RCD-inducing agent but also on specific features of dying cells and intrinsic characteristics of the host.[23–26]

Here, we outline the molecular and cellular factors underlying the efficient activation of adaptive immunity by cells undergoing ICD, with a specific focus on the antigenic landscape of dying cells, the adjuvant signals emitted by the latter, as well as the microenvironmental conditions that shape ICD-driven immune responses. We also discuss the main implications of ICD for cancer therapy and potential ways for ICD to be therapeutically manipulated in support of anticancer immune responses in patients.

ANTIGENICITY

Antigenicity refers to the ability of cells to present major histocompatibility complex (MHC) class I molecules loaded with antigenic epitopes that can be recognized by circulating naïve T cell clones in a specific host. Such reactive antigens can be: (a) neoepitopes originating from somatic cancer-associated mutations;[27,28] (b) viral epitopes expressed upon the reactivation of latent endogenous retroviruses;[29,30] (c) self epitopes for which low-affinity reactive T cell clones have escaped thymic selection;[31–34] and (d) conformational neoepitopes derived from post-transcriptional or post-translational modifications (PTMs) occurring in malignant cells or the tumor microenvironment (TME).[35–37]

Healthy cells usually display minimal antigenicity and hence have limited ability to initiate adaptive immune responses, as most of their antigens have been presented by the thymic epithelium during T cell development, resulting in the deletion of high-affinity T cell clones in the context of central tolerance.[38,39] At odds with their normal counterparts, both infected and malignant cells typically display a high antigenicity (and thus have an elevated potential to initiate adaptive immunity) as they generally express mutated proteins that are not covered by central tolerance.[40–42] The antigenicity of infected cells mostly originates from proteins encoded by the pathogen genome.[43,44] At least in part, the same is true for neoplastic malignant cells from tumors of viral origin. However, such tumors (which constitute a minority of all human neoplasms) generally undergo considerable immunoediting before emerging, implying that most antigenic epitopes of viral origin are lost or suppressed via epigenetic mechanisms or that robust local immunosuppression is established.[45–48] Moreover, malignant cells from nonviral cancers often express a variety of the so-called tumor neoantigens, that is, novel antigenic epitopes originating from somatic mutations in protein-coding DNA regions that are expressed and normally processed by the antigen-presentation machinery for exposure on MHC class I molecules.[49–51]

Tumor neoantigen (TNA)-generating mutations include nonsynonymous point mutations and frameshift mutations generated by small insertions and deletions (indels), ultimately altering the amino acid sequence of a specific protein.[27,41,52–54] Once exposed on the cell surface, TNAs can be recognized as "non-self" (and hence potential initiate anticancer immunity) as they were not presented by the thymic epithelium during T cell maturation (meaning that they could not elicit central tolerance, and thus failed to cause the deletion of TNA-specific naïve T cell clones). Of note, the mutational rate of progressing tumors is higher than that of healthy tissues, endowing malignant lesions with the potential to generate numerous TNAs.[49,50]

An additional source of antigenicity in cancer cells reflects the expression of wild-type antigens not entirely covered by T cell tolerance, which can be relatively leaky for low-affinity T cell clones.[31,32] Thus, even though these antigens are "self" from a strictly immunological perspective, they may initiate adaptive immune responses, especially when expressed to supraphysiological levels or at ectopic locations. In addition to underlying the pathogenesis of at least some autoimmune disorders,[55–57] such a loss in peripheral tolerance explains why wild-type epitopes can be harnessed to initiate tumor-targeting immune responses in the presence of appropriate adjuvant signals and microenvironmental conditions.[32] Such antigenic entities, which in oncological settings are commonly referred to as "tumor-associated antigens" (TAAs), include tissue differentiation antigens such as CD19, CD20, melan-A (MLANA, best known as MART-1) and premelanosome protein (PMEL, best known as gp100), oncofetal antigens such as α-fetoprotein (AFP) and carcinoembryonic antigen (CEA), the so-called cancer-testis antigens (CTAs) such as cancer/testis antigen 1B (CTAG1B, best known as NY-ESO-1), as well as multiple members of the melanoma-associated antigen A (MAGE-A) family, and preferentially expressed antigen in melanoma (PRAME).[32,33,58] Of note, based on their frequency and absent coverage by central tolerance, TNAs generally dominate ICD-driven anticancer immunity as compared to TAAs and viral antigens.[31]

Antigenic epitopes can also be derived from post-transcriptional modifications (e.g., noncanonical splicing) and by PTMs, which can be mediated by enzymatic or nonenzymatic reactions (e.g., acetylation, phosphorylation, oxidation, and ubiquitination).[42,59] PTMs can impose structural changes to proteins and lipids, and hence impact their processing by the molecular machinery for antigen presentation, as well as the probability to be recognized by a naïve T cell clone.[60] Of note, both enzymatic and nonenzymatic PTMs are significantly altered under stressful conditions, and neoepitopes generated by PTMs have been causally linked to the etiology of autoimmune diseases, including type 1 diabetes and rheumatoid arthritis.[61,62] However, the relative contribution of PTM-derived antigens to the initiation of anticancer immune responses downstream of ICD remains to be clarified.

The antigenic potential of cancer cells is heterogeneous across and within tumors and changes under the influence of the TME, potentially affecting ICD-driven immune responses.[63] In particular, a wide range of genomic studies indicates that hematological malignancies usually display a low mutational burden (~1 mutation/Mb), while solid tumors present a heterogeneous mutational burden, with a subset displaying a so-called hypermutator phenotype (> 10 mutations/Mb).[64–66] Moreover, solid neoplasms acquire high levels of intratumoral heterogeneity as they progress, and their mutational landscape evolves both in distinct areas of the tumor (spatial evolution) and at distinct stages of disease progression (temporal evolution), largely as a means to cope with the selective pressure imposed by microenvironmental factors and the host immune system.[50,67,68] This seems to hold true also for the TNA landscape during disease progression and in response to antitumor immunity.[67–70] In particular, antigen loss and subclonal antigen evolution enable the expansion of cancer cells that do not present reactive neoepitopes, ultimately resulting in reduced antigenicity.[67] Thus, not only distinct tumors but also distinct regions of the same malignant lesion can exhibit differential antigenicity and hence a differential capacity to elicit anticancer immunity downstream of ICD.[63]

Not surprisingly, the antigenicity of cancer cells is also influenced by defects in the antigen presentation machinery. As they enable immunoevasion, such alterations confer an evolutive advantage to neoplastic cells at virtually all stages of oncogenesis.[47,71] In this setting, low antigenicity can arise from genetic or epigenetic alterations of a variety of key components of the antigen-presenting machinery, including (but not limited to) MHC class I molecules, β-2-microglobulin (B2M), transporter 1, ATP-binding cassette subfamily B member (TAP1), transporter 2, ATP-binding cassette subfamily B member (TAP2), calreticulin (CALR), and components of the proteasome machinery.[70,72–74] Of note, some of these alterations are particularly common in neoplasms characterized by an elevated mutational burden and T cell infiltrate.[70,75]

A high mutational burden has been associated with increased sensitivity to immune checkpoint blockers (ICBs) in multiple, although not all, oncological settings.[76–78] Similarly, the link between mutational load and ICD sensitivity is still a matter of investigation. On the one hand, malignant lesions that are abundantly infiltrated by immune cells often display ICD-related transcriptional signatures.[79] On the other hand, a relatively low mutational load appears to suffice for cancer cells succumbing to ICD to initiate anticancer immunity.[80] Clinical studies investigating the impact of mutational burden on the efficacy of ICD-inducing anticancer regimens are therefore urgently awaited. Moreover, it will be important to elucidate the impact of ICD inducers on the antigenicity of malignant cells. Indeed, some of these drugs, including DNA-damaging agents, have been suggested to boost not only the adjuvanticity but also the antigenicity of cancer cells, either by increasing their mutational burden or by altering the antigenic landscape presented by cancer cells via reactivation of endogenous retroviruses, stimulation of TAA/TNA expression, up-regulation of MHC class I molecules, or proteasome deregulation.[81–87]

In conclusion, the antigenicity of cancer cells depends on the efficient presentation of epitopes not covered by central tolerance in a specific host (Figure 13.1). Together with a robust adjuvanticity and a permissive microenvironment, antigenicity is a *sine qua non* for neoplastic cells succumbing to RCD to initiate adaptive anticancer immunity.

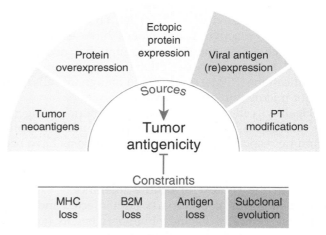

Figure 13.1 Major determinants of cancer cell antigenicity. Cancer cells present a variety of antigenic epitopes that are not covered by central tolerance in a specific host (implying that epitope-specific naïve T cell clones are available in such a host), which is a *sine qua non* condition for their demise to be perceived as immunogenic. Such epitopes can originate from spontaneous or therapy-driven somatic mutations resulting in the expression of tumor neoantigens, overexpression or ectopic expression of wild-type proteins for which central tolerance is leaky, (re-)expression of (latent) viral proteins, or PTMs altering the structure of an otherwise wild-type peptide. The overall antigenic landscape of malignant cells evolves in response to the local immunological pressure as specific cancer cell subclones dominate over others, at least in part as they lose highly antigenic epitopes or limit antigen presentation on MHC class I molecules.

B2M, β-2-microglobulin; PTM, post-translational modification.

ADJUVANTICITY

Adjuvanticity refers to the ability of a biological entity to deliver costimulatory signals that drive the maturation of antigen-presenting cells (APCs), ultimately enabling them with immunostimulatory (as opposed to immunosuppressive) functions upon the uptake of potentially antigenic material.[88–90] All cells, including healthy cells, can emit adjuvant signals in response to stress, which (as least in some circumstances) explains the initiation of autoimmune responses of pathological significance.[55] Most often, however, the antigenicity of healthy cells is insufficient for the activation of adaptive immunity even in the context of robust adjuvanticity (see above).

Adjuvant signals that support antigen-specific immune responses encompass microbe-associated molecular patterns (MAMPs), damage-associated molecular patterns (DAMPs), and immunostimulatory cytokines. A variety of microbial products including nucleic acids like viral double-stranded (ds) RNA and bacterial CpG-rich DNA, and surface components like flagellin, lipopolysaccharide, and peptidoglycans, can serve as MAMPs. Once emitted, MAMPs support immune responses by engaging specific sensors within infected cells or APCs, which are cumulatively known as pattern recognition receptors (PRRs).[91–93] Key PRRs include cytosolic nucleic acid sensors, including (but not limited to) cyclic GMP-AMP synthase (CGAS) and RIG-I-like receptors (RLRs), as well as a panel of sensors with broad distribution and/or binding ligand specificity such as Toll-like receptor (TLR) and NOD-like receptor (NLR) family members.[94,95] PRR engagement by MAMPs is followed by the production of immunostimulatory signals that recruit and activate APCs, ultimately resulting in the cross-presentation of antigenic material to naïve T cells and hence the elicitation of adaptive immune responses.[96]

Along similar lines, the adjuvanticity of cancer cells succumbing to RCD arises from the spatiotemporally coordinated exposure or secretion of endogenous molecules that normally are not available for interaction with PRRs. These danger signals include (a) ATP;[97,98] (b) endoplasmic reticulum (ER) chaperones, such as CALR, heat shock protein family A (Hsp70) member 1A (HSPA1A, best known as HSP70), Hsp90 α-family class A member 1 (HSP90AA1, best known as HSP90), and protein disulfide isomerase family A member 3 (PDIA3, also known as ERp57);[99–101] (c) cytosolic/mitochondrial nucleic acids;[102,103] (d) high mobility group box 1 (HMGB1);[104,105] (e) annexin A1 (ANXA1);[106] (f) F-actin;[107] as well as reactive oxygen species (ROS) and mitochondrial lipids.[108] Finally, some cytokines, such as type I interferon (IFN), C-C motif chemokine ligand 2 (CCL2), C-X-C motif chemokine ligand 1 (CXCL1), and C-X-C motif chemokine ligand 10 (CXCL10) also act as adjuvant signals during anticancer immune responses-initiated ICD.[102,109,110] As shown in preclinical studies, DAMPs and immunostimulatory cytokines are generally emitted by stressed or dying cells as a consequence of the unsuccessful activation of stress response pathways upstream of the execution of RCD.

Unsuccessful cytoprotective pathways causally linked to the emission of specific DAMPs during ICD include the following: (a) macroautophagy (herein referred to as autophagy), a lysosomal pathway contributing to the physiological preservation of cellular homeostasis via degradation of superfluous or potentially dangerous cytosolic materials and organelles,[111,112] and (b) the so-called integrated stress response (ISR), a molecular cascade responsible for the preservation of cellular homeostasis in response to ER stress.[113] A large body of evidence indicates that autophagy is required for the preservation of lysosomal ATP in the course of stress responses.[97,114] The release of lysosomal ATP to the extracellular space during ICD occurs via the translocation of lysosomal-associated membrane protein 1 (LAMP1) to the plasma membrane area and the opening of pannexin 1 (PANX1) channels, resulting in cellular blebbing.[115,116] Once released, ATP exerts adjuvant functions by binding to distinct PRRs on APC precursors. In particular, ATP can favor the recruitment of APCs and their precursors to sites of active RCD upon interaction with purinergic receptor P2Y2 (P2RY2) and stimulate APC activation and release of interleukin (IL)-1β upon binding to purinergic receptor P2X7 (P2RX7).[97,98,117] The exposure of ER chaperones on the surface of cells succumbing to ICD mechanistically relies on the ISR.[118–121] For example, anthracycline (which are prototypical activators of ICD) stimulates the inactivating phosphorylation of eukaryotic translation initiation factor 2 subunit α (EIF2S1, best known as eIF2α) by eukaryotic translation initiation factor 2 α kinase 3 (EIF2AK3, best known as PERK).[122] This is followed by the activation of caspase 8 (CASP8), which promotes the translocation of ER chaperones including CALR to the plasma membrane through the cleavage of B cell receptor-associated protein 31 (BCAP31) and activation of proapoptotic BCL2 family members.[100,118,123] In some settings, the ICD-related exposure of ER chaperones on the cell surface also requires ROS production[124] and anterograde ER-to-Golgi transport via vesicle-associated membrane protein 1 (VAMP1) and synaptosomal-associated protein 25 (SNAP25).[118,125,126] Of note, CALR exposure in the context of ICD is also regulated by an autocrine/paracrine cascade driven by C-X-C motif chemokine ligand 8 (CXCL8),[125] as well as (a) reticular Ca^{2+} levels,[127] and (b) caspase 2 (CASP2) activation, at least in the case of ICD initiated by high hydrostatic pressure.[128] Once exposed on the cell surface, CALR (and possibly other ER chaperones) stimulates the phagocytosis of dying cells by APCs upon interaction with LDL receptor-related protein 1 (LRP1) on the latter, at least in some experimental setting.[123,129] Notably, surface-exposed CALR also seems to drive the production of type I IFN by APCs, resulting in potent antitumor T cell immunity.[130,131] That said, it should be noted that malignant cells succumbing to hypericin-based photodynamic therapy secrete ATP and expose CALR during ICD independent of autophagy activation and eIF2α phosphorylation, respectively,[123,132] while cancer cells succumbing to necroptotic variants of ICD expose low levels of CALR in a manner that does not depend on the ISR.[133,134] These experiments indicate the existence of ICD modalities that do not exhibit complete mechanistic overlap with each other.

Importantly, the adjuvanticity of cells undergoing ICD is also governed by molecular circuitries that are normally activated by cellular responses to pathogen infection.[135] Indeed, immunogenic variants of chemotherapy and radiotherapy have been shown to induce an innate immune response driven by the accumulation of nucleic acids in the cytosol of dying cancer cells and their microenvironment.[109,136,137] In the context of immunogenic chemotherapy, endogenous RNAs appear to activate a cell-intrinsic molecular cascade upon recognition by endosomal TLR3, culminating with the release of type I IFN.[109] Conversely, radiotherapy-driven ICD appears to rely on type I IFN production downstream of the activation of CGAS by cytosolic dsDNA.[94,136–139]

Type I IFN delivers robust immunostimulatory cues by binding to heterodimeric IFN α and β receptors (IFNARs) on APCs and effector T cells.[140] Type I IFN also promotes a paracrine cascade resulting in the expression of interferon-stimulated genes (ISGs), including CXCL10 by cancer cells, ultimately promoting effector T cell recruitment.[109] When co-released with CXCL1 and CCL2, CXCL10 also stimulates the recruitment of neutrophils, which in some experimental settings contribute to ICD-driven antitumor responses by operating in an antigen-independent manner.[102] Finally, nucleic acids derived from cancer cells can also exert a direct immunostimulatory effect upon (most likely exosome- or gap junction-dependent) transfer to APCs, where they stimulate type I IFN secretion.[137,139]

Of note, the stress response pathways involved in the secretion of other ICD-related DAMPs such as ANXA1 and HMGB1 are still unknown. As for their mechanisms of adjuvanticity: (a) ANXA1 is released by cancer cells undergoing RCD to facilitate the homing of APCs upon interaction with formyl peptide receptor 1 (FPR1) on the latter,[106] and (b) HMGB1 exits dead cancer cells to exert multipronged immunostimulatory functions upon interaction with advanced glycosylation end-product specific receptor (AGER, also known as RAGE) and TLR4.[104,105,141,142]

The critical role of DAMP emission on the activation of adaptive immunity downstream of ICD has been demonstrated by a large number of preclinical studies. The involvement of intracellular stress pathways in DAMP emission has been experimentally proven by inhibiting these cascades in cancer cells by pharmacological or genetic means, for instance through the stable depletion of components of the autophagic machinery (e.g., ATG5 or ATG7)[116] or expression of a nonphosphorylatable variant of eIF2α.[118] Alternatively, intracellular stress pathways (e.g., ISR) have been artificially activated in neoplastic cells via the administration of specific agents (e.g., ER stressors) as a means to render immunogenic RCD driven by an otherwise nonimmunogenic agent.[143,144] Second, the adjuvanticity of DAMPs has been verified with experiments in which specific DAMPs have been neutralized/blocked/deleted to interrupt anticancer immunity downstream of RCD (e.g., upon overexpression of an enzyme degrading cytosolic dsDNA in irradiated cancer cells)[104,136,145] or exogenously complemented to convert nonimmunogenic RCD into bona fide ICD (e.g., using recombinant CALR in cancer cells responding to chemotherapy in the absence of endogenous CALR exposure).[99,118,146,147] Finally, DAMP-dependent PRR signaling has been mechanistically involved in the immunogenicity of RCD by knocking-out or knocking-down PRR-coding genes in the host (e.g., Fpr1, P2ry2, or P2rx7)[98,106,117] by blocking PRRs with specific monoclonal antibodies (e.g., LRP1 or type I IFN receptors)[109,123] or by stimulating antagonistic processes (e.g., CD47 expression which inhibits CALR-dependent phagocytosis).[148–150]

In conclusion, the adjuvanticity of ICD is ensured by a set of danger signals that are sequentially emitted by dying cells to enable the recruitment, maturation, and functional activation of immune effector cells in support of adaptive immunity (Figure 13.2).

MICROENVIRONMENT

The initiation and execution of adaptive immunity downstream of ICD require a microenvironment that allows for the infiltration and activation of immune effector cells.[151] Thus, the ultimate immunogenicity of RCD, be it driven by chemical, physical, or biological (e.g., microbial) insults, depends not only on the antigenicity and adjuvanticity of dying cells but also on their microenvironment. Importantly, all these ICD determinants are not intrinsic to dying cells or the host but originate from the interaction between dying cell- and host-intrinsic features.[152–154] Supporting the key role of microenvironmental features in the immunogenicity of RCD, progressing tumors not only evade antigenicity and adjuvanticity (e.g., by becoming resistant to RCD initiation, losing key antigenic determinants, or avoiding

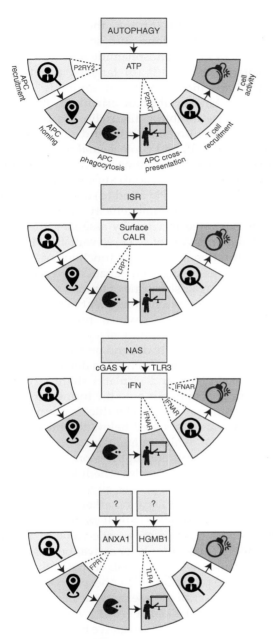

Figure 13.2 Major determinants of cancer cell adjuvanticity. Intracellular responses to stress including autophagy, the ISR, and NAS support immunostimulatory processes including (but not limited to) ATP secretion, CALR exposure on the cell surface, and type I IFN production, as well as ANXA1 and HMGB1 release. Upon binding to cognate receptors on APCs or effector T cells, these molecules favor each of the steps that are required for cancer cell death to be perceived as immunogenic.

ANXA1, annexin A1; APC, antigen-presenting cell; CALR, calreticulin; CGAS, cyclic GMP-AMP synthase; FPR1, formyl peptide receptor 1; HMGB1, high mobility group box 1; IFN, interferon; ISR, integrated stress response; NAS, nucleic acid sensing; LRP1, LDL receptor related protein 1; P2RX7, purinergic receptor P2X 7; P2RY2, purinergic receptor P2Y2; TLR3, Toll-like receptor 3; TLR4, Toll-like receptor 4.

the emission of DAMPs by dying cells)[154,155] but establish a microenvironment that prevents the infiltration or activation or immune effector cells.[45,156,157]

Several microenvironmental factors can compromise antitumor immunity, driven by ICD. Indeed, immune infiltration differs quantitatively and qualitatively not only across different tumors but also in different regions of the same neoplasm.[158] Thus, tumors (or tumor areas) exhibiting an elevated infiltration by immune effector cells, including APCs or their precursors and CTLs (the so-called hot tumors), are permissive for the activation of adaptive tumor-targeting immune responses downstream of ICD induction (provided that dying cells exhibit sufficient adjuvanticity and antigenicity). On the contrary, the ability of RCD to elicit adaptive immune responses is compromised in neoplasms (or neoplastic areas) in which the immune infiltrate is either scarce, due to poor infiltration by immune effector cells (the so-called cold tumors) or confined to stromal areas and excluded from tumor nests (the so-called excluded tumors).[19,159] In this context, immune cell infiltration (and thus the ability of RCD to initiate anticancer immunity) can be compromised by vascular defects and/or a dense fibrotic stroma, acting as a physical and functional barrier to access by immune cells.[160,161]

Along with this, tumor-infiltrating CTLs can undergo functional exhaustion on chronic stimulation,[162–164] often upon expression of coinhibitory receptors, including (but not limited to) programmed cell death 1 (PD-1), CTL-associated protein 4 (CTLA4), and hepatitis A virus cellular receptor 2 (HAVCR2, best known as TIM-3).[165–168] Interestingly, TIM-3 can also affect anticancer immunity downstream of RCD by directly binding to HMGB1 or phosphatidylserine, an immunosuppressive "eat me" signal exposed by dying cells.[103,169] In addition, both APCs and tumor-infiltrating CTLs can be actively suppressed by malignant cells or other immune cell subsets of the TME.[153] Thus, beyond expressing immunosuppressive ligands such as CD274 (the main ligand for PD-1, best known as PD-L1), cancer cells can compromise ICD-driven immune responses through the release of a variety of immunosuppressive molecules. These include DAMPs exerting inhibitory rather than stimulatory effects, such as adenosine and prostaglandin E_2,[88,170–172] as well as immunostimulatory DAMPs that acquire immunosuppressive functions in some settings. For example, extracellular HMGB1 may exert anti-inflammatory effects depending on its redox state or the PRR it engages.[173–175] Moreover, extracellular HMGB1 in its oxidized form has been linked to the overexpression of coinhibitory ligands by cancer cells, at least in the context of a form of RCD involving gasdermin and inflammasome activation (i.e., pyroptosis).[1,176] Likewise, chronic type I IFN secretion appears to mediate immunosuppressive, rather than immunostimulatory, functions.[126,177,178] Finally, the TME is characterized by a harsh cellular competition for nutrients and oxygen.[179–184] This results in an extensive metabolic rewiring of cancer cells, potentially affecting CTL functions. On the one hand, an increased utilization of glucose and amino acids by cancer cells limits the availability of these key nutrients for effector T cells de facto inhibiting anticancer immune responses. On the other hand, some metabolic byproducts overproduced by cancer cells, such as kynurenine and lactate, exhibit direct immunosuppressive effects.[185–187]

The heterogeneity of the TME and its evolution over time can also influence the initiation and execution of anticancer immune responses downstream of ICD. Indeed, the microenvironment of progressing tumors is populated (and often dominated) by distinct populations of immunosuppressive cells, including CD4+CD25+FOXP3+ regulatory T (T$_{reg}$) cells, M2-polarized tumor-associated macrophages (M2-like TAMs), and/or myeloid-derived suppressor cells (MDSCs).[188–195] These cells antagonize the activity of effector immune cells (and thus impair the initiation and execution of anticancer immunity) as they produce immunosuppressive cytokines and metabolites including (but not limited to) IL-10, transforming growth factor beta 1 (TGF-β1), lactate, and kynurenine.[191,196–199] Moreover, the immunosuppressive cells of TME overexpress enzymes catalyzing the degradation of immunostimulatory DAMPs, such as ectonucleoside triphosphate diphosphohydrolase 1 (ENTPD1; best known as CD39) and 5'-nucleotidase ecto (NT5E; best known as CD73), which catalyze the conversion of extracellular ATP into adenosine.[170,200–205] Of note, multiple therapeutic regimens, which are purported to induce ICD, also modulate the immune response by acting directly on distinct immune cell subsets,[206,207] which complicates the dissection of their mechanisms of action. The therapeutic "off-target" effects of these agents include the depletion of immunosuppressive cells (e.g., cyclophosphamide, doxorubicin) or the activation of CTLs and other immune effector cells (e.g., 5-fluorouracil and oxaliplatin).[208,209]

In conclusion, the propensity of RCD to drive efficient anticancer immunity is dictated by specific features of the TME, including its accessibility to APCs and effector T cells, the abundance of immune cell subsets, and the overall balance between immunosuppressive versus immunostimulatory cues (Figure 13.3).

IMPLICATIONS FOR CANCER THERAPY

Preclinical and clinical evidence accumulating over the past two decades indicate that multiple agents commonly employed in the clinical management of oncological disorders induce bona fide ICD.[20,210] The agents encompass the following: (a) conventional chemotherapeutic, such as the anthracyclines doxorubicin, epirubicin, idarubicin, and mitoxantrone, the antimitotic agents docetaxel and patupilone, and some DNA-damaging agents, such as cyclophosphamide and oxaliplatin (but not cisplatin);[99,101,145,211–213] (b) targeted agents, such as the EGFR-specific monoclonal antibody cetuximab, the tyrosine kinase inhibitor crizotinib, the cyclin-dependent kinase inhibitor dinaciclib, the Bruton's tyrosine kinase inhibitor ibrutinib, and poly-(ADP-ribose) polymerase (PARP) and proteasomal inhibitors;[214–217] (c) multiple physical interventions including (but not limited to) distinct types of ionizing radiation and photodynamic therapy;[120,207,218–224] and (d) oncolytic viruses and peptides.[225–232] The immunogenicity of these agents has been demonstrated in vitro, by assessing their capacity to drive the emission of ICD-relevant DAMPs, as well as the maturation and effector functions of APCs, and/or in vivo, by assessing their capability to activate adaptive immunity against murine or human tumors injected, respectively, into immunocompetent syngeneic hosts or into immunodeficient mice with a "humanized" immune system.[20,233] Of note, the ability of a given agent to induce ICD does not necessarily depend on the molecular structure or cytotoxic mode of action, as demonstrated by the fact that oxaliplatin and cisplatin share structure and mechanism of action, but only the former drives ICD.[145] Moreover, in most cases, ICD inducers promote anticancer immunity at doses well below the maximum-tolerated dose (MTD), which in many instances cause at least some degree of immunosuppression, especially when delivered according to precise schedules.[206,234]

Several retrospective studies support the clinical relevance of ICD. In particular, biomarkers of functional ICD-associated stress responses in malignant lesions have been associated with positive prognostic value in a variety of neoplasms.[155] Thus, autophagy activation has been associated with improved prognosis in patients with breast cancer,[235] while proficient eIF2α phosphorylation has been correlated to superior disease outcome in patients affected by acute myeloid leukemia (AML), non-small-cell lung cancer (NSCLC), and triple-negative breast cancer.[236–238] Of note, in patients with NSCLC, eIF2α phosphorylation is also associated with elevated CALR levels.[238] Along similar lines, a negative prognostic and/or predictive impact has been reported for (a) limited CALR exposure in patients with AML,[121,237] ovarian cancer, or NSCLC;[121,237–239] (b) low HMGB1 expression, in patients with breast cancer;[155] and (c) up-regulation of DAMP-antagonizing factors such as CD39, CD73, and/or CD47, in patients affected by AML, esophageal squamous cell carcinoma, or ovarian carcinoma.[240–242] Finally, loss-of-function polymorphisms in genes encoding DAMP receptors, such as P2RX7, TLR4, or FPR1, as well as defects in type I IFN signaling, have been associated with limited therapeutic responses and poor prognosis in patients with breast carcinoma and head and neck cancer.[104,243,244]

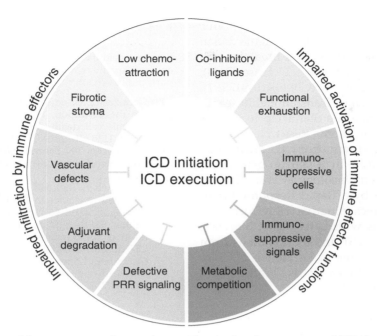

Figure 13.3 **Microenvironmental factors preventing anticancer immunity downstream of ICD.** Progressing neoplasms harness a variety of mechanisms to prevent the initiation or execution of anticancer immunity downstream of ICD, including processes that limit tumor infiltration by immune effector cells as well as pathways that block immune effector functions.

ICD, immunogenic cell death; PRR, pattern recognition receptor.

Given the clinical success of ICBs in a variety of oncological indications including melanoma, NSCLC, and urothelial carcinoma,[245–250] these agents stand out as promising combinatorial partners for ICD-inducing therapeutics, especially for the treatment of "cold" tumors, based on complementary mode of action. At least in theory, ICD inducers could indeed initiate a wave of RCD in the "cold" TME (as the cytotoxicity of these agents is not influenced by immune infiltration), driving the recruitment of APCs, uptake of antigenic material, migration of APCs to tumor-draining lymph nodes, cross-priming of tumor-specific CTLs, and, ultimately, influx of such CTLs into the TME, where therapeutic efficacy would be maximized by limiting CTL exhaustion with ICBs.[251,252] Combinatorial regimens involving one ICD inducer and one or more ICB(s) are being extensively investigated in both preclinical and clinical settings,[213,216,253] and some particularly promising combinations (e.g., doxorubicin plus nivolumab in patients with triple-negative breast cancer) have been already translated to the clinic.[254] However, additional work is needed to harness the full therapeutic potential of ICD inducers plus ICBs for cancer therapy.

full clinical potential of ICD inducers for cancer therapy remains to be unfolded. One major obstacle in this sense is the lack of suitable humanized mouse models enabling the investigation of tumor-targeting immunity driven by cancer cell death in the context of a fully immunocompatible system.[20,255] Moreover, at the mechanistic level, it appears urgent (a) to identify the complete repertoire of adjuvant-like signals emitted by dying cancer cells in support of ICD; (b) to elucidate the relevance of key RCD players such as caspase 3 (CASP3, the executor of intrinsic and extrinsic apoptosis)[256,257] and mixed-lineage kinase domain-like pseudokinase (MLKL, the mediator of necroptosis).[6,258] in the emission of DAMPs during ICD; and (c) to explore the contribution of immunosuppressive DAMPs, such as adenosine, phosphatidylserine, and prostaglandin E_2, in the context of ICD.[1,88] Finally, the precise impact of ICD inducers on the host immune system, at both the cellular and the organismal levels, remains to be clarified. Solving these and other outstanding issues will foster the development of effective therapeutic strategies based on the manipulation of ICD to promote or reinstate anticancer immune responses in patients.

CONCLUSION

Although it is now clear that ICD has considerable implications for the management of patients with cancer, the

ACKNOWLEDGMENTS

IV is supported by the Associazione Italiana per la Ricerca sul Cancro (AIRC, IG 2017 grant number 20417)

and a startup grant from the Italian Institute for Genomic Medicine (Candiolo, Turin, Italy) and Compagnia di San Paolo (Torino, Italy). LG is supported by a Breakthrough Level 2 grant from the U.S. Department of Defense (DoD), Breast Cancer Research Program (BRCP; #BC180476P1), by the 2019 Laura Ziskin Prize in Translational Research (#ZP-6177, PI: Formenti) from the Stand Up to Cancer (SU2C), by a Mantle Cell Lymphoma Research Initiative (MCL-RI, PI: Chen-Kiang) grant from the Leukemia and Lymphoma Society (LLS), by a startup grant from the Department of Radiation Oncology at Weill Cornell Medicine (New York, US), by a Rapid Response Grant from the Functional Genomics Initiative (New York, US), by industrial collaborations with Lytix (Oslo, Norway) and Phosplatin (New York, US), and by donations from Phosplatin (New York, US), the Luke Heller TECPR2 Foundation (Boston, US), Onxeo (Paris, France), and Sotio a.s. (Prague, Czech Republic).

KEY REFERENCES

Only key references appear in the print edition. The full reference list appears in the digital product on Springer Publishing Connect: connect.springerpub.com/content/book/978-0-8261-3743-2/part/part01/chapter/ch13

20. Galluzzi L, Vitale I, Warren S, et al. Consensus guidelines for the definition, detection and interpretation of immunogenic cell death. *J Immunother Cancer*. 2020;8(1):e000337. doi:10.1136/jitc-2019-000337
41. Schumacher TN, Schreiber RD. Neoantigens in cancer immunotherapy. *Science*. 2015;348(6230):69–74. doi:10.1126/science.aaa4971
47. O'Donnell JS, Teng MWL, Smyth MJ, et al. Cancer immunoediting and resistance to T cell-based immunotherapy. *Nat Rev Clin Oncol*. 2019;16(3):151–167. doi:10.1038/s41571-018-0142-8
151. Salmon H, Remark R, Gnjatic S, et al. Host tissue determinants of tumour immunity. *Nat Rev Cancer*. 2019;19(4):215–227. doi:10.1038/s41568-019-0125-9
257. Galluzzi L, López-Soto A, Kumar S, et al. Caspases connect cell-death signaling to organismal homeostasis. *Immunity*. 2016;44(2):221–231. doi:10.1016/j.immuni.2016.01.020

14

Cancer Cell-Intrinsic Pathways of Immune Resistance

Emanuela Romano, Hua Yu, and Kim Margolin

KEY POINTS

- Significant and lasting clinical responses with immunotherapy provide a new breakthrough treatment for a variety of refractory cancer histologies.

- Although immune checkpoint inhibitors are promising for achieving longer-term efficacy, their benefits in the overall population are still low (i.e., low frequency of response in common tumor types such as breast and prostate cancer and heterogeneity in the degree of response among different tumor lesions in the same patient).

- Most patients do not respond to immunotherapy or inevitably develop resistance to treatment after a period of treatment (primary versus acquired resistance).

- The mechanisms of resistance to immune checkpoint inhibitors are very complex and involve multiple aspects such as oncogenic pathways, metabolism, inflammation, and stromal features.

- This chapter sheds light on the intricate interplay between oncogenic pathways and resistance to immune checkpoint inhibitors with the goal of understanding that such mechanisms may help in identifying new therapeutic targets for expanding the efficacy of cancer immunotherapies.

INTRODUCTION

Immunotherapy has established an important role over the past decade for most solid tumors or their subsets, but the rates of clinical benefit from immunotherapeutic interventions—largely based on immune checkpoint blocking (ICB) antibodies alone or in combination with cytotoxic or molecularly targeted agents—vary widely, from extremely modest in the 12% to 15% clinical benefit rate range (most epithelial cancers) to moderately

high with a chance of durable response and possible cure (40% to 55% response rates for Merkel cell carcinoma, melanoma, colorectal and other cancers with germline or somatic microsatellite instability, and urothelial cancer with high programmed death-ligand 1 [PD-L1] expression).[1,2] The two major challenges to improving these outcomes are to better understand the reasons for resistance to immunotherapy—which may have common mechanisms across tumor types but will also likely vary by disease and immune tumor microenvironment (iTME)—and to identify optimal regimens for subsets of patients so that all outcomes can be improved.

The majority of efforts to elucidate mechanisms of intrinsic or acquired resistance to immunotherapy have been directed at understanding common elements of the iTME and the vast array of interacting cellular and soluble factors that limit the development and maintenance of effective immune-mediated cytotoxicity. Mounting evidence over the past two decades supported the concept that tumor-intrinsic signaling alterations, not only in genes associated with oncogenic drivers (i.e., BRAFv600) but also in essential intracellular pathways (i.e., Phosphatase and tensin homolog [PTEN], Wnt/β-Catenin), may limit the benefits of immunotherapy. Importantly, identification of the roles of these oncogenic drivers in suppressing antitumor immune responses and mediating resistance to immunotherapies also provides opportunities to explore therapeutic vulnerabilities. Many of these oncogenic drivers are also targetable with drugs that may be safely and effectively combined or sequenced with immunotherapeutic agents.

Although the oncogenic drivers are mostly tumor-specific or applicable to a limited number of tumors, many of the oncogenic and immunosuppressive molecules are either upstream or downstream of STAT3, a signal transducer and transcription factor that is persistently activated in diverse tumor cells and in the tumor-associated immune cells (Figure 14.1). In addition to many tyrosine kinases and other kinases that are overactivated in tumor cells, STAT3 is activated by a myriad of cytokines and growth factors known to be immunosuppressives. More recently, it has also been shown that PD-1

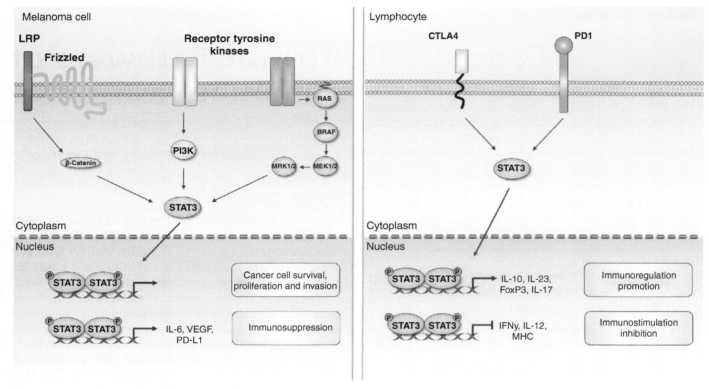

Figure 14.1 Many oncogenic drivers converge on STAT3 in both melanoma tumor cells and tumor-associated immune cells to promote immunosuppression. Multiple oncogenic signaling pathways important for melanoma tumor cell growth and immunosuppression require STAT3, a signal transducer and transcription activator, to exert their effects. In particular, a number of the receptor tyrosine kinases, through their mediators, such as RAS/BRAF and MEK1/2 and ERK1/2, or PI3K that are frequently activated in melanoma, activate STAT3. Activated STAT3 in turn upregulates the expression of many molecules underlying tumor cell survival and proliferation, as well as invasion. In particular, STAT3 in tumor cells is also responsible for the upregulation of many factors critical for tumor immunosuppression in the tumor cells. In the tumor-associated lymphocytes, both PD-1 and CTLA-4 can lead to STAT3 activation, in addition to several cytokine and growth factor receptors, and activated STAT3 is known to promote the expression of multiple immunosuppressive factors. In addition, STAT3 has been shown to inhibit an array of multiple molecules produced by lymphocytes that are necessary for antitumor immune activities.

Source: Illustration created with data from Herrmann A, Lahtz C, Nagao T, et al. CTLA4 promotes Tyk2-STAT3-dependent B-cell oncogenicity. *Cancer Res.* 2017 September 15;77(18):5118–5128. doi:10.1158/0008-5472.CAN-16-0342; Zhang C, Yue C, Herrmann A, et al. STAT3 activation-induced fatty acid oxidation in CD8+ T effector cells is critical for obesity-promoted breast tumor growth. *Cell Metabolism.* 2019 November 21;31(1):148–161.E5. doi:10.1016/j.cmet.2019.10.013.

IFN, interferon; IL, interleukin; MHC, major histocompatibility complex; PD-L1, programmed death-ligand 1; VEGF, vascular endothelial growth factor.

and cytotoxic T-lymphocyte-associated protein 4 (CTLA-4), the two most well-known checkpoints, activate STAT3 in tumor-associated T cells and/or B cells. As a transcription factor, STAT3 also upregulates numerous immunosuppressive factors such as interleukin (IL)-10, IL-23, vascular endothelial growth factor (VEGF), PD-L1, and FOXp3, among many others. Although it was not quite expected from a transcription factor, STAT3 has been shown to inhibit the expression of many Th-1-stimulating molecules, notably interferon (IFN)-γ, IL-12, and major histocompatibility complex (MHC) molecules. Consequently, persistently activated STAT3 in both tumor cells and in the tumor-associated immune cells plays a key role in mediating immunosuppression and

immunotherapy resistance. Although an important role of STAT3 in mediating resistance to therapy, including immunotherapy, is known, due to the lack of well-studied direct small-molecule STAT3 inhibitors for evaluation of immune responses in the clinic, we will focus our review on select tumor-intrinsic oncogenic drivers with clinically evaluated inhibitors for their impact on cancer immunotherapies.

In the first part of this chapter, we will review selected tumor-intrinsic oncogenic drivers and pathways, which are targetable, on antitumor immune responses. Inhibitors of many of the selected targets result in beneficial immunomodulatory effects in patients. Many of these oncogenic drivers cross talk with STAT3 and/or activate STAT3, and they include but are not limited to BRAF, MEK/mitogen-activated protein kinase (MAPK), EGFR, PI3K/Akt pathway, and Wnt/β-Catenin pathway. We have also selected for inclusion in this chapter these key oncogenic drivers in tumor cells in promoting immune resistance and the effects of their inhibitors in reducing the resistance to frontline immunotherapies. In the second part, we will discuss the most important immune cell determinants of treatment outcomes and how the molecular determinants of immune cell–tumor cell–iTME interactions contribute to both oncogenesis and therapeutic outcomes, with a focus on pathways that may be targeted therapeutically.

IMMUNOLOGICAL EFFECTS AND THERAPEUTIC TARGETING OF SELECTED ONCOGENIC DRIVER MUTATIONS

BRAF Mutation in Melanoma and Other Solid Tumors

Oncogenic BRAFv600 mutations activate the MAPK pathway by bypassing the requirement for BRAF dimerization or weakening the interaction with MEK1.[3] While the hyperactivation of this MAPK pathway is neither necessary nor sufficient for all forms of melanomagenesis,[4] these mutations can be strong drivers of melanoma biology and also contribute to the behavior of several other adult solid tumors, including colorectal, non-small cell lung, and thyroid malignancies (Figure 14.2).[5] In all of these instances, other molecular alterations also contribute to the biology of the tumor as well as its therapeutic vulnerabilities. Melanoma, however, is the tumor in which most of the immunological effects of BRAF mutations—occurring in about half of the common cutaneous cases[6]—and MAPK pathway inhibition were first elucidated and where the fortuitous and nearly simultaneous development of effective immunotherapy and highly active BRAF inhibitors led to critical insights on their interactions.

Multiple studies in melanoma with activating BRAF mutations showed the unfavorable impact of this mutation on the iTME and immune responses against melanoma. These include reports in humans and mice demonstrating diminished T cell activity against melanoma differentiation antigens and decreased tumor expression of these antigens, with both effects reversible with BRAF inhibition.[7–9] Khalili et al.[10] showed that BRAF-mutated melanoma cells secrete IL-1α and IL-1β that induce tumor-associated fibroblasts to upregulate COX-2 and PDL-1/2, leading to the suppression of antigen-specific T cell cytotoxicity, which can be reversed by BRAF inhibition. Liu et al.[11] showed that BRAF inhibition increased melanoma tumor infiltration by adoptively transferred T cells in vivo and enhanced the antitumor activity of these cells, which in the presence of BRAF-mutant melanoma express increased levels of the suppressive or exhaustion markers PD-1 and TIM-3. The increased T cell infiltration was primarily mediated by the ability of the BRAF inhibitor to block the production of VEGF by melanoma cells through a reduction in the binding of the c-myc transcription factor to the VEGF promoter.

These immunological effects of the strong oncogenic driver BRAF in melanoma cells were demonstrated to be reversible with BRAF inhibition. Although MEK inhibitors, which enhance the effects of BRAF inhibition by inhibiting downstream ERK phosphorylation, are generally immunosuppressive to T cells, the combination of BRAF plus MEK inhibitors retained their immunomodulatory benefits, including an increased CD8+ T cell infiltration and upregulation of melanoma antigens in the tumors of patients treated with BRAF and MEK inhibitors.[12] MEK inhibition may also paradoxically enhance the effector T cell response by inhibiting the apoptosis associated with chronic T cell receptor stimulation by antigens.[13] Other reports also described the increase of intratumoral CD4+ T and cytotoxic CD8+ T cells following BRAF inhibition, along with increased granzyme B production, tumor regression, and tumor necrosis.[14] Cooper et al. demonstrated an increase in the clonality of tumor-infiltrating lymphocytes from pretreatment to on-treatment biopsies of metastases from patients with BRAF-mutant melanoma treated with a BRAF inhibitor,[15] and Hu-Lieskovan demonstrated, in a murine model system, additional immunomodulatory effects of BRAF plus MEK inhibition that included a decrease in two populations of immunosuppressive cells in the iTME—tumor-associated macrophages and regulatory T (T_{reg}) cells—as well as increased IFN-γ and tumor antigen presentation.[16]

Some of these findings were corroborated by a clinical translational study of tumor biopsies from 39 patients before therapy, on treatment, and at the time of resistance development to either MAPK inhibition or PD-1 blockade.[17] The results indicated that in comparison with pretreatment levels of CD8 T cell infiltration, targeted therapy was associated with an increase in CD8 cells shown in the biopsies of patients during therapy, but at the time of progression, the CD8 infiltrate had diminished significantly. In contrast, for patients receiving PD-1 blockade, CD8 T cell infiltrates were higher than baseline when assessed both during treatment and at the time of progression. Although definitive comparisons could not be made due to the modest sample size, nonrandomized design, and, most importantly, lack of BRAF mutation information in the tumors from patients treated with PD-1 blockade, the study results support the concept of important fluctuations in the interactions among immune cells and tumor cells of the iTME in response to MAPK inhibitor-based targeted therapy versus immune checkpoint blockade.

Most recently, a newly described mechanism for the favorable immunomodulatory effects of MAPK

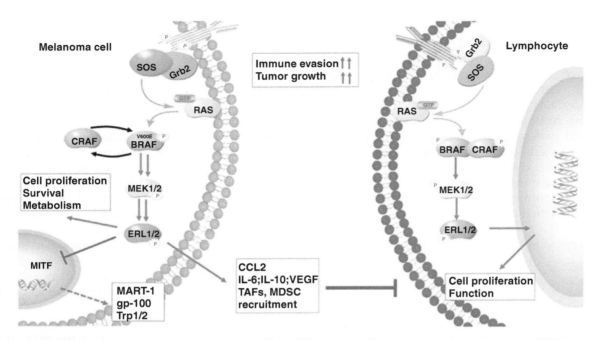

Figure 14.2 BRAF^{V600E} oncogene promotes melanoma cell proliferation and immune evasion. Mutations in BRAF oncogene cause constitutive activation of the MAPK pathway and lead to the uncontrolled proliferation of tumor cells by various mechanisms including induced anti-apoptosis, increased invasiveness, and metastatic behavior. However, activation of MAPK pathway leads to a marked reduction in TAAs (MART-1, gp-100, and Trp1/2) through inhibiting transcriptional expression of MITF. Meanwhile, the activation of the MAPK pathway could contribute to increased immunosuppressive regulators such as IL-6, IL-10, VEGF, IL-1, and CCL2, as well as enhanced recruitment of TAF and MDSCs. Both downregulation of antigens and upregulation of immunosuppressive factors contribute to immune evasion.

CCL2, chemokine ligand 2; IL, interleukin; MAPK, mitogen-activated protein kinase; MDSC, myeloid-derived suppressor cells; MITF, Melanocyte Inducing Transcription Factor; TAA, tumor-associated antigen; TAF, tumor-associated fibroblasts; VEGF, vascular endothelial growth factor.

Source: Reproduced from[24] Yu C, Liu X, Yang J, et al. Combination of immunotherapy with targeted therapy: theory and practice in metastatic melanoma. *Front Immunol.* 2019;10:990. doi:10.3389/fimmu.2019.00990

inhibition was demonstrated by Erkes et al., who developed a novel model of BRAF-mutant melanoma cell lines rendered more immunogenic by UV irradiation. In this model, the optimal response to MAPK inhibition required CD4 and CD8 T cells; was associated with the elaboration of immunogenic molecules high–mobility group box 1 (HMGB-1), calreticulin, and IL-1α; and was also accompanied by increased expression of MHC Class II molecules on tumor-resident dendritic cells. These investigators also showed that a recently described form of tumor cell death, termed "pyroptosis" for its association with acute inflammatory cytokines, was mediated in part by the immunogenic effects of MAPK inhibition and that this pathway was triggered by the cleavage of the pore-forming protein gasdermin by caspase-3.[18]

Further exploration of the potential rationale for combining BRAF inhibition with immune checkpoint blockade was provided in two recent reports addressing possible therapeutic synergy. Yue et al.[19] conducted an exhaustive study of the impact of BRAF and MEK inhibitors on T cell activation by nivolumab, demonstrating that while BRAF inhibition caused increases in type 1 cytokines IFN-γ, TNF-α, and IL-2, there was less impact on the expression of other

markers of T cell activation, including Ki67, CD25, CD69, and granzyme B. The addition of MEK inhibition markedly reduced T cell activation, likely due to interactions between MEK and the PI3K/AKT pathway required for T cell activity, which is upregulated in response to PD-1 blockade (Figure 14.2).[19] The authors of this report concluded that the variability from patient to patient in these responses to combined PD-1, BRAF, and MEK inhibition, together with the demonstrated impairment of T cell function, failed to support the use of these combinations in the clinic. In contrast, Atay et al. studied the impact of BRAF inhibition on melanoma cell lines and patient-derived xenografts and reported that melanoma cells resistant to BRAF and MEK inhibition could be sensitized to cytotoxic T cells by re-exposing them to BRAF inhibitor, which leads to upregulation of the mannose-6-phosphate receptor for granzyme B.[20] Additional data in support of the immunomodulatory effects of BRAF mutation and the potential for combining MAPK inhibitors and immunotherapy include those of Jiang[21] and Kakavand,[22] who showed upregulation of PD-L1 expression on both tumor cells and infiltrating immune cells, a variant of the so-called adaptive resistance that may enhance tumor sensitivity to PD-1/PD-L1 blockade (Figure 14.3).[23]

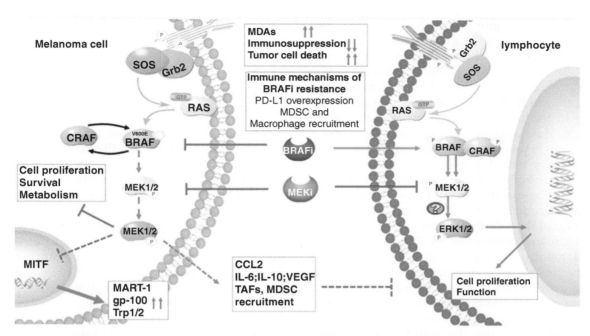

Figure 14.3 **MAPK inhibitors induce melanoma cell death and regulate immune microenvironment.** BRAF and MEK inhibitors induce melanoma cell death through suppression of the MAPK pathway. The expression of TAAs will be increased by upregulated transcription of MITF when MAPK pathway is blocked. In addition to affecting melanoma cells, MAPK pathway blockade can also abolish the tumor immunosuppressive microenvironment, including inhibition of TAFs and downregulation of immunosuppressive factors. Treatment of selective BRAF inhibitors in BRAF wild-type lymphocytes leads to paradoxical activation of the MAPK pathway by the transactivation of CRAF, thus promoting cell proliferation and function. Although MEK inhibitors may impair T cell function in vitro via MAPK pathway blockade, combination with BRAF inhibitors increased expression of antigens and suppressed the immunosuppressive environment. Immune microenvironment also contributes to acquired resistance to BRAF inhibitors.

CCL2, chemokine ligand 2; IL, interleukin; MAPK, mitogen-activated protein kinase; MDSC, myeloid-derived suppressor cells; MITF, Melanocyte Inducing Transcription Factor; TAA, tumor-associated antigen; VEGF, vascular endothelial growth factor.

Source: Reproduced from Yu C, Liu X, Yang J, et al. Combination of immunotherapy with targeted therapy: theory and practice in metastatic melanoma. *Front Immunol.* 2019;10:990. doi:10.3389/fimmu.2019.00990

Preclinical studies also provided data in support of combining BRAF inhibition with immune checkpoint blockade rather than sequencing therapy at the time of resistance development. Using a model of a BRAFV600E/PTEN(−/−) syngeneic tumor graft into an immunocompetent syngeneic mouse, Cooper et al.[25] also observed prolonged antitumor effects when combining anti-PD1/PD-L1 with a BRAF inhibitor. Similarly, in a BRAF wild-type colon carcinoma mouse model, the antitumor effects and CD8+ T cell infiltration were enhanced by combining PD-1 blockade with MEK inhibition (Figure 14.3).[11]

Since the predominance of the data—and a strong need to improve the outcomes of both targeted and immunotherapy modalities for patients with advanced BRAF mutant melanoma—supported the clinical exploration of combination therapies, studies were initiated using vemurafenib and ipilimumab, the prototypes of each modality, which had both been approved as single agents for melanoma in 2011. Early experience with this combination was cut short by the occurrence of excessive hepatotoxicity,[26] and combinations remained on hold until the advent of PD-1 blockade—far more active and less toxic than CTLA-4 blockade—and MAPK inhibitor combinations (using both BRAF and MEK inhibitors, which were also more effective and less toxic than BRAF inhibition alone), which proved to be tolerable in a series of combination Phase I studies that also demonstrated encouraging response rates,[27,28] setting the stage for two recently completed Phase III studies to evaluate double MAPK inhibitor therapy with and without PD-1 or PD-L1 blockade as first-line therapy in patients with advanced melanoma carrying a BRAFv600-activating mutation.

The first of these studies, Keynote-022 by Ascierto et al.,[29] was a Phase II trial for patients with untreated advanced melanoma carrying a BRAFv600E or K mutation, in which 60 patients were randomized to the BRAF inhibitor dabrafenib and the MEK inhibitor trametinib plus the PD-1 antibody pembrolizumab, all at standard doses, and 60 patients received the same MAPK inhibitors plus placebo. The results of this trial showed superiority for the combination in the primary endpoint of progression-free survival (PFS; medians 16 and 10 months, hazard ratio .66). Other important results included the longer duration of response (medians 19 and 12 months, hazard ratio .41) and a trend toward a late separation of the overall survival (OS) curves that did not reach statistical significance, possibly limited by the small, Phase II nature of the study. Toxicities were for the most part attributable to the targeted agents, which are readily managed with dose adjustments, although there was a higher incidence of pneumonitis in the triplet arm.

A similar study was designed with the power of a large, placebo-controlled Phase III study (514 patients randomized) to assess the contribution of the PD-L1 antibody atezolizumab to the backbone MAPKi doublet, consisting of the BRAF inhibitor vemurafenib plus the MEK inhibitor cobimetinib. In this trial, a run-in period of 1 month on vemurafenib plus cobimetinib preceded the first dose of atezolizumab, with the goal of assessing toxicity and tolerance as well as initiating the development of immunomodulatory effects in the tumor microenvironment. Also, the vemurafenib dose was reduced by 25% (with the appropriate placebo/blinding to maintain the atezolizumab blinding) in the triplet arm to reduce toxicities. The results of this trial,[30] (30 = placeholder), reported by McArthur et al. at the AACR 4/27/20—likely to be published before chapter in press—included identical ORRs (66% and 65%), a statistically significant improvement in investigator-assessed PFS for the triplet that was borderline on the independent review committee's assessment, and a late separation of both the OS curves and the duration of response curves (medians 20 versus 13 months), not yet statistically significant but potentially significant after a longer follow-up period. The toxicities that occurred at an increased rate among patients randomized to the triplet regimen included fever, arthralgias, transaminase elevations, and thyroid disturbances, but the overall rate of treatment discontinuation for toxicity was similar between the treatment arms (13% with the triplet, 16% with MAPK inhibitors alone) as was the percentage of fatal toxicities (seven patients in each arm, 3% of total). These results appear to confirm an important and favorable immunomodulatory interaction between double MAPK inhibition and immune checkpoint blockade, and additional combinations of targeted agents with immune checkpoint blockade have been initiated or are in development (clinicaltrials.gov NCT02967692).

For BRAF-mutant tumors other than melanoma, the impact of the oncogene on immune responsiveness has not been determined. Interestingly, an association of BRAFv600 mutation with microsatellite instability and with increased tumor expression of PD-L1 was noted in colon cancer, but the impact of this finding on responsiveness to immunotherapy remains unproven,[31] and in other tumor types with subsets that carry BRAF mutations, including lung, thyroid, and hepatocellular cancers, there is also no information on the impact of this molecular alteration on immune responsiveness.

EGFR PATHWAY ACTIVATION AND RESPONSIVENESS TO IMMUNOTHERAPY IN NON-SMALL CELL LUNG CANCER

EGFR mutations occur in the tumors of approximately 15% of patients with non-small cell lung cancer (NSCLC), predominantly in adenocarcinoma in nonsmokers, and a growing number of molecularly targeted agents has been highly effective against this subset of NSCLC.[32] A series of preclinical studies suggest that activation of EGFR-stimulated signaling pathways is associated not only with enhanced tumor growth and survival but also with the modulation of antitumor immune responses. For example, skin cancer-bearing mice treated with EGF-like growth factors showed an increased suppressive T_{reg} activity[33] and loss of CCL27 expression, a T cell chemokine.[34] Numerous studies have been performed to understand the potential association between EGFR mutation and expression of PD-L1, which has been considered a predictive factor for benefit from immune checkpoint blockade in patients with advanced, EGFR-unmutated (wild-type) lung cancer. For patients with EGFR-mutated tumors, the predictive value of PD-L1 expression varies widely, possibly in part due to differences in the assay methodologies for PD-L1.[35] The effects of other cells of the iTME in tumors with EGFR mutation will also require further elucidation (Figure 14.4).

To date, the clinical outcomes of treatment with ICB for patients with EGFR-mutated advanced NSCLC have been unfavorable, not only due to low PD-L1 expression but also attributed to a non-inflamed or cold TME with low CD8+ T cell infiltrates.[36,37] There is no consistently reported relationship between TMB/neoantigen load, EGFR mutation, and immunoresistance in lung cancer, likely due to the wide variability of other mutations impacting the biology and resistance to immunotherapy,[35] including MDM2/MDM4 and STK11.[38,39] Further, different activating mutations of EGFR may have different impact on the likelihood of response to immunotherapy, which might also vary depending on prior exposure to EGFR-directed tyrosine kinase inhibitors (TKIs).[35] Finally, other oncogenic drivers of lung cancer biology, including alterations of ALK, ROS1, RET, ERBB2, and MET, have as yet unknown effects on immunotherapy benefits, and BRAF-activating mutations, which are associated with increased expression of PD-L1, may confer immunoresponsiveness on the small subset of BRAF-mutated NSCLC (Figure 14.4).[40] EGFR mutations in lung cancer may also impact the response to other therapies with immune-related mechanisms, including radiotherapy, the effects of which can lead to the promotion of cellular proliferation and apoptosis evasion.[41]

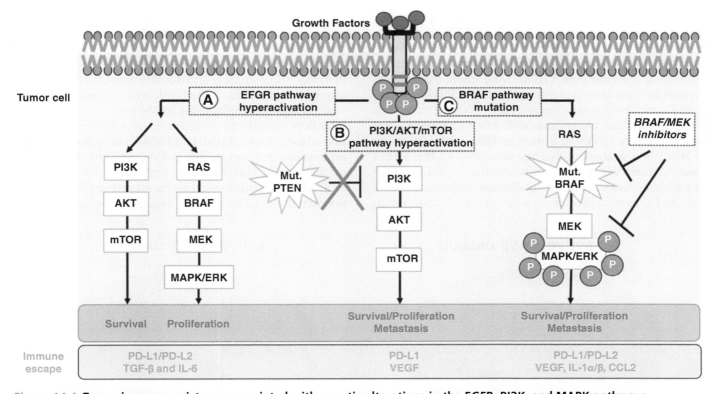

Figure 14.4 Tumor immune resistance associated with genetic alterations in the EGFR, PI3K, and MAPK pathways.
Representative scheme from collective studies describing tumor mutations found in the canonical EGFR, PI3K, and MAPK pathways.
(A) Mutations responsible for EGFR pathway hyperactivation lead to increased proliferation and survival of tumor cells, while immune escape mechanisms are triggered by PD-L1/L2 upregulation, and the release of TGF-β and IL-6. **(B)** PTEN LOF induces hyperactivation of the PI3K/AKT/mTOR pathway, resulting in enhanced tumor growth and spreading and immune escape mechanims via PD-L1 upregulation and VEGF secretion. **(C)** Activating BRAF mutations can lead to increased tumor growth and metastasis. Several strategies targeting activating BRAF mutations have been tested. However, a significant percentage of patients present acquired resistance to BRAF inhibitors, in which upregulation of PD-L1/L2 and increased production of VEGF, IL-1-α, and CCL2 emerge as acquired immune escape mechanisms.

IL, interleukin; LOF, loss of function; MAPK, mitogen-activated protein kinase; mTOR, mechanistic target of rapamycin; PD-L1, programmed death-ligand 1; VEGF, vascular endothelial growth factor.

Source: With permission from Mario M, Romano E. *Mechanisms of Drug Resistance in Cancer Therapy.* Springer International Publishing; 2018.

IMPACT OF UPREGULATED PI3K/AKT/ MTOR PATHWAY IN CANCER RESISTANCE TO IMMUNOTHERAPY

While not representing the effects of a single driver oncogene analogous to the BRAF and EGFR mutation stories that were previously detailed, many tumors feature alterations of the PI3K/AKT/ mechanistic target of rapamycin (mTOR) pathway resulting either from loss of function (LOF) alterations of PTEN (most often due to hypermethylation rather than genetic deletion) or, less commonly, from signaling through receptor tyrosine kinases, downstream growth factor receptors, cytokine receptors, B and T cell receptors and G-protein-coupled receptors (Figure 14.4).[42] PTEN LOF alterations often occur in combination with other driver oncogenes, for example, in melanoma with BRAFv600 mutations.

The effects of this pathway activation range widely and include augmentation of the cell cycle and different cellular functions such as cell growth, metabolism, proliferation, and survival, all key cellular processes participating in the initiation and the maintenance of cancer (Figure 14.4).[43]

The loss of *PTEN* has been associated with immunosuppressive mechanisms in some tumors, depending on other pathways driving the biology of those tumors, and consequently, the impact of pathway inhibitors on immunotherapy responsiveness is variable. As in the case of the BRAF and EGFR pathway effects that were previously detailed, the impact of oncogenic alterations on tumor sensitivity to immunotherapy depends on their effects on elements and functions in the iTME. A comprehensive preclinical study by Peng et al.[44] investigated the impact of this pathway on T cell responses to melanoma and demonstrated that tumors lacking intact PTEN pathways were more resistant to T cell-mediated killing in vitro and in vivo. In patients, they observed that tumors with lack of PTEN (defined as PTEN expression lower than 10% by immunohistochemistry [IHC]), had lower CD8+ T cell infiltration, and tumor infiltrating lymphocytes (TILs) were more difficult to expand in vitro than patients with normal PTEN expression. Using The Cancer Genome Atlas (TCGA) data, they also observed that melanomas with low *PTEN* copy numbers had lower T cell infiltration by IHC, with expression of IFN-γ and granzyme B. They also showed that PTEN loss increased VEGF expression and that blocking VEGF in a mouse model increased infiltration of the tumor by T cells and that treatment of mice bearing melanomas with

a PI3Kβ inhibitor improved the efficacy of anti-PD-1 and anti-CTLA4 antibodies. Importantly, PI3K signaling in myeloid cells can block tumor progression in experimental tumor models,[45] and there are numerous other examples of PI3K/AKT signaling and downstream effects having an impact both on cells of the iTME and on the tumor itself, with therapeutic implications for the series of PI3K isoform inhibitors recently approved or in development.[46] In support of these preclinical data, a Phase I study demonstrated an impressive response rate of 73% with the combination of ipatasertib, atezolizumab, and paclitaxel in patients with advanced triple-negative breast cancer (TNBC), independent of PD-L1 or *PI3CKA/AKT/PTEN* status.[47,48]

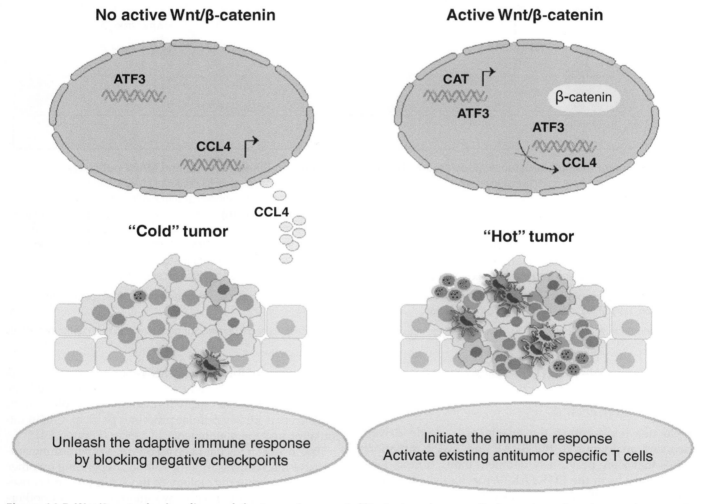

Figure 14.5 Wnt/β–catenin signaling and the tumor immune infiltrate. In melanoma cells, β-catenin mediates immune ignorance in the TME through the induction of transcriptional repressor ATF3, which in turn inhibits CCL4 production via the transcriptional silencing of the *CCL4* gene. Lack of CCL4 secretion results in poor recruitment of CD103 dendritic cells, associated with an impaired cross-priming of antitumor T cells. In addition, the intratumoral T cells show predominantly a naïve phenotype with low PD-1, PD-L1, and LAG3 expression. Knockdown of β-catenin or ATF3 restores CCL4 production in these cells, which in turn leads to a T cell-inflamed melanoma, characterized by the presence of Batf3-lineage dendritic cells as well as transcripts encoding IDO, PD-L1, and Foxp3.

IDO, indoleamine-2, 3-dioxygenase; PD-L1, programmed death-ligand 1.

Source: With permission from Mario M, Romano E. *Mechanisms of Drug Resistance in Cancer Therapy.* Springer International Publishing; 2018.

THE WNT/β-CATENIN PATHWAY AND IMMUNE RESPONSE

Tumor-cell-intrinsic Wnt/β-catenin signaling in melanoma is specifically associated with one of the cardinal manifestations of tumor resistance to immunotherapy, the T cell noninflamed TME that is of particular importance in resistance to PD-1 blockade (Figure 14.5). The mechanism for these effects was elegantly worked out by Spranger et al.[49] and depends on the transcriptional repression of chemokines, particularly CCL4, responsible for recruiting a subset of dendritic cells to the TME that are critical for priming and recruitment of effector T cells. Thus, the consequence of elevated Wnt/β-catenin pathway signaling (Figure 14.5)[43] is the resistance to a variety of immunotherapies, and recent data from analyses across multiple tumor types in TCGA demonstrated a range of inflamed to noninflamed TME that correlated well with the known activity of PD-1/PD-L1 blockade in those tumor types. High β-catenin-in-expressing tumors exhibited a noninflamed TME and were intrinsically resistant to ICBs.[50] The mechanisms for immune modulation of dendritic cell (DC) functions by β-catenin are consistent with the observation that activation of β-catenin signaling in DCs inhibited cross-priming of CD8+ T cells by mTOR-mediated upregulation of IL-10, a DC-suppressive cytokine.[51]

CONCLUSION

In this chapter, we discussed the mechanisms of how oncogenic signaling mediates tumor immune escape, which includes decreased immune infiltration and effector functions and increased levels of immunosuppressive cells in the tumor microenvironment, hence inducing primary or secondary resistance to immune checkpoint inhibitors. The understanding of tumor-intrinsic signaling pathways in patients with tumor progression/recurrence is critical, as targeting these pathways is a promising strategy for cancer treatment. As recent preclinical studies and clinical trials of targeting oncogenic signaling have shown encouraging results, we anticipate that combinatorial treatments targeting oncogenic signaling pathways and mediators of the antitumor immune response will be used for cancer patients in the future.

KEY REFERENCES

Only key references appear in the print edition. The full reference list appears in the digital product on Springer Publishing Connect: connect.springerpub.com/content/book/978-0-8261-3743-2/part/part01/chapter/ch14

7. Boni A, Cogdill AP, Dang P, et al. Selective BRAFV600E inhibition enhances T-cell recognition of melanoma without affecting lymphocyte function. *Cancer Res.* 2010;70(13):5213–5219. doi:10.1158/0008-5472.CAN-10-0118
8. Ho PC, Meeth KM, Tsui YC, et al. Immune-based antitumor effects of BRAF inhibitors rely on signaling by CD40L and IFNγ. *Cancer Res.* 2014;74(12):3205–3217. doi:10.1158/0008-5472.CAN-13-3461
17. Cooper ZA, Reuben A, Spencer CN, et al. Distinct clinical patterns and immune infiltrates are observed at time of progression on targeted therapy versus immune checkpoint blockade for melanoma. *Oncoimmunology.* 2016;5(3):e1136044. doi:10.1080/2162402X.2015.1136044
35. Santaniello A, Napolitano F, Servetto A, et al. Tumour microenvironment and immune evasion in EGFR addicted NSCLC: hurdles and possibilities. *Cancers.* 2019;11(10):1419. doi:10.3390/cancers11101419
36. Gainor JF, Shaw AT, Sequist LV, et al. EGFR mutations and ALK rearrangements are associated with low response rates to PD-1 pathway blockade in non-small cell lung cancer: a retrospective analysis. *Clin Cancer Res.* 2016;22(18):4585–4593. doi:10.1158/1078-0432.CCR-15-3101
38. Skoulidis F, Goldberg ME, Greenawalt DM, et al. STK11/LKB1 mutations and PD-1 inhibitor resistance in KRAS-mutant lung adenocarcinoma. *Cancer Discov.* 2018;8(7):822–835. doi:10.1158/2159-8290.CD-18-0099
44. Peng W, Chen JQ, Liu C, et al. Loss of PTEN promotes resistance to T cell-mediated immunotherapy. *Cancer Discov.* 2016;6(2):202–216. doi:10.1158/2159-8290.CD-15-0283

Chemokines and Chemokine Receptors: Regulators of Tumor Immunity

James J. Mulé, Michelle M. Appenheimer, Sharon S. Evans, and Michael T. Lotze

KEY POINTS

- The chemokine/chemokine receptor family dates to ~650 million years ago and includes in humans 18 receptors and 42 chemokines (C, CC, CXC, and CX3C families); most receptors are encoded on chromosome 3 with the rest on chromosomes 2, 17, 6, 11, and X in order of frequency.

- The chemokine superfamily is an important collective mediating the migration and positioning of immune cells. They coordinate the circulation as well as attraction and retention of leukocytes to sites of infection, tissue injury, or malignancy, regulated in part by posttranslational modifications and binding partners such as high mobility group box-1 (HMGB1).

- Chemokine receptors are seven-transmembrane G-protein-coupled receptors (GPCRs) and are thus susceptible to small-molecule drugs to inhibit their function; chemokines are small (~8,000 daltons) proteins that can be produced and utilized as transgenes or as recombinant proteins/muteins.

- Chemokines serve important functions as co-stimulatory molecules during T cell activation as well as signaling hubs involving individual leukocytes and between T cells and their tumor targets.

- There is substantial evidence that malignant tumors have defects in the chemokine system, thereby escaping immunosurveillance and promoting progression and metastasis.

- Chemokines are natural candidates for therapeutic targeting in anticancer immunotherapy serving as prognostic indicators of outcome.

- Chemokine-targeting therapeutic approaches are under investigation to diminish immunosuppressive tumor microenvironments and increase the intratumoral infiltration of effector T cells and associated inflammatory cells.

"Out of intense complexities, intense simplicities emerge."
—Winston Churchill

INTRODUCTION

The degree of T cell accumulation at tumor sites correlates with better patient prognosis and outcomes.[1] Indeed, T cell infiltration is a better predictor of survival[2–16] than conventional staging methods based on tumor size and metastatic status in colorectal, breast, ovarian, esophageal, kidney, lung, and pancreatic cancer.[17–22] Moreover, it has become clear that therapeutic outcomes are also dictated by localization of other immune cell types that can mediate both anti- and protumorigenic activities.[17,19–22] These "secret differing springs" found within tissues arise with now better-understood drivers. Accordingly, understanding the mechanisms that regulate immune cell trafficking and the strategies used by tumors to influence immune cell influx are fertile grounds for the development of new therapeutic approaches to tip the balance for antitumor immunity.

The chemokine superfamily of low molecular weight chemotactic cytokines has emerged as an important factor, mediating the migration and positioning of immune cells.[23] Based on studies performed in the immune system, the functions of chemokines include coordination of homeostatic circulation of leukocytes as well as attraction and retention of leukocytes to sites of infection, tissue injury, or developing malignancy.[24,25] Chemokine receptors are seven-transmembrane G-protein-coupled receptors (GPCRs) that bind to several different classes of chemokines. Approximately 20 chemokine receptors have been identified, along with 50 chemokines that are subdivided into four families (C, CC, CXC, CX3C) according to the number of conserved cysteine (C) residues and any intervening amino acid (X) between these cysteines in the N-terminus of the protein (Figure 15.1A). The additional complexity of the chemokine network stems from the redundancy of chemokines and chemokine receptors, whereby most chemokines interact with more than one chemokine receptor and vice versa. This inherent complexity is belied by the fact that chemokine

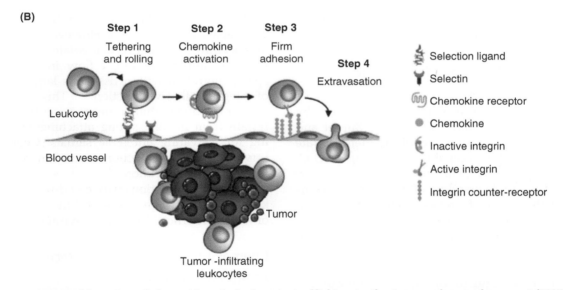

Figure 15.1 Structure and function of chemokines in leukocyte trafficking to the tumor microenvironment (TME).
(A) Schematic diagram of the N-terminal structure of the four chemokine classes and their respective members. Black indicates polypeptide chain; red indicates the eponymous cysteine residues that distinguish each class; blue indicates disulfide linkages. **(B)** Schematic illustrating the chemokine-dependent multistep adhesion cascade by which leukocytes gain access to the TME. Individual types of trafficking molecules are indicated.

receptors often converge on common downstream signaling pathways to coordinate diverse biological responses. It is now well established that chemokines and their receptors contribute significantly to both immune-mediated tumor rejection and tumor architecture, and multiple aspects of tumor progression, including tumorigenesis, growth/survival, angiogenesis, organ-specific metastasis, and immune evasion.

From an evolutionary perspective, zebrafish have the most chemokines, 63, as well as chemokine receptors, 24. Fruit flies, sea squirts, and sea urchins have no chemokines nor chemokine receptors.[26] Plants have no migratory leukocytes, no obvious chemokines, and utilize small-molecule mediators of pathogen containment[27] although plant homologues have been identified that activate human CXCR4.[28] The tumor microenvironment

(TME) contains innate immune cells (i.e., macrophages, dendritic cells [DCs], natural killer [NK] cells, natural killer T [NKT] cells, neutrophils, eosinophils, myeloid-derived suppressor cells [MDSCs]), and adaptive immune cells (i.e., αβ and γδ T cells, NKT, NK and B lymphocytes), as well as cancer cells and their surrounding stroma (i.e., endothelial cells, fibroblasts, and mesenchymal cells).[29] Chemokine production and surface expression of chemokine receptors by diverse immune cells shape the delicate TME, which, in turn, determines the aggressiveness of cancer. Thus, new information regarding the mechanisms by which chemokines and chemokine receptors either inhibit or promote tumor progression will provide perspectives for the development of new immunotherapeutic approaches to cancer treatment. Here, we discuss how chemokines/chemokine receptors regulate anti- and protumorigenic immune responses, mechanisms controlling chemokine/chemokine receptor expression in the tumor at diverse levels, and ongoing preclinical investigation and clinic trials that target the chemokine network in solid malignancies. The reader is referred to recent comprehensive reviews for additional information about chemokine/chemokine receptor contributions to host immunity, response to cancer immunotherapy, and roles in the pathology of hematological diseases.[30–36]

CHEMOKINES NETWORK IN ANTITUMOR IMMUNE RESPONSE

Tumor immunosurveillance was first conceived by Ehrlich in 1909.[37] In the mid-20th century, Burnet and Thomas used transplantation models to demonstrate that the immune system is capable of targeting cancer.[38] Seminal studies by Robert Schreiber and colleagues further advanced our understanding of tumor immunosurveillance with the advent of mouse models and molecular reagents to directly interrogate the role of specific molecular and cellular immune networks in controlling cancer,[39] positing the tumor editing triad of elimination, equilibrium, and escape. The chemokine network has emerged as a master regulator of tumor immunosurveillance and the antitumor immune response at all levels.

Chemokines were initially identified based on their ability to regulate the spatiotemporal distribution of immune cells by activating motility and guiding the movement of cells along chemokine gradients, a process known as "chemotaxis" (in the soluble phase) or "haptotaxis" (in the solid phase). Immune cell trafficking occurs through a cascade of coordinated steps that integrates information streams between tissue sites and circulating immune cells (Figure 15.1B).[40] Leukocytes moving through the bloodstream must rapidly sense and interpret signals presented by vascular endothelial cells and use this information to modify their trafficking behavior within target tissues.[23,41,42] The first step of the trafficking cascade

involves members of the selectin family of glycoproteins. Selectins mediate short-lived tethering and rolling behavior and slow the movement of the leukocyte in the blood flow, allowing cells to scan the endothelial substrata for chemokine signals.[23] Differential leukocyte trafficking at various tissue sites is largely dependent on the expression of chemokine/chemokine receptor pairs such that if the cell does not encounter activating chemokines, it will dislodge from the vessel wall and rejoin the fast-moving circulation within seconds. However, if chemokine receptors engage cognate chemokines on the vascular surface, they rapidly signal via their associated G-protein molecules through intracellular second messengers, including inositol phosphates, phospholipase C, and mobilization of intracellular Ca^{2+} stores.[43–45] These second messengers collectively lead to subsequent activation of protein kinase B (PKB, also known as AKT), protein kinase C (PKC), and the guanine exchange factor Rap.[43–45] Chemokine signaling stimulates rapid cytoskeletal-mediated clustering of leukocyte integrin adhesion molecules as well as conformational changes in integrin structure, thereby increasing their affinity for endothelial counter-receptors that leads to leukocyte extravasation.[45–47]

Within tissues, chemokines contribute to the migratory capacity of leukocytes. However, whereas chemokines act through integrins to mediate leukocyte adhesion under conditions of blood flow in the intravascular space, migration within tissues is largely independent of integrin adhesive function.[46,48] This stands to reason, since migration within tissues requires that lymphocytes refrain from making strong attachments while searching for activating antigenic signals. Chemokines also serve an important function as co-stimulatory molecules during T cell activation, as well as signaling conduits that control interactions between different types of leukocytes and between T cells and their tumor targets, all of which are crucial for an effective antitumor response.

Chemokines and Chemokine Receptors in Innate Antitumor Immunity

NK, NKT, and γδ T cells are among the innate immune cells that form the first line of immune defense during infection or cancer development. Intratumoral infiltration of these cells has been associated with a favorable prognosis in patients with multiple types of cancer and accumulating evidence documents their important protective function in tumor immunosurveillance. The innate immune response is initiated by the recognition of damage-associated molecular pattern molecules (DAMPs) present on the malignant cells or subcellular debris by pattern recognition receptors (PRR) on DC precursors and tissue-resident macrophages (Figure 15.2). DAMP recognition jump-starts the release of chemokines from the DCs and macrophages. NK, NKT, and γδ T

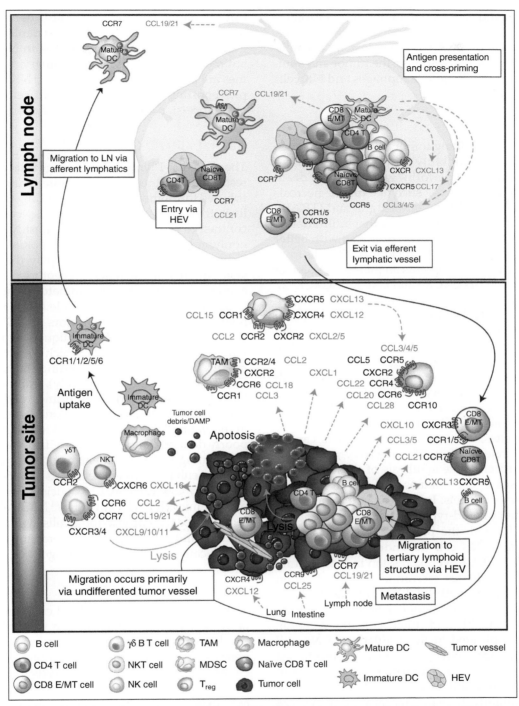

Figure 15.2 Chemokine network in the antitumor and protumor immune response. Upon the recognition of tumor-derived DAMPs by DCs and macrophages, chemokine release is triggered to recruit and activate γδ T, NKT, and NK cells that can lyse tumor cells. Tumor cell debris is engulfed by immature DCs, leading to downregulation of tissue-specific chemokine receptors and upregulation of CCR7 that directs their migration toward CCL19/21 expressed in the afferent lymphatics and draining LN. In the LNs, mature DCs present processed tumor antigens to naïve CD4+ and CD8+ T cells, as well as B cells that enter LNs via HEVs. Primed CD8+ T cells upregulate chemokine receptors in response to specific chemokines from tumors and leave LNs via lymphatic vessels and travel to a tumor site through undifferentiated tumor vessels and HEVs. Ideally, the activated T cells can clear the malignant cells; however, the TME is also rich in chemokines that recruit immunosuppressive immune cells, including TAMs, MDSCs, and T_{reg} cells, which potentially promote tumor progression.

DAMP, damage-associated molecular patterns; DC, dendritic cell; HEV, high endothelial venule; LN, lymph node; MDSC, myeloid-derived suppressor cell; NK, natural killer; NKT, natural killer T; TAM, tumor-associated macrophage; T_{reg}, regulatory T.

cells are recruited and activated to inhibit tumor proliferation and kill tumor cells.[49–51] Among these chemokines, CXCL10, CXCL9, and CXCL11 are angiostatic chemokines that block neovascularization in the tumor and stimulate the cytocidal activity in macrophages and NK cells entering the tumor.[52]

Natural Killer Cells

NK cells are capable of killing tumor cells lacking expression of major histocompatibility complex (MHC) class I molecules via secretion of perforin/granzyme and death receptor-mediated pathways, such as tumor necrosis factor (TNF)-related apoptosis-inducing ligand (TRAIL) and FasL. Clinical studies demonstrate that infiltration of NK cells in some tumor biopsies is correlated with better prognosis in cancer patients.[53] Trafficking of NK cells from bone marrow to the blood depends on their expression of the chemokine receptors CXCR3 and CXCR4.[53] CXCL12/ SDF1 is the predominant ligand interacting with CXCR4. It is also evolutionarily the most ancient chemokine, only differing between mouse and man by a single amino acid interacting with CXCR4. CXCR4/CXCL12 play critical roles in multiple organ systems including the brain, the circulatory system, and embryonic stem cells, and both CXCR4 and CXCL12 are embryonic lethal when knocked out.[54–56] Furthermore, the corresponding CXCR3 ligands CXCL9, CXCL10, and CXCL11 mediate NK cell recruitment to tumor sites, as attraction of NK cells can be enhanced by the release of interferon-γ (IFN-γ), which is an upstream inducer of the synthesis of these chemokines. Other classes of chemokines also recruit NK cells in preclinical tumor models. In a liver carcinoma mouse model, restoration of wild-type p53 increases tumor cell secretion of CCL2 with the potential to recruit CCR5+ NK cells, leading to NK cell–dependent elimination of local tumor cells.[57] CCL2-overexpression in human lung cancer cells also facilitates recruitment and activation of NK cells, correlating with inhibition of metastasis in the severe combined immunodeficient (SCID) mouse model.[58] CCL19/CCL21 and their cognate receptor, CCR7, are also implicated in the regulation of NK cell trafficking into lymph nodes. Transgenic mouse breast cancer cells engineered to overexpress CCL19 recruit NK cells to the tumor site, resulting in tumor rejection by the host.[57] Similarly, transduction of CCL21 in CT26 murine colon adenocarcinoma cells reduces their tumorigenicity in vivo, which is abrogated by depletion of NK cells or CD8+ T cells.[59] Intratumoral injection of CCL27-expressing adenovirus also induces the accumulation of CCR10+ NK cells and synergistic antitumor activity when combined with IL-12-expressing adenovirus.[60] The CX3CR1/CX3CL1 axis facilitates the binding of NK cells to activated endothelial cells, which results in the elimination of YAC-1 tumor cells in mouse lung tumor models.[61] Further, CXCL14-transgenic mice show decreased tumor volume and lung metastasis, which is attenuated by anti-asialo-GM1 antibodies that deplete NK cells, suggesting the importance of CXCL14 in NK cell-mediated antimetastatic activity.[62] In summary, diverse chemokines are potent chemoattractants for NK cells, and therapies boosting the recruitment of NK cells via chemokine overexpression could be of clinical interest.

Natural Killer T Cells

These unique T lymphocyte lineage cells express a highly restricted T cell receptor repertoire. They are widely distributed throughout the body, including the bone marrow, liver, thymus, lymph nodes (LNs), spleen, and lung.[63] In contrast to conventional T cells, most NKT cells express nonlymphoid tissue-homing chemokine receptors, and individual NKT cell subsets display distinctive expression patterns of chemokine receptors.[63] Most NKT cells express receptors for inflammatory chemokines (e.g., CCR2, CCR5, and CXCR3), while few NKT cells express homeostatic chemokine receptors (CCR7 and CXCR5).[63] CCR4, CCR1, and CCR6 are uniquely expressed by individual subsets of NKT cells, which are preferentially chemoattracted to their corresponding chemokines (CCL17, CCL3, and CCL20, respectively). Although NKT cells have been implicated in antitumor and antimetastatic responses, the roles of chemokine receptor expression in regulating NKT cell–mediated tumor rejection remain poorly defined. The CXCR6/CXCL16 axis mediates NKT cell homing and activation in response to glycolipid antigens, as enhanced liver metastasis of B16-F10 melanoma caused by CXCR6/CXCL16 deficiency can be overcome by systemic NKT cell activation.[64] NKT cells are also chemoattracted to neuroblastoma cells in a CCL2-dependent manner and infiltrate CCL2-expressing tumors lacking amplification of the MYCN oncogene.[65]

γδ T cells

These cytolytic innate lymphoid cells also participate in antitumor immune defense. The γδ T cells limit cancer incidence in models of carcinogen-induced skin carcinogenesis[66] and a transgenic model of prostate adenocarcinoma.[67] Dermal-resident γδ T cells express CCR8 that promotes their skin residence, whereas circulating γδ T cells express a series of inflammatory chemokine receptors, including CCR1, CCR2, CCR3, CCR5, CXCR1, CXCR2, and CXCR3. In the B16 melanoma model, the CCR2/CCL2 axis promoted intratumoral infiltration of γδ T cells in vivo, as evidenced by significant reduction of γδ T cell infiltrates in $Ccl2^{-/-}$ and $Ccr2^{-/-}$ mice and overall higher tumor growth rates in $Ccr2^{-/-}$ mice.[68] In this study, a subset of human γδ T cells expressing CCR2 migrates in response to CCL2, whose expression is strongly deregulated in multiple human tumors of diverse origins. An independent study illustrates that adoptive transfer of one subset of γδ T cells inhibits the growth of HT29 tumors, which is blocked by the anti-CCR3 monoclonal antibody, indicating that CCR3-mediated migration is necessary for the antitumor activity of γδ T cells.[69] In some infectious diseases and wound healing models, γδ T cells are involved in the recruitment of macrophages and facilitate their differentiation into inflammatory macrophages,[70] which could theoretically promote rather than retard tumor progression. In this regard, it should be noted that at early phases of tumorigenesis, macrophages can initiate the immune response against transformed cells, but may also contribute to tumor progression when the immune surveillance is not sufficient, which will be discussed in subsequent sections.[71] Thus, application of γδ T cells in novel anticancer immunotherapies warrants further investigation. Certainly, substantial effort is starting to define sites of recognition in MHC-like molecules, the butyrophilins, and the major role of these cells coupling both innate and adaptive properties.[72–82] CCR5 and CXCR3 expression has been noted on these cells that is consistent with their tumor-homing capability,[83] suggesting that deeper understanding of the protumor versus antitumor activity of γδ T cells is needed to maximize therapeutic response.

Chemokines and Chemokine Receptors in Adaptive Antitumor Immunity

Efficient cancer immunosurveillance requires coordinated activation of both the innate and adaptive arms of the immune response. In addition to direct effector functions, the innate immune response serves as a bridge to adaptive immunity, with professional antigen-presenting cells (APCs) of the innate system (e.g., macrophages, DCs) informing and directing antitumor cytotoxic T cell responses. Cellular positioning is crucial for both the priming and effector phases of adaptive immunity, so it is not surprising that chemokines have emerged as central regulators of antitumor T cell function. Because cytolytic T cells that can respond to a given antigen are rare (existing at a frequency of only ~1 in 10^5–10^6),[84] chemokine-dependent trafficking ensures that sufficient numbers of T cells colocalize with antigen-bearing DCs within lymphoid organs that provide a supportive environment favoring T cell activation and proliferation. Additionally, chemokines direct the delivery of activated effector T cells to tumor targets in distal organs.

The priming phase of adaptive immunity begins with the release of cellular debris generated as a result of tissue damage or injury, as well as immune cell–mediated cancer cell death. Following tumor lysis, the debris is engulfed by immature DCs, which then undergo a maturational process characterized by the reciprocal loss of selected chemokine receptors (CCR1, CCR2, CCR5, and CCR6) and acquisition of CCR7.[46,85–88] This leads to CCL19/CCL21-driven unidirectional migration of mature DCs through the afferent lymphatic vessels and into draining LNs (Figure 15.2). CCR7 is necessary for integrin-independent DCs trafficking into LNs via the lymphatic vascular network that drains surrounding tissue sites.[86,89,90] In the absence of CCR7 or its ligands, the DCs ferrying tumor antigens fail to migrate from tumors to draining LNs, and thus are unable to deliver activating signals driving CD8+ T cell-mediated antitumor adaptive immunity.[91] Once DCs have reached the LN, they continue to follow CCR7-dependent chemokine cues to migrate deeper into the T cell zone, maximizing their chances of encountering and activating cognate T cells.[92] The obligate requirement for CCR7 in antitumor immunity is revealed by preclinical studies showing that tumor-derived oxidized cholesterol (oxysterols) reduces CCR7 expression by resident DCs, which then fail to traffic to draining LNs and initiate adaptive immunity.[93] CXCL14 is a potent chemoattractant of immature DCs.[94] In head and neck squamous cell carcinoma (HNSCC), loss of CXCL14 correlated with decreased infiltration of DCs.[94] Furthermore, restoration of CXCL14 increased tumor infiltration by DCs in vivo in chimeric animal models.[94]

Malignant cells expressing tumor-associated antigens (TAAs) can be specifically recognized and eliminated by the immune system before they are clinically apparent. Naïve and central memory CD8+ T cells continually traffic from the blood circulation into LNs, where they search for targets by quickly scanning DCs distributed throughout the T cell region of the node. CCR7 ligands direct T cell exit from the blood, their migration within the node in search of antigen, and their retention or ultimate egress from the node. T cell trafficking into LNs takes place at morphologically and functionally distinct postcapillary vessels termed "high endothelial venules" (HEVs) that uniquely express the array of trafficking molecules required to direct the extravasation of naïve and central memory T cells.[40,41,95] Initial tethering and short-lived rolling interactions between circulating T cells and HEVs are mediated by lymphocyte CD62L (L-selectin) and its glycoprotein ligands, collectively known as peripheral node addressin (PNAd), presented by HEVs.[96–98] CD62L-dependent slow rolling enables T cells to sample the local environment for the presence of chemokines. In HEVs, CCR7/CCL21 interactions drive the conformational changes that increase the affinity of lymphocyte integrin molecules for their endothelial counter-receptors, resulting in lymphocyte arrest, firm adhesion, and subsequent extravasation into the stroma of the LN (Figure 15.2).[99–104] Once inside the LN, CCL21 guides T cells in their integrin-independent migration toward the DC-enriched areas, where they then undertake random, CCR7-dependent exploration, scanning for cognate antigen, and priming co-stimulatory signals.[48,90,105] Naïve B cell entry across LN HEVs also occurs via a CCR7-dependent mechanism, whereas their migration to follicles where tumor-specific antibody production occurs is guided by CXCR5/CXCL13.[106,107] Interestingly, tumor-draining LNs (TdLNs) in both humans and mice have reduced levels of CCL21 mRNA or protein, suggesting that multiple steps are necessary for productive DC–T cell or T–B cell interactions and may be disrupted in cancer.[108,109] Indeed, in a murine melanoma model, CCL21 presentation is deficient on HEVs in TdLNs, corresponding to substantially reduced naïve T cell trafficking.[110]

Within the LN, chemokines not only guide the movement and subanatomical localization of naïve lymphocytes but also play a role in the activation of T cell responses. CCR7 ligands presented by LN DCs to T cells form an antigen-independent physical "tether" that potentiates the priming of naïve T cells, making them more sensitive to subsequent antigen-dependent interactions with DCs.[111,112] One early priming step of an effector CD8+ cytotoxic T lymphocyte (CTL) response is the antigen-dependent licensing of DCs by CD4+ helper T cells through CD40 ligand (CD40L)/CD40 interactions.[113] Upon the binding of CD4+ T cells with DCs presenting their cognate antigen, both DCs and CD4+ T cells produce the CCR5 ligands CCL3, CCL4, and CCL5. Following LN entry, a subset of naïve CD8+ T cells acquires the expression of CCR5 that facilitates their migration toward CD4+ T cell/DC clusters, resulting in classical cross-priming.[114,115] Alternatively, DCs licensed by NKT cells produce CCL17, which attracts naïve CCR4-expressing CD8+ T cells.[116] CXCR3-expressing T cells within the LN are also driven by CXCL9 and CXCL10 to migrate into regions populated by DCs that promote Th1 polarization.[117] Following T cell receptor (TCR) engagement, CXCR4/CD184 and CCR5/CD195 become sequestered within the immunological synapse, where they contribute to antigen-dependent IL-2 production and resultant T cell proliferation.[118,119]

Upon productive engagement with cognate antigen and co-stimulatory molecules, naïve antigen-specific CD8+ T cells undergo a multilogarithmic clonal expansion and differentiation to either effector cells that search out and destroy tumor target cells or memory T cells that contribute to host protection from future tumor challenge.[120] To perform their antitumor function, most effector T cells must exit the LN and migrate to distant tumor sites, where they recognize and kill tumor cells expressing cognate antigens. Each of these steps again relies on chemokines (Figure 15.2), as well as expression of sphingosine-1-phosphate (S1P), and its receptor (S1PR1) on T cells, B cells, and macrophages.[121–125] Fibroblastic reticular cells (FRCs) expressing CCL19 and CCL21 recruit and retain T cells in lymph nodes (LNs).[121] Retention appears to be driven by downregulation of the S1PR, which is greater on B than on T cells. One mechanism by which regulatory T (T$_{reg}$) cells present within the lymph node regulate T cell responses is by downregulating the expression of SIPR1 on effector T cells, thus promoting T cell retention within the LN.[125] After activation within LNs, effector T cells downregulate CCR7, enabling them to resist the retention signals delivered by CCL21, and leave the LN under the influence of S1P, which guides newly activated lymphocytes back to the blood circulation via the efferent lymphatics.[126,127] Concomitant with the CCR7 loss, effector T cells upregulate chemokine receptors that are typically associated with homing to peripheral sites; for example, CCR1, CCR2, CCR3, CCR5, and CXCR3.[128]

Several studies have reported a positive correlation between patient outcomes and expression of specific chemokine receptors by immune cells, chemokine production at tumor sites, and effector cell infiltration within tumors (Figure 15.2).[17,129–131] For example, in colon (CX3CL1,[132] CXCR3),[130] lung (CCL5),[133] kidney (CXCL9, CXCL10, CCL4, and CCL5),[134] melanoma (CXCR3),[131,135] and ovarian (CCL3, CCL5, CXCL9, CXCL10)[86] cancers, chemokine or chemokine receptor expression is linked to better patient outcomes and antitumor immune responses. Conversely, in a retrospective analysis of melanoma patients, loss of CXCR3 or CCR6 on circulating T cell subsets is associated with skin or LN metastases, loss of CXCR4, CXCR5, and CCR9 correlates with lung involvement, and increased CCR10 correlates with widespread dissemination.[136] These observations are in agreement with the widely accepted view that multiple chemokine/chemokine receptor pairs cooperatively support T cell trafficking across tumor blood vessels and into the tumor parenchyma. However, it is worthwhile noting that the majority of these correlative studies typically present a snapshot of the TME at a single time point during cancer progression. Thus, it has been unclear whether one or more chemokine/chemokine receptor pairs guide trafficking across the vessel wall, or instead act within the tumor parenchyma to support lymphocyte survival, proliferation, or retention.[23,135,137]

Recent work has shed light on this question by investigating the hierarchy of chemokine requirements for trafficking at tumor vascular checkpoints in murine and human preclinical melanoma models for adoptive T cell transfer immunotherapy.[135,137] Intravital microscopy revealed that despite expression of multiple functional chemokine receptors (i.e., CXCR3, CCR2, CCR5) by adoptively transferred T cells and availability of cognate ligands in the TME, only CXCR3 is necessary and sufficient for trafficking of adoptively transferred CD8+ effector T cells across tumor vessels and destruction of tumor targets.[135,138] In the context of immune checkpoint inhibitor (ICI) therapy, CXCR3 appears to be less important for CD8+ T cell migration into tumors in murine models, but rather is critical for the antitumor activity of intratumoral cytotoxic T cells.[139] Substantial homologous correlatives in human tumor and murine tumor derangements and chemokine-driven therapies provide confidence that targeting tumors can be effective by engaging suitable chemokines and their receptors.[140–146] While CCR2 and CCR5 do not contribute to extravasation, they could instead play a role in retaining T cells within the intratumoral space or in lowering the threshold for T cell activation, as has been shown in nonmalignant systems.[103,147,148] This unexpected disconnect between proteomic expression profiling for chemokine receptors/chemokines and functional readouts for T cell trafficking raises a cautionary note that in vivo endpoints are important for drawing conclusions about the contributions of individual chemotactic molecules to antitumor immunity. Multiple cell types produce CXCR3 ligands within the TME, including tumor cells and CD103[+] DC, with the latter emerging as key chemokine providers to support the efficacy adoptive T cell therapy and ICI therapy.[34,138,139,149] Moreover, elevated plasma levels of CXCL9 and CXCL10 correlated with clinical response to ICI therapy in melanoma patients.[139] Collectively, these observations have raised speculation that CXCR3 ligands and CD103[+] DC could serve as important biomarkers of response to T cell–based immunotherapy.

Formation of Immune-Stimulating Tertiary Lymphoid Structures

Trafficking of CXCR3[hi] CD8[+] effector T cells to tumors in preclinical mouse models predominantly occurs at undifferentiated blood vessels by virtue of endothelial display of inflammatory chemokines (CXCL9, 10, 11).[135,150] As a result, CXCR3[lo] CCR7[hi] naïve T cells are largely excluded from trafficking via the vasculature in the TME.[150] However, in a subset of cancers in patients and mouse models, the formation of intratumoral ectopic lymphoid aggregates known as tertiary lymphoid structures (TLSs) that resemble the characteristics of peripheral LNs have been observed.[151–155] Many TLSs exhibit an organizational architecture that includes B cell–T cell segregation and HEVs, suggesting that TLSs may be an entry site for naïve lymphocytes and a component of an active host immune response to growing tumors (Figure 15.2).[156,157] There is evidence showing that TLS presence correlates with a favorable clinical outcome of patients with certain types of cancer[143,151,156,158–160] and their response to ICI therapy.[161–163] The chemokines necessary for initiation of TLSs are at least partially identical to those required for LN formation, given that the administration of CCL21 and CXCL13 on their own can induce TLSs within tumor tissues as well as in normal organs in mouse models.[153,164–166] As in LNs, PNAd and CCL21 expressed on intratumoral HEVs are thought to be important for the entry of naïve and memory T cells expressing the cognate ligands L-selectin and CCR7, respectively, and subsequent differentiation into cytotoxic CD8[+] T cells in situ.[154,155,167] Additionally, a recent study suggests that it is possible that these TLS's recruit and activate effector T cells based on observations that CXCR3[+] T cells colocalize with CXCL10-expressing activated DCs within murine melanomas.[154] A potential caveat is that the presence of TLS's is not necessarily beneficial, as the ectopic CCL21 expression by melanomas in mice is also reportedly associated with induction of immunosuppressive "disorganized" TLSs, which facilitate tumor progression by shifting from an immunogenic to tolerogenic host immune response.[110,168]

A 12-chemokine gene expression signature (12-CK GES; *CCL2, CCL3, CCL4, CCL5, CCL8, CCL18, CCL19, CCL21, CXCL9, CXCL10, CXCL11,* and *CXCL13*) has been identified that accurately predicts the presence of TLSs in stage IV melanoma metastases, which is also associated with better overall survival in a subset of melanoma patients.[143] The use of this unique 12-CK GES may potentially improve the identification and selection of melanoma patients most suitable for immunotherapy. Similar results were observed in other cancer types, such as human primary colorectal carcinoma (CRC).[169] Most recently, the fidelity of this 12-CK GES in identifying TLSs has been confirmed by others in a variety of solid tumors[169] as well as for its potential clinical use and in identifying better patient outcomes in CRC using integrated data of resected 975 CRC cases within three independent cohorts from France, Japan, and the United States.[170–172] Another specific gene expression signature that includes *CCL19, CCL21, CXCL13, CCL17, CCL22,* and some adhesion molecules has been observed in TLSs within non-small cell lung cancer (NSCLC), while the T cells residing in TLS's show expression of the corresponding chemokine receptors.[173] These findings collectively suggest that TLS-associated chemokines are important for recruiting lymphocytes to the tumor and generating an active and functional response.[153] However, whether TLSs are a consequence of or a crucial contributor driving antitumor immunity remains an important question to be investigated further.

Chemokine Receptors and Angiostatins

Angiogenesis promotes the development of new capillaries from existing blood vessels, which involves activation of endothelial cells, degradation of extracellular matrix, and migration and proliferation of endothelial cells into so-called tuft cells.[174] The roles of chemokines in angiostasis and angiogenesis in various cancer types were comprehensively reviewed previously.[175] CXCR3 expressed on endothelial cells is considered a major chemokine receptor that mediates angiostasis.[176] The

CXCR3 ligands CXCL9, CXCL10, and CXCL11 inhibit migration of human microvascular endothelial cell (HMEC) in response to CXCL8, a known angiogenic chemokine.[177] Further studies indicate that these chemokines block HMEC proliferation in vitro, which can be abrogated by an anti-CXCR3 antibody.[178] Two distinct splice variants of CXCR3 exist which exert distinct influences on angiogenesis: CXCR3A (the "classical" receptor for CXCL9-11) and CXCR3-B (functional receptor for CXCL4 as well as CXCL9-11). Overexpression of CXCR3-A increases HMEC survival, whereas overexpression of CXCR3-B dramatically promotes apoptotic HMEC death.[179] Interestingly, a recent study in wound healing demonstrates that treatment with CXCL10 during the resolving phase of wound healing causes regression of newly formed blood vessels, whereas mice lacking CXCR3 express more vessels at injury sites compared to wild-type mice.[180] Neutralization of CXCL10 also enhances tumor-derived angiogenic activity and tumor growth, whereas reconstitution of intratumoral CXCL10 leads to significant inhibition of tumor growth, neovascularization, and spontaneous lung metastases.[181] The E3 ubiquitin ligase, Pellino-1, which promotes chemokine expression in response to inflammatory signaling,[182] has been shown to play a role in driving angiogenesis in myocardial infarction, suggesting that this molecule could also be critical in vascular remodeling in cancer.[183] Viral vector-mediated CXCL4 transduction similarly inhibits endothelial cell proliferation in vitro and tumor-associated angiogenesis and prolongs mouse survival.[184] Furthermore, the CXCL4 analog CXCL4L1 displays potent suppression of tumor growth and metastasis of melanoma through inhibition of angiogenesis.[185,186] High mobility group box-1 (HMGB1) enhances CXCR4/CXCL12 binding by interacting with the ligand SDF1/CXCL12, as well as markedly enhancing its affinity for CXCR4 and CXCR7, promoting angiogenesis and lymphangiogenesis.[187,188] CXCR4 is expressed on many cancer cells, whereas CXCR7 is expressed on tumor-associated endothelium. Collectively, these findings suggest that CXCR3/CXCL9-11, HMGB1/CXCL12/CXCR7, and CXCL4/4L1 could be promising angiostatic targets in cancer treatment.

CHEMOKINE NETWORK IN PROTUMOR IMMUNE RESPONSE

During immunosurveillance against solid tumors, the immune system can initiate innate immunity that directly recognizes and lyses malignant tumor cells, as well as the subsequent adaptive immune response that is mediated by specific TAA-targeting CTLs allowing eradication. However, the stark reality is that the immune system frequently enters an equilibrium followed by escape and cancer progression. This failure is partially attributed to the dual host-protective versus tumor-sculpting actions of the immune system in cancer, termed "cancer immunoediting."[52] There is now strong evidence that cancer cells with poor immunogenicity or high metastatic capacity manipulate the chemokine system to escape immunosurveillance. Additionally, tumors secrete chemokines that recruit immunosuppressive cells to maintain the tolerogenic microenvironment that fosters tumor progression.

Chemokines and Chemokine Receptors in Protumorigenic Immunity

There are compelling data indicating that infiltration by tumor-associated macrophages (TAMs), T_{reg} cells, and MDSCs is associated with a worse prognosis for a number of different tumor types, making targeting chemokines truly complex.[189,190] TAMs exist in almost all solid neoplasms and play an important role in cancer inflammation. There are two types of TAMs: (1) M1 macrophages that are activated by IFN-γ and are capable of killing pathogens and priming antitumor immune responses and (2) M2 macrophages that are induced by IL-4, IL-10, and IL-13 and promote tumor growth and angiogenesis, invasion, and metastasis.[29] M2 macrophages produce various immunosuppressive factors, such as TNF-α, IL-6, and IL-17, to dampen antitumor immunity of immune effector cells.[191] In a mouse model of liver metastasis, CXCL16-expressing SL4 colon carcinoma cells promoted tumor accumulation of M1 macrophages, which then enhanced apoptosis of SL4 cells by secreting TNF-α, thereby resulting in inhibition of metastasis.[192]

CCL2 is one of the TME-derived chemokines that recruit TAMs with the M2 immunoregulatory phenotype (Figure 15.2).[24] The recruitment of TAMs that express CCR2 is dependent on synthesis of its ligand CCL2 by the tumor and stroma, given that blocking CCL2–CCR2 impairs the recruitment of TAM and metastasis in vivo and prolongs the survival of tumor-bearing mice.[193–195] Ccr2 deletion in murine breast tumors promotes better adaptive immune responses, less MDSCs, and enhanced CD103+ Batf3+ antigen cross-presenting DCs.[196] Similarly, CCL2 overexpression in a human prostate cancer cell line PC-3 increases the growth of transplanted xenografts and accumulation of macrophages in vivo and enhances bone metastasis.[197] Knockout of the formyl peptide receptor 2 (FPR2), which is expressed on macrophages[198] in mice, decreased survival that correlates with increased myeloid cell infiltration and angiogenesis at the tumor site. The macrophages from Fpr2−/− mice display a more potent chemotactic response to tumor-derived supernatant and CCL2, which is likely due to increased expression of CCR4, which is another receptor for CCL2. In another conditional genetic mouse model of lung adenocarcinoma, injection of a lipid nanoparticle containing CCR2-silencing siRNA leads to the reduction of TAMs and tumor progression, providing further evidence that TAMs are recruited via CCR2.[199] A distinct population of CCR2[+] macrophages, termed "metastasis-associated macrophages" (MAMs), has also been identified that requires CCL2 for recruitment to tumor sites and interaction with metastasizing tumor cells.[193,195] Furthermore, MAMs secrete another chemokine, CCL3, and genetic deletion of CCL3 or its receptor CCR1 in macrophages reduces the number of lung metastasis foci, and MAMs accumulate in mammary adenocarcinoma cell-challenged lung in mice.[193]

Other chemokine receptors are also implicated in the recruitment of TAMs, such as CCR6, CXCR2, CXCR3, and CX3CR1 (Figure 15.2). CCR6-deficient mice show diminished spontaneous intestinal tumorigenesis, which may be due to decreased macrophage infiltration into the intestine, as well as the proliferation of neoplastic epithelial cells.[200] Furthermore, infiltration of CCL18[+] TAMs is positively associated with increased microvascular density, metastasis, and a worse prognosis in breast cancer patients.[201] Accordingly, blocking the CCR6 ligand CCL18 with neutralizing antibody inhibits the promigratory effects of TAMs. Macrophage-induced migration of mammary epithelial cells and human breast cancer cells in vitro is also blocked by the CXCR2 pharmacologic inhibitor SB225002, suggesting that targeting CXCR2 may be a novel therapeutic strategy for breast cancer with high levels of infiltrating macrophages.[202] In a study of necroptosis (programmed necrosis) in pancreatic ductal adenocarcinoma (PDA), the macrophage-induced immunosuppressive microenvironment partially depends on signaling of the CXCR2 ligand, CXCL1, triggered by necroptosis, and CXCL1 blockade protects against PDA progression in mice[203] with important correlatives in patients.[204] Gemcitabine treatment in murine models increased CCL/CXCL chemokines and TGF-β-associated inhibition of T cells, which, when ablated, enhanced antitumor effects.[205] Interestingly, CXCR3-deficient mice injected orthotopically with polyoma middle T antigen (PyMT)-transformed breast cancer cells display increased M2 polarization of macrophages in the tumors and spleen, which is accompanied by larger tumor development.[206] This study further demonstrated that $Cxcr3^{-/-}$ macrophages have a greater predisposition toward M2 polarization that contributes to a tumor-promoting environment. Further investigation demonstrated that CX3CR1-mediated survival of angiogenic macrophages leads to tumor metastases in colorectal cancer, based on evidence that CX3CR1 deficiency significantly impairs hepatic metastasis and tumor angiogenesis in association with enhanced macrophage apoptosis in metastatic tumors.[207]

T_{reg} cells defined by a CD4[+]CD25[+]Foxp3[+] phenotype is yet another type of immunosuppressive immune cell that is used by tumors to escape TAA-specific immunity. The mechanisms of T_{reg}-induced immunosuppression include production of immunosuppressive cytokines (IL-10, TGF-β, IL-35) and indirect downregulation of co-stimulatory molecules on APCs via cytotoxic T-lymphocyte-associated protein-4 (CTLA-4).[208] A high frequency of T_{reg} cells in solid tumors is reported for a growing list of cancer patients, including breast cancer, colorectal cancer, esophageal cancer, gastric cancer, hepatocellular carcinoma, lung cancer, prostate cancer, melanoma, ovarian cancer, and pancreatic cancer.[209] Accumulating evidence revealed that the homing of T_{reg} cells to tumor sites is mediated through CCR4 expressed on T_{reg} cells and its ligand CCL22 produced by both tumor cells and TAMs (Figure 15.2).[157,210–212] Furthermore, T_{reg} cell migration can be abrogated through the CCR4 blockade in vitro. Differentiation of T_{reg} cells involved in CCR4-dependent migration to metastatic mammary and melanoma tumors is promoted by regulatory B (B_{reg}) cells and immunosuppressive B_{regs} (CD38[hi]CD24[hi]CD5[+]CD1d[hi]CD24[hi]CD27[+]IL-10[+]), frequently infiltrate patient tumors, and are associated with a poor prognosis.[3,213–215] Human breast tumors overexpress CXCL13, which supports migration of CXCR5[+] B cells,[216] and promising avenues of investigation are exploring the therapeutic benefits of exploiting the CXCR5/CXCL13 axis to shift the balance between B_{reg} and immunostimulatory B cells (Figure 15.2).[217] CCR10 has also been implicated in T_{reg} cell control, whereby hypoxia upregulates CCL28 in human ovarian cancer cells. CCL28 is responsible for the recruitment of T_{reg} cells expressing the cognate receptor CCR10, leading to immune tolerance and angiogenesis.[218]

Additional chemokine/chemokine receptor partners are also emerging as regulators of T_{reg} cell recruitment, such as CCL5/CCR5, CCR6/CCL20, and CXCR2/CXCL1. For example, in both human pancreatic adenocarcinoma and a murine pancreatic tumor model, CCR5/CCL5 signaling disruption, either by reducing CCL5 production from tumor cells or systemic administration of a CCR5 inhibitor, impairs T_{reg} cell migration to tumors and reduces tumor growth.[219] Nuclear focal adhesion kinase (FAK) upregulates $Ccl5$ transcription that is crucial for the recruitment of T_{reg} cells, favoring the development of an overall immunosuppressive microenvironment.[220] In a colorectal cancer model, both cancer cells and TAMs produce large amounts of CCL20, which is the sole ligand of CCR6 found to be predominantly expressed on the T_{reg} cells.[221] In this study, intratumoral injection of recombinant mouse CCL20 promoted tumor development with marked recruitment of T_{reg} cells. Conversely, decreased CCL20 levels as a result of conditional ablation of macrophage populations block T_{reg} cell recruitment and inhibit tumor growth. Ectopic expression of miR141 in tumor cells reduces mRNA level of CXCL1 and also significantly inhibits tumor growth and metastasis in an immune-competent mouse model in association with decreased migration of T_{reg} cells.[222] Moreover, CXCL1-neutralizing antibody suppresses miR141-specific inhibitor-induced migration of T_{reg} cells. Blocking of CXCR2 on T_{reg} cells also strongly inhibits CXCL1-induced migration of T_{reg} cells.

MDSCs are another type of immunosuppressive immune cell that is present in murine tumors and various human cancers, such as glioblastoma, urothelial carcinoma, pancreatic adenocarcinoma, and breast cancer.[223] MDSCs can suppress both innate and adaptive antitumor immunity via inhibiting CD4[+], CD8[+], NK, and NKT cell activities, blocking DC maturation, and inducing T_{reg} cells.[224] MDSCs are actively recruited to primary and metastatic tumor sites via chemokines and HMGB1[198,225–230] produced at tumor sites (Figure 15.2).[223] In addition to chemo-attracting TAMs, CCL2 also mediates homing of the CCR2[+] monocytic-MDSC subset, given that the absence of CCL2-CCR2 signaling impairs both MDSC migration and MDSC-promoted tumor growth.[231] CCR2-deficient MDSCs exhibit reduced trafficking to tumor sites, blood, and spleen, but retain equivalent suppressive capability on a per-cell basis compared to MDSCs purified from wild-type mice.[232] In a spontaneous mouse model of colitis-associated colorectal carcinoma, deletion of CCL2 suppresses progression from dysplasia to adenocarcinoma and reduces the number of colonic MDSCs, while CCL2 neutralization reduces tumor numbers and MDSC accumulation and function.[233] CCR2-expressing MDSCs from various types of cancer patients also migrate toward CCL2 secreted from breast, ovarian, and gastric human tumors cultured in vitro.[223] Tumor-infiltrating MDSCs secrete CCL3, CCL4, and CCL5, which recruit high numbers of CCR5[+] T_{reg} cells, revealing a novel immune-suppressive role of MDSCs in tumor development.[234] Furthermore, CCL5-deficient mice are remarkably resistant to the growth of highly aggressive triple-negative mammary tumors. This resistance is attributed to the aberrant generation of MDSCs with impaired capacity for suppressing cytotoxicity of CD8[+] T cells in both orthotopic and spontaneous mammary tumors.[235] In this same mammary tumor model, antibody-mediated systemic blockade of CCL5 inhibits tumor progression and improves the efficacy of therapeutic vaccination.

Additional chemokine–chemokine receptors are also reportedly involved in the regulation of MDSCs. In an orthotopic xenograft mouse model of human colorectal cancer, loss of SMAD4 is associated with increased CCL15 expression, which recruits CCR1[+] cells with an MDSC phenotype (i.e., CD11b[+]CD33[+]HLA-DR[-]) and results in aggressive tumor growth.[236] There is also strong evidence that the CXCR2-expressing granulocytic MDSC subset is essential for colitis-associated tumorigenesis, based on findings that CXCR2 deficiency dramatically suppresses colonic inflammation and colitis-associated tumorigenesis, while adoptive transfer of wild-type MDSCs into $Cxcr2^{-/-}$ mice restores tumor progression.[237-241] A causal link between CXCR2-mediated MDSC recruitment and chemotherapeutic drug resistance has been established in murine breast cancer.[242] CXCR2-deficiency or CXCR2 antagonists prevent MDSCs trafficking to multiple tumor types in murine models, leading to an enhanced antitumor effect of checkpoint blockade immunotherapy targeting programmed-death 1 (PD-1) molecules.[243] Notably, the CXCR2-binding chemokines CXCL1, CXCL2, and CXCL5 recruit MDSCs to both tumor sites and the premetastatic niche.[237,244] In addition, CXCR1 and CXCR2 chemokine receptor agonists produced by tumors induce extrusion of neutrophil extracellular traps (NETs) by intratumoral neutrophils and granulocytic MDSC that coat tumor cells, thereby providing protection from cytolytic attack by NK cells and CD8[+] T cells during checkpoint blockade immunotherapy.[245] Prostaglandin E2 (PGE2) controls the expression of both CXCL12 and CXCR4, which attract MDSCs into the ascites of ovarian cancer patients.[246] Furthermore, inhibition of inflammation using COX2 or PGE_2 receptor antagonists suppresses the expression of CXCR4 by MDSCs, as well as their responsiveness to CXCL12 from ovarian cancer ascites. CXCR5–CXCL13 crosstalk is also reportedly essential in the migration of CD40[+] MDSCs toward gastric tumors.[247]

Chemokines and Metastasis

Metastasis is a complex multistep process that involves exit of cancer cells from the original tumor site, migration to other organs including regional LNs, and outgrowth in metastatic niches within distant organs.[248] Chemokines and their corresponding receptors regulate cancer metastasis through three main mechanisms: (a) chemokines secreted by tumors attract immunosuppressive immune cells, such as TAMs, T_{reg} cells, and MDSCs; (b) chemokine-directed organ-specific metastasis manipulates normal cellular highways that guide the travel of cells to specific sites; and (c) chemokine-associated signaling promotes tumor growth and manipulates metastasis-related genes in tumor cells.[248]

With regard to the first mechanism, as mentioned in the prior sections, the CCL2–CCR2 axis contributes to multiple steps in TAM-mediated functions leading to the metastatic occurrence in mouse models of human prostate cancer and breast cancer.[193,195,197,249] Direct contact between macrophages and tumor cells leads to invasion and egress of tumor cells into the blood vessels, supporting the hypothesis that macrophages aid and abet tumor cell intravasation at this initial stage of the metastatic process.[249] Additionally, a subpopulation of CCR2-expressing monocytes is recruited by CCL2 synthesized by metastatic tumor cells and by the target-site tissue stroma, leading to enhanced extravasation of tumor cells at metastatic sites.[195] Incubation of hepatocellular carcinoma cells (HCCs) with IL-8/CXCL8 activates expression of the transcription factor forkhead box C1 (FOXC1) via PI3K–AKT and hypoxia-inducible factor 1α (HIF-1α), leading to transactivation of CCL2 and CXCR1 that promotes TAMs infiltration and metastatic activities of HCC cells.[250] Knockdown of host CXCR2 decreases tumor growth and metastasis, correlating with reduced Gr1+ tumor-associated granulocytes, TAMs, and MDSCs.[251] Macrophage infiltration mediated by CXCR3 and CXCL4/CXCL4L1 is also observed in hepatic metastasis of colon cancer cells.[207] Similarly, CXCR3 deficiency in host cells in a 4T1 mammary tumor model significantly decreases metastases, accompanied by reduced IL-4, IL-10, inducible nitric oxide synthase (iNOs), and arginase-1 (Arg-1) production in myeloid cells, which correspond to increased T cell responsiveness.[252] Adding to the complexity are observations that in livers of nude mice, SMAD4-deficient human colorectal cancer cells upregulate CCL15, which recruits CCR1+ myeloid cells to promote tumor invasion and metastasis, suggesting that reagents that block CCL15-mediated recruitment of CCR1+ cells can prevent metastasis of colorectal cancer cells to the liver.[253] The CCL5 deletion in an MMTV–PyMT transgenic mouse model results in reduced primary tumor burden and pulmonary metastasis, which is associated with deficiency of Th2 cells.[254] Further study shows that CCL5 activates CCR3 expression on CD4+ T cells to induce Th2 polarization, which facilitates the prometastatic activity of tumor-associated myeloid cells.[254]

For the second mechanism, the regulation of organ-specific metastasis by homeostatic chemokine receptors has been extensively discussed in a prior review.[248] In brief, cancer cells expressing specific chemokine receptors can manipulate the cellular highways mediated by corresponding chemokine gradients in the body to reach different sites or organs. For instance, inhibition of the CXC12–CXCR4 axis blocks pulmonary metastasis of diverse cancer types such as breast cancer, prostate, colorectal cancer, and glioblastoma in orthotropic tumor mouse models.[255–260] Along the same lines, de novo expression of CXCR4 in a B16 melanoma cell line is linked to a propensity for metastasis to the lung. One provocative study uncovered complex contributions of the CXCR4/CXCR7–CXCL12 axis to organotropic metastasis in neuroblastoma.[261] Specifically, this study established that CXCR4 expression guides neuroblastoma cell dissemination to the liver and the lungs. CXCR7 strongly promotes neuroblastoma cell homing to the adrenal gland and the liver. Co-expression of CXCR4 and CXCR7 selectively increases neuroblastoma dissemination toward

the bone marrow. In a classic example of malignancy coopting normal mechanisms of immune cell migration, CXCR7 expression is positively correlated with regional LN metastasis and deeper lymphatic invasion in a variety of solid tumors, such as breast cancer, cervical cancer, melanoma, colorectal carcinoma, and squamous cell carcinoma.[262] Clinical studies have further revealed that high CCR9 expression on melanoma cell lines isolated from small intestinal metastases is associated with selective expression of the CCR9 ligand, CCL25, in the small intestine.[263]

The third mechanism has been addressed in numerous studies. Overexpression of CCR6 in colorectal cells increases their proliferation, migration, and colony formation in vitro and promotes metastatic spread in vivo, likely via activation of AKT signaling, upregulation of metastasis-promoting genes, and downregulation of metastasis-suppressor genes.[264] Similarly, CCL2 secreted from prostate cancer cells in a paracrine/autocrine fashion is implicated in promoting cell survival and growth via the PI3 kinase/ AKT signaling pathway.[265] The intrabone injection of a murine breast cancer cell line with enhanced expression of CCL4 generates larger tumors than that of the parental cells, accompanied by an increase in CCR5+ fibroblasts expressing connective tissue growth factor (CTGF) that supports tumor proliferation under hypoxic culture conditions.[266] In a breast cancer mouse model, the introduction of miR-101 suppresses tumor growth and lung metastasis in vivo.[267] This is possibly due to miR-101 directly targeting CXCR7 followed by downregulation of genes in the STAT3 signaling pathway, including cyclin D1, Mcl-1, Bcl-2, E-cadherin, Snail, matrix metalloproteinase 2 (MMP2), and MMP9. The CXCR4 ligand CXCL12/SDF1 stimulates HCC migration through the extracellular signal-regulated kinase 1/2 pathway, and pharmacological inhibition of CXCR4 reduces HCC cell migration stimulated by MMP10.[268] Notably, incubation of human breast cancer cells with CXCL12 and CCL21 stimulates the formation of pseudopodia that is necessary for invasion by malignant cells and efficient formation of metastasis.[269]

Dysregulation of Chemokine and Chemokine Receptors Within the Tumor Microenvironment

Accumulating evidence from mouse and human studies indicates that the TME manipulates the expression and activity of chemokines and their receptors, resulting in the exclusion of immune effector cells from the tumor or, conversely, in the recruitment of immune cells that promote metastasis. Although the underlying molecular mechanisms warrant further investigation, it is clear that conditions within the TME (hypoxia, acidosis, and hyperglycemia) as well as radiation and chemotherapeutic agents can regulate chemokines and chemokine receptors at the transcriptional, posttranscriptional, and posttranslational levels.[24,270]

The overall consensus from multiple studies is that cancer-associated signaling proteins and transcriptional regulators, including oncogene and tumor suppressor proteins, have a major impact on the chemokine system. Oncogenic Ras activation induces expression of CXCR2 and its ligands CXCL1 and CXCL8, as well as CXCR3 and its ligand CXCL10 in tumors of diverse origins, including cervical,[271] breast,[272] colorectal,[273] thyroid,[274] and alveolar epithelial neoplasia.[275]

In contrast, loss of the tumor suppressor protein von Hippel–Lindau (pVHL) upregulates CXCR4 through transactivation by hypoxia-induced factor-1α (HIF-1α) in renal cell carcinoma,[276] while the tumor suppressor p53 indirectly represses CXCR4 via ATF-1 and cJUN-binding elements on the CXCR4 promoter in breast cancer cells.[277] Furthermore, the CXCL8 promoter contains consensus binding sites for NF-κB, AP-1, C-EBP, β-catenin, and HIF-1α transcription factors, suggesting that the effect of tumor-associated genes on the chemokine network may be broader than expected.[278] Extracellular factors associated with cancer can also regulate the chemokine system. For example, accumulation of adenosine at immunosuppressive concentrations in murine melanoma tumors reduces local production of CXCR3 ligands (CXCL9, CXCL10) in melanoma lesions.[279–281]

Expression of chemokines/chemokine receptors may also be under epigenetic control, as a recent study investigating the mechanisms of loss of CXCL14 in prostate cancer cells identified hypermethylated CpG island sequences within the CXCL14 gene promoter and found that the demethylating agent 5-aza-2-deoxycytidine (5AC) restored CXCL14 expression.[282] Similarly, oncogenic mechanisms involving epigenetic silencing by the polycomb repressive complex 2 (PRC2) and demethylase JMJD3-mediated histone H3 lysine 27 trimethylation (H3K27me3) have been identified as a key mediator of intratumoral immunosuppression through repression of CXCL9 and CXCL10 expression in colon cancer cells.[283] Posttranscriptional mechanisms may also control chemokine/chemokine gene receptor expression. Expression of several gain-of-function tumor-associated p53 isoforms causes increased stabilization of CXCL1 and CXCL8 mRNA, resulting in increased angiogenic potential.[284] Furthermore, mRNA for both CXCR4 and CXCL8 is stabilized by the RNA-binding protein HuR, which is frequently upregulated in tumors.[285,286]

Perhaps the most interesting and therapeutically targetable level of regulation of the chemokine system is at the level of posttranslational modifications. Increased expression of the protease CD26 (also known as dipeptidyl peptidase-4; DPP4) is observed in malignant transformation[287,288] and has recently been implicated in diminishing the functional activity of chemokines, including CXCL10,

CXCL12, CCL5, CCL11, and CCL21.[289–291] CD26 cleaves CXCL10, forming a truncated product that can bind CXCR3 but cannot signal, resulting in suppressed trafficking of cytotoxic CD8+ T cells to melanomas in mice.[289,292] Use of sitagliptin, a U.S. Food and Drug Administration (FDA)-approved DPP4/CD26 inhibitor, enhances antitumor effects, in part, by enabling infiltration with inflammatory cells including eosinophils.[289,293,294] Another line of investigation revealed that the prometastatic HER2 oncoprotein[14,295] enhances CXCR4 protein synthesis and protects this chemokine receptor against CXCL12-induced degradation.[296] Further, reactive nitrogen species (RNS), which are enriched in the TME, have been shown to modify chemokine bioactivity. Specifically, nitration of CCL2 within tumors renders it incapable of recruiting T cells, while leaving intact its ability to attract immunosuppressive myeloid cells to the TME.[297]

Chemokine Receptors and Angiogenesis

CXCR1/CXCR2 and their corresponding chemokines, including CXCL1-3 and CXCL5-8, are considered major angiogenic chemokines.[175] CXCR2 is required for endothelial cell chemotaxis, while neutralization of CXCR2 blocks the response of human endothelial cells to CXCL8. CXC chemokine-mediated angiogenesis has been demonstrated in multiple cancer types, including melanoma, pancreatic cancer, ovarian cancer, gastrointestinal cancer, bronchogenic cancer, prostate cancer, glioblastoma, head and neck cancer, and renal cell cancer.[175] The CC chemokine family also participates in the angiogenesis of solid tumors.[298] CCL2 plays a crucial role in mediating hemangioma growth and angiogenesis, which is dependent on type 1 MT1-MMP. Furthermore, neutralizing antibody to CCL2 significantly inhibits the growth of lung micrometastases and increases survival in immune-deficient mice bearing human breast carcinoma cells. Additional CC chemokine family members, such as CCL11 and CCL16, promote angiogenesis in vitro and in vivo.

EMERGING IMMUNOTHERAPIES TARGETING CHEMOKINE RECEPTORS AND CHEMOKINES

Chemokines are natural candidates for therapeutic targeting in anticancer immunotherapy in light of evidence that they are prognostic indicators of cancer patient outcome and observations that chemokine expression and function can be dysregulated in the TME. Indeed, there is ample correlative and experimental preclinical evidence supporting therapeutic targeting of the chemokine system as an adjuvant to a comprehensive immunotherapy approach in order to enhance the efficacy of T cell–based therapies such as DC vaccination, immune checkpoint blockade strategies, or adoptive T cell transfer immunotherapy. The traditional chemokine-targeting immunotherapy approaches include intratumoral delivery of chemokines, small-molecule antagonists, neutralizing antibodies, and RNA-induced transcriptional silencing against chemokines or chemokine receptors. In addition, novel methods such as epigenetic agents and chemokine receptor-modified chimeric antigen receptor (CAR) T cell therapeutics are emerging.

Preclinical Immunotherapy Augmenting the Chemokine Network

The concept that chemokines are limiting factors for effective antitumor immune responses is supported by various gain-of-function approaches showing that delivery of chemokines into tumor lesions has a therapeutic benefit (summarized in Table 15.1). One informative experimental approach has been to genetically modify tumor cell lines to express selected chemokines. Specifically, forced expression of chemokines in tumors from various origins such as myeloma (CCL1),[299] colon (CCL3),[301]

colorectal (CXCL16),[192] ovary (CCL3, CXCL8),[300] lung (CCL5),[302] breast (CCL16, CCL19),[303,305] fibrosarcoma (CCL5),[140,302] and pancreas (CXCL12)[318] is associated with reduced tumor growth and increased leukocyte infiltration into tumors. More clinically relevant approaches to increasing local chemokine availability have yielded similar results. Direct intratumoral injection of chemokine into the murine lung (CCL21,[307,308] CXCL10)[315] and kidney (CXCL9)[314] cancer models results in reduced tumor growth and metastasis, diminished infiltration of MDSCs and T_{reg} cells, and enhanced intratumoral infiltration by T cells and DCs. Parallel results are observed following treatment of colon (CCL17),[304] melanoma (CCL20),[306] and lung (CCL20, CCL21, CCL22)[306,312,313] tumors with chemokine-encoding adenoviral vectors, which suppress tumor growth and increase CD8+ T cell infiltration into tumor lesions. Similarly, treatment with DCs genetically modified to express CCL21 reportedly reduces tumor burden and increases intratumoral infiltration of T cells in melanoma[141,309] and lung cancer.[310,311] A recent advance involves manipulation of the functionality of a chemokine receptor

Table 15.1 Preclinical Immunotherapy Augmenting the Chemokine Network

CHEMOKINE	RECEPTORS	THERAPEUTIC APPROACH (MOUSE [M] OR HUMAN [H])	TUMOR MODEL (MOUSE [M] OR HUMAN [H])	IMMUNE RESPONSE	TREATMENT OUTCOME	REFERENCES
CCL1	CCR8	Tumor cells transduced with CCL1; intratumoral injection CCL1	Myeloma (M)	Lymphocyte-independent antitumor activity and tumor-specific immunity	Tumor regression	299
CCL3	CCR1 CCR5	Tumor cells transfected with CCL3 (H&M) or CXCL8 (H)	CHO ovarian carcinoma (M)	Neutrophil infiltration	Tumor regression	300
CCL3	CCR1 CCR5	Tumor cells transfected with CCL3 (H&M)	CT26 colon carcinoma (M)	Infiltration of macrophages and neutrophils	Tumor regression	301
CCL5	CCR1 CCR5	Tumor cells transduced with CCL5 (H)	Lung adenocarcinoma (M); fibrosarcoma (M)	Enhancement of CD8+ T cell activation	Tumor regression	140,302
CCL16/LEC/HCC4	CCR1 CCR3	Tumor cells transduced with CCL16 (H)	TSA mammary adenocarcinoma (M)	Increased monocyte, DCs, T cells, and granulocytes influx into the tumor	Tumor regression	303
CCL17	CCR4	Intratumoral injection of adenovirus encoding the chemokines CCL17 (M)	CT26 colon carcinoma (M)	Increased tumor infiltration of macrophages and CD8+ T cells	Tumor regression	304
CCL19/Cuba-11	CCR7	Tumor cells transduced with the retroviral vector CCL19 (H)	Breast cancer cell line C3L5 (M)	Infiltration of NK and CD4+ T cells	Tumor regression	305
CCL20/(MIP-3α)	CCR6	Intratumoral injection of adenovirus-CCL20 (H)	B16 melanoma, CT26, CL25, 3LL Lewis lung carcinoma (M)	Infiltration of DCs and increased tumor-specific cytotoxic T-lymphocyte activity	Tumor regression	306

(continued)

Table 15.1 Preclinical Immunotherapy Augmenting the Chemokine Network (*continued*)

CHEMOKINE	RECEPTORS	THERAPEUTIC APPROACH (MOUSE [M] OR HUMAN [H])	TUMOR MODEL (MOUSE [M] OR HUMAN [H])	IMMUNE RESPONSE	TREATMENT OUTCOME	REFERENCES
CCL21/LEC/6C-kine	CCR7	Intratumoral injection of recombinant CCL21 (M)	L1C2 lung adenocarcinoma, 3LL Lewis lung carcinoma (M)	Increased infiltration of CD4 and CD8 T cells and DCs to the tumor and the draining LN	Tumor regression	[307]
		Intratumoral injection of CCL21 (M)	A549 lung cancer (H)	No differences in the infiltration of leukocyte subpopulations	Tumor regression	[308]
		Intratumoral injection of CCL21-overexpressing DCs	B16 melanoma (M)	Increased infiltration of IFN-γ producing T cells into the tumor	Tumor regression	[141,309]
		Intratumoral injection of CCL21-overexpressing DCs	L1C2 lung carcinoma (M)	Increased CD4$^+$, CD8$^+$, and DCs; reduced CD4$^+$CD25$^+$ T$_{reg}$ infiltration	Tumor regression	[310]
		Intrapulmonary-administered DC-AdCCL21	Spontaneous bronchoalveolar cell carcinoma (M)	Extensive mononuclear cell infiltration of the tumors	Tumor regression	[311]
		Intratumoral delivery of CCL21-Vault nanocapsule (H&M)	3LL Lewis lung carcinoma (M)	Enhanced leukocytic infiltration, reduced MDSCs, T$_{reg}$ cells, and IL-10$^+$ T cells	Tumor regression	[312]
CCL22/MDC	CCR4	Intratumoral injection of adenovirus-CCL22 (H)	3LL Lewis lung carcinoma (M)	Infiltration of DCs, increased IL-4 production in tumor	Tumor regression	[313]
CXCL8	CXCR1 CXCR2	Tumor cells transfected with CXCL8 (H)	CHO ovarian carcinoma (M)	Neutrophil infiltration	Tumor regression	[300]
CXCL9	CXCR3	Systemic IL-2 with an intratumoral CXCL9 (M)	Renal cell carcinoma (M)	Increased intratumor infiltration of CXCR3$^+$ mononuclear cells	Tumor regression	[314]
CXCL10/IP-10	CXCR3	Intratumoral injection of CXCL9 (H)	A549 lung cancer (H)		Inhibited lung metastasis	[315]
CXCL9/10	CXCR3	Systemic administration of epigenetic modulators DZNeP and 5-Aza-dc with anti-PD-1 Ab	AT-3 triple negative breast cancer (M)	Increased production of CXCL9/10 by intratumoral CD11c$^+$MHCII$^+$ DCs	Delayed tumor growth, enhanced survival	
CXCL12	CXCR4	Photo-activatable CXCR4 expressing tumor-targeting cytotoxic T cells	B16/ovalbumin (OVA) melanoma (M)	Infiltration of CTLs improved the efficacy of adoptive T cell transfer immunotherapy	Tumor regression	[316]
CX3CL1	CX3CLR	Genetically modified CX3CLR-expressing T cells (H)	NCI-H630 colorectal cancer cells (H)	Enhanced the homing of adoptively transferred T cells toward CX3CL1-producing tumors	Tumor regression	[317]
CXCL16	CXCR6	Tumor transduced with CXCL16 (M)	SL4 colorectal cancer cells (M)	Accumulation of M1 macrophages releasing TNF-α	Reduced liver metastasis	[192]
CXCL12	CXCR4 CXCR7	Tumor transduced with CXCL12 (H)	MiaPaCa2 pancreatic cancer cells (H)		Lower tumor burden	[318]

CHO, Chinese hamster ovary; CTL, cytotoxic T lymphocyte; DCs, dendritic cells; IFN, interferon; LN, lymph nodes; MDSC, myeloid-derived suppressor cell; NK, natural killer; OVA, ovalbumin; TNF, tumor necrosis factor; T$_{reg}$, regulatory T.

independent of ligand availability.[316,317] In this proof-of-principle study, CXCR4 was engineered to be photoactivatable such that it can transmit intracellular chemokine signals in response to light stimulation irrespective of chemokine availability, thereby augmenting adhesion of T cells at the tumor vessel wall.[316] Application of this approach in an adoptive cell transfer model of immunotherapy revealed that local delivery of light to melanomas increases intratumoral accumulation of transferred T cells bearing photoactivatable CXCR4 and reduces tumor growth. Human T cells genetically modified to express CX3CR display enhanced homing toward CX3CL1-producing tumors, resulting in increased T cell infiltration in tumor tissues and decreased growth of human colorectal tumors in a mouse xenograft model.[317]

Suppression of Chemokine Networks by Preclinical Immunotherapy

The chemokine receptors or chemokines contributing to protumorigenesis have emerged as attractive targets of immunotherapy. Traditional immunotherapy approaches include neutralizing antibodies, small-molecule antagonists, and RNA-induced transcriptional silencing of chemokines or chemokine receptors (summarized in Table 15.2), while novel methods such as epigenetic agents offer promising new directions for therapeutic intervention.

Neutralizing antibodies have been used effectively in a loss-of-function approach to limit the protumorigenic activities of chemokines in preclinical studies. Therapeutic antibodies have advantages over small molecules and peptides, including long-circulating half-life, specificity, and high-affinity interactions with targets, as well as relatively low toxicity.[36] Systemic delivery of anti-CCL2 neutralizing antibody attenuates tumor burden in a prostate cancer mouse model[197,320] and reduces the number of metastatic nodules in a mammary carcinoma mouse model.[195] Similarly, blockade of CCL2/CCR2 signaling with a peptide antagonist of CCR2 (RDC018) in a mouse model of hepatocellular carcinoma reverses immunosuppression in the TME, thereby inhibiting malignant growth, metastasis, and postsurgical tumor recurrence and improving overall survival.[319] Limited efficacy and only transient diminution of CCL2 with potent neutralizing monoclonal administration have been identified alone and in combination with chemotherapy.[328,329,330] CCL4-neutralizing antibody also significantly blocks macrophage-mediated protumorigenic signaling in prostate tumors.[331] Treatment with CCL5-neutralizing antibody induces tumor regression and reduces lung metastasis in the mouse 4T1 mammary tumor model.[235] Antibodies against CXCL8 have also demonstrated tumor-suppressive activity in xenograft murine models of bladder cancer and melanoma.[231,322] CXCR2 neutralizing antibody treatment reduces tumor volume, angiogenesis, and neutrophil infiltration into the TME in a human pancreatic tumor xenograft model.[324] Furthermore, anti-CXCR7 nanobodies (i.e.,

Table 15.2 Preclinical Immunotherapy-Suppressing Chemokine Network

CHEMOKINE	RECEPTORS	THERAPEUTIC APPROACH	MOUSE (M) OR HUMAN (H) TUMOR MODEL	IMMUNE RESPONSE	TREATMENT OUTCOME	REFERENCES
CCL2	CCR2	CCR2-antagonist RDC018	Hepatocellular carcinoma (M)	Inhibited recruitment of inflammatory monocytes, infiltration, and M2-polarization of TAMs	Inhibited growth, metastasis, and enhanced survival	319
		Lipid nanoparticle that contains CCR2-silencing siRNA	Lung adenocarcinoma (M)	Reduced TAMs to tumor	Tumor regression	199
		Inhibition of the CCL2 nitration by AT38	EG7-OVA lymphoma (M)	Improved infiltration of CTL to tumor	Tumor regression	297
		CCL2 neutralizing antibodies (H&M)	PC3 prostate cancer (H)	Reduced TAMs to tumor	Tumor regression	197,320
		CCL2 neutralizing antibodies (H&M)	Mammary carcinoma Met-1 (M)	Inhibited recruitment of inflammatory monocytes	Reduced metastasis burden	195

(continued)

Table 15.2 Preclinical Immunotherapy-Suppressing Chemokine Network (*continued*)

CHEMOKINE	RECEPTORS	THERAPEUTIC APPROACH	MOUSE (M) OR HUMAN (H) TUMOR MODEL	IMMUNE RESPONSE	TREATMENT OUTCOME	REFERENCES
CCL5	CCR5	Systemic administration of a CCR5 inhibitor	Pancreatic adenocarcinoma (H&M)	Reduced T_{reg} migration to tumor	Tumor regression	219
		Oral CCR5 antagonist (maraviroc)	Prostate epithelial cells transformed with the v-Src oncogene (M)		Reduced metastatic cancer burden	321
		CCL5 neutralizing antibody	4T1 mammary tumor (M)	Significant number of antigen-specific IFN-γ-producing T cells in the spleen	Tumor regression and reduced lung metastasis	235
CCL20	CCR6	Anti-CCR6 antibody (H)	CMT93 and CT26 colorectal tumor (M)		Tumor regression	264
CXCL8/IL-8	CXCR2	Anti-CXCL8 antibody ABX-IL-8 (H)	Bladder transitional cell carcinoma (H)		Tumor regression	322
		Anti-CXCL8 antibody ABX-IL-8 (H)	Melanoma cells (H)		Suppressed tumor growth and metastasis	323
		CXCR2 neutralizing antibody	Pancreatic cancer (M)		Reduced tumor volume and microvessel density	324
CXCL1, CXCL2, CXCL8/IL-8	CXCR1, CXCR2	Noncompetitive CXCR1/2 allosteric antagonist reparixin	Triple negative breast cancer (M)		Inhibited intratumoral NETs, reduced metastasis, and increased responsiveness to checkpoint blockade immunotherapy	245
CXCL12	CXCR4	Selective CXCR4 antagonist	BR5-1 ovarian cancer cells (M)	Reduced intratumoral T_{reg} cells	Increased tumor death and reduced intraperitoneal dissemination	325
		CXCL12 neutralizing antibody	A549 lung cancer cells (H)		Reduced metastasis	326
	CXCR7	Tumor cells expressing shCXCR7	4T1 mammary tumor (M)		Tumor regression and reduced metastasis	267
		CXCR7-specific nanobodies	Head and neck cancer (H)	Reduced secretion of CXCL1 from cancer cells	Tumor regression	327

CTL, cytotoxic T lymphocyte; IFN, interferon; TAM, tumor-associated macrophage; T_{reg}, regulatory T.

single-domain antibody fragment) suppress growth and angiogenesis of CXCR7+ head and neck tumors in a xenograft mouse model.[327] Taken together, the large body of evidence in preclinical tumor systems supports the merit of targeting chemokine systems for therapeutic benefit in the context of cancer immunotherapy.

Clinical Experience Targeting the Chemokine Landscape in Cancer

Chemokines are currently under intense investigation in cancer therapy, with more than 100 U.S. trials registered in the clinicaltrials.gov database in 2020. While a variety of approaches are under study, interventional studies mainly fall into three major categories: (a) chemokine blockade, (b) cellular modifications and vaccines, and (c) reprogramming the chemokine profile of the TME to reduce immunosuppression and/or increase trafficking of effector CD8[+] T cells. Clinical investigation of chemokine-directed therapeutics in cancer has benefited substantially from extensive prior experience using similar agents in the treatment of autoimmune disorders or infectious diseases.

Chemokine/chemokine receptor blockade in a clinical setting traditionally has been implemented using neutralizing antibodies,[328,329] although small-molecule antagonists and peptide inhibitors are also actively under investigation (a list of selected chemokine/chemokine receptor modulating therapies is summarized in Table 15.3). CCR2 targeting with a humanized neutralizing antibody (MLN1202) showed efficacy in a Phase 2 clinical trial for metastatic bone cancer (ClinicalTrials.gov identifier: NCT01015560). Despite these observations

Table 15.3 Clinical Trials Targeting Chemokine Network

CHEMOKINE	RECEPTORS	THERAPEUTIC APPROACH	CONDITION	TREATMENT OUTCOME	CLINICALTRIALS. GOV ID	REFERENCES
CCL2	CCR2	Anti-CCL2 monoclonal antibody (Carlumab)	Metastatic castration-resistant prostate cancer patients	Did not block the CCL2/CCR2 axis or show antitumor activity as a single agent	NCT00992186	329
		Anti-CCL2 monoclonal antibody (CNTO 888)	Solid tumors	No long-term suppression of serum CCL2 or significant tumor responses	NCT01204996	328
		CCR2 antagonist (PF-04136309)	Metastatic pancreatic ductal adenocarcinoma	Safety profile raised concern for synergistic pulmonary toxicity and did not show an efficacy signal above nab-paclitaxel and gemcitabine.	NCT02732938	332
		Anti-CCR2 monoclonal antibody (MLN1202)	Metastatic cancer	Urinary N-telopeptide (uNTx) response rate, 14/43 patients; serious adverse events developed in 7% of patients	NCT01015560	333
CCL3 CCL4 CCL8	CCR5	CCR5 antagonist (maraviroc)	Liver metastases of advanced refractory colorectal cancer	Antitumor effect	NCT01736813	334
CCL21	CCR7	GM-CD40L vaccine with H1944 cells expressing CCL21	Lung cancer adenocarcinoma	No significant associations between vaccine immunogenicity and outcomes; in limited biopsies, one patient treated with GMCD40L. CCL21 displayed abundant tumor-infiltrating lymphocytes.	NCT01433172	335
		Autologous dendritic cell-adenovirus CCL21 vaccine	Melanoma	Completed, results not reported	NCT00798629	
			Lung cancer	Completed, results not reported	NCT00601094	
			Non-small cell lung cancer	4/16 patients had stable disease; intratumoral CD8[+] T cell infiltration induced in 7/13 patients (54%); patients with increased CD8[+] T cells following vaccination showed significantly increased PD-L1 mRNA expression in tumors	NCT01574222	336

(continued)

Table 15.3 Clinical Trials Targeting Chemokine Network (*continued*)

CHEMOKINE	RECEPTORS	THERAPEUTIC APPROACH	CONDITION	TREATMENT OUTCOME	CLINICALTRIALS. GOV ID	REFERENCES
XCL1	XCR1	Neuroblastoma cells expressing XCL1	Neuroblastoma	Active, not recruiting; no results reported	NCT00703222	
CXCL1-3 CXCL5-8	CXCR1 CXCR2	Inhibitor of CXCR1 and CXCR2 (Reparixin)	Metastatic breast cancer	Completed, safe, well-tolerated, 30% response rate	NCT02001974	[337]
		CXCR2-transduced tumor-infiltrating lymphocytes	Melanoma	Active, not recruiting; no results reported	NCT01740557	
CXCL12	CXCR4	CXCR4 antagonist (LY2510924)	Solid tumor	Acceptable safety and tolerability; overall response of stable disease observed in 4/9 patients (44.4%), one patient had unconfirmed partial response	NCT02737072	[338]
		CXCR4 inhibitor (USL311)	Solid tumors (Phase 1) relapsed/recurrent glioblastoma multiforme (Phase 2)	Terminated; business reasons unrelated to safety	NCT02765165	
		CXCR4 antagonist (BKT140)	Multiple myeloma (Phase 1/2)	Safe and efficient stem cell mobilizer	NCT01010880	[339]
CXCL9/10/11	CXCR3	Chemokine modulation therapy targeting CXCL9/10/11 by triple combination with celecoxib, recombinant interferon alfa-2b, and rintatolimod		Completed	NCT02151448	
CXCL9/10/11	CXCR3	Chemokine modulation therapy targeting CXCL9/10/11 by triple combination with celecoxib, recombinant interferon alfa-2b, and rintatolimod	Early stage triple negative breast cancer	Ongoing	NCT04081389	

and promising preclinical results, Phase 2 studies in metastatic castration-resistant prostate cancer patients revealed that monoclonal antibody targeting of CCL2 (using the antibody CNTO 888) does not have sustained effects on diminishing circulating CCL2, nor does it show clinical benefit when administered as a single agent, suggesting that other strategies may be necessary to disrupt the CCL2/CCR2 axis in cancer.[328] One concern regarding this approach is raised by unexpected adverse outcomes

in preclinical mouse metastatic breast tumor models in which cessation of antibody-based CCL2 therapy accelerated metastasis by stimulating local angiogenesis as well as macrophage influx.[340]

CCR5 has also been targeted for the blockade, with several clinical trials and preclinical studies focusing on the small-molecule CCR5 antagonist maraviroc, which is FDA approved as an entry inhibitor in HIV infection. Administration of maraviroc alleviated tumor burden in mouse models of the prostate[321] and gastric cancer.[341] In a Phase 1 clinical trial, the antitumor effects of a CCR5 antagonist were confirmed in patients with liver metastases of advanced refractory colorectal cancer.[334] Ongoing clinical trials of maraviroc are focused on colorectal cancer (NCT01736813).

There is a strong rationale for targeting the protumorigenic activity of CXCR4 and CXCR1/2. Administration of the CXCR4 antagonist, AMD3100 (plerixafor, FDA-approved for stem cell mobilization in non-Hodgkin lymphoma and multiple myeloma), has shown antitumor efficacy in a mouse model of ovarian cancer, which was associated with increased tumor apoptosis and reduced intratumoral accumulation of T_{reg} cells.[325] Further, in an autochthonous immunotherapeutic model of PDA, AMD3100 stimulated T cell infiltration into tumors and acted synergistically with an anti-PD-L1 antibody to control tumor growth.[342] A Phase 1 study (NCT02737072) is currently underway for another CXCR4 peptide antagonist (LY2510924) in combination with anti-PD-L1 checkpoint inhibitor immunotherapy in solid tumors,[343] while yet another CXCR4 antagonist (BKT140) is in trials for multiple myeloma (NCT01010880).[339] Additionally, preclinical studies demonstrating attenuation of angiogenesis and tumor growth in mice treated with CXCR1/2 antagonists in breast cancer and colorectal cancer xenograft mouse models[278] have led to a current Phase 1 clinical trial (NCT02001974) investigating a CXCR1/2 antagonist, Reparixin, in breast cancer patients.

The use of modified cellular agents is yet another promising therapeutic strategy. Indeed, several ongoing clinical trials are evaluating the efficacy of chemokine-expressing tumor cells or viral vectors as an anticancer vaccine. In this regard, cellular vaccines engineered to express the DC-attracting chemokines CCL21[86] (NCT01433172) and XCL1 (lymphotactin; NCT00703222)[344] are under investigation for the treatment of lung cancer and neuroblastoma, respectively. Moreover, there is the potential to exploit the chemokine-rich TME by genetically modifying CAR T cells to express chemokine receptors, although this has not reached the stage of clinical trials. CAR T cell therapy is a novel cancer immunotherapy that involves genetic engineering of a patient's own T cells to express CARs that recognize TAAs on tumor cells. Preclinical reports have shown that co-expression of a TAA-directed antigen receptor and CCR2 enhances CAR T cell infiltration of tumors and increases the efficacy of this therapy in mouse models of mesothelioma[193] and neuroblastoma.[195]

A promising complementary approach aims to modify the chemokine signature of the TME to improve host and/or therapeutic antitumor immune responses. Recent preclinical studies have begun investigating the antitumor effects of epigenetic agents that potentially target chemokines. Administration of the histone deacetylase inhibitor (HDACi) romidepsin (which is FDA approved for treatment of lymphoma) in a lung adenocarcinoma mouse model increases T cell chemokine expression, promotes T cell infiltration, and results in T cell-dependent tumor regression.[345] In a human ovarian cancer mouse model, treatment with epigenetic modulators (3-deazaneplanocin A and 5-aza-2-deoxycytidine) and the methyltransferase inhibitor GSK126 increases T helper 1 (Th1)-type chemokines CXCL9 and CXCL10, and stimulates intratumoral infiltration of effector T cells, correlating with suppressed tumor progression.[346] Evidence from preclinical studies that CXCR3 ligands can be enzymatically inactivated within the TME (i.e., by CD26/DPP4) further suggests that CXCR3 ligand activity may have to be rescued by therapeutic intervention in a cancer setting.[289] This hypothesis is currently being tested in a small-scale (14 patients) pilot clinical study in hepatocellular carcinoma patients undergoing resection (NCT02650427), which investigates whether the DPP4 inhibitor sitagliptin (FDA-approved as an antidiabetic drug used by more than 30 million people worldwide) has an impact on CXCL10 truncation, circulating CXCR3$^+$ cells (as a surrogate for T cell trafficking), and immune cell infiltration at tumor sites. No data are available from this completed study.

Another attractive strategy to modify the chemokine landscape of tumors is to reprogram the inflammatory state of the TME. Preclinical studies have shown that a combination of type I IFN and Toll-like receptor-3 (TLR3) agonistic "danger signals" enhances production of CCL5 and CXCL10 in tumor lesions and suppresses the production of CCL22 in human tumor explants.[149,347] These observations are in line with preclinical observations that the Stimulator of Interferon Genes (STING) pathway responsible for the synthesis of type I IFNs is necessary for DC activation and intratumoral production of CXCR3 ligands (CXCL9, CXCL10), together with T cell-mediated antitumor immunity.[348,349] Results will be of interest for a recently completed Phase 1/2 clinical trial (NCT02151448) that investigated the safety, impact on CD8$^+$ T cell infiltration, and efficacy of a chemokine-modulating regimen of interferon-α2b (a TLR3 agonist) and Celecoxib during DC vaccination of cancer patients.

CONCLUSION

During the first two decades of this millennium, we have witnessed remarkable progress in understanding the complex role of chemokine systems in tipping the balance between antitumor immunity versus protumorigenic immune functions leading to aggressive disease.

Armed with this information, the field is now poised to test whether chemokine networks can be exploited for clinical benefit in solid malignancies. Groundbreaking advances are most likely to emerge through combinations of molecular diagnostics employing Clinical Laboratory Improvement Amendments (CLIA)-certified, chemokine gene expression signatures and therapeutics that dually target chemokine/chemokine receptors together with T cell-based cancer immunotherapies.

KEY REFERENCES

Only key references appear in the print edition. The full reference list appears in the digital product on Springer Publishing Connect: connect.springerpub.com/content/book/978-0-8261-3743-2/part/part01/chapter/ch15

18. Fridman WH, Pagès F, Sautès-Fridman C, Galon J. The immune contexture in human tumours: impact on clinical outcome. *Nat Rev Cancer.* 2012;12(4):298–306. doi:10.1038/nrc3245

49. Tang D, Kang R, Coyne CB, Zeh HJ, Lotze MT. PAMPs and DAMPs: signal 0s that spur autophagy and immunity. *Immunol Rev.* 2012;249(1):158–175. doi:10.1111/j.1600-065X.2012.01146.x

107. Okada T, Ngo VN, Ekland EH, et al. Chemokine requirements for B cell entry to lymph nodes and Peyer's patches. *J Exp Med.* 2002;196(1):65–75. doi:10.1084/jem.20020201

143. Messina JL, Fenstermacher DA, Eschrich S, et al. 12-Chemokine gene signature identifies lymph node-like structures in melanoma: potential for patient selection for immunotherapy? *Sci Rep.* 2012;2:765. doi:10.1038/srep00765

150. Fisher DT, Chen Q, Skitzki JJ, et al. IL-6 trans-signaling licenses mouse and human tumor microvascular gateways for trafficking of cytotoxic T cells. *J Clin Invest.* 2011;121(10):3846–3859. doi:10.1172/JCI44952

187. Shakir M, Tang D, Zeh HJ, et al. The chemokine receptors CXCR4/CXCR7 and their primary heterodimeric ligands CXCL12 and CXCL12/high mobility group box 1 in pancreatic cancer growth and development: finding flow. *Pancreas.* 2015;44(4):528–534. doi:10.1097/MPA.0000000000000298

346. Peng D, Kryczek I, Nagarsheth N, et al. Epigenetic silencing of TH1-type chemokines shapes tumour immunity and immunotherapy. *Nature.* 2015;527(7577):249–253. doi:10.1038/nature15520

16

Role of the Tumor Microenvironment

David H. Munn and Vincenzo Bronte

KEY POINTS

- The immune response to therapy is constrained in most patients by the immunosuppressive tumor microenvironment .

- Suppression of tumor-specific effector T cells is orchestrated by a variety of inhibitory myeloid and lymphoid cells in the tumor milieu.

- These suppressive mechanisms are often the same natural regulatory mechanisms that enforce self-tolerance and protect against excessive immune activation, but in the tumor microenvironment these become exaggerated and dominant.

- Specific suppressive mechanisms that may be targets for therapy include cytotoxic T-lymphocyte-associated protein 4 (CTLA-4), programmed cell death protein 1 (PD-1)/ PD-ligand, indoleamine 2,3-dioxygenase (IDO), transforming growth factor beta (TGF-β), activated regulatory T cells (T_{reg} cells), inhibitory myeloid-derived suppressor cells, and the activation state of tumor-associated dendritic cells (immunogenic versus immunosuppressive).

- One important choice that may be controlled by the nature of the tumor microenvironment is the fundamental decision as to whether to remain tolerant to dying tumor cells or undergo protective immune activation.

- If it is possible to create a milieu that promotes immunogenic responses to dying tumor cells, then this could have a far-reaching impact on the combination of immunotherapy with conventional chemotherapy and radiation and on the long-term response to immunotherapy itself.

TUMORS DEPEND ON SUPPRESSIVE MECHANISMS IN THE TUMOR MICROENVIRONMENT FOR SURVIVAL

Malignant cells are immunogenic and are visible to the immune system.[1] DNA mutations and altered protein processing give rise to neoantigens, while chronic stress, aneuploidy, and constant cell turnover can cause even shared self-antigens to be displayed in an immunogenic fashion. To evade immune surveillance, the tumor must evolve mechanisms to suppress the immune response.[2–4] To achieve this suppression, the tumor does not invent new mechanisms but exaggerates and hijacks the normal regulatory mechanisms that enforce self-tolerance and immune control. However, within tumors, these normal control pathways become pathological mechanisms of immune escape and suppression (Figure 16.1).

CTLA-4 AND PD-1 PATHWAYS: THE CLASSIC IMMUNE CHECKPOINTS

CTLA-4

CTLA-4 and PD-1 are inhibitory molecules expressed by T cells. Blocking antibodies against these molecules can enhance T cell antitumor activity, particularly when patients already have a robust spontaneous T cell response prior to therapy. Anti-CTLA-4 antibody was the first checkpoint inhibitor to be approved for use.[5,6] When used as a single agent, responses have been rather limited, but the efficacy is enhanced when combined with blockade of the PD-1/PD-ligand pathway.[7,8]

When used as a single agent, CTLA-4 blockade appears most beneficial when tumors have a high mutational burden, and hence many likely neoantigens.[9–11] CTLA-4 blockade may increase the ability of the host immune system to respond to tumor antigens. In one study, patients showed a significant increase in the frequency of T cells reacting with a panel of defined melanoma antigens.[12] This was due in large part to the emergence of new T cells reactive with additional antigens (epitope spreading). Of note, the antigens tested were not mutational neoantigens but were simply self-antigens overexpressed by melanomas. Thus, blocking CTLA-4 appeared to help break functional tolerance to shared self-antigens in the tumor.

Exactly how this improved antigen response arises is not yet defined, because the mechanism of action of CTLA-4 blockade is not fully elucidated.[5,13,14] Blocking CTLA-4 may lower the activation threshold and render

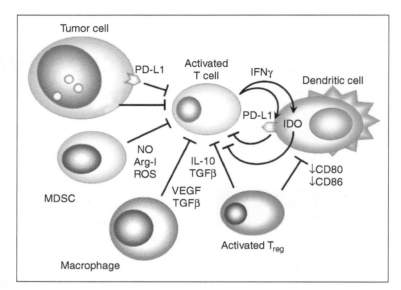

Figure 16.1 Constitutive and inducible suppressor mechanisms in the tumor microenvironment. T cells attempting to activate in the tumor microenvironment may face expression of PDL-1 and IDO by the tumor cells themselves. MDSCs may produce immunosuppressive NO, arginase-I, or reactive oxygen species. TAMs may produce TGF-β and VEGF, which can be inhibitory for both T cells and DCs. Activated T_{reg} cells can produce IL-10 and TGF-β, which can directly suppress T cells. T_{reg} cells may also inhibit the expression of costimulatory ligands CD80 and CD86 on local DCs, thus rendering them ineffective and tolerizing antigen-presenting cells. As effector T cells attempt to activate, their production of IFN-γ and other proinflammatory cytokines may actively upregulate expression of IDO and PDL-1 by DCs, thus eliciting counter-regulatory suppression. Many tumor cells may also respond to IFN-γ by upregulating IDO and PDL-1.

DCs, dendritic cells; IDO, indoleamine 2,3-dioxygenase; IFN-γ, interferon-γ; IL-10, interleukin 10; MDSC, myeloid-derived suppressor cell; NO, nitric oxide; ROS, reactive oxygen species; TAMs, tumor-associated macrophage; TGF-β, transforming growth factor beta; T_{reg}, regulatory T; VEGF, vascular endothelial growth factor.

effector T cells more responsive to antigen, and it may deplete or inhibit regulatory T cells (T_{reg} cells), which express high levels of CTLA-4.[14–16] T_{reg} cells, in turn, can potently suppress the function of antigen-presenting cells (APCs) in the tumor.[17–19] Therefore, CTLA-4 blockade might indirectly enhance cross-presentation of tumor antigens. Whatever the mechanism may be, an encouraging message from these studies is that the baseline T cell response against tumor antigens is not fixed and immutable, and it can be increased by immunotherapy if the right suppressive mechanisms can be removed.

The PD-1/PD-Ligand Pathway

PD-1 is another inhibitory molecule expressed on activated T cells—in particular, on those T cells that have become "exhausted" by chronic antigen exposure.[20,21] PD-1 exerts its suppressive effect when engaged by one of its counter-ligands, PDL-1 or PDL-2. In some tumors, PDL-1 may be expressed constitutively; in other cases, PDL-1 may not be spontaneously expressed but can be upregulated on tumor cells in response to inflammatory signals.[22,23] This latter point is important when considering combination immunotherapy regimens, because PDL-1 expression may be collaterally induced by other immunotherapies, even when tumors were initially PDL-1–negative.

In addition to expression by tumor cells, host antigen-presenting cells (APCs) may express PDL-1 or PDL-2 (or both). It is not yet clear which site of PD-ligand expression—host or tumor—is more important for immunosuppression, and both may contribute.[24] Although expression of PD-ligands on host APCs and stromal cells may be more difficult to detect than the more obvious expression on tumor cells, the host cells may be the more predictive of outcome.[25] However, this issue needs further research to be clarified.

Clinically, blocking either PD-1 or PDL-1 can trigger some striking clinical responses, especially in melanoma and lung cancer. Like CTLA-4 blockade, response to single-agent therapy was found to be more likely in patients who already had a strong antitumor response at baseline[22,25,26] and/or who had a high mutational burden in the tumor genome.[27] In some studies, response to PD-1 blockade appeared to correlate with constitutive PDL-1 expression in the tumor.[28] However, since PDL-1 expression is inducible by T cell–derived signals such as IFN-γ, the presence of PDL-1 at diagnosis may be acting as a proxy for the degree of upstream T cell response. In one combination trial, when CTLA-4 blockade was added to enhance T cell responses, blocking PD-1 in this setting provided benefit even in those patients who lacked PDL-1 expression at diagnosis.[8] This study did not perform on-treatment biopsies to ask whether the addition of CTLA-4 blockade increased T cell activation in the tumor and upregulated PDL-1, but this is a testable hypothesis.

Overall, the results from the initial trials of CTLA-4 and PD-1 blockade are encouraging, especially when used in combination. However, from the patient's perspective, it is important to remember that most types of tumors do not respond to checkpoint blockade, and of those that do, in many cases, individual patients will not show a long-term response. At present, clinical responses appear confined to those lucky enough to have the most immunogenic tumors and who are already mounting the most robust spontaneous immune response. Thus, additional strategies are needed that can build upon these encouraging beginnings.

DEFECTIVE ANTIGEN-PRESENTING CELLS IN THE TUMOR MILIEU

One of the fundamental immunological defects in the tumor microenvironment is the failure of immunogenic antigen presentation.[29] We have seen previously that when stimulated with something as simple as single-agent CTLA-4 blockade, many patients' T cells have the potential to recognize far more antigens on their own tumors than was evident at baseline.[12] These antigens do not even have to be non-self-neoantigens in order to be immunogenic.[30] But if these antitumor T cell responses were potentially available, why were they not elicited spontaneously? This implies that either the tumor-associated APCs did not effectively cross-present tumor antigens or the antigens were presented in an actively suppressive and tolerogenic fashion.

APCs in tumors are known to display multiple defects.[29,31] As discussed in the text that follows, the kinds of APCs recruited by tumors, such as "M2" polarized macrophages, may be ideally suited for supporting tissue remodeling and wound-healing, but they are ineffective at cross-presenting tissue antigens. Indeed, this type of APC may actively suppress T cell responses as part of their natural physiology. Virchow observed that tumors resemble "wounds that never heal,"[32,33] and tumors display the same angiogenesis, constant tissue remodeling, and accumulation of fibroblasts and reparative macrophages as seen in wound-healing.[34-36] In the context of normal tissue repair, the host must dispose of many apoptotic cells and self-antigens, and it is critical to maintain strict tolerance to these self-antigens. Thus, while a sterile wound (or a growing tumor) may be inflamed, it is not a type of inflammation that permits T cell activation.

Tumor-Associated Macrophages

As discussed in more detail in Chapter 11, tumor-associated macrophages (TAMs) are drivers of tumor-promoting angiogenesis, fibrous stroma deposition, and metastasis formation.[37-39] TAMs are also inhibitory for T cell responses.[40,41] This immunosuppressive phenotype may in part simply recapitulate the "reparative" phenotype of macrophages during tissue remodeling.[35] However, signals in the tumor such as acidosis and hypoxia may further drive their phenotype and function.[42,43] Molecular mechanisms of TAM-induced T cell immune suppression are not yet well defined but likely include the production of VEGF and TGF-β, both of which inhibit T cell responses.[40,41,44] One important undesirable effect of TAMs is to protect tumor cells from damage by other antitumor therapies.[45] In certain tumors, destabilization of the tumor-promoting macrophage pool, for example, by blocking the colony-stimulating factor 1 (CSF-1) receptor, can significantly impair tumor growth and enhance antitumor immune responses, although this effect is model-specific.[46-48] More broadly, conversion of immunosuppressive macrophages into proinflammatory "M1"-like macrophages may promote antitumor immune activation.[37]

Myeloid-Derived Suppressor Cells

While the macrophage population in tumors may resemble normal tissue-reparative macrophage seen in other settings, in reality, the myeloid lineage in tumors is profoundly disordered.[38,49] Systemically, myelopoiesis in the bone marrow is altered by factors such as GM-CSF and IL-6 secreted by the tumor. This affects the production and differentiation of both the monocytic and granulocytic lineages.[50] These circulating immature myeloid cells then become further altered when they are recruited into the tumor microenvironment, with its low-grade inflammation, hypoxia, excessive free-radical production, and constant metabolic stress.[51] The presence of indoleamine 2,3-dioxygenase (IDO) and activated T_{reg} cells in the tumor may enhance the recruitment of these cells and render them even more suppressive.[52] Once in place, this heterogeneous population of myeloid-derived suppressor cells (MDSCs) creates an immunosuppressive milieu via the elaboration of NO, arginase, and reactive oxygen species.[38,53] Much of the research on these cells has focused on mouse models, but relevant counterparts appear to exist in human tumors.[54,55]

A variety of strategies have been proposed to circumvent suppression by MDSCs.[56] Chemotherapy can cause depletion of MDSCs;[57,58] however, chemotherapy can also cause a paradoxical rebound of suppressive MDSCs,[59] so this approach is not straightforward. Other strategies have attempted to block the production or suppressive mechanisms of these cells.[56] A more recently proposed approach is to promote the maturation of MDSCs into nonsuppressive immunogenic APCs.[60] This approach arises from the observation that MDSCs share many similarities with the normal immunogenic inflammatory myeloid cells seen during infection.[61] In mouse models, inflammatory cytokines such as IL-12, IFN-γ, or IFN-α/β can promote the maturation of intratumoral myeloid cells into immunogenic APCs.[62–64] In certain tumor models, immunogenic chemotherapy (e.g., anthracyclines or oxaliplatin) may by itself drive the maturation of MDSCs.[65] Thus, a number of potential strategies exist, although few of these have yet been evaluated in the clinic.

Dendritic Cells in Tumors

The immune system treats tumors like an indolent, chronic wound; yet they ought to receive as much attention as a life-threatening viral infection. This failure does not seem to be due simply to an absence of foreign antigens on the tumor. It is now clear that tumors have many non-self neoantigens.[66–68] Indeed, a mutated tumor genome may have far more neoantigens than a cell infected with a small virus. Yet most viruses generate robust immune activation and their antigens are effectively cross-presented to activate CD8$^+$ T cells, while tumors do not. The mechanisms of this difference in response to the "altered self" of a virus-infected cell and the "mutated self" of a tumor cell are not yet entirely clear, but these point to a failure of immunogenic antigen cross-presentation by dendritic cells (DCs).

At the conceptual level, it seems clear that tumors actively inhibit the recruitment and differentiation of effective antigen-presenting cells (APCs).[3,31,69] The molecular mechanisms are likely diverse and may include cytokines such as IL-10, TGF-β, and VEGF, which favor tolerogenic DCs.[69] In part, the paucity of immunogenic DCs may also relate to the inability of myeloid cells in tumors to appropriately differentiate into activated, immunogenic DCs in response to inflammation.[60,61] Although immunogenic CD103$^+$ "cDC1" DCs have been identified in tumors and can be potent cross-presenting APCs for tumor antigens,[70,71] in most tumors these cells are rare. Even worse, the mature cross-presenting DCs that are constitutively resident in tumors may be actively immunosuppressive, rather than immune-activating.[72] Oncogenic drivers such as the WNT/β-catenin signaling pathway may exclude proinflammatory immunogenic DCs from the tumor environment.[73] Thus, identifying the local factors that block the recruitment, differentiation, and activation of immunogenic DCs in the tumor microenvironment is a priority for the field.

One reason that DC-targeted therapy is important is because DCs appear to be centrally positioned "gate-keepers" for the response to other forms of immunotherapy.[71,74,75] Creating an activated, proinflammatory DC population in the tumor may thus be a precondition for successful antitumor immune activation.[76] The conventional PD-1 or CTLA-4 checkpoint-blockade strategies do not address this need, since they do not directly activate DCs. Thus, additional strategies are needed to specifically target DCs.[77] Although still at the discovery phase, such strategies may include DC growth factors such as FMS-related tyrosine kinase 3 ligand (FLT3-L),[78] activating signals that target DCs such as CD40 ligation,[79] or inhibition of local factors that antagonize DC function such as tumor-associated TGF-β, IDO, or T$_{reg}$ cells.

TGF-β AND THE "COLD" TUMOR MICROENVIRONMENT

TGF-β is a complex cytokine with multiple roles in tumor biology.[80] Emerging evidence suggests that TGF-β may be an important contributor to the local immunosuppressive milieu in "cold" tumors.[81] TGF-β can be produced by tumor cells themselves or by cells of the immune system (macrophages, T$_{reg}$ cells, and others). TGF-β can directly suppress tumor-specific T cells[82] and can inhibit innate immune inflammation and activation of stromal cells.[83] Expression of TGF-β in the tumor milieu has been identified as an independent prognostic factor predicting response to PDL-1 checkpoint blockade.[84] In preclinical models, blocking TGF-β signaling using the inhibitor galunisertib[85] allowed T cell penetration into the otherwise cold, immune-excluded tumors and restored responsiveness to checkpoint blockade.[84,86] Clinical trials are in progress to test the effects of galunisertib in combination with chemotherapy or checkpoint inhibitors.

INDOLEAMINE 2,3-DIOXYGENASE AND TOLERANCE TO TUMOR CELLS

Physiological Role of Indoleamine 2,3-Dioxygenase

IDO is a tryptophan-degrading enzyme that plays a regulatory and tolerogenic function in the immune system.[87] The biological role of IDO is more focused and restricted than CTLA-4 or PD-1, but in certain specific settings, it can be critical for creating acquired peripheral tolerance. Thus, in contexts as different as pregnancy,[88] mucosal tolerance,[89] tissue transplantation,[90–92] and tolerance to apoptotic cells,[93,94] disrupting the IDO pathway could convert a normally tolerizing antigen exposure (when IDO was active) into an immunogenic and activating immune response (when IDO was blocked).[95] In all of these models, it is important to note that it was not the nature of the antigens that dictated tolerance versus immunity but rather the presence or absence of IDO and the regulatory signals it elicited.

IDO is also upregulated by exposure to apoptotic cells. Mice with a genetic deletion of the *IDO1* gene rapidly develop lethal lupus-like autoimmunity when challenged with injections of apoptotic self cells.[93,94] Here again, the antigens on the apoptotic cells were the same, but in the absence of IDO, these antigens were immunogenic and caused autoimmunity, whereas in the presence of IDO (and its downstream T$_{reg}$ cell activation) they were tolerizing. As will be discussed further in the text that follows, this concept has important implications for settings such as chemotherapy and radiation.

Indoleamine 2,3-Dioxygenase in Tumors

In tumors, IDO can be expressed by the tumor cells themselves, or by host stromal cells (DCs, macrophages, endothelial cells, and others). Often, both tumor and host cells may express IDO. IDO in tumors can exert several effects that contribute to the suppressive tumor microenvironment: it can contribute to activation of suppressive T$_{reg}$ cells;[96–98] it may create a local milieu that is deficient in tryptophan, and thus inimical to T cell activation;[99] and it can produce elevated levels of kynurenine and downstream metabolites, which can themselves affect the immune system by activating the aryl hydrocarbon receptor (AhR).[100] IDO may also help recruit MDSCs into the tumor, thereby increasing suppression in the tumor milieu.[52]

In some tumors, the expression of IDO may be a constitutive feature of the tumor. But IDO is also highly inducible, in both host cells and tumor cells, and can be upregulated in response to local inflammation. This may help explain why IDO in certain tumors can be paradoxically associated with increased T cell infiltration[23,101,102]—in this case, IDO is elicited as a counter-regulatory suppressive response, rather than being a primary inhibitory mechanism. (In these tumors, IDO would still be a target for immunotherapy, because it is immunosuppressive, but its presence might indicate a more favorable subset of patients because it could be a proxy for the underlying T cell response.) The inducible nature of IDO also has implications for screening patients for clinical trials. Unlike driver oncogenes, IDO expression may initially be negative at diagnosis but may rapidly become positive when the tumor comes under immune attack. Clinical trials targeting the IDO pathway suffered a setback with the failure of the first Phase 3 trial of the IDO inhibitor drug epacadostat, but trials of other IDO inhibitors with different mechanisms of action are ongoing.[103,104]

OVERCOMING THERAPY-INDUCED COUNTER-REGULATION

Some of the immunosuppressive mechanisms used by tumors may actually be reactive or counter-regulatory, that is, mechanisms whose expression is induced by the inflammatory signals that they are intended to suppress. The immune system naturally contains many such feedback loops that protect the host from excessive immune activation. Thus, for example, proinflammatory IFN-γ upregulates anti-inflammatory IDO and PD-ligands,[23] and activation of effector T cells simultaneously recruits suppressive T$_{reg}$ cells.[105,106] In the tumor milieu, these natural counter-regulatory mechanisms are often pathologically exaggerated to create a chronically suppressive milieu.[22] This potential for exaggerated counter-regulation becomes particularly relevant in the setting of active immunotherapy. Any successful immunotherapy will create inflammation in the tumor; yet, this desirable inflammation may itself elicit intensified counter-regulation—for example, by upregulating PD-1 ligands or IDO.[22,23] Similarly, potent and effective vaccine adjuvants such as TLR-ligands or STING agonists may also be inadvertent inducers of counter-regulatory IDO.[107,108] Thus, some immunotherapies may unwittingly sacrifice a portion of their efficacy to induced counter-regulation, unless agents are added to block this suppression. Conversely, however, this offers a potential opportunity for synergy—for example, by combining an IDO inhibitor drug or PD-1 ligand blockade with other, inflammation-inducing immunotherapy.

ACTIVATED REGULATORY T CELLS INDUCED BY TUMORS

T$_{reg}$ cells are an important suppressive population in tumors.[109] Depleting T$_{reg}$ cells[110] or inhibiting signaling pathways that they require[111] can at least partially rescue immune surveillance against the tumor. However, it remains unclear how T$_{reg}$ cells exert their suppressive function. T$_{reg}$ cells are known to produce local IL-10, IL-35, and TGF-β, all of which are important immunosuppressive cytokines in tumors.[112] An additional important mechanism of T$_{reg}$ cell suppression is their inhibitory effect on DCs.[17,18] In the presence of T$_{reg}$ cells, tumor-associated DCs lose costimulatory ligands and cannot support T cell activation.[17] T$_{reg}$ cells can also induce immunosuppressive IDO expression in DCs, via CTLA-4/B7 interaction.[113]

One important unanswered question is why T$_{reg}$ cell activity is so excessive and dominant in tumors. In part, this may be due to new specificities of T$_{reg}$ cells that arise against tumor neoantigens.[114] However, this seems unlikely to be the major explanation, since tumor neoantigens are relatively rare, and many of the T$_{reg}$ cells in tumors appear to recognize the same self-antigens that are found in the tissue of origin.[115] Thus, the exaggerated degree of T$_{reg}$ cell activity in tumors may reflect more aggressive recruitment to the tumor, for example, via receptors such as CCR4[116] and a higher degree of functional suppressor activity once they reach the tumor. This concept of enhanced functional activation of T_{reg} cells in tumors is important, but the mechanisms are still not well understood.

Some upstream pathways have been identified that activate T_{reg} cell function in tumors. These include IDO[97,98,117] and neuropilin-1.[118] When T_{reg} cells are activated by exposure to IDO, they upregulate the expression of PD-1 receptor; PD-1 then functions to perpetuate the suppressive T_{reg} cell phenotype by signaling via the Phosphatase and TENsin homolog (PTEN) phosphatase.[96] PTEN acts to limit the activity of the RAC-alpha serine/threonine-protein kinase 1 (Akt1)/mechanistic Target of Rapamycin (mTOR) pathway, which helps to stabilize the suppressive T_{reg} cell phenotype and prevents conversion into inflammatory "ex-T_{reg} cells."[96,97,119] Neuropilin-1 also activates PTEN in T_{reg} cells,[118] and PTEN has been recently implicated in maintaining function and stability of T_{reg} cells to prevent autoimmunity.[119,120] Thus, PTEN is emerging as an important pathway for T_{reg} cell activation in tumors. Consistent with this possibility, genetic ablation of the PTEN pathway in T_{reg} cells, or its pharmacological inhibition, prevents tumors from creating an immunosuppressive local microenvironment, and markedly enhances immune responses to dying tumor cells after chemotherapy.[96]

Overall, however, the biology of T_{reg} cells in tumors remains incompletely understood, and strategies to circumvent them are still at an early stage. Nonspecific depletion with toxins has proved difficult to achieve and may need to be finely balanced to create enough depletion to promote antitumor immunity, and yet not create collateral autoimmunity. Alternative strategies include functional inhibition of the IL-2-receptor with daclizumab,[121,122] and depletion/inhibition of recruitment using CCR4 antibodies.[123] T_{reg} cells are a major inhibitory pathway in the tumor microenvironment, and hence an important target for immunotherapy, but more research is needed to identify the pathways that can selectively target T_{reg} cell activity in tumors.

THE TUMOR MICROENVIRONMENT AS A TARGET FOR THERAPY

In the following section, we will consider how the inflammatory and antigen-presenting milieu of the tumor microenvironment may have a far-reaching impact on the efficacy of anticancer therapy. To date, most immunotherapy has focused on blocking a single pathway with a single agent. But the more fundamental goal of immunotherapy is to empower the endogenous host immune system to respond spontaneously to the entire array of antigens released from the patient's own tumor. Mellman et al. have termed this the "cancer-immunity cycle,"[124,125] in which tumor cells killed by exogenous treatment (chemotherapy, radiotherapy, or immunotherapy of whatever kind) then serve as a source of antigen to activate more T cells, which kill more tumor cells

and release more antigen. In essence, this self-amplifying cycle represents a restoration of antitumor immune surveillance,[1,126–128] with progressive broadening and tailoring of the antitumor T cell repertoire. And, unlike a time-limited exogenous intervention, it is an inherently self-sustaining process.

Achieving this self-amplifying endogenous T cell response is a more complex task than simply blocking a single pathway, because it requires all the different elements of checkpoints, costimulation, antigen presentation, inflammation, and counter-regulation discussed previously. The entire tumor microenvironment needs to be reconfigured from a suppressive milieu into an immunogenic milieu. But there is emerging evidence that—at least in the most highly responsive patients—this virtuous circle of amplification and diversification is beginning to emerge.[12,129,130] Now the task is to reliably create this in all patients and drive it to become self-sustaining and curative.

This focus on activating the patient's own endogenous T cells represents something of a shift in thinking. In the past, the tacit assumption has been that the endogenous immune response must be hopelessly overwhelmed by the tumor (anergic, exhausted, evaded, and escaped). However, experience with immunotherapy trials shows that this is not correct. Indeed, the patient's own preexisting level of spontaneous T cell activation (i.e., prior to treatment) has frequently turned out to be a major predictor of response to therapy.[11,22,25 26,130,131] Using checkpoint blockade alone, only the most highly mutated tumors seem to spontaneously trigger a robust T cell response prior to therapy.[9–11,27,131] However, it seems likely that these are just the tip of the iceberg. Far more tumor antigens are probably able to be immunogenic than was previously thought,[132] if the local tumor-induced immune suppression can be overcome.[133,134] Increasing evidence suggests that tumors contain a pool of tumor-specific T cells that are quiescent but capable of reactivation with immunotherapy.[74,135–138] Thus, if patients can be suitably stimulated with immunotherapy that renders the tumor microenvironment immunogenic, then more than just the fortunate few can probably mount an effective immune response. One goal of immunotherapy is to restore and enable the powerful—but often suppressed—endogenous immune response.

The Tumor Milieu Dictates Tolerance Versus Immunity to Dying Tumor Cells

In this regard, one of the most fundamental immunologic decisions that must be made in the tumor microenvironment is how to respond to dying tumor cells.[139–141] As previously reviewed, data from both IDO-KO mice[94] and T_{reg}-specific PTEN^{Treg}-KO mice[96] show that the immunological response to the same, identical apoptotic cells can be either tolerogenic or immunogenic, depending on whether these suppressive mechanisms are active or not. If generally applicable, this implies a fundamental conceptual shift in how we think about tumor cell death. The traditional understanding has been that apoptotic cell death is immunologically "silent" and leads to tolerance,[142] whereas when certain tumor models are treated with certain chemotherapy drugs, they can undergo a different form of cell death that is spontaneously immunogenic.[65,143] But the assumption to date has been that these are intrinsic properties of the cell-death pathway—not that they might be flexible, changeable responses dictated by external signals from the tumor milieu.

However, data from IDO and PTEN-T$_{reg}$ models now imply that tumor cell death might be an inherently more mixed process, as summarized in Figure 16.2. Under this model, whenever tumor cells are killed, some cells will die in a chaotic and highly immunogenic fashion, releasing proinflammatory factors such as high mobility group box 1 (HMGB-1) and adenosine triphosphate (ATP) and activating the Stimulator of Interferon Genes (STING) sensor of DNA.[144–149] At the same time, other tumor cells will undergo conventional apoptotic cell death, and this apoptosis elicits a set of dominant tolerogenic signals such as IDO, PTEN-T$_{regs}$, and TGF-β. These are the normal suppressive signals elicited by any apoptotic cells, but the tumor milieu is particularly primed to overproduce all of these, so the tolerogenic response is exaggerated and dominant. This makes it seem (incorrectly) that true "immunogenic" cell death is rare and occurs only under certain circumstances.[150] In reality, tumor cell death may be always immunogenic, but the inducible inhibitory pathways frequently overwhelm this. However, as drugs become available to target IDO, PTEN, TGF-β, and other relevant pathways, this overlay of suppression may be removable, and the underlying immunogenic cell death exploited for therapy.

Chemotherapy and Radiation as Immunological Adjuvants

If dying tumor cells could be rendered consistently immunogenic, then this might have major implications for the efficacy of conventional chemotherapy and radiation. Immunotherapy can be strikingly effective for certain patients with certain tumors, but the vast majority of patients are not cured by immunotherapy. Thus, almost all patients still rely on conventional chemotherapy and radiation as frontline treatments. Fortunately, there is the potential for significant synergies between standard-of-care chemotherapy or radiation and the addition of innovative immunotherapies. We will first consider the case of chemotherapy and immunotherapy and then describe analogous opportunities with radiation and immunotherapy.

Bidirectional Synergy: Chemotherapy as a Vaccine and the Immune System as a Cytolytic Mechanism

In theory, chemotherapy has the potential to function as an endogenous "vaccine" when it releases a wave of antigens from dying tumor cells.[151–154] By itself, however, conventional chemotherapy is typically not highly immunogenic.[155] This may change, however, as we become able to block the inhibitory mechanisms that

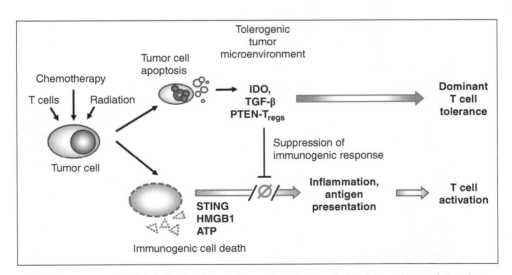

Figure 16.2 Two responses to tumor cell death. This figure summarizes the possibility that two sets of signals are created simultaneously during tumor cell death: some death occurs by apoptosis (top), and thus triggers suppressive mechanisms (IDO, TGF-β, T$_{reg}$ cells) and elicits tolerance. Simultaneously, some tumor cell death is disordered and uncontrolled death (immunogenic cell death) with inflammatory mediators. In the usual suppressive tumor milieu, the inhibitory pathways are exaggerated and dominant, so the immunogenic component is suppressed. If these inhibitory signals can be blocked by therapy, however, then the immune system becomes able to cross-present and respond to the underlying tumor antigens.

suppress immunogenic antigen presentation and T cell activation after chemotherapy. When these pathways are identified and inhibited, then even standard chemotherapy agents may be revealed as much more immunogenic than previously thought.

Reciprocally, given the right setting, the immune system may become a potent effector mechanism for conventional chemotherapy. Historically, when immunogenic cell death was first discovered, there was some speculation that perhaps all chemotherapy—by itself—might recruit the immune system to mediate tumor regression.[156] This turned out to be too optimistic,[157] but it is quite possible that all chemotherapies release antigens that could *potentially* be used by the immune system to attack the tumor. If the immune system can be empowered by blocking the tumor-associated suppressive pathways, then reactivated T cells may provide additional antitumor effector mechanisms—essentially, the immune system becomes a downstream effector arm for the chemotherapy. This effect has been modeled in preclinical mouse systems,[71,96,158] and there are some encouraging suggestions that chemo-immunotherapy may be translatable to the clinic as well.[159–163]

Local Radiation as an Endogenous "Vaccine"

Radiation kills tumor cells by damaging DNA and generating free radicals. This is highly inflammatory, and dying tumor cells after radiation are potentially immunogenic.[139,164] Thus, radiation releases a wave of tumor antigens and creates local inflammation—in essence, creating a "vaccine" against endogenous tumor antigens.[165] The problem, however, is similar to chemotherapy: tolerogenic mechanisms usually dominate, and radiation is rarely able to break tolerance to tumor antigens. The tolerogenic checkpoints after radiation appear similar to those following chemotherapy.[166,167] Hence, the immunogenic effects of radiation may become much more pronounced when combined with suitable targeted immunotherapy.[153,166,168,169]

Thus, for example, anecdotal evidence suggested that local radiation combined with concurrent CTLA-4 blockade could trigger immune-mediated regression of distant lesions ("abscopal effect").[170] Similar effects have been reported with other immunotherapy, and clinical trials have been initiated.[168,171] As a source of antigens and inflammation, hypofractionated radiation (e.g., stereotactic radiosurgery or stereotactic body radiotherapy) may be more immunogenic than a conventional hyperfractionated schedule.[165] In another approach, local irradiation of isolated tumors has been combined with intralesional injection of inflammatory Toll-like receptor (TLR) ligands; in lymphomas, this was able to elicit abscopal responses at distant sites.[172,173] Thus, at least in principle, local irradiation has the potential to make an important contribution to multimodal chemo/radio/immunotherapy regimens.

Practical Considerations

Is Chemotherapy Immunosuppressive for T Cells?

Many chemotherapy drugs are myelosuppressive. However, myelosuppression (primarily manifesting as reduced neutrophil, platelet, and red-cell production) does not necessarily imply antigen-specific T cell immunosuppression (which is the relevant attribute immunotherapy). Recovery from transient lymphopenia may actually be a congenial milieu for stimulating antitumor T cells.[174] In practice, the timing and dose-intensity of chemotherapy relative to immunotherapy must be optimized to avoid inadvertently suppressing the desired immune response, but this can be done.[175] Thus, chemotherapy is in principle a receptive context for immunotherapy and a potential opportunity for synergy.[152,153]

Using Immunotherapy to Reduce Dose and Toxicity of Chemotherapy

Chemotherapy regimens have become progressively more effective, but this success is often purchased at the price of higher dose intensity, especially in patients with high-risk or relapsed disease. This dose intensity contributes greatly to the morbidity, cost, and impact on quality of life. Most of the toxicity of chemotherapy occurs as the dose approaches the maximum tolerated level; hence, even a modest reduction in dose can have a major impact on toxicity. The tendency toward more dose-intensive regimens has been driven by the fact that moderate doses are often not effective against high-risk disease. However, this may in part reflect the fact that chemotherapy is being asked to function as a single modality. When chemotherapy is used alone, the only route to more efficacy is often greater dose intensity. However, if immunotherapy can be added and contribute synergistic efficacy, then it may not be necessary to push the chemotherapy component to highly toxic levels. Indeed, for purposes of immunogenic antigen release, an intermediate dose of chemotherapy may be more potent than a higher, more immunosuppressive dose.[175]

Choosing the Right Immune Modulator for Combination With Chemotherapy

Much attention has been given to the standard checkpoint inhibitors targeting the CTLA-4 or PD-1/PD-ligand pathways, because these are approved for therapy. Mechanistically, however, both CTLA-4 and PD-1 are checkpoint molecules expressed on T cells. Thus, they primarily come into play when the T cell encounters antigen or after T cell activation. In the case of chemotherapy, this may be too late: the key decision point may lie upstream, in deciding the nature of the APC that will present antigen in the first place, and whether this will be in a tolerogenic or immunogenic fashion. In contrast, immunotherapy agents such as CD40 agonists, STING/TLR agonists, IDO inhibitors, T_{reg}-depleting agents, TGF-β inhibitors, and others may exert a large part of their action at the level of the APC and by altering the antigen-presenting milieu (i.e., local inflammation and cytokines). Thus, when selecting which immunomodulatory agents to combine with chemotherapy, it may be ideal to incorporate agents that directly activate the APCs, and/or create an immunogenic tumor microenvironment. Once the T cells are activated, then conventional checkpoint blockade may become relevant and beneficial.

CONCLUSION

This chapter has focused on certain suppressive immunoregulatory pathways in the tumor microenvironment, with an emphasis on how they may be exploited in the clinic. Additional inhibitory pathways also exist and have been reviewed elsewhere.[2,3,38,53,176–178] From a therapeutic standpoint, however, the most important question may be which of these suppressive pathways need to be targeted in order to change the tumor from an immunosuppressive and tolerizing milieu into an immunogenic milieu. The ability of the patient's immune system to cross-present endogenous tumor antigens in an immunogenic fashion, and thus activate the full spectrum of endogenous T cell responses, may be key in creating a long-term, curative antitumor immune response.

ACKNOWLEDGMENTS

This work was supported by grants from the Italian Ministry of Health; the Italian Ministry of Education, Universities and Research (FIRB cup: B31J11000420001); the Italian Association for Cancer Research (AIRC 6599, 12182, and 14103); the Italian Ministry of Health (FINALIZZATA 2011-2012 RF-2011-02348435 cup: E35G1400019001); and NIH grants R01CA211229 and R01CA103320.

KEY REFERENCES

Only key references appear in the print edition. The full reference list appears in the digital product on Springer Publishing Connect: connect.springerpub.com/content/book/978-0-8261-3743-2/part/part01/chapter/ch16

3. Spranger S, Gajewski TF. Impact of oncogenic pathways on evasion of antitumour immune responses. *Nat Rev Cancer.* 2018;18(3):139–147. doi:10.1038/nrc.2017.117
31. Wculek SK, Cueto FJ, Mujal AM, et al. Dendritic cells in cancer immunology and immunotherapy. *Nat Rev Immunol.* 2020;20(1):7–24. doi:10.1038/s41577-019-0210-z
40. Denardo DG, Ruffell B. Macrophages as regulators of tumour immunity and immunotherapy. *Nat Rev Immunol.* 2019;19(6):369–382. doi:10.1038/s41577-019-0127-6
55. Veglia F, Perego M, Gabrilovich D. Myeloid-derived suppressor cells coming of age. *Nat Immunol.* 2018;19(2):108–119. doi:10.1038/s41590-017-0022-x
76. Moussion C, Mellman I. The dendritic cell strikes back. *Immunity.* 2018;49(6):997–999. doi:10.1016/j.immuni.2018.12.007
86. Tauriello DVF, Palomo-Ponce S, Stork D, et al. TGFβ drives immune evasion in genetically reconstituted colon cancer metastasis. *Nature.* 2018;554(7693):538–543. doi:10.1038/nature25492
124. Chen DS, Mellman I. Oncology meets immunology: the cancer-immunity cycle. *Immunity.* 2013;39(1):1–10. doi:10.1016/j.immuni.2013.07.012

Cancer-Immune Exclusion: An Enigmatic Phenomenon

Violena Pietrobon, Jakob Nikolas Kather, and Francesco M. Marincola

KEY POINTS

- T cell immune-exclusion defines a paradoxical phenomenon—From an immunologic standpoint, human solid tumors occur in three landscapes distributed at approximately equal frequency across most cancer types: "*immune active, infiltrated, or hot*"; "*immune silent, desert, or cold*"; and "*immune excluded.*" The third is characterized by T cells teeming at the periphery of cancer nests but incapable of penetrating them. While lack of immunogenicity may explain the immune desert phenotype, the determinism of immune exclusion remains enigmatic. The presence of T cells at the periphery of tumor nests suggests that chemoattraction recruits circulating T cells and an immunogenic stimulus promotes their persistence. What prevents then the T cells from penetrating the tumor nest?

- Relevance of immune exclusion—Cancer-immune exclusion is more prevalent than previously recognized, affecting about a third of solid cancers. It represents a distinct biology compared to the other two immune phenotypes and, therefore, offers distinct opportunities for intervention.

- Immune infiltration is a hallmark of anticancer-immune surveillance—The infiltration of tumors CD+ T cells has been shown to be the strongest harbinger of good prognosis and positive outcomes in response to immunotherapy. However, the infiltration needs to be reaching the internal component of the cancer nests, while immune-excluded tumors do not bear the same favorable connotation. Thus, understanding the reasons for the dichotomy between chemoattraction at the tumor site and the lack of penetration to exert antitumor effects may represent a unique opportunity to understand the mechanisms of cancer-immune resistance.

- Several mechanisms may cause immune exclusion—A better understanding of the dominant mechanisms leading to immune exclusion, and their causation, may lead to a better rationale for drug development and the selection of sound combination therapies. Currently, the frequency and weight that postulated mechanisms play in human cancer are unknown. The following categories will be discussed in this chapter: (a) mechanical barriers defined as physical impediments preventing contact between T cells and cancer cells; (b) functional barriers as preexisting biological and/or metabolic interactions between cancer, stromal, and immune cells limiting the migration, function, and/or survival of T cells; and (c) dynamic barriers as biological interactions between cancer and T cells that result in limited function.

THE ENIGMA OF IMMUNE EXCLUSION

It is increasingly appreciated that from an immunologic standpoint, human solid tumors occur in three landscapes distributed at approximately equal frequency across most cancer types: "immune active, infiltrated, or hot"; "immune silent, desert, or cold"; and "immune excluded."[1,2] The third is characterized by T cells teeming at the periphery of cancer nests but incapable of penetrating them.

Immune-infiltrated tumors are characterized by genetic instability and high mutational rate.[3,4] The latter corresponds to powerful immunogenicity promoted by catastrophic cancer cell death that leads to Immunogenic Cell Death (ICD) and release of DAMPs[5–8] and/or the induction of adaptive immune responses in the presence of neo-antigens.[9–11] As a consequence of immunogenicity, the evolutionary survival of these tumors in the immune component host depends upon the presence of powerful compensatory mechanisms of immune resistance.[8,12] Conversely, immune desert tumors are genetically stable, do not release Damage Associated Molecular Patterns (DAMPs), bear low mutational rates, are not immunogenic, and do not depend upon immune-suppressive mechanisms to survive in the immune-competent host.

While lack of immunogenicity due to low tumor mutational burden[13,14] and/or loss of the antigen processing and presentation capability[15] may explain the immune desert phenotype, the determinism of immune exclusion remains enigmatic. The presence of T cells at the periphery of tumor nests suggests that chemo-attraction recruits circulating T cells and an immunogenic stimulus promotes their persistence. What prevents the T cells from penetrating the tumor nest? A concentric gradient of increasing chemo-repulsion or decreasing chemo-attraction from the periphery to the center must draw the "do not trespass" line. This gradient may be related to the intrinsic biology of cancer cells that may deviate from an orderly non-immunogenic Cancer Stem Cell (CSC) phenotype endowed with immune-suppressive properties to progressively become more immunogenic and prone to excite ICD.[16–20] Indeed, transcriptional signatures of ICD are tightly associated with immune infiltration and immune activation.[12] This transition could be, in turn, dependent upon preferential localization of CSCs in hypoxic niches at the center of the cancer nests.[21]

Alternatively, a disorderly architecture of the tumor microenvironment (TME) may alter in a centripetal direction cancer and surrounding stromal cell metabolism, which, in turn, may affect the function of immune cells. Several experimental models propose determinants of immune exclusion that could be broadly classified into physical, functional, or dynamic barriers (Table 17.1). However, no consensus exists at present over the weight that any of them plays in human cancers.

Table 17.1 Hypotheses Raised to Explain Immune Exclusion (N.B. Mechanisms Are Not Mutually Exclusive)

MECHANICAL BARRIERS	PHYSICAL IMPEDIMENT TO A DIRECT CONTACT BETWEEN T CELLS AND CANCER CELLS	
Stromal fibrosis	Extracellular matrix	(22–32)
	Filaggrin and desmosomal proteins	(33)
	Endothelin B Receptor	(34–36)
	Defects in physical interaction between immune cells and TME	(37)
	Hypoxia/Transforming growth factor (TGF)-β-induced fibrosis	(27,31,33, 37–55)
	Epithelial-mesenchymal transition	(56–60)
Vascular access	Vascular endothelial growth factor (VEGF) and angiopoietin 2	(52,55,61–65)
Cancer cell coating	Platelet aggregation	
	CAFs-mediated biosynthesis of CXCL12	(31,66–68)
FUNCTIONAL BARRIERS	BIOLOGICAL OR METABOLIC INTERACTIONS BETWEEN CANCER, STROMAL, AND IMMUNE CELLS LIMITING MIGRATION, FUNCTION, AND/OR SURVIVAL OF T CELLS	
Metabolic barriers	Nutrient depletion by cancer cells	(69–71)
	Warburg and reverse Warburg effect (lacto-genesis)	(71–76)
	Metabolic reprogramming of immune cells	(77,78)
	Altered lipid metabolism	(79)
	Hypoxia	(80–84)
	K+ levels	(72,85)
	Glutaminase-dependent metabolism	(86,87)

(continued)

Table 17.1 Hypotheses Raised to Explain Immune Exclusion (N.B. Mechanisms Are Not Mutually Exclusive) (*continued*)

FUNCTIONAL BARRIERS	BIOLOGICAL OR METABOLIC INTERACTIONS BETWEEN CANCER, STROMAL, AND IMMUNE CELLS LIMITING MIGRATION, FUNCTION, AND/OR SURVIVAL OF T CELLS	
	Metabolic inhibitors	(69,87–92)
	Cyclooxygenase and prostaglandin metabolism	(93–95)
Soluble factors	Cytokine/chemokine gradients	(37,39,96,97)
	Vascular endothelial factor (VEGF)-α-mediated immune suppression	(63,98)
	Transforming growth factor-β	(38,39,99,100)
	Tumor-associated immune and stromal infiltrate-suppressive mechanisms	(74,101–108)
Danger sensing	Tolerogenic cell death/absent immunogenic cell death	(109–111)
	Adenosine signaling	(101,112–114)
	TAM receptor tyrosine kinases	(115–118)
	"Don't eat me" signals (CD47/signal regulatory protein (SIRP)-α axis)	(119–121)
Tumor cell-intrinsic signaling	Tumor cell-intrinsic β-catenin/ signaling	(122–127)
	Extended PI3K pathway signaling	(125–132)
	Tumor cell-intrinsic STAT-3 activation	(133–136)
	Tumor cell-intrinsic MAPK signaling	(3,4)
	Tumor cell-intrinsic NF-kB signaling	(137–142)
	Tumor cell-intrinsic p53 signaling	(143–146)
DYNAMIC BARRIERS	INTERACTIONS BETWEEN CANCER AND T CELLS RESULTING IN LIMITED FUNCTION	
	Checkpoint/ligand interaction	(77,147,148)

CLINICAL RELEVANCE OF IMMUNE EXCLUSION

Cancer treatment has been revolutionized by *immune-oncology (IO)* approaches, particularly checkpoint inhibitor therapy (CIT) and adoptive cell transfer (ACT). However, clinical benefit is derived in only a subset of cancer types (such as melanoma, lung cancer, and renal cell cancer, among others). Even in these cancer types, only a subset of patients responds, highlighting the need for clinically applicable predictive biomarkers based on functional understanding. The next frontier in cancer immunotherapy is to unveil mechanisms of immune resistance that limit the efficacy of therapy in the majority of patients.[8] CIT, in particular, is most effective in immunogenic tumors,[149,150] where high frequency of expression of inhibitory checkpoints is observed.[8,12] When CIT is not effective in this context, it is because compensatory immune resistance due to the presence of

other immune regulatory mechanisms not targeted by the therapeutic overrules its effect. Lack of response in other immune landscapes is instead due to other mechanisms. Another mechanism of immune resistance is an absent dialogue between cancer and immune cells.[151] This occurs in the context of "immune silent"[149,152] and, perhaps, "immune-excluded" tumors.[115,151,153] Since T cells do not come in direct contact with cancer cells, CIT is rendered immaterial unless the TME can be reprogrammed to facilitate T cell homing and infiltration.[12]

Similarly, ACT may be affected by immune exclusion that limits direct T cell contact with targeted antigen-expressing cancer cells. *Pockaj et al.*[154] observed that adoptively transferred *tumor-infiltrating lymphocytes (TIL)* labeled with radioactive [111]Indium to track them in vivo, often, did not localize at metastatic sites. Lack of TIL trafficking corresponded to total absence of tumor regression as an absolute requirement for the success of ACT.

Furthermore, successful homing of TILs to the tumor site was not consistently sufficient as only a proportion of patients responded to therapy underlying the multiple ways in which tumors can evade immune recognition.[155] We observed in patients with melanoma that response to TIL therapy is associated with the expression of CXCR3 and CCR5-ligand chemokines capable of recruiting activated T cells to the metastatic site.[96] These observations highlight the multifactorial requirements for an effective antitumor immune response. One may hypothesize that in the case of successful trafficking of TILs to the target lesions without accompanying tumor regression, immune exclusion may prevent them from infiltrating the tumor nest and deploy their full effector functions.

IMMUNE INFILTRATION AS THE HALLMARK OF IMMUNE SURVEILLANCE

It is well established that the infiltration of cancers by CD8+ T cells bears a favorable prognostic connotation,[3,156,157] whereas a high density of *tumor-associated macrophages (TAMs)* is associated with poor survival.[158] As a consequence, high ratios of CD8+ T cells over CD68+ myeloid cells or CD163+ TAMs bear favorable predictive and prognostic implications.[159,160] When morphological descriptions are combined with transcriptional analyses, a functional characterization of immune infiltrates provides deeper insights.[149,161,162] Transcriptional patterns such as the *immunologic constant of rejection (ICR)*[161,163] or the *tumor inflammation signature (TIS)*[149] demonstrated that the activation of *interferon (IFN)*-γ signaling, immune effector mechanisms, and the expression of CCR5 and CXCR3-ligand chemokines stand as independent prognostic and predictive biomarkers. The ICR predicts prolonged survival in several independent data sets of breast[3,164,165] and other cancers (*Roeland et al.'s manuscript in press*). Moreover, the ICR is a predictor of responsiveness to the systemic administration of human recombinant *interleukin (IL)*-2 and to TIL administration.[96,162] The presence of the ICR is consistently accompanied by the expression of ICD marking immune activation and by immune regulatory functions implying immune resistance.[12] The congregation of immune effector and immune regulatory mechanisms within the same cancer landscape suggests that an evolutionary balance is required for the survival of antigenic tumors in the immune-competent host that depends on offsetting immunogenicity with compensatory mechanisms of tolerance.[12] In this case, resistance of tumors to IO agents and, in particular, CIT, maybe due to the multiple immune-suppressive forces that operate within the TME; this may explain why targeting a single pathway with monotherapy by CIT may not always suffice to induce tumor rejection; a phenomenon that we described as *compensatory immune resistance*.[12,166] Whether

other mechanisms determine cancer resistance to IO agents in immune-excluded tumors remains unknown.

PREVALENCE OF IMMUNE EXCLUSION IN HUMAN CANCERS

Immune exclusion has been described by several investigators.[1,115,151,153,33,38,167–170] Galon et al.[156] observed that the infiltration of CD8 T lymphocytes within tumor nests prognosticates improved survival of patients with colorectal cancer,[157] whereas T cells presence limited at the periphery of tumor nests does not,[156,157,171,172] suggesting that immune exclusion is a distinct biological entity with different clinical implications.

The prevalence of immune exclusion in different cancer types has not been extensively characterized although the information is critical for the stratification of patients during clinical trials.[168,173–177] A recent study systematically measured by *immunohistochemistry (IHC)*, the pattern of immune infiltration ("*topography*") of approximately 1,000 histological tissue slides from patients bearing cancers of different histology.[1] Tissue specimens were categorized according to the presence of immune cells in three compartments: *outer invasive margin* (0–500 μm outside the tumor invasion front), *inner invasive margin* (0–500 μm inside the tumor invasion front), and *tumor core* (>500 μm inside the invasion front). A strong correlation was observed between the infiltration of the tumor core and the inner invasive margin and, therefore, these categories were combined to define immune active or "*hot*" tumors. Tumors with high frequency of immune cell density limited to the outer invasive margin were defined as immune excluded. Low density in all compartments characterized cold tumors. Cancers considered sensitive to IO agents, such as melanoma, lung adenocarcinoma, lung squamous cell carcinoma, and *head and neck squamous cell carcinoma (HNSSC)*, displayed a high frequency of immune infiltration (Figures 17.1 and 17.2). The immune-excluded phenotype was quite common among most cancers of epithelial derivation. Several reciprocally exclusive behaviors were observed: while CD3 and CD8-expressing T cell infiltrates were generally concordant, inverse correlations were observed between CD8 and Foxp3 expressing T cells or CD68 expressing TAMs infiltrates. The critical point of this study is the demonstration that immune-excluded cancers are more prevalent than generally perceived.

Tsujikawa et al.[168] studied *human papillomavirus (HPV)* positive HNSCC, known to be associated with an immunogenic gene signature,[178,179] sub-classifying them into tumors expressing only lymphoid signatures and tumors that included a mixture of lymphoid and myeloid cell signatures. The worst prognostic connotation was the presence of a strong myeloid infiltrate independent of

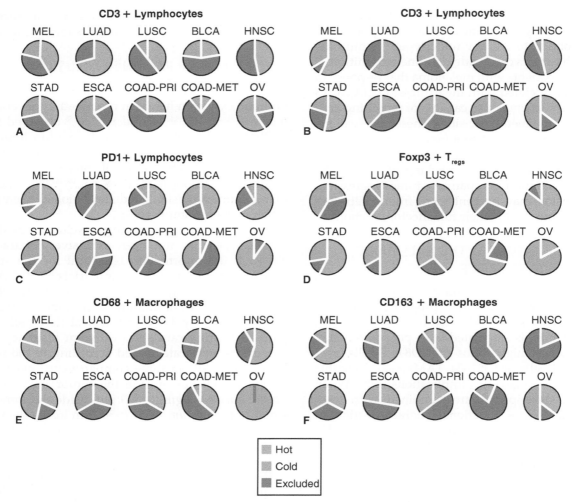

Figure 17.1 Distribution of immune topography phenotypes among different tumor types in the pan-cancer cohort. Analysis for all six immune cell types (A–F) and for all analyzed tumor types. These data comprise all $N = 965$ tissue slides from $N = 177$ patients. MEL through HNSC are to some degree sensitive to approved immunotherapies and predominantly have 'hot' phenotypes for most immune cells. However, among these tumor types, different phenotypes for immunosuppressive immune cells (Foxp3+ regulatory T cells [T_{reg} cells]) and CD163+ macrophages prevail.

BLCA, bladder; COAD-MET, colorectal liver metastasis; COAD-PRI, colorectal primary; ESCA, esophageal squamous; HNSC, head and neck squamous; LUAD, lung adeno; LUSC, lung squamous; MEL, melanoma; OV, ovarian; STAD, stomach adeno; T_{reg}, regulatory T.

Source: Reproduced from Kather JN, Suarez-Carmona M, Charoentong P, et al. Topography of cancer-associated immune cells in human solid tumors. *Elife.* 2018;7:e36967.

the lymphoid infiltrate.[168] Unfortunately, this study was performed on tissue microarrays that did not allow spatial discrimination of invasive margins versus tumor core assessment. Thus, it remains unknown whether lymphoid to myeloid ratios are also affected by spatial distribution.

We propose that the biology of immune-excluded tumors is partially similar to that of immune-active tumors as compared to the immune-silent phenotype. This hypothesis is based on the premise that in both phenotypes, chemo-attraction can recruit the T cells to the tumor periphery and that some immunogenic stimulus

can preserve their persistence. The biological mechanisms determining the two phenotypes diverge at this point; in inflamed tumors no chemo-repulsive signals hamper penetration but immune suppression affects the function of T cells. Immune exclusion could be determined by chemo-repulsive mechanisms not present in hot tumors that limit contact between T cells and cancer cells, while immune-suppressive mechanisms directed against T cell function may play a limited role.

In the case of HNSCC, immune-excluded cancers are transcriptionally indistinguishable from the immune-active ones. By applying the ICR signature to HNSCC

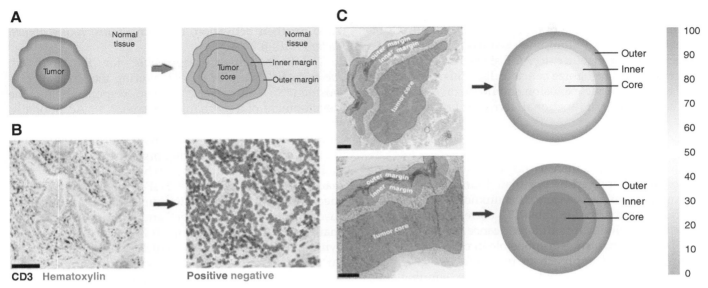

Figure 17.2 **Immune Exclusion**—Semiautomatic image analysis defines immune cell topography. (A) Manual delineation of three compartments: outer 500 μm invasive margin, inner 500 μm invasive margin, tumor core. (B) Example of automatic cell detection in a CD3-stained gastric carcinoma slide. Left: original image, right: after cell detection and classification. (C) Cell counts in all three compartments can be used to create a 'target plot' (visualization resembling a shooting target) where the color of each compartment corresponds to the percentile-normalized cell density. Here, two examples of CD3-stained gastric carcinoma tissue slides are shown. The upper sample has an immune-excluded phenotype while the lower sample has an inflamed phenotype. Unit on the color scale: percentile-normalized cell density. Scale bar in B is 100 μm, scale bars in C are 1 mm.

samples, we observed that both immune-excluded and immune-infiltrated tumors display an immune-effector Th1-like polarization of T cells,[3,4,165,180,181] combined with the presence of immune-suppressive mechanisms (*Pai SI. et al., ASCO 2018, Abstract # 6052*). Thus, the distinction between the immune-excluded versus the immune-active phenotypes is primarily centered around the spatial localization of immune cells.[1] The ICR signature includes Th1 polarization markers such as IFN-γ-related transcripts, granzyme, and perforin that are detectable upon cognate activation of T cells by antigen exposure. Thus, CD8 T cells come into contact with and recognize cancer cells at the border of the tumor nest but some functional barrier prevents their infiltration. This conclusion may not apply across the board. For instance, we observed that the expression of genes regulating physical barriers was in some cases inversely correlated with the ICR signature.[33] This observation suggests that when mechanical barriers prevent T cell infiltration, no direct contact occurs between cancer cells and T cells and, therefore, no activation of immune effector gene signatures can be observed. Since this latter study did not include extensive histological examination of the samples, it remains unknown whether the inverse correlation relates to immune silent or represents a functionally distinct sub-type of immune-excluded cancers. Thus, we suggest that immune exclusion may be dependent on separate categories of determinants. In some cases, T cells

reach the tumor side and engage a dialogue with cancer cells but functional mechanisms block their penetration and expansion within the tumor core. We define this category as *functional barriers*. Alternatively, T cells may be prevented from engagement with cancer cells by structural components of the stroma that build a mechanical separation. We refer to the latter as *mechanical barriers*.

Functional barriers may not be present in baseline conditions, but they may be induced only when contact occurs between T cells and cancer cells, preventing subsequent infiltration into tumor nests.[77,147,148] As discussed later, we refer to this concept as dynamic barriers.

In summary, we propose that determinants of immune exclusion can be grouped into three categories: (1) mechanical barriers that pose a physical impediment, preventing engagement between T cells and cancer cells; (2) functional barriers that consist of constitutive biological and/or metabolic interactions between cancer, stromal, and immune cells limiting the migration, function, and/or survival of T cells; and, lastly, (3) dynamic barriers that are induced upon the interaction between cancer and immune cells, preventing further T cell recruitment, migration, and/or survival.

Distinguishing these three mechanisms of immune exclusion has important implications in guiding novel IO therapeutics aimed at overcoming immune resistance. Lack of chemo-attraction of T cells to the tumor site may not be the rate-limiting factor for successful antitumor immune response in immune-excluded tumors as it is for immune-silent cancers as suggested by the [111]Indium-labelled TIL study.[115] Immune-excluded tumors may be susceptible, for instance, to ACT since T cells reach the cancer site and recognize cancer cells. Thus, the focus in the case of immune exclusion should be on overcoming mechanical and/or functional/dynamic barriers.[182-184]

MECHANISMS OF IMMUNE EXCLUSION

To our knowledge, there is no integrated understanding of the role played by postulated models of immune exclusion in human cancers. It is unknown whether the plethora summarized in Table 17.1 corresponds to a random distribution across different cancer types or a predominant mechanism is responsible in most cases.

An integrated approach to resolving the enigma of immune exclusion should include the simultaneous analysis of biomarkers that are representative of the distinct mechanisms of immune exclusion. This approach can identify associations that may have similar upstream mechanistic determinants. To further improve upon this, a topographical analysis, surveying the centripetal gradients within individual tumor nests, should be included. Such comprehensive analyses have never been done on human cancer samples, and we encourage such efforts as part of the systematic.[8] A better understanding of the dominant mechanisms leading to immune exclusion, and their causation, may lead to a better rationale for drug development and the selection of sound combination therapies.

Here, we separate the potential mechanisms according to three main categories (Table 17.1):

Mechanical Barriers

Physical Impediment Preventing Contact Between T Cells and Cancer Cells

The *extracellular matrix* (ECM) is a dynamically organized molecular network, comprised of proteoglycans and fibrous proteins.[185] Changes in the composition of the ECM during tumor progression have been well documented and reflect both its biological and biophysical significance.

In tumor tissue, the most common ECM alteration is the increase in collagen deposition, which leads to tumor fibrosis that can act as a physical barrier to T cell infiltration[22-27,186] (Figure 17.3). Collagen fibers make up around 90% of the ECM and confer structural integrity to the molecular mesh.[28] Moreover, they regulate the physical and biochemical properties of the TME, which modulates cancer cell polarity, migration, and signaling.[29,30]

Studies have shown that tumor fibrosis is caused by the activation of recruited and resident fibroblasts and myofibroblasts. Cancer cells secrete molecules responsible for their activation, including *transforming growth factor (TGF)-β*.[31]

TGF-β is largely responsible for the *epithelial-mesenchymal transition (EMT)*, altering the stromal composition.[56,57] This process is also responsible for the development of a mechanical barrier.[33,58-60] Additionally, this pleiotropic cytokine is essential for the induction of fibrotic responses through a cross talk among extracellular matrix components during organ tissue regeneration.

EMT is not the only way in which TGF-β activity may lead to fibrosis in cancer.[37-39] TGF-β is critical for TME to mediate resistance to the immune surveillance mechanism through several direct and indirect mechanisms that restrict T cell trafficking. TGF-β also stimulates the synthesis of ECM proteins, which remodel the molecular network, and acts on the modulation of various cell populations contributing to the development of mesenchymal stromal cells,[38,40] and *cancer-associated fibroblasts (CAFs*; Figure 17.3B).[39]

CAFs bear several immune regulatory properties beyond the generation of fibrous material, contributing simultaneously to the development of both physical and functional barriers. The first mechanism through which CAFs can mediate physical exclusion is through the extracellular matrix that they produce.[187] The second mechanism involves the biosynthesis of CXCL12, which binds and shields cancer cells (Figure 17.3C). Studies have shown that CXCL12 binds to pancreatic ductal adenocarcinoma, colorectal cancer, and ovarian cancer cells.[66,67,68] Accumulation of stromal cells and CXCL12 coating physiologically occurs in non-tumorigenic inflammatory lesions, probably as a means by which injured epithelial cells protect themselves from the adaptive immune system.[188-190]

For its multiple roles in mediating resistance to immune surveillance mechanisms, TGF-β is considered a promising therapeutic target, particularly for immune-silent cancers. However, its role in determining immune exclusion remains indeterminate.[191]

TGF-β is produced by many different cell types and is induced by a variety of factors. An interesting environmental condition in which TGF-β is upregulated is under hypoxic conditions.[41] Hypoxia is an environmental occurrence in which the demand of oxygen exceeds supply. Hypoxia occurs in the majority of solid tumors, where cellular proliferation outgrows its blood supply. Indeed, solid tumors display regions that are permanently or transiently subjected to hypoxia.[42] A family of transcriptional factors called *hypoxia-inducible factors (HIFs)* are stabilized in hypoxia and are responsible for the hypoxic response.[43] HIF-dependent signaling promotes cancer progression, favoring the adaptation and selection of both cancer and stromal cells to the surrounding conditions.[44]

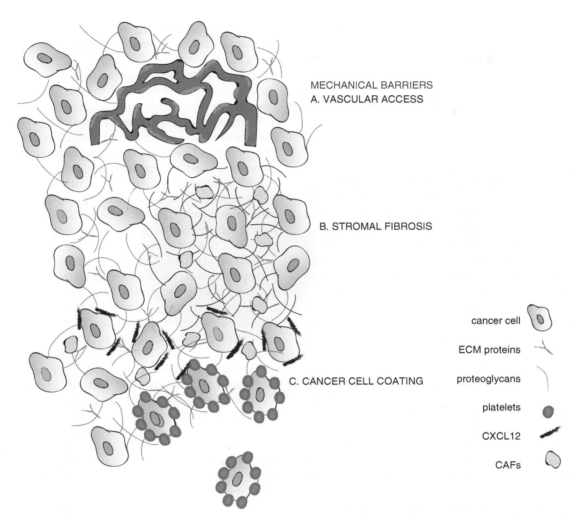

MECHANICAL BARRIERS
A. VASCULAR ACCESS

B. STROMAL FIBROSIS

C. CANCER CELL COATING

cancer cell

ECM proteins

proteoglycans

platelets

CXCL12

CAFs

Figure 17.3 **Mechanical barriers**—Visual representation of the main categories of physical barriers. T cells accessibility can be challenged by a suboptimal vascular structure, an excessive stromal fibrosis, and/or cancer coating molecules. These latter impede the physical accessibility of T cells to cancer cells rather than the infiltration into the tumor nest itself.

CAFs, cancer-associated fibroblasts; ECM, extracellular matrix.

Evidence demonstrates increased TGF-β dependent and independent ECM deposition in hypoxic tumor regions.[45,46] Hypoxia drives the recruitment of fibroblasts and myofibroblasts to the site of pathological fibrosis and induces an increase in collagen gene expression.[47–50] Studies have shown that HIF proteins activate a transcriptional program that results in the degradation of the basement membrane, while simultaneously increasing de novo synthesis of fibrillary collagens.[27] Reducing the levels of HIF-1, but not HIF-2, in vivo results in decreased fibrosis in orthotopic tumors in immune-deficient mice.[51,192]

Cell adhesion molecules are involved in cell-cell and cell-extracellular matrix binding, creating a continuum between the TME and the cell surface. In an effort to identify genes encoding for proteins with mechanical barrier functions, Salerno et al. identified eight genes in two independent cohorts that included 114 metastatic melanoma and 186 ovarian cancer samples.[33]

The expression of the identified genes was inversely correlated with the Th1-like ICR immune signature, and was associated with worse prognosis in patients with melanoma.[33] Specifically, the expression of the desmosomal protein *dystonin* (*DST*) marked cancers lacking the expression of the Th1 immune signature, suggesting that no interactions between T cells and cancer cells were present in these tumors. The other seven genes demarcated a set of cancers characterized by reduced and variable expression of the ICR signature, suggesting that some functional interactions were occurring. Importantly, expression of the latter barrier molecules occurred independently of the expression of endothelin receptor B and, in a mutually exclusive manner, with the activation of the β-catenin signaling pathway, both reported to interfere with T cell infiltration into human cancers. [34,122–124] These observations suggest that several mechanisms of immune exclusion may shape cancer-immune landscapes, and that such mechanisms may at times be mutually exclusive.

Interestingly, expression of DST identified a subset of melanoma cases in which absolute absence of CD8+ gene signatures was observed, but this was not associated with decreased patient survival. Indeed, a stromal mechanical barrier (thick layer of desmoplastic stroma around the tumor) has been linked to a favorable outcome in colorectal liver metastases[193] and to checkpoint inhibitor response in melanoma.[194] Thus, the stroma may affect tumor growth and responsiveness to immunotherapy in different ways by on one hand slowing down tumor growth in a lymphocyte-deprived environment while promoting immune escape in a lymphocyte-enriched environment.[32] This supports the concept that the absolute presence of T cells within a given TME is not a singular prognostic determinant and possibly the ratio between lymphoid over myeloid, or other cellular infiltrate may better define prognostic significance.[159,160,168] This hypothesis, however, was not explored by this study. Limited IHC analyses validated the expression of the barrier molecules at the protein level. In addition, IHC analyses suggested that the expression of proteins that could function as physical barriers was predominantly observed in cancer cells. The expression of these markers was associated morphologically with the cold or immune-silent TME, which is consistent with the exclusion of transcriptional ICR signatures. This suggests that mechanical barriers are more likely to be relevant to the immune-silent than the immune-excluded landscape. Conversely, the truly immune-excluded landscape is likely due to functional rather than physical barriers. More extensive analyses, combining histological with functional methods, are needed to test this hypothesis.

Another mechanism of physical exclusion of T cells could be related to the process of tumor vascularization. Since the proliferation of cancer cells depends on an adequate supply of nutrients and oxygen, angiogenesis is essential for tumor growth. Most solid tumors experience hypoxic conditions as cellular proliferation outgrows blood supply.[195] HIF-1 proteins bind and induce transcription of genes involved in angiogenesis including *vascular endothelial growth factor (VEGF family)*,[52] stromal cell-derived factor 1 (CXCL12), *angiopoietin 2 (ANG2)*,[61] platelet-derived growth factor (CTGF),[53] and stem cell factor (SCF).[54,55] It is likely that hypoxia gives rise to increased levels of VEGF family members, including VEGF-A, -C, and -D, in the TME.[62] VEGF family members play complex and pleiotropic roles in the TME by regulating lymphangiogenesis. Although, intuitively, VEGF should increase lymphocyte infiltration in tumors, due to increased angiogenesis, most studies refute this

concept, demonstrating that anti-angiogenic and vascular normalization therapies enhance immune infiltration of T cells.[63,64,98,196]

Indeed, although tumor angiogenesis is meant to create a new vascular network for the tumor, the resulting vessels are often chaotically organized, leaky, immature, and thin-walled[197] (Figure 17.3A). Newly formed blood vessels are often blunt-ended, unstable, and have inconsistent blood flow.[198] These suboptimal blood vessels are also prone to collapse and diminish the perfused area, creating once again hypoxic conditions.[199]

Therefore, both the lack of vascularization and aberrant vessels morphology have been shown to lead to profound depression of T cell function that, on its own, is sufficient to lead to immune exclusion.[80–84]

Independent of specific receptors mediating T cell transposition across the vascular structures, VEGF seems to play a prominent role by mediating not only the access of immune cells into tumors but also their function.[63,65] In addition, various endothelial receptors may play either facilitator or inhibitor roles by mediating the translocation of immune cells into the extravascular space.[34–36]

Tumor angiogenesis can also be induced by the release of platelet-derived growth factor D.[200] Recent studies in vivo and in vitro show that primary tumors express thrombin, inducing *platelet activation and aggregation*[201,202] In renal cancer cells with high GAL3ST-1 sulfatide expression (HIF-target gene), platelets bind more efficiently to cells, thereby protecting them from natural killer mediated cytotoxicity[203] (Figure 17.3C). Moreover, selective inhibition of platelet activity in patients with malignant tumors reduced tumor growth.[204–206] The role of platelets in shielding tumor cells from the immune system could be another layer of complexity added to this overview of physical barriers.

Functional Barriers

Pre-Existing Biological and/or Metabolic Interactions Between Cancer, Stromal, and Immune Cells Limiting the Migration, Function, and/or Survival of T Cells

The mechanisms limiting immune infiltration through adaptive or innate interactions are extensive. Additionally, other mechanisms may indirectly confer immune exclusion by dampening the production of pro-inflammatory and/or chemo-attractive signals. For example, innate immune cells may be inefficient at processing and presenting apoptotic cancer cells for immune activation because of the presence of *"don't eat me signals,"*[119–121] and/or other tolerogenic mechanisms in which cancer cells may die as discussed later.

A comprehensive discussion about individual theories, proposed to explain a functional basis for immune exclusion, is beyond the purpose of this chapter, and we refer to the content arranged into sub-categories in Table 17.1. Here, we are limiting the discussion to principles that reflect similar biological facets.

A first category of functional barriers is represented by metabolic alterations specific to the TME (Figure 17.4A). Schwartz et al.[121] suggested that most of the hallmarks of cancer can be attributed to the *Warburg effect*, where, even under aerobic conditions, cancer cells favor glycolysis over oxidative phosphorylation. According to this view, the metabolic impairment of oxidative phosphorylation triggers a cascade of events that include the fractal shape of tumors, the secretion of collagen by CAFs, and the production of lactic acid. These events trigger the induction of an acid TME with direct and indirect effects of innate and adaptive immune functions. Furthermore, this can induce an increase in intracellular alkalosis in cancer cells and can alter functions of the mitochondria. This phenomenon can lead to dysregulation of the ion concentration in the TME, with its increasingly recognized effects on T cell function.[72,73,85] Whether this hypothesis or modifications of it, including the reverse Warburg effect, whereby cancer cells induce aerobic glycolysis in neighboring CAFs,[74] is correct is debatable as discussed by Xu et al.[207] However, its weight is not as important as the general concept suggested by the authors that efforts should be placed to identify convergent views regarding this otherwise chaotic portrait of immune exclusion. We propose that functional barriers could be categorized into those determined by metabolic alterations specific to the TME, as illustrated previously for example by the Warburg effect.[72,75,76]

Like the Warburg effect, hypoxia itself may represent a principal component of immune exclusion, mediating direct and indirect immune infiltration and function. VEGF has been shown to mediate direct and indirect immune suppression through a series of distinct mechanisms,[65] once again pointing out that the border between physical and functional barriers is not always well demarcated. Often, the same pathways may lead to contrasting effects due to the pleiotropic properties of the cells involved and the factors that they secrete. To complicate things, it has been shown that VEGF family members can be overexpressed constitutively by cancer cells independent of hypoxic conditions.[97,208,209]

Chemo-attraction (and lack thereof) is a factor that regulates immune infiltration (Figure 17.4B). While several chemokines have been implicated in the recruitment of T cells and other immune effector cells to the TME, it appears that CXCR3 and CC5 ligand chemokines play a dominant role in immune surveillance, and significantly correlate with CD8 T cell infiltration as part of the ICR signature.[96,161,163,210] The central role that these two families of cytokines play in immune surveillance has been clearly established for both immune-active and immune-silent cancers, as they are tightly correlated to these two phenotypes.[12] However, the question about the role they may play in the context of immune-excluded tumors remains unclear. Intuitively, these or other T cell-attracting chemokines should be present to attract T cells at the periphery of tumor nests, although this presumption has never been tested. As such, it is possible that, for unknown reasons, an abrupt reduction in the gradient of chemo-attraction from the center to the periphery, such as expression of CXCR3 and CCR5 associated chemokines, may reduce the chemo-attractive propulsion that occurs at the periphery. For instance, it has recently been suggested that chemokine expression in melanoma is modulated by cancer cell-intrinsic pathways, such as microphthalmia-associated transcription factor, whose expression is associated with that of CXCL-10.[211] Alternatively, while the expression of these chemokines is stably maintained within the concentric circles of the tumor nest, additional overpowering repulsive mechanisms, emanated from the center, may counterbalance the attractive signals gradually limiting the progression of T cells.

An increasing gradient of repulsing signals is best exemplified by TGF-β. As previously mentioned, this extremely pleiotropic factor exercises effects on the TME way beyond the stimulation of the production of fibrotic material.[38,39] Beyond its effects on stromal cells including CAFs, TGF-β acts directly on immune cells, in particular CD4+ T cells.[99,100]

Evolving patterns of cell death from the germinal center to the periphery may create a gradient of increasing chemo-attraction. At the periphery, cancer cells may rapidly dedifferentiate from a stem cell-like core to a degenerate progeny prone to ICD.[109–111] This could be tested by surface expression of calreticulin or other ICD markers.[212] Alternatively, cancer cell death might occur only at the periphery while the "germinal" centers continue to actively proliferate, and this could be tested using proliferation markers. Thus, *DAMPs* may be present only at the periphery. To our knowledge, this possibility has never been assessed and remains only speculative. One option is that various mechanisms affecting the processing of stressed or dying cells may play a significant role by dampening pro-inflammatory signals. These mechanisms include adenosine signaling,[101,112–114,213] TAM receptor tyrosine kinases,[115–117,214] and the *"don't eat me"* signals through the CD47/signal regulatory protein (SIRP)-α interactions.[114,119–121]

Extracellular adenosine is an almost ubiquitous component of tissues exposed to stress. It is generated in response to pro-inflammatory conditions, in particular hypoxia,[114] when stressed cells release ATP. The latter is then degraded by CD39 into AMP and subsequently turned into adenosine by CD73. Adenosine, in turn, interacts with several G-protein-coupled receptors that are ubiquitously expressed on the surface of most immune

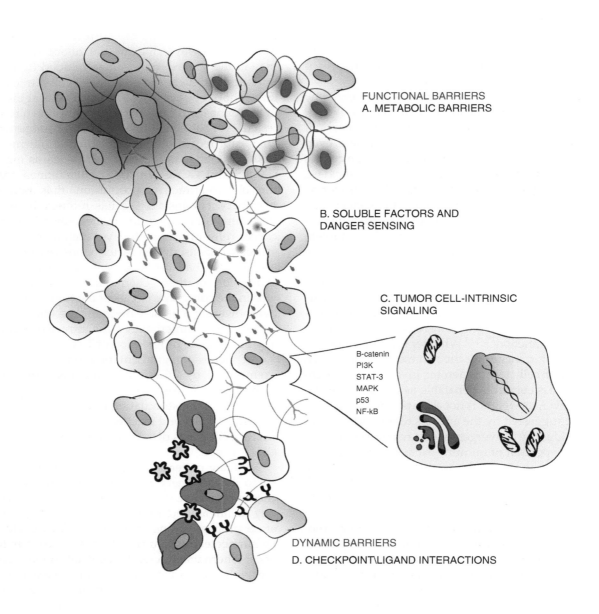

FUNCTIONAL BARRIERS
A. METABOLIC BARRIERS

B. SOLUBLE FACTORS AND
DANGER SENSING

C. TUMOR CELL-INTRINSIC
SIGNALING

B-catenin
PI3K
STAT-3
MAPK
p53
NF-kB

DYNAMIC BARRIERS

D. CHECKPOINT\LIGAND INTERACTIONS

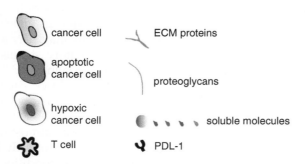

cancer cell

apoptotic
cancer cell

hypoxic
cancer cell

T cell

ECM proteins

proteoglycans

soluble molecules

PDL-1

Figure 17.4 Functional and dynamic barriers—Visual representation of the main categories of functional and dynamic barriers. Among functional barriers are listed metabolic barriers, soluble factor and danger sensing molecules, and tumor cell-intrinsic signaling. Dynamic barriers are consequence of the first encounter between T cells and cancer cells, for example, the inducible activation of PDL-1 in response to IFN-γ signaling.

ECM, extracellular matrix; IFN, interferon.

cells. These receptors promote anti-inflammatory responses as described by Young A et al.[213] Similarly, TAM receptors (Tyro3, AXL, and Mertk) are tyrosine kinases that orchestrate a prominent regulatory role, particularly on innate immune cell functions by promoting the phagocytosis of apoptotic cells and inhibiting inflammation.[214] Through this process, TAM receptors inhibit natural dendritic cell and macrophage maturation signals. Consequently, their targeting promotes the activation of immune responses against cancer as exemplified by the potentiation of radiation effects by the inhibition of Mertk.[117] Similar to TAM receptors, other cancer cell/immune checkpoint interactions may occur as exemplified by CD47/SIPR-α interactions.[119–121,215,216] Although CD47 interacts with its ligand, which is expressed by cells of the myeloid lineage, inhibiting phagocytosis and clearance of dying cells, it also has a direct anti-inflammatory role through the activation of innate immune effector cells. Thus, it could be considered a cell surface checkpoint molecule that can be a target for immunotherapy.

A final category of potential functional mechanisms of immune exclusion is represented by the direct effect that cancer-intrinsic signaling pathways can play in modulating chemo-attractive signals and immune-modulatory responses (Figure 17.4C). Among them, the role played by tumor cell-intrinsic signal transducer and activator of transcription (STAT)-3[133–136] and phosphatidylinositol-4, 5-bisphosphate 3-kinase (PI3K)[125,128–132,136] signaling have been extensively described. In addition, the contribution of alterations in β-catenin[122–124,126,127] and MAPK[3,4] signaling have been described. Interestingly, both PI3K and STAT-3 signaling are prominent features of myeloid cell activation,[135,136,143,217] and their role in immune modulation is often confused with the genuine alteration of intrinsic cancer pathways. Interestingly, most studies on the dysregulation of the PI3K pathway refer to mutations of genes involved in cancer cell signaling. However, the same pathway is critical in the activation of myeloid suppressor dendritic cell function downstream of TAM receptor signaling.[117] This functional signature is totally independent of the cancer cells' mutational status and is purely related to immune cell functions determined by other signaling mechanisms. For instance, we noticed that transcriptional signatures associated with activation of the PI3K pathway were most frequently observed in immune-active cancers.[12,166] This activation was likely due to the myeloid cells. However, in those tumors, no specific somatic mutations relevant to cancer cell biology were noted, particularly related to STAT-3 and PI3K. Conversely, β-catenin and MAPK activation have been associated with the mutational status of genes within the respective pathways and are, therefore, considered to be purely related to activation of cancer cell-intrinsic pathways.[180,181] However, we believe that both mechanisms are not likely to be relevant to immune exclusion as both

are tightly associated with the immune-silent cancer phenotype and the absolute lack of expression of the ICR signature.[12] Roelands et al. recently validated this observation in a set of 9,282 tumor samples in a Pan-cancer analysis of cancer of 31 different histologies (Roelands et al., in press), but no specific analysis attempting to match morphologic features with transcriptional activation have been done to verify this assumption.

Other interesting cancer-intrinsic signaling pathways with potential roles in immune exclusion are p53 and NF-kB signaling. Intact p53 pathway is associated with the recruitment and activation of innate immune cells.[144] However, somatic mutations involving TP53 have been detected in more than 50% of human solid tumors, and p53 mutations represent an early event in carcinogenesis.[145] An in vivo study, using a mouse model of liver carcinoma, showed that tumor regression associated with inducible re-expression of wild-type p53 was dependent on the activation and recruitment of NK cells.[146] Moreover, a close correlation between wild-type p53 and the presence of T cells in the TME of triple-negative breast cancer cells was detected in a study testing the interaction between TP53 mutations and integrative cluster analysis in 1,420 breast tumors.[137]

The contribution of NF-kB signaling to the immune-excluded phenotype seems to be more elusive. Several studies show how the impact of NF-kB activation on host immunity may depend on the cellular context. Indeed, activation of this pathway in cancer cells has been associated both with tumor progression[138,139] and with activation of cytotoxic immune cells against early stage cancer cells.[140] Treatment with the NF-kB inhibitor DHMEQ reversed the immunosuppression of human dendritic cells and macrophages cultured in the supernatant of epithelial ovarian cancer cells.[141,142] It has also been shown that NF-kB signaling pathways increase the production of cytokines and regulate adhesion molecules involved in T cell recruitment within the TME.[218]

Dynamic Barriers

Biological Interactions Between Cancer and T Cells That Result in Limited Function

As previously described, the regulatory interactions that limit T cell infiltration into tumor nests may not be present in baseline conditions but develop as a consequence of the first encounter between T cells and cancer cells. This is well exemplified by the inducible activation of PDL-1 in response to IFN-γ signaling.

In head and neck squamous cell carcinoma, programmed cell death protein-1 (PD-1) is observable in functionally anergic PD-1 expressing TILs at the periphery of tumor nests. The latter are flanked by tumors and/or CD68+ TAMs that express programmed death ligand-1

(PD-L1). This suggests that a functional cross-check occurs dynamically at the initial encounter between T cell and cancer cells, possibly triggered by the production of IFN-γ by T cells upon exposure, to cognate stimulation (Figure 17.4D). This, in turn, induces expression of PD-L1 by either cancer cells or TAMs that serve as a negative feedback loop to limit the function of CD4[+] and CD8[+] T cells[147] (Figure 17.1). Similarly, close dynamic interactions between PD-1[+] CD8[+] T cells and PD-L1 expression cancer cells, and/or CD68[+] TAMs, were reported in human papillomavirus-associated HNSSC.[148] Finally, a cross talk between T cells and dendritic cells expressing PD-L1 in response to IFN-γ and IL-12 stimulation plays a critical role in modulating immune responsiveness.[77] Whether these dynamic interactions may be at the basis of immune exclusion of T cells has not been sufficiently investigated. We believe that future studies should include extensive analyses integrating transcriptional with morphological description of cancer-immune phenotypes. Finally, future studies are needed to more closely investigate the interaction between T cells and B lymphocytes, which are often clustered in extratumoral lymphoid aggregates called tertiary lymphoid structures (TLS).[219] Like the T cell excluded phenotype, TLS can be observed and quantified in IHC histological images. Whether there is an added predictive clinical value of quantifying T cell topography and TLS together remains to be tested in clinical cohorts.

CONCLUSION

Improved understanding of the mechanisms that drive immune exclusion has important clinical implications in the development of novel therapeutic strategies aimed to overcome immune resistance against IO agents, including ACT. It remains to be clarified whether a predominant biology is at the basis of most immune-excluded cases.

Future studies may reveal that a complex combination of mechanical, functional, and dynamic barriers may shape the immune biology of individual tumors. In particular, future studies may clarify the prognostic and predictive role of immune topographies across human solid tumors. This would attest to the need for more in-depth precision medicine-based molecular and histological characterization to be implemented for the selection of appropriate monotherapy or combination therapeutics.

KEY REFERENCES

Only key references appear in the print edition. The full reference list appears in the digital product on Springer Publishing Connect: connect.springerpub.com/content/book/978-0-8261-3743-2/part/part01/chapter/ch17

1. Kather JN, Suarez-Carmona M, Charoentong P, et al. Topography of cancer-associated immune cells in human solid tumors. *Elife*. 2018;7:e36967. doi:10.7554/eLife.36967
2. Pai SI, Cesano A, Marincola FM. The paradox of cancer immune exclusion: immune oncology next frontier. *Cancer Treat Res*. 2020;180:173–195. doi:10.1007/978-3-030-38862-1_6
8. Bedognetti D, Ceccarelli M, Galluzzi L, et al. Toward a comprehensive view of cancer immune responsiveness: a synopsis from the SITC workshop. *J Immunother Cancer*. 2019;7(1):131. doi:10.1186/s40425-019-0602-4
12. Turan T, Kannan D, Patel M, et al. Immune oncology, immune responsiveness and the theory of everything. *J Immunother Cancer*. 2018;6(1):50. doi:10.1186/s40425-018-0355-5
89. Munn DH, Bronte V. Immune suppressive mechanisms in the tumor microenvironment. *Curr Opin Immunol*. 2016;39:1–6. doi:10.1016/j.coi.2015.10.009
154. Pockaj BA, Sherry RM, Wei JP, et al. Localization of [111]indium-labeled tumor infiltrating lymphocytes to tumor in patients receiving adoptive immunotherapy. Augmentation with cyclophosphamide and correlation with response. *Cancer*. 1994;73(6):1731–1737. doi:10.1002/1097-0142(19940315)73:6<1731::AID-CNCR2820730630>3.0.CO;2-H
156. Galon J, Costes A, Sanchez-Cabo F, et al. Type, density, and location of immune cells within human colorectal tumors predict clinical outcome. *Science*. 2006;313(5795):1960–1964. doi:10.1126/science.1129139

18

Cancer Biomarkers: Tumor-Infiltrating T Cells, Programmed Death-Ligand 1, and Tumor Mutation Burden

Colt Egelston, Weihua Guo, and Peter P. Lee

KEY POINTS

- Early work profiling the immune tumor microenvironment (TME) demonstrated the importance of preexisting T cell infiltration into tumors for response to immune checkpoint blockade (ICB).

- Programmed death-ligand 1 (PD-L1) expression, likely as a marker of T cell effector activity and interferon-γ (IFN-γ) production within tumors, is currently the main biomarker used to predict patient response to ICB.

- Elevated tumor IFN-γ-pathway-related transcriptomic signatures are associated with response to ICB in a variety of cancers.

- Somatic mutation-based "neoantigens" are thought to be a key component in generating antitumor T cell responses. High tumor mutation burden (TMB) and microsatellite instability high (MSI-H) tumors have demonstrated the greatest benefit to ICB.

- No biomarker is perfect. Current ICB biomarkers, when predictive, may apply to most, but not all, patients. Disease and tumor-specific features must also be carefully considered going forward.

- Integrating tumor, systemic, and dynamic features of response will be important toward the development of improved biomarkers for ICB.

INTRODUCTION

The immune contexture of tumors is now undisputed as a critical determinant of patient survival. As immunotherapy-based treatments have exploded over the last decade, exploration of various tumor immune components has expanded from understanding their role in prognosis to harnessing them for improved patient outcomes via immunotherapy. Continued efforts today focus on further understanding the mechanisms that drive response to immunotherapy, especially in the context of either durable responses or therapeutic resistance.

In this chapter we summarize the current knowledge regarding tumor immune biomarkers of response to immune checkpoint blockade (ICB) and look to the future as next generation biomarkers are developed. We will discuss general features of the antitumor immune response, especially in the context of biomarkers of prognosis. We will then discuss the application of these concepts in understanding mechanisms of ICB efficacy and identifying immune biomarkers of response. Finally, we will examine tumor mutation burden (TMB) as a key driver of immune responses and present the current state of TMB-based predictive biomarkers for ICB.

IMMUNE BIOMARKERS FOR IMMUNE CHECKPOINT BLOCKADE

Evidence for the Survival Benefit of Antitumor Immunity in Treatment of Naïve Patients

T cell infiltration into tumors has long been associated with positive prognostic outcomes in numerous cancer types. Pretreatment tumors with higher levels of tumor-infiltrating lymphocytes (TILs) have been associated with longer overall survival and response to chemotherapy. Accumulation of these findings in a variety of cancer types provided significant evidence for de novo antitumor immune activity in patients. Thus, boosting these immune responses, especially antitumor T cells, became the focus of modern ICB-based immunotherapy.

Early immunohistochemistry-guided research studies identified the prognostic impact of T cells, specifically CD8+ T cells, in a variety of carcinomas. The presence of intratumoral CD8+ T cells has been linked to improved survival in esophageal, lung, breast, melanoma, colorectal, and renal cell carcinoma (RCC), among others.[1-6] This evidence, coupled with clinical efforts to treat cancer patients with IL-2 to augment antitumor T cell function or expand autologous T cells ex vivo for therapy with adoptive cell transfer, accelerated modern immunotherapy approaches.[7,8]

As evidence for the positive impact of TILs on survival of cancer patients accumulated, more sophisticated techniques to assess lymphocyte subsets and their spatial localization within tumors developed. Such efforts were necessary not just to address heterogeneity of the tumor infiltrate immune contexture, but also to address heterogeneity of immune cell localization.[9] In a prominent example of this, the Immunoscore assay defines tumors based on the densities of both CD3+ and CD8+ T lymphocytes within the tumor center and tumor invasive margin. Using automated quantitative imaging software, Immunoscore highlights the positive correlation of patient survival and tumor infiltration by CD8+ T cells.[10] Large scale validation of such an approach has shown Immunoscore to successfully prognosticate colorectal cancer patients and has led to the suggestion that immune classification of tumors may add significantly to traditional tumor staging.[11] Such seminal work highlights the importance for immune biomarkers in the cancer setting and laid the groundwork for implementation of assessment of other immune biomarkers in the tumor microenvironment (TME).

With the evolution of multiplex immunohistochemistry and immunofluorescence technologies, a deeper understanding of specific CD3+ TIL subsets on patient survival grew. Early Immunoscore work provided evidence that tumors infiltrated with CD45RO expressing memory T cells were those that provided survival benefits to colorectal cancer patients.[12] Other groups demonstrated that CD103-expressing CD8+ T cells were found to be a major component of TILs that positively correlated with patient survival in a variety of cancer types.[13-16] Later these CD103+ T cells were defined as resident memory T cells with long-lived tumor tissue retention and found to be heavily enriched within the cancer islands of patient tumors.[17] Together these findings highlighted the importance of understanding both the type and location of TILs within the TME.

Preexisting T Cell Infiltrate Predicts Response to Immune Checkpoint Blockade

Current ICB therapies primarily rely upon monoclonal antibodies that inhibit the engagement and signaling of checkpoint molecules and their ligands. Checkpoint molecules may be activating or inhibitory. Inhibitory checkpoints act as cellular "brakes" to reduce immune cell effector functions. Although there are many recent U.S. Food and Drug Administration (FDA) approvals for monoclonal antibody pharmaceuticals in several cancer types, their targets are still limited to cytotoxic T lymphocyte-associated protein 4 (CTLA-4), programmed cell death protein-1

(PD-1), and programmed death ligand 1 (PD-L1). While distinct targets, both PD-1- and CTLA-4-mediated inhibition of T cells are thought to primarily act by inhibiting T cell receptor signaling and therefore act to limit antitumor T cell responses. PD-L1-mediated engagement of PD-1 on T cells suppresses T cell receptor and CD28 signaling pathways via a series of phosphorylation events.[18-20] Blockade of PD-1/PD-L1 engagement via PD-1 or PD-L1 targeting antibodies allows for enhanced T cell cytokine production, proliferation, and target cell killing.[21,22]

As understanding of the mechanisms of immune checkpoint molecules matured in the field of basic immunology, attention in tumor immunology turned toward characterizing the presence of these molecules within the TME.[23] Studies showed that the majority of TILs expressed PD-1, often at high levels, and could demonstrate tumor specificity[24,25] In parallel, PD-L1 expression was found to be elevated in human tumor samples, both on cancer cells and tumor-infiltrating myeloid cells.[26,27] Furthermore, tumor-associated PD-L1 was shown to inhibit tumor-infiltrating T cells and this could be reversed with PD-1 or PD-L1 blocking antibodies.[28,29] Other studies characterized tumor-infiltrating T cells as overexpressing various checkpoint molecules and as dysfunctional, with reduced cytokine production and cytolytic capacity.[30-32] Mechanistically, ICB antibodies demonstrated the ability to reverse this T cell "exhaustion" and enable antitumor T cell function.[22] In a culmination of this work, the clinical potential for enhancing antitumor immunity by ICB became clear and resulted in several breakthrough clinical trials for the treatment of melanoma, non-small cell lung cancer (NSCLC), and RCC.[33,34] As such, efforts toward gaining a detailed understanding of immune infiltration in the context of immunotherapy outcomes accelerated.

Early clinical correlates of response to ICB suggested that preexisting T cell infiltrates determined clinical efficacy of CTLA-4 and PD-1 blockade in melanoma patients.[35,36] Similar observations were later made in the setting of NSCLC, head and neck squamous cell carcinoma (HNSCC), colorectal cancer, and Merkel cell carcinoma (see Table 18.1).[43,59,65,81] Together these findings have led to a current conceptual framework for immune classification of tumors based on the degree and localization of T cell infiltration: immune-inflamed, immune-excluded, and immune-desert.[82] Immune-inflamed tumors are characterized by infiltration of T cells into and around the tumor parenchyma (cancer islands), while immune-excluded tumors are defined as those with T cell infiltration restricted to the periphery of the tumor. Immune-desert tumors have little T cell infiltration into either the tumor center or tumor margins.

Exploration of mechanisms for immune-exclusion and immune absence from tumors is currently an active area of research, with the goal of identifying combinatorial therapeutic strategies to enhance response to ICB. In

Table 18.1 Classical Biomarkers for Checkpoint Blockade Response

CANCER TYPE	T CELL INFILTRATION		PD-L1 EXPRESSION	
	SURVIVAL PROGNOSTIC	ICB RESPONSE	SURVIVAL PROGNOSTIC	ICB RESPONSE
Breast (TNBC)	↑[5]	–	↑[37,38]	↑F[39]
Cervical	↑[40]	–	✕[41]	↑F[42]
CRC (MSI-H)	↑[2]	↑[43]	↓[44,45]	✕[46]
Cutaneous SCC	–	–	–	–
Endometrial	↑[47]	–	↑[48]	↑F[49]
Gastric/Esophageal	↑[3,50]	–	↓[51,52]	↑F[53]
HCC	↑[54]	–	↓[55]	↑↓[56,57]
HNSCC	↑[58]	↑[59]	↑[60]	↑[61]
Melanoma	↑[4]	↑[35,36]	↑[62]	↑[63]
Merkel	↑[64]	↑[65]	↑[66]	✕[67]
NSCLC	↑[6]	↑[49]	↑[68]	↑F[69,70]
Renal cell	↓[1]	↑[71]	↓[72]	↑[71,73]
SCLC	–	–	–	✕[74]
Urothelial	↑↓[75,76]	–	↑↓[77,78]	↑F[79]
PMBCL	–	–	–	↑[80]
Hodgkin lymphoma	–	–	–	↑[80]

↑Indicates improved survival. ↓Indicates worse survival. ↑↓Indicates mixed evidence for survival association. ✕ Indicates no observed correlation. F Indicates FDA companion diagnostic.

CRC, colorectal carcinoma; HCC, hepatocellular carcinoma; HNSCC, head and neck squamous cell carcinoma; ICB, immune checkpoint blockade; MSI-H, microsatellite instable-high; NSCLC, non-small cell lung cancer; PD-L1, programmed death ligand 1; PMBCL, primary mediastinal B-cell lymphoma; SCC, squamous cell carcinoma; SCLC, small cell lung cancer; TNBC, triple-negative breast cancer.

addition to a multitude of immunosuppressive features associated with the TME, drivers of tumor immune-exclusion and immune escape may also be cancer cell intrinsic.[83] Increased Wnt-β-catenin pathway signaling, for instance, has been shown to limit immune cell infiltration into tumors.[83] Furthermore, loss of MHC molecule expression, impaired antigen presentation machinery, and loss of interferon-γ (IFN-γ) responsiveness by cancer cells have been demonstrated to be significant means of resistance to ICB therapy.[84–86] In parallel, immune-inflamed tumors are actively being investigated to identify both biomarkers and mechanisms of response to ICB. In general, these tumors display several features of immune activation, including increased IFN-γ-pathway signaling, higher PD-L1 expression, and increased infiltrate of other immune cell subsets.

Tumor Programmed Death Ligand 1 Expression as a Predictor of Response to Immune Checkpoint Blockade

PD-L1 expression is a key mediator of tumor escape from immunosurveillance. In general, PD-L1 protein expression is limited to cancer tissues, with the exception of immune cell rich tissues such as lymph nodes, liver, and lung tissues.[23] When expressed by cancer cells, PD-L1 enables resistance to T cell-mediated cytotoxicity.[87] Additionally, PD-L1 expressed by dendritic cells in the TME suppresses T cell proliferation and tempers the antitumor T cell response.[88] In the fashion of an immune response negative feedback loop, PD-L1 expression is upregulated by IFN-γ signaling.[26] IFN-γ in the TME has primarily been attributed to infiltration of activated CD8+ T cells.[89] Thus, via IFN-γ-mediated PD-L1 expression, CD8+ TILs act to inhibit themselves, allowing for tumor escape.[62] PD-1/PD-L1 blocking antibodies interfere with this immune resistance, allowing for both the expansion and cytolytic activity of antitumor T cells.[90]

PD-L1 expression in the TME is an FDA-approved diagnostic indication for several ICB modalities in various cancer settings (see Table 18.1). However, PD-L1 expression is an imperfect biomarker. FDA indications for what is considered PD-L1 "positive" range in both the degree of expression (positive staining) and cell type to be considered (immune stroma, cancer cells, or both).[91]

For example, while PD-L1 staining is assessed on cancer cells in NSCLC, it is assessed on immune stroma in triple-negative breast cancer (TNBC). In addition, technical issues specific to immunohistochemistry contribute to the discordance in tissue assessment of PD-L1. These may include difficulties in obtaining suitable tumor biopsy tissue, including the use of archival primary tumor rather than metastatic tissue, inconsistencies in tissue storage and fixation, and large interpatient variabilities in time of tissue biopsy acquisition and treatment. In addition to differing scoring techniques, different anti-PD-L1 antibodies are used for different indications (clones 22C3, 28-8, SP142, SP263, 73-10). Together, these technical issues have hampered a clear understanding of PD-L1 biology and response to ICB. Efforts to harmonize the pathology evaluation of PD-L1 expression by immunohistochemistry are ongoing in an effort to improve clinical diagnostics.[92,93] In parallel, more sophisticated multiplex immunofluorescence techniques are being considered as diagnostic tools for immune biomarkers.[94] Finally, RNA sequencing-based approaches to identify PD-L1 expression are being developed in hopes of developing a more accurate detection method.[95]

As a predictive biomarker, tumor PD-L1 expression is generally accepted to reflect two key features of the TME. Most obviously, PD-L1 expression represents the presence of the therapeutic target for anti-PD-1 and anti-PD-L1 antibodies. Secondly, PD-L1 expression signifies the presence of activated T cells and their IFN-γ production. Immunohistochemistry of melanoma tumors has shown PD-L1 upregulation to be most significant in areas enriched with TILs.[62] It is still unclear whether the ICB-induced antitumor T cell response develops within the tumor itself, tumor draining lymph nodes, or both. Early evidence from clinical specimens identified increased T cell mitosis in tumors after ICB.[35] Furthermore, in a murine model in which T cell egress from lymph nodes was inhibited, preexisting TILs were sufficient to reduce tumor burden in response to ICB.[96] However, recent work examining peripheral blood and tumor tissues of patients undergoing ICB has provided evidence for the importance of newly generated T cell clones to infiltrate tumor and replace preexisting T cell clones.[97,98] In light of this, PD-L1 expression in the tumor may more indirectly reflect the capacity of the host immune system or T cell repertoire to respond to tumor antigen. Further work is needed to dissect the connection between systemic immune surveillance and local antitumor activity.

Although initial research efforts on disrupting the PD-1/PD-L1 pathways focused on interactions between T cells and cancer cells, it has long been shown that PD-L1 expression on myeloid cells also plays an important role in attenuating T cell function.[27] Recent evidence suggested that the majority of TME PD-L1 expression is found on myeloid cells, specifically macrophages.[99] Indeed, PD-L1 expression specifically by tumor-infiltrating immune cells has been recognized as a biomarker of ICB response in clinical correlates across several tumor types.[100] While macrophage expression of PD-L1 appears to be a key biomarker predictive of response to ICB, accumulating research suggests that PD-L1+ dendritic cells may be a more critical mechanistic driver of antitumor T cell activity.[88,101] Taken together, it seems that PD-L1 expression by cancer cells primarily provides resistance to T cell killing.[87] More importantly, PD-L1 expression by immune cells, and specifically dendritic cells, tempers the magnitude of the antitumor T cell response which can be amplified by ICB.[102,103]

Despite the clear connection between T cell IFN-γ production and PD-L1 upregulation, mechanisms for PD-L1 expression in the TME are nuanced. It is still perhaps underappreciated that PD-L1 can be upregulated via numerous pathways other than IFN-γ signaling, including GM-CSF, TNF-α, IL-4, and hypoxia.[104] Additionally, constitutive PD-L1 expression may be triggered by genomic alterations, including oncogenic kinase pathway activities, chromosomal translocations, DNA damage, and overactive mutant growth factor receptor pathways.[105–109] Cancer cell intrinsic features such as these result in several cancer type specific features of PD-L1 expression. In colorectal cancer, mutant BRAF drives PD-L1 expression in a subset of tumors. Alterations in the AKT-mTOR pathway, such as epidermal growth factor receptor (EGFR) mutations, generate constitutive PD-L1 expression in a subset of NSCLC tumors.[108,110] In classical Hodgkin lymphoma and PMBCL, chromosomal amplification results in increased PD-L1 copy numbers.[111] Clearly, a variety of cancer cell intrinsic and extrinsic factors may contribute to PD-L1 upregulation, all of which must carefully be considered to infer meaning from tumor PD-L1 expression assays.

Differing clinical outcomes result due to heterogeneity in both mechanisms driving PD-L1 upregulation and the cell types expressing PD-L1. In the context of general survival outcomes, PD-L1 expression is less well-established to benefit patient prognosis as compared to T cell infiltration (see Table 18.1). Tumor PD-L1 expression correlates with improved outcomes in TNBC, endometrial cancer, HNSCC, melanoma, Merkel cell carcinoma, and NSCLC.[37,38,48,60,62,66,68] In contrast, tumor PD-L1 expression correlates with worse outcomes in colorectal cancer, gastric cancer, hepatocellular carcinoma (HCC), and RCC.[44,51,52,55,72] In fact, a subset of colorectal tumors with high PD-L1 expression is associated with poor clinical outcomes despite also having high CD8+ T cell infiltration and other features of immune activation, perhaps reflecting an immune overdrive state.[45] These seemingly contradictory findings likely reflect differing driving forces for PD-L1 expression and demonstrate that tumor PD-L1 can reflect either a potent antitumor T cell response or a more aggressive tumor phenotype. Indeed, tumors enriched in PD-L1 expression driven by macrophage produced cytokines and independently of T cell activation demonstrate poor response to chemotherapy agents.[112] Complementary evidence points to the important role PD-L1 signaling plays in promoting cancer cell survival, proliferation, and metabolic fitness via altered mTOR and autophagy pathways.[113–115] As a result, disruption of PD-L1 activity may also sensitize cancer cells to chemotherapy-mediated cytotoxicity in a T cell independent fashion.[116] Intriguingly, NSCLC tumors with apparent T cell independent PD-L1 expression on cancer cells appear to respond well to anti-PD-L1 ICB.[117] Together these findings remind us that anti-PD-L1 and anti-PD-1 monoclonal antibodies will have differing biological consequences and mechanisms of action in tumor therapy.

In summary, the clinical significance of PD-L1 expression is complex. PD-L1 upregulation may be driven by a variety of different factors, both T cell dependent and independent, and result in mixed downstream consequences for tumor progression. Adding to the difficulty in connecting PD-L1 expression with ICB blockade response is the transient nature of PD-L1 expression within the TME.[118] Currently our view of PD-L1 as a biomarker is limited to generalities of patient response. Clinical observations that both ICB-responsive PD-L1-tumors and ICB nonresponsive PD-L1+ tumors occur indicate a need for improved understanding of ICB mechanisms and checkpoint molecule expression.[119] An integrated perspective of the tissue, cell, and temporal specifics of PD-L1 expression will be necessary for an increased understanding of mechanisms for response to ICB going forward.

Transcriptional Signatures of Response to Checkpoint Blockade

With the complex variety of mechanisms for PD-L1 expression and challenges with its assessment via immunohistochemistry, efforts have been taken toward identifying genomic signatures of response to ICB.[120] This has been enabled thanks to the increasingly common genomic sequencing of patient tumor biopsies prior to initiation of therapy. RNA sequencing offers the ability to rapidly assess numerous biomarkers, while offering similar detection sensitivity as immunohistochemistry approaches.[121] As clinical responses to ICB emerged, it became clear that in addition to elevated T cell infiltration and PD-L1 expression, responsive tumors had a distinct gene expression pattern. This knowledge has enriched our understanding of the immune-inflamed TME and provided numerous insights into mechanisms of response and resistance to ICB.

Initial results of transcriptional profiling of patient tumors set out to identify mechanisms that drive immune-inflamed tumor profiles. Lymphocyte prevalence in melanoma tumor samples was found to correlate with expression of several chemokine genes, including *CCL4, CCL5, CXCL9,* and *CXCL10.*[122] Similar findings have been made in other tumor types, including RCC, HCC, and colorectal cancer.[123–125] In contrast, several gene networks were found to associate with T cell exclusion from tumors. Overactivation of the Wnt/β-catenin pathway in melanoma cancer cells was shown to result in diminished tumor chemokine levels, altered dendritic cell recruitment, and reduced T cell activation.[126] Increased activation of the Wnt/β-catenin, which may result from somatic mutations or copy number variations, was validated to be a major mediator of tumor immune exclusion across several cancer types.[127] Similar evidence for the critical role of Batf3+ dendritic cells (CD103+ dendritic cells in mice) in promoting antitumor T cell responses was found in several other studies.[128,129] A genomic signature of Batf3+ dendritic cells was found to correlate with both lymphocyte infiltration and patient prognosis in HNSCC, breast cancer, and lung cancer.[130] Observations for these have highlighted the tight interplay between cancer cells, myeloid cells, and lymphocytes in the generation of an immune-inflamed TME.

T cell infiltration into tumors is generally correlated with gene expression for checkpoint molecules, such as PD-L1, TIM-3, and LAG-3.[131] In the context of ICB, pre-existing genomic signatures of T cell activation in tumor tissues were quickly shown to correlate with clinical responses. Anti-CTLA-4 responsive melanoma tumors display higher levels of *GZMA* and *PRF1,* both involved in cytotoxicity, and *CTLA-4* itself.[132] Given the relationship between T cell activation, IFN-γ production, and PD-L1 upregulation, it was no surprise that IFN-γ signaling pathway genes were commonly found elevated in tumor biopsies of ICB-responsive patients. IFN-γ-related genes have been correlated with response to ICB in melanoma, HNSCC, NSCLC, and RCC.[100,133–135] Furthermore, tumor transcriptional profiling using the Nanostring platform has identified an 18-gene IFN-γ-related signature which includes *IFNG, STAT1, CCR5, CXCL9, CXCL10, CXCL11, IDO1, PRF1, GZMA,* and *HLA-DRA.* The Nanostring IFN-γ signature has demonstrated predictive value for anti-PD-1-treated melanoma, gastric, and HNSCC patients and is seeking FDA approval as a companion diagnositic.[135] In contrast to an IFN-γ signature, increased TGF-β signaling in bladder tumors imparts T cell exclusion features and resistance to anti-PD-L1 therapy.[136] Similarly, loss of IFN-γ response elements, antigen presentation machinery, and HLA molecules is a major mechanism of resistance to ICB.[85,137,138] Along with immune centric signatures, other gene expression patterns have been correlated with response to ICB. *PTEN* loss in melanoma cancer cells is correlated with reduced response to ICB, apparently due to increased production of immunosuppressive cytokines.[139] Genes associated with mesenchymal cell transition and wound healing contribute to a tumor innate anti-PD-1 resistance (termed IPRES) phenotype in melanoma patients.[140]

In addition to the increase in whole transcriptome sequencing of patient samples, other technical and bioinformatic advances have greatly enabled an expanded view of the TME. Nanostring technology, which enables rapid and accurate gene expression detection using FFPE tissue, has allowed for a wealth of data to be extracted from archived tissue samples.[141] As sequencing data became widely accessible, this facilitated assessment of tumor-infiltrating immune cells in greater detail. Deconvolution algorithms such as Cibersort and xCell have become popular tools to rapidly identify a general picture of the immune tumor contexture.[142,143] T cell receptor (TCR) sequencing, which can assess the clonality of a T cell response, is now widely available to researchers through several commercial platforms. Varied evidence for preexisting TIL clonality and ICB responses has been observed, and may depend greatly on the modality of ICB therapy.[35,144] Assessment of the TCR repertoire before and after initiation of ICB therapy may be helpful to understanding the dynamics of the antitumor T cell response, as oligoclonal T cell expansion has been identified in ICB responders.[145,146] More recent advancements with single-cell sequencing technology, which allows for assessment of gene expression and TCR sequencing in the same cell, will continue to improve our understanding of T cell dynamics in response to ICB. Genomic sequencing information has rapidly advanced our understanding of ICB mechanisms and provided several potential biomarkers of response. Machine learning and artificial intelligence techniques to harness such data are also quickly advancing. As an example of this, an "immunophenoscore" demonstrated significant predictive power across multiple ICB treatment cohorts.[147] Ongoing bioinformatic efforts such as these will undoubtedly continue to disentangle the complexity of the TME and mechanisms of ICB response.

Upcoming Immune Tumor Biomarkers of Response to Checkpoint Blockade

As our understanding of the antitumor response grows, new potential biomarkers of ICB response are emerging (see Table 18.2). In recent years, much focus has been paid to detailing facets of antitumor CD8+ T cell biology in the context of ICB. CD8+ T cells that accumulate in tumors often become "exhausted," which includes loss of function, terminal differentiation, and loss of memory cell potential.[158] ICB has widely been viewed as "reinvigorating" exhausted T cells due to the induction of more effective antitumor T cell immunity.[158] Perhaps as a marker of significant antitumor

Table 18.2 Upcoming Biomarkers for Checkpoint Blockade Response

POTENTIAL BIOMARKER	CANCER TYPE EVIDENCE OBSERVED IN
IFN-γ signature	Gastric, HNSCC, melanoma, RCC[133,148]
B cell/CXCL13	Melanoma, RCC, urothelia[149,150]
Exhausted T cell subsets	HNSCC, melanoma, NSCLC[151–153]
Innate anti-PD-1 resistance signature (IPRES)	Melanoma[140]
PTEN loss	Melanoma[139]
Lower TGF-β signature	Urothelial[136]
T cell receptor oligoclonality	Melanoma[35,144]
Microbiome diversity	Melanoma[154,155]
Circulating classical monocyte levels	Melanoma[156]
Circulating effector memory T cell levels	Melanoma[157]

HNSCC, head and neck squamous cell carcinoma; IFN-γ, interferon gamma; NSCLC, non-small cell lung cancer; RCC, renal cell carcinoma; TGF-β, transforming growth factor beta.

activity, increased tumor infiltration of exhausted CD8+ T cells expressing high levels of PD-1 and a unique transcriptomic signature have been found to correlate with ICB response in NSCLC patients.[151] However, similar T cell subsets have been associated with reduced response to ICB in HPV viral negative HNSCC patients.[152] Sophisticated single-cell analysis of melanoma tumor samples has identified transcription factor TCF7+ CD8+ T cells as important precursors to exhausted T cells and as a key determinant of ICB response.[153] In parallel, other research has shown that ICB induces tumor infiltration by new T cells with distinct clonality from preexisting exhausted T cells found in the tumor, suggesting that preexisting exhausted T cells may not play a direct role in antitumor activity.[98] Together this data suggests that T cell responses to ICB are highly dynamic at the transcriptional and clonal level. Further dissection of such mechanisms will be critical toward understanding durable responses to ICB.

Evidence has suggested that features of the immune tumor landscape other than T cells also play an important role in therapeutic response. Mounting evidence points toward intratumoral B cell activity as a significant biomarker of response to ICB in a number of cancer types. Several groups have identified upregulation of the B cell chemoattractant CXCL13, increased numbers of tumor-infiltrating B cells, and matured tertiary lymphoid structures (TLSs) in the ICB responsive tumors of bladder cancer, RCC, melanoma, and sarcoma patients.[149,150,159]

Notably, CXCL13 has been found to be highly expressed by exhausted CD8[+] T cells, perhaps connecting the antitumor T cell and B cell response.[160] Preclinical research suggests tumor-infiltrating B cells may be critical to ICB efficacy, and not just a biomarker of response.[161] While mechanisms for B cell contribution to the antitumor response have not been fully elucidated, the capacity for antibody-producing B cells to contribute to a durable, long-lasting antitumor immune response is intriguing. Given the apparent antitumor role of infiltrating B cells, it is surprising that follicular-like CD4[+] T cells seem to mediate suppressive function and correlate with worse prognosis in ICB-treated melanoma patients.[162] Conversely, peripheral expanding ICOS[+] CD4[+] T cells have been noted as a biomarker of response to anti-CTLA-4 therapy in melanoma patients.[163] Efforts to understand features of the TME that drive antitumor T cell responses are ongoing. As one example, clusters of dendritic cells and natural killer (NK) cells in melanoma patient tumors appear to be critical for efficacy of ICB.[164] CD4[+] T cells likely play a similar role in promoting dendritic cell function in the TME.[165] Thus, current evidence suggests that a concerted effort between T cells, B cells, and dendritic cells is required to generate immune-inflamed tumors associated with ICB response (see Figure 18.1).

Moving beyond the tumor, systemic features of host immune activity in ICB-treated patients are being examined. Peripheral blood correlates have found preexisting levels of circulating effector memory T cells and nonclassical monocytes to correlate with response to ICB in melanoma patients.[156,157] Samples collected over the course of treatment provide valuable dynamic data and show rapid

expansion of peripheral T cells.[166–168] The impact of the gut microbiome on ICB response and on systemic immune function in general is now becoming more appreciated. Although evidence for the impact of individual bacterial strains has not been identified, the diversity of patient microbiome correlates with anti-PD-1 and anti-CTLA-4 efficacy in melanoma patients.[154,155] Preclinical research has found modulating the gut microbiome may improve responses to ICB, but currently clinical evidence of this is still lacking.[169] Clearly, the role of the local and systemic immune responses in promoting response to ICB is multifaceted. Continued co-evolution technological advances, basic tumor immunology research, and therapeutic development will rapidly accelerate therapeutic successes in the clinic.

TUMOR MUTATION BURDEN IN CANCER IMMUNOTHERAPY

As an emerging, promising, and the latest FDA-approved biomarker for immune checkpoint inhibitor (ICI) therapy, TMB has been validated to be associated with patient outcomes and clinical responses in multiple clinical trials. In this subsection, we will first introduce the basic principles of TMB and other related genetic markers (i.e., microsatellite instability and neoantigen loading), basis in TMB measurement and calculation, and the association between TMB and other biomarkers. We will also present a comprehensive comparison across different technical platforms (panels) for TMB. In addition, we will summarize the clinical applications of TMB in ICI therapy, presented in Table 18.3 based on cancer types.

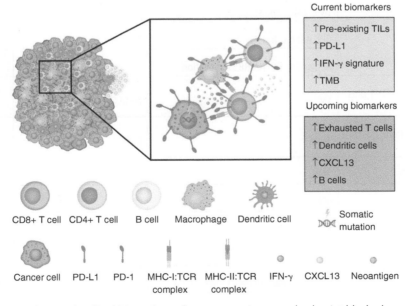

Figure 18.1 Schematic summary of tumor localized biomarkers of response to immune checkpoint blockade.

Source: Illustration created with Biorender.com.

Table 18.3 Summary of Published Studies on the Clinical Relevance of Tumor Mutation Burden and Other Genetic Markers to Cancer Immunotherapies

ICI THERAPY	GENETIC BIOMARKER	CANCER TYPE	CLINICAL BENEFITS		
			RR	PFS	OS
Ipilimumab (anti-CTLA-4)[170]	TMB, neopeptide signature	Melanoma	−	−	↑
Ipilimumab (anti-CTLA-4)[132]	TMB, neoantigen loading	Melanoma	−	↑	↑
Pembrolizumab or nivolumab (anti-PD-1)[140]	TMB	Melanoma	−	−	↑
	BRCA2 mutation		↑	−	↑
Pembrolizumab or atezolizumab (anti-PD-1 or anti-PD-L1)[171]	TMB	Melanoma	↑	↑	↑
Anti-CTLA-4 plus anti-PD-1[144]	TMB	Melanoma	×	−	−
	Copy number loss		↓	−	−
Ipilimumab (anti-CTLA-4)[146]	TMB	Melanoma	↑	↑	↑
Nivolumab (anti-PD-1)[146]	Clonal persistence	Melanoma	↓	↓	↓
Ipilimumab (anti-CTLA-4)[63]	TMB	Melanoma	↑	−	×
	CGP (response score)	Melanoma	↑	−	↑
Pembrolizumab (anti-PD-1)[172]	TMB, neoantigen	NSCLC	↑	↑	−
Anti-PD-(L)1 or plus anti-CTLA-4[173]	TMB (+ PD-L1)	NSCLC	↑	↑	−
	CNA, EGFR variants, STK11 variants		↓	−	−
Nivolumab plus ipilimumab (anti-PD-1 plus anti-CTLA-4)[174]	TMB	NSCLC	↑	↑	−
Anti-PD-(L)1[175]	TMB, FAT1 mutation	NSCLC	↑	↑	−
	CPL related to ITGA9		−	↓	↓
	Activating EGFR/ERBB2 mutation		−	↓	−
Nivolumab plus ipilimumab (anti-PD-1 plus anti-CTLA-4)[176]	TMB	NSCLC	↑	↑	−
Nivolumab plus/or ipilimumab (anti-PD-1 plus/or anti-CTLA-4)[177]	TMB	SCLC	↑	↑	[1]↑
Anti-PD-1 plus/or anti-CTLA-4[178]	TMB	SCLC	×	↑	↑
Atezolizumab (anti-PD-L1)[179]	bTMB	NSCLC	×	↑	↑
Anti-PD-1 and anti-PD-L1[180]	bTMB	NSCLC	↑	↑	−
Anti-PD-(L)1[181]	ctDNA mutation	NSCLC	−	[2]↓	[2]↓
	Mutant allele frequency (MAF)		−	[2]↓	↓

(continued)

Table 18.3 Summary of Published Studies on the Clinical Relevance of Tumor Mutation Burden and Other Genetic Markers to Cancer Immunotherapies (*continued*)

ICI THERAPY	GENETIC BIOMARKER	CANCER TYPE	CLINICAL BENEFITS		
			RR	PFS	OS
Camrelizumab (anti-PD-1)[182]	TMB	Gastric and GEJ cancer	³↑	–	–
		ESCC	↑	–	–
Nivolumab (anti-PD-1)	MSI	Gastric cancer	↑	↑	–
Pembrolizumab (anti-PD-1)[183]	MSI	Gastric cancer	↑	↑	–
	PIK3CA mutation		↑	–	–
Atezolizumab (anti-PD-L1)[79]	TMB	UC	↑	–	–
Atezolizumab (anti-PD-L1)[184]	TMB	UC	↑	–	↑
Nivolumab (anti-PD-1)[185]	TMB	UC	↑	↑	↑
Nivolumab or atezolizumab[186]	DDR mutation	UC	↑	↑	↑
Pembrolizumab (anti-PD-1)[187]	MSI, TMB	CRC	↑	↑	↑
Ipilimumab (anti-CTLA-4)[188]	TMB	Melanoma	–	↑	↑
		Lung cancer	↑	↑	–
Cancer immunotherapy[189]	TMB	21 cancers	↑	↑	×
Pembrolizumab (anti-PD-1)[190]	TMB	22 cancers	↑	↑	–
JS001 (anti-PD-1)[191]	TMB	UC, melanoma, CRC	↑	–	–
ICI therapies	TMB	10 cancers	–	–	↑

Notes: 1, positive correlation only existed in nivolumab plus ipilimuman treatment; 2, not validated in the independent validation cohort; 3, not statistically significant.

↓, negative correlation with the genetic marker; ×, no significant correlation; ↑, positive correlation with the genetic marker.

BRCA2, breast cancer 2 (DNA repair associated); bTMB, blood-based tumor mutation burden; CGP, comprehensive genomic profiling; CNA, copy number alteration; CNL, copy number loss; CRC, colorectal carcinoma; ctDNA, circulating tumor DNA; ctDNA, circulating tumor DNA; CTLA-4, cytotoxic T lymphocyte-associated protein 4; DDR, DNA damage response and repair; EGFR, epidermal growth factor receptor; ERBB2, Erb-B2 Receptor Tyrosine Kinase 2; ESCC, esophageal squamous cell carcinoma; FAT1, FAT atypical cadherin 1; GEJ, gastroesophageal junction; ICI, immune checkpoint inhibitor; ITGA9, integrin subunit alpha 9; mCRC, metastatic colorectal cancer; MSI, microsatellite instability; NA, not applicable (not tested); NSCLC, non-small cell lung cancer; OS, overall survival; PD-1, programmed cell death protein-1; PD-L1, programmed death ligand 1; PFS, progression-free survival; PIK3CA, phosphatidylinositol-4,5-bisphosphate 3-kinase catalytic subunit alpha; RR, response rates; STK11, serine/threonine kinase 11; TMB, tumor mutation burden; UC, urothelial carcinoma

Besides TMB, we will also review the applications of TMB-included biomarkers (i.e., combinational biomarkers and advanced) and other genetic markers. Lastly, we will discuss the limitations of TMB as a biomarker in cancer immunotherapy with current attempts to overcome these, as well as future directions for TMB as a biomarker.

Basic Principles of Tumor Mutation Burden and Genetic Biomarkers

Tumor Mutations and Neoantigens

Mutations are generally defined as abnormal DNA sequences from DNA damage or replication errors without correct repair. Based on the heritability of mutations, there are two major types of mutations (i.e., germline mutations and somatic mutations). Somatic (or acquired) mutations, as opposed to germline (or hereditary) mutations, are alterations in DNA that occur in cells other than the germ cells (sperm and egg).[192] These alterations are not only caused by exogenous factors (e.g., exposure to ultraviolet radiation or certain chemicals), but also by endogenous factors (e.g., aldehydes and reactivate oxygen species).[193] While most somatic mutations do not have noticeable effects, some mutations confer selective cell-proliferation advantages (termed as "driver mutations"). Progressive accumulation of such mutations throughout life can lead to cancer, with autonomous clonal expansion of abnormal cells.[192]

The determinative role of mutations in cancers has been demonstrated via the malignant transformation of normal cells upon introduction of specific DNA fragments from cancer cells. Responsible genes for such malignant transformation were termed "oncogenes."[194] In addition, inactivation of tumor suppressor genes via either somatic or germline mutations has also been found to play a critical role in tumor progression.[195] While highly variable somatic mutations have been well recognized as the major drivers for progressive tumors, they also lead to products (e.g., abnormal peptides) that may be recognized by the immune system to distinguish cancer cells from noncancer cells.[196]

Neoantigens are abnormal proteins or peptides that may be processed and presented on the surface of cancer cells[197] and capable of triggering the immune system.[196,198] Antigen-processing machinery is involved to process mutation-derived peptides that are then loaded onto major histocompatibility complex (MHC) molecules for presentation on the cell surface. As modified self-antigens, neoantigens on tumor cells are recognized by cytotoxic T cells and likely killed.[199–202] However, generation of immunogenic neoantigens is intrinsically insufficient to lead to effective tumor recognition and elimination.[202] Inactivating mutations often arise in antigen-processing or presenting pathways, which can impair the efficiency and efficacy of the immune surveillance process, as well as the efficacy of cancer immunotherapy.[203,204]

Tumor Mutation Burden Definition and Measurement

TMB is generally defined as the number of nonsynonymous single nucleotide variants (SNVs) per megabase (Mb) of sequenced genome. It quantifies the accumulated somatic mutations and has emerged as an independent and promising biomarker for ICI therapy response in cancer patients.[205] Over the past decade, the rapid development and widespread use of DNA sequencing technology, especially next-generation sequencing (NGS), has enabled precise quantification of tumor mutations (i.e., TMB) in a fast and comprehensive manner.[206] As the first detailed investigations of tumor genome heterogeneity, whole-genome sequencing (WGS) and whole exome sequencing (WGS) were applied to tumor tissues for quantifying the prevalence of somatic mutations (i.e., TMB).[207,208] Both studies found that TMBs across different cancer types could vary by more than 1000 folds. It was also found that TMBs from WES are highly consistent with the TMBs from WGS. Compared to WGS, WES only sequences the exome region, which represents only ~1% of the whole genome. This confers multiple advantages to WES, including faster sequencing procedures, less computational burden, and lower cost. More importantly, WES sequences the coding fraction, which is directly related to neoantigen production, with a greater sequencing depth to provide both clonal and subclonal variants.[209] Due to the previously noted advantages, WES has replaced WGS to become the "golden standard" for TMB measurement in cancer immunotherapy.[198]

The bioinformatic analysis pipeline also significantly impacts the accuracy of TMB measurement.[210] In general, sequencing quality is controlled by quantifying several key quality parameters, and low-quality bases are labeled for the following analysis. Next, reads from DNA sequencing are aligned to the latest human genome data following several quality control steps (e.g., marking duplicated reads from PCR and recalibrating base quality scores).[211] With aligned reads, somatic variants are called and the TMB is calculated with well-established bioinformatic tools. Within this general procedure, there are several key steps which directly impact TMB accuracy. First, including synonymous SNVs in TMB measurements varied from different TMB panels.[205] A synonymous mutation is a substitution of codon with a synonymous codon, that is, a change in the DNA sequence that does not alter the encoded amino acid in a protein sequence. This mutation was once considered as having no phenotype consequences and referred to as "silent," but is now increasingly acknowledged to have substantial impact on precursor mRNA splicing, RNA stability, and RNA folding—as such, it is now accepted that synonymous mutations frequently contribute to human cancer.[212,213] However, in the common procedures, TMB measurements do not include synonymous mutations, even though TMBs including synonymous mutations are highly concordant with ones with nonsynonymous mutations only.[214] In addition, another key step to accurately measure TMBs is to filter germline mutations including nontumor and benign mutations. To remove germline mutations from TMBs, there are two approaches: (a) based on population sequence databases (e.g., The 1000 Genome Project[215] and dbSNP),[216] or (b) based on tumor-paired normal samples (including both tumor-adjacent normal tissue and peripheral blood monocyte cells). As a more economical method, using multiple population databases can filter out common germline mutations based on epidemiological information. However, patient-specific germline mutations cannot be captured in such databases, which leads to an overestimation of TMBs.[205] Therefore, the second approach with tumor-paired normal samples is preferred currently, and several bioinformatic tools or automated pipelines can clean germline mutations of normal samples from tumor samples.[217–219]

Microsatellite Instability and Other Potential Genetic Markers

In normal cells, microsatellites (MSs) are short stretches of DNA (1–6 nucleotides long or longer) tandemly repeated thousands of times throughout the whole genome, generally located within introns.[220] MSs can also be found in regions related to coding genes (e.g., promoter section and terminal regions[221]). Abnormal expansion or reduction of the repeated bases in MSs has been defined as MS instability (MSI), which is normally corrected by the DNA mismatch repair (MMR) system. Therefore, when germline and/or somatic mutations develop in key proteins related to MMR systems (including MLH1, MSH2, PMS2, MSH6, or epithelial cellular adhesion molecules), MSI will be significantly increased (referred to as MSI-H) and results in tremendous unorganized repetitive DNA sequences. In contrast, tumors with intact MMR systems do not exhibit MSI (or low MSI) and are termed "microsatellite stable" (MSS; or MSI-L). Due to the key genomic locations of some MSs, MSI is generally associated with increased nonsynonymous SNV, hypermethylation status, and prevalent immune infiltrations.[222] Thus, it is proposed that the MSI tumors express more neopeptides from somatic mutations, which increases the opportunity for the immune system to recognize these as neoantigens and trigger an immune response with more TILs.[187] As such, MSI has been recognized as a predictor for efficacy of ICI therapies.[223,224]

Since the basis of MSI-H is a deficient MMR system, lower expression of MMR-related mRNA or proteins could reflect MSI status. Therefore, two conventional assays have been widely used in clinics: immunohistochemically (IHC) staining-based assay and PCR-based assay. For the IHC-based assay, the key proteins in MMR systems are selected as the IHC markers, and samples with cells lacking these MMR-related markers are identified as MSI-H.[225] Although this IHC-based method is fast and cheap, it may lead to false-negative results because it cannot detect MSI caused by point mutations or small indel mutations which may not significantly reduce the expression of MMR proteins. A PCR-based assay overcomes this limitation by directly measuring MMR gene expressions with sensitive and well-designed primers.[226] With emerging NGS techniques, the latest assays for MSI determination are directly based on DNA sequencing and bioinformatic analysis, and provide the highest accuracy for MSI quantification (e.g., MSIPlus[227] and ColoSeq).[228]

Besides MSI, there are several novel NGS-based genetic biomarkers associated with responses to ICI therapies. As an alternative biomarker for tumor TMB (tTMB), blood TMB (bTMB) has been shown to be predictive for ICI therapies with multiple advantages, such as less invasive and easily accessible diagnostic materials with minimum sampling bias from tissue biopsies.[229] In addition to the general tumor mutation profile, mutation profiles of a single gene with critical functions or impact in oncogenic pathways can also be considered as biomarkers (e.g., STK11, KEAP1, PTEN, B2M, etc).[230]

By integrating DNA sequencing and RNA sequencing with optional proteomic data, the neoantigen load can be quantified recently as a biomarker for ICI therapies.[231] In general, DNA sequencing is still used to identify genomic alterations, while RNA sequencing is used to confirm the mutated genes (or DNA fragments) having been transcribed. The confirmed mutated gene with high mRNA expression can be directly considered as neoantigens,[232,233] while the neoantigens can also be either predicted based on in silico methods[234,235] or identified with mass spectrometry data.[236]

Targeted Sequencing Panels for Tumor Mutation Burden

U.S. Food and Drug Administration-Approved Pan-Cancer Targeted Sequencing Panels

WES provides comprehensive measurements of TMB as the "gold standard." However, it cannot fit into community oncology as a routine test due to its long turn-over time and high price. To overcome such limitations, multiple targeted sequencing panels have been developed which attempt to provide TMB estimations with high accuracy and similar predictivity to ICI therapies compared to WES-derived TMB.[198] Among the targeted TMB panels with published data, currently two products (i.e., FoundationOne CDx [F1-CDx] assay and MSK-IMPACT) have been approved by the FDA to profile the pan-cancer genome (>10 cancer types) and to facilitate the identification of cancer patients who may benefit from cancer immunotherapy.[196]

Covering most of the solid tumors, F1-CDx detects substitutions, indels, and copy number alteration for more than 320 genes in the full coding exonic regions and gene rearrangement for 36 genes in selected intronic regions. Along with the previously noted genomic profiles, MSI, loss of heterozygosity, and TMB are also analyzed to help identify patients who may benefit from targeted therapies for specific tumors or benefit from pembrolizumab for all solid tumors. F1-CDx has been validated to be a predictive marker for ICI therapies for multiple types of solid tumors (including NSCLC[176,237] and MSI-H colorectal carcinoma [CRC][238]).

The other FDA-approved targeted tumor-sequencing test is MSK-IMPACT, Integrated Mutation Profiling of Actionable Cancer Targets, developed by Memorial Sloan Kettering Cancer Center. By sequencing and analyzing 10,000 cancer patients with coverage of 18 different cancer types, MSK-IMPACT includes 468 genes which play important roles in tumor progression.[239] Similar to F1-CDx, MSK-IMPACT measures not only TMB but also other tumor-related molecular alternations in targeted genes (e.g., MSI) to provide an inclusive picture of the tumor genome. The predictive power of

MSK-IMPACT for ICI therapies has also been proved for both primary and metastatic solid tumors across different cancer types.[173,240] By inclusively characterizing the genomic alterations, such approaches are collectively denoted as comprehensive genomic profiling (CGP).[241]

Major Limitations in Targeted Sequencing Panels and Potential Solutions

In addition to these two pan-cancer FDA-approved CGP panels, multiple targeted sequencing panels are being developed and validated for clinically predictive values for ICI therapies in various types of solid tumors. These are well summarized in a recent review focusing on targeted sequencing panels for TMB measurements in cancer immunotherapy.[198] Although targeted sequencing panels can reduce time, labor, and cost, and provide greater sequencing depth for more comprehensive characterizations of tumor-related genomic alternations, several key concerns have been realized in recent studies.

First, due to low coverage of the whole exome in targeted sequencing panels, one of the major concerns is measurement consistency compared to WES. It has been found that the size of the NGS panel (i.e., coverage lengths of the exome) significantly impacts TMB accuracy. Coefficient of variances of TMB estimation was shown to be negatively correlated with the size of the NGS panel. Specific thresholds (i.e., 0.5~1 Mb) were also found as the watershed for reliable TMB estimation from targeted sequencing panels.[241,242] In other words, an extremely high variance of TMB estimation was observed with panels sequencing less than 0.5 Mb, and a rapid increase of variance was observed with panels sequencing less than 1 Mb. In this case, 300 genes and/or 1 Mb are recommended as the minimum size for NGS panels to guarantee the accuracy of TMB estimation from the targeted sequencing panel.[243] And as an encouraging result, computational analyses have demonstrated that there was an acceptable consistency comparing targeted sequencing panel-derived TMB and WES-derived TMBs.[244]

Another major limitation for community-level application of targeted sequencing panels is the variable settings crossing different panels or products. First, the sequencing panel design impacts the precision of TMB measurements from different targeted sequencing panels. For example, different selections of tumor-associated genes among targeted sequencing panels produce variable TMB measurements, and exclusion of key genes related to tumor progression may lead to severe biases in TMB results.[245] In addition, sequencing depth also influences detection sensitivity for genetic mutations, which directly impacts TMB calculation.[239,246] Besides sequencing parameters, distinguished in-house bioinformatic pipelines for targeted sequencing panels also significantly influence the final results of TMB

estimation. As mentioned in the last subsection, removal of germline mutations with tumor-paired normal samples help to improve the precision of TMB calculation. However, some of the targeted sequencing panels do not include the germline mutation removal step, or use a population-based DNA database to filter germline mutations, which both lead to major variances in TMB estimation. As mentioned, some of the targeted sequencing panels also include synonymous mutations in TMB calculations.[231,239,241] Different mutation callers with different mutation counting rules are used among target sequencing panels, which directly impact the TMB value. Precise TMB measurement should involve more comprehensive counting procedures; therefore, TMB from a combination of different callers should be considered as the optimal solution.

To overcome these limitations, two standardization and harmonization efforts for TMB panels across sequencing panels and cancer types are underway in the United States (i.e., Friends of Cancer Research) and Germany (i.e., Quality Assessment Service for Pathology).[245] In general, both efforts aim to assess variations between WES-derived TMBs and targeted-panel-derived TMBs, as well as interassay and interlaboratory variabilities with their sources.[247] TMB variants between WES and targeted sequencing panels will facilitate the design of targeted sequencing panels with reliable TMB estimations. Then interassay and interlaboratory variabilities of TMB estimations will be used to minimize and/or correct the variants of TMB estimations and reports across different targeted sequencing panels. To achieve these aims with Friends of Cancer Research as an example, there are three phases to harmonize a TMB report with sufficient predictive power for cancer immunotherapy. First, in silico analysis is used to learn the variants between WES-derived TMBs and targeted-panel-derived TMBs by correlating these two TMBs in a TCGA database (Phase 1, completed).[248] Next, to align the panel-derived TMB estimates into a standard reference, patient-derived tumor cell lines are used to establish such universal standards with WES (Phase 2, ongoing).[247] Lastly, cutoffs for TMB estimations for predicting clinical outcomes will be developed from published trials (Phase 3, proposed). To this end, a harmonized TMB report regardless of sequencing panel design and subsequent bioinformatic analysis will be available for cancer patients with different types of tumors.

Clinical Association and Application of Tumor Mutation Burden and Genetic Biomarkers in Immunotherapy

As an emerging and promising biomarker for ICI therapies, TMB has been widely examined for its predictive power in clinical outcomes or therapeutic responses

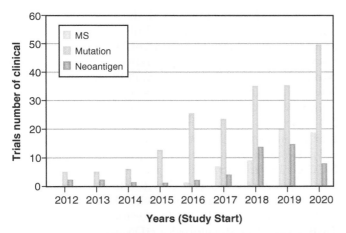

Figure 18.2 Increasing clinical trials related to mutation, microsatellite, and neoantigen and cancer immunotherapy since 2012. The number of clinical trials collected through clinicaltrials.gov by searching with "cancer" as condition or disease, and "immunotherapy" plus the corresponding searching keywords (i.e., "mutation," "microsatellite," and "neoantigen") as other terms. All metrics are updated as of August 25, 2020.

among different cancer types. TMB-related clinical trials have exponentially increased in recent years (Figure 18.2). Several comprehensive reviews and chapters have been published to summarize the latest studies and clinical trials with TMB as a biomarker for ICI therapies from various aspects.[196,198,240,249–252] In this section, we provide a summary of key studies and clinical trials using TMB and/or other genetic biomarkers to predict responses of ICI treatments based on cancer types (Tables 18.1 and 18.2). At the end, we summarize the limitations of TMB as a biomarker for cancer immunotherapy and outlooks for TMB and other genetic biomarkers.

Application in Melanoma

As perhaps the earliest study investigating the relationship between tumor genomics and clinical benefits of ICI therapies, Snyder et al. found that more mutations were associated with long-term benefits and longer overall survival (OS) in both their discovery set and validation set for anti-CTLA-4 (i.e., ipilimumab)-treated melanoma patients.[170] With genome-wide somatic neoepitope analysis and patient-specific HLA type, some potential tumor neoantigens were identified for each patient and neoantigens related to a strong response to anti-CTLA-4 treatments were found and validated as a predictive marker. In a subsequent study with a larger cohort, Van Allen et al. investigated the genomic factors associated with clinical outcomes of >100 metastatic melanoma patients with ipilimumab monotherapy. Strong correlations of TMB, neoantigen loads, and expression of cytolytic markers with clinical benefits (i.e.,

>6-month progression free and >2-year overall survival) were found, suggesting the clinically predictive value of genomic factors in ICI therapies.[132] For anti-PD-1 treated metastatic melanoma patients, Hugo et al. found that the TMB predicted improved OS, but not clinical response to anti-PD-1 treatments, while BRCA2 mutation profile was associated with anti-PD-1 clinical response.[140] Johnson et al. developed a targeted sequencing panel with 315 genes for TMB estimation. This panel-derived TMB was highly concordant with WES-derived TMB, and by using two independent cohorts, TMB was validated to be significantly associated with higher response rates, as well as longer PFS and OS for melanoma patients with anti-PD-(L)1 treatments.[171] By implementing comprehensive genome profiling, Roh et al. found that higher copy-number loss (CNL) was observed in nonresponders of anti-CTLA-4 plus anti-PD-1 treated melanoma patients.[144] However, there were no statistical differences of TMB between responder and nonresponder groups for either pre-anti-CTLA-4 or pre-anti-PD-1 treatment samples. By integrating TMB with CNL for ICI response prediction, additive effects were observed indicating a potentially stronger predictive power from combinatorial biomarker than with TMB or CNL alone. Similar to the finding from Snyder et al., Riaz et al. found a strong correlation between TMB and clinical benefits of ipilimumab-treated melanoma.[146] Interestingly, Riaz et al. discovered that ICI treatments (i.e., anti-PD-1 therapy) also impacted the TMBs in melanomas by examining the genomic changes in advanced melanoma before and after nivolumab treatment (CA209-038). After nivolumab treatments, more genome contraction (i.e., lost clone/subclones in the pretreatment tumor) was found in the responder group, while more genome persistence was found in the nonresponder group.[146] To systemically evaluate the prediction powers of biomarkers of ICI treatment for melanoma, Morrison et al. compared the predictive sensitivities and specificities of different biomarkers (including TMB) for ICI-treated melanoma patients.[63] Higher TMB was associated with response of ICI-treated patients, but not with overall survival. The sensitivity of TMB was closed to PD-L1 expression but lower than the comprehensive immune profile.

Application in Lung Cancers

As one of the earliest studies on the correlation between TMB and lung cancer, Rizvi et al. found that both high nonsynonymous mutation burden and high neoantigen loading were associated with significantly improved objective response, durable clinical benefit, and progression-free survival in two independent cohorts of NSCLC patients treated by pembrolizumab.[172] In a trial with both ICI therapy and chemotherapy in advanced or recurrent NSCLC (CheckMate 026), Carbone et al. discovered that within high TMB patients, higher response rates in the nivolumab group with longer PFS were observed when comparing them to the chemotherapy group, while similar OS was found between the nivolumab group and chemotherapy group.[253] Modest correlation between PD-L1 expression and TMB was found, while higher response rates were observed in TMB-high and PD-L1-high patients in the nivolumab group compared to each single stratification factor. In a study with ICI therapy only, Rizvi et al. found that TMB derived from the MSK-IMPACT panel was correlated with WES-derived TMBs. Within advanced NSCLC patients treated with anti-PD-(L)1 therapy, higher TMB was observed in the DCB group compared to the NDB group.[173] Longer progression-free survival (PFS) was observed in the high TMB group with median of TMB as the threshold. Higher fraction of copy number alteration was found in the NDB group and variants in EGFR and STK11 were associated with lack of benefit. Although TMB was found to be independent of PD-L1 expression, incorporation of TMB with PD-L1 was shown to have greater predictive power for anti-PD-(L)1 therapy. Similarly, Fang et al. validated that a customized targeted sequencing panel (including 422 genes) for TMB estimation was strongly correlated with WES-derived TMBs and associated with improved clinical outcomes in NSCLC patients treated with anti-PD-(L)1 therapies.[175] Similar findings were published by Hellmann et al., showing that high TMB from WES was associated with efficacy of PD-1 plus CTLA-4 inhibitors in advanced NSCLC patients.[174] Several mutation profiles and copy number loss with specific genes were also found to be highly predictive for clinical outcomes (i.e., PFS and ORR). As one of the most recent completed trials, the CheckMate 568 Phase 2 study was designed to examine the efficacy of nivolumab plus low-dose ipilimumab as first-line treatment for advanced or metastatic NSCLC, as well as the association between panel-derived TMB (F1-CDx) and clinical outcomes.[176] In this trial, it was observed that patients with higher TMB (10 or more mut/Mb) had higher objective response rate (ORR) and longer PFS regardless of PD-L1 expression.

For small-cell lung cancer (SCLC), Hellmann et al. observed that high TMB was correlated with efficacy of nivolumab regardless of ipilimumab treatments, and SCLC patients with higher TMB had greater benefit from combinatorial therapy with both nivolumab and ipilimumab compared to nivolumab monotherapy (CheckMate-032).[177] However, Ricciuti et al. did not find significant differences in the ORR between TMB high and low cohorts with ICI treated SCLC patients when using a targeted sequencing panel for TMB estimation and median TMB as the threshold.[178] In that study, longer PFS and OS were found to be correlated with higher TMB.

Besides tTMB, Gandara et al. derived a bTMB assay, and the predictive power for clinical benefits (i.e., PFS and OS) of atezolizumab (anti-PD-L1) therapy in NSCLC patients was validated with a retrospective analysis of two large randomized trials (i.e., POPLAR and OAK).[179] It was also found that bTMB was significantly correlated with tTMB. When this bTMB assay was combined with PD-L1 expression, the predictive power in PFS was further improved by 38.7% compared to the PD-L1 assay only. Wang et al. utilized a targeted sequencing panel NCC-GP150 to show that higher bTMB (>6 mut/Mb) was significantly associated with clinical benefits (i.e., PFS) of anti-PD-1 and anti-PD-L1 therapy in patients with advanced NSCLC.[180] In addition to blood-based TMB, Chae et al. developed a ctDNA-based TMB assay for predicting clinical outcomes from ICI treatments in NSCLC patients. This ctDNA-based TMB was not correlated with RECIST TMB, but was significantly associated with progression-free survival and overall survival; however, this was not validated in a small independent cohort.[181]

Application in Gastrointestinal Cancer

Compared to lung cancer and melanoma, studies for ICI therapy genetic biomarkers of other cancers, such as gastrointestinal cancer, started later. In an early study, Janjigian et al. found that TMB and MSI scores were correlated to each other in esophagogastric cancer patients, and patients with MSI-H, who were resistant to chemotherapy, were more likely to have durable clinical responses (overall survival) to immunotherapy.[254] Huang et al. presented results of two clinical trials of anti-PD-1 antibody treatment for advanced esophageal squamous cell carcinoma (ESCC) and gastric/gastroesophageal junction (GEJ) cancer.[182] For the ESCC study, WES-derived TMB was found to be significantly associated with better responses. However, for gastric and GEJ study, patients with higher TMB tended to have better responses but not significantly. By using an IHC-based assay, Mishima et al. reported higher overall response rates of nivolumab treatment in the MSI-H advanced gastric cancer patients, and longer PFS was observed in MSS patients.[183] Similar positive findings have also been reported by Overman et al. in a Phase 2 trial for nivolumab-treated MSI-H CRC patients.[46] Schrock et al. demonstrated that TMB was strongly associated with the objective response rate and PFS within MSI-H metastatic CRC patients treated with anti-PD-(L)1 therapy.[238] Recently, results of two clinical trials for examining the efficacy of pembrolizumab in MSI-H tumors were published. Although pembrolizumab could benefit both MSI-H metastatic CRC[255] and MSI-H non-CRC tumors,[256] about 60% of MSI-H patients from both trials did not respond to pembrolizumab treatment, indicating that MSI-H was not necessarily a reliable biomarker for ICI therapies.[257]

Application in Urothelial Carcinoma

Rosenberg et al. demonstrated the efficacy of aterolizumab in treating advanced and metastatic urothelial carcinoma (UC), and The Cancer Genome Atlas (TCGA) subtypes and TMB could be used as predictive biomarkers for response to atezolizumab.[79] A subsequent clinical trial also found an association between TMB and response to atezolizumab in advanced and metastatic UC patients.[184] For anti-PD-1 therapy, Galsky et al. found that higher TMB was significantly associated with ORR, PFS, and OS within urothelial cancer patients treated with nivolumab.[185] Since alterations in DNA damage response and repair (DDR) genes are associated with increased TMB, Teo et al. found that alterations in DDR genes were associated with RRs, PFS, and OS of advanced urothelial cancer patients treated with anti-PD-(L)1 therapies.[186]

Pan-Cancer Applications

In addition to focusing on one specific cancer type, several studies investigated the genetic biomarkers of ICI therapies for multiple cancer types. As one of the early studies, Le et al. reported on a Phase 2 trial to investigate the association of pembrolizumab efficacy and MMR status (MSI) in metastatic carcinomas.[187] They found that high deficiency of MMR system (high MSI) was associated with higher ORRs and longer PFS for CRC patients treated with pembrolizumab. For MSI-H non-colorectal carcinoma patients, ICI response rates were similar to the response rates of MSI-H CRC patients. As expected, significantly higher TMB was observed in MSI-H patients compared to MSS/MSI-L patients.[187] In another pan-cancer study, Roszik et al. developed a predicted total mutation burden (PTMB) from WES-derived TMB of melanoma and lung cancer samples, which included 170 genes. High concordance between PTMB and WES-derived TMB was found in both cutaneous melanoma and lung adenocarcinoma validation cohorts. In addition, PTMB was also significantly correlated with clinical benefits of anti-CTLA-4 treated melanoma patients (three cohorts) and anti-PD-1 treated lung cancer patients.[188] Goodman et al. subsequently reported on a large-scale pan-cancer study (including 151 patients with 21 cancer types) to better understand the correlation between TMB and clinical benefits from ICI therapies. High TMB was significantly associated with higher RR and longer PFS for all included cancer types, but not significantly with OS.[189] Another large-scale study involving >300 patients across 22 different cancer types has been implemented to examine the predictive power of TMB and T cell-inflamed gene expression profile (GEP) for pembrolizumab treatments.[190] TMB presented an independent predictive power for responses across the KEYNOTE clinical data sets, with longer PFS associated with TMB. The joint application of TMB and GEP could stratify human cancers based on clinical responses to pembrolizumab monotherapy. Results from clinical trials of a new anti-PD-1 antibody (JS001) for advanced melanoma, urothelial cancer, and RCC showed that TMB was associated with clinical responses for all three cancer types.[191] Recently, another comprehensive study was implemented by associating the genomic profiles from MSK-IMPACT with clinical data of 1,662 advanced cancer patients with ICI treatments and 5,371 without ICI treatments.[240] TMB was associated with improved overall survival but the optimal thresholds for high TMB were highly varied and crossed different cancer types.

Challenges and Outlooks in Tumor Mutation Burden as a Biomarker in Clinical Applications

As an FDA-approved pan-cancer biomarker for ICI therapies with a wealth of supportive results, TMB nonetheless still faces challenges for community-level application in cancer immunotherapy.[249] As mentioned in the "Targeted Sequencing Panel" section, standardization and harmonization of various TMB panels is one of the biggest challenges for TMB. Tumor genomic heterogeneity is another issue for the universal application of TMB.[240] It is well-known that TMB is dramatically varied crossing different cancer types based on large-scale pan-cancer studies, which leads to a serious issue for determining TMB thresholds. TMB thresholds could directly impact the reproducibility of clinical predictions from TMB. It is difficult to generate universal or cancer-specific TMB thresholds. Also, there are still conflicting results of the association between TMB and ICI clinical benefits crossing different cancer types and/or different ICI therapies. From the practical aspect, while targeted sequencing has improved turnaround time and reduced cost dramatically, total time-cost for TMB is still less favorable to other assays (e.g., PD-L1 expression). As such, a TMB assay with shorter turnaround time and lower costs is still required, and without impairing its prediction accuracy.

As we move into the age of precision medicine, application of TMB and other genetic biomarkers for cancer therapies will generate petabyte-level data.[258] We are looking forward to even more data-driven diagnostic tools with combinational biomarkers and higher prediction accuracies for cancer immunotherapy. Such tools must harness the latest techniques in artificial intelligence and "Big Data" analysis. In conclusion, TMB and other genetic biomarkers are promising predictive biomarkers for ICI therapies among various cancer types (especially melanoma and lung cancers). The major limitation for wider applications of TMB is the standardization and harmonization of TMB results across different panels and various cancer types.

CONCLUSION

Rapidly growing understanding of the mechanisms of ICB response have yielded numerous biomarkers over recent years. These range from those approved as FDA companion diagnostics (PD-L1) to upcoming biomarkers that need wider validation. As technologies for interrogating local and systemic antitumor responses advance, we will rely increasingly on bioinformatic tools to distill a wealth of information into clinically actionable biomarkers. Furthermore, as clinical application of ICB continues to exponentially increase, it will be critical to sort out the context specificities of immune biomarkers given combinatorial treatment approaches with chemotherapy, radiation therapy, and other therapeutics. Future predictors of response to immunotherapy will need to integrate and fine-tune multiple biomarkers including tumor genomic components, systemic immune features, and dynamic host responses to therapeutic intervention. Care will need to be taken to sort out correlation versus causation as we work to understand and improve response to ICB.

KEY REFERENCES

Only key references appear in the print edition. The full reference list appears in the digital product on Springer Publishing Connect: connect.springerpub.com/content/book/978-0-8261-3743-2/part/part01/chapter/ch18

33. Topalian SL, Hodi FS, Brahmer JR, et al. Safety, activity, and immune correlates of anti-PD-1 antibody in cancer. *N Engl J Med.* 2012;366:2443–2454. doi:10.1056/NEJMoa1200690
35. Tumeh PC, Harview CL, Yearley JH, et al. PD-1 blockade induces responses by inhibiting adaptive immune resistance. *Nature.* 2014;515:568–571. doi:10.1038/nature13954
100. Herbst RS, Soria J-C, Kowanetz M, et al. Predictive correlates of response to the anti-PD-L1 antibody MPDL3280A in cancer patients. *Nature.* 2014;515:563–567. doi:10.1038/nature14011
132. Van Allen EM, Miao D, Schilling B, et al. Genomic correlates of response to CTLA-4 blockade in metastatic melanoma. *Science.* 2015;350(6257):207–211. doi:10.1126/science.aad0095
140. Hugo W, Zaretsky JM, Sun L, et al. Genomic and transcriptomic features of response to anti-PD-1 therapy in metastatic melanoma. *Cell.* 2016;165:35–44. doi:10.1016/j.cell.2016.02.065
172. Rizvi NA, Hellmann MD, Snyder A, et al. Mutational landscape determines sensitivity to PD-1 blockade in non–small cell lung cancer. *Science.* 2015;348(6230):124–128. doi:10.1126/science.aaa1348
248. Merino DM. Establishing guidelines to harmonize tumor mutational burden (TMB): in silico assessment of variation in TMB quantification across diagnostic platforms: Phase I of the Friends of Cancer Research TMB harmonization project. *J Immunother Cancer* 2020;8:e000147. doi:10.1136/jitc-2019-000147

Role of the Microbiota in Carcinogenesis and Cancer Therapy

Ernesto Perez-Chanona and Giorgio Trinchieri

KEY POINTS

- The relationship between the microbiota, cancer, and immunotherapeutics is tested using metagenomic, *16S rRNA* gene, and metatranscriptomic sequencing followed by analysis using specialized algorithms.

- Microbes maintain homeostasis at the sites of barrier function through immune cell maturation, pathogen exclusion, and metabolism of nutrients.

- Microbes contribute to carcinogenesis through the modulation of proliferation-inducing pathways and oncogene expression, the induction of inflammatory responses, and through secretion of toxins.

- Dysbiosis of commensal microbes contributes to carcinogenesis through faulty metabolic processes that modulate local immunity, expansion of pathobiont niches, and direct inhibition of antitumor immune responses.

- The microbiota fosters the immunogenic clearance of tumors, thereby enhancing the therapeutic efficacy of chemotherapy and immunotherapies by promoting lymphocyte development and infiltration into the tumor where they exert antitumor immune responses.

INTRODUCTION

The epithelial barrier sites of our body, exposed to the external environment, are colonized by microorganisms, including archaea, protozoa, fungi, bacteria, their respective viruses and bacteriophages, and human viruses, which support the development of important host physiological functions.[1] These microbes, defined as the human microbiota, modulate metabolism, neurological and cognitive functions, inflammation, and hematopoiesis, as well as toning of innate resistance effector cells

and of adaptive immune cells.[2,3] The systemic effects of the microbiota are highlighted by their ability to modulate cancer progression and immunotherapeutic and chemotherapeutic efficacy.

The first description of the bacteria and other microbes living as commensals in our body was due to the pioneering microscopy work of Antony van Leeuwenhoek in the late seventeenth century.[4] Progress in the characterization of the microbiota, however, was slow due to our inability to isolate and grow most of the commensal microbes in culture. The field has been recently revolutionized by our ability to characterize the microbiota using the advanced high-throughput sequencing technology to identify the entire microbial genomes, their RNA transcripts, and the amplicons of the 16S ribosomal RNA (*16S rRNA*) gene followed by bioinformatic analysis (Figure 19.1). By sequencing entire microbial genomes using metagenomic shotgun sequencing, reliable taxonomic identification and the abundance of each taxa can be determined using programs such as MetaPhlAn.[5,6] To understand the meaning behind the changes observed in the biota, other tools such as HUManN are used to infer the metabolic potential of a microbial community using the short DNA sequences.[7,8] An alternative approach to community profiling is the sequencing of specific highly variable regions or the full-length bacterial *16S rRNA* gene. Unlike meta genomic sequencing, this approach allows researchers to sequence hundreds of samples simultaneously through the creation of a library of sequences that are barcoded using a unique DNA sequence identifier.[9] This process is called multiplexing and requires downstream separation of the sequences by sample using bioinformatic tools that recognize the barcodes embedded in the sequences. Through this approach, the resolution of taxa identification is limited, offering reliable information at higher levels of phylogeny but dubious identification at the species and strain levels, although a better resolution is obtained when the full-length *16 rRNA* gene is sequenced.[9] Using software packages such as QIIME or Mothur, bioinformaticians process the raw sequences, filter low-quality reads, and map them to reference genomes in public databases such as Green Genes and the Ribosomal

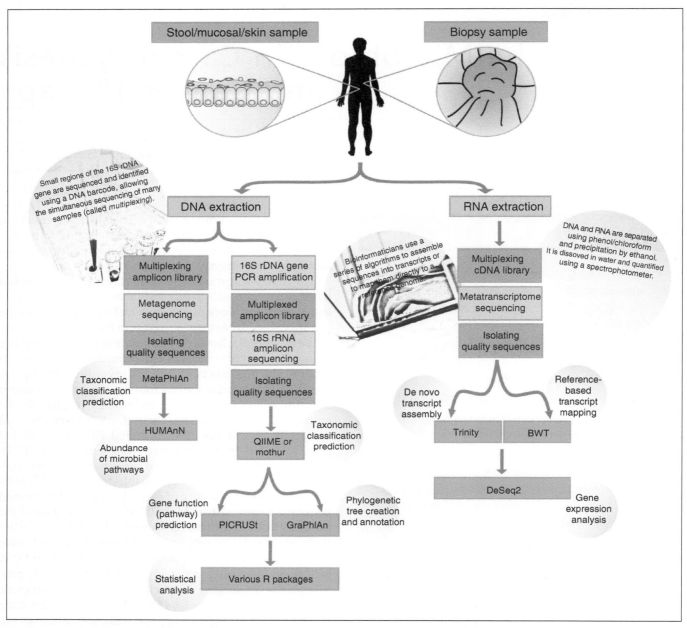

Figure 19.1 Pipelines for next-generation sequencing of DNA and RNA. Researchers using stool, mucosal samples, or biopsies can obtain information regarding the microbial composition of the sample, as well as gene expression information using different methods of next-generation, high-throughput sequencing. The experimental steps (purple boxes) performed in the laboratory are followed by bioinformatic analysis using algorithms (green boxes) that generate specific types of data (beige bubbles). For example, microbial DNA sequences can be used as input to certain algorithms, such as PICRUSt, that predict the metabolic pathways active in the microbial community. More detailed information is available in the text.

Database Project.[10–13] The 16S rDNA sequences can also be used to predict the metabolic pathways present in a group of microbes using the software PICRUSt or graphed into phylogenic trees using GraPhlAn.[14,15] To find true changes in gene expression between microbial groups, microbial RNA can be sequenced using shotgun sequencing called metatranscriptomic sequencing.

The RNA is converted to complementary DNA (cDNA), and then multiplexed in a similar way to DNA sequencing. The sequences can be assembled into transcripts de novo, whereby large transcripts and alternatively spliced isoforms can be analyzed even in the absence of a reference genome using the program Trinity.[16] Other algorithms such as the Burrows–Wheeler transform can map cDNA sequences to a reference genome in a database.[17] Then, tools such as DESeq2 can be used to analyze these large data sets containing gene expression data in quantitative and interpretable ways.[18]

While sequencing is useful to test the impact of cancer progression or of drug treatment on the gut microbiota, the contribution of a specific microbe or set of microbes on carcinogenesis and the therapeutic efficacy of a drug can also be tested. In parallel with the development of the new omics technologies for the characterization of the microbiota, major advances have been made in our ability to culture and identify most unknown bacteria in the human microbiota as a part of the rebirth of culture techniques in microbiology. Using well-defined culture conditions, combined with the rapid identification of bacteria, thousands of new microorganisms have now been cultured and characterized, enabling a much deeper understanding of the host–bacteria relationship.[19] Using gnotobiotic techniques, germ-free (GF) mice (raised from birth in conditions devoid of any microbes) are colonized with a specific microbe, or a group of microbes, from murine and/or human origin. These studies can test the contribution of selected microbes to cancer progression.[20] When fecal transplantations are performed in GF murine hosts and are coupled to high-throughput sequencing, associations can be made between human microbes and diseases, including cancer.[20] By harnessing the power of these technologies, great advances have been made to understand the relationship between the microbiota, host genetics, and disease progression.

IMMUNE SYSTEM TONING BY THE MICROBIOTA

Microbial Detection Occurs Through Pattern-Recognition Receptors

The development of the immune system relies on the environmental cues provided by commensal microorganisms colonizing the epithelial barriers of our body (Figure 19.2). The sensing of the microbiota relies on the detection of microbial-associated molecular patterns (MAMPs) by pattern recognition receptors (PRRs) expressed on a wide variety of cells. These PRRs include the Toll-like family of receptors (TLRs), the nucleotide-binding oligomerization domain (NOD)-like receptors (NLRs), RNA helicases, C-type lectin receptors, and cytosolic DNA sensors.[21] TLRs, the most extensively studied of the PRRs, specialize in recognizing bacterial components such as lipopolysaccharide (LPS), peptidoglycans, flagella, CpG-containing DNA, and viral double-stranded RNA and envelope proteins.[21] Upon detecting MAMPs from commensals and pathogens, these receptors activate intracellular signaling pathways regulating the synthesis and release of cytokines and chemokines that orchestrate the development of an immune response. The importance of TLR signaling in regulating the microbial composition of the colon is highlighted when the TLR and IL-1 receptor adapter protein myeloid differentiation gene 88 (MyD88) is deleted in mice.[22] These MyD88-deficient B6 mice demonstrate dysregulation of adaptive and innate immune responses, dysbiosis, and also, in C57Bl6 mice, the reactivation of the endogenous murine leukemia retrovirus.[23–25]

At barrier sites—the lung, skin, and gastrointestinal tract—our first line of defense against microbes are the epithelial cells and physiochemical boundaries, such as keratin and mucous layers. These structures aid in maintaining microbial homeostasis not only by providing a mechanical barrier but also by secreting soluble factors that regulate bacterial growth, in part, through MAMP detection by PRRs. In the gut, for example, specialized epithelial cells known as Paneth cells, located in the small bowel, secrete a variety of antimicrobial peptides, including C-type lectins. Regenerating islet-derived protein 3γ (RegIIIγ), in particular, binds to Gram-positive bacterial cell walls and exerts bactericidal effects.[26] Microbial sensing through TLRs on the surface of epithelial cells spurs the secretion of these peptides, enhances wound-healing mechanisms, and leads to the proliferation of the epithelium.[22,27–29] Bacteroides thetaiotaomicron induces the expression of RegIIIβ and RegIIIγ, although the identification of the producer cell type remains elusive.[30] Lactobacillus plantarum, a human commensal, was shown to fortify the intestinal epithelium by upregulating the expression of tight-junction proteins to form a paracellular seal between epithelial cells and prevent microbial translocation and dissemination.[31] Another mechanism used by microbes to modulate local immune responses is through the fermentation of dietary carbohydrates, specifically indigestible starches and dietary fiber, into short-chain fatty acids (SCFAs). Detection of these metabolic products by G protein-coupled receptors located on the apical surface of intestinal epithelial cells promotes the production and secretion of IL-18, a cytokine that promotes barrier function.[32–34]

Microbial Signals Drive Immune Homeostasis at Barrier Sites

Immunological homeostasis induced by the microbiota is essential for a functional immune system. Early studies on GF mice revealed that microbial colonization was essential for the development of lymphoid tissues, such as the spleen and lymph nodes, gut-associated lymphoid tissues (GALTs), and the maturation of T cells.[35] Unlike conventionally derived mice, GF mice also do not develop lymphoid follicles in the small bowel and are

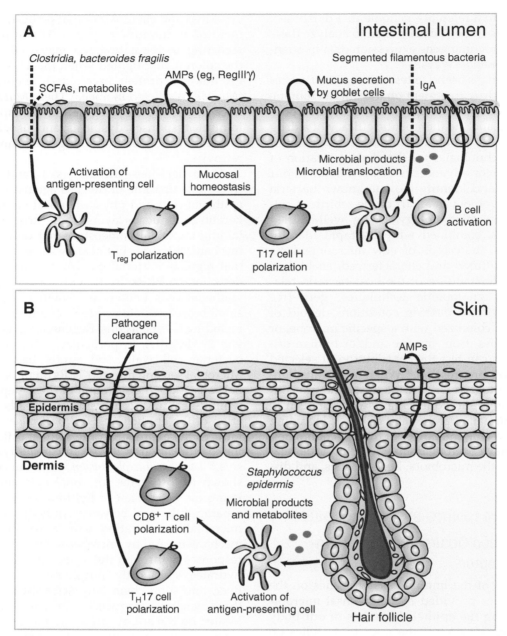

Figure 19.2 **Control of immunity by host microbiota at barrier sites.** (A) The intestinal epithelium is composed of a single cell-layer sheet of epithelial cells, including absorptive and secretory cells such as mucus-producing goblet cells. Specific microbes, like *Clostridia* and *Bacteriodes fragilis*, and microbial metabolic products such as SCFAs support the activation of APCs and the subsequent polarization of naïve T cells to T_{reg} cells. Other microbes, such as segmented filamentous bacteria, support the polarization of T helper 17 (Th17) cells and induce IgA secretion from resident B cells. These immune cells maintain microbial homeostasis along side intestinal epithelial cells which produce AMPs like RegIIIγ. (B) The skin epidermis is several cell layers deep stitched together by secreted lipids. Underneath the epidermis lies the dermis that contains innate and adaptive immune cells. The microbiota that reside in the hair follicles, sebaceous glands, and sweat glands induce the production of AMPs by keratinocytes, and induce the activation of APCs and the subsequent recruitment and polarization of adaptive immune cells, such as CD8+ T cells and Th17. These cells serve to maintain homeostasis by protecting against invasive pathogens.

AMP, antimicrobial peptide; APC, antigen-presenting cell; SCFA, short-chain fatty acid; T_{reg}, regulatory T.

deficient in immunoglobulin A secretion. Colonization of GF animals promotes neutrophils homing to the gut through microbial-induced expression of serum amyloid A, typically expressed by intestinal epithelial cells.[36,37] T helper type 1 (Th1) immune responses are also deficient in GF mice, increasing their susceptibility to infection by

Shigella flexneri.[38,39] Upon colonization with conventional microbes, GF mice demonstrate an increase in IL-10, IL-1, IL-18, IFN-γ, TNF, and the restoration of the complement system in the intestine.[22] In contrast, the systemic delivery of TLR ligands to GF mice does not induce the expression of inflammatory genes such as *Ifnb1*, *Tnf*, and *Il6*.[40] This finding suggests that microbial signals in conventional mice are required to prime cells for TLR signaling in part by epigenetic alteration of chromatin conformation of genes coding for the inflammatory cytokines.[40]

The absence of the gut microbiota increases the susceptibility to influenza virus infection in the lung and to *Listeria* infection in the mouth.[41–43] Similarly, in experimental models of autoimmunity, GF animals do not develop autoimmune diseases, such as multiple sclerosis and arthritis.[44–46] Recently, the gut microbiota was shown to foster efficacious anticancer responses upon treatment with immunotherapy and chemotherapy, while in the absence of microbes, the therapies are inefficient.[47–50]

Through the advent of next-generation sequencing and gnotobiotic technology, recent studies have linked specific microbial niches to immune cell development. When GF mice are colonized with *Bacteriodes fragilis* in combination with other commensals, the balance between Th1 and Th2 type responses is restored.[51] Pro-inflammatory signals such as IFN-γ from Th1 cells and IL-17 from Th17 cells are maintained at homeostasis by the anti-inflammatory signals from regulatory T cells (T_{reg} cells). When the intestine is colonized with segmented filamentous bacteria (SFB), these microbes promote the polarization of Th17 and, to lesser degree, Th1 cells.[37,52,53] SFB also promotes the exclusion of pathogens such as *Citrobacter rodentium* and *Salmonella spp.*, as well as increases IgA production.[54] SFB can penetrate the thick mucus layer and interact closely with the intestinal epithelium. There, dendritic cell sampling and antigen presentation in the lamina propria results in the differentiation of Th17 cells from T-helper precursors.[53] Hence, upon monocolonization with SFB, GF animals reestablish susceptibility to experimental models of arthritis and allergic encephalomyelitis through a Th17-mediated autoimmune response.[45,46] Remarkably, these microbial species are so influential on immune cell responses that they alone are enough to trigger autoimmunity. In humans, colonization of SFB has been shown to occur mostly within the first three years of life, correlating with the maturation of the immune system. The SFB community is significantly reduced in most individuals older than 36 months.[55–57]

Unlike SFB, monocolonization of GF mice with *B. fragilis* promotes the differentiation of T_{reg} cells in the colon through its capsular polysaccharide A, which binds TLR2 on CD4[+] T cells.[35,58] Other microbes that support anti-inflammatory responses include *Clostridia* clusters IV, XIVa, and XVIII. These promote the development of T_{reg} cells

by promoting TGF-β1 release from intestinal epithelial cells in the lamina propria.[59] SCFAs produced by microbial fermentation of dietary fibers, specifically butyrate, drive CNS1-dependent differentiation of extrathymic T_{reg} cells. Luminal concentrations of SCFAs correlate with the number of T_{reg} cells in the colon.[60–62] SCFAs are protective in preventing experimental autoimmune encephalomyelitis and contact hypersensitivity reactions in the skin.[63,64] Through induction of T_{reg} cells, SCFAs also limit the antitumor effect of CTLA-4 blockade in cancer patients.[65]

In the small intestine, isolated lymphoid follicles comprised of B cells and T cells do not develop in GF mice.[66] However, spleen marginal zone B cells are unaffected in GF mice, suggesting that lymphoid structures at barrier sites rely more heavily on microbial cues. Interestingly, mice with a stable, distinct community of resident bacteria preferentially promote the expansion of CD8[+] cytotoxic T cells (CTLs) relative to mice with a stable, but different microbial composition at the species to family levels.[67] In the same study, CTLs were found to impair B-cell development in the marginal zone through a perforin-dependent cytolytic mechanism.[67]

The skin contains a microbial community that controls the balance between T_{reg} cells and effector cells through IL-1 and MyD88 signaling. However, in contrast to the gut, the skin microbiota is not required for the development of secondary lymphoid tissues.[68,69] The skin of GF mice has subdued IFN-γ and IL-17 production from T cells and demonstrates a greater abundance of T_{reg} cells compared to conventional mice. Remarkably, mono-association of the skin with *Staphylococcus epidermis* was sufficient to restore IFN-γ and IL-17 responses.[70] However, the restoration of local immunity on the skin has no effect on the immune maturation of other organs.

Although the gut microbiota has been shown to have systemic effects, attributed to its large biomass and diversity, the biomes of organs such as the skin display a compartmentalized modulation of local inflammation and immunity and appear to play a smaller role in systemic immunity.[68] However, it is plausible that the contribution of the microbes at all barrier sites, combined, contributes to systemic homeostasis. The regulation of systemic immunity by the gut microbiota to infection was demonstrated in studies that described a link between the gut microbiota and the immune response to influenza virus infection in the lung.[41,71] Antibiotic-treated mice were limited in their capacity to control viral replication due to a reduction in the constitutive expression of pro-IL-1β and pro-IL-18 genes. In addition, IFN-γ production by immune cells was also inhibited. Remarkably, the systemic administration of TLR ligands rescued the immune response necessary to clear the infection.[71] The gut microbiota has also been shown to be indispensable for the extravasation of neutrophils to remote sites of injury, a response mediated by MyD88-dependent signaling.[36,72]

Microbes Regulate the Composition of Their Community Through Colonization Resistance Mechanisms

In addition to toning their local immune environment, microbial populations also regulate the expansion of other niches along the gastrointestinal tract through competition for nutrients, secretion of inhibitory peptides, and through the modulation of local immune responses. These mechanisms could serve as potential therapeutic targets to modulate the microbial composition of the gut, thereby fostering the therapeutic efficacy of immunotherapeutic agents. Indeed, outgrowth of *Lactobacilli* in mice treated with antibiotics has been shown to negatively correlate with TNF expression in flank tumors treated with CpG-ODN. Impaired TNF expression likely contributed to the poor outcome of anticancer responses in antibiotic-treated mice.[48] Like *Lactobacilli*, vancomycin-resistance *enterococci* (VRE) may expand to 10^7 bacteria per gram of luminal content in some antibiotic-treated hosts; 10,000-fold higher than in untreated hosts.[73] Interestingly, recolonization of the antibiotic-treated infected mice by fecal transplant eliminated the VRE infection and efficient elimination was shown to correlate with the abundance of *Barnesiella intestihominis,* a dominant colonic anaerobe.[74] The mechanism by which this occurs is unclear; however, it is likely due to a combination of the reestablishment of microbial homeostasis and the induction of local host immune response. The observation that VRE growth is reduced in the cecal contents of untreated mice, but not in filtered or sterilized cecal contents, excludes depletion of nutrient as a likely cause for these findings.[75] Therefore, soluble factors secreted by the microbiota or the host are more likely to mediate the response against VRE and limit its expansion. While a direct role of *B. intestihominis* remains based on correlative evidence, it has been shown that a four-strained consortium of commensal bacteria that contains a strain of *Blautia producta* can reverse antibiotic-induced susceptibility to VRE infection.[76] This was mediated by the ability of *B. producta* to reduce growth of VRE by secreting a lantibiotic that is similar to the nisin-A produced by *Lactococcus lactis.*[77] In patients, the high abundance of the lantibiotic gene reduces the risk of VRE infection.[77] In other cases of opportunistic infection by pathobionts, microbes compete for the same nutrients, as in the case of *B. thetaiotaomicron* which directly competes with the *Citrobacter rodentium* for plant-derived monosaccharides and subsequently leads to its clearance.[78] *B. thetaiotaomicron* also secretes molecules that inhibit production of shigella toxin by enterohaemorrhagic *Escherichia coli.*[79] To combat viral intruders, *B. thetaiotaomicron* and *Bifidobacterium longum* increased the expression of antiviral GTPase-induced type I interferon responses.[30] Interestingly, the administration of anti-CTLA-4 antibodies to mice bearing MCA205 sarcomas increases the abundance of *B. thetaiotaomicron* and *B. fragilis* in the gut.[49] When these microbes were administered into tumor-bearing mice, the therapeutic efficacy of anti-CTLA4 increased through a mechanism involving the differentiation of Bacteroides-specific Th1 cells.[49] *B. fragilis* also stimulates dendritic cells in the gut, which present polysaccharide A (PSA) cell wall components to naïve T cells, inducing their differentiation to T_{reg} cells that secrete IL-10 and anti-inflammatory cytokines.[51,80] This results in a state of mucosal tolerance to *B. fragilis* that allows the outgrowth of this commensal bacterium. These examples are part of a multitude of effects driven by commensal microbes to promote homeostasis at barrier sites by regulating the abundance of specific microbial niches and by preventing pathogens' dominance either through direct inhibition, nutrient competition, and/or regulation of adaptive immune responses.

The Immunology of Carcinogenic Pathogens

Microbial-driven cancers account for about 16% of cancer cases worldwide.[81] Of the human skin commensal polyomaviruses, the recently characterized Merkel cell polyomaviruses are regarded as a causal factor in Merkel cell carcinoma, an aggressive and often lethal skin cancer, and they have also been suggested to be a possible cause of bladder cancer.[82,83] Of the human herpesviruses, Epstein-Barr virus (EBV) is associated with Burkett's lymphoma, gastric cancer, and nasopharyngeal carcinoma.[84] In addition, Kaposi's sarcoma-associated herpesvirus type 8 causes the development of Kaposi's sarcoma in immunosuppressed individuals.[85] Hepatitis viruses that are known to account for approximately 80% of hepatocellular carcinoma include hepatitis B virus (HBV) and hepatitis C virus (HCV).[86,87] In addition to cervical cancer, a proportion of head and neck cancers, anogenital cancers, and skin cancers are also induced by oncogenic strains of human papilloma viruses (HPVs).[88,89] One aspect that links many of these viruses is their ability to immortalize cells through genetic alterations of tumor-suppressors and signaling pathways. Viral oncogenes, regulated by alternative RNA splicing, are expressed by HPV, adenovirus, and polyomavirus, while some DNA tumor viruses encode microRNAs in order to modulate the host cell's replication mechanisms.[90]

In addition to the transforming effects of the virus, the environment in which the virus is infecting host cells also impacts tumor progression. For example, during infection of the urogenital tract, vaginal inflammation and dysbiosis have been associated with enhanced tumor progression induced by HPVs.[91,92] In the case of HBV and HCV, the development of hepatocellular carcinoma is directly related to the magnitude and the extent of the inflammatory response to the virus. HCV inhibits the antiviral signaling cascade by suppressing type I interferon production and interferon-regulated immune responses.[93] HBV, on the other hand, was linked to intestinal dysbiosis caused by an increase in fungal biodiversity, including *Candida* spp., an increase in the abundance of *Bifidobacterium dentium,* but a decrease in *Bifidobacterium catenulatum.*[94,95]

Helicobacter pylori is the only human bacterial species categorized as a class I carcinogen and is a known risk factor for gastric cancer, the fifth-leading cause of cancer-related deaths worldwide.[96] The remarkable adaptation of this Gram-negative microbe allows it to survive for prolonged periods of time in the harsh environment of the stomach, where it induces inflammation through the production of virulence factors, resulting from epithelial injury and IL-1β secretion by infected dendritic cells.[97] Long-term, sustained inflammation likely contributes to the changes in microbial composition in gastric tissues and to the *KRAS* and *p53* mutations observed in gastric adenocarcinomas.[98,99] The microbial niche deteriorates to the extent that *H. pylori* is no longer detected at the sites of atrophic body gastritis, supporting the hypothesis that *H. pylori* may also facilitate the expansion of other cancer-inducing pathobionts.[100]

In some cases of colorectal cancer, certain microbes have been identified within the tumor microenvironment. *Streptococcus gallolyticus* sequences have been found in approximately 20% of colon tumors, compared to control tissue where the abundance is less than 5%.[101,102] Though the contribution of *S. gallolyticus* to carcinogenesis is still under investigation, in a small number of cases co-infection of the colon tumor and bloodstream does occur, suggesting that *S. gallolyticus* contributes to the disintegration of the barrier function.[101–105] A more virulent colonic pathogen, enterotoxigenic *B. fragilis* (ETBF), is a leading cause of morbidity and mortality from diarrheal illnesses in developing countries. Its virulence factor, *B. fragilis* toxin fragilysin, a zinc-metallo-protease, weakens the structure of the intestinal epithelium through digestion of E-cadherin, a structural protein involved in cell-cell adhesion junctions. E-cadherin also has an intracellular function by triggering cellular division via activation of the *Wnt/*β-catenin pathway, leading to activation of the protooncogene *MYC* and colon carcinogenesis.[106,107] Murine models of spontaneous colorectal cancer show that ETBF rapidly induces colorectal carcinoma (CRC) by inducing an IL-17 response, similar to those observed in human CRC.[108]

Recently, microbes have been identified within solid tumors that originate or reside in tissues not in direct contact with the epithelial barrier surfaces on which commensal microbes reside, such as pancreatic cancer, lung cancer, and colorectal carcinoma metastases.[109–112] These tumor-associated microbes are hypothesized to modulate cancer progression and susceptibility to therapy.

In murine pancreatic ductal adenocarcinoma models, tumor-associated gammaproteobacteria produce cytidine deaminase that inactivate the cytotoxic drug gemcitabine. The antibiotic ciprofloxacin eliminates these proteobacteria and re-establishes sensitivity to gemcitabine.[110] High microbial species diversity (α-diversity) in the tumors predicts longer overall survival of pancreatic cancer patients.[112] An opposite correlation was described in non-small-cell lung cancer patients: in this case, progression-free and disease-free survival correlates with lower α-diversity in nontransformed tumor-adjacent lung tissues (but not in the tumor).[111] *Fusobacterium* spp. and their associated microbiota are frequently associated with human colon carcinomas; they are also detected in distant metastases and persisted for several passages when the metastatic tumors are transplanted in immunocompromised mice.[109] Antibiotics that eliminate *Fusobacteria* slow tumor growth, suggesting the possibility to target cancer-associated bacteria for cancer therapy.[109] Tumor-associated bacteria in different types of tumors including breast, lung, ovary, pancreas, melanoma, bone, and brain tumors have been recently characterized using a novel sequencing method analyzing five regions of the *16S rRNA* gene, microscopy, and cell culture.[113] Most cancer types contain bacteria, mostly present intracellularly inside either tumor cells or infiltrating immune cells. The microbiome composition is distinct in each type of tumor and is most rich and diverse in breast cancers. The tumor-associated bacteria and their predicted functions correlate with tumor types, patients' smoking status, and the response to immunotherapy.[113]

Several studies have also studied the presence of intratumoral microbes (particularly bacteria but also viruses and fungi) by analyzing publicly available cancer whole-genome sequences or RNA sequences (e.g., The Cancer Genome Atlas [TCGA]) for the presence of non-human microbial sequences.[114–116] Owing to the very low microbial biomass in samples derived from tumors or healthy tissues; however, these studies have been hampered by the overwhelming presence of contaminants and by substantial "batch" effects of the sequencing methodology used in different institutions.[114,116] The sources of contamination include handling of surgical specimens by surgeons and laboratory technicians, contamination of molecular biology reagents, and cross-contamination during sequencing. In addition to the surgical biopsy samples, microbial DNA can be detected in blood and cell-free plasma. Although, in the absence of septicemia, blood was thought to be sterile, low levels of microbial DNA can be detected either as free fragments or microbes or in some cases carried inside blood cells. It seems to be constantly present in the blood, probably due to transitory exchanges through the mucosal or skin epithelial barriers or from cancer tissue that, because of their abnormal vasculature, metabolic characteristics, and low oxygen level, may offer a thriving environment for certain types of bacteria.[117,118]

A recent study analyzed microbial sequences in TCGA samples from more than 10,000 patients with 33 different tumor types, including tumor biopsies, non-neoplastic tumor-adjacent tissue, blood samples, and matching tissues from individuals without cancer.[116] Novel algorithms were applied to recognize and discard contaminant bacterial sequences and machine learning was used to identify microbial signatures. It was found that the microbial composition associated with the tumor and blood samples not only discriminated between tumor and non-neoplastic tissues but also allowed the identification of the tumor type.[116] The data obtained using total blood sequences from TCGA were validated using plasma from a confirmation cohort including patients with prostate, lung, or skin cancer as well as healthy donors.[116] The use of a blood test for cancer detection and prediction of recurrence after therapy would represent an important progress in cancer diagnosis. Liquid tumor biopsies that present tumor biomarkers, including cell-free DNA, have been reported to allow the identification, the presence, and the type of cancer with some accuracy.[119] The report showing that the analysis of microbial DNA found in blood may distinguish patients with cancer from individuals without cancer and, moreover, identifies the tumor type adds a possible new dimension to liquid biopsy-based diagnostics that could facilitate a practical and accurate implementation in cancer screening.[116]

The Contribution of Commensal Microbes to Carcinogenesis

The disruption of the intestinal ecosystem, either through alterations in host immunity, unbalanced diet, or inflammatory damage to the epithelium, can result in dysbiosis and may foster carcinogenesis induced by commensal microbes.[120] The secretion of IL-18 by intestinal epithelial cells and myeloid cells is dependent on an intricate pro-inflammatory signaling and inflammasome activation by SCFAs.[121,122] IL-18 has been shown to be integral to intestinal homeostasis by promoting pathogen clearance and barrier integrity.[122] When different components of the inflammasome are missing in genetically manipulated mice, the interruption of IL-18 production, detection, and signaling ensues. For example, mice deficient in the NLR-related protein 6 inflammasome, which cleaves and activates IL-18, exhibit faulty mucus-producing goblet cells which may harbor persistent enteric infections like C. rodentium.[123] The immunological deficiencies in these mice also include intestinal dysbiosis, marked by the expansion of the bacterial phyla Bacteroidetes (Prevotellaceae) and TM7, as well as an increased susceptibility to colorectal cancer. In fact, the colitogenic

microbes are transmissible and induce intestinal inflammation in healthy, wildtype hosts.[124] Concomitantly, recipients of these microbes are also more susceptible to chemically induced colitis-associated colorectal cancer.[23,24,124–126] Yet, in other models, microbe fermentation of dietary fibers to produce SCFAs has been shown to prevent carcinogenesis. SCFAs act directly on intestinal epithelial cells through inflammasome activation to help produce IL-18, which promotes the production of IL-22 from type 3 innate lymphoid cells and blocks the production of the IL-22 antagonist IL-22BP from myeloid cells. IL-22, in turn, promotes antibacterial peptide secretions as well as epithelial proliferation; however, its role in carcinogenesis remains controversial.[23,126,127] On the other hand, T_{reg} cells produce the anti-inflammatory cytokine IL-10, which suppresses inflammation and carcinogenesis.[32] SCFAs promote the expansion of colonic T_{reg} cells in GF animals, demonstrating the importance of microbial function in the differentiation of these cells.[60–62] These T_{reg} cells are inducible or peripherally derived T_{reg} cells, that do not undergo regulator effector differentiation in the thymus like natural T_{reg} cells.[62] When genes encoding key inflammation regulatory molecules, such as IL-10, or T and B cell developmental factors, such as Rag2, are genetically ablated in mice, the mice become susceptible to colitis and colorectal cancer.[107] Moreover, the dysbiosis observed in the gut of these animals is transferrable to healthy, wildtype hosts, potentially increasing their susceptibility to carcinogenesis.

Colorectal carcinoma (CRC) in humans has been shown to be associated with particular bacterial species that may form biofilms on the neoplastic lesions or adjacent mucosa.[128,129] Fusobacterium spp., Bacteroidetes, Lachnospiraceae, and proteobacteria have been described as enriched in patients with CRC and are probably the expression of dysbiosis that is responsible for inflammation leading to tumor initiation or progression.[128,129] Fusobacterium nucleatum, an oral commensal, was recently found to reside in the microenvironment of colorectal tumors, where it activates tumor-promoting myeloid cells and cell division in colon epithelial cells.[130,131] Within the tumor microenvironment, F. nucleatum is able to inhibit natural killer (NK) cells, which would otherwise mediate an antitumor response.[132] This interaction is mediated by the microbial protein Fap2 which binds the NK cell receptor called T cell immunoreceptor with Ig and ITIM domains (TIGIT) present on human, but not mouse, NK cells.[132] Within the proteobacteria involved in both experimental and clinical colon carcinogenesis, particularly relevant are E. coli strains expressing the gene cluster (pks island) encoding nonribosomal peptide and polyketide synthases leading to the synthesis of colibactin—a bacterial genotoxin that alkylates DNA at adenosine residues inducing double-stranded breaks in the eukaryotic cells with a defined mutational signature.[133–136]

This mutational signature was described in over 20% of CRCs, suggesting pks-positive strains of *E. coli* may play an important role in CRC tumor initiation.[135] In several experimental models of colitis-associated colon carcinogenesis, *pks+ E. coli* strains have been shown to promote polyps formation.[134,137] Anti-TNF therapy, a well-established treatment for inflammatory bowel disease, also prevents colitis-associated colon cancer in mice and likely in human patients by altering the gut microbiota composition and transcriptional activity, including that of the genes in *E. coli* that control colibactin synthesis.[137]

The microbes associated with colon carcinogenesis also increase carcinogenesis by modulating the microbial composition of the tumor microenvironment through quorum-sensing mechanisms, competing for nutrients, and secreting antimicrobial peptides.[107] In addition, it is likely that cancer-promoting microbes traverse the epithelium at the sites where adenomas are present, due to the barrier defects present at those sites.[138] The inflammation invoked by the translocating microbes has been shown to be necessary for tumor progression whereas sampling of these microbes by tumor-infiltrating myeloid cells likely induces cancer-promoting cytokines such as IL-23, IL-17, TNF, and IL-1 that drive polyp formation.[138,139] By changing the microbiota of neoplasm-prone mice, through antibiotic treatment, the development of serrated polyps was markedly decreased.[139]

In addition to the local effects on tumor formation at the barrier sites on which the microbiota resides, like in the colon, certain gut commensals may also affect carcinogenesis at distant sterile sites. *Helicobacter hepaticus*, for example, not only enhances tumorigenesis in the gut of mice in chemically induced and spontaneous models of colorectal cancer but also induces a systemic inflammatory response that increases the susceptibility of APC$^{min/+}$ mice to prostate cancer and mammary carcinoma.[127,140–144] In another instance, *H. hepaticus* was shown to promote the development of liver carcinogenesis in mice exposed to carcinogenic chemicals and hepatitis virus transgenes.[145]

The Contribution of the Microbiota to Cancer Therapy Efficacy

After decades of discovery, testing, and demonstrating the anticancer potential of immunomodulatory drugs in preclinical settings, immunotherapeutics (treatments designed to modulate immune responses) have become a new weapon in the arsenal against these malignancies. Long-lasting responses were observed in a high percentage of patients with lung cancer and metastatic melanoma treated with these therapies.[146] One of the limitations of the use of immunotherapeutics is the variable nature of the patients' immune response to different types of cancer.[147] By harnessing the potential of the gut microbiota in stimulating the immune system, the therapeutic efficacy of these drugs could be boosted, thereby improving clinical outcomes.

Adoptive T Cell Transfer

The adoptive transfer of cancer-specific cytotoxic T cells was one of the earliest immunotherapeutic strategies in which the importance of the gut microbiota in the clinical outcomes of the treatment was identified. Upon total body irradiation, the translocation of the microbiota from the intestinal lumen to the mesenteric lymph nodes supports the anticancer effects of the transferred cytotoxic T cells.[148] These effects are mediated by TLR4 signaling, as demonstrated by the abrogated effects in *Tlr4*-deficient mice. Remarkably, the therapeutic efficacy in antibiotic-treated mice, which demonstrate poor outcomes upon T cell transfer, is rescued by the administration of the TLR4 agonist, LPS. These findings are supported by clinical data which show that patients with metastatic melanoma respond better to treatment if the myeloablative radiotherapy is used in conjunction with adoptive cell transfer.[149]

Cyclophosphamide

Cyclophosphamide (CTX) is an alkylating drug that has been used to target cancer cells over the last five decades. Furthermore, the immunosuppressive properties of CTX, at high doses, are efficacious in the treatment of bone marrow transplant recipients and autoimmune disorders, including lupus erythematosus and rheumatoid arthritis. At low doses, CTX inhibits T$_{reg}$ cell functions and enhances immune responses.[150] In addition, CTX induces the immunogenic cell death of tumors, and activates antitumor adaptive immunity.[151]

The importance of the gut microbiota in the chemotherapeutic efficacy of CTX was demonstrated by comparing the efficacy of the drug in conventional mice and in GF mice. The antitumor effects of the drug were also tested in mice administered wide-spectrum non-absorbable antibiotics that depleted the gut microbiota. When GF mice with developing MCA205 sarcomas were treated with CTX, they showed poor therapeutic responses compared to conventional mice.[47] The efficacy of CTX was also reduced in mice administered the Gram-positive bacteria selective antibiotic, vancomycin A. These mice harbored fewer "pathogenic" Th17 (pTh17) cells (expressing markers of Th1 cells such as transcription factor T-bet, IFN-γ, and the chemokine receptor CXCR3) and Th17 cells (expressing RORγt and CCR6 and secreting IL-17). Together with cytotoxic T lymphocytes, these cells drove the immunogenic clearance of tumors. The insult to the intestinal epithelium, induced by CTX, enhanced the transmucosal translocation of specific Gram-positive bacteria, *Lactobacillus johnsonii* and *Enterococcus hirae*. These microbes were key to fostering the development of an immunological response, including activation of pTh17 cells, which maximized the therapeutic efficacy of CTX by invoking antitumor adaptive immunity.[47]

Platinum-Based Drugs

The chemotherapy drugs oxaliplatin and cisplatin induce genotoxicity and apoptosis of tumor cells. Oxaliplatin, but not cisplatin, also activates programmed cell death. Upon treatment with these drugs, platinum binds DNA to form intrastrand cross-linking adducts. The resulting DNA damage triggers the activation of apoptosis.[152] The administration of antibiotics to tumor-bearing mice significantly reduces the therapeutic efficacy of these platinum compounds.[48] Similarly, GF mice with subcutaneous tumors and administered oxaliplatin and cisplatin are unable to effectively combat the growing tumor. The contribution of the microbiota toward the efficacy of these chemotherapeutics was, in part, mediated by the activation of tumor-infiltrating myeloid cells. These cells contributed to the DNA damage induced by oxaliplatin by releasing reactive-oxygen species (ROS). In microbe-deficient animals, subcutaneous EL4 lymphomas demonstrated attenuated oxaliplatin-induced DNA damage and reduced the expression of ROS-responsive genes. Therefore, the therapeutic efficacy of oxaliplatin depends upon the priming of the myeloid cells by the gut microbiota for the release of ROS that contribute to the genotoxicity that drives tumor cell apoptosis.[48]

CpG Oligonucleotides and Anti-Interleukin 10 Receptor Immunotherapy[148,149,152]

CpG-ODN are Toll-like receptor 9 (TLR9) agonists, which mimic the unmethylated CpG motifs present in microbial DNA. They enhance the body's immune responses to vaccines against malaria and hepatitis B virus, for example, by inducing the expression of pro-inflammatory cytokines.[153] In humans, synthetic CpG-ODN are able to bind TLR9 on plasmacytoid dendritic cells and B cells, thereby enhancing the body's immune response to tumors, particularly when used in conjunction with peptide vaccines.[154] In mice, the antitumor efficacy of CpG-ODN was enhanced when combined with anti-interleukin-10 receptor antibodies (α-IL-10R ab). This combination reactivated tumor-infiltrating dendritic cells, triggering de novo synthesis of IL-12 and eliciting antitumor immune memory.[155] This combination therapy induces a rapid hemorrhagic necrosis of treated tumors dependent on the release of pro-inflammatory cytokines such as tumor necrosis factor (TNF) and nitric oxide by tumor-infiltrating macrophages followed by the activation of tumor-specific cytotoxic T lymphocytes.[156] Remarkably, tumor-bearing GF mice and antibiotic-treated mice are refractory to this treatment, revealing

the importance of the gut microbiota in immunotherapy.[48] In the microbiota-deficient animals treated with CpG ODN/α-IL-10R ab, various subsets of tumor-infiltrating myeloid cells show a reduction in IL-12 and TNF production. This response is partially rescued by the administration of LPS to microbiota-deficient mice.

The microbiome analysis of animals treated with CpG-ODN/α-IL-10R ab identified bacterial species that positively and negatively correlated with the antitumor response. The abundance of Gram-negative bacteria of the *Alistipes* genus in the intestinal lumen positively correlated with TNF production in the tumor and gavage of microbiota-depleted animals with LPS induced a recovery of TNF production and therapy effectiveness.[48] On the other hand, the abundance of *Lactobacillus* genera was negatively correlated. When the microbe-depleted mice were administered *Alistipes shahii*, the number of TNF-producing myeloid cells in the tumor increased to the levels observed in the controls and was significantly higher than that observed in the antibiotic-treated mice. A reduction in the TNF response was observed when the animals were gavaged with *Lactobacillus fermentum*. Therefore, the training by the microbiota of tumor-infiltrating myeloid cells, in part through TLR4, enables the production of TNF by myeloid cells in response to CpG-ODN. At the site of the tumor, this culminates in hemorrhagic necrosis of the tumor, activation of cytotoxic T lymphocytes, and eradication of the tumor.[48]

Anti-CTLA-4 Immunotherapy

Monoclonal antibodies against lymphocyte-associated antigen 4 (CTLA-4), the programmed cell death protein 1 (PD1), and its ligand, PDL-1, are immune checkpoint inhibitors with significant clinical efficacy in patients with advanced melanoma, renal cell cancer, and lung cancer.[157] Antibodies against CTLA-4 block the interaction of CTLA-4 with its ligands, thereby bypassing the inhibition checkpoint and instead proceeding on with T cell proliferation and additionally depleting T_{reg} cells from the tumor microenvironment. Similar to other immunotherapeutics, anti-CTLA-4 therapy of subcutaneous tumors is not effective in GF mice or in mice treated with antibiotics.[49] Indeed, the efficacy of anti-CLTA-4 depended on the abundance of the intestinal microbiota species *Bacteriodes*, such as *B. thetaiotaomicron* and *B. fragilis*, and the proteobacteria *Burkholderia cepacia*. Interestingly, anti-CLTA-4 antibodies altered the microbial composition of both patients and mice due to the intestinal injury caused by the drug. However, GF mice became responsive to the therapy after being colonized with any of the three species that were previously mentioned. The microbiota in these models was required for activating dendritic cell functions necessary for the antitumor immune responses that are boosted by the anti-CTLA-4 treatment. In addition, the presentation of antigens derived from these microbes by dendritic cells to T cells was shown to be an important mechanism of antitumor immunity as demonstrated by the ability of *B. fragilis*-specific Th1 cells to rescue the antitumor efficacy of anti-CTLA-4 therapy when adoptively transferred into GF mice.[49] Remarkably, the toxicity to the intestinal epithelium induced by anti-CTLA-4 treatment was abrogated in GF mice gavage with a combination of *B. fragilis* and *B. cepacia*, indicating that modification of the microbiota composition could improve therapy effectiveness while ameliorating immune-related adverse reactions.[49]

Anti-PD1/PD-L1 Immunotherapy

Tumor-infiltrating T cells produce IFN-γ that stimulates the expression of PD-L1 in many cells in the tumor microenvironment, including the tumor cells. Once PD-L1 binds to the PD-1 receptor on activated T cells, they become exhausted and their tumoricidal capabilities are diminished. Antibodies against PD-L1 and PD-1 prevent their interaction, thereby prolonging the cytotoxic capacity of T cells.[157] Unlike anti-CTLA-4 treatment, an absolute requirement of the microbiota in licensing the therapeutic efficacy of anti-PD-L1 treatment in mice was not consistently observed. However, mice from different vendors and with different microbial compositions showed differences in tumor growth rates and ability to respond to anti-PD-L1.[50] *Bifidobacterium* spp. were found to be more abundant in the responding mice and able to promote antitumor immunity against the B16 transplantable melanoma. In the group of mice without *Bifidobacterium* spp., anti-PD-L1 treatment reduced tumor growth but the therapeutic efficacy was lower than in those that contained the microbe in their intestinal niche. Upon supplementing the mice with a cocktail of *Bifidobacterium* spp., the antitumor effects of anti-PD-L1 were significantly increased, whereupon tumor growth was almost completely abrogated.[50]

Recently, several studies have addressed the role of the microbiota in patients treated with anti-PD1. It has been shown that patients treated with anti-PD1, particularly lung and kidney cancer patients, that have received antibiotics treatment before or soon after anti-PD1 treatment have a significantly decreased progression-free and overall survival.[158–161] Studies in anti-PD1 treated patients with melanoma, lung, or kidney cancer have identified bacterial species in the patients' gut that correlated with a successful antitumor response. When transferred alone or as part of a more complex microbiota, in bacteria-depleted mice, it conferred responsiveness to anti-PD1 treatment leading to a series of subsequent experimental mechanistic studies.[161–164] However, the different studies identified a wide variety of bacterial species and clear unifying mechanisms have not yet been uncovered. In lung cancer patients, an antitumor promoting role for the mucin-degrading bacterial species *Akkermansia muciniphila* was identified.[161] A higher frequency of *Staphylococcus haemolyticus* and *Corynebacterium aurimucosum* was found in nonresponder patients and a higher representation of *Enterococcus hirae* in responder patients were also identified. In melanoma patients, one study demonstrated an enrichment of *Clostridiales*, *Ruminococcaceae*, and *Faecalibacterium* in responder patients and in Bacteroidales in nonresponder patients.[164] A favorable composition of gut microbiota at treatment baseline was associated with enhanced cytotoxic CD8+ T cell infiltration in the tumor bed and evidence of preexisting anticancer immune responses.[164] Another study identified an increased abundance of *Bifidobacterium longum* (confirming the murine data), *Colinsella aerofaciens*, and *Enterococcus faecium* in melanoma patients responding to anti-PD1.[50,163] Together, these studies based on correlative clinical data and strong, mechanistic experimental animal evidence strongly support the conclusion that the gut microbiota modulates the response to inhibitors of the PD1-PD-L1 axis. While the composition of the human microbiota is quite resilient and changes little during adult life, a change in lifestyle such as diet, the use of drugs and medications, early childhood exposure, stress, and antibiotic use may result in major changes in microbial composition.[165] Thus, the discrepant data from the different studies may be due to the reduced size of the patient cohorts, their geographical localization, and the different endpoints for therapy response. Also, the accuracy of taxonomic identification both by 16 rRNA gene sequencing or by shotgun meta genomics is limited by the current incomplete databases of full bacterial genomic sequences. However, rapid progress is being made in the isolation and deposition of the genomes of new species and the development of new pipelines for genomic analysis. It should also be considered that the observed effects on immunotherapy may not be due to the single species but rather to the overall contribution of the gut microbiota ecology and metabolism. The species or group of species identified in the different studies may represent biomarkers of the ecological and metabolic status of the gut microbiota. Due to the heterogeneity and limited size of the clinical cohorts analyzed, different species reached significance in the various trials. Better standardized studies in terms of sample collection, DNA purification, sequencing, and bioinformatic analysis, together with larger clinical cohorts correcting for the population difference, will allow a more accurate identification of the composition and metabolic characteristics of the microbiota able to promote favorable clinical responses.

The recent clinical results have generated much interest in targeting the microbiota to increase the number of patients that can benefit from the therapy. There are ongoing studies of transplanted fecal microbiota from patients that responded to anti-PD1 treatment into anti-PD1 refractory patients with cautiously promising results being reported.[166] Also, clinical trials are ongoing using different formulations of single bacterial species or combination of species that have been shown, in clinical trials and in experimental animals, to correlate with successful anti-PD1 therapy.[167,168]

Allogenic Bone Marrow Transplant

Allogenic hematopoietic stem cell transplantation and bone marrow transplantation following chemotherapy or chemoradiotherapy is a common treatment used to eliminate a wide variety of cancers, including multiple myeloma, chronic and acute leukemia, and solid tumors. The graft used to restore hematopoiesis to patients, however, can elicit graft-versus-host-disease (GvHD), as well as systemic infections.[169] Paneth cells, which secrete antimicrobial peptides in the small bowel, are targeted by GvHD and stop producing α-defensins, which kill pathogens. The treatment and, in particular, the prophylactic use of antibiotics is associated with a decrease in the phylogenic diversity of the gut and a notable bloom of *E. coli*.[170,171] Patients with low microbial diversity at the time of engraftment showed higher mortality rates than those with higher diversity.[172] In patients, the microbiota changed substantially during GvHD due to the antibiotics given as part of the treatment regimen, typified by the loss of *Clostriadiales* and the bloom of *Lactobacillales*.[170,173–175] Similar to humans, mice also demonstrated a bloom of *Lactobacillales*. The elimination of *Lactobacillales* before the transplant exacerbated GvHD in mice, whereas reintroducing it conferred protection against the disease. In other clinical studies, some antibiotics fostered the expansion of *Enterococcus*, *Streptococcus*, and *Proteobacteria*, increasing the risk of vancomycin-resistant *Enterococcus* bacteremia.[176] In two additional patient cohorts, the abundance of the genus *Blautia* correlated with the survival of GvHD.[172] These examples demonstrate that even though antibiotics are necessary for the prevention of infection, the selection of pathogen and pathobionts may hinder the survival of the patients after the engraftment. The use of probiotics and autologous fecal preparations, collected from the patients before therapy initiation, may provide support for the patients after transplantation, thereby preventing GvHD and other related toxicities.

CONCLUSION

The body of information regarding the importance of the microbiota in carcinogenesis, tumor progression, and the response to therapy continues to grow. Microbes act locally, either by promoting immune cell polarization, modulating the toxicity of the tumor environment, or altering barrier function. They also produce extraintestinal effects, through the secretion of microbial products and by translocating to other organs, thereby altering systemic immunity and the response to extraintestinal tumors and the efficacy of therapy. These findings are paving the way for clinical approaches such as the use of probiotics and diets, prebiotics, and microbial transplants, to foster therapeutic outcomes by boosting the anticancer responses and cancer[177] therapy, as well as ameliorating cancer comorbidities. It is important to note, however, that studies have shown that even genetically identical mice show differences in cancer susceptibility and responses to immunotherapeutics. This may be due to the development of dysbiosis, either through diet or co-housing with immunodeficient mice, or changes in the fungal, viral, or protozoan communities, as well as the reactivation of endogenous retroviruses.[25,34,124,178–184] Similarly, using antibiotics changes the microbial composition of the gut so drastically that it compromises the efficacy of immunotherapeutics. Analyzing the precise effects of different antibiotics in the clinical setting will help strategize which antibiotics to use without hindering anticancer therapeutic outcomes.[177]

It is also important to consider that the immunology of a rodent is, in some respects, different from that of a human. *Bifidobacterium*, for instance, induces the immune response against tumors and increases the efficacy of anti-PD-L1 therapy.[50] TLR9 is the receptor by which *Bifidobacterium* triggers an inflammatory response, and it is expressed on all myeloid and dendritic cells in mice. In humans, however, TLR9 is primarily expressed on B cells and plasmacytoid dendritic cells;[185] therefore, the effects of *Bifidobacterium* on cancer therapy in humans requires further clinical studies. Though these differences need to be addressed, it is becoming increasingly apparent that targeting the microbiota in cancer is likely to become the next step toward personalized medicine.

KEY REFERENCES

Only key references appear in the print edition. The full reference list appears in the digital product on Springer Publishing Connect: connect.springerpub.com/content/book/978-0-8261-3743-2/part/part01/chapter/ch19

47. Viaud S, Saccheri F, Mignot G, et al. The intestinal microbiota modulates the anticancer immune effects of cyclophosphamide. *Science.* 2013;342(6161):971–976. doi:10.1126/science.1240537
48. Iida N, Dzutsev A, Stewart CA, et al. Commensal bacteria control cancer response to therapy by modulating the tumor microenvironment. *Science.* 2013;342(6161):967–970. doi:10.1126/science.1240527
49. Vetizou M, Pitt JM, Daillere R, et al. Anticancer immunotherapy by CTLA-4 blockade relies on the gut microbiota. *Science.* 2015;350(6264):1079–1084. doi:10.1126/science.aad1329
50. Sivan A, Corrales L, Hubert N, et al. Commensal *Bifidobacterium* promotes antitumor immunity and facilitates anti-PD-L1 efficacy. *Science.* 2015;350(6264):1084–1089. doi:10.1126/science.aac4255

107. Sears CL, Garrett WS. Microbes, microbiota, and colon cancer. *Cell Host Microbe.* 2014;15(3):317–328. doi:10.1016/j.chom.2014.02.007

161. Routy B, Le Chatelier E, Derosa L, et al. Gut microbiome influences efficacy of PD-1-based immunotherapy against epithelial tumors. *Science.* 2018;359(6371):91–97. doi:10.1126/science.aan3706

163. Matson V, Fessler J, Bao R, et al. The commensal microbiome is associated with anti-PD-1 efficacy in metastatic melanoma patients. *Science.* 2018;359(6371):104–108. doi:10.1126/science.aao3290

164. Gopalakrishnan V, Spencer CN, Nezi L, et al. Gut microbiome modulates response to anti-PD-1 immunotherapy in melanoma patients. *Science.* 2018;539(6371):97–103. doi:10.1126/science.aan4236

Synthetic Biology for the Immunotherapy of Cancer

Victor Tieu and Lei S. Qi

KEY POINTS

- Synthetic biology uses engineering approaches to study and manipulate complex biological systems at a molecular–cellular level.

- The chimeric antigen receptor (CAR) T cell is a breakthrough treatment for hematologic cancers but faces specific challenges in solid tumors and beyond.

- Synthetic immunology is an emerging field that addresses clinical unmet needs in CAR T cell therapy by combining synthetic biology approaches with immunological engineering.

- A growing toolkit of synthetic sensors, processors, and actuators has enabled us to engineer more powerful proof-of-concept immune cell therapies.

- The future of synthetic immunology presents significant promise, exciting opportunities, and open questions.

INTRODUCTION TO THE FIELD

The field of synthetic biology is built upon the core idea that engineering approaches can be used to study and manipulate complex biological systems at a molecular–cellular level. Broadly defined, synthetic biology is the rational design of novel molecules, genetic circuits, biological pathways, and whole cells to encode arbitrary, desirable functions. The resulting technologies developed by synthetic biologists are being used to answer fundamental biological questions and address key unmet needs in human health, the environment, and beyond.

Examples of engineering methodologies that are commonly leveraged in synthetic biology include the following: the iterative cycle of design-build-test, the abstraction and black-boxing of phenomena, the emphasis on modular frameworks and closed-loop systems, the systematic perturbation of unknowns, and the development of data-driven computational models. These methods enable us to form a deeper, quantitative understanding of biology that can be used to better predict system behavior and inform the development of useful tools and devices.

The development of new molecular cloning techniques and ever-improving DNA synthesis and sequencing technologies gave birth to the field of modern synthetic biology at the turn of the 21st century.[1] Borrowing concepts from electrical, computer, and systems engineering, early work in the field sought to recapitulate the behavior of common motifs in circuit design and control systems using living cells. For example, various logic gates—which compute simple input–output Boolean operations such as *AND*, *OR*, and *NOT*—were implemented in *Escherichia coli* using synthetic transcriptional regulation and could be composed into larger, combinatorial circuit designs for advanced computing.[1-3]

Other seminal work focused on building and characterizing dynamic circuits that exhibited system-level behavior. The *toggle switch* uses two different chemical inputs to switch between two stable states of gene expression.[4] The *repressilator* is an oscillating circuit generated by closed-loop feedback of transcriptional repressors with a certain frequency.[5] Finally, the *pulse generator* is a circuit that utilizes temporal delay in an incoherent feed-forward loop to sequentially turn a gene *ON* and then *OFF*.[6] These studies demonstrated that complex, arbitrary behavior and synthetic circuits mimicking endogenous processes could be rationally designed, encoded, and executed in living cells using recombinant DNA.

Abstracting Biology

Biological systems are inherently complex and stochastic, which makes them hard to engineer. Early work in synthetic biology has given us a foundation for how to approach the engineering of biology in a systematic way through the use of *abstraction hierarchies* (Figure 20.1).[7,8] In this framework, a system is broken down into distinct

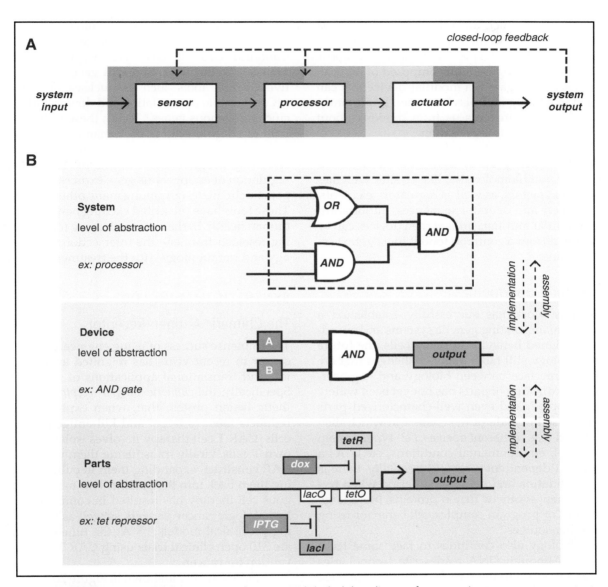

Figure 20.1 **An abstraction hierarchy for an example system.** (**A**) Black-box diagram for a generic sensor-processor-actuator architecture. Arrows denote inputs and outputs. (**B**) Different levels of abstraction for an example processor module. Abstraction "barriers" separate each layer, simplifying and limiting the scope of the engineer.

dox, doxycycline; IPTG, isopropyl β-d-1-thiogalactopyranoside; lacI, lactose repressor; lacO, lactose operator; tetO, tetracycline operator; tetR, tetracycline repressor.

simplified layers that effectively reduce complexity by limiting the scope of the engineer.

At the topmost layer, a system can be represented by a *generic system architecture*, such as the "black-box" diagram shown in Figure 20.1A. This example system uses a modular, sensor-processor-actuator framework. The *sensor* detects arbitrary inputs and feeds the signal to the processing unit, which computes logic. The signal from the *processor* is then sent to the *actuator* unit, which outputs an action. Occasionally, the action may feedback to the processor unit and influence future outputs. This flow of information is often used in other engineering

disciplines and is, for example, analogous to the way a house thermostat works. Sensors detect the ambient room temperature, which is compared with the set temperature by the processor. The decision to heat or cool the room is then sent to the actuator, which physically changes the temperature of the air. Finally, the sensor closes the loop by detecting the new ambient temperature. In the following sections, we discuss how this system-level architecture can be readily applied to the engineering of living cells.

In Figure 20.1B, we can see that to implement such a system, we must delve one layer lower in the abstraction hierarchy to *devices*, which are functional, composable modules that have a specified input–output function. For example, to implement a processor, we might choose to use a combinatorial logic circuit composed of Boolean logic gates. Each logic gate is a modular device that can be combined in a "plug and play" manner. Importantly, the *abstraction barrier* prevents us from thinking about any specific biological implementation.

Finally, at the lowest level of abstraction, we have *parts*. Examples of biological parts include the DNA elements encoding functional biomolecules, like specific enzymes and transcription factors, as well as regulatory elements, such as promoters and operator sequences. Importantly, if parts are modular and *standardized* then devices can be easily assembled from a common toolkit in a context-independent manner.

Challenges and Opportunities

While previous work has successfully established a framework for manipulating genetic systems and encoding human-designed behavior in living cells, the future of synthetic biology still faces many challenges that are unique to the interface between biology and engineering. The standardization of parts has not yet been widely nor strictly adopted, and even well-characterized parts can fail when used outside of the context in which they were developed (e.g., different species, cell type, protein expression level, environmental conditions, etc.).[3] As a result of context-dependent *parts interoperability*, there is a necessary validation and debugging period when trying to express new synthetic fusion proteins, build large genetic circuits, or program complex cell behavior using parts from other sources.[1]

Synthetic biology also continues to face some technical hurdles. Although DNA read–write technologies have greatly advanced in the past few decades, the idea of printing new plasmid DNA from scratch remains quite futuristic. Instead, most laboratories rely on traditional molecular cloning techniques to generate new DNA constructs—this is a major bottleneck to the types of rapid prototyping and testing routinely seen in other engineering fields.[1] Improvements in DNA synthesis will be instrumental to the realization of high-throughput construct designs for applications in protein and circuit engineering. Limitations in our ability to introduce foreign DNA of any size into any cell type (e.g., through transfection or transduction) also pose a challenge, and significant efforts are underway to improve and optimize these protocols.

Despite these challenges, synthetic biology has observed an unprecedented acceleration in growth and progress within the past decade. Notably, the advent of technologies such as clustered regularly interspaced short palindromic repeats (CRISPR) has thoroughly reshaped mammalian synthetic biology by enabling us to engineer and manipulate the genome of living cells. Canonical CRISPR/Cas9 uses a synthetic guide RNA molecule to cut DNA and edit genes, whereas alternative CRISPR tools such as nuclease-deactivated Cas9 (dCas9) enable upregulation and downregulation of specific endogenous genes.[9] Today, these technologies facilitate rapid gene-editing of human cells (e.g., primary T cells), systematic genetic perturbations for genome-wide screening, programmable transcriptional and epigenetic regulation of endogenous gene expression, and complex genetic circuit design among many other applications.[3,9,10] These tools have presented exciting new opportunities in human health. In the next section, we focus on an emerging research frontier—the intersection of synthetic biology and immunology—for the treatment of cancer.

SYNTHETIC IMMUNOLOGY

The Chimeric Antigen Receptor

The immense success of using engineered T cells to treat cancer in recent years has reignited an interest in clinical and translational applications of synthetic biology. Specifically, the *chimeric antigen receptor (CAR)* is a synthetic fusion protein that, when expressed on T cells, redirects them to target and kill antigen-specific tumor cells. CAR T cell therapy involves isolating the patient's own T cells, virally transducing them with the synthetic CAR construct, expanding them in culture, and reinfusing them back into the patient. This new class of autologous cell therapy has resulted in complete remission in hematologic cancer patients as well as in many promising preclinical models.[11–13] At the time of writing, there are 310 open clinical trials using CAR T cells as an intervention for cancer.

The CAR molecule shown in Figure 20.2A is composed of an extracellular single-chain variable fragment (scFv) that recognizes specific tumor surface antigens, linked via a flexible hinge-transmembrane region to intracellular co-stimulatory and endogenous T cell receptor (TCR) activation domains. Notably, from an engineering perspective, the CAR is made of modular and interchangeable parts. While the overall architecture of the CAR remains the same, each domain can be swapped out to achieve distinct functionality (Figure 20.2B).

Assembly of the CAR from its constituent parts results in a single-input, single-output signal transduction device (represented by a *BUFFER* gate). The CAR recognizes a specific surface antigen as its input, and its output is the downstream T cell activation and signaling that parallels, but does not recapitulate, recognition of peptide-bound MHC by the endogenous TCR–CD3 complex. The "truth table" in Figure 20.2A describes CAR function in the context of its input and output: *IF* antigen

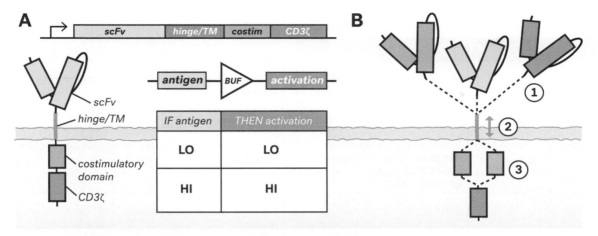

Figure 20.2 Structure and function of the chimeric antigen receptor. (A) Top: Linear DNA map of a representative CAR construct. Left: The CAR is a fusion protein consisting of four domains. Right: The function of the CAR resembles a BUFFER (BUF) gate. **(B)** The structure of the CAR is modular: (1) Different scFvs can be used interchangeably to target different surface antigens. (2) The hinge/transmembrane domain can be lengthened or shortened to tune CAR sensitivity. (3) The co-stimulatory domain most commonly consists of the CD28 or 4-1BB signaling domain.

CAR, chimeric antigen receptor; scFv, single-chain variable fragment; TM, transmembrane.

is HI, *THEN* T cell signaling and activation will be HI, and vice versa.

While the simple BUFFER gate CAR T cell has already proven to be a breakthrough cancer therapy, there are still many challenges that must be addressed. Notably, limited progress has been made in treating solid tumors with CAR T cells.[11,13,14] Furthermore, even in established clinical targets, achieving an effective response using CAR T cells is a balancing act: insufficient CAR T activity results in tumor relapse and outgrowth, whereas overactive CAR T cells can promote lethal systemic toxicity and dysfunction.[12,15] Recent experimental and clinical data have shed light on key barriers to progress, mechanisms of tumor resistance, and drivers of poor clinical outcomes, which are summarized in Table 20.1.

Engineering Immune Cell Therapies

Immune cells are an attractive candidate for biological engineering due to their (a) natural role in whole-body surveillance, (b) ability to compute and execute complex tasks, (c) enhanced motility and trafficking to nearly every organ system, (d) capacity to proliferate, and (e) persistent circulation and formation of long-term memory.[15] In the new and emerging field of *synthetic immunology*, we use recent advances in synthetic biology and genome engineering technologies to encode useful, human-defined genetic programs in immune cells. Within the context of cancer, we can expand the simple BUFFER gate functionality of the conventional CAR T cell to more complex behaviors that address many of the challenges facing CAR T cell therapy in the clinic.[15,42,43]

In Figure 20.3, we apply the powerful generic system architecture of sensing, processing, and actuation to the CAR T cell to define a new therapeutic modality. Biological sensors detect external inputs, such as tumor-associated antigens, cues from the tumor microenvironment, or the physician-controlled administration of synthetic drugs. These inputs are wired to the processor module, which uses encoded circuits to compute whether an action should occur. This information is then sent to the actuator in order to execute a vast and diverse array of biological functions. If the output is fed back into either the cell's sensing or the processing modules, then self-regulation can occur. This "closed-loop" behavior is a major goal of synthetic immunology: engineered feedback systems enable immune cells to evaluate their own performance in real-time and adjust their behavior accordingly. Examples of sensors, processors, and actuators to address clinical unmet needs in CAR T cell therapy are summarized in Table 20.1. In the following sections, we discuss these implementations in greater detail.

SENSING INPUTS

Sensors are devices that detect inputs to the system in real-time and generate signals which are transduced to downstream modules. Examples of naturally occurring sensors in biology include surface receptors, enzymes, transcription factors, and DNA response elements. Biological sensors span a wide range of speeds and sensitivities. The strength of the output signal may be digital-like (approximately binary ON/OFF states with

Table 20.1 Current Synthetic Biology Solutions to Address Clinical Unmet Needs in CAR T Cell Therapy

UNMET NEED[11-13,15]	DESCRIPTION	SYNTHETIC BIOLOGY APPROACHES	REF.
Specificity	Lack of abundant tumor-restricted neoantigen targets, "on-target off-tumor" effects, and tumor heterogeneity	Boolean logic gates, universal CAR designs, combination therapies	16–19
Antigen escape	Tumors exhibit a functional loss of the recognized antigen epitope due to protein downregulation or alternative splicing of isoforms	Boolean logic gates, universal CAR designs, combination therapies	16–19
T cell exhaustion	CAR T cell dysfunction (reduced cytokine secretion, proliferation, and killing) due to tonic signaling	Overexpression of c-Jun, transient "rest" using a drug-regulatable CAR, therapeutic CRISPR gene knockouts, endogenous gene regulation at the *TRAC* locus	20–25
Excessive toxicity	Lethal systemic inflammation and neurotoxicity due to CRS or tumor lysis syndrome	Control systems to regulate CAR expression, ON/OFF switch, kill switch	26–28
Immunosuppression within the tumor microenvironment	Accumulation of cellular signals, biochemical factors, and metabolites in solid tumors that suppress CAR T activity	Sensors to detect the tumor microenvironment, rewiring immunosuppressive signals to activate CAR T cells, metabolic engineering, combination therapies	29–37
Poor trafficking and tumor infiltration	Inability of CAR T cells to infiltrate solid tumors	Sensors to detect solid tumor ECM, local secretion of pro-inflammatory cytokines and degradative enzymes, synthetic chemotaxis	37–41

CAR, chimeric antigen receptor; CRISPR, clustered regularly interspaced short palindromic repeats; CRS, cytokine release syndrome; ECM, extracellular matrix; TRAC, T cell receptor alpha constant.

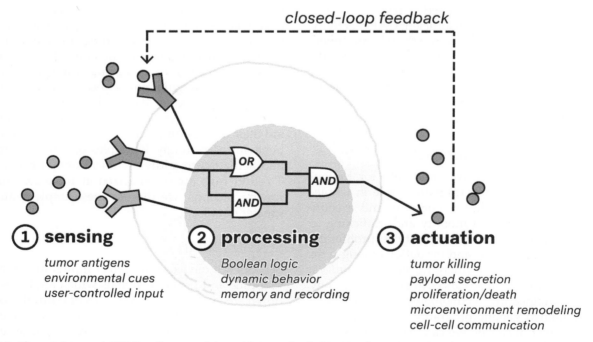

Figure 20.3 The engineered CAR T cell, as envisioned by synthetic immunology, is a new therapeutic modality for the treatment of cancer. A combination of synthetic sensors, processors, and actuators enables "smarter" cells to potentiate a safe and effective antitumor response.

a sharp transition curve) or engineered to vary continuously with input strength. Sensors play a crucial role in engineered immune cells for cancer immunotherapy: input information is integral to the cell's ability to sense its environment, its own state, and the identity of neighboring cells. In the following section, we discuss the design and function of various synthetic sensors—these details are summarized as a schematic diagram in Figure 20.4.

Chimeric Antigen Receptor Engineering

The canonical CAR is a sensor-actuator device that detects the presence of a custom antigen input and wires it to downstream T cell activation (Figure 20.2A). The choice of targeted surface antigen is dictated by the extracellular scFv domain, which can recognize a virtually limitless repertoire of possible epitopes. While the canonical "gold-standard" CAR targets CD19, many other CARs have been generated from this scaffold by swapping out the anti-CD19 scFv for one that targets other tumor-associated antigens, including CD20, CD22, Her2, mesothelin, and B7-H3, among many others.[11,44,45] However, the development of these CARs requires experimental validation and optimization to ensure that the new scFv domain does not interfere with proper protein folding, membrane trafficking, and overall effector function.

Mechanism of Chimeric Antigen Receptor Activation

Current models of TCR and CAR signaling suggest that antigen-dependent activation largely depends on the extent of receptor clustering and mechanotransduction.[46,47] In these models, the extracellular scFv binds strongly to antigens displayed on the surface of target cells. If the antigen density is above a threshold level, the CAR molecules are physically brought together, facilitating receptor clustering, membrane deformation, and phosphorylation of intracellular signaling domains. Interestingly, certain scFvs like the GD2-targeting 14g2a(E101K) can promote antigen-independent CAR aggregation, which drives tonic signaling and exhaustion-related T cell dysfunction.[20,48]

Soluble antigens usually can provide neither the clustering nor the mechanical tensile force needed for CAR activation, limiting targeting to surface antigens. Notably, the development of a CAR targeting soluble TGF-β, a cytokine found in the tumor microenvironment, enables robust rewiring of a normally immunosuppressive soluble signal to instead trigger T cell activation and proinflammatory cytokine secretion.[33] Because TGF-β is naturally homodimeric, crosslinking of the TGF-β-CAR and consequent receptor clustering enables sensing and signal transduction.

Tuning Chimeric Antigen Receptor Sensitivity

Recent studies have shown that the CAR antigen density recognition threshold can be raised or lowered by tuning biophysical parameters of the CAR molecule. For example, the affinity/avidity of the CAR can determine its sensitivity: a low-affinity CD19–CAR selectively targets tumor cells with high antigen density while sparing healthy cells with low antigen expression,[49] and the affinity of the ROR1–CAR affects its ability to sense ROR1$^+$ target cells and to trigger effector function.[50] Structural modifications to the hinge-transmembrane region also affect sensing: tuning the length and composition of this domain affects ROR1–CAR function and enables the CD19–CAR to sense and respond to otherwise undetectable tumor cells with low antigen density.[50,51] Finally, the intracellular signaling domains affect antigen recognition: enhancing the intensity of the CD19–CAR response by increasing the number of immunoreceptor tyrosine-based activation motifs (ITAM) or using a "stronger" co-stimulatory domain enables targeting of antigen-low cells.[51,52]

While we have begun to elucidate the many interdependent factors determining CAR sensitivity, these results are also likely to be context-dependent.[53] Much work is still needed to understand the underlying mechanism of CAR activation and to identify generalizable design principles for CAR engineering.

Alternative Chimeric Antigen Receptor Targeting Moieties

Alternative CAR designs have utilized molecules other than scFvs to target specific antigens. A CAR with an extracellular, single-domain anti-PD-L1 antibody (nanobody) has exhibited antitumor efficacy in preclinical models.[54] Nanobodies are more compact and stable than scFvs, which could facilitate CAR engineering by minimizing the time and effort spent on fusion protein optimization.[55] Other CARs have incorporated ligands as an extracellular domain to target specific receptors upregulated on tumor cells. The IL-13Rα2–CAR currently in a Phase 1 clinical trial for the treatment of glioblastoma uses a mutated IL-13(E13Y) molecule as its targeting domain.[56] Another glioblastoma-targeting CAR uses the small peptide chlorotoxin (CLTX), which is derived from the deathstalker scorpion, as its extracellular targeting domain to broadly sense and destroy malignant glial cells expressing surface MMP-2.[57] This innovative repurposing of ligands that naturally bind to tumor cells as novel CAR targeting domains highlights the modularity and permissiveness of the general CAR architecture.

Universal Chimeric Antigen Receptor Designs

Beyond targeting a single fixed antigen, a variety of "universal" CARs have also been developed. Rather than

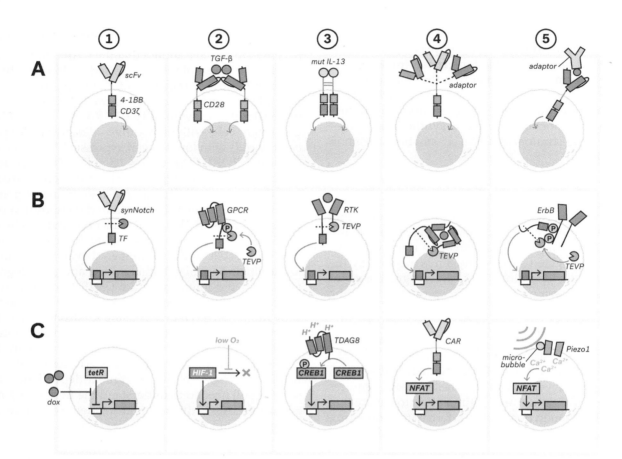

Figure 20.4 **Examples of engineered biological sensors for CAR T cell therapy.** (**A**) CAR engineering. (1) CAR molecular architecture. (2) TGF-β CAR detects soluble antigens. (3) IL-13Rα2- and CLTX-CARs use small ligand ectodomains. (4) Universal SUPRA-CAR and SNAP-CAR use interchangeable targeting adaptors. (5) Universal FITC-CAR and AT-CAR bind to labeled tumor-targeting adaptors. (**B**) Generic and composable sensors. (1) SynNotch receptor. (2) GPCR-based Tango receptor. (3) RTK-based Tango receptor. (4) Intrabody-based Tango receptor. (5) RASER recognizes intracellular signaling via phosphorylation. (**C**) Promoter-based sensors. (1) Dox-inducible promoter. (2) Hypoxia-inducible promoter. (3) pH-sensing promoter. (4) T cell activation-inducible promoter. (5) Mechanoresponsive ultrasound promoter.

CAR, chimeric antigen receptor; CREB1, cyclic AMP-responsive element-binding protein 1; dox, doxycycline; GPCR, G-protein–coupled receptor; HIF-1, hypoxia-inducible factor 1; mut IL-13, mutated interleukin-13; NFAT, nuclear factor of activated T cells; RTK, receptor tyrosine kinase; scFv, single-chain variable fragment; TDAG8, T cell death–associated gene 8; tetR, tetracycline repressor; TEVP, tobacco etch virus protease; TGF-β, transforming growth factor beta.

covalently linking an extracellular targeting domain to the CAR through protein fusion, these approaches rely on noncovalent binding of the CAR to an antigen-targeting adaptor molecule. For example, the split universal programmable (SUPRA)-CAR uses leucine zippers to bring the CAR signaling domains and the soluble scFv adaptor component together.[18] In addition to being able to easily swap out adaptors to target different antigens, orthogonal leucine zipper combinations also enable multiplexed antigen targeting. Another universal CAR approach involves the secondary binding of an anti-FITC CAR to tumor cells through FITC-conjugated, tumor-specific small molecule ligands such as FITC-DUPA and FITC-AZA.[58] Finally, the high-affinity interactions between

biotin and streptavidin have also been exploited for universal CAR applications. In these studies, avidin/streptavidin CAR T cells bind specifically to tumor cells coated with biotinylated antibodies against EGFRvIII, CD19, or CD20.[59,60]

Universal CAR designs already begin to decouple the function of the CAR as a sensor and as an actuator—in these concepts, the adaptor molecule is the sensor and the CAR is the actuator. Binding of the CAR to the adaptor bridges antigen sensing and actuation of downstream T cell signaling by the CAR. This concept complements the development of "off-the-shelf," allogeneic CAR T cells,[61] which envisions a future where a bank of CAR T cells prepared from healthy donors or genetically engineered induced pluripotent stem cells (iPSCs)[62] can be mixed with various targeting adaptors to easily generate antigen-specific, personalized therapies for multiple cancer patients.

Practically, these designs enable interchangeable antigen specificity as well as rapid prototyping and testing without the need for cloning and protein engineering. The addition of a secondary binding interaction also introduces more kinetic parameters to tune, which may enhance our ability to precisely control CAR function, though not without the cost of greater complexity and context dependence. The antitumor activity of these CAR T cells also requires constant dosing of the adaptor molecule, which may present challenges regarding pharmacokinetics and biodistribution. Recent work addresses this concern by covalently linking the adaptor to CAR molecules expressed on the cell surface using the SNAPtag self-labeling enzyme system.[63] Altogether, these approaches enable flexible antigen targeting with a single CAR construct, which may better address antigen escape in the clinic.

Generic and Composable Receptors

Unlike the conventional CAR molecule, true sensors in the sensor-processor-actuator architecture do not perform an action at the systems level (e.g., triggering T cell activation). This is the job of the actuator. Instead, sensors detect input signals and simply wire the output to downstream processing or actuation modules. This is known as *generic signal transduction,* which allows sensor devices to "talk" to other modules in order to compose larger systems. By enforcing sensing and actuation as functions that are executed separately and distinctly, we can begin to move away from single-molecule effector designs, which are limited in scope to simple input–output devices, and engineer more complex behavior into immune cells.

The most well-studied class of sensors in the context of immune cell engineering is the diverse family of transmembrane receptors. These proteins bind to extracellular ligands and either undergo a conformational change or oligomerize in order to transduce a signal. The type of signal that these receptors output can also vary. Some receptors signal through phosphorylation cascades; for example, the ITAM domains in the TCR, TIR domains in the Toll-like receptors (TLR), and the C-terminal tail of G-protein–coupled receptors (GPCR). Others, like the Notch receptor, release transcription factors to directly modulate gene expression when bound to ligand. The direct use of these receptors as sensors has been limited by the inherent complexity of endogenous signaling pathways—however, the development of synthetic receptors that co-opt natural signaling mechanisms has enabled flexible and programmable sensing.[64]

Receptor engineering often relies on the assumption that receptors are protein devices composed of modular domains. While we previously discussed this in the context of the CAR, many other receptors can also be engineered in a similar manner. The generic receptor architecture is an extracellular ligand-binding ectodomain, a transmembrane region, and intracellular signaling domains. In the following discussion, we outline novel receptors with composable output (i.e., regulation of transgene expression). These synthetic sensors are generated by swapping out one domain for another to introduce new human-defined functions or by rewiring the behavior of natural endogenous receptors.

Detecting Surface Markers

The synthetic Notch (synNotch) receptor is an example of an agnostic biological sensor.[65] It detects arbitrary surface antigens and conditionally outputs a transcriptional signal. The structural design of synNotch reflects the generic transmembrane receptor architecture. An extracellular scFv acts as the ligand-binding domain (validated cancer-relevant target antigens include CD19, EpCAM, B7-H3, Axl, and apelin among others).[18,66–68] This is linked to a cytosolic signaling domain (a synthetic transcription factor) by a transmembrane linker consisting of endogenous Notch receptor components. *IF* the ligand is bound, *THEN* a mechanical force triggers spontaneous proteolytic cleavage of the Notch region, freeing the transcription factor to traffic from the membrane into the nucleus to regulate transgene expression. Notably, transcriptional regulation is the output signal, rather than a native program like T cell activation. This enables us to couple the output of synNotch to other genetic modules such as processing (combinatorial logic circuits)[17] and actuation (custom cell behavior).[37]

Detecting Soluble Ligands

While the sensors we have discussed are generally designed to detect the presence of surface antigens on tumor cells, there is also a significant need to target soluble antigens. For example, the tumor microenvironment is a hostile workplace for CAR T cells—an overabundance of immunosuppressive cytokines and metabolites generated within the tumor milieu dampens T cell effector activity and antitumor response.[14] Here, we outline recent developments in receptor engineering that enable CAR T cells to sense and respond to these soluble cues.

GPCRs are multipass transmembrane receptors that detect a wide variety of ligands, including small molecules, peptides, hormones, cell surface adhesion molecules, protons, and light.[69] Sensor frameworks such as Tango, CRISPR ChaCha, and dCas9-synR all utilize endogenous GPCRs as a front end for sensing soluble cues.[70–72] In the Tango system, the GPCR is fused to an arbitrary transcription factor cargo via a cleavable linker. Upon ligand binding, a viral protease is recruited to the GPCR via the cytosolic adaptor molecule β-arrestin, which enables cleavage and release of the cargo. Building upon this concept, the CRISPR ChaCha and dCas9-synR approaches utilize analogous scaffolds with the CRISPR activator molecule dCas9-VPR as the cargo to flexibly regulate the expression of either transgenes or endogenous genes.

Natural single-pass transmembrane receptors that detect soluble cues, such as receptor tyrosine kinases (RTK) and cytokine receptors, most likely dimerize or oligomerize upon ligand binding in order to transduce signal.[73] Synthetic single-pass transmembrane receptors must co-opt this ligand-dependent crosslinking mechanism in order to sense soluble ligands. The Tango and dCas9-synR approaches have also been developed using RTKs. In these systems, the ligand-binding ectodomain and transmembrane region of an RTK are fused to either a viral protease or a synthetic cargo with a protease cleavage site. Upon ligand binding, these constructs hetero dimerize, bringing the viral protease and cargo together for cleavage and release. Modular extracellular sensor architecture (MESA) receptors use a similar approach, though instead of having endogenous RTK ectodomains, the heterodimers utilize two different extracellular scFvs that target two nonoverlapping epitopes on the same molecule.[74]

Engineered sensors can also detect soluble cues within the cell using a two-component, intrabody-based synthetic receptor based on the Tango architecture.[75] A membrane-bound intrabody is fused to a synthetic transcription factor by a cleavable linkage, whereas another cytosolic intrabody is fused to the viral protease. Like MESA, the two intrabodies detect nonoverlapping epitopes. When the ligand crosslinks the two intrabodies, the viral protease can cleave the linkage and free the transcription factor.

Detecting Cell Signaling

Rewiring of aberrant signaling to effector release (RASER) is another example of a composable sensor technology.[76] Rather than detecting extracellular antigens, however, RASER senses intracellular cues. A proof-of-concept demonstration of RASER detects aberrant cancer cell signaling via hyperactivation and constitutive phosphorylation of ErbB, a family of receptor tyrosine kinases that include HER2 and EGFR. Recruitment of a sequence-specific viral protease to autophosphorylated sites in the ErbB cytoplasmic domain enables cleavage of arbitrary membrane-bound synthetic cargos such as transcription factors and effector molecules. Thus, RASER can act as a generic signal transducer of endogenous receptor signaling. While the technology is currently demonstrated

in tumor cells to sense a specific input (ErbB phosphorylation), the modular nature of the components may one day enable the detection of other intracellular cues in immune cells (e.g., aberrant phosphorylation of T cell signaling proteins in dysfunctional cells).

Promoter-Based Sensors

Promoter engineering builds upon early foundational work in synthetic biology, which used DNA elements from naturally occurring operons in E. coli to build synthetic gene regulatory networks. For example, the tet operon naturally regulates the expression of the antibiotic resistance gene, tetA, in response to doxycycline, a small-molecule input. Normally, the transcriptional repressor tetR binds to tetO operator sequences within the promoter region to block transcription initiation. When doxycycline is present, however, it binds allosterically to tetR. This results in a conformational change that prevents tetR from binding to DNA, which allows tetA to be expressed in a dox-inducible manner. By engineering synthetic DNA regulatory elements like those derived from the tet operon, we can enable immune cells to sense a broad range of inputs. Furthermore, because the output of these sensors is conditional gene expression, this method is both generic and composable.

Sensing the Tumor Microenvironment

As previously mentioned, the tumor microenvironment (TME) is a complex and heterogeneous milieu found within solid tumors that poses major challenges to engineered immune cell therapies. Key characteristics of the TME include metabolic imbalance, hypoxia, increased acidity, nutrient deficiency, irregular vasculature and dysregulated angiogenesis, recruitment of immunosuppressive cell types, and a dense and rigid extracellular matrix (ECM).[14] These factors often block immune cell infiltration and suppress effector function.

Promoter engineering enables cells to sense and respond to the TME. To sense low oxygen levels, for example, hypoxia response elements (HRE) within the promoter region upstream of the desired output gene can be used to control transcription.[30] Hypoxic conditions stabilize the protein structure of the endogenous HIF-1 transcription factor, which can then bind to HRE to activate gene expression. To sense the rigidity of the tumor ECM, we can use a mechanoresponsive promoter driven by the YAP/TAZ transcriptional activator.[38] Endogenous signaling pathways control the nuclear localization of YAP/TAZ in response to stiffness. Finally, to sense the acidity of the TME, a pH-inducible system can be used, which senses high extracellular proton levels through a constitutively expressed GPCR and a promoter with c-AMP response elements.[29] Once the cell senses these and other TME components, it can send signals to downstream processing and actuation modules to respond accordingly (e.g., integrate signals for targeting specificity, secrete proinflammatory cytokines, stimulate T cell activation, upregulate CAR expression, alter metabolic programs, etc.).

Sensing Internal Cell State

In addition to sensing extracellular cues, promoter-based sensors can also sense internal signals that may correspond to a specific cell state. In the context of immunotherapy, T cell activation is a particularly interesting cell state to feed into downstream computation: we might want to engineer a CAR T cell to upregulate the expression of a certain gene or gene program only in response to antigen-dependent activation.

The CAR is known to signal through canonical pathways that upregulate the production of molecules like CD69 and IL-2 upon activation. The promoters that control the expression of these activation markers contain binding motifs for key transcription factors such as NFAT and NF-κB among others. When we place these core regulatory elements upstream of a minimal constitutive promoter, we can create synthetic promoters that enforce conditional transgene expression only upon T cell activation.[77,78,79] In addition, this approach could conceptually be used to sense other cell states as well—coupling the expression of a transgene to that of a gene upregulated in response to altered metabolism, or differentiation into exhausted or memory phenotypes, may be an interesting and powerful application of promoter engineering.

Sensing Synthetic Inputs

Promoter engineering can also be used to sense synthetic exogenous inputs for human-defined behavior. The transcriptional output of these sensors is commonly linked to processing and actuation modules that enable "remote control" of cell trafficking, localization, and gene expression. The characteristics of these inputs determine the spatiotemporal resolution of sensing, enabling a wide range of applications with varying utility.

Promoter-based sensors often detect soluble, small-molecule inputs through allosteric binding to regulators of transcription. For example, the antibiotic doxycycline blocks binding of the synthetic activator tTA to the promoter in the Tet-Off system and enables binding of the activator rtTA in the Tet-On system.[80] Rapamycin, abscisic acid, and gibberellin are other small molecules that can induce the dimerization of synthetic heterodimeric transcription factors to activate or repress genes.[81] These chemical sensors are often useful to detect systemic changes, such as intravenous administration of a drug inducer.

Promoter-based sensors can also detect light, sound, and heat as inputs, which offer greater spatiotemporal resolution over diffusion-limited small molecule administration. Engineered CAR T cells can respond to rapid blue-light stimulation using a promoter that responds to synthetic transcription factors incorporating heterodimeric CRY2/CIB1 proteins from the flowering plant *Arabidopsis thaliana*.[82] However, the clinical utility of blue-light inducible systems is generally limited due to poor tissue penetration. To address this, mechanoresponsive sensors use a two-step process to detect acoustic inputs such as high-frequency ultrasound, which can reach deep tissues and achieve up to single-cell resolution.[83] These CAR T cells constitutively express Piezo1, an ion channel that transduces mechanical ultrasound signal to a signal in calcium influx. An NFAT-responsive promoter is then used to couple calcium signaling to transgene expression. Recent work also demonstrates the versatility of these sensors to detect heat—the promoter for human heat-shock protein HSPB can be used to drive thermally-responsive gene expression.[84]

PROCESSING AND CONTROL

The processor is the computational hub of the engineered cell. Processing units continuously receive inputs from sensors and integrate these signals together, and the logical outputs are then sent to downstream actuator modules. In other words, we give the processor information in the form of inputs, and the output "tells" the cell what to do. In biology, signal integration can take on many different forms. Here, we outline the current implementations of immunological processing in engineered CAR T cells as well as modes of generic signal processing in synthetic biology—these details are summarized as a schematic diagram in Figure 20.5.

Regulating Chimeric Antigen Receptor Expression

A common application of processing in the context of CAR T cell therapy is the ON/OFF switch, which enables exogenous inputs to regulate CAR expression. CAR ON/OFF switches can be implemented in many different ways. Transcriptional switches utilize promoter-based sensors to activate CAR expression upon detection of small molecules, light, or sound.[82,83,85] However, transcriptional regulation is generally slow, and the outputs of these switches resemble binary states.[15]

Alternatively, faster kinetics and greater dose dependency can be achieved with regulation at the protein level. A split ON/OFF CAR design uses the inducible FKBP–FRB heterodimerizing system to bring together two inactive receptor halves in the presence of the small-molecule rapalog.[28] Only the heterodimerized CAR contains both the co-stimulatory and the signaling

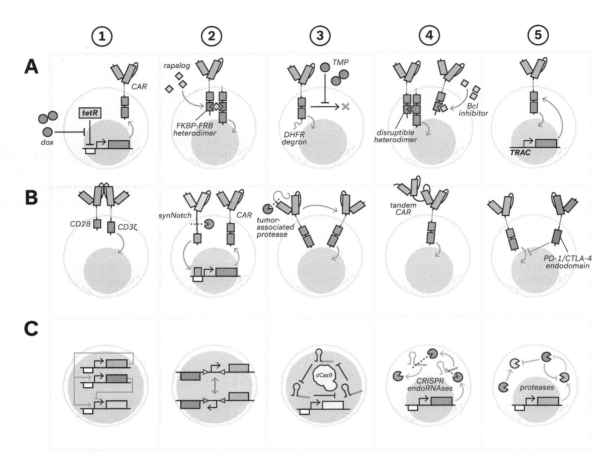

Figure 20.5 Examples of processing and control systems for engineered CAR T cells. (**A**) Regulating CAR expression. (1) Drug-inducible transgene expression. (2) Drug-induced dimerization. (3) Drug-induced protein stabilization. (4) Drug-induced heterodimer disruption. (5) Endogenous regulation at the *TRAC* locus. (**B**) Immunological logic gates. (1) AND gate via dissociated CAR signaling domains. (2) AND gate via synNotch priming of CAR expression. (3) AND gate via proteolytic cleavage of a masking peptide by an extracellular protease. (4) OR gate via tandem scFvs. (5) NIMPLY gate via inhibitory CAR co-expression. (**C**) Programming genetic circuits. (1) Pulse-generating transcriptional circuit. (2) Memory storage via DNA inversion. (3) CRISPR-based repressilator. (4) RNA-level repression cascade using the PERSIST framework. (5) Band-pass filter using the CHOMP protease framework.

Bcl, B cell lymphoma; CAR, chimeric antigen receptor; CRISPR, clustered regularly interspaced short palindromic repeats; CTLA-4, cytotoxic t-lymphocyte protein 4; dCas9, nuclease-deactivated Cas9; DHFR, dihydrofolate reductase; dox, doxycycline; FKBP, FK506-binding protein; FRB, FKBP-rapamycin binding; PD-1, programmed cell death protein 1; rapalog, rapamycin analog; tetR, tetracyline repressor; TMP, trimethoprim; TRAC, T cell receptor alpha constant.

domains needed for total CAR function. Small molecules that stabilize protein degradation are also interesting candidates for CAR ON/OFF switch control.[86,87] Recent work has shown that fusing the DHFR degron to the CAR enables regulatable expression using the U.S. Food and Drug Administration (FDA)-approved stabilizing drug trimethoprim.[23] Universal CAR designs can also be turned ON/OFF with the adaptor molecule.[20]

Advances in computational tools for protein design have also informed new CAR ON/OFF switches. The STOP-CAR approach uses a stable, computationally designed heterodimer consisting of Bcl-XL bound to a BH3 domain synthetically engrafted onto the human apolipoprotein E4.[29] Addition of a high-affinity Bcl

small-molecule inhibitor causes the heterodimer to dissociate, separating the CAR signaling domains and disrupting receptor function. Exciting work in de novo protein design also holds the potential to expand the CAR regulation toolkit—for example, degronLOCKR is a new and completely synthetic switch that can degrade an arbitrary protein-of-interest when bound to a small peptide inducer.[88,89]

The "remote control" enabled by these ON/OFF switches addresses significant safety concerns raised by engineered cell therapies.[15] For example, CAR T cells can be turned OFF after infusion into the patient in the event of an uncontrolled immune response to prevent toxicity associated with cytokine release syndrome. Depending on the spatiotemporal resolution of the input, these CAR T cells can also be selectively turned ON in specific areas, such as within the tumor mass, to further prevent on-target off-tumor effects.

ON/OFF switches can also improve the efficacy of CAR T cell therapy. Achieving optimal antitumor activity is a balancing act—too little effector function results in tumor outgrowth, whereas too strong of a response can lead to systemic toxicity.[26] Inducible systems can actively tune the CAR T cell response in a dose-dependent and physician-guided manner to better optimize tumor-killing behavior. Furthermore, the transient "rest" afforded by turning OFF the CAR can reinvigorate dysfunctional exhausted cells to improve overall antitumor activity.[21]

Finally, besides synthetic control, CAR expression can also be regulated through cell-intrinsic mechanisms. When the CD19–CAR transgene is knocked into the T cell receptor alpha constant (TRAC) locus using CRISPR gene-editing, the resulting CAR T cells demonstrate more uniform CAR expression and better tumor-killing and persistence.[25] This suggests that endogenous regulation of the CAR transgene (mimicking that of the endogenous TCR) can generate more potent CAR T cells and better cell therapies.

Immunological Logic Gates

While the canonical CAR sensor–actuator resembles a simple BUFFER gate, new receptor designs have implemented more complex logic-gated behavior such as AND, OR, and NOT. This added layer of receptor-based processing (in addition to sensing) addresses many critical challenges facing CAR T cell therapy in the clinic such as specificity and antigen escape. However, because processing is coupled to actuation in these approaches, logical complexity quickly reaches an upper-bound, and the output is generally limited to immune function. Despite these drawbacks, immunological logic gates are a powerful demonstration of how synthetic biology approaches have already impacted patient treatment in clinical studies and how they can begin to further improve engineered cell therapies.

AND Gate

Immunological AND gates enable CAR T cells to sense multiple antigens and only trigger activation when all antigens are present. For example, in a two-input system with antigens A and B, AND-gated CAR T cells will only signal upon recognition of A *AND* B simultaneously. This added specificity addresses toxicity issues and can mitigate "on-target, off-tumor" effects. Furthermore, cancers that express a single unique, tumor-specific neoantigen marker are rare.[15] AND-gated CAR T cells can selectively target a wider range of cancers that express two or more upregulated tumor-associated antigens.

Implementations of AND-gated CARs use two-component systems that only trigger activation when both receptors are engaged. For example, CAR T cells that co-express a poorly signaling PSCA–CAR and an anti-PSMA chimeric costimulatory receptor only signal when bound to PSCA⁺PSMA⁺ prostate cancer cells.[90] The presence of both PSCA and PSMA on the surface of the target cell brings the CAR and chimeric costimulatory receptor together, boosting CAR signaling above a threshold level to trigger T cell activation. Another split approach uses two incomplete CARs with dissociated signaling domains.[91] Signaling occurs when the mesothelin CAR (with the CD3z signaling domain) and the a-folate receptor CAR (with the CD28 co-stimulatory domain) are brought together.

Pseudo-AND gate behavior can be achieved using the synNotch receptor.[17] *IF* antigen A is present, *THEN* synNotch will transcriptionally activate CAR expression. The CAR can then recognize antigen B to trigger T cell activation. Notably, because the synNotch is "priming" CAR expression, both target cells that express either antigen B alone or antigen A and B together are killed. This temporal behavior has advantages in the context of tumor heterogeneity, where not all cancer cells express both antigens A and B. However, this system can also exhibit unintended toxicity and "on-target, off-tumor" effects—when an anti-EpCAM synNotch primes ROR1–CAR expression to target EpCAM⁺ROR1⁺ tumor cells, normal cells expressing ROR1 in adjacent healthy tissues are also killed.[66]

Other CAR designs that detect soluble cues from the tumor microenvironment can also behave as pseudo-AND gates. For example, in the "masked" CAR approach, *IF* tumor-associated extracellular proteases are present, *THEN* a masking peptide is cleaved, revealing the antigen-targeting scFv.[32] In an engineered hypoxia-sensing CAR, *IF* oxygen levels are low, *THEN* the HIF-1α oxygen-dependent degradation domain is stabilized, which stabilizes CAR expression.[31]

OR Gate

OR-gated CAR T cells enable broader targeting and killing of cancer cells that express antigen A *OR* antigen B. This is useful in the context of tumor heterogeneity, where cells isolated from the same tumor have markedly different surface marker expression profiles. Moreover, OR-gated CAR T cells can prevent antigen escape, which is a major obstacle to established CAR T therapies like the CD19–CAR[12,92–95]—it is more improbable for a tumor cell to generate double antigen loss variants against the dual selection pressure enabled by OR-gated CAR T cells. However, these approaches can be susceptible to systemic toxicity due to a more permissive antigen specificity.[96]

The implementation of OR-gated CAR T cells is more straightforward than the AND-gated counterparts. CAR T cells specific to single antigens can be simply pooled together in a cocktail mixture, though these cells are usually outperformed by their dual CAR (either through co-transduction or expression via bicistronic vector) counterparts.[97] Notable examples of multivalent CAR T cells include dual targeting of CD19/CD123 for relapsed or refractory B-cell acute lymphoblastic leukemia (B-ALL)[92] and triple targeting of HER2/IL-13Rα2/EphA2 for glioblastoma.[98]

The bispecific, "tandem" CAR approach utilizes a single CAR molecule with two extracellular scFvs[16] and is favorable for cell manufacturing due to greater transduction efficiency and expression consistency over co-transduced CARs or polycistronic vectors. The bispecific CD19/CD20 CAR is currently in Phase I clinical trials for the treatment of non-Hodgkin lymphoma,[93,99] while the bispecific CD19/CD22 CAR is in Phase I for the treatment of B-ALL.[94,100] Tandem CARs have also been developed for glioblastoma (IL-13Rα2/HER2)[101] and multiple myeloma (BCMA/CS1).[102]

NOT Gate

The NOT gate is a signal inverter. Immunological NOT gates tell surface antigen inputs on healthy cells to suppress T cell signaling rather than trigger activation. When used in conjunction with a conventional CAR, the overall system behaves as a NIMPLY gate (i.e., antigen A *AND NOT* antigen B). NOT-gated CAR T cells add an additional layer of safety and regulation to prevent the "on-target, off-tumor" effect.[15] The inhibitory chimeric antigen receptor (iCAR) is an example of such a device—rather than using activating or co-stimulatory domains, the intracellular component of the iCAR consists of dominant suppressive cytosolic domains from the inhibitory receptors PD-1 and CTLA4.[103]

Another conceptual variant of the NOT gate is the immunomodulatory fusion protein (IFP), which rewires inhibitory signals that normally suppress CAR T activity into activating signals.[34] This device inverts the inhibitory signal that CAR T cells receive upon binding to upregulated CD200 on leukemia cells using a synthetic CD200 receptor (CD200R) with a cytoplasmic CD28 co-stimulatory domain.

Programming Genetic Circuits

Processing in CAR T cell therapy has been tied to sensing and/or actuation by engineering simple switches and Boolean logic gate behavior into synthetic receptors. However, advances in tool development and mammalian synthetic biology are beginning to build more powerful and decoupled processing units. These technologies utilize transcriptional regulation, post-transcriptional regulation, or protein-protein interactions to build composable genetic circuits that can perform combinatorial logic, store state memory, and execute other complex behaviors.[3] While few genetic circuits have been implemented in CAR T cells to date, we envision a future where such technologies will enable better clinician-driven control over engineered cell behavior and the realization of fully autonomous, self-regulating, and decision-making cells.

Transcriptional Regulation

Foundational work in synthetic biology established transcriptional regulation as a framework for the construction of combinatorial Boolean logic gates[2] and dynamic circuit engineering.[4–6] In this concept, the flow of RNA polymerase (RNAP) on DNA is analogous to the flow of electricity through a circuit wire. To implement digital logic, DNA-binding proteins such as transcription factors can interact with operator sites within promoter DNA to conditionally recruit or block RNA polymerase activity and regulate transgene expression.[104–106] Transcription factors can also be used to implement feedback and feed-forward loops, which enable complex behaviors like analog computation,[107] signal processing,[108] event counting,[109] edge detection,[110] hysteresis,[111] memory storage,[112–114] and dynamic circuits across bacterial, plant, and mammalian systems.[3] Some devices, like the toggle switch, have been implemented using synthetic transcription factors that induce epigenetic modifications.[115]

Other DNA-binding proteins, such as recombinases, have also been used to regulate RNAP activity. Serine integrases (a class of site-specific recombinases) can amplify logic gates and store rewritable digital memory by flipping the physical orientation of DNA encoding promoters or transcriptional terminators.[116,117] Building on this principle, Boolean logic and arithmetic through DNA excision (BLADE) technology uses orthogonal recombinases to compute more than 100 distinct, arbitrary large multi-input multi-output Boolean logic circuits.[118] Moreover, chemical- and light-inducible recombination can couple varied modes of sensing to these circuits.[119] However, due to the nature of DNA excision, BLADE computation is irreversible—each circuit has a lifetime of exactly one use, and unlike serine integrase switches, stored memory is read-only. As such, potential applications of BLADE in CAR T therapy might include event recording and sustained gene expression in specific, terminally differentiated effector cell types.

Unlike synthetic transcription factors that bind to specific operator sequences, CRISPR-based genetic circuits harness the RNA-mediated programmability of CRISPR effector molecules such as Cas9 and Cpf1/Cas12a. In these approaches, a constitutively expressed CRISPR repressor (dCas9 or dCas9-KRAB) molecule acts as a "shared resource," enabling circuit behavior to be driven by guide RNA expression alone.[120–122] This alleviates the need for multiple orthogonal TF-operator pairs since specificity is solely determined by guide RNA complementary to the target promoter. Furthermore, existing RNA regulatory strategies can be used to modulate dCas9 activity,[123,124] and orthogonal dCas9 homologues can be used for limited multiplexing.[125] Higher-order multiplexing can be achieved using dCpf1/Cas12a, an alternative CRISPR effector that can process multiple guide RNAs from a single transcript for multi-input, multi-output processing.[126–129] New anti-CRISPR proteins further expand this toolkit by repressing Cas activity to build dynamic circuit behavior, such as pulse generation.[130]

Post-Transcriptional Circuits

Genetic circuits can also be implemented at the RNA level.[131–133] The first RNA circuits co-opted the endogenous RNA interference (RNAi) mechanism to build combinatorial logic gates and mammalian cell classifiers.[131] Modern circuits utilize RNA-binding proteins in conjunction with RNA–RNA interactions to build complex regulatory networks and drug-inducible systems.[132,133] Recent work has also demonstrated that RNA circuits utilizing CRISPR endoRNAses (including Csy4 and the Cas13 family of CRISPR effectors) resist epigenetic silencing.[134] This is especially attractive for CAR T cell therapies since long-term persistence is key to good clinical outcomes.[11]

Protein-level circuits are a relatively new class of genetic circuit that uses protein–protein interactions to represent connective wires. Circuits of hacked orthogonal modular proteases (CHOMP) create a framework with parts consisting of viral proteases, cleavage sites, degrons, and leucine zippers.[135] By combining these parts strategically, we can compute Boolean logic, construct synthetic regulatory networks, and engineer dynamic analog signal-processing function. This approach is generally faster and more compact than transcriptional circuits, and entire systems can be expressed on a single transcript. However, protein structure optimization and the limited pool of orthogonal protease-cleavage site pairs are potential bottlenecks for programmability and scalability. Finally, phosphorylation-based circuits can theoretically offer speed and sensitivity akin to endogenous signaling pathways. However, these circuits are still in the early stages of development due to their overall complexity and our limited ability to manipulate tertiary protein structure.[136,137]

ACTUATION AND OUTPUT

The actuator of a system is responsible for outputting a specific action in response to an input. Biological actuators cause functional, system-level changes in cell behavior. For example, the CAR is an actuator because it triggers T cell activation and downstream effector function (e.g., cell growth and proliferation, cytokine production, and target cell killing).

Custom actuation by engineered CAR T cells remains a relatively unexplored research area in comparison to sensing and processing. This is partly due to the complexity of engineering novel biological function, but also because the native T cell program has already proven to be extremely effective in clearing tumors for cancer immunotherapy. Here, we outline examples of novel cell function as well as current approaches to improve endogenous T cell behavior—these details are summarized as a schematic diagram in Figure 20.6.

Engineering Synthetic Functionality

A handful of actuators have been developed that execute functions beyond canonical CAR T cell activation. For example, some actuators activate black-box endogenous signaling pathways that affect cell-level behavior. The inducible caspase 9 (iCasp9) kill-switch uses a small-molecule drug to activate the endogenous caspase cascade and trigger cell apoptosis.[28,138] Inducible cell death addresses safety concerns by enabling selective ablation of CAR T cells in patients that experience adverse effects (such as cytokine release syndrome) after infusion. Another actuator mediates cytoskeletal rearrangement via synthetic GPCR signaling to increase cell motility and facilitate trafficking and chemotaxis toward a bioinert chemical ligand.[41] This technology may address current challenges in solid tumor infiltration. Integrated CRISPRa/CRISPRi systems can also be used to programmatically modulate the expression of endogenous immune-relevant genes and custom gene programs to improve anti-tumor activity.[10,139]

Secretion of Soluble Factors

CAR T cells can be engineered to release synthetic soluble factors into the local tumor microenvironment to improve antitumor efficacy in a synergistic manner. For example, CAR T cells can constitutively secrete small scFvs and nanobodies that bind to molecules normally targeted in immune checkpoint blockade strategies, such as PD-1, CTLA-4, and CD47.[36,37,140] Other CAR T cells secreting bispecific T cell engagers (BiTEs) can recruit endogenous T cells to clear heterogeneous tumors without antigen escape.[19] Preclinical studies show that "armored" CAR T cells, which are genetically modified to express cytokines such as the pro-inflammatory IL-12[39,141] or the engineered IL-2 variant super-2,[142,143] can overcome immunosuppression in the tumor microenvironment. CAR T cells can also secrete degradative enzymes such as heparanase, which breaks down extracellular matrix components, to facilitate infiltration into stroma-rich solid tumors.[40] Preliminary studies using CAR T cells to deliver oncolytic viruses may

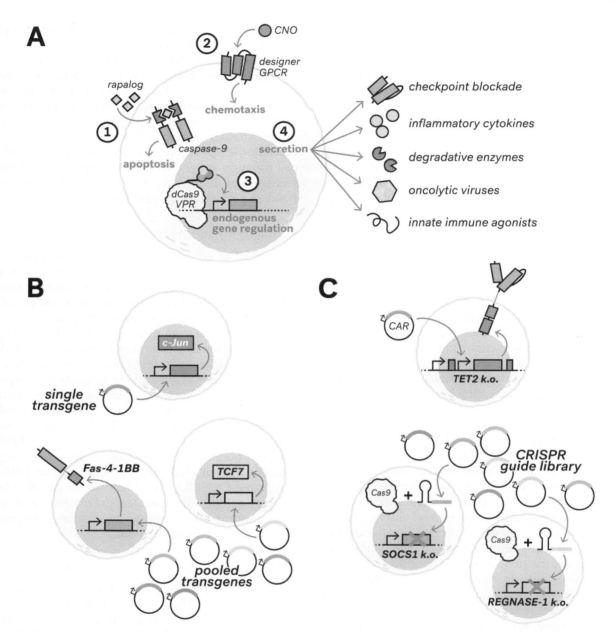

Figure 20.6 Examples of current approaches to program or modulate CAR T cell function. (A) Engineering synthetic functionality. (1) Inducible apoptosis using a caspase-9 kill switch. (2) Chemotaxis toward a synthetic bioinert ligand. (3) Endogenous gene regulation using CRISPRa/CRISPRi. (4) Secretion of immune-relevant payloads. **(B)** Enhancing the natural T cell response via transgene expression. Top: Transgenic overexpression of c-Jun ameliorates T cell exhaustion. Bottom: CRISPR screen using a small library of pooled transgenes identifies Fas-4-1BB and TCF7 as top hits for enhanced antitumor activity. **(C)** Enhancing the natural T cell response via gene knockout. Top: Random lentiviral integration of the CAR transgene disrupted TET2 and enhanced therapeutic efficacy. Bottom: High-throughput CRISPR screens identify SOCS1 and REGNASE-1 as key negative regulators of T cell activity.

CAR, chimeric antigen receptor; CNO, clozapine-*N*-oxide; CRISPR, clustered regularly interspaced short palindromic repeats; dCas9, nuclease-deactivated Cas9; GPCR, G protein-coupled receptor; k.o., knockout; Rapalog, rapamycin analog; REGNASE-1, regulatory RNase 1; SOCS1, suppressor of cytokine signaling 1; TCF7, transcription factor 7; TET2, Tet methylcytosine dioxygenase 2; VPR, VP64-p65-Rta.

open the door to synthetic combination therapies that attack tumors from multiple angles.[144] Finally, the secretion of custom, immune-relevant payloads (including cytokines, cytotoxic molecules, TLR agonists, blocking scFvs, etc.) can be linked to upstream sensing and processing via synNotch.[37]

Enhancing the Natural T Cell Response

There is significant interest in using synthetic biology to augment the endogenous antitumor activity triggered by CAR actuation. For example, the intensity and character of the CAR response can be tuned by swapping out different co-stimulatory domains. The CD28 domain triggers faster and stronger signaling, which results in more effector cell differentiation and exhaustion compared to the slower and more moderate co-stimulation by 4-1BB.[48,145,146] Other co-stimulatory domains, including OX-40, ICOS, CD27, and MyD88/CD40, have exhibited varying effects on T cell metabolism, persistence, cytokine secretion, differentiation, proliferation, and survival.[147]

Transgenic expression of immunostimulatory proteins can also potentiate the CAR T cell response. Synthetic overexpression of the transcription factor c-Jun has been shown to ameliorate T cell exhaustion,[20] while ectopic expression of receptors that provide "signal 3" (cytokine signaling), such as the modified erythropoietin receptor[148] or synthetic cytokine receptors (SyCyR),[149] can boost CAR T cell effector function. Recent work has demonstrated that a CRISPR-based knock-in approach in T cells can be used to screen a small library of synthetic proteins for potential therapeutic benefit.[150]

New studies have also begun to generate mathematical models using in vitro killing assay data to predict CAR T cell persistence, exhaustion, and their ability to clear solid tumors.[151] Further development of these models may provide some insight on new parameters to tune in an iterative design process to enhance CAR T cell antitumor activity.

Systematic Genetic Perturbations

A previous clinical study using CD19-CAR T cells to treat chronic lymphocytic leukemia revealed, surprisingly, that most of the patient's CAR T cells had expanded from a single cell.[24] Later analysis confirmed that random lentiviral integration of the CAR transgene disrupted the *TET2* gene, which consequently enhanced the performance of the clone and resulted in its enrichment. Multiple studies have since identified single genes like *TET2* that, when knocked-out, can improve antitumor activity.[22,23,152] With the advent of better CRISPR screening technologies, a new and fast-growing area of research in synthetic immunology seeks to systematically perturb the genome of engineered CAR/TCR T cells to scale-up the discovery of these therapeutic gene targets.

For example, a genome-wide in vitro CRISPR screen in primary human T cells has identified new candidate gene hits, such as *SOCS1*, that enhance endogenous T cell effector function when ablated.[153] Alternatively, an in vivo CRISPR screen has shown that knocking out *REGNASE-1*, a metabolic regulator of T cells, can enhance therapeutic efficacy in mouse models of leukemia and melanoma.[35] Significant strides in the improvement

of CRISPR-based gene-editing techniques for primary human T cells should facilitate the translation of these findings to the clinic.[154,155] Indeed, a recent landmark Phase 1 clinical trial has shown that multiplexed CRISPR knockouts of *TRAC*, *TRBC*, and *PD-1* in T cells for cancer immunotherapy are both safe and feasible.[156]

FUTURE PERSPECTIVE

The field of synthetic immunology is still very new, which presents us with many exciting opportunities as well as open questions to address (Figure 20.7A). In the past few years, we have begun to assemble a working toolbox of proof-of-concept parts and devices, and we have gathered promising data from clinical and preclinical studies. Now, we are just beginning to envision the blueprints for a novel class of biomedical device: the engineered immune cell. Here, we outline some key considerations as we think about shaping the future of synthetic immunology (Figure 20.7B).[157]

1. **Deeper mechanistic understanding of CAR structure and function for rational design**

   The CAR is a wholly synthetic receptor, yet we continue to have a limited understanding of its mechanism of action and how different, interrelated parameters affect overall receptor functionality. Current studies are highly context-dependent and rely on swapping out different modular protein domains. However, it is likely that these observed effects alter some biophysical property of the receptor that cannot be directly modified or easily measured—for example, the physical length and flexibility of the ectodomain, the diffusivity of the receptor within the cell membrane, or the spatial arrangement of antigen-bound receptor clusters that dictate signaling. Mechanistic studies are needed in order to improve our ability to rationally design CAR constructs, whether through protein fusion or de novo computational methods.

2. **Expanded framework of composable parts and devices**

   While our informal synthetic immunology toolbox has seen accelerated growth in the past few years, the parts and devices being developed have not yet been well-characterized, standardized, or shared to a central repository. Because of this, few systems have been developed that use more than two different parts. Unfortunately, the high biological variability of donor-derived cells poses a major challenge to parts standardization and parts interoperability. In the future, the development of "off-the-shelf" allogeneic cell therapies may offer a solution by using engineered iPSCs from a single healthy donor that would mitigate the effects of genetic variation on device performance. Alternatively, advancements in DNA read–write technologies may enable rapid parameter

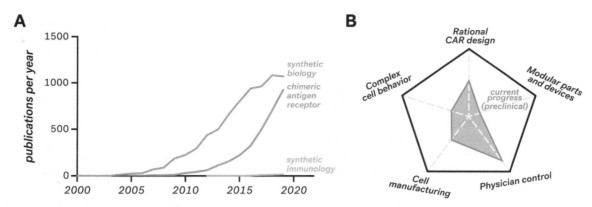

Figure 20.7 The field of synthetic immunology is currently at a nascent stage—the work of today will likely have a significant impact on the ideas of tomorrow. (A) Trends in the number of publications per year by topic on PubMed up until 2019[158]. Data were generated from a search for keyword matches in either the title or abstract of PubMed entries. **(B)** Current progress and future goals for synthetic immunology.

tuning and customization of functional parts for individual patients, either through high-throughput testing or automated, machine-learning assisted methods using genomic data.

3. **Enhanced physician control of CAR T cell therapy**
Once CAR T cells are infused into the patient, the therapy becomes a black-box process. Physicians can closely monitor the patient for cytokine release syndrome (CRS) and other forms of systemic toxicity, but treatment usually addresses critical symptoms such as hypotension and seizures rather than the causative CAR T cell immune response.[157] Immunosuppressive drugs like the IL-6 receptor antagonist tocilizumab have successfully treated CRS, but their effect on antitumor efficacy remains unclear,[157] while kill-switches permanently terminate the therapy.[138] Near-term goals for synthetic immunology seek to increase physician-mediated control of CAR T cell therapy to enable precise titration of the immune response. For example, in the future, sensors built into CAR T cells may enable high spatiotemporal control, allowing the physician to "drive" CAR T cells postinfusion.

4. **Modular design of complex cellular behavior**
While external control is useful, the ultimate long-term goal of synthetic immunology is to build autonomous, self-regulating CAR T cells that can learn to adapt and control themselves. The engineering of complex behavior is limited by our current toolkit, which generally consists of orthogonal devices that cannot "talk" to one another. Many of these devices are also incompatible because their sensing, processing, and actuating functions are not decoupled. As such, they act as single molecule effectors that cannot fully take advantage of the cell as a machine. Future parts and devices must be built in a composable manner such that we can wire them together to

build larger systems. Notably, reliance on analogies to electrical and systems engineering, while useful, can also be limiting—as synthetic immunology grows and develops, we can begin to define our own flexible system architectures that may be more applicable to biological engineering and immunology.

Moving forward, we hope to encode useful synthetic functions that do not rely entirely on black-boxed natural signaling pathways to avoid cross-talk with endogenous processes. Examples of complex behavior might include: solid tumor edge-detection to avoid the immunosuppressive TME, CAR T cells that "learn" using an inducible reward system, and autonomous formation of immune "islands" within compartmentalized tumors that correlate to better prognoses,[158] among others.

5. **Better cell manufacturing to scale-up cell-based immunotherapies**
As our engineered cell systems become increasingly complex, the CAR T cell manufacturing process will likely present major bottlenecks to clinical translation. There are currently limited protocols for genetic manipulation of primary human T cells in comparison to cultured cell lines such as HEK293T (the workhorse of mammalian synthetic biology). Larger recombinant DNA cargo from added "bells and whistles" will also necessitate more efficient delivery methods. Finally, in the current manufacturing workflow, donor-derived cells experience a limited time frame for ex vivo expansion and manipulation—this does not allow for iterative cycles of tweaking and fine-tuning of synthetic constructs. Overall, better cell manufacturing protocols, along with the development of "off-the-shelf" cells, will facilitate immune cell engineering and help accelerate the bench-to-bedside-to-bench design cycle.

CONCLUSION

CAR T cell therapy has already demonstrated immense success in clearing hematologic malignancies and shows remarkable promise as a new therapeutic modality to treat many other types of cancer. However, recent clinical studies have outlined key limitations of the canonical, BUFFER gate CAR T cell that diminish its overall therapeutic utility. Meanwhile, advances in synthetic biology have endowed us with the capacity to manipulate the genome of living cells and control a variety of cellular and molecular processes to encode rational, human-designed behavior. The emerging field of synthetic immunology is a natural intersection of these two spaces—where biological tool development meets clinical application—and presents us with many new and exciting opportunities. In this chapter, we reviewed the growing toolkit of sensors, processors, and actuators that have been developed to independently address shortcomings in the current CAR T cell paradigm. Looking to the future, we envision combining these parts and devices to build multicomponent systems that potentiate a "smarter" CAR T cell response.

KEY REFERENCES

Only key references appear in the print edition. The full reference list appears in the digital product on Springer Publishing Connect: connect.springerpub.com/content/book/978-0-8261-3743-2/part/part01/chapter/ch20

3. Brophy JA, Voigt CA. Principles of genetic circuit design. *Nat Methods*. 2014;11(5):508–520. doi:10.1038/nmeth.2926
11. Shah NN, Fry TJ. Mechanisms of resistance to CAR T cell therapy. *Nat Rev Clin Oncol*. 2019;16(6):372–385. doi:10.1038/s41571-019-0184-6
15. Roybal KT, Lim WA. Synthetic immunology: hacking immune cells to expand their therapeutic capabilities. *Annu Rev Immunol*. 2017;35(1):229–253. doi:10.1146/annurev-immunol-051116-052302
42. Lim WA, June CH. The principles of engineering immune cells to treat cancer. *Cell*. 2017;168(4):724–740. doi:10.1016/j.cell.2017.01.016
147. Labanieh L, Majzner RG, Mackall CL. Programming CAR-T cells to kill cancer. *Nat Biomed Eng*. 2018;2(6):377–391. doi:10.1038/s41551-018-0235-9

Cancer Immunotherapy Targets
and Classes

Howard L. Kaufman

21

Introduction to Principles of Cancer Immunotherapy

Jon M. Wigginton

KEY POINTS

- Cancer immunotherapy mobilizes the host immune system to treat cancer.

- Major divisions of the immune system include innate and adaptive immunity, with multiple potential targets for therapeutic intervention.

- Strategies for cancer immunotherapy span multiple technology platforms and classes of therapeutics.

- Tumor vaccines and other antigen-directed therapies seek to mobilize and focus the immune response to cancer.

- Cytokines, T cell agonist antibodies, and targeted inducers of innate immunity can activate and drive the antitumor immune response.

- Multiple cell surface receptor-ligand interactions can modulate the activity of key effector cell populations, including T, natural killer (NK), and dendritic cell (DC) populations.

- Tumors exert multiple mechanisms to evade and/or suppress the host immune system.

PREMISE FOR CANCER IMMUNOTHERAPY

Recognition of the intrinsic ability of the host immune system to identify and destroy cancer has existed since the era of William Coley, a New York surgeon in the late 1800s. Coley astutely observed that some cancer patients experienced tumor regression in conjunction with episodes of infection, and that bacteria or bacterial products (Coley's toxins) could be isolated and injected to mediate tumor regression.[1,2] Several studies suggest that patients can mount an immune response to their cancer in the absence of treatment, and that the nature of this response may be significant prognostically.[3,4] Nonetheless, this response is ineffectual, as overt tumors grow, invade

locally, and metastasize despite this response. Informed by deepening understanding of the organization of the immune system, powerful new tools have emerged to mobilize, focus, and amplify the host immune response for the treatment of cancer.

The field of cancer immunotherapy has experienced a true renaissance over the past decade, leading to transformative changes in the treatment of patients with many cancers, including both solid tumors and hematologic malignancies. The dramatic advances and regulatory approvals achieved with checkpoint inhibitors (CPI), chimeric antigen receptor T cells (CAR T), CD3-based bispecific molecules, oncolytic viruses, and cytokines emerged from foundational basic, translational, and clinical observations gathered over several decades. These insights more clearly defined the critical components and key mechanistic nodes that regulate the antitumor immune response, and in turn enabled the development of new therapeutics to deliver meaningful, long-term clinical benefit for patients with cancer. In addition, the clinical success of cancer immunotherapy has led to efforts to integrate these regimens with standard-of-care, including surgery, radiotherapy, chemotherapy, and small molecule targeted drugs. Clinicians have now hypothesized, and established in randomized clinical trials, that immunotherapy can be safely and effectively combined with chemotherapy to improve outcomes over chemotherapy alone.[5,6] Further, in selected patients with squamous cell carcinoma of the head and neck (SCCHN)[5] or non-small cell lung cancer (NSCLC),[6] whose tumors express programmed cell death ligand 1 (PD-L1), anti-programmed cell death 1 (PD-1) monotherapy alone can outperform standard chemotherapy. Although this reality was arguably unthinkable little more than 10 years ago, similar questions are now being investigated in other cancers as well.

With the advent of broadly effective agents such as CPI, the use of cancer immunotherapy has expanded rapidly beyond the treatment of "sensitive" tumors like melanoma and renal cell carcinoma (RCC), and is now part of the standard of care for solid tumors including carcinomas of the skin, head/neck, breast, lung, esophagus, stomach, colon, kidney, and bladder, as well as melanoma, Merkel cell carcinoma, and hematologic malignancies, including both leukemias and lymphomas.[7,8] To provide context for these clinical advances, the broad spectrum of approaches under investigation, and future opportunities for the use of cancer immunotherapy, it is important to consider the general architecture of the tumor-host interface, and key elements of the human immune response to cancer.

KEY COMPONENTS OF THE ANTITUMOR IMMUNE RESPONSE: GENERAL CONSIDERATIONS

The immune response to cancer is mobilized by surveillance mechanisms that detect the tumor and initiate a cascade of events leading to activation, expansion, and trafficking of critical effector cell populations into the tumor microenvironment (TME), culminating in the execution of cytolytic mechanisms by these cells (Figure 21.1A). Aside from the high degree of specificity conferred by mechanisms that govern T cell recognition of tumor antigen(s), the antitumor immune response is exquisitely tuned by coordinated interactions between cell populations including CD4+ "helper" and CD8+ "cytotoxic" T cells, CD4+CD25+Foxp3+ regulatory T cells, natural killer (NK) and natural killer T (NKT) cells, and monocyte/macrophage and dendritic cell (DC) populations, among others. The functions of these cell populations are integrated via soluble factors such as cytokines and chemokines (discussed in Chapters 15 and 24), intercellular receptor-ligand interactions (including activating agonist receptors and inhibitory checkpoint receptors; discussed in Chapters 8, 27, and 28), downstream intracellular signal transduction pathways (e.g., JAK/STAT), and various cytolytic mechanisms (including receptor-dependent and granule-dependent) that mediate destruction of the tumor (see Chapter 12). The goal of cancer immunotherapy is to harness and potentiate the endogenous host immune system to destroy cancers, or alternatively, to engraft a potent immune response using molecularly engineered adoptive cellular therapy strategies (discussed in Chapters 25 and 26).

TUMOR RECOGNITION AND THE INTEGRATION OF INNATE AND ADAPTIVE IMMUNITY

The immune system can be divided into two major arms, innate and adaptive immunity. The innate immune system is a nonspecific, front-line defense mechanism that senses and responds to danger signals consisting of infection, inflammation, injury, and/or tumor. It is mediated primarily by NK, NKT, and gamma-delta (γδ) T cells, as well as monocyte/macrophage and DC populations (discussed in Chapters 10–12). In the setting of cancer,

effector cells of the innate immune system, in particular NK cells, may detect tumor cells and become activated. The activation and function of NK cells is regulated by cytokines including IL-2, IL-12, IL-15, IL-18, IL-21, and type 1 interferons,[9] as well as positive and negative receptor-ligand interactions between the NK cell and target cells (Figure 21.1A and 21.1B; discussed in Chapters 12 and 22). These cell surface receptors enable NK cells to detect abnormal or distressed cells to be targeted for killing, including virus-infected and/or malignant cells. Activating receptors on NK cells include NKG2D, DNAM-1, NKp30, NKp44, NK46, and activating KIR molecules, among others, while inhibitory receptors include several KIR molecules, as well as NKG2A and ILT2.[10,11] Normal healthy cells express HLA class I molecules that can bind to inhibitory KIR receptors on NK cells, and deliver a negative signal that protects these normal cells from recognition and destruction by NK cells. In contrast, tumor (or virus-infected) cells may downregulate HLA class I expression,[12–14] thus diminishing the self-protective signal delivered via binding to inhibitory KIR receptors on NK cells. Many cancers, including both solid tumors and hematologic malignancies, overexpress ligands including MICA, MICB, and ULBP1-4.[15,16] Ligands such as MICA can activate NK cells via NKG2D and facilitate NK cell cytotoxicity directed against the tumor.[17]

NK cells can react rapidly, in a non-antigen-restricted manner, to mediate direct cytolytic activity against malignant cells, and can do so via granule-dependent (perforin, granzyme B) and receptor-mediated (FAS/FAS-L, TRAIL/TRAIL-R) pathways.[18] Further, innate effector cells (including NK cells, monocyte/macrophage populations, and granulocytes) express activating Fc receptors (CD16A and CD32A) that can bind to the Fc domain of endogenously produced or exogenously administered antibodies bound to antigen(s) on tumor cells, and mediate antibody-dependent cellular cytotoxicity (ADCC). Activated NK cells also produce cytokines (including IFN-γ, TNF-α, and granulocyte-macrophage colony-stimulating factor [GM-CSF]) and chemokines that can exert direct antitumor activity, promote M1 macrophage polarization, support DC maturation, and upregulate the expression of HLA class I on target cells.

DCs are a central component of innate immunity and play a key role in integration of the immune system[19] (Figure 21.1A and 21.1C; see Chapters 5, 22, and 23). Dendritic cells differentiate from bone marrow progenitor cells into distinct subsets including plasmacytoid DC, conventional DC (including cDC1 and cDC2 subpopulations), and monocyte-derived, inflammatory DC. These DC subsets express distinct cell surface phenotypic markers and have complementary functional roles. Conventional DC populations (especially the cDC1 subset) are particularly effective antigen-presenting cells

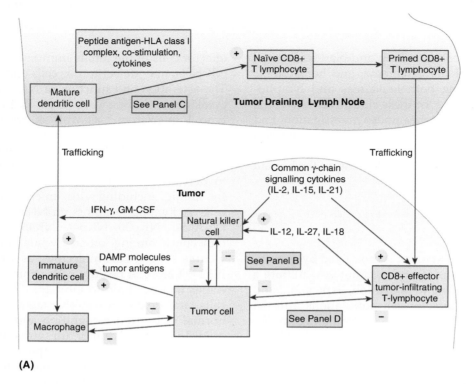

(A)

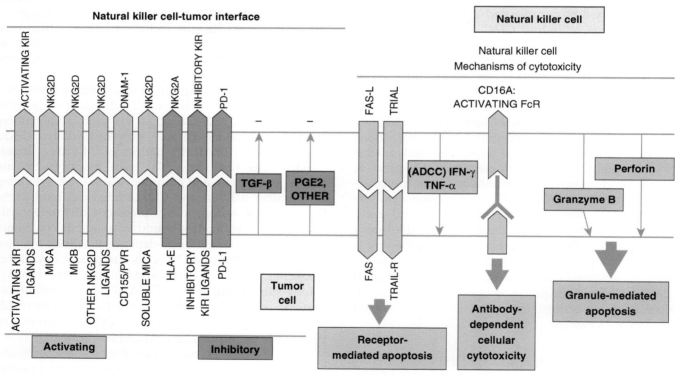

(B)

Figure 21.1 **Components of the antitumor immune response.** (**A**) General organization; (**B**) Key interactions in the interface between NK cells and tumor cells. (*continued*)

DAMP, danger-associated molecular pattern; DNAM-1, DNAX accessory molecule-1, CD226; FcR, Fc receptor; GM-CSF, granulocyte-macro; HLA-E, HLA Class I histompatibility antigen, alpha chain E; IFN-γ, interferon-gamma; KIR, killer cell immunoglobulin-like receptor; MICA, MHC Class I polypeptide-related sequence A; MICB, MHC Class I polypeptide-related sequence B; NKG2a, natural killer group 2a receptor; NKG2D, natural killer group 2D receptor; PD-1, programmed cell death protein-1; PD-L1, programmed death ligand-1; PGE2, prostaglandin E2; PVR, poliovirus receptor; TGF-β, transforming growth factor beta; TNF-α, tumor necrosis factor alpha; TRIAL, TNF-related apoptosis-inducing ligand; TRIAL-R, TNF-related apoptosis-inducing ligand receptor.

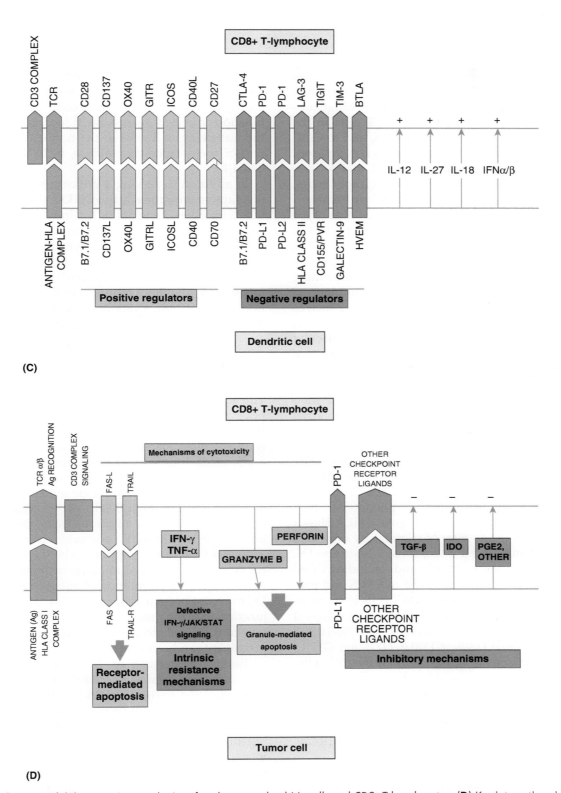

Figure 21.1 (*continued*) (**C**) Interactions at the interface between dendritic cells and CD8+ T lymphocytes; (**D**) Key interactions in the interface between effector CD8+ T lymphocytes and tumor cells.

BTLA, B- and T-lymphocyte attenuator; CTLA-4, cytotoxic T-lymphocyte-associated protein 4; GITR, glucocorticoid-induced TNF-R related protein; GITR-L, GITR-ligand; HLA, human leukocyte antigen; HVEM, herpes virus entry mediator; ICOS, inducible T cell co-stimulator; ICOS-L, ICOS-ligand; IDO, indoleamine-pyrrole 2,3-dioxygenase; IL-12, interleukin-12; IL-27, interleukin-27; IL-18, interleukin-18; IFN-α/β/γ, interferon-alpha/beta/gamma; JAK, Janus kinase; LAG-3, lymphocyte-activation gene 3; PD-1, programmed cell death protein 1; PD-2, programmed cell death protein 2; PD-L1, programmed death ligand 1; PD-L2, programmed death ligand 2; PGE2, prostaglandin E2; PVR, polio virus receptor; STAT, signal transducer and activator of transcription; TCR, T cell receptor; TGF-β, transforming growth factor beta; TIGIT, T cell immunoreceptor with Ig and ITIM domains; TIM-3, T cell immunoglobulin and mucin domain-containing protein 3.

(APC) and are critical for initiation and expansion of an antigen-specific T cell-mediated immune response. These DC detect, internalize, and process exogenous antigens for cross-presentation to CD8+ T cells in the context of peptide-HLA class I complexes, and to CD4+ T cells in the context of peptide-HLA class II complexes.

DCs may be found in the peripheral blood, lymphoid organs including tumor-draining lymph nodes, and various normal tissues. "Immature" or "mature" DC are classified based on their cell surface phenotype and functional properties. Immature DC are effective at endocytosis and antigen uptake, but express low levels of HLA class I and co-stimulatory molecules, and are ineffective at antigen-cross presentation and the priming of T cells. Immature DC may be activated and matured by cytokines, and via the interaction of receptors such as Toll-like receptors (TLR) and NOD-like receptors (NLR) expressed by DC with pathogen-associated molecular pattern (PAMP) or danger-associated molecular pattern (DAMP) molecules that are expressed and/or released by pathogens and stressed, dead, or dying cells, respectively.[19] Tumor cells may express or release DAMP molecules including nucleic acids such as mitochondrial DNA (detected by the cGAS-Stimulator of Interferon Genes [STING] pathway), calreticulin, heat-shock proteins (HSP70 and HSP90), adenosine triphosphate (ATP), high mobility group protein B1 (HMGB1), and type 1 interferons[19-22] (see Chapters 11, 13, and 22).

As DC transition to a mature phenotype, they downregulate endocytosis and upregulate HLA class I expression and the production of stimulatory cytokines (including IL-12 and Type 1 interferons).[19] Maturing DC also upregulate the expression of ligands including CD80 (B7.1) and CD86 (B7.2) that can bind to CD28 and provide critical co-stimulation to activate T cells in conjunction with antigen presentation.[19] Other receptor-ligand interactions, including CD137 (4-1BB)/CD137(4-1BBL), CD40/CD40L, OX40/OX40L, CD70/CD27, and GITR/GITRL can deliver activating signals from the DC to the T cell, while soluble factors such as IL-10, and receptor-ligand interactions including cytotoxic T-lymphocyte-associated protein 4 (CTLA-4)/B7.1, CTLA-4/B7.2, PD-1/PD-L1, and VISTA can mediate inhibitory signals to tune the kinetics and intensity of the antigen-specific T cell response.[19]

Mature DC can migrate to tumor-draining lymph nodes, facilitated by increased expression of the chemokine receptor, CCR7.[23] In the draining lymph node, DC cross-present processed antigen-HLA complexes to prime and support the expansion of naïve T cell populations, including both CD4+ and CD8+ T cells. Although tumor-draining lymph nodes appear to be the predominant location for priming of naïve tumor-specific CD8+ effector T cells, DC within the local TME can also prime naïve T cells. Activated CD8+ T cells are the dominant effector cell in the host immune response to tumor, and after activation in the draining lymph node, these cells traffic to the tumor site to execute cytolytic effector functions directed against the tumor. DCs also support the trafficking of T cells to the tumor via local production of chemotactic chemokines, including CXCL9 and CXCL10.[24]

In addition to serving a critical role in the initiation of adaptive immunity, activated DC also maintain crosstalk with other elements of the innate immune system, including NK cells, and can produce a diverse range of potent immunoregulatory cytokines including IL-12 family members (IL-12, IL-23, IL-27) and IL-18.[19,25-27] These cytokines serve as key mechanistic links between innate and adaptive immunity, and regulate the activation, proliferation, cytokine production, and cytolytic function by both T and NK cell populations.[10,25-27]

ADAPTIVE IMMUNITY AND THE T CELL-MEDIATED IMMUNE RESPONSE

The adaptive immune system consists of T and B lymphocyte populations. Relative to innate immunity, the adaptive immune response may take longer to fully mobilize mechanistically, but in turn can confer a powerful, highly specific immune response, as well as long-lasting, durable capacity to react to an antigen upon re-exposure (immunologic memory; see Chapters 4, 6, and 33). Although B cells play a critical role in the immune response to infectious pathogens, and in the immunopathogenesis of various autoimmune disorders, activated CD8+ T cells appear to be the dominant effector cell in the adaptive immune response to cancer. In addition to the presentation of antigens to CD8+ T cells, DC may also present antigens to CD4+ T cells, and in conjunction with the production of IL-12, drive the polarization of these cells to a Th1 phenotype characterized by prominent production of IFN-γ.

Tumor antigens may be classified into categories including tumor-associated antigens (TAA) and tumor-specific antigens (TSA)[28-31] (see Chapters 4, 5, 23, 36, and 37). These respective categories may have important differences in patterns of antigen expression, potential cross-reactivity with antigen also expressed in normal tissues, and intrinsic immunogenicity. TAA include self-antigens that are overexpressed in cancer cells compared with normal cells, as well as antigens that are expressed in a tissue-specific manner (differentiation antigens), including antigens otherwise restricted to expression in the testes (cancer testis antigens). Examples of overexpressed TAA include EGFR, hTERT, p53, HER2, and survivin. These molecules also contribute to the neoplastic phenotype of the tumor cell and, as a consequence, may be less prone to the emergence of antigen-loss variant subclones within the tumor under the selective pressure of antigen-directed cancer immunotherapy. Nonetheless, because these antigens are also expressed in normal tissue, unintended immunologic cross-reactivity with normal tissues may contribute to additional toxicity. Further, in that TAA are self-antigens, the physiology of immunologic tolerance may limit reactivity of the existing T cell pool to respond to these antigens. Examples of tumor-associated differentiation antigens include tyrosinase, Melan-A/MART-1, gp100 and tyrosinase-related proteins 1 and 2, prostate-specific antigen (PSA), and carcinoembryonic antigen (CEA). Cancer testis antigens include various MAGE family members, such as PRAME, NY-ESO1, SSX2, and GAGE. These differentiation antigens and cancer testis-antigens generally do not contribute to maintenance of the neoplastic phenotype, and consequently are subject to the emergence of antigen-loss variant subclones in the tumor. As targets, these self-antigens are also subject to immunologic tolerance by the host immune system, but may have reduced potential for normal tissue cross-reactivity due to more limited patterns of expression than other TAA.

More recently, tremendous attention has focused on TSA as targets for cancer immunotherapy. Tumor-specific antigens arise from proteins expressed as a consequence of mutations in the tumor DNA (neoantigens), or proteins derived from viral oncogenes (oncoviral antigens) or from tumor-specific endogenous retroviruses (TERVs).[28–31] Neoantigens are truly tumor- and patient-specific, and may arise from point-mutations, frame-shift mutations, or insertion/deletion mutations. These unique neoantigens could have improved potential for immunogenicity compared with TAA, and reduced potential for cross-reactivity with normal tissue, unlike TAA. Notably, patients whose tumors have a greater tumor mutational burden (TMB) score have a greater propensity to harbor tumor neoantigens, and in some settings an increased probability of objective clinical response to T cell-directed, checkpoint inhibitor immunotherapy.[32,33]

As previously described, DC play a central role in presenting tumor antigens to the T cell receptor (TCR) complex on T cells. For the majority of T cells, known as αβ T cells, the heterodimeric T cell receptor consists of alpha (α) and beta (β) polypeptide chains that are responsible for recognition of specific peptide-HLA complexes[34,35] (discussed in Chapters 4–6). Alternatively, the T cell receptor may consist of variant gamma (γ) and delta (δ) chains, as seen in γδ T cells. Although the TCR provides the machinery for antigen recognition, it does not directly mediate signal transduction. Instead, intracellular signaling is delivered via CD3, a polypeptide complex that associates with the heterodimeric TCR. CD3 is a polypeptide comprised of δ, γ, ε, and ζ chains, each containing signaling motifs known as immunoreceptor tyrosine-based activation motifs (ITAMs) in their intracellular cytoplasmic domains. These signaling components serve as the critical interface between engagement of the TCR complex by APCs, and mobilization of key intracellular signal transduction pathways that activate T cell function.

The overall outcome of antigen presentation, with induction of tolerance (in the absence of adequate co-stimulation), or the activation and execution of a productive T cell-mediated immune response to cancer, is also highly regulated by cytokines, and the integration of signals delivered to receptors on T cells via cell-surface ligands expressed by DC, tumor cells, and other elements of the TME (Figure 21.1A, 21.1C, and 21.1D)[19,36,37] (discussed in Chapters 8, 24, 27, and 28). These include activating receptors (OX-40, CD137/4-1BB, CD28, ICOS, CD40L, GITR) and several inhibitory checkpoint molecules (PD-1, CTLA-4, LAG-3, TIM-3, BTLA, TIGIT, adenosine A2a receptor, CECAM-1). Normal tissue expression of ligands for these inhibitory receptors, in particular PD-L1, can contribute to immune privilege in selected normal tissues and protection of these sites from autoreactive T cells. T cell checkpoint receptors can be differentially expressed during the evolution of an immune response and deliver incremental inhibitory signals that fine-tune the function of activated T cells. CTLA-4 and PD-1 appear to be particularly important in this regard, and upregulation of these and other checkpoint molecules on the surface of activated T cells can contribute to incremental inhibition of T cell function and, ultimately, T cell exhaustion.[38–42]

Malignant cells can constitutively overexpress PD-L1 and co-opt the PD-1/PD-L1 pathway as a major mechanism of tumor self-defense.[43–45] Tumor cells can also adaptively upregulate PD-L1 expression in response to effector cytokines including IFN-γ that are produced locally by infiltrating T and NK cells within the TME. The interaction of PD-L1 expressed on tumor cells can engage PD-1 on the surface of T cells within the TME, and in so doing, suppress the function of these T cells. Blockade of the PD-1/PD-L1 interaction can mediate profound clinical activity across a broad range of cancers (discussed in Chapters 8 and 27 and Section 4). In turn, consistent with their role in maintaining immune privilege in normal tissues, the blockade of T cell checkpoints in cancer patients treated with anti-PD-1/PD-L1 or anti-CTLA-4 antibodies can manifest with side effects including immune-mediated hypophysitis, uveitis, thyroiditis, pneumonitis, colitis, and hepatitis, among others.[46]

T cell function is also regulated by several cytokines, including members of the common γ-chain signaling family (IL-2, IL-7, IL-15, IL-21), the IL-12 family (IL-12, IL-23, IL-27), and IL-18.[25–27,47] Of these, IL-12 is particularly important in driving T cells toward a so-called Th-1 type phenotype, characterized by IFN-γ, an important antitumor effector cytokine. Inputs to the T cell via antigen presentation, cytokines, co-stimulation, and other receptor-ligand interactions at the cell surface are integrated by intracellular signal transduction pathways that regulate the overall intensity, kinetics, and duration of the ensuing T cell-mediated immune response.

Activated, primed T cells need to traffic into the tumor to engage tumor cells and exert their cytolytic function. The trafficking of CD8+ T cells into the tumor and trans-migration across the vascular endothelium is regulated by several chemokines, including CXCL9 and CXCL10,[24] and interaction between integrins such as lymphocyte function-associated (LFA-1) T cells and adhesion molecules such as very-late antigen-4 (VLA-4), as well as intercellular adhesion molecule 1 (ICAM-1) on vascular endothelial cells.[48] Within the TME, cytolytic CD8+ T cells can recognize tumor antigen in the context of HLA class I expressed on the surface of tumor cells, and mediate destruction of the tumor via the elaboration of effector cytokines such as IFN-γ and, similar to NK cells, mobilization of both granule-mediated (perforin, granzyme B) cytotoxicity and the induction of receptor-mediated apoptosis via the FAS/FAS-L or TRAIL/TRAIL-R pathways.[49]

THE TUMOR FIGHTS BACK: EVASION AND SUBVERSION OF THE HOST IMMUNE RESPONSE

Tumors can elaborate a diverse spectrum of mechanisms to evade detection by the immune system, and to suppress the antitumor immune response, including the function of tumor-infiltrating T cells. The PD-1/PD-L1 pathway (described previously) is perhaps the most extensively studied mechanism of tumor self-defense[43–45] (discussed in Chapters 8 and 27). Tumors can also evade detection of the immune response by virtue of downreg-ulation of HLA class I expression,[13,14] the enzymatic activity of indoleamine 2,3-dioxygenase (IDO)[50,51] within the TME, and the release of soluble factors that directly or indirectly suppress T cell function, including arachidonic acid metabolites such as PGE2,[52] transforming growth factor beta (TGF-β),[53] and soluble MICA (sMICA),[54–58] among others (discussed in Chapters 41 and 46).

TGF-β is overexpressed by various solid tumors and can suppress both innate and adaptive immunity.[53] TGF-β contributes to the expansion of immune-suppressive regulatory T cells (T_{reg} cells) and can also inhibit the function of antigen-presenting DC, as well as T cell activation, proliferation, and effector function. TGF-β can also inhibit innate immunity, including NK cell function. Many tumors produce proangiogenic factors such as vascular endothelial growth factor (VEGF) to support tumor vascularization, and VEGF can also support the tumor via suppression of the antitumor immune response, in particular via inhibition of DC maturation and antigen presentation.[59] Tumor cells may also release immuno-suppressive cytokines such as IL-10,[60] and aberrant

chemokine/chemokine receptor expression can disrupt the trafficking of T cells into the local tumor site. Tumor cells also can develop molecular alterations that confer intrinsic resistance to mechanisms that govern cell death (discussed in Chapter 14). These include activation of Wnt/β-catenin signaling,[61] defects in IFN-γ signaling including mutations in downstream JAK-STAT signaling pathways,[62] and overexpression of antiapoptotic molecules including cFLIP,[63,64] bcl-2,[65] and survivin.[66]

The diverse mechanisms that mediate immune evasion and suppression by the tumor highlight the complex considerations that influence mobilization of a productive antitumor immune response, and, in turn, potential challenges in the development of successful approaches to cancer immunotherapy. Collectively, these strategies must overcome the spectrum of suppressive mechanisms of tumor self-defense, and support detection of the tumor, antigen processing and presentation, priming of T cells, and, ultimately, the activation and trafficking of cytolytic CD8+ T cells into the tumor to deliver immune-mediated tumor regression.

THERAPEUTIC STRATEGIES FOR CANCER IMMUNOTHERAPY

Armed with an improved understanding of the mechanisms that regulate the antitumor immune response, and innovative therapeutic tools to target these mechanisms, there has been explosive growth in efforts to leverage the human immune system for the treatment of cancer. The majority of these strategies are designed to mobilize and potentiate the patient's own immune response to their cancer. Cellular therapy emphasizes the isolation and ex vivo engineering of effector cells including T cells, NK cells, or macrophage populations to more effectively arm these cells to recognize and destroy cancer. Once modified, these autologous or allogeneic engineered effector cells are reinfused with or without other therapeutics to mediate the destruction of hematologic malignancies and/or solid tumors (discussed in Chapters 25 and 26). To frame the discussion here, strategies for cancer immunotherapy are categorized as follows:

- enhancing immune surveillance
- mobilizing and focusing the antitumor immune response
- activating and driving the antitumor immune response
- taking the brakes off the immune response
- reversal of tumor-mediated immunosuppression

It is worth noting that this review is not intended to be exhaustive. Further, given the complex and dynamic interplay in regulation of the host immune response, and the integration of mechanisms of innate and adaptive immunity, it is important to recognize that modulation of one mechanism inevitably can impact other mechanisms positively or negatively, either directly or indirectly. In addition, the role of some pathways in regulating the immune response may be highly context dependent. As a result, some of this categorization is artificial in nature but is designed to enable this discussion. Lastly, clinical outcomes achieved with these respective approaches are generally not discussed here, as they are covered in detail elsewhere in this textbook.

ENHANCING IMMUNE SURVEILLANCE

As previously described, the innate immune system represents the front-line of the host immune response, and key contributors include NK, NKT, and γδ T cells, as well as monocyte/macrophage and DC populations[9–11,16–18] (discussed in Chapters 10–12). Cytokines including IL-2, IL-12, IL-15, IL-18, and IL-21 have been investigated clinically,[67–71] and can enhance the activation, proliferation, cytokine production, and cytolytic function of NK cells.[9,25–27,47,72] These and other cytokines also play a critical role in regulating the function of T cells,[25–27,47] and, in the case of IL-12 family members and IL-18, in the integration of innate immune surveillance and mobilization of an antigen-specific T cell-mediated immune response.[19,25,27] With the re-emergence of interest in cytokines for cancer immunotherapy, a wide variety of new cytokine-based molecules, including engineered variants of recombinant IL-2, IL-7, IL-12, IL-15, and IL-18, are now in development.

In addition to cytokines, NK cell function is regulated via integrated inputs from various activating or inhibitory cell surface receptors[10–12,17] (discussed in Chapters 10 and 12). Antibodies that block inhibitory NK receptors, such as NKG2A (monalizumab) and inhibitory KIR molecules (lirilumab, lacutamab), are designed to potentiate NK cell function, and are being investigated for the treatment of hematologic malignancies and/or solid tumors. Activating NK cell receptors such as NKG2D bind to MICA or MICB on the surface of stressed or transformed target cells, and this facilitates recognition and killing of these target cells by the NK cell.[17] Tumors can proteolytically cleave and shed soluble MICA and MICB to disrupt NKG2D binding to MICA/MICB on the surface of intact tumor cells, and, as a decoy, inhibit NK-mediated killing of these cells.[54–58] In several retrospective studies, elevated levels of circulating sMICA have been associated with adverse clinical outcomes,[73,74] including in patients with elevated sMICA levels at baseline prior to treatment with CPI.[54] Several antibodies are now in development to target the NKG2D-MICA interaction, including CLN-619, a molecule that both inhibits the cleavage and shedding of sMICA by tumor cells and potentiates NK-mediated ADCC. Bispecific (BiKEs) and trispecific (TriKEs) antibody-based multispecific molecules are in

development and are designed to redirect NK cells to mediate cytotoxicity that is not HLA-restricted but is directed against tumor cells that express specific antigen(s).[75] NK cell-based adoptive cellular therapy, including both autologous and allogeneic NK chimeric antigen receptor (CAR) cells, is under investigation, including cells engineered to recognize target antigens such as CD19 or CD33, and to co-express activating molecules such as IL-15.[76] Early in clinical development, other CAR-based approaches utilize innate effector cells including NKT cells, macrophages, and γδ T cells.

Macrophages are important contributors to innate immunity, both as participants in antigen presentation and as mediators of ADCC and phagocytosis[77] (discussed in Chapters 11, 12, and 22). Recently, the CD47/signal regulatory protein alpha (SIRP-α) pathway has emerged as an important macrophage checkpoint pathway and a new target for cancer immunotherapy.[78,79] Receptor ligand interaction between CD47 (expressed by several cell types, including various tumors) and SIRP-α (expressed on the surface of macrophages, monocytes, DCs, and granulocytes) mediate an inhibitory "don't eat me" signal that inhibits macrophage activation and the phagocytosis of tumor cells by macrophages. Agents that block the interaction between CD47 and SIRP-α have demonstrated preclinical antitumor activity,[80,81] and clinical activity in patients with hematologic malignancies.[82,83]

MOBILIZING AND FOCUSING THE ANTITUMOR IMMUNE RESPONSE

Strategies to mobilize and focus the endogenous antigen-specific immune response to cancer represent some of the earliest approaches to cancer immunotherapy and have evolved dramatically over time. In the infectious disease setting, numerous vaccines have demonstrated the capability to induce and expand B and/or T cell immune responses that confer protective immunity to prevent various bacterial and/or viral infections. As a consequence, many investigators have hypothesized that patients similarly could be vaccinated with tumor antigens to treat or prevent cancer. Early strategies began with peptide-based vaccines with or without various chemical or biological adjuvants, and evolved over time to include full-length peptides, nucleic acids, or even whole-cell lysates[28,29,84–86] (discussed in Chapters 4, 5, and 23). Features of the various classes of tumor antigens targeted with tumor vaccines were previously described.

Although the success of first-generation tumor vaccines in inducing T cell responses to treat established cancers has been limited, one of the most impactful examples of cancer prevention has utilized a vaccine-based approach to raise antibody production directed against human papillomavirus (HPV) oncoviral antigens. Infection with HPV, particularly HPV serotype 16 (HPV-16), is common world-wide, and is well-recognized as a significant risk factor for HPV-associated cancers including cervical, vaginal, endometrial, anal, and penile carcinomas, as well as SCCHN.[87–89] HPV-16 encodes viral oncogenes, including E6 and E7, that can interfere with the function of tumor suppressor genes that regulate the cell cycle in infected cells, and in so doing lead to uncontrolled cell proliferation and cancer. HPV vaccines have been developed based on the use of non-infectious virus-like particles (VLP) to induce the production of antibodies directed against antigens found on the surface of intact HPV, and the induction of antibody production directed against L1 appears to account for the protection from infection. HPV vaccines including GARDASIL (quadrivalent HPV-6, -11, -16, and -18), GARDASIL 9 (9-valent vaccine), and Cervarix (HPV-16 and -18) are effective in the prevention of various HPV-associated precancerous/dysplastic lesions and cancer. These vaccines have achieved regulatory approvals and broad implementation in the standard of care for children and adolescents.[90–92] Nonprotective CD4+ T cell responses have been demonstrated in some patients that receive preventative HPV vaccines,[93] and vaccines designed to mobilize a T cell response for the treatment of established HPV-associated cancers are being explored.[94,95]

Optimal T cell priming and activation require signals beyond interaction of the antigen-HLA complex with the T cell receptor (Signal 1), including co-stimulation such as that mediated by the interaction of CD28 with B7.1 and B7.2 (Signal 2) and soluble factors including immunoregulatory cytokines such as IL-12 (Signal 3)[19,96] (see Chapters 6, 24, and 28). Given their importance as APCs, producers of potent immunoregulatory cytokines, and central integrators of innate and adaptive immunity, several studies have investigated the use of DC-based tumor vaccines[19,28,29,84–86,97] (discussed in Chapters 5 and 23). DCs can provide all three classes of signals, and therapeutic strategies designed to leverage the biology of DC are under investigation, including loading of DC with tumor antigen(s) using peptides or other protein-derived antigens or cellular lysates, and engineering of DC to overexpress T cell co-stimulatory molecules and/or cytokines such as IL-12. Indeed, Provenge® is an autologous DC that is loaded with the prostate acid phosphatase (PAP) antigen and GM-CSF, and is approved for the treatment of asymptomatic or minimally symptomatic metastatic hormone refractory prostate cancer.

A variety of other vaccine-based approaches to deliver these complementary signals concurrently with tumor antigen(s) have been investigated, including viral vectors, DNA and RNA constructs, and engineering and vaccination with tumor cells, fibroblasts, and/or various cellular lysate preparations[28,29,84–86] (discussed in Chapters 4, 5, and 23). Although these approaches have demonstrated the ability to potentiate trafficking of

effector cells into the tumor site, and in some instances enhancement of antigen-specific T cell responses, the ability to deliver durable tumor regression broadly in patients with solid tumors using these approaches has been limited to date.

DCs can also be activated and matured via pathways including toll receptors, cGAS-STING, and FLT3[19] (see Chapter 22). Toll-like receptor (TLR) agonists can potentiate DC activation and maturation, and are under investigation as therapeutics to enhance DC function and the antitumor immune response.[98–100] These include systemic, peritumoral, or intratumoral administration of agonists for TLR3 (poly-ICLC), TLR7/8 (NKTR-262, CV8102, LHC-165), and TLR-9 (SD-101, CMP-001, IMO-2125). Imiquimod is a TLR7 agonist that can be applied topically, and is U.S. Food and Drug Administration (FDA) approved for use in the treatment of superficial basal cell carcinomas. cGAS-STING has been identified as an important pathway for sensing intracellular DNA, and activation of this pathway enhances the production of type 1 interferons.[101] In turn, type 1 interferons enhance the function of several contributors to the immune response, including DCs, as well as T and NK cells. Synthetic agonists for the STING pathway, including ADU-S100 and MK-1454, have been tested as intratumoral therapeutics, but have demonstrated limited activity in studies to date. Fms-like tyrosine kinase 3 ligand (FLT-3L) can promote DC expansion and upregulate HLA class II expression.[102] Recombinant FLT-3L (CDX-301) is under investigation as a monotherapy, and in combination with other immunotherapeutic agents, chemotherapy and stereotactic radiotherapy are being explored for the treatment of patients with advanced cancer.

A number of oncolytic viruses are being explored as tools for cancer immunotherapy, including adenovirus, measles virus, Newcastle disease virus, reovirus, and herpes simplex virus[103–106] (discussed in Chapter 30). Talimogene laherparepvec (IMLYGIC®, T-VEC), an oncolytic, attenuated herpes simplex virus-type 1 (HSV-1) that is engineered to replicate selectively in tumor cells and to overexpress GM-CSF, has been approved by the FDA for the local treatment of patients with unresectable cutaneous, subcutaneous, and nodal melanoma lesions.[107] It is delivered directly into tumor deposits, replicates selectively in tumor cells, and induces cell lysis. The resulting cell death and release of tumor antigen(s) may contribute to the priming of T cells, and the overexpression of GM-CSF can enhance DC recruitment and maturation within the tumor.

ACTIVATING AND DRIVING THE ANTITUMOR IMMUNE RESPONSE

The initial sensing of tumor via immune surveillance mechanisms initiates a cascade of events that integrate innate and adaptive immunity and mobilize the T cell-mediated immune response. Cytokines including members of the common γ-chain family (IL-2, IL-7, and IL-15), the IL-12 family (IL-12 and IL-27), and IL-18 are key orchestrators of these mechanisms[25–27,47] (discussed in Chapter 24). Cytokines coordinate the activation, proliferation, differentiation, cytokine production, and cytolytic activity of both T cells and NK cells. In turn, common γ-chain signaling cytokines (IL-2, IL-7, IL-15, and IL-21) can induce the upregulation of PD-1 on the surface of T cells,[108] and regulatory cytokines such as IL-12 and IL-18 can potently enhance the production of IFN-γ,[109,110] a key downstream effector cytokine that can upregulate the adaptive expression of PD-L1 on tumor cells.[43] Some cytokines, in particular IL-2, can drive the expansion of suppressive cell populations, including T_{reg} cells.[111,112] Despite the complex biology that is integrated by these cytokines, they can deliver pronounced monotherapy antitumor activity in preclinical models.[25,47,113–115] Further, combinations of IL-2 with IL-12, IL-18, or IL-27 can mediate synergistic antitumor activity in preclinical tumor models.[116–118]

Recombinant IL-2 entered the clinic in the 1980s, and was FDA approved for the treatment of patients with metastatic kidney cancer and melanoma in the 1990s. Multiple immunoregulatory cytokines, including IL-2, IL-7, IL-12, IL-15, IL-18, and IL-21, have been investigated in patients with cancer[67–71,119] (discussed in Chapter 24), although only IFN-α and IL-2 have achieved regulatory approval to date. Although several of these cytokines have demonstrated pronounced biologic activity in treated patients, and the ability to mediate tumor regression in some tumor types, the development of each of these cytokines (other than IL-2) was largely abandoned after the early stages of clinical development. In retrospect, early clinical strategies may have been suboptimal from several perspectives, including an emphasis on highly dose-intensive monotherapy regimens focused on definition of a maximum tolerated dose (MTD), rather than the maximum biologically effective dose. In addition, many trials enrolled unselected, relapsed/ refractory, metastatic patients who were heavily pretreated with immunosuppressive cytotoxic chemotherapy that may have compromised the ability of patients to mount an immune response to cytokine monotherapy. Further, despite several lines of evidence that cytokine combinations can additively or synergistically enhance T and/or NK cell function in vitro, and deliver synergistic antitumor activity in preclinical models, relatively limited investigation of these cytokine combinations was undertaken in the clinic, other than initial studies with the combination of IL-2 and IL-12. Lastly, the clinical development of cytokines was also compromised by toxicity due to broad systemic activation of the immune system, and the significant expertise that was required to provide the necessary supportive care for patients treated with high-dose cytokine regimens.

Fortunately, with improved understanding of cytokine biology, dramatic advances in the supportive care of patients being treated with cancer immunotherapy, and new clinical development paradigms, multiple new cytokine-based molecules are now in active development. These include engineered recombinant cytokines with differential affinity for subunits of the IL-2 receptor to diminish toxicity and/or undesirable expansion of T_{reg} cell populations,[120,121] or more selectively target and/or retain cytokines within the TME after local or systemic administration.[121,122] Many of these novel molecules are focused on delivery of the biology of cytokines such as IL-2, IL-12, IL-15, or IL-18, and, in some cases, combinations of cytokines to deliver an immunotherapy combination in one molecule.[120,123,124]

It is widely recognized that CD28-mediated co-stimulation is critical for T cell priming and activation. Other receptor-ligand pairs that can potentiate the activation of T cells include ICOS/ICOS-L, CD137 (4-1BB)/CD137L (4-1BBL), OX40/OX40L, CD27/CD70, GITR/GITR-L, and CD40L/CD40[19,36] (discussed in Chapters 6 and 28). To leverage these pathways, agonistic monoclonal antibodies to activate these receptors on T cells are now undergoing clinical investigation as monotherapy, and in combination with other immunoregulatory agents, including checkpoint inhibitors.[36,125] Further, several multispecific molecules that combine agonistic targeting of these pathways with moieties that mediate PD-1/PD-L1 blockade, or targeting to PD-L1⁺ tumors, are advancing to the clinic.

Numerous CD3-directed, antibody-based multispecific molecules have been developed to engage and redirect T cells to kill malignant target cells expressing a specific cell surface antigen.[126,127] Many molecules utilize a bispecific format with a CD3-binding arm, and a distinct arm to bind the specific tumor antigen of interest. The bispecific molecule brings CD3⁺ T cells and tumor cells into close proximity, and potently enhances T cell activation, proliferation, cytokine production, and cytolytic activity directed against the tumor cell. In that redirected killing is non-HLA-restricted, any T cell can be redirected in principle to mediate cytotoxicity. Blinatumomab, a CD3xCD19 bispecific BITE® molecule, is the most advanced agent in this class, and is FDA approved for the treatment of children and adults with B cell precursor acute lymphoblastic leukemia (ALL).[128] Several next-generation multispecific structural platforms including DART®, XmAb®, Multiclonics®, and VelociBi® have advanced molecules into the clinical setting, including molecules with an extended half-life that obviates the need for a continuous infusion treatment regimen, as required for blintumomab. Several platforms have developed agents with altered affinities for CD3, as a strategy to ameliorate the cytokine-release syndrome

(CRS) that is commonly observed in patients treated with CD3-based bispecific molecules. The use of CD28 rather than CD3 in T cell-directed bispecific molecules has also been established,[129] and preclinical studies suggest that these molecules can be combined with CD3-based bispecific molecules to achieve synergistic antitumor activity without inducing cytokine storm.[130] Although a large number of CD3-based bispecific molecules have been evaluated in patients with various hematologic malignancies or solid tumors, clinically significant efficacy to date has largely been restricted to patients with hematologic malignancies including acute lymphoblastic leukemia (CD3xCD19),[131,132] lymphoma (CD3xCD20),[133] and acute myelogenous leukemia (CD3xCD123).[134] Trispecific molecules are in development to more selectively target specific effector cell subsets or to improve the selectivity of binding to tumor cells.

TAKING THE BRAKES OFF THE IMMUNE RESPONSE

Along with dramatic new observations utilizing chimeric antigen receptor T (CAR T) cells for the treatment of patients with hematologic malignancies,[134–138] regulatory approvals for checkpoint inhibitor monoclonal antibodies including anti-CTLA-4,[139] anti-PD-1,[7,8] and anti-PD-L1[140] for the treatment of patients with a variety of solid tumors and hematologic malignancies have revolutionized the field of cancer immunotherapy. Aside from CTLA-4 and PD-1, T cells can express several other inhibitory cell surface checkpoint receptors that contribute to modulation of T cell function, including LAG-3, TIM-3, BTLA, TIGIT and CECAM-1[141,142] (discussed in Chapter 27).

In 2010, investigators reported for the first time that ipilimumab (YERVOY®), an anti-CTLA-4 antibody, could prolong the survival of metastatic melanoma patients compared with standard-of-care chemotherapy.[143] Shortly thereafter, Phase 1 studies demonstrated that anti-PD-1 and anti-PD-L1 antibodies had pronounced clinical activity in patients with solid tumors[144–146] or hematologic malignancies.[147] These studies highlighted both the central importance of PD-1/PD-L1 and CTLA-4 in regulating T cell function, and potential opportunities that could be afforded by targeting other T cell checkpoints alone or in combination. Despite the exciting clinical results achieved with CPI in patients with solid tumors, it is important to recognize that most patients treated with checkpoint inhibitors do not respond clinically, and few patients are cured of their disease. Blocking antibodies designed to block other T cell checkpoint receptor-ligand interactions are now in clinical development (discussed in Chapter 27) and are being investigated both as monotherapy regimens and in numerous combination studies. These include various CPI combinations (in particular, those containing anti-PD-1 or anti-PD-L1 antibodies), as well as combinations of CPI with other distinct classes of immune modulators, including agonist antibodies, cytokines, CD3-based bispecifics, tumor vaccines, and modulators of innate immunity and cellular therapy (discussed in Chapters 27 and 32). The most advanced regimen to date is the combination of anti-PD-1 and anti-CTLA-4 antibodies,[148] which has demonstrated clinical efficacy supporting FDA approvals for the treatment of patients with melanoma, NSCLC, mesothelioma, RCC, colorectal carcinoma, and hepatocellular carcinoma.[7] Another checkpoint inhibitor combination of interest is the combination of tiragolumab (anti-TIGIT) and atezolizumab (anti-PD-L1) antibodies.[149] This combination achieved FDA breakthrough-therapy designation based on encouraging clinical observations in patients with NSCLC whose tumors express PD-L1, and this approach is now undergoing investigation in several other solid tumors. In addition to numerous antibody combination studies, multiple platforms are advancing various bispecific constructs that incorporate checkpoint inhibitor combinations (e.g., PD-1 x CTLA-4, PD-1 x LAG-3, PD-1 x TIM-3) or checkpoint-agonist combinations (e.g., PD-1 or PD-L1 x CD137), among others.

An important consideration in the clinical development of regimens containing CPI is patient selection using various biomarkers (discussed in Chapters 18, 44, and 45). Although the expression of PD-L1 as determined by immunohistochemical staining of pretreatment tumor specimens is useful for the identification of patients who are more likely to respond to PD-1/PD-L1 blockade for some tumor types treated with some anti-PD-1 or anti-PD-L1 antibodies, patient selection based on tumor expression of PD-L1 does not appear to be necessary in all settings.[7,8,140] Further, the cut-point for defining PD-L1 positivity may vary based on the assay and on the specific tumor type. The presence of elevated TMB also has been a patient selection marker of interest, with the rationale that patients with elevated mutational burden may harbor a greater number of tumor-neoantigens, and that these patients may be more likely to mobilize an endogenous immune response to their tumors.[31–33] Patients who have microsatellite instability high (MSI-H) or mismatch repair deficient (dMMR) colorectal and other carcinomas are highly sensitive to treatment with checkpoint blockade. As a consequence of these molecular alterations, these tumors appear to have an increased mutational burden and neoantigen load that may render these tumors more immunogenic and poised to respond to checkpoint blockade.

REVERSAL OF TUMOR-MEDIATED IMMUNE SUPPRESSION

Despite the diverse array of mechanisms that can be leveraged to potentiate the host immune response to mediate tumor regression, tumor cells and elements of the associated microenvironment can exploit a range of mechanisms to allow the tumor to evade detection by the immune system, and to suppress the antitumor immune response (discussed in Chapters 27, 41, and 46). Informed by advancements in understanding the complex interplay between the host and tumor, many new therapeutic strategies have emerged to attenuate or reverse tumor-mediated immunosuppression.

Antibody blockade of PD-1/PD-L1 interaction is perhaps the most intensively studied and clinically successful strategy to reverse tumor-mediated immunosuppression to date. Several strategies to inhibit the expression or release of soluble immunosuppressive mediators such as TGF-β are also under active investigation.[53] Agents designed to target TGF-β include small molecule inhibitors of TGF-β signaling (galunisertib, vactosertib, LY3200882, PF-06952229), monoclonal antibodies directed against TGF-β (SAR-439459, GC1008), TGF-β-trap (AVID200), or bispecific molecules containing moieties designed to neutralize or inhibit TGF-β function in combination with other immune modulators, including TGF-β trap x anti-PD-L1 (bintrafusp alfa).[53] The IDO pathway has been shown to be capable of inhibiting T cell function, and can be upregulated by IFN-γ, suggesting that this pathway could play a role in tuning T cell function within the TME.[50,51] Although preclinical studies provided supportive proof-of-mechanism, IDO inhibitors demonstrated limited clinical activity as monotherapy.[150] Further, although early clinical studies suggested that the combination of IDO inhibition and checkpoint inhibition could achieve antitumor activity greater than either agent alone,[151] subsequent randomized studies failed to demonstrate a benefit for the addition of IDO inhibitors over checkpoint inhibitors alone.[152]

As previously noted, many cancers, including both solid tumors and hematologic malignancies, can overexpress MICA,[15,16] a ligand for NKG2D[17] (see Chapters 22 and 41). Tumors can cleave and shed soluble MICA (sMICA) as a consequence of the cleavage of cell surface MICA by matrix metalloproteinases.[54–58] The ability of sMICA to serve as a decoy to disrupt NK cell function suggests that neutralization of sMICA could potentiate NK cell function and enhance the immune response to cancer. This concept has been demonstrated using anti-MICA antibodies in preclinical models,[57,153] and it is anticipated that these agents that neutralize sMICA or inhibit the shedding of MICA will move into clinical testing in the future. Activation of β-catenin signaling can contribute to immune exclusion and confer intrinsic resistance by tumors to treatment with checkpoint inhibition,[61,154,155] and has led to the suggestion that inhibitors of β-catenin could be used to reverse this resistance and extend the clinical activity of CPI.[156–158] Given the diversity and potential redundancy of mechanisms by which tumors can suppress the host immune response, it is likely that the dominant mechanism(s) of suppression may differ across distinct tumor types. In addition, the possibility for patient-to-patient variability and intratumoral heterogeneity may complicate future efforts to target and systematically reverse tumor-mediated immune suppression. To achieve clinical success, these approaches may require well-defined biomarker strategies to enable proper patient selection and combination with other immunotherapeutic agents to leverage the full potential of targeting these suppressive mechanisms.

CONCLUSION

Cancer immunotherapy has come of age as a result of the dogged perseverance and sustained commitment and innovation by a relatively small number of groups that navigated the complexity of the immune system and frequent doubts within the broader scientific community to lay the foundation for the field. These efforts set the stage for the incredible advancements that are now occurring broadly across the entire field of oncology, transforming the treatment of many cancers. Nonetheless, despite tremendous progress over the past decade, it remains true that the majority of patients do not respond to cancer immunotherapy, and a limited number of patients are cured. Fortunately, there is an extensive and ever-expanding spectrum of possibilities for mechanism-based therapeutic intervention, and a rapidly expanding toolkit of reagents to target these mechanisms. Sustained progress in the field of cancer immunotherapy will necessitate ongoing broad investment in basic, translational, and clinical science. The execution of rigorous, hypothesis-driven translational medicine and clinical studies will benefit from close collaboration between basic scientists and clinicians, and between industry and academia, as new targets are identified, and novel therapeutics are designed and advanced through clinical development. Armed by rapidly expanding scientific insights, innovative therapeutic tools, improved supportive care, and the evolution of new strategies for clinical development and patient selection, opportunities to expand and refine the use of mechanism-based strategies for cancer immunotherapy should continue for many years to come.

KEY REFERENCES

Only key references appear in the print edition. The full reference list appears in the digital product on Springer Publishing Connect: connect.springerpub.com/content/book/978-0-8261-3743-2/part/part02/chapter/ch21

6. Mok TSK, Wu YL, Kudaba I, et al. Pembrolizumab versus chemotherapy for previously untreated, PD-L1-expressing, locally advanced or metastatic non-small-cell lung cancer (KEYNOTE-042): a randomised, open-label, controlled,

Phase 3 trial. *Lancet*. 2019;393(10183):1819–1830. doi:10.1016/S0140-6736(18)32409-7

19. Wculek SK, Cueto FJ, Mujal AM, et al. Dendritic cells in cancer immunology and immunotherapy. *Nat Rev Immunol*. 2020;20(1):7–24. doi:10.1038/s41577-019-0210-z

33. Rizvi NA, Hellmann MD, Snyder A, et al. Cancer immunology. Mutational landscape determines sensitivity to PD-1 blockade in non-small cell lung cancer. *Science*. 2015;348(6230):124–128. doi:10.1126/science.aaa1348

39. Leach DR, Krummel MF, Allison JP. Enhancement of antitumor immunity by CTLA-4 blockade. *Science*. 1996;271(5256):1734–1736. doi:10.1126/science.271.5256.1734

61. Spranger S, Bao R, Gajewski TF. Melanoma-intrinsic β-catenin signalling prevents anti-tumour immunity. *Nature*. 2015;523(7559):231–235. doi:10.1038/nature14404

62. Nowicki TS, Hu-Lieskovan S, Ribas A. Mechanisms of resistance to PD-1 and PD-L1 blockade. *Cancer J*. 2018;24(1):47–53. doi:10.1097/PPO.0000000000000303

143. Hodi FS, O'Day SJ, Mcdermott DF, et al. Improved survival with ipilimumab in patients with metastatic melanoma. *N Engl J Med*. 2010;363(8):711–723. doi:10.1056/NEJMoa1003466

146. Topalian SL, Hodi FS, Brahmer JR, et al. Safety, activity, and immune correlates of anti-PD-1 antibody in cancer. *N Engl J Med*. 2012;366(26):2443–2454. doi:10.1056/NEJMoa1200690

Manipulating Innate Immune Pathways for Cancer Immunotherapy

Olivier Demaria, Thomas F. Gajewski, and Eric Vivier

KEY POINTS

- The innate immune system plays an essential role in bridging the gap between acute inflammation and adaptive immune responses.

- In the cancer context, both innate lymphoid cells and myeloid cells contribute to immune recognition and the modulation of adaptive immunity.

- A key role for Batf3 dendritic cells (DCs) and type I interferon (IFN) signaling in the generation of spontaneous CD8+ T cell responses against tumor antigens has been suggested.

- Therapeutic strategies for manipulating, boosting, or mimicking innate immune processes have given promising results in preclinical models and have entered clinical testing.

- The TLR7 agonist imiquimod is approved by the U.S. Food and Drug Administration (FDA) for the treatment of basal cell carcinomas and actinic keratosis, and IFN-α has been utilized for the treatment of several types of cancer.

- Stimulator of Interferon Genes (STING) agonists and the adoptive transfer of innate lymphoid populations are currently being tested in clinical trials as cancer therapies.

- Blockade of inhibitory receptors on natural killer (NK) cells or their direct activation with natural killer cell engagers (NKCEs) is opening up new opportunities for therapeutic interventions.

INTRODUCTION

The innate immune system provides the first line of defense against infectious pathogens. Various cell types produce cytokines and other factors following the binding of fixed, nonvariable receptors to pathogen-derived ligands. Innate immune cells also participate in immune homeostasis, and they bridge the gap to the generation of an adaptive immune response against specific antigens. In the context of cancer, evidence of spontaneous CD8+ T cell priming against tumor-associated antigens in a subset of cancers has generated renewed interest in the innate immune pathways potentially involved in this process. The manipulation of endogenous T cell responses for therapeutic purposes has already yielded impressive clinical results, most notably through the use of blocking antibodies inhibiting cytotoxic T lymphocyte-associated protein 4 (CTLA-4) engagement and programmed cell death 1/programmed cell death ligand 1 (PD-1/PD-L1) interactions. An understanding of the innate immune mechanisms underlying this T cell response is thus of considerable clinical relevance, particularly with a view toward the recruitment of immune responses into non–T cell–inflamed tumors. Defined innate immune interactions in the context of cancer include tumor recognition by innate cell populations (innate lymphoid cells [ILCs], a population comprising natural killer [NK] cells, $\gamma\delta$ T cells, natural killer T [NKT] cells, mucosal-associated invariant T [MAIT] cells), and also by dendritic cells (DCs) and macrophages, in response to damage-associated molecular patterns (DAMPs). Advances in our knowledge of the clinically relevant innate immune pathways involved in tumor recognition are opening up new therapeutic opportunities for cancer treatment. The novel approaches to treatment being developed include the intratumoral application of pharmacological activators of innate immune receptors, treatment with innate cytokines, and the blockade of inhibitory receptors on NK cells or their direct activation with natural killer cell engagers (NKCEs).

Improvements in our understanding of immune regulation within the tumor microenvironment (TME) have led to the identification of new targets for cancer immunotherapy. Following the initial molecular identification of tumor antigens, it was broadly assumed that most cancers were nonimmunogenic, and the main emphasis in immunotherapeutic development was active immunization or adoptive T cell therapy, to increase the frequency of tumor antigen-specific CD8+ T cells.[1] However, analyses of the TME in patient biopsy specimens rapidly made it clear that most tumors display evidence of the spontaneous generation of an antitumor T cell response. This response is revealed by transcriptional profiling, in which a subset of tumors can be observed to display the expression of T cell–specific genes and of a panel of chemokine and interferon (IFN)-induced genes that appear to be coordinately expressed.[2,3] The presence of CD8[+] T cells has been confirmed by immunohisto-chemistry, and analyses of antigen specificity in selected patients have revealed that tumor-associated antigens are recognized by at least a subset of these T cells.[4–6] T cell receptor (TCR) deep sequencing has shown these populations to be oligoclonal, implying antigen specificity.[7–10] In addition, the in vitro expansion of T cell cultures from melanoma metastases has revealed the recognition of mutational neoepitopes in many cases, supporting the idea that a significant proportion of this T cell infiltrate represents an active antitumor immune response.[11] Such immune responses do not appear to be completely effective, as they do not eradicate the tumor, but the presence of an immune infiltrate has been reported to be of positive prognostic value in multiple types of cancers, as exemplified by the pioneering "Immunoscore" work in colorectal cancer.[12] The incomplete nature of tumor elimination appears to result from the coordinate activity of multiple immune regulatory processes limiting the function of tumor-infiltrating T cells.[13] Indeed, tumors may have high levels of Forkhead box protein P3 (Foxp3)[+] regulatory T cells (T_{reg} cells), PD-L1 (the major ligand of inhibitory receptor PD-1 on activated T cells), and indoleamine-2,3-dioxygenase (IDO), the tryptophan-catabolizing enzyme associated with peripheral tolerance.[14] Thus, T cells appear to be spontaneously activated and recruited to the microenvironment of many tumors, where they are subsequently incapacitated by immune regulation.

The targeting of these and other immune regulatory pathways in preclinical models, either alone or in combination, has been shown to mediate potent therapeutic effects in multiple tumor models.[15] The clinical application of these therapies has driven a revolution in cancer therapeutics, with anti-CTLA-4 and anti-PD-1/PD-L1 monoclonal antibodies (mAbs) leading the charge. The antibody-mediated blockade of these pathways has yielded remarkable therapeutic results in multiple human cancers, with U.S. Food and Drug Administration (FDA) approval obtained for squamous cell head and neck cancer, melanoma, Merkel cell carcinoma, cutaneous squamous cell carcinoma, hepatocellular carcinoma, advanced renal cell carcinoma, cervical cancer, small cell lung cancer (SCLC) and non-small cell lung cancer (NSCLC), triple-negative breast cancer, bladder cancer, and Hodgkin lymphoma and any microsatellite instability high/deficient mismatch repair (MSI-H/dMMR)

cancers.[16] Combination immunotherapy may be even more effective, with the first combination regimen of the anti-CTLA-4 mAb ipilimumab plus the anti-PD-1 mAb nivolumab approved for melanoma,[17] NSCLC,[18] and pleural mesothelioma.[19] Studies of predictive biomarkers for these immunotherapies have revealed a greater clinical response in patients who have a T cell–inflamed TME phenotype at baseline,[9,20] and also with a higher mutational load indicative of an increased prevalence of neoantigens.[21] Thus, a working model has emerged in which the blockade of negative regulatory pathways can reactivate dysfunctional T cells within the TME, translating into a restoration of immune-mediated tumor control.

Conversely, a non–T cell–inflamed TME is generally predictive of a lack of clinical efficacy of anti-PD-1 therapy. Thus, understanding the biological basis of the presence or absence of spontaneous immune cell activation and infiltration into the TME is crucial for understanding resistance to immunotherapies. It is thought that converting non-T cell–inflamed tumors into a T cell–inflamed phenotype (or increasing endogenous immune cell infiltration) could potentially expand the fraction of patients responding to immunotherapies that aim to restore T cell function within the TME. Innate immunity provides one key to understanding and influencing this process.

Preclinical model studies have identified many of the key early fundamental steps involved in the spontaneous activation of antitumor CD8[+] T cells in vivo. Most of the available evidence suggests that T cells are initially activated in the tumor-draining lymph node, via the cross-presentation of antigens by host DCs.[22] The dominant subset of DCs mediating this process in mice is that driven by the basic leucine zipper transcription factor cyclic AMP-dependent transcription factor-3 (ATF3)-like 3 (Batf3). These DCs express the CD8α, CD103, and XCR1 surface markers in mice.[23,24] The key role of these DCs in antitumor immunity was demonstrated in Batf3[−/−] mice, which do not reject immunogenic tumors and fail to prime tumor antigen-specific CD8[+] T cells in vivo.[22,25,26] Human DCs do not express CD8α, but gene expression profiling has indicated that the human equivalent of murine Batf3 DCs is a cell population expressing blood DC antigen 3 (BDCA3, also known as CD141).[27,28] This DC subset is referred to as cDC1 thereafter. Like murine Batf3 DCs, human CD141[+] DCs express the transcription factors interferon response factor 8 (IRF8) and Batf3, together with C-type lectin domain family 9 member A (Clec9A, also known as DNGR1), which potentiates the cross-presentation of antigens derived from necrotic cells.[29,30] Recent data have indicated that non-T cell–inflamed human tumors lack the markers of cDC1s,[31] suggesting that the absence of this antigen-presenting cell (APC) subset may be the key to the lack of spontaneous T cell infiltration in patients with this phenotype of tumors.

Additional support for a key role of cDC1s in antitumor immunity was provided by the demonstration that CD103+ DCs in the lung internalize membrane-bound cytoplasmic material released into the lung vasculature by circulating tumor cells.[32] Seventy-two hours after the injection of ovalbumin (OVA)-expressing tumor cells, these CD103+ DCs were detected in mediastinal lymph nodes, clustering together with adoptively transferred OT-I TCR-transgenic T cells. The ability of these CD103+ DCs to activate OT-I cells was confirmed conclusively ex vivo and with bone marrow chimeras.

Thus, one critical population of innate immune cells (cDC1s) appears to be crucial for spontaneous immune priming against cancers. cDC1s play an important role not only in the priming of tumor-specific CD8+ T cells but also in the infiltration of these cells into tumors. The recruitment of tumor-specific T cells to the tumor is driven by two molecules produced by cDC1s: CXCL9 and CXCL10, which engage the chemokine receptor CXCR3.[33] The presence of a cDC1 signature has been identified as a strong prognostic factor in humans and is associated with both better survival[34] and greater responsiveness to anti-PD-1 treatment.[35] The demonstration of the important role of cDC1s raised a number of new questions. These include the identification of the innate immune sensors and signaling pathways mediating DC activation during endogenous antitumor immune responses and the possibility of the direct activation of a

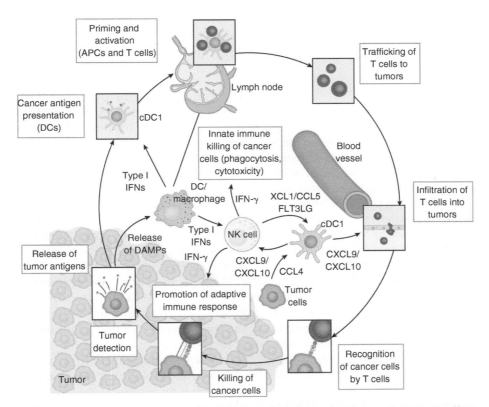

Figure 22.1 **Innate immune cells participate in tumor killing and lead to adaptive antitumor T cell responses.** In the TME, dying tumor cells can express and release DAMPs. Tumor-infiltrating APCs sense DAMPs and produce type I IFNs and other factors. Type I IFNs promote the recruitment and activation of inflammatory cells, including NK cells, at the tumor site. Ligands expressed by transformed cancer cells activate NK cells and induce cytotoxicity and the production of IFN-γ, which promotes innate and adaptive antitumor immune responses. Activated NK cells also produce chemoattractant factors such as XCL1, CCL5, or FLT3LG, promoting the recruitment of cDC1. CCL4 produced by tumor cells also contributes to cDC1 recruitment at the tumor site. After tumor antigen uptake, cDC1 cells migrate to secondary lymphoid organs to cross-present tumor antigens and prime tumor-specific CD8 T cells. In addition, cDC1 cells in the tumor produce CXCL9 and CXCL10, two chemoattractants essential for tumor-specific CD8 T cell infiltration into the tumor and killing activity. CXCL9 and CXCL10 also induce NK cell recruitment, which promotes tumor killing and sustains T cell response.

APCs, antigen-presenting cells; CCL, CC chemokine ligand; CXCL, C-X-C motif chemokine ligand; DAMPs, damage-associated molecular patterns; DCs, dendritic cells; FLT3LG, Fms-related tyrosine kinase 3 ligand; IFNs, interferons; NK, natural killer; TME, tumor microenvironment; XCL1, X-C motif chemokine ligand 1.

particular innate sensing pathway as a therapeutic strategy to "push" de novo T cell responses and immune cell infiltration into the TME. Other innate lymphoid cells, such as NK cells, may also facilitate cDC1 infiltration into tumors, through their production of CCL5, XCL1,[36] and FLT3 ligand.[35] Tumor-site NK cell activation, therefore, can participate in antitumor immunity via direct cytotoxicity and by promoting adaptive responses through IFN-γ secretion and cDC1 regulation. A schematic representation of the contribution of innate immunity in direct antitumor activity and in antitumor T cell responses is provided in Figure 22.1. Preclinical studies, along with correlative assays in cancer patients, have already led to the development of therapeutic strategies aiming to initiate or amplify innate immune pathways to improve immune-mediated tumor control in vivo.

INNATE IMMUNE PATHWAYS MEDIATING HOST ANTIGEN-PRESENTING CELL ACTIVATION IN THE TUMOR CONTEXT

Central Role for Type I Interferons

A clue that innate immune pathways might be activated in the tumor context and correlated with spontaneous T cell priming was provided by gene expression profiling in melanoma metastases. These studies showed that T cell–associated transcripts were associated with the expression of genes known to be induced by type I IFNs.[2,22,37] Like T cell infiltration, a type I IFN gene signature has been shown to be predictive of a favorable clinical response to therapeutic cancer vaccines.[38] Type I IFNs have been reported to act at several levels during the generation of an adaptive T cell response, promoting the cross-priming of antigens by APCs and the migration of these cells to lymph nodes, enhancing the effector functions of cytotoxic T lymphocytes (CTLs), and supporting memory CTL survival.[39] Based on previous studies of antiviral immunity, mouse models were used to investigate whether host type I IFN signaling was important for the spontaneous generation of antitumor T cell responses. In fact, an impairment of immunogenic tumor rejection was observed in vivo in type I IFNR[-/-] mice.[22] Studies in several mouse transplantable tumor models showed that host type I IFN signaling was necessary for the early priming of tumor antigen-specific CD8[+] T cells. Mixed bone marrow chimera and conditional knockout mouse studies revealed that type I IFN signaling was necessary specifically in Baft3-lineage DCs, and IFN-β production by CD11c[+] DCs was detected. Thus, as in most viral infections, host type I IFN signaling appears to be crucial for the induction of an adaptive immune response against tumors. This implication of type I IFNs in the antitumor response prompted deeper investigations of the innate immune-sensing pathways

and ligands potentially acting upstream from the induction of this cytokine by host DCs.

Acute transient type I IFN production appears to provide positive support for antitumor immunity, but other model systems have provided evidence to suggest that chronic or high levels of type I IFN production may contribute to immune suppression. In the chronic lymphocytic choriomeningitis virus (LCMV) model, anti–type I IFNR mAb treatment has been shown to improve immune-mediated viral clearance in vivo.[40] Type I IFN action has also been reported to upregulate the expression of PD-L1 and IDO,[41,42] which inhibit T cell function. High doses of IFN-β can have a therapeutic effect against established murine tumors, mediated by an anti-angiogenic effect with no increase in CD8[+] T cell priming.[43] Thus, the level and duration of type I IFN production and signaling may be a critical determinant of the ability to support adaptive immune responses directed against tumors.

The Stimulator of Interferon Genes Pathway of Cytosolic DNA Sensing

The evaluation of the dominant innate signaling pathways and candidate ligands mediating the induction of IFN-β production by host APCs in response to tumor implantation has been investigated with in vivo mouse models. These studies were enabled by the use of mice with engineered genetic deficiencies of specific innate immune pathway molecules. Based on discoveries made in infection models, the major candidate pathways were the Toll-like receptor (TLR) pathways that signal through MyD88 and/or TIR-domain-containing adapter molecule 1 (TRIF), cytosolic RNA sensing via mitochondrial antiviral-signaling protein (MAVS), and cytosolic DNA sensing via the Stimulator of Interferon Genes (STING) pathway.[44] These candidate pathways are illustrated in Figure 22.2. Interestingly, no apparent impairment of the spontaneous priming of antitumor CD8[+] T cells was observed in mice deficient for TLR pathways or cytosolic RNA sensing. In contrast, a striking decrease was observed in STING[-/-] mice.[45] A similar blunting of IFN-β production by tumor-infiltrating APCs was observed in the absence of host STING, suggesting a possible proximal defect in innate immune recognition of tumors. The STING signaling pathway begins with cyclic GMP-AMP synthase (cGAS), the major cytosolic DNA sensor, which catalyzes the generation of the second messenger cyclic GAMP (cGAMP). This cGAMP binds to STING, inducing the aggregation and intracellular relocalization of this molecule. The downstream TANK-binding kinase 1 (TBK1), which undergoes autophosphorylation on interaction with STING and also phosphorylates the transcription factor IRF3, is then translocated to the nucleus, where it regulates the transcription of various genes, including the IFN-β gene (Figure 22.2). Defective spontaneous T

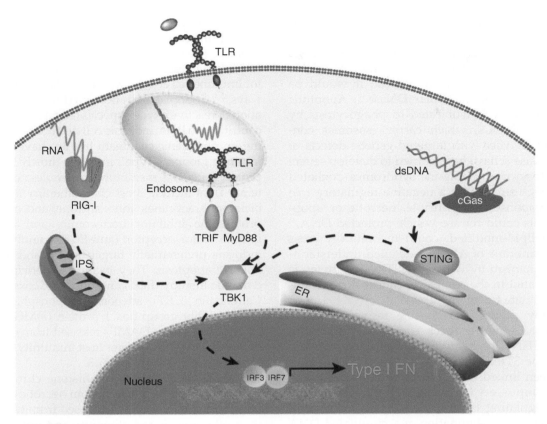

Figure 22.2 Innate immune-sensing pathways that can lead to type I IFN production by APCs. TLRs (e.g., TLR3, TLR7/8) can induce type I IFN gene expression through the adapter molecule TRIF. Cytosolic RNA is recognized via RIG-I, and cytosolic DNA can induce the generation of cyclic dinucleotides by cGAS and initiate a signaling event via the STING protein. The subsequent activation of TBK1 and IRF3 or IRF7 leads to IFN-β transcription.

APC, antigen-presenting cell; cGAS, cyclic GMP-AMP synthase; dsDNA, double-stranded DNA; ER, endoplasmic reticulum; IFN, interferon; IPS, interferon-beta promoter-stimulator; IPS, Interferon-beta promoter-stimulator (aka MAVS); IRF3, interferon regulatory factor 3; RIG-1, retinoic acid–inducible gene I protein; STING, stimulator of interferon genes; TBK1, TANK-binding kinase 1; TLRs, Toll-like receptors; TRIF, TIR-domain-containing adapter inducing interferon-β.

cell priming and IFN-β production in response to tumors were also observed in IRF3$^{-/-}$ mice, and evidence for a functional role for cGAS and TBK1 was obtained from in vitro knockdown studies. In addition, a single-cell analysis of tumor-infiltrating immune cells identified labeled tumor-derived DNA within the cytosol of APCs, placing the known ligand in the expected compartment.[45] These data suggest that the STING pathway activated in host APCs is a major innate immune pathway mediating the sensing of implanted tumors.

The protective role of STING signaling in tumorigenesis has been confirmed in several additional in vivo tumor models. In a model of colitis-associated carcinogenesis induced by azoxymethane/dextran sodium sulfate (AOM/DSS), STING-deficient hosts were found to be more susceptible to both colitis and tumor formation.[46,47] AOM causes DNA damage, triggering STING signaling, which, in turn, induces the production of wound repair-initiating cytokines, such as interleukin-1β (IL-1β)

and IL-18, and suppresses the production of growth-inhibitory IL-22 binding protein. By contrast, the colons of animals with defective STING signaling produced larger amounts of the proinflammatory cytokines IL-6 and keratinocyte chemoattractant (KC), and displayed higher levels of active signal transducer and activator of transcription 3 (STAT3). Persistent STAT3 activation was associated with an amplification of inflammation and the promotion of colon tumorigenesis.

In an inducible model of glioma generated with the Sleeping Beauty transposon system, brain-infiltrating CD11b$^+$ cells in STING-mutant mice were found to produce lower amounts of type I IFNs, and to have weaker immune-mediated tumor control.[48] In transplantable models of melanoma and lymphoma, cryoablation of the tumor was found to activate the STING pathway in CD11c$^+$ cells, leading to the production of type I IFNs and the generation of an adaptive immune response directed against tumor-associated antigens.[49]

The mechanism by which tumor-derived DNA gains access to the cytosol of host APCs is incompletely understood and is currently under investigation. Naked DNA in the extracellular space would presumably be unable to activate the immune system because it would be rapidly degraded by extracellular DNase I. Apoptotic cells would probably be subjected to phagocytosis by macrophages and DCs, which carry lysosomes containing DNase II. Mice with targeted genetic defects of DNase I or DNase II have been shown to develop severe proinflammatory or autoimmune syndromes mediated by type I IFNs,[50] suggesting a negative regulatory role in immune responses. In principle, necrotic or apoptotic tumor cells could release vesicle-protected DNA,[51] which, being lipid-modified, could theoretically cross the plasma membrane of APCs. A detailed understanding of the mechanism by which the STING pathway is naturally activated in the context of cancer might highlight new candidate treatment targets.

As in many aspects of immune responses, there must also be negative feedback events leading to the inhibition of STING pathway activation. Inappropriate activation of the STING pathway and type I IFN generation have been linked to Aicardi–Goutières syndrome and systemic lupus erythematosus.[51-54] Several mechanisms downregulating the STING pathway have been described, such as the elimination of accumulated DNA by DNases[55] and the posttranslational modification of proteins in the signaling pathway after stimulation.[56] Recent studies have also suggested another level of regulation: the simultaneous stimulation of two innate immune pathways by the same ligand, with opposite functional consequences. In particular, cytosolic DNA can activate both the STING pathway and the absent in melanoma 2 (AIM2) inflammasome in APCs. AIM2 senses DNA and forms a heterocomplex between the adaptor protein apoptosis-associated speck-like protein (ASC) and caspase-1. Inflammasome formation leads to the activation of caspase-1, which then generates processed forms of IL-1β and IL-18, and also causes a type of cell death known as pyroptosis.[57] APCs lacking the AIM2 inflammasome display a marked overactivation of the STING pathway,[58] mostly due to reduced caspase-1-dependent induction of cell death. This result indicates that cross-talk between different innate immune pathways can potentially lead to unexpected outcomes, providing new opportunities for the targeting and modulation of immune responses.

Evidence for Innate Immune Pathways During Immunogenic Cell Death

Although the STING pathway appears to be a major innate immune-sensing pathway involved in spontaneous antitumor T cell responses at steady state, there is evidence for the involvement of additional pathways in the response to immunogenic cell death induced by chemotherapy agents.[59] The tumor cell death triggered by chemotherapy is thought to result in the expression or release of DAMPs for immune cell activation via specific innate sensing pathways.[60,61] Endoplasmic reticulum (ER) stress and the generation of reactive oxygen species (ROS) have been shown to contribute to immunogenic cell death. The agents promoting immunogenic cell death in vitro have been classified into two groups.[62] Type I inducers mostly target cytosolic proteins, plasma membrane molecules, or nuclear proteins. They include most chemotherapy agents (doxorubicin, anthracyclines, mitoxantrone, and oxaliplatin), the proteasome inhibitor bortezomib, and anti–epidermal growth factor receptor (anti-EGFR) antibodies. Type II inducers preferentially target the ER and induce immunogenic apoptosis. They include hypericin-based photodynamic therapy (PDT) and oncolytic coxsackie virus B3. Calreticulin (CRT), adenosine triphosphate (ATP), and high-mobility group box 1 protein (HMGB1) have been identified as major DAMPs released from dying cells that can potentially help trigger host immunity.[59] These factors are summarized in Figure 22.3.

HMGB1 is a nuclear nonhistone chromatin-binding protein that can be released from necrotic cells. In mouse tumor models, HMGB1 is released from tumor cells after chemotherapy or radiotherapy, and appears to engage TLR4 on DCs, thereby promoting an antitumor immune response.[61] Polymorphisms of the *TLR4* gene have also been shown to be associated with clinical outcome in breast cancer patients. However, in another study, HMGB1 was found to increase the survival of human malignant mesothelioma cells in vitro, and its blockade with an mAb-suppressed tumor growth in immunodeficient mice.[63] Another report suggested that high levels of HMGB1 were associated with a poor prognosis in human bladder cancer patients.[64] Interactions between the T cell immunoglobulin domain and mucin domain 3 (TIM-3) and HMGB1 have also been reported to inhibit innate immune sensing by tumor-associated DCs.[65] These discrepancies in different experimental systems may be explained by different roles of HMGB1 in different redox states.[66] Fully oxidized HMGB1 is inactive, whereas the reduced form has chemoattractant properties. Thus, the role of released HMGB1 in antitumor immunity is complex but could be positive in some contexts.

Calreticulin (CRT) is resident in the ER lumen.[67] CRT translocation across the membrane has been observed in anthracycline-treated tumor cells and has been implicated in uptake by DCs and the antitumor immune response.[68] Oncolytic virus (coxsackievirus B3) treatment in a human NSCLC model enhances CRT expression, and the intratumoral administration of this virus markedly inhibits tumor growth.[69] CRT expressed at the cell surface appears to interact with CD91 on phagocytic cells, facilitating

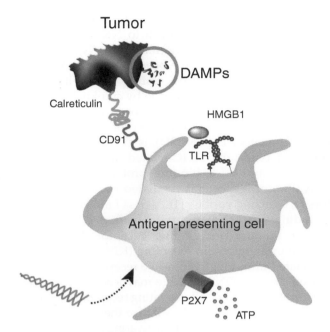

Figure 22.3 Suggested role of DAMPs for innate immune activation in response to tumor cell stress or death. Surface CRT expression on tumor cells facilitates the uptake of these cells through interaction with CD91 on APCs. The increase in tumor antigen uptake presumably enhances cross-presentation to specific T cells. ATP released from dying tumor cells can, in principle, bind to the P2X7R on APCs, leading to the activation of cytoplasmic inflammasome pathways, and the production of IL-1β, which may play a role in the induction of antitumor immune responses. The HMGB1 released from dying tumor cells may bind to TLR4 on APCs, leading to DC maturation, and may contribute to the antitumor T cell response. Tumor-derived nucleic acids can activate TLRs or cytosolic nucleic acid–sensing pathways. The activation of this pathway probably contributes to antitumor immune responses, presumably by inducing the production of type I IFNs.

APCs, antigen-presenting cells; ATP, adenosine triphosphate; CRT, calreticulin; DAMPs, damage-associated molecular patterns; DCs, dendritic cells; HMGB1, high-mobility group box 1 protein; IFN, interferon; IL-1β, interleukin 1β; P2X7R; P2X purinoceptor 7; TLR4, Toll-like receptor 4.

phagocytosis, and potentially delivering tumor-derived antigens. CD91 activation has also been shown to induce the maturation of APCs, which may contribute to immune-mediated tumor control.[70] Surface CRT expression has been reported to be mediated by eIF2α phosphorylation by the protein kinase R (PKR)-like ER kinase (PERK) and caspase 8-dependent proteolysis of the ER-sessile protein BAP31 after chemotherapy.[71] The transient knockdown of CRT pathway components with small interfering RNA (siRNA) approaches before tumor cell–based vaccination decreased therapeutic effects in mouse models in vivo. In human myeloid leukemia patients, the overall survival of patients is higher for

patients with CRT-expressing malignant cells.[72] In colon cancer patients, higher levels of surface CRT expression in tumor tissue have also been reported to be associated with prolonged survival.[73] Thus, surface CRT is probably involved in a mechanism for the host sensing of dying tumor cells.

Chemotherapy agents can also promote the release of ATP from tumor cells in vitro.[74] Extracellular ATP contributes to the recruitment of monocytes, macrophages, and DCs, by binding to P2Y2 purinergic receptors.[75] ATP can also contribute to activation of the nucleotide-binding oligomerization domain, leucine-rich repeat, and pyrin domain-containing 3 (NLRP3) inflammasome, leading to the production of IL-1β and IL-18 by DCs expressing P2X7 receptors.[76] In one model, tumor growth control and CD8+ T cell priming were shown to be defective in IL-1R−/−, NLRP3−/, or Casp-1−/− mice after oxaliplatin treatment. However, ATP can be hydrolyzed by the ecto-nucleotidases CD39 and CD73.[77,78] A high concentration of ATP is required for the activation of P2X7 receptors (EC_{50} >100 µM), and the adenosine generated by ATP degradation has an immunosuppressive effect. CD73-deficient mice display better tumor growth control in the methylcholanthrene (MCA)-induced cancer system or transgenic adenocarcinoma mouse prostate (TRAMP) model of prostate cancer.[79] Adenosine 2A receptor (A2A)-deficient mice also display better tumor growth control in vivo.[80] These data indicate that extracellular ATP probably plays a complex role in the induction of antitumor immunity, and the positive or negative nature of its net effect may depend on the degree of implication of adenosine in the biological activity of the tumor.

Regardless of whether additional innate immune-sensing pathways play a functional role in natural immune responses directed against tumors in vivo, treatments targeting these pathways directly may deliver an antitumor effect. For example, specific TLR agonists engaging TLR3, TLR7, and TLR9 have all been shown to enhance adaptive immunity to tumors, and are being explored clinically. These advances are discussed in the text that follows, specifically in the section on therapeutic interventions.

INNATE LYMPHOID CELL POPULATIONS

The contributions of innate lymphoid cell populations to immune recognition and control have also been studied. Evidence for NK cell involvement has been obtained for tumors with a T cell–inflamed microenvironment.[81] NKT cells and γδ TCR-expressing T cells also have been studied in this respect.[82,83] Both positive and negative immune regulatory functions have been attributed to these cell populations, but the net effect is often positive, and innate immune cells may contribute to tumor control either directly (via ligand recognition) or indirectly (through DC activation or the production of cytokines supporting effector T cell differentiation). In addition to the well-described NK, NKT, and γδ T cell subsets, the potential role of the more recently defined helper ILCs[84,85] has only recently begun to be investigated. A brief discussion of these cell populations follows, as a background to early therapeutic strategies currently in clinical trials.

Innate Lymphoid Cells

ILCs may be considered to be counterparts of T lymphocytes in innate immunity.[86–88] These cells do not carry adaptive antigen receptors formed through the recombination of genetic elements. In terms of function, ILC1s, ILC2s, and ILC3s share cytokine secretion capacities with CD4$^+$ T helper (Th)1, Th2, and Th17 cells, respectively, whereas NK cells can be seen to correspond to innate counterparts of CD8$^+$ cytotoxic T cells. ILCs act at early stages of the immune response. They react rapidly to the cytokines produced by tissue-resident cells or to other signals emitted by these cells.

The role of NK cells in cancer has been investigated in detail, but the roles of the other ILC subsets remain unclear, with reported functions including both tumor promotion and cancer immune surveillance. There may be several reasons for the gaps in our knowledge of the functions of these cells in cancer. First, an absence of specific markers has impeded the detection of non-NK ILCs in tumors by immunohistochemical or transcriptomic means. It is currently possible to detect these cells reliably only by flow cytometry analysis with staining for a set of nonspecific ILC markers and lineage exclusion. There is, therefore, a need for refined methods for assessments of ILC heterogeneity and investigations of the role of ILC subsets in cancer. Second, the phenotype and function of ILCs seem to depend on their "contexture," the tissues, and microenvironments in which they are found.[89] Third, the interconversion of ILC subsets has been reported, with changes in both phenotype and functions.[90] This plasticity renders the situation much more complex, making it harder to understand the precise role of particular subsets in cancer.

Natural Killer Cells

NK cells can infiltrate the solid-TME, and this infiltration has been associated with favorable prognosis in cancer patients.[91,92] NK cells have been shown to contribute to the control of tumor growth in several tumor models.[93–95] Activated NK cells secrete membrane-disrupting proteins (perforin and granzymes) and IFN-γ, mediating cytotoxicity. They also express TRAIL (TNF-related apoptosis-inducing ligand) and Fas-L, which induce the apoptosis of target cells by binding to TRAIL-RII and the death domain receptor Fas, respectively. The activation of NK cells depends on a delicate balance between activating and inhibitory signals, which determines the susceptibility of the target cell to NK-mediated lysis.[96] Three natural cytotoxicity receptors (NCR) involved in NK cell activation have been identified: NKp46 and NKp30 are expressed by resting NK cells, whereas expression of NKp44 is induced by cytokine stimulation. Additional receptors have also been implicated in NK cell activation. One of these receptors, the natural killer group 2 member D (NKG2D), is expressed by most NK cells and binds the MHC-related antigens (MIC)-A/B molecules and UL16-binding proteins (ULBP1-4). The activation of NK cells is regulated by inhibitory receptors recognizing various HLA-class I molecules (HLA-I), including CD94/NK group 2 member A (NKG2A), leukocyte immunoglobulin-like receptor B1 (LILRB-1), killer immunoglobulin receptors (KIRs), and leukocyte-associated immunoglobulin-like receptor 1 (LAIR-1).[97,98]

Cell stress or DNA damage may lead to an increase in the expression of NK cell-activating receptor ligands on the surface of tumor cells. NK cells are then activated by the binding of these ligands to the activating receptors. The dysregulation of tumor cell proliferation associated with Ras pathway activation has been shown to result in increased levels of retinoic acid early transcript 1 (RAE1) and UL16-binding proteins (ULBP1-3). RAE1 upregulation has also recently been shown to depend on E2F transcription factors, which controls progression through the cell cycle.[99] The DNA-damage response (DDR) induced by replication stress and the development of DNA double-strand breaks in tumor cells also enhances the expression of NKG2D ligands in mice and humans (ULBP1-3 and MICA/B). This occurs via the Rad3-related (ATR)/ATM and checkpoint kinases 1/2 (CHK1/CHK2) and ataxia telangiectasia mutated (ATM) pathways.[100] It has also been shown, in vitro, that various anticancer treatments upregulate the expression of stress-inducible ligands on cancer cells, rendering them susceptible to NK cell-mediated cytolysis. Indeed, human cell lines derived from multiple myelomas display an enhancement of MICA expression following treatment with epigenetic drugs, such as BET (bromodomain and extraterminal motif) inhibitors, increasing the efficiency of NK cell cytotoxicity.[101] In addition, many standard antitumor drugs have been shown to upregulate B7-H6 on tumor cells.[102] This molecule is a ligand of the NK cell-activating receptor NKp30, and its expression identifies the cell as a target for NK cells. Chemotherapy may also lead to a nonlethal type of growth arrest known as senescence, which may alert the innate immune system to the presence of the tumor. For example, the treatment of tumor cells with MEK and CDK4/6 inhibitors in vivo causes these cells to become senescent, selectively triggering the antitumor functions of NK cells.[103] The NK cells interact with the tumor, killing their target cells and secreting cytokines, such as IFN-γ and TNF-α, together with growth factors, such as granulocyte-macrophage colony-stimulating factor (GM-CSF).

Type 1 Innate Lymphoid Cells

ILC1s secrete IFN-γ and TNF-α. They express the Tbet transcription factor, and can be distinguished from NK cells on the basis of their lack of dependence on the Eomes transcription factor. Their functions and plasticity are affected by the cytokines present in the microenvironment of solid tumors. IL-15 drives the expansion of granzyme B- and TRAIL-expressing CD49a[hi] ILC1-like cells in a breast tumor model. CD49a[hi] ILC1-like cells have been shown to display cytolytic activity and to control tumor growth in mice.[104] Cytotoxic ILC1-like cells have been detected in AML patients, with this population being deficient at diagnosis and restored during remission.[105] By contrast, TGF-β can trigger the conversion of NK cells into CD49a[+]CD49b[−]Eomes[int] or CD49a[+]CD49b[+]Eomes[+] ILC1-like cells in a fibrosarcoma model, resulting in a loss of ability to control tumor growth and, even, potentially, the promotion of metastasis.[106] In NK cells, SMAD4 deficiency leads to an upregulation of canonical TGF-β signaling and confers an ILC1-like gene expression signature. In this context, the conversion of NK cells into ILC1-like cells decreases IFN-γ production and increases the levels of regulatory molecules, resulting in weaker metastasis control.[107] The growth of TGF-β rich tumors may, therefore, be facilitated by the conversion of cytotoxic NK cells into noncytotoxic ILC1s.

Type 2 Innate Lymphoid Cells

ILC2s express higher levels of GATA3 than the other ILC subsets, and their development and function are disrupted by the absence of this transcription factor. These cells are a major source of IL-4, IL-5, IL-9, and IL-13, and they respond to IL-25, thymic stromal lymphopoietin (TSLP), and IL-33. The cytokine most frequently implicated in the triggering of ILC2 function in cancers is IL-33, but both TSLP and IL-25 have also been detected in tumors. ILC2s have been reported to have both pro- and antitumor effects. They are present in large numbers in various types of tumors, including acute promyelomonocytic leukemia, breast, gastric, bladder, and prostate cancers, and high levels of these cells have been correlated with high rates of tumor growth and a poor prognosis.[108] The production of IL-4 and IL-13 by ILC2s is thought to be responsible for these protumorigenic functions. These two cytokines are involved in recruiting and activating monocytic myeloid-derived suppressor cells (M-MDSCs), which downregulate the antitumor immune response.[109] The protumorigenic effects of ILC2s may also result from their ability to promote the accumulation and functions of T$_{reg}$ cells[110] and to inhibit the antitumor effects of NK cells.[111] However, ILC2s have also been reported to have antitumor activities, mediated by the production of factors inducing both innate and adaptive immune

responses to tumors. ILC2s can recruit eosinophils to tumor sites by producing IL-5, which can result in a limitation of tumor growth.[112,113] They may also enhance T cell immunity by recruiting cDC1s to tumors, thereby promoting the priming and activation of antitumor CD8[+] T cells.[114] Finally, the direct targeting of ILC2s with anti-PD-1 treatments can also participate in antitumor immunity.[114]

Type 3 Innate Lymphoid Cells

ILC3s are typically activated by IL-1β and IL-23, resulting in the secretion of IL-17, IL-22, and GM-CSF. ILC3s may be natural cytotoxicity receptor (NCR) or NCR[+], as they can express NKp46 and NKp44.[115–117] In humans, only the NCR[+] ILC3 subset produces IL-22, and the production of IL-17 is limited to NCR[−] ILC3s, which are absent from RORC-deficient humans.[118] In mice, the generation and function of ILC3s require the nuclear hormone receptor RORgT.[117,119,120] The role of ILC3s in cancer is, like that of other groups of ILCs, unclear. High levels of NCR[+] ILC3 infiltration are observed in human NSCLC[121] and colorectal cancer.[122] NCR[+] ILC3 numbers are correlated with the presence of tertiary lymphoid structures (TLS), suggesting a possible role in the formation of these protective structures, and their frequency decreases as the disease advances and prognosis worsens.[121,122] IL-12 produced at the tumor bed has been shown to repress growth of subcutaneous B16 mouse melanomas, through the effects of NKp46[+] ILC3 cells. IL-12 recruits NKp46[+] ILC3s to the tumor, and the effects of these cells on the vasculature lead to leukocyte invasion and tumor suppression.[123] ILC3s have also been reported to promote tumor progression. In humans, high levels of IL-23, IL-22, and IL-17A, potentially produced by ILC3s, may promote tumor development and have been associated with poor prognosis.[124–126] A subset of regulatory IL-22-producing NKp46[+] ILCs controlling tumor-infiltrating lymphocyte (TIL) responses has also been implicated in high-grade serous cancer (HGSC), with the presence of these cells associated with a shorter time to relapse.[127] CCR6[+] ILC3s were identified as the major source of IL-22 in an IL-22-driven mouse model of colon cancer induced by *Helicobacter hepaticus*, and were shown to contribute to tumorigenesis.[128] IL-23 seems to promote tumor growth and development by inducing the production of IL-17 by ILC3s.[129] This cytokine was found to stimulate NCR[−] ILC3s, which were identified as the principal source of IL-17, in a mouse model of hepatocellular carcinoma (HCC), thereby promoting CD8[+] T cell inhibition and favoring tumor development.[130] In the 4T1 mouse model of breast cancer, NKp46[−] ILC3s have been shown to be recruited to tumors in a CCL21-dependent manner and to participate in metastatic migration to the lymph nodes.[131]

Natural Killer T Cells

NKT cells recognize the lipid-based antigens presented by CD1d, which is a β2microglobulin (B2M)-associated nonclassical MHC class-I-like molecule.[132] NKT cells have been reported to contribute to the immune recognition of tumors and, in some settings, to tumor control. MCA induces sarcomas more readily in CD1d$^{-/-}$ or Jα18$^{-/-}$ mice, and the rates of lymphomas and sarcomas in p53-heterozygous mice were also higher in mice with these backgrounds.[133,134] NKT cells can be classified into two major functional types. Type I NKT (iNKT) cells express the invariant Vα14Jα18 TCR in mice and Vα24Jα18 in humans. They recognize glycolipid antigens presented by CD1d.[135,136] The best-characterized glycolipid antigen is α-galactosylceramide (α-GalCer), which originated from a marine sponge.[137] Isoglobotrihexosylceramide (iGB3), glycophosphatidylinositol, and phosphatidylcholine have been identified as endogenous antigens.[135,136] Type II NKT cells have more variant TCRs and recognize antigens different from those recognized by iNKT cells. Type II NKT cells are frequently reported to have immunoregulatory functions.[138]

iNKT cells can be activated directly by the recognition of glycolipid antigens presented by CD1d. Exogenous antigens from different bacteria can activate iNKT cells directly, but the tumor-derived ganglioside GD3 and the endogenous antigen iGb3 have been shown to act as ligands for iNKT cells.[135,136] Activated iNKT cells rapidly produce cytokines and acquire cytotoxic activity.[139] Indirect iNKT cell activation has been shown to be mediated by DCs producing IL-12 and expressing CD1d-presented self-antigens.[139] IFN-β also can contribute to iNKT cell activation by upregulating CD1d expression on DCs and macrophages.[140] Activated iNKT cells induce the upregulation of co-stimulatory molecules, such as CD40, CD80, and CD86, on DCs, and this may indirectly promote conventional T cell activation.[141,142]

An immunosuppressive role has been suggested for type II NKT cells. The underlying mechanism seems to involve the production of IL-13 and activation of STAT6 pathways, as shown by studies in mouse tumor models.[143] Thus, NKT cells may have a positive or negative effect on antitumor immunity, and the polarity of the effect may depend on their antigen specificity and differentiation state in specific inflammatory contexts.

γδ T Cells

γδ T cells have been implicated in antitumor immune responses and γδ T cell transcriptomic signatures were associated with good prognosis in cancer patients.[144] Most circulating human γδ T cells express Vγ9Vδ2$^+$ TCRs, whereas a Vδ1 segment is expressed by tissue-resident γδ T cells. γδ T cell–deficient (TCRδ$^{-/-}$) mice display a higher incidence of tumor development in both the MCA-induced sarcoma and DMBA/TPA-induced skin tumor models.[145,146] A potent antitumor activity of Vγ9Vδ2 T cells has been reported in combination with chemotherapy.[147] Vγ9Vδ2 T cells recognize the natural phosphoantigens (PAgs) expressed by tumor cells.[148] The butyrophilin (BTN) surface protein BTN3A1 is expressed on the cells of various types of tumor[149] and plays a key role in the recognition of PAg by Vγ9Vδ2 T cells.[150] BTN3A1 associates with BTN2A1 at the cell surface.[151,152] A dysregulated mevalonate cholesterol biosynthesis pathway may be responsible for pAg production in tumor cells, and these antigens may bind to the intracellular B30.2 domain of BTN3A1. This interaction triggers a change in the conformation of the BTN3A1/BTN2A1 complex,[153,154] enabling it to bind to the Vγ9Vδ2 TCR and inducing γδ T cell activation.[151,152] In addition, Vγ9Vδ2 T cells can be activated by the recognition of stress-induced molecules, such as MICA, MICB, ULBP 1–4, and RAET1, by NKG2D receptors.[155] Activated γδ T cells may produce cytotoxic granules containing perforin and granzymes, and can be cytolytic. They can also produce effector cytokines, such as IFN-γ and TNF-α, together with Fas-L and TRAIL. The expression of CD16 on γδ T cells can also facilitate antibody-dependent cellular cytotoxicity (ADCC). Thus, multiple effector mechanisms exist for the direct killing of tumor cells. Furthermore, stimulated γδ T cells can activate DCs, indirectly supporting the activation of αβ T cells. Interactions with CD8$^+$ T cells or NK cells can regulate the proliferation of γδ T cells in a positive or negative manner, depending on the experimental setting.[156,157]

An immunoregulatory role has also been reported for γδ T cells. Tumor-infiltrating γδ T cells in breast and prostate tumor tissues have been shown to have a suppressive function against conventional T cells.[158] Thus, like CD4$^+$ αβ and NKT cells, γδ T cells may be able to differentiate into cells with a regulatory phenotype. Thus, whether γδ T cells exert a tumor-promoting or immunostimulatory effect in individual cases may depend on the functional phenotype of the cells and the other factors present within the TME.

Mucosal-Associated Invariant T Cells

MAIT cells and their ligands were discovered only recently, and tools for their identification and targeting have, therefore, only recently become available. Immunologists and clinicians have developed a particular interest in MAIT cells, due to their high abundance in humans and their particular specificity for microbial vitamin B antigens presented by the major histocompatibility complex (MHC) class I–like protein MR1. Many key aspects of these cells remain unexplored, but several studies have suggested a possible role for MAIT cells in tumor immunity. In a large study of diverse tumor samples, *KLRB1* (encoding CD161, a MAIT cell-specific surface receptor) was identified as the gene most significantly associated with a good prognosis.[144] The gene encoding the Vα7 of the MAIT cell TCR was among the very small number of TCR Vα region-encoding genes consistently detected in TILs from patients with glioma, melanoma, brain lesions, and kidney tumor lesions.[159]

Despite the role in tumor immunity suggested by these studies, MR1-deficient mice were found to have lower levels of tumor initiation, growth, and experimental lung metastasis, suggesting a possible protumoral effect of MAIT cells through a suppression of NK cell effector functions.[160] Further studies are required to develop a full understanding of the contribution of these cells to tumor immunity.

MR1-restricted T cells can also recognize nonmicrobial antigens presented by MR1.[161] MR1-restricted T cell clones from human PBMCs have been shown to mediate pan-tumor recognition via a mechanism that seems to involve the presentation by MR1 of tumor metabolic derivatives. TCR transfer from these clones to the T cells of patients led to the killing of autologous and nonautologous melanoma cells,[162] identifying MR1 T cells as a potential candidate for use in broadly reactive T cell therapy for cancer.

INFLUENCE OF THE HOST MICROBIOTA

Given the importance of early DC activation and type I IFN production in the activation of T cells against tumor-associated antigens, attention has recently focused on the potential contribution of the commensal microbiota in shaping antitumor immunity. In addition to the ability of gut bacteria to influence mucosal immunity within the intestine,[163,164] the host microbiome can influence APC activation state systemically, in turn, regulating overall adaptive immune responses. The composition of the commensal bacterial flora has been shown to modulate the threshold of activation of APCs, affecting their responsiveness to systemic viral infection.[165] It is thought that peripheral APCs may detect microbial products in a TLR-dependent manner, leading to the production of low levels of type I IFNs. The constant type I IFN autocrine loop may keep these APCs in a tonic state, ready to boost an effective adaptive immune response in the presence of a viral challenge.

Recent evidence suggests that the intestinal microbiota can also modulate the immune response against distant tumors. In a subcutaneous tumor model, commensal bacteria were found to regulate the response to treatment with an immunotherapeutic combination of CpG + anti-IL-10R, or with the alkylating agent oxaliplatin, which has previously been shown to cause immunogenic cell death. The pretreatment of mice with antibiotics, or the use of germ-free mice, resulted in a lower level of myeloid cell infiltration into implanted tumors, as well

as the production of smaller amounts of cytokines by these cells, which was associated with poorer tumor control.[166] Gut microbes have also been reported to regulate the immune-mediated tumor control induced by cyclophosphamide (CTX). This chemotherapy drug causes dysbiosis and the translocation of gram-positive bacteria to lymph nodes, leading to the generation of Th17 cells, which, in turn, contribute to the therapeutic efficacy of the drug. Thus, a deficiency of gut bacteria has a negative impact on the antitumor effect of CTX by impairing the generation of Th17 cells.[167] These results highlight the importance of the intestinal microbiota in regulating the response to chemotherapy by modulating the innate and adaptive immune response.

Recent studies have demonstrated that the intestinal microbiota can also regulate systemic antitumor immune responses in concert with checkpoint blockade immunotherapy. Genetically similar C57BL/6 mice from two different vendors, Jackson (JAX) and Taconic (TAC), with different gut microbiotas,[163,164] were found to have strong and weak spontaneous T cell responses to tumors, respectively. This difference was correlated with the rate of tumor growth in the two cohorts of mice.[168] Cohousing of the mice was sufficient to eliminate the difference in phenotype, and the transfer of fecal material from JAX mice (which had superior antitumor immunity) to TAC mice had a therapeutic effect, increasing tumor antigen-specific T cell frequencies and slowing tumor growth in TAC mice. Sequencing of the gut microbiome of TAC mice, JAX mice, and TAC mice receiving JAX fecal material revealed multiple reproducible differences in bacterial species, with some increasing and others decreasing in abundance, in the mice with superior tumor control. One of the commensal organisms present at higher frequency in mice with superior tumor control was *Bifidobacterium*, which was markedly more abundant in mice with stronger antitumor immune responses. The administration of a cocktail of *Bifidobacterium* strains to tumor-bearing TAC mice improved tumor control in vivo, and acted in synergy with anti-PD-L1 mAb to deliver maximal therapeutic benefit. Mechanistic studies demonstrated that DCs isolated from either JAX mice or *Bifidobacterium*-treated TAC mice were better able to stimulate antigen-specific T cells in vitro. Gene expression profiling of these DCs provided evidence for a modest pre-activation of DCs in the presence of *Bifidobacterium*, consistent with an innate immune mechanism underlying this improvement in immune activation.[168] In a separate study, the tumors of germ-free mice and antibiotic-treated mice were found to be relatively resistant to anti-CTLA-4 treatment in vivo.[169] The oral transfer of *Bacteroides fragilis* or *Bacteroides thetaiotaomicron* restored the therapeutic effects of anti-CTLA-4 treatment, demonstrating that these bacteria were sufficient to account for the greater efficacy. In this model, anti-CTLA-4 treatment may induce subclinical colitis, promoting bacterial translocation and systemic effects on immune activation. Together, these studies demonstrate how different commensal flora compositions can affect the basal state of endogenous innate immune cells, either favoring or impeding antitumor immune responses.

Based on these preclinical observations, bacterial sequencing from stool samples of advanced cancer patients being treated with checkpoint blockade immunotherapy was pursued by several groups and correlated with efficacy.[170–172] Indeed, bacterial sequences were identified that were enriched in responder patients, and distinct bacterial sequences were enriched in nonresponder patients. To determine causality, fecal transplantation into germ-free mice was performed, and efficacy of checkpoint blockade was tested in vivo against implanted mouse tumors. In the majority of cases, fecal transfer from responder patients led to therapeutic efficacy in the corresponding mice, whereas fecal transfer from nonresponder patients led to lack of response in mice. Favorable gut microbiota was associated with augmented innate and adaptive immune responses, indicating a systemic immune-potentiating effect.

Based on these mouse model data supporting a therapeutic effect of fecal transplantation, clinical trials are being pursued in patients who initially fail to respond to anti-PD-1. Typically, fecal material from patients with a major clinical response is collected and prepared for administration into the GI tract of patients who were nonresponders, combined with repeated administration of anti-PD-1. Initial results have been encouraging, with several patients demonstrating clinical response when fecal transplantation was added to anti-PD-1 therapy.[173] Fecal transplantation was also associated with favorable immune changes within the TME. While this approach is still in its infancy, these early data suggest that it may be possible to favorably impact the innate myeloid cell composition and activation state within the TME through the use of gut microbiota manipulations.

THERAPEUTIC INTERVENTIONS BASED ON THE MANIPULATION OF INNATE IMMUNITY

With the increasing use of T cell-modulatory cancer immunotherapy in clinical practice (e.g., with anti-PD-1 Abs), it is becoming clear that only a subset of patients derives clinical benefit from these interventions. Deeper investigations of the mechanisms of treatment failure are pointing to modulators of innate immunity as important candidates for clinical development, with the hope of expanding the proportion of patients benefiting from checkpoint blockade therapy.

Stimulator of Interferon Genes Agonists

Based on the evidence indicating a crucial role for endogenous STING pathway signaling in the generation of spontaneous antitumor T cell responses, pharmacological stimulation of this pathway has been explored for cancer treatment. Serendipitously, an older anticancer compound, 5,6-dimethylxanthenone-4-acetic acid (DMXAA),[174,175] was found to interact directly with mouse STING.[176] In vivo studies were, therefore, performed with DMXAA considered a candidate STING agonist. A single intratumoral injection of DMXAA was sufficient to promote the rejection of B16 melanoma in most of the treated mice, and was associated with a marked increase in the frequency of tumor-specific CD8$^+$ T cells in the spleen and the tumor.[177] This therapeutic effect was completely abolished in STING$^{-/-}$ hosts, suggesting an indirect effect via host immune cells. CD8$^+$ T cells were required for maximal tumor control, but partial antitumor effects were seen with DMXAA even in the absence of T cells, suggesting that innate immunity alone could have a mechanistic effect, perhaps through an anti-angiogenic effect of secreted cytokines. The mice that completely rejected tumors were completely protected against a second challenge, indicating an induction of long-lived immunological memory. In addition, when two tumors were implanted, the injection of DMXAA into one lesion led to distant regression of the other lesion, suggesting a potent induced downstream immune response. Such potent antitumor effects were seen in multiple transplantable tumor models.[177]

These studies with DMXAA confirm the therapeutic potential of STING agonists. However, DMXAA does not interact with human STING because of differences in key amino-acid residues in the drug-binding site.[176] This difference may account for the negative results obtained in a Phase 3 clinical trial of DMXAA in patients with NSCLC.[178] Novel STING agonists interacting with the human molecule have been developed, based on cyclic dinucleotide (CDN) structures and also having other chemical designs. An analysis of the 1000 Genome Project database identified five human STING variants: the wild-type (WT) allele, the reference (REF) allele (R232H), the HAQ allele (R71H, G230A, R293Q), the AQ allele (G230A, R293Q), and the Q allele (R293Q). It would be desirable to develop compounds active against all the known polymorphic variants. The first rationally designed synthetic CDN agonist, ML RR-S2-CDA, has moved through Phase 2 clinical trials. It has enhanced stability, is capable of activating human STING, and displays greater cellular uptake, lower reactogenicity, and greater antitumor efficacy than the natural STING ligands produced by bacteria or host cells (via cGAS). Rp, Rp (R,R) dithio-substituted diastereomer CDNs were found to be resistant to digestion with phosphodiesterase, stimulated high levels of IFN-β production in cultured human cells, and induced more potent antitumor immunity than CDNs without dithio modifications. Affinity for the human STING was increased by developing ML RR-S2 CDA, which contains a noncanonical structure defined by a phosphate bridge with one 2′-5′ and one 3′-5′ mixed phosphodiester linkage (2′, 3′-CDNs). The 2′, 3′ mixed linkage structure confers a higher affinity for STING.[179] ML RR-S2 CDA broadly activated all known human STING alleles in a human embryonic kidney HEK293T cellular STING signaling assay, and induced dose-dependent IFN-β expression in human peripheral blood mononuclear cells (PBMCs) isolated from multiple donors with different STING genotypes, including a donor homozygous for the REF allele, which is known to be refractory to signaling induced by 3′,3′-CDNs produced by bacteria. ML RR-S2 CDA was evaluated in multiple syngeneic mouse tumor models, including B16.F10 melanoma, 4T1 mammary carcinoma, and CT26 colon carcinoma: in each of these models, a potent antitumor immune response and significant tumor regression were observed.[177] Potent abscopal effects and an induction of immunological memory were also observed. The intratumoral injection of STING agonists presumably promotes the induction of specific antitumor T cell responses in a type I IFN-dependent manner, mediating both local tumor rejection and distant antitumor effects, due to the circulation of a subset of the activated T cells.[177,180]

Numerous additional STING agonists are in various phases of development. The compound BMS-986301 was also developed to activate human STING variants in addition to mouse STING. BMS-986301 achieved >90% rejection of tested transplantable tumors while causing low cytotoxicity to CD8+ T cells and less inhibition of their proliferation, compared with ADU-S100 (Society for Immunotherapy of Cancer Annual Meeting 2018 Poster P525). An additional compound was identified (SB11285) that displayed antitumor activity when delivered via the IV, IP, and IT routes (American Association for Cancer Research 2017 Conference on Tumor Immunology and Immunotherapy Poster A25).

Several groups have performed chemical compound screens to identify nonnucleotide STING agonists with systemic antitumor activity.[181,182] Such compounds can be selected for increased cell permeability and also resistance to hydrolysis by ENPP1.[183] One such screen identified several amidobenzimidazole (ABZI)-based compounds. The investigators linked two of these to create a dimeric ligand with even higher STING binding affinity. This compound demonstrated efficacy in the CT-26 colorectal model when administered IV.[184]

Packaging cGAMP in liposomal nanoparticles has demonstrated improved cellular uptake and better tumor control in transplantable and genetically engineered triple-negative breast cancer models as well as the B16.

F10 melanoma model.[185] Another study found that liposomal formulated STING agonist can cause loss of APC viability, so the authors chose to load a STING agonist ex vivo into exosomes instead (designated ExoSTING). ExoSTING induced superior IFN-β production compared to soluble STING agonists, and the responding mice were protected against tumor re-challenge (Society for Immunotherapy of Cancer Annual Meeting 2018 Poster P618).

Modifying bacteria is an alternative strategy for developing novel STING agonists that can be delivered systemically. The SYN-STING method introduces a di-nucleotide cyclase gene into *Esherichia coli* Nissle to generate cyclic-di-AMP in the hypoxic TME. SYN-STING demonstrated robust antitumor responses to transplanted tumors and immunologic memory when re-challenged 40 days after the initial complete response (Society for Immunotherapy of Cancer Annual Meeting 2018 Poster P624). Another bacterial approach utilizes a highly attenuated strain of *Salmonella typhimurium* that localizes to tumor due to auxotrophic consumption of immunosuppressive adenosine and delivers TREX1 RNAi to block degradation of cytosolic DNA (STACT-TREX1). Following IV delivery, these bacteria were found to be 1000-fold enriched in the tumor compared to liver and spleen, and demonstrated CD8-dependent tumor growth inhibition and regression in multiple tumor models (Society for Immunotherapy of Cancer Annual Meeting 2018 Poster P235).

Other novel preclinical strategies activate the STING pathway by targeting regulatory components that indirectly activate STING. For example, ENPP1 inhibitors reduce cGAMP degradation, thus improving STING pathway activation. They can be delivered systemically to increase sensitivity to endogenous STING agonists (Society for Immunotherapy of Cancer Annual Meeting 2018 Poster P410). Blocking endolysosome acidification with bafilomycin A1 (BaFA1) can also support STING signaling by preventing STING degradation. Intratumoral injection of cGAMP and BaFA1 in B16 subcutaneous tumors resulted in improved tumor control compared with cGAMP alone.[186]

Early Clinical Trials With Stimulator of Interferon Genes Agonists

The initial STING agonist to enter clinical development was ADU-S100/MIW815 with first results reported at the Society for Immunotherapy of Cancer meeting in 2018. The study was a Phase 1, single-arm dose-escalation study evaluating ADU-S100/MIW815 as an intratumoral (IT) injection 3 weeks out of four per cycle. The eligibility population included patients with advanced solid tumors, age of 18 years or older, Eastern Cooperative Oncology Group (ECOG) performance status of 0 to 1, and at least two cutaneous or subcutaneous tumor lesions that could be biopsied, with one accessible for injection. Pre- and posttreatment biopsies were obtained from both the injected and non-injected lesions. A total of 41 patients received a dose of ADU-S100/MIW815 with four patients still with ongoing treatment at the time of data lock. All but three (7.3%) patients had one or more prior lines of treatment with 82.9% having had two or more prior treatments and 53.7% having had prior exposure to checkpoint blockade immunotherapy. Melanoma (excluding uveal) was the most common tumor type, making up 19.5% of patients, and the most common adverse events included headache, injection site pain, and pyrexia. No maximum tolerated dose was established, with elevated lipase being the only grade 3 or higher treatment-related adverse event reported in more than one patient ($n = 2$; 4.9%). Best treatment response by Response Evaluation Criteria in Solid Tumors (RECIST) was partial response observed in two patients (parotid gland adenocarcinoma, PD-1 antibody-refractory; Merkel Cell carcinoma, PD-1 antibody-naïve) with four patients continuing on treatment more than 6 months. Translational analysis was described in the context of two patients who had demonstrated clinical benefit. The first was a patient with collecting duct carcinoma continuing on treatment more than 8 months at the 800 µg dose level. In this patient, increases in systemic cytokine levels (i.e., IL-6) were observed consistently following injection, and a more than two-fold increase in gene expression for pre- to posttreatment injected tumor biopsy was observed for IFN-γ, PD-L1, CD8A, and an NK cell gene set. In the non-injected lesion, an increase in CD8+ TIL and PD-L1 stromal staining was also observed. A second vignette included a patient with esophageal cancer treated with 800 µg for three cycles with best response of stable disease. In this patient, increased levels of IFN-β were observed following each injection. Within the injected tumor, biopsy demonstrated more than two-fold increased expression of CD8A and the NK cell gene set as well as an increase in the staining of CD8+ TIL and PD-L1 stromal staining.

Data for a second STING agonist administered IT (MK-1454) were disclosed at the 2018 European Society for Medical Oncology meeting. The study was a Phase 1, multi-arm dose-escalation study evaluating MK-1454 alone (arm 1; IT injection weekly for 9 weeks, then every 3 weeks thereafter) or in combination with pembrolizumab (arm 2; 200 mg IV every 3 weeks). The eligibility population included subjects with advanced solid tumors, an age of 18 years or older, and ECOG 0-1 who had at least two tumor lesions with one accessible for injection. Pre- and posttreatment biopsies were obtained from both of the lesions. Accelerated dose titration was pursued using patient dose cohorts of MK-1454 as monotherapy from 1090 µg, then three patients at 270 µg, followed by modified toxicity probability interval

(MTPI) design including three to six patients through 3,000 µg. In combination with pembrolizumab, accelerated titration was performed for 90 to 270 µg, then MTPI through 2,000 µg. Crossover of patients from monotherapy to combination was allowed after initial progression. Results of the study included 26 patients treated with monotherapy and 25 patients treated in combination (nine patients crossed over and were not included in the 25). Most patients had one or more lines of treatment, though some were treatment naïve, including 19.2% and 40% in arm 1 and arm 2, respectively. The most common tumor types were triple-negative breast cancer and head and neck squamous cancer jointly making up 42.2% in arm 1 and 36.0% in arm 2. The most common adverse events included low-grade pyrexia, injection site pain, chills, and fatigue. No maximum tolerated dose was established, although three dose-limiting toxicities were observed including vomiting at 1,500 µg monotherapy as well as erythema multiforme at 540 µg and injection site pain/tumor necrosis at 1,500 µg in combination. No RECIST responses were observed in monotherapy with best response of stable disease being observed in a patient with leiomyosarcoma treated with 30 µg for 4 months. In combination with anti-PD-1, 24% of patients experienced RECIST response ($n = 6$; 3 HNSCC, 1 TNBC, 2 anaplastic thyroid), with most of these ongoing more than 6 months at the time of data cut-off. Pharmacokinetic analysis demonstrated dose-dependent increase in exposure of MK-1454 with a systemic half-life of 1.5 hours. Peripheral blood cytokine analysis demonstrated approximately two-fold induction of IP-10 at 90 µg and apparent plateau of four- to eight-fold induction between 270 to 1,500 µg. Similarly, a STING-induced 20-gene signature was induced nearly three-fold at 90 µg and showed a possible plateau between approximately six- to 15-fold induction for the 270 to 1,500 µg dose levels.

Intratumoral Application of Other Innate Immune Activators

The TLR pathways were arguably the first innate immune pathways to be pursued as drug targets in clinical practice. The first agent was developed by 3M, by screening for compounds with antiviral properties in vitro. A potent agent was identified and found to activate innate immune pathways that indirectly controlled viral infection. With the further discovery and definition of TLR signaling pathways, this novel agent was found to be a TLR7 agonist. Clinical trials were then pursued and this agent, imiquimod, was tested as a 5% cream for use as a topical treatment for genital warts, gaining FDA approval in 1997. For superficial cancer indications, it was found to be effective for the treatment of actinic keratoses (a precursor lesion to squamous cell carcinoma) and primary basal cell carcinomas

(BCCs).[187,188] In two Phase 3 studies of 364 subjects with BCC, 75% had durable tumor elimination on repeat biopsy at 12 weeks. Durable responses at 2 years were also confirmed in independent studies, leading to FDA approval for this indication in 2004. An analysis of post-treatment biopsy specimens revealed an upregulation of numerous innate immune system transcripts, and increases in CD4[+] and CD8[+] T cell levels, supporting an immunological mechanism.[189] These data established imiquimod as an effective immunotherapy for primary BCC, and it is typically used in cases that are difficult to resect surgically.

The successful development of imiquimod led to the evaluation of other TLR agonists as potential cancer treatments. Initial testing has often been based on systemic administration, but attention is increasingly being focused on intratumoral application. CpG-rich oligodeoxynucleotides (CpG ODN, PF-3512676), as a TLR9 agonist, were injected into 15 subjects with advanced non-Hodgkin lymphoma, who also received low-dose radiotherapy, in a Phase 1/2 clinical study.[190] The treatment was generally well-tolerated and resulted in significant reductions of both treated and distal lesions in several subjects, with 13 of the 15 subjects displaying clinical responses. Intratumoral administration of SD-101 (a TLR9 agonist), in combination with a PD-1 inhibitor, has beneficial effects on the TME and increases type I IFN production and infiltration of CD8[+] T cells into tumors. These effects are correlated with durable tumor responses,[191] with an overall response rate (ORR, $n = 45$) of 71% in metastatic melanoma.[192] Several other TLR ligands are currently under clinical evaluation, including the TRL3/retinoic acid-inducible gene-1 (RIG-I) agonist polyinosinic-polycytidylic acid (poly I:C)-LC (Hiltonol®), the TLR4 agonist glucopyranosyl lipid adjuvant (GLA), and the TLR8 agonist, VTX-2337. A list of the active clinical trials testing intratumoral injections of innate immune agonists appears in Table 22.1.

Multiple clinical trials have also been conducted with oncolytic viruses, which may function, in part, through innate immune activation. Talimogene laherparepvec (T-VEC) is a recombinant engineered herpes simplex virus-1 (HSV-1), a double-stranded DNA virus encoding GM-CSF that, when administered by intratumoral injection, has clinical activity against metastatic melanoma. It received FDA approval in 2015. Interestingly, the STING pathway has been identified as an important innate immune-sensing pathway for the induction of IFN-β in response to HSV-1,[193,194] raising the possibility that T-VEC efficacy may be partly STING-dependent. A Phase 3 trial of T-VEC plus the anti-PD-1 mAb pembrolizumab for melanoma has completed accrual.

Table 22.1 Innate Immune System Agonists Currently Tested in Clinical Trials Involving Intratumoral Delivery

TARGET	DRUG	DEVELOPER	CLINICAL TRIAL ACTIVE PHASE IN ONCOLOGY	CLINICAL TRIALS.GOV LOCATOR REFERENCE
TLR3	BO-112	Highlight Therapeutics	2	NCT04570332
	Poly-ICLC	Oncovir	1/2	NCT01976585
TLR7	NKTR-262	Nektar Therapeutics	1,2	NCT03435640
	LHC165	Novartis	1	NCT03301896
TLR9	IMO-2125 / Tilsotolimod	Idera Pharmaceuticals	3 2	NCT03445533 NCT03865082
	SD-101	Dynavax	1 1 1/2 2	NCT03410901 NCT04050085 NCT02927964 NCT03007732
	CMP-001	Checkmate Pharmaceuticals	1 1 1 1/2 1/2 2 2 2 2/3	NCT03507699 NCT03084640 NCT02680184 NCT04387071 NCT03983668 NCT04633278 NCT04698187 NCT03618641 NCT04695977
	AST-008	Exicure	1,2	NCT03684785
STING	MIW815 / ADU-S100	Aduro Biotech, Novartis	1 1 2	NCT03172936 NCT02675439 NCT03937141
	MK-1454	Merck	1 2	NCT03010176 NCT04220866
	E7766	Eisai	1	NCT04144140
TLR4	G100	Immune Design	2	NCT02406781
TLR8	VTX-2337/ Motolimod	Celgene, VentiRx Pharmaceuticals	Early phase 1 1	NCT04272333 NCT03906526
RIG-I	MK-4621/ RGT100	Merck, Rigontec	1	NCT03739138
	CV8102	CureVac	1	NCT03291002
NLRP3	BMS-986299	BMS, IFM Therapeutics	Early phase 1	NCT04541108

NLRP3, NOD-like receptor family, pyrin domain-containing 3; RIG-I, retinoic acid-inducible gene I; STING, Stimulator of Interferon Genes; TLR, Toll-like receptor.

Manipulation of Innate Lymphoid Cells

Not only can ILCs interfere with T cell activity, but they also have antitumor effector functions that, like those of T cells, can be manipulated through the targeting of activating receptors or the blockade of inhibitory pathways.

Fc Receptors

Fc receptors (FcRs) are receptors with specificity for the Fc fragments of different antibody types. The binding of antitumor antibodies to FcRs provides most myeloid cells and some ILCs with genuine antigen-specific receptors able to mediate tumor recognition. Therapeutic antibodies directed against tumor antigens can, therefore, destroy cancer cells by making use of cytotoxic (for example, NK cells) and/or phagocytic (for example, macrophages) cells expressing immunoreceptor tyrosine-based activation motif (ITAM)-containing activating FcRs.

Most of the existing therapeutic antibodies targeting tumors are human IgG1 antibodies binding FcRs for IgG (FcγRs). Activating FcγRs include FcγRIIA (CD32A) and FcγRIIC (CD32C), which are single-chain receptors, and FcγRIIIA (CD16A) and FcγRI (CD64), which have multiple chains. The tissue distributions and biological effects of these FcγRs differ. FcγRIIAs are present on monocytes, macrophages, mast cells, platelets, and polymorphonuclear cells. By contrast, FcγRIICs are found in the NK cells of 20% of the human population. FcγRIIIAs are expressed by monocytes, macrophages, DCs, and NK cells, and FcγRIs are present on DCs, monocytes, and macrophages. The expressing cell types, FcγRs, and underlying mechanisms of action differ between antibodies. The anti-CD20 mAb rituximab, used to treat chronic B-lymphocyte leukemia and non-Hodgkin lymphoma, provides a historical example. It destroys malignant B lymphocytes through binding to the ITAM-containing FcγRs on monocytes and macrophages.[195] A new generation of therapeutic mAbs has been engineered, with improved selective binding to activating FcγRs of various types.[196–198] A prospective clinical study is currently underway to assess the impact of FcγRs on the therapeutic efficacy of antibodies. This trial is comparing margetuximab, an Fc-engineered anti-HER2 antibody, with trastuzumab (Herceptin; NCT02492711 Phase 3 SOPHIA clinical trial). Immune responses are influenced by FcγR polymorphisms, and the Fc moiety of margetuximab has been engineered to increase its affinity for the activating CD16A and decrease its affinity for the inhibitory CD32B. The preliminary results of this trial indicate that progression-free survival (PFS) is longer in patients with pretreated HER2-positive metastatic breast cancer treated with margetuximab than in those treated with trastuzumab. They also suggest that it might be possible to manipulate ADCC or ADCP mechanisms in solid tumors, as it is already the case in hematological malignancies.

Antitumor antibodies are elicited by both experimental tumors in mice and spontaneous tumors in humans.[199–201] These antibodies may protect against cancer, like passively administered therapeutic antibodies. However, they may also promote tumor growth. Protection is probably primarily due to the engagement of activating FcRs on innate cells, but most myeloid cells also express activating and inhibitory FcγRs. FcγRIIBs (CD32B) are inhibitory and have the same specificity for human IgG1 and IgG3 as FcγRIIA and FcγRIIIA, respectively. They are single-chain receptors with an ITIM, but no ITAM. The co-engagement, on the same cell, of ITIM-containing and ITAM-containing receptors inhibits cell activation.[202] The tissue distributions of FcγRIIBs and FcγRIIAs are similar, with FcγRIIBs being thought to attenuate the FcγRIIA-mediated protection induced by antitumor antibodies. FcγRIIBs may also be involved in the enhancement of experimental tumor growth induced by antibodies.[203]

FcγRIIB seems to act as an immune checkpoint in tumor immunity.[204] Anti-FcγRIIB antibodies prevent IgG antibodies from interacting with FcγRIIB, but not FcγRIIA; they should, therefore, increase the protection afforded by antitumor antibodies.[205] Indeed, they have been shown to abolish the inhibitory effects of FcγRIIB in several cell types. These antibodies may constitute a new class of immune checkpoint inhibitors (ICIs) with the potential to increase the efficacy of both endogenous antitumor antibodies involved in immunosurveillance and exogenous antitumor antibodies used in cancer immunotherapy.

Broad-Spectrum Immune Checkpoint Inhibitors

Broad-spectrum ICIs can be used to target NK cells and/or myeloid cells in addition to T cells. These innovative treatments are based on a rationale of releasing the multiple brakes on T cells and harnessing the beneficial effects of unleashing innate immunity and T cell functions.

NK cells and T cells expressed the inhibitory receptor NKG2A, which recognizes HLA-E. Unlike classical MHC class I molecules, HLA-E expression is normal or abnormally strong in tumors. Monalizumab is an IgG4-blocking mAb directed against NKG2A. In concert with anti-PD-1 antibody, it promotes effector T cell responses and enhances NK cell effector functions and ADCC. This antibody is the prime example of an ICI capable of unleashing both NK and T cell responses.[206] The CD8+ T cell responses induced by a peptide-based cancer vaccine are enhanced by antibody-mediated NKG2A blockade in a mouse model of HPV16-induced carcinoma.[207] The clinical potential of monalizumab is currently being assessed in several studies, focusing particularly on its use with durvalumab, an anti-PD-L1 antibody, in solid-tumor treatment, and with the anti-EGFR antibody cetuximab for the treatment of head and neck cancers. Signs of efficacy against head and neck cancers were detected in a Phase 2 clinical trial reporting an ORR of 31%, well above the value of 13% reported in a previous study for cetuximab alone.[206]

TIGIT (T cell immunoglobulin and ITIM domain) is an inhibitory receptor expressed on NK cells and T cell subsets.[208,209] It interacts with CD155 (PVR) and CD112 (PVRL2, nectin-2) on APCs, T cells, and various nonhematopoietic cells, including tumor cells and downregulating antitumor responses. Tumor growth is significantly slower in TIGIT-deficient mice than in wild-type mice.[208] Building on preclinical data demonstrating antitumor treatment by the blockade of TIGIT and PD-L1 to be effective,[210] these two molecules were blocked in CD8+ T cells from melanoma patients, resulting in additive improvements in cell proliferation, cytokine production, and degranulation.[211,212] MK-7684, an anti-TIGIT antibody, has been evaluated in a Phase 1 trial (NCT02964013), both as a monotherapy and in combination with anti-PD-1, for the treatment of 68 patients with advanced solid tumors and treatment failure on standard regimens. The preliminary data revealed clinical responses, with a manageable safety profile, but it is still too soon for any firm conclusions to be drawn.

TIM-3 (T cell immunoglobulin and mucin-domain containing-3) is an inhibitory receptor expressed on various immune cells, including T cells, NK cells, NKT cells, DCs, and macrophages. It recognizes several ligands: galectin-9, HMGB1, carcinoembryonic antigen cell adhesion molecule 1 (CEACAM1), and phosphatidylserine on the surface of apoptotic cells. It regulates T cell and NK cell functions, and is associated with the exhaustion of these cells and with the immunosuppressive capacity of T_{reg} cells and tumor-associated macrophages.[213] TIM-3 also inhibits the sensing of tumor nucleic acids, thereby preventing detection of the tumor by DCs.[65] TIM-3 thus inhibits antitumor immune responses and promotes tumor tolerance. The targeting of TIM-3 with mAbs has been shown to be effective in preclinical models of several types of tumor.[214] Preliminary data from studies evaluating TIM-3-targeting antibodies in solid tumors (TSR-022 Phase I NCT02817633 and MBG453 Phase I-Ib/2 NCT02608268) show the safety profile to be manageable, as for other checkpoint inhibitors, and have revealed early signs of activity (even after treatment with PD-1 or PD-L1 inhibitors). However, further studies are required to determine the mechanisms of action of the molecules targeting this pathway.

The inhibitory receptor lymphocyte activation gene-3 (LAG-3) was first described as a suppressor of T cell activation and cytokine secretion.[215] It inhibits cellular functions after the recognition of several molecules produced by cancer cells present in the TME: MHC-II,[216] galectin-3,[217] LSECtin,[218] and fibrinogen-like protein 1 (FGL1).[219] LAG-3 is present on CD4+ T cells, including T_{reg} cells, and on CD8+ TILs. However, it is also expressed on B cells, NK cells, NKT cells, and plasmacytoid DCs, and it has been shown to downregulate the functions of these cells. Clinical studies have identified LAG-3 as a promising new checkpoint. Indeed, several molecules targeting the LAG-3 pathway have been developed. These molecules, including blocking anti-LAG-3 antibodies (relatlimab) and soluble LAG-3–Ig fusion proteins, showed some activity in early-stage clinical trials, when administered as a monotherapy or in combination (NCT02720068; NCT01968109). A randomized Phase 2/3 study comparing a combination of relatlimab and nivolumab to nivolumab alone is currently being performed in patients with previously untreated metastatic or unresectable melanoma (NCT03470922).

Administration of Innate Cytokines

The key role of innate immunity in promoting T cell effector functions has led to multiple attempts to manipulate innate immune cells in cancer. Few of these approaches have yet been clinically validated, but interesting preclinical results have been reported for the induction of APC proliferation and maturation and for NK cell activation with cytokines, such as FLT3L (Fms-like tyrosine kinase 3 ligand), GM-CSF, type I IFNs, IL-2, and IL-15.

FLT3L promotes the commitment of hematopoietic progenitors to the DC lineage and enhances DC survival and proliferation. Its injection in mice enhances the expansion of cross-presenting DC populations and responses to intratumoral TLR3 agonists. These effects are mediated by increases in the number of tumor-infiltrating antigen-specific CD8+ T cells and the CD8+ T cell-to-T_{reg} cell ratio in the tumor.[220] The combination of an intratumoral vaccine consisting of FLT3L and a TLR3 agonist with local radiotherapy has been shown to promote tumor-specific CD8+ T cell priming, induce abscopal effects, and increase the efficacy of checkpoint blockade, by increasing the number and activation of cross-presenting DCs at the tumor site.[221]

GM-CSF also plays a key role in DC recruitment and differentiation. It enhances tumor antigen presentation through the recruitment of NK cells and myeloid cells, such as DCs. GM-CSF injection into the tumor site stimulates immunity, generating durable responses in mice.[222,223] The injection of recombinant GM-CSF into melanoma tumors in patients increases the number of tumor-infiltrating DCs.[224] Tests are currently being performed to assess the value of GM-CSF for use in various cancer vaccine approaches, in association with tumor peptide vaccines or in vaccine platform formulations, such as GVAX (in which irradiated, allogeneic cancer cells are modified to express GM-CSF) and T-VEC (talimogene laherparepvec, an engineered oncolytic virus, in this case harboring the GM-CSF gene). Intratumoral T-VEC has been shown to outperform subcutaneous GM-CSF in cases of advanced melanoma.[225] T-VEC has obtained FDA approval for use in the local treatment of unresectable melanoma recurring after initial surgery. Effective T-VEC treatment leads to an increase in the number of tumor-specific T cells in regressing metastases and a decrease in the number of T_{reg} cells in treated lesions, consistent with systemic antitumor immunity.[225] A Phase 1b study assessing a combination of T-VEC with approved ICIs showed such combinations to be potentially more effective than each of the treatments used independently.[226,227] A Phase 3 study has completed accrual, with a combination of T-VEC and pembrolizumab.

Type I IFNs have pleiotropic effects on innate immune cells. In addition to promoting tumor-specific CD8⁺ T cells[22,26,228] by enhancing APC cross-presentation and presentation of antigens from dead cells,[39] as described earlier, type I IFNs also modulate the activity of NK cells and the attraction of these cells to tumor sites, by inducing the production of CXCL9 and CXCL10.[229] Mice lacking IFNAR1, IFN-β, or downstream components of the type I IFN pathway present impairments of tumor surveillance by NK cells and poor NK cell cytotoxicity.[230] IFNa2a and IFNa2b have been used, either in their unmodified recombinant form or as PEGylated variants, in the treatment of various types of cancer. However, they are no longer widely used for these indications due to their toxicity and controversy surrounding their overall benefits in terms of survival. Type I IFN-based immunocytokines (mAb–cytokine fusion proteins) have been generated as a way of delivering type I IFNs to the tumor site, and the results of preclinical trials with these drugs are promising.[231–233] However, given the widespread expression of type I IFN receptors throughout the body, engineered type I IFN molecules may rapidly become undetectable in the bloodstream before ever reaching their targets. The delivery of low-affinity type I IFNs, developed to overcome this problem, to cross-presenting DCs by an immunoconjugate targeting CLEC9A leads to antitumor activity without toxicity.[234]

IL-2 induces T cell proliferation and activation, ultimately leading to the generation of effector and memory T cells. It also stimulates other cells, such as ILC2s and NK cells.[235,236] IL-2 binds to CD25 with low affinity, the CD122–CD132 complex of resting NK cells and CD8⁺ T cells with moderate affinity, and the CD25–CD122–CD132 complex on activated lymphocytes with high affinity. T_{reg} cells are very sensitive to IL-2, as they bear the high-affinity CD25–CD122–CD132 receptor. Recombinant IL-2 treatment induces a marked regression of established metastases in mouse models. By contrast, its efficacy in humans is limited to a small proportion of patients with advanced melanoma or renal cell cancer,

probably due to expansion of the T_{reg} cell population in nonresponders.[237,238] IL-2 has a short half-life, another matter of concern because it necessitates the use of high doses, potentially causing high levels of toxicity due to cytokine outburst and capillary leak syndrome. New forms of IL-2 are being engineered to circumvent these problems, and methods based on fusion proteins, immunoconjugates, and PEGylation are being considered as ways of extending the half-life of this molecule and preventing T_{reg} cell activation by limiting binding to CD25. One PEGylated form of IL-2, NKTR-214, was found to be effective against metastatic melanoma and urothelial carcinoma when combined with PD-1 blockade for first-line treatment.[239] Phase 3 randomized studies of NKTR-214 plus nivolumab are currently underway in patients with previously untreated advanced renal cell carcinoma (NCT03729245)[240] and patients with previously untreated, unresectable, or metastatic melanoma (NCT03635983).[241]

IL-15 signaling occurs via the heterodimeric CD122–CD132 receptor. Like IL-2, it promotes the activation and expansion of CD8⁺ T cells, NK cells, gδ T cells, and NKT cells. IL-15Ra⁺ hematopoietic or nonhematopoietic cells must *trans*-present IL-15 to CD122–CD132-expressing cells for full potency. IL-15 treatment promotes the proliferation and survival of T cells and NK cells, together with the generation of cytotoxic lymphocytes.[242] IL-15 has been shown to have a more favorable toxicity profile than IL-2, with robust antitumor activity in preclinical studies in mice. Both IL-15 and IL-2 enhance immunity, but IL-15 does not interact with CD25 or stimulate T_{reg} cell expansion. It, therefore, has no immunosuppressive activity and does not cause capillary leak syndrome. The stronger biological activity of *trans*-presented IL-15 has led to the development of methods for achieving super-agonist effects by mimicking *trans*-presentation in vivo.

Next-Generation Immunotherapies Targeting Innate Immunity

By extension of engineered chimeric antigen receptor (CAR) T cell strategies that have reached FDA approval based on efficacy against B cell malignancies, CARs are also being introduced into innate immune cell populations for therapeutic testing. Briefly, CARs are generated by fusing a mAb fragment recognizing a tumor antigen with T cell receptor (TCR) modules capable of transducing activation signals in T cells. Several studies of non-T cells carrying CARs are currently underway. In particular, clinical trials of infusions of off-the-shelf cord-blood-derived CAR-NK cells for the treatment of several types of leukemia have been launched, based on the absence of graft-versus-host disease observed after the injection of allogeneic NK cells.[243,244] CAR-NK cells have been generated from induced pluripotent stem cells, and these cells have levels of antitumor activity at least as high as those of CAR T cells, but with lower toxicity, in preclinical models.[245] Finally, CAR-macrophages are also being produced and tested. The underlying rationale here is that, as monocytes and macrophages are actively recruited to solid tumors, engineered CAR-macrophages could be polarized toward an antitumor phenotype (M1), which would enhance the activation and recruitment of other immune cells, including T cells, to the TME.[246]

Another potential tool for immune system manipulation in cancer patients is multifunctional molecules generated by assembling various mAb components. Bispecific T cell engagers (BiTEs) acting via the antigen receptor complex, BiKEs (bispecific killer cell engagers), which engage CD16, and TriKEs (trispecific killer cell engagers), which contain IL-15 and engage CD16, have been developed as a way of targeting solid-tumor antigens, such as EpCAM and CD133.[247] BiKEs and TriKEs are highly effective both in vitro and in preclinical models. The recently developed trifunctional natural killer cell engagers (NKCEs), which engage NKp46 and CD16 on NK cells, together with a tumor antigen, have stronger antitumor activity in preclinical situations than approved mAbs, such as rituximab, obinutuzumab, and cetuximab.[248] NK cells infiltrating solid tumors display a downregulation of activating receptors, such as CD16 and most NCRs. Conversely, NKp46 is strongly expressed on many solid tumors, and the engagement of this receptor could be used to promote NK cell function against these tumors. Multifunctional CD16-NKp46 engaging antibodies may thus present the advantage of activating tumor-infiltrating NK cells with low levels of CD16 expression.[249] These findings support the clinical development of NKCEs as a complementary approach for cancer immunotherapy.

Decreases in inhibitory signals for NK cells, in the form of HLA-class I downregulation and the loss of b2-microglobulin expression, may underlie the development of resistance to T cell-mediated lysis after treatment with ICIs.[250] Tumors presenting these features would be good targets for therapies involving NK cell engagement.

Sialylation is one of the most widely observed glycosylation changes in tumor cells and is associated with a poor clinical outcome in several types of cancer.[251] Siglecs (sialic acid–binding immunoglobulin-like lectins) bind sialic acids in a specific manner. There are 16 known members of the Siglec family, 10 of which generate inhibitory signals and carry intracellular ITIM motifs. Based on both the distribution of Siglecs (principally expressed on

immune cells) and their inhibitory signaling functions, a role for sialylation in immune escape has been suggested. Siglec targeting in cancer patients might, therefore, inhibit the changes in glycosylation that promote tumor growth. Siglec-15 is upregulated in tumor-infiltrating myeloid cells and macrophages. It strongly inhibits the antitumor effects of T cells, by creating an immunosuppressive environment.[252] This suppression is abolished by mAb-mediated Siglec-15 blockade, which enhances antitumor responses.[252] Siglec-7 and Siglec-9 are also potential targets of particular interest, given their inhibitory function and the diversity of cells on which they are expressed, including myeloid cells and cytotoxic lymphocytes such as NK cells and T cells in cancer patients.[253–255]

CONCLUSION

New immunotherapy approaches for the treatment of cancer are making significant inroads in the clinic and are transforming patient care. Along with interventions modulating adaptive T cell responses to tumor-specific antigens, improvements in our understanding of innate immune pathways and their interface with adaptive immunity are opening up new opportunities for therapeutic interventions.

KEY REFERENCES

Only key references appear in the print edition. The full reference list appears in the digital product on Springer Publishing Connect: connect.springerpub.com/content/book/978-0-8261-3743-2/part/part02/chapter/ch22

25. Hildner K, Edelson BT, Purtha WE, et al. Batf3 deficiency reveals a critical role for CD8alpha+ dendritic cells in cytotoxic T cell immunity. *Science*. 2008;322(5904):1097–1100. doi:10.1126/science.1164206
36. Bottcher JP, Bonavita E, Chakravarty P, et al. NK cells stimulate recruitment of cDC1 into the tumor microenvironment promoting cancer immune control. *Cell*. 2018;172(5):1022–1037. doi:10.1016/j.cell.2018.01.004
45. Woo SR, Fuertes MB, Corrales L, et al. STING-dependent cytosolic DNA sensing mediates innate immune recognition of immunogenic tumors. *Immunity*. 2014;41(5):830–842. doi:10.1016/j.immuni.2014.10.017
204. Clynes RA, Towers TL, Presta LG, Ravetch JV. Inhibitory Fc receptors modulate in vivo cytotoxicity against tumor targets. *Nat Med*. 2000;6(4):443–446. doi:10.1038/74704
228. Dunn GP, Bruce AT, Sheehan KC, et al. A critical function for type I interferons in cancer immunoediting. *Nat Immunol*. 2005;6(7):722–729. doi:10.1038/ni1213
248. Gauthier L, Morel A, Anceriz N, et al. Multifunctional natural killer cell engagers targeting NKp46 trigger protective tumor immunity. *Cell*. 2019;177(7):1701–1713. doi:10.1016/j.cell.2019.04.041

Cancer Vaccines: Considerations of Antigen, Formulation, and Delivery

Alena Donda, Mathias Wenes, Margaux Saillard, and Pedro Romero

KEY POINTS

- Neoantigen-based vaccines using either synthetic peptides or mRNAs have been successfully tested in cancer patients.
- T cell memory formation following antigen priming may be modulated by pharmacological intervention.
- Biomaterials and nanoparticles provide promising platforms for efficient delivery of subunit vaccine components.

INTRODUCTION

The development of therapeutic cancer vaccines is an essential goal in oncology, both for medical and economic aspects. First, subunit vaccines can be developed at reasonable costs and applied to all patients, in contrast to adoptive cell therapies, which involve expensive individualized procedures. Second, the development of cancer vaccine formulations able to break T cell tolerance, promote robust memory T cell development and favor the homing of the antigen to the draining lymph nodes would be essential to allow long-term tumor control and prevent tumor recurrence.

After our contribution to the first edition dedicated to *Cancer Immunotherapy Principles and Practice* (doi:10.1891/9781617052736), we will focus in this second edition on the following topics:

1. The state of the art in neoantigen-based cancer vaccines
2. Promoting memory T cell development during therapeutic cancer vaccination
3. Novel delivery vehicles to promote antigen uptake by pro-inflammatory dendritic cell (DC) populations

TUMOR NEOANTIGEN-BASED CANCER VACCINES

The clinical success of therapeutic cancer vaccines involving different formulations of tumor-associated antigens (TAA) has remained poor, mainly due to the mechanisms of central and peripheral tolerance, which tolerize T cells against self-antigens.[1] In this context, tumor neoantigens resulting from various genetic modifications that occur during tumor progression may offer new antigen candidates that will efficiently prime naïve T cells. On the one hand, these neoantigens will be seen as foreign by the immune system, which may result in much stronger T cell responses and T cell memory development. On the other hand, these mutated antigens would prevent target toxicities that are sometimes seen when using self-antigens.[2]

Large-Scale Integrative Genomic and Epigenomic Studies

The increasing power of computational tools has allowed systematic whole genome sequencing (WGS) and whole exome sequencing (WES) of large cohorts of cancer patients. Due to well-known environmental carcinogens, such as smoke and ultraviolet (UV) light, melanoma and lung tumors have been characterized by a high tumor mutational burden (TMB), which made them good candidates to profit from immune checkpoint blockade (ICB) immunotherapy,[3,4] as well as from neoantigen-based vaccines.[5] However, more recent WGS and WES studies of other types of cancers have revealed that even cancers so far known to have a low TMB and poor T cell infiltration, such as prostate, head and neck, and ovarian cancers, may also develop a collection of defined neoantigens susceptible to generate T cell responses.[6–8] Moreover, recent genomic studies in prostate cancer patients have shown that ethnic-specific genetic predispositions and/or different environmental carcinogens may increase the complexity of TMB, as shown by qualitatively different TMB in tumor samples from Asian and Western populations.[9]

From Tumor Mutational Burden Data to In Silico Epitope Prediction

Neoantigens may arise from multiple genetic and epigenetic mechanisms, such as missense somatic mutations, gene deletion/insertion, frameshifts,[7,10] alternative splicing,[11,12] or gene fusion caused by genomic rearrangements.[8] Moreover, several posttranslational modifications, such as protein methylation, acetylation, and phosphorylation, can be altered during tumor progression, which can also result in the appearance of tumor-specific neoantigens.[13,14] Despite all these mechanisms that are able to create tumor neoantigens, only a few epitopes will be of immunological significance, and despite powerful computational tools, there is still no clear strategy as to how to select and validate these relevant epitopes.

Briefly, the digestion of tumor cell debris within the immunoproteasome of pro-inflammatory DCs will deliver only a minority of epitopes able to bind to the major histocompatibility complex (MHC) I or MHC II presenting molecules, and even fewer will be recognized by a specific TCR in the patient. In the text that follows, we describe two strategies used to identify tumor neoantigens.

Computational Epitope Prediction From Whole Exome Sequencing/Whole Genome Sequencing and Their In Vitro Experimental Validation

A large number of computational tools have been developed to search for neoantigens, such as algorithms and artificial intelligence networks, which can scan mutation-containing DNA, RNA, and protein sequencing and predict peptides with MHC I or MHC II binding activity based on biochemical and biophysical properties. Several steps are required, which include checking the quality of the DNA sequences and their alignment with the reference sequence. RNA-Seq data from the same tumor sample are also very precious for confirming the potential mutations and exclude, as much as possible, false positives. An extensive review of these computational tools has been recently published by Roudko et al. in early 2020.[15] Although the approach described earlier can efficiently identify a myriad of potential tumor neoepitopes, the hard work resides in their in vitro validation for their MHC I and MHC II binding, as well as for their recognition as antigens by specific T cells from cancer patients. Previous studies have estimated that only 2% to 3% of all exact length MHC I epitopes predicted from a given protein can be expected to be MHC binders,[16] and even fewer will be recognized by epitope-specific T cells. Altogether, these considerations render this computational approach highly time-consuming for relatively modest success rates.

Ex Vivo Immunoprecipitation and Elution of Major Histocompatibility Complex I and II Binding Peptides by Mass Spectrometry

Immunopeptidomics represents a promising alternative to a purely computational prediction of neoepitopes. This approach was pioneered in the group of HG Rammensee,[17,18] and is now being exploited by a growing number of laboratories. It consists of the immunoprecipitation of MHC class I and class II from body fluids, cell suspensions, or small tumor fragments, followed by the acid elution of the MHC-bound peptides. The recovered peptides are then analyzed by liquid chromatography/mass spectrometry (LC-MS/MS) and their amino acid sequences are compared to the WGS data for identifying neoepitopes. Garcia-Garijo et al.[19] have recently made a "complete overview of the different existing strategies to identify candidate neoantigens and evaluate their immunogenicity." This immunopeptidomics approach considerably narrows down the number of candidate epitopes to be screened, as compared to the in silico approach. Immunoprecipitation of HLA-bound peptides is also the only approach that directly reveals the naturally processed epitopes that could be presented on MHC molecules, including neoepitopes resulting from posttranslational modifications, alternative open reading frames, or novel exon–exon junctions resulting from DNA translocations. A major limitation, however, is the intrinsic sensitivity of MS, which was much improved in the recent year and further improvements are likely expected in the near future. For instance, the use of nano-ultra performance liquid chromatography, coupled with high-resolution mass spectrometry (nUPLC-MS/MS), was recently reported to deliver thousands of peptides with a turnaround time of 2 to 3 days.[20] Among others, the group of Bassani-Sternberg has recently demonstrated that MS-identified tumor epitopes are an extremely rich source of so-called tumor-rejection mediating neoepitopes (TRMNs), which are very promising for personalized cancer vaccine development.[21] Figure 23.1 is taken from another publication of the same group, which illustrates well the different steps of this procedure.[22]

Neoantigen Vaccine Trials in Cancer Patients

A number of studies have shown that tumor-infiltrating T cells, including neoantigen-specific T cells, have an exhausted phenotype characterized by high levels of programmed cell death 1 (PD-1).[23,24] As mentioned earlier, the use of ICB has revealed promising clinical effects in patients suffering from various solid malignancies,[3,4,25-27] and this may be related to high TMB, which also has implications for neoantigen-based vaccines.[8] Therefore, the development of neoantigen vaccine, combined with

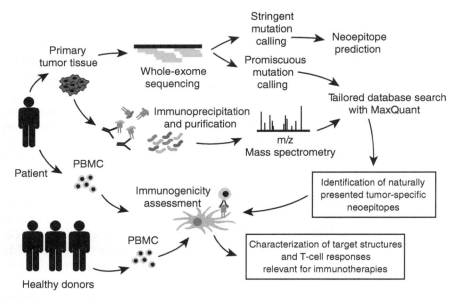

Figure 23.1 **Overview of the experimental approach to personalized neoantigen identification.** Patient tumor tissue was used for MS analysis and exome sequencing. Mutations were called and matched with MS data. Mutated peptide ligands were then further evaluated for recognition by the patient's autologous and matched allogeneic T cells.

MS, mesoporous silica; PBMC, peripheral blood mononuclear cell.

Source: Reproduced with permission from Bassani-Sternberg M, Braunlein E, Klar R, et al. Direct identification of clinically relevant neoepitopes presented on native human melanoma tissue by mass spectrometry. *Nat Commun.* 2016;7:13404. doi:10.1038/ncomms13404

ICB, holds great promise, and several clinical trials have already been completed (Table 23.1).[8,28–35]

For instance, a large Phase 1b trial was recently published.[28] Eighty-two patients were enrolled in this study, 34 with melanoma, 27 with NSCLC, and 21 with bladder cancer. Sixty patients were enrolled in the trial based on a minimum of 50 nonsynonymous point mutations or gene fusions. A total of 30 neoantigen peptides were selected based on MHC I presentation scores, which included predicted high binding affinity, allele-specific expression, proteasomal cleavage potential, and high expression of the neoepitopes. Finally, the NEO-PV-01

Table 23.1 Clinical Trials Involving Neoantigen-Based Vaccines or Adoptive Cell Transfer of Neoantigen-Specific Tumor-Infiltrating Lymphocytes

REFERENCES	TITLE	YEAR
8	Immunogenic neoantigens derived from gene fusions stimulate T cell responses	2019
28	A phase 1b trial of personalized neoantigen therapy plus anti-PD-1 in patients with advanced melanoma, non-small cell lung cancer, or bladder cancer	2020
29	An immunogenic personal neoantigen vaccine for patients with melanoma	2017
30	Personalized RNA mutanome vaccines mobilize poly-specific therapeutic immunity against cancer	2017
31	Neoantigen vaccine generates intratumoral T cell responses in Phase 1b glioblastoma trial	2019
32	Detection of neoantigen-specific T cells following a personalized vaccine in a patient with glioblastoma	2019
33	Mining exomic sequencing data to identify mutated antigens recognized by adoptively transferred tumor-reactive T cells	2013
34	Immune recognition of somatic mutations leading to complete durable regression in metastatic breast cancer	2018
35	Novel and shared neoantigen derived from histone 3 variant H3.3K27M mutation for glioma T cell therapy	2018

vaccine was made of at least 20 peptides in four pools and was formulated with poly-ICLC, a TLR3 agonist, as adjuvant. Anti-PD1 (Nivolumab) was administered during the 3 months needed for the generation of the vaccine as well as during the vaccine and boost period and was continued for up to 2 years. Of the 60 enrolled patients, 26 with melanoma, 14 with non-small cell lung cancer (NSCLC), and 11 with bladder cancer completed the study. The response rate as seen by a decrease in tumor lesions was 59%, 39%, and 27%, respectively, in melanoma, NSCLC, and bladder cancer patients. Moreover, increased frequencies of effector memory T cells with increased TCR clonality and presence of tumor-infiltrating TCF7+CD8+ T cells correlated with increased progression-free survival (PFS) at 9 months in the melanoma cohort. Importantly, epitope spreading was evident in two melanoma patients with peripheral T cell responses to three and four non-immunizing peptides, respectively.

Melanoma Neoantigen-Based Vaccine Trials

In 2017, two clinical trials were published that involved neoantigen-based vaccines in melanoma patients. One study consisted of a pool of up to 20 synthetic long peptides combined with the TLR3 ligand, polyinosinic:polycytidylic acid (poly I:C).[29] Six patients were involved and four of them had no tumor recurrence for up to 25 months postvaccination. Of note, the two patients who experienced tumor recurrence showed complete tumor regression upon combination with anti-PD-1 treatment, which confirms the potency of ICB to revive the functionality of neoantigen-specific T cells. The second clinical trial in melanoma patients involved an mRNA vaccine encoding 5 to 10 MHC I- and MHC II-restricted neoepitopes selected by exome sequencing and RNA-Seq and predicted to be high-affinity MHC binders.[30] Among the 13 patients involved, only two died by 15 months, while 11 patients showed significantly longer PFS correlating with highly reduced metastatic events. As for the peptide vaccine, one patient experienced complete objective response only upon combined programmed cell death-1 (PD-1) therapy. Of note, one patient developed a late relapse resulting from the outgrowth of beta2-microglobulin-deficient melanoma cells.

Glioblastoma Neoantigen-Based Vaccine Trials

In contrast to melanoma, glioblastoma tumors are considered to have a low TMB. Strikingly, one recent study in early 2019, involving WES and RNA-Seq of 10 GBM patients, revealed a median of 116 single nucleotide mutations per tumor sample.[31] Neoantigens were identified by WES, RNA-Seq, and bioinformatic analysis of tumor samples. Patients were immunized with up to 20 long synthetic peptides administered in nonrotating pools of three to five peptides combined with polyinosinic-polycytidylic acid-poly-l-lysine carboxymethylcellulose (poly-ICLC), a synthetic double-stranded RNA complex that serves as a ligand for Toll-like receptor-3 and melanoma differentiation-associated protein 5 (MDA-5). Unfortunately, most patients required dexamethasone to treat cerebral edema, which likely impacted the success of the vaccine, and no objective clinical response was obtained.

A case report was published shortly after, in which one GBM patient was treated with an autologous tumor lysate-DC vaccine followed by a personalized neoantigen vaccine made of eight synthetic long peptides (SLPs) encompassing seven neoantigens.[32] After each procedure, the patient demonstrated pseudo-progression as seen by magnetic resonance imaging (MRI), which led to a subtotal resection. Strikingly, histopathology revealed extensive T cell infiltration and T cell reactivity to 3 MHC I and 5 MHC II-restricted neoantigens. Although the patient succumbed 21 months after diagnosis, secondary to several complications, these two clinical studies demonstrate the feasibility and relevance of neoantigen vaccination in GBM patients and the need to find alternative treatments to treat intracranial edema, without the use of steroids.

Adoptive Cell Transfer of Neoantigen-Specific Tumor-Infiltrating Lymphocytes

In parallel to the development of neoantigen-specific therapeutic vaccines, several trials have evaluated the feasibility and efficacy of adoptively transferred tumor-infiltrating lymphocytes (TILs) in which neoantigen-specific T cells had been characterized.[34,36] Based on the success of TIL therapy in melanoma patients in which 40% of patients developed a complete regression of all measurable lesions for at least 5 years,[37] exomic sequencing and biocomputing studies established an association between clinical success and the presence of neoantigen-specific T cells in the tumor biopsies.[33] This approach was then extended to other types of cancers. For instance, a metastatic breast cancer patient was successfully treated with TILs that were reactive against mutant versions of four proteins, in conjunction with interleukin-2 (IL-2) and checkpoint blockade. A 49-year-old patient demonstrated a durable complete response for more than 22 months.[34] Similar to T cell transfer, a preclinical study has shown the feasibility of transducing T cells with a selected glioma neoantigen-specific TCR for adoptive transfer.[35]

Concluding Remarks

Neoantigen-based cancer vaccines likely represent the most attractive approach to generate a long-lasting antitumor immune response. The "foreign" nature of tumor neoantigens combined with ICB may efficiently overcome immunosuppressive mechanisms in the tumor environment (TME). Finally, epitope spreading, which was correlated with prolonged PFS, should greatly contribute to a sustained antitumor response with the aim of restoring tumor immunosurveillance.

PROMOTING MEMORY T CELL DEVELOPMENT DURING THERAPEUTIC CANCER VACCINATION

When naïve T cells encounter their cognate antigen and receive the appropriate co-stimulatory signals, they undergo multi-log clonal expansion and differentiate into specialized cells that release effector cytokines and acquire cytolytic activity. Upon antigen clearance, this initial activation phase is quickly followed by a contraction phase, in which most of the effector cells die by apoptosis. However, a fraction of the T cells persist and form a pool of memory cells that persist as quiescent lymphocytes for prolonged periods of time in an antigen-independent fashion and are characterized by increased activation kinetics and amplitude upon secondary antigen encounter.[38] It has become clear that the generation of potent memory T cells during vaccination and immunotherapy is crucial for establishing durable clinical responses.[39-41] However, current therapeutic cancer vaccines are often not able to amplify the dysfunctional, exhausted memory T cell subsets and induce functional antitumor immunological memory, resulting in poor efficacy.[42] Indeed, persistent antigen stimulation during both chronic viral infections and cancer has shown to drive an exhaustion program in T cells, with some exhausted T cell subsets that are hard to reinvigorate with current vaccines and other immunotherapeutic modalities.[43] It has, therefore, become clear that the efficacy of a therapeutic vaccine will, by and large, depend on its potential to rejuvenate these often exhausted T cells, and ideally induce a rather stem-cell-like memory phenotype.

Pathways Regulating Memory T Cell Differentiation and Maintenance

Memory T cells undergo antigen-independent slow homeostatic proliferation. Both the generation and the homeostasis as well as long-term survival of memory T cells are dependent on the cytokines IL-7 and IL-15.[44-47] A balance of transcription factors is determining the expression of effector versus memory genes. A terminally differentiated effector phenotype is induced by T-bet, BLIMP-1, ID2, and STAT4, while the expression of memory genes depends on FOXO1, Eomes, BCL-6, ID3, and STAT3.[48] T cell factor 1 (TCF1) is a key transcription factor regulating both memory CD8 T cell differentiation and longevity.[49] TCF1 acts downstream of the Wnt signaling pathway, which has been shown to be involved in effector versus memory T cell differentiation. Upon activation of the canonical Wnt pathway, glycogen synthase kinase-3β (GSK-3β) activity is inhibited, allowing the accumulation of β-catenin, which forms an active transcription factor complex with TCF1.[50] It was found that overexpression of β-catenin leads to an increased generation of memory CD8 T cells upon bacterial or viral infection.[51] Alternatively, inhibition of GSK-3β blocks effector T cell differentiation and promotes the differentiation into CD44[low]CD62L[high]Sca-1[high]CD122[high]Bcl-2[high] self-renewing multipotent CD8 memory stem cells.[52] Stem cell-like memory CD8 T cells are the least differentiated cells in the memory T cell pool with proliferative and antitumor capacities exceeding those of central and effector memory T cell subsets.[53] However, doubts have been raised about the specificity of the GSK3b inhibitor used in these experiments. Indeed, TWS119 was found to also efficiently inhibit mammalian target of rapamycin (mTOR) complex 1 (mTORC1) signaling in both mouse- and human-activated T cells.[54] As explained in the text that follows, inhibition of mTORC1 signaling during T cell activation and expansion is a robust pharmacological procedure to favor memory CD8 T cell differentiation.

Another central signaling hub regulating T cell differentiation is the Notch pathway. The activation of Notch cell surface receptors leads to the cleavage of the Notch intracellular domain (NICD), which then migrates to the nucleus and activates transcription.[55] The role of Notch in effector versus memory T cell differentiation is controversial, and likely depends on the cell type, inflammatory context, and/or experimental design. Upon TCR activation, Notch1 is upregulated in both CD4 and CD8 T cells.[56] Deletion of Notch1 dramatically abrogates CD8 T cell activation and blocks Eomes expression, as well as subsequent cytolytic effector function.[57,58] Since Eomes expression is also important for correct memory T cell differentiation, Notch1 signaling was initially believed to be important for memory T cell induction. Indeed, Notch pathway was shown to protect CD4 T cells from apoptosis, thus stimulating their longevity.[59] However, deletion of both Notch1 and Notch2 in CD8 T cells dramatically repressed effector gene expression and terminal effector T cell differentiation, while memory gene expression and memory precursor cell differentiation were induced.[60] The authors found that Notch expression was induced in activated T cells via mTOR signaling and T-bet transcriptional activity. Notch pathway, however, further amplified mTOR activity and created a positive feedback loop. mTOR, being a central metabolic hub integrating environmental cues and regulating cellular growth and proliferation, has indeed been shown to be involved in all aspects of T cell activation and differentiation. Constitutive mTORC1 activation locked CD8 T cells in an effector phenotype and inhibited memory T cell differentiation. Conversely, mTORC1 genetic inhibition prevented effector T cell differentiation and induced a memory phenotype that was, however, dysfunctional in its recall capacities.[61] In contrast to genetic inhibition of mTORC1, pharmacological inhibition by rapamycin did induce functional CD8 memory T cells.[62] This was also the case for activated human naïve CD4 and CD8 T cells.[54] Moreover, mTORC2 deletion induces memory T cell differentiation by inhibiting downstream AKT activation, allowing for the unphosphorylated form of FOXO1 to migrate to the nucleus and induce memory gene transcription.[63]

The discovery of a role for mTOR during T cell differentiation is among the first studies linking cellular metabolism with T cell phenotypes. Since then, T cell metabolism became an emerging field unveiling that different T cell subsets are characterized and can be regulated by specific metabolic processes.[64] Upon activation, T cell clonal expansion requires a tremendous activation of cellular metabolism. Glycolysis, pentose phosphate pathway, and glutamine oxidation are drastically increased, while fatty acid oxidation is suppressed.[65] In contrast, fatty acid oxidation and mitochondrial metabolism are characteristics of memory T cells, induced by IL-7 and IL-15.[66,67]

Pharmacological Interventions to Promote Memory Differentiation During Vaccination

Several decades of discoveries in the pathways regulating memory T cell differentiation allowed for the identification of druggable targets that might stimulate memory formation during vaccination against pathogens or for cancer treatment (see Figure 23.2). While the stimulation of Wnt signaling induces potent stem-cell-like memory T cells,[52] this is not an attractive target for therapeutic cancer vaccination, because the Wnt/β-catenin pathway is often upregulated in cancer, and further boosting this pathway might aggravate cancer progression. Additionally, Wnt signaling has a strong antiproliferative effect in activated T cells, thus hampering antitumor immunity. In contrast, induction of Notch pathway does not have antiproliferative effects and has been shown to induce stem cell-like memory T cells in vitro, with improved antitumor activity when adoptively transferred into tumor-bearing mice.[68] However, inducing Notch signaling during therapeutic vaccination might have detrimental systemic side effects, also resulting from the oncogenicity of the Notch pathway in several cell types.[69]

The mTOR inhibitor rapamycin is an immunosuppressive drug mainly used to prevent transplant rejection in humans. Following the observation that rapamycin treatment increases memory T cell differentiation when administered in mice upon acute viral infection,[62] several studies have explored the potential of mTOR inhibitors to improve the efficacy of vaccines. In a mouse model, mTOR inhibition in combination with an OX40 agonist during recombinant adenovirus vaccination enhanced memory CD8 T cell differentiation and favored protection against multiple viral challenges.[70] Also, in nonhuman primates, rapamycin treatment during vaccinia virus vaccination

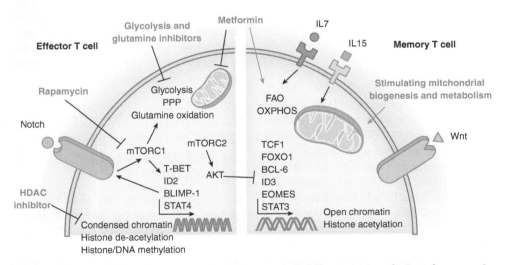

Figure 23.2 Pharmacological interventions for inducing memory T cell differentiation during therapeutic cancer vaccination. Overview of the major pathways driving effector versus memory differentiation. Effector T cells are characterized by high mTOR activity that stimulates a glycolytic and glutaminolytic metabolism, and activates effector transcription factors. In effector T cells, the chromatin is more condensed due to histone de-acetylation and methyl deposition on histones and DNA. Memory T cells are characterized by a mitochondrial oxidative metabolism and display an open chromatin conformation. Several strategies intervening with these pathways have been shown to drive memory T cell differentiation in preclinical models and clinical studies (shown in red).

FAO, fatty acid oxidation; HDAC, histone deacetylase; OXPHOS, oxidative phosphorylation; PPP, pentose phosphate pathway.

enhanced the quantity and quality of memory CD8 T cell formation.[71] The protective effect induced by mTOR inhibition can also occur independently of the effects on CD8 T cell differentiation. For instance, rapamycin inhibits germinal center formation upon influenza vaccination, thereby blocking IgM to IgG class switching, resulting in a broader spectrum antibody production, with one vaccine enabling enhanced protection against various subtypes of influenza virus.[72,73] In a Phase 2a study in humans, mTOR inhibitors were shown to enhance the immune function in older adults and induce improved responses to influenza vaccination.[74] These promising results in improving viral vaccine efficacy have ignited a strong interest to test mTOR inhibition during therapeutic cancer vaccination. Indeed, as with viral vaccines, mTOR inhibition in mice during both recombinant protein and RNA vaccination against kidney cancer and melanoma induced a more potent antitumor response and memory T cell formation.[75,76] Dosing regimen appears to be crucial, since short-term high-dose mTOR inhibition during vaccination increased memory CD8 T cell differentiation and antitumor activity, while long-term high-dose mTOR inhibition was detrimental for memory T cell differentiation.[77] However, mTOR inhibition does not improve antitumor immunity in every preclinical therapeutic vaccination model and has even been shown to impair antitumor activity of a cervical cancer vaccine.[78] This can be partially explained by the induction of regulatory T cells, an effect that can be prevented by cotreatment with a CCR4 antagonist.[79,80] In addition, the broad-spectrum activity of mTOR inhibition may limit its antitumor potential. Specifically targeting activated T cells by conjugating a small interfering RNA (siRNA) against the mTORC1 component, raptor, to an aptamer that binds 4-1BB generated a potent memory response and enhanced vaccine-induced antitumor activity in mice.[81] However, mTOR inhibition in cells other than T cells might also be beneficial. Inhibiting mTOR in dendritic cells has proven to enhance their survival, induce maturation markers, and improve CD8 T cell activation and cytolytic activity.[82,83] This extensive preclinical work has led to the design of several clinical trials in humans to test the efficacy of mTOR inhibitor administration during vaccine therapy (ClinicalTrials.gov Identifiers: NCT01522820 and NCT02833506). Unfortunately, no data has been reported so far, while the latter study has been discontinued due to adjuvant production issues.

Finally, the antidiabetic drug metformin is also a potent molecule able to induce memory T cell differentiation. Its mode of action remains unclear, although memory differentiation is likely induced by the upregulation of fatty acid oxidation.[84] Alternatively, through its inhibition of complex 1 of the electron transport chain, metformin treatment increases AMP levels, thereby activating AMPK and thus inducing a memory phenotype by inhibiting mTOR.[62] Despite its "dirty" profile, metformin is an interesting memory-inducing drug due to its highly favorable safety profile. A clinical trial testing the effect of metformin treatment on the efficacy of a flu vaccine in older adults has recently been initiated (ClinicalTrials.gov Identifier: NCT03996538).

Future Perspectives

The successful induction of memory T cells and improved antitumor activity upon mTOR inhibition during therapeutic cancer vaccination in preclinical animal models hold great promise for its clinical translation. However, at the same time, choosing the right dose regimen and improving cellular target specificity appear to be critical. Since mTOR is a central hub in the regulation of cellular metabolism, downstream metabolic targets might prove to be more specific in inducing the desired memory T cell phenotype. Inhibition of glycolysis and the induction of a mitochondrial oxidative metabolism are strategies that have been shown to induce a memory T cell phenotype and that could have synergistic antitumor activity by interfering with the metabolism of cancer cells.[67,85] More recently, the epigenetic events driving terminal effector versus memory T cell differentiation are being elucidated. Memory T cells are characterized by an open chromatin conformation favored by histone posttranslational modifications.[86] Drugs interfering with those posttranslational modifications, such as histone deacetylase inhibitors, could potentially improve the memory T cell differentiation and efficacy of therapeutic cancer vaccines.[87] When carefully balancing systemic side effects with therapeutic benefit, these emerging metabolic and epigenetic modulators hold the potential to provide long-lasting immune memory combined with direct antitumor activity in the therapeutic vaccination setting.

NANOPARTICLE VACCINES AS NOVEL DELIVERY VEHICLES TO PROMOTE ANTIGEN UPTAKE BY PRO-INFLAMMATORY DENDRITIC CELL POPULATIONS

Draining lymph nodes (LNs) are the primary site of action for initiating adaptive immunity where lymphocyte accumulation, activation, and proliferation are organized. Because of their crucial role in the immune response to antigens, many studies focused on delivering vaccines directly to the draining LNs. Indeed, targeting LNs with peptide vaccines can promote tumor-reactive T cells able to lyse tumor cells to treat cancer. However, it remains challenging to target LN-specific cell populations by simply delivering subcutaneously free antigens and adjuvant.[88] Moreover, peptide-based vaccines, as well as other subunit vaccines, have shown no or only modest clinical benefit, primarily because of their susceptibility to rapid enzymatic degradation, and because of their poor loading on antigen-presenting cells (APCs), resulting in low immunogenicity. Since the immune response is primarily initiated in LNs, tumor antigens must be efficiently delivered to the LNs in order to effectively induce an anticancer immune response.[89] Therefore, the optimization of the subunit vaccines is essential to achieve therapeutic efficacy. Nanoparticles (NPs) as carriers for vaccines are a promising solution to these hurdles. NPs can be conjugated or loaded with specific adjuvants, tumor-associated antigens, or neoantigens in order to optimize the priming of naïve T cells within lymphoid organs.[90,91] To induce tumor immunity, tumor antigens must be efficiently loaded and presented by APCs.[92] APCs, such as DCs, are able to capture, internalize, and process proteins expressed by tumor cells into short peptides.[93] NPs efficiently protect tumor antigens from degradative enzymes in the body and promote their selective delivery to the LNs. As a matter of fact, upon in vivo delivery, NPs with encapsulated or surface-loaded cancer antigens are efficiently internalized into APCs, thereby enhancing the immunogenicity of antigens and modulating immune cell activities.[89] NPs can be composed of silica, liposomes, polymeric micelles, or even gold, which are all ideal vehicles to penetrate tissue barriers and reach LNs, where they are taken up by DCs.[89,91] It was shown that NP size and shape play an important role for their accumulation in LNs. Indeed, small spherical NPs of 20 nm were found in higher amounts in LNs, as compared to larger and nonspherical NPs.[94] Moreover, there was a relatively low accumulation in nonlymphoid organs. The surface charge and hydrophobicity of NPs can also interfere with their delivery to LNs and may affect their uptake by APCs. Generally, positively charged NPs generate a higher immune response than neutral or negatively charged NPs.[95] In addition, the route of administration is critical and subcutaneous; intradermal, or intramuscular routes are preferred in order to facilitate the drainage of NPs to LNs for their DC uptake and presentation.[90,93,96] It has also been suggested that targeting the tumor-draining LN increases the antitumor activity of NP-delivered vaccines. Indeed, these vaccines can reshape the local immune microenvironment to promote tumor antigen-specific effector immune responses.[97,98] NPs can be loaded with an adjuvant, such as a TLR ligand, to potentiate DC maturation and antigen immunogenicity. Moreover, NP-adjuvant conjugates can also enhance activation of DCs and promote a cytolytic phenotype of effector and memory CD8+ T cells, resulting in protection against syngeneic tumor challenges.[99]

In the following sections, we describe several strategies that have been developed to enhance the NP-mediated peptide and RNA vaccines. Table 23.2 provides an overview of the various types of nanomaterials.

Inorganic Material-Based Nanoparticles

Gold Nanoparticles

Gold NPs (AuNPs) represent an attractive nanomaterial in view of their therapeutically beneficial physiochemical properties and their high biocompatibility.[100] It has been shown that AuNP vaccines less than 50 nm in diameter can preferentially drain, and thus effectively deliver antigens, to a local LN.[91] For instance, Almeida et al. synthesized AuNPs in order to facilitate delivery of the ovalbumin (OVA) peptide antigen and the CpG adjuvant, and to enhance their therapeutic effect in a B16-OVA tumor model. In this study, AuNPs induced a significantly stronger antigen-specific immune response than the delivery of free OVA. This response resulted in

Table 23.2 Characteristics and Advantages of Various Nanoparticles Used as Vaccine Delivery System

	INORGANIC MATERIAL-BASED NANOPARTICLE		ORGANIC MATERIAL-BASED NANOPARTICLES	
	Gold NP (AuNPs)	Mesoporous silica NP (MSNs)	Liposome	Polymeric micelle
Size	20–50 nm	100–200 nm	40–1,000 nm	10–100 nm
Characteristics	Safe platform vaccine delivery system	Can have large pore to load protein antigen with high molecular weight	Spontaneously assembled lipid-bilayer membrane vesicles containing an aqueous core	Self-assembled formation of synthetic amphiphilic block in an environment
Advantages	• Reduce the need for high doses of adjuvants • Reduce toxicities • High biocompatibility	• Can act as adjuvant themself • High biocompatibility	• Low toxicities • Protected from early degradation	• Long circulation time in blood • Easily modifiable • Highly stable

significant tumor inhibition associated with significant prolonged survival, demonstrating that AuNPs can be an effective carrier of peptide cancer antigens and adjuvants for cancer treatment. In addition, delivery with AuNPs may reduce the need for high doses of adjuvants, thereby reducing possible toxicities, such as spleen enlargement and systemic cytokine release.[101] Similarly, Kang et al. also synthesized AuNPs conjugated with OVA, in order to explore the effect of these NPs on the efficiency of delivery to draining LNs and antigen-specific T cell immunity. They observed that tumor-specific T cells induced by 22 nm OVA-gold NPs were capable of recognizing and killing their corresponding antigen-bearing tumor cells in mice.[102] Therefore, AuNP-based vaccines could serve as a safe platform delivery for inducing polyfunctional T cell responses to eliminate tumors.

Mesoporous Silica Nanoparticles

Mesoporous silica NPs (MSNs) represent another promising material for cancer vaccines because of their delivery properties and their biocompatibility. MSNs can act as adjuvant by themselves and, when loaded with cancer antigen(s), they can significantly enhance anticancer immunity in vivo in mice.[103] An et al. developed an MSN that can efficiently target and activate the APC to lead to tumor regression.[104] They showed that cationic MSNs can efficiently co-load adjuvant, TLR-9, and OVA antigen, which provides a multivalent presentation that can more strongly engage and enhance immunogenic responses. This approach also greatly reduces vaccine-induced toxicity by minimizing systemic exposure.[104] Similarly, Cha et al. synthesized extra-large pore MSNs; these NPs have a size of 100 to 200 nm and pore around 25 nm, which are beneficial for loading protein antigens with high molecular weight.[105] In vitro culture with extra-large pore MSNs loaded with OVA and a TLR-9 agonist led to enhanced DC activation, antigen presentation, and increased secretion of pro-inflammatory cytokines. In vivo, the authors demonstrated a significantly higher loading of OVA, when loaded with the TLR-9 agonist, resulting in efficient targeting to draining lymph nodes and a higher immune response. Moreover, they demonstrated efficient suppression of tumor growth in prevention settings when B16-OVA tumor cells were grafted after two immunizations, possibly due to a significant generation of memory T cells. These results suggest that mesoporous silica NPs can be used as an attractive delivery system of peptides and proteins for cancer vaccination.

Organic Material-Based Nanoparticles

Liposomes

Barati et al.[106] used AE36, a HER2 peptide associated with high-affinity binding to multiple DR alleles, from the intracellular part of the protein. AE36 was encapsulated in liposomal NPs. Liposomes are spherical lipid vesicles that contain one or more phospholipid bilayers. Because of their low toxicity, ease of preparation, and scale-up, liposomes have been extensively investigated as a drug delivery system.[107] In this study, liposomes encapsulating HER2 AE36 peptide were prepared from 1,2-dioleoyl-3-trimethylammoniumpropane (DOTAP) and dioleoylphosphatidylethanolamine (DOPE), which are two phospholipids well known for the formulation of liposomes.[108] Similar to the previously described silica NPs,[105] CpG was also used as an adjuvant in combination with liposomes loaded with HER2 AE36 peptide. Female mice were grafted subcutaneously with TUBO tumor cells, a mouse mammary carcinoma overexpressing the HER2 protein, before three immunizations subcutaneously in the flank at 2-week intervals with the AE36-CpG liposomes. Two mice out of five became tumor free and were completely cured while survival was significantly prolonged in the other mice. This liposomal formulation has significantly enhanced the antitumor function of HER2 AE36 peptide in mice. Along this line, Zamani et al. developed a nanoliposomal vaccine containing P5 peptide, a HER2-derived protein conjugated on the surface of a liposomal formulation and monophosphoryl lipid A as adjuvant.[109] This liposomal NP therapeutically reduced tumor growth in the HER2-overexpressing TUBO breast cancer mouse model. This liposomal NP formulation can be considered as a potential candidate for developing therapeutic breast cancer vaccines.

Cationic Liposomes

Cationic liposomes are based on a double emulsion solvent of the cationic surfactant dimethyldioctadecylammonium (DDA) and the immunopotentiator trehalose 6,6'-dibehenate (TDB). Liposomes based on DDA can promote immunogenic responses, but they are unstable and form aggregates. The addition of TDB increases the stability and the efficacy of these particles, making them a promising vaccine delivery system.[110] Cationic liposomes are used as carriers for nucleic acid TLR agonists. Indeed, Nordly et al.[111] developed a stable DDA/TDB liposomal complex with poly(I:C) and they confirmed with in vivo studies that CD8+ T cell responses can be induced by the cationic liposome vaccine adjuvant in a poly(I:C) dose-dependent manner. Varypataki et al.,[112] for their part, used them as carriers of SLPs. They showed that poly(I:C) adjuvanted-DOTAP-based liposomes loaded with an SLP, harboring the model epitope SIINFEKL, can be a successful vaccine candidate for the induction of a functional CD8+ CTL response that is required for tumor eradication. Then, they showed in another study that cationic liposomes loaded with well-defined tumor-specific SLPs and a TLR3 ligand as adjuvant can strongly activate functional, antigen-specific CD8+ and CD4+ T cells and induced in vivo cytotoxicity against target cells after intradermal vaccination.[113] In addition, Salomon et al.[114] used cationic liposomes as carriers of mRNA-based vaccines in tumors as lipoplexes. Indeed, RNA-based poly-neo-epitope can be used as an approach to mobilize immunity against cancer to implement a vaccine.[30] Here, they reported that tumor rejection is augmented in a CD8+ T cell-dependent manner by a lipoplex-formulated RNA (RNA-LPX) vaccine that encodes CD4+ T cell-recognized neoantigens. Mice were primarily immunized against the immunodominant gp70 antigen, then, they are treated with local radiotherapy plus the CD4 neoantigen vaccine. They observed that mice rejected gp70-negative tumors and were protected from rechallenge with these tumors, indicating a potent polyantigenic CD8+ T cell response and T cell memory. Antigen-encoding RNA-LPX enables systemic delivery to lymphoid compartments and promotes immunogenic responses.

Finally, very recently, Sahin et al.[115] developed a lipid nanoparticle (LNP)-formulated RNA vaccine containing the BNT162b1, which encodes the receptor-binding domain (RBD) of the SARS-CoV-2 protein, a key target of neutralizing antibodies. They observed after vaccination an increase of pro-inflammatory CD4+ and CD8+ T cell responses in almost all participants, with Th1 polarization of the helper response, suggesting that it has the potential to protect against COVID-19 through multiple beneficial mechanisms.

Polymeric Micelles

The physicochemical characteristics of tumor peptides can largely impact their efficient loading on APCs, and therefore on their immunogenicity. In a recent study, Lynn et al.[116] developed charge-modified peptide and TLR-7/8 agonist conjugates able to self-assemble into NPs independently of the physicochemical properties of tumor antigens. Indeed, in addition to the adjuvant TLR-7/8 agonist, they introduced a charge-modifying group to the N-terminus of peptide antigens that improves the solubility of hydrophobic peptide antigens during synthesis and purification and induces the self-assembly of conjugates into nanoparticle micelles of a small, optimal size for APC targeting and T cell immunity. This self-assembling NP (SNP) enabled the loading of diverse peptides and enhanced their uptake by APCs leading to superior CD8 T cell induction over similar conjugates without peptide charge modification. Moreover, they observed a tumor regression in mice bearing TC-1 and B16 tumors after treatment with antigen as SNP in combination with an anti-PD-L1 delivered by the intraperitoneal route.

Nanoparticle Vaccines in Combination With Immune Checkpoint Blockade

Of note, antibodies against cytotoxic T-lymphocyte antigen 4 (CTLA-4), programmed cell death-1 (PD-1), and programmed cell death ligand-1 (PD-L1) have been approved as standard of care for an increasing number of cancer types.[117] In preclinical studies, when cancer antigen delivery-based NPs are combined with ICB, the anticancer immune response can be further improved. For instance, Li et al.[118] have developed an NP made of micelles based on the tumor-penetrating Linear TT1 (Lin-TT1) peptide conjugated with cholesterol and histidine, which allowed the delivery of siRNA able to block PD-L1 synthesis in tumor cells and improved antitumor response. This tumor-penetrating peptide assembling NP is capable of accumulating in the breast cancer tumor site. siPD-L1 is locally released in the tumor environment and favors the survival and activation of cytotoxic lymphocytes, resulting in the killing of breast cancer cells.

NP-based vaccines have been claimed to have several advantages and can enhance vaccine immunity with codelivering multiple antigens and adjuvants. In addition, NPs provide better stability for poorly soluble peptide antigens and improve low immunogenicity of certain antigens.

CONCLUSION

Over the last 40 years, a series of nanoparticle drug delivery systems have been developed and are currently being tested in clinical trials, both in infectious diseases and cancer. For instance, the mRNA-based SARS-Cov-2 lipid nanoparticle vaccine has provided promising results in mice and is now being tested in clinical trials.[115,119–121] Nanomaterial can promote the targeting of the antigen to lymphoid organs, favor their cellular uptake and codeliver the danger signals to promote an optimal immune response.[115] This approach will also be very attractive when applied in the context of tumor. As the science of nanomaterials develops, platforms that are more sophisticated are designed and tested as carriers for vaccines. Here, we have decided to focus solely on nanoparticles. However, other nanomaterials such as polymeric wafers, biomaterials including biopolymers, and various fusion proteins offer a myriad of opportunities for innovative vaccine designs. Future clinical studies will tell whether and how the use of these platforms do increase the therapeutic efficacy of nanovaccines in cancer patients.

KEY REFERENCES

Only key references appear in the print edition. The full reference list appears in the digital product on Springer Publishing Connect: connect.springerpub.com/content/book/978-0-8261-3743-2/part/part02/chapter/ch23

28. Ott PA, Hu-Lieskovan S, Chmielowski B, et al. A Phase Ib trial of personalized neoantigen therapy plus anti-PD-1 in patients with advanced melanoma, non-small cell lung cancer, or bladder cancer. *Cell.* 2020;183(2):347–362. doi:10.1016/j.cell.2020.08.053

30. Sahin U, Derhovanessian E, Miller M, et al. Personalized RNA mutanome vaccines mobilize poly-specific therapeutic immunity against cancer. *Nature.* 2017;547(7662):222–226. doi:10.1038/nature23003

43. McLane LM, Abdel-Hakeem MS, Wherry EJ. CD8 T cell exhaustion during chronic viral infection and cancer. *Annu Rev Immunol.* 2019;37:457–495. doi:10.1146/annurev-immunol-041015-055318

54. Scholz G, Jandus C, Zhang L, et al. Modulation of mTOR signalling triggers the formation of stem cell-like memory T cells. *EBioMedicine.* 2016;4:50–61. doi:10.1016/j.ebiom.2016.01.019

62. Araki K, Turner AP, Shaffer VO, et al. mTOR regulates memory CD8 T-cell differentiation. *Nature.* 2009;460(7251):108–112. doi:10.1038/nature08155

63. Zhang L, Tschumi BO, Lopez-Mejia IC, et al. Mammalian target of rapamycin complex 2 controls CD8 T cell memory differentiation in a foxo1-dependent manner. *Cell Rep.* 2016;14(5):1206–1217. doi:10.1016/j.celrep.2015.12.095

88. Schudel A, Francis DM, Thomas SN. Material design for lymph node drug delivery. *Nat Rev Mater.* 2019;4(6):415–428. doi:10.1038/s41578-019-0110-7

116. Lynn GM, Sedlik C, Baharom F, et al. Peptide-TLR-7/8a conjugate vaccines chemically programmed for nanoparticle self-assembly enhance CD8 T-cell immunity to tumor antigens. *Nat Biotechnol.* 2020;38(3):320–332. doi:10.1038/s41587-019-0390-x

T Cell Modulatory Cytokines

Emanuela Romano and Kim Margolin

KEY POINTS

- Interleukin (IL)-2, IL-4, IL-7, IL-9, IL-15, IL-21, and thymic stromal lymphopoietin (TSLP) are cytokines that bind through unique cytokine-specific α and/or β chains to a common γ chain ($γ_c$) receptor on T lymphocytes and are termed "$γ_c$ cytokines." Additional cytokines that play critical roles in antitumor cytotoxicity, in part by mediating communication and functions of innate and adaptive immune responses, include IL-12 and interferon-γ.

- The cytokine-specific α and/or β chains of the $γ_c$ cytokines control different aspects of cytokine biology such as the site(s) of production, target cell(s), and functional interactions with other cytokines (e.g., IL-4 and IL-13, the latter a non-$γ_c$ cytokine that shares an α receptor chain with IL-4), while IL-12 mediates important signals between antigen-presenting cells (APCs) and other cells of the innate immune system such as natural killer (NK) cells and the adaptive immune system such as T and B cells.

- Actions of the $γ_c$ cytokines are related to the proliferation and differentiation of T lymphocytes, as well as their trafficking from thymus to lymph nodes to non-nodal tissues and to tumors.

- $γ_c$ cytokines and the transcription factors they control contribute substantially to the plasticity of CD4+ T lymphocytes, which can differentiate into a wide spectrum of different subsets with different activities and roles in the immune system, ranging from allergy and inflammation to organ rejection and control of malignancy as well as protection against autoimmune disease.

- NK and CD8+ T cells depend on $γ_c$ cytokines for proliferation, cytotoxicity, protection against apoptosis, and, for some cytokines, protection against activation-induced cell death (AICD).

- IL-2, the most intensively studied $γ_c$ cytokine, was the first of this class of cytokines to demonstrate robust antitumor activity in animal models and humans when given in high doses that were also associated with multiorgan toxicities. Nevertheless, high-dose IL-2 (HD-IL-2) was U.S. Food and Drug Administration (FDA)-approved in the 1990s for advanced renal cancer and melanoma based on the achievement of durable tumor regressions and long survival plateaus in a small fraction of treated patients. Although HD-IL-2 has been almost completely eclipsed by immune checkpoint-blocking antibodies (ICB), new engineered IL-2 formulations with enhanced effector cell activation and reduction of regulatory T cell (T_{reg} cell) stimulation are now in clinical trials seeking improved therapeutic index and safe combinations that potentiate ICB.

- Therapeutic potential for $γ_c$ cytokines other than IL-2, particularly the homeostatic cytokines IL-7 and IL-15, which support lymphopoiesis and induce memory T cells as well as broadening of the antigen repertoire, is now being investigated in a broad range of disease settings and therapeutic combinations.

- IL-4, a pleiotropic cytokine with important effects on B cell maturation and function, is associated with mainly suppressive effects on T cells but promotes the maturation of dendritic cell (DC) subsets that are in current trials as APCs for selected tumor vaccines.

- The most important roles for all of the $γ_c$ and other T cell modulatory cytokines are likely to be in combinatorial regimens developed to optimize antigen-specific T cell responses as well as innate immune system elements in the control of malignancy.

INTRODUCTION

Cytokines are secreted molecules that mediate communication among cells of the innate and adaptive immune systems as well as between tissues, including tumor cells, and their surrounding microenvironment. Cytokines may also contribute to the pathogenesis of malignancy, mainly by participating in chronic inflammatory but immunosuppressive circuits that promote tumorigenesis and escape from immune control. However, a number of cytokines are immunopotentiating and contribute to the control of cancer by promoting both innate and adaptive immune responses against tumors. Many of the latter cytokines have shown great potential for the treatment of human tumors, and interleukin (IL)-2 as a single agent is U.S. Food and Drug Administration (FDA) approved for the treatment of metastatic melanoma and advanced renal cell carcinoma. Some of these cytokines also have important functions when used ex vivo in the preparation of a therapeutic lymphocyte product for adoptive cell transfer (ACT). One important group, consisting of cytokines that share a common γ chain (γ_c) receptor subunit and, thus, has selected effects on T cells, contains IL-2, IL-7, IL-9, IL-15, IL-21, and thymic stromal lymphopoietin (TSLP). Several members of this group have demonstrated a role in the treatment of human malignancy but appear insufficiently active to be used alone and are currently under investigation in combinations that exploit their unique functions and interactions in vivo. In the first edition of this text, we summarized the most important immunologic and clinical data for each of the γ_c receptor cytokines that showed immunotherapeutic activity, and in the present edition, we will update this information to reflect the current state of the science, as well as translational, and clinical data.

T cells are the foundation of protection against many pathogens, autoimmune disorders, and cancer, as well as being the mediators of rejection in solid organ transplants and graft-versus-host syndromes in allogeneic hematopoietic transplantation. T cells are also responsible for protection against a broad variety of viral-mediated malignancies, in which the oncogenic drive may result from a whole virus infection and a complex inflammatory response (as in chronic viral hepatitis B or C and hepatocellular cancer, human papilloma virus, and squamous cancer of the cervix or head and neck, and Epstein–Barr virus and B cell lymphomas or nasopharyngeal cancer). Oncogenesis may alternatively be driven by viral-derived oncogene sequences within epithelial cells, as in the case of Merkel cell cancer and the Merkel cell polyoma virus, and perhaps others. Successful T cell activation to effector function as well as control of the complex immune responses that protect against the emergence of malignancy but also against the damaging results of uncontrolled activation depend on a large number of T cell subsets and a complex network of signaling and regulation of gene expression. Beyond viral-related cancers, oncogene-driven cancers derived from mutational and epigenetic events also are now known to be capable of driving T cell responses and to be amenable to immune-mediated destruction.

Other immune and inflammatory cells that interact with T cells in the control of these processes are also tightly controlled physiologically, and alterations of these regulatory processes are often characteristics of pathologic states such as cancer.

CYTOKINE OVERVIEW

Cytokines are essential for the orchestration of rapid and effective immune responses to pathogens and foreign tissue and against antigens of malignant cells arising during oncogenesis. Early studies of these molecules provided insight into their cellular effects and potential for successful immunotherapy. Table 24.1 lists, for all of the γ_c cytokines and IL-12 that are detailed in this chapter, their cell source, target cell(s), molecular weight, receptor structure, signaling mechanisms, and predominant cellular functions.

The earliest immunotherapeutic cytokine used for malignancy was interferon-α (IFN-α) in patients with indolent B cell lymphoma and hairy cell leukemia, as well as in chronic myelogenous leukemia, renal cell carcinoma, and the adjuvant therapy of melanoma, but the use of this highly pleiotropic type I IFN has largely been supplanted by more powerful agents with improved therapeutic index in each disease and in many others. The subsequent discovery of the first T cell cytokine, IL-2—originally known as T cell growth factor for its property of supporting the proliferation of T cells in vitro—expanded the field by providing an immunomodulatory agent exerting potent, durable antitumor effects in a subset of advanced melanoma and renal cancer patients. Recombinant cytokine molecules for a wide range of biologic investigation and potential therapeutic use soon followed, which led to the identification of many of the mechanisms of action of IL-2 and additional T cell cytokines and their receptors.

Currently, the cytokines as a whole are grouped into families based on commonly shared receptor subunits that mediate partially overlapping but also unique responses. The largest such family—and the predominant focus of the chapter—consists of the γ_c cytokines that, in addition to IL-2, include IL-4, IL-7, IL-9, IL-15, IL-21, and TSLP[1] (see Figure 24.1).

Another important family of inflammatory cytokines, composed of uniquely heterodimeric structures that determine the responding cell type(s), receptor binding, signal transduction, and transcriptional response (Figure 24.2[2]) includes IL-12, -23, -27, and -35, with the figure showing schematically the relative position of each of these cytokines along the spectrum of pro-inflammatory to inhibitory functions. To date, IL-12 is the only member of this cytokine family that has shown a potential for clinical application in cancer therapy and will be discussed later in this chapter.

Table 24.1 T Cell Immunomodulatory Cytokines

CYTOKINE	CELL SOURCE	TARGET CELL	MOLECULAR WEIGHT	RECEPTOR STRUCTURE	SIGNALING MECHANISMS	PREDOMINANT CELLULAR FUNCTIONS
IL-2	Th/c cells; DC and NK cells	T, B, NK cells; monocytes	15 kD	IL-2Rα IL-2/15Rb γ$_c$	STAT1 STAT3 STAT5	Potent lymphoid cell growth factor Promotes proliferation, differentiation, cytotoxicity of all Th, Tc, T$_{reg}$, and NK cells. Involved in the elimination of autoreactive T cells. Supports proliferation, differentiation of B cells
IL-4	T and NK cells; mast cells; eosinophils	T, NK, and B cells; mast cells; basophils	15 kD	IL-4/IL-13Rα γ$_c$	STAT5 STAT6	Differentiation of naïve CD4$^+$ T cells into helper Th2 cells; suppression of Th1 development; proliferation and differentiation of B cells, isotype switching; induction and promotion of chemotaxis of mast cells and basophils switching; promotion of chemotaxis of mast cells and basophils
IL-7	Epithelial and stromal cells; fibroblasts	T, pre-B cells, DCs	20 kD	IL-7Rα γ$_c$	STAT1 STAT3 STAT5	T cell development and homeostasis; T cell growth factor and critical antiapoptotic survival factor for naïve and memory T cells
IL-9	T cells	T cells, epithelial and mast cells, eosinophils	14 kD	IL-9R γ$_c$	STAT5	Mitogen of lymphoid cells and other immune cells, including mast cells, Th2 cells, and eosinophils; immunoglobulin production
IL-15	Neutrophils, monocytes, DCs, mast cells, B cells, fibroblasts	T, NK, and B cells; PMNs; Mph; fibroblasts	15 kD	IL-15Rα IL-2/15Rb γ$_c$	STAT5	T cell activation, cytotoxicity, memory, maintenance; NK cell maturation, activation, cytotoxicity; B cell activation; neutrophil activation; macrophage activation/suppression (dose dependent); B cell differentiation, activation, isotype switching; fibroblast activation
IL-21	Th cells (TFH, Th17), NKT cells	T, NKT, and B cells; DCs	15 kD	IL-21R γ$_c$	STAT1 STAT3 STAT5	T cell homeostasis, promotion of CD8$^+$ T cell and NK cell cytotoxicity; differentiation of B cells into plasma cells
TSLP	Keratinocytes, fibroblasts, stromal cells, mast cells, basophils	T, NKT, B, and DC cells; mast cells	15 kD	IL-7Rα TSLPR	STAT3 STAT5	DC maturation, activation; mast cell co-stimulation; B cell expansion and differentiation
IL-12	APC—DC, macrophages, B cells	NK, CD8$^+$, Th1 CD4$^+$ cells; B cells	75 kD	IL-12R β1β2	JAK2, Tyk2, STAT4	Type I immune responses, IFN-γ secretion from NK and T cells.

APC, antigen-presenting cells; DC, dendritic cell; IL, interleukin; JAK, Janus kinase; NK, natural killer; NKT, natural killer T cells; PMNs, polymorphonuclear leukocytes; STAT, signal transducers and activators of transcription; TFH, T follicular helper; Th1, T helper cell 1; T$_{reg}$, regulatory T; TSLP, thymic stromal lymphopoietin; TSLPR, TSLP receptor.

Other families of cytokines that do not target T cells directly have also been exploited therapeutically to support ACT and DC-based cancer vaccines. Remarkably, despite encouraging preclinical data supporting a therapeutic role for most of the γ$_c$ cytokines—particularly IL-7, IL-15, and IL-21—their activity as single agents or in vivo as part of multi-agent regimens remains undefined. In particular, IL-15, with its complex structure and physiologic functions, is considered to have the greatest potential for a supportive role in many immunotherapeutic strategies, including combinations with ICB, with tumor vaccines, with ACT, and with other cytokines or

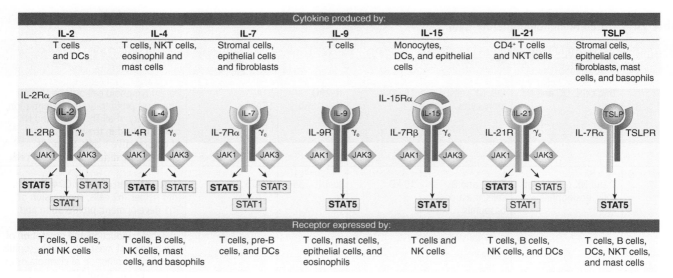

Figure 24.1 **Receptors for γ_c family cytokines and TSLP**. IL-2, IL-4, IL-7, IL-9, IL-15, IL-21, and TSLP and their receptor chains are shown. IL-2 and IL-15 share IL-2Rβ, whereas IL-7 and TSLP share TSLPR, and of the cytokines shown, only TSLP does not share γ_c. There are three classes of IL-2 receptors, binding IL-2 with low affinity (IL-2Rα alone), intermediate affinity (IL-2Rβ+ γ_c), and high affinity (IL-2Rα+ IL-2Rβ+ γ_c), with the high-affinity receptor containing all three subunits αβγ_c. Each γ_c family cytokine activates JAK1 and JAK3. The major STAT proteins activated by these cytokines are shown. STAT5 refers to both STAT5A and STAT5B.

DC, dendritic cell; IL, interleukin; JAK, Janus kinase; NK, natural killer; NKT, natural killer T cells; STAT, signal transducers and activators of transcription; TSLP, thymic stromal lymphopoietin; TSLPR, TSLP receptor.

Source: Adapted from Rochman Y, Spolski R, Leonard WJ. New insights into the regulation of T cells by gamma(c) family cytokines. *Nat Rev Immunol*. 2009;9(7):480–490. doi:10.1038/nri2580

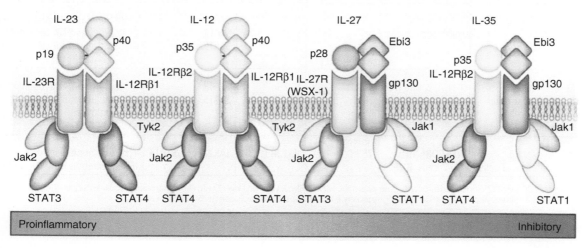

Figure 24.2 **Members of the IL-12 family of cytokines are presented together with their receptors and Jak-STAT signaling partners**. Key (bottom) indicates the functional spectrum of these cytokines, from most proinflammatory (IL-23) to most inhibitory (IL-35). Tyk2, kinase of the Jak family.

Source: Adapted from Vignali DA, Kuchroo VK. IL-12 family cytokines: immunological playmakers. *Nat Immunol*. 2012;13(8):722–728. doi:10.1038/ni.2366

immunomodulatory agents.[3] Other γ_c cytokines may play distinct supportive roles—for example, IL-4, generally considered a type 2 or a T cell-suppressive cytokine, with granulocyte-macrophage colony-stimulating factor (GM-CSF). GM-CSF is a highly pleiotropic myeloid/monocytic growth factor and chemotactic molecule used in the clinic to enhance recovery from myelosuppressive chemotherapy and for the ex vivo elicitation of therapeutic DC from peripheral blood mononuclear cells (PBMCs) in selected cancer vaccine strategies. GM-CSF has also been used as a component of cancer vaccines produced from tumor cells transduced with the GM-CSF gene (GVAX) as well as attenuated herpesviruses carrying the gene for GM-CSF that are injected intratumorally as a form of oncolytic virotherapy (talimogene laherparepvec, approved for melanoma, and others under investigation). IL-21, which had an unfavorable therapeutic index when used alone or with CTLA-4 blockade in early studies, is now being used in some laboratories to support T cell expansion for ACT, including tumor-infiltrating lymphocytes (TIL), transgenic T cell receptor (TCR) or chimeric antigen receptor (CAR)-expressing T cells, or antigen-specific autologous circulating T cells—all forms of ACT that are expanded ex vivo to provide an autologous therapeutic product. Most of these ACT regimens include a pre-infusion administration of lymphodepleting chemotherapy, which enhances expansion of the therapeutic T cells and may promote epitope spreading y eliciting the γ_c cytokines IL-7 and IL-15, which act as homeostatic growth factors that broaden the T cell repertoire (IL-7) and promote T cell memory (IL-15 predominantly). Finally, the elaboration of certain cytokines by tumor cells or inflammatory and immune cells, either unprovoked or in response to immunotherapeutic interventions (particularly IL-6, in myeloma and renal cell cancer), is a remarkable example of the role of cytokines in oncogenesis and the control of tumor immunity.[4,5]

TYPE 1 AND TYPE 2 CYTOKINES AND CELL-MEDIATED CYTOTOXICITY

Cytokines produced by T cells have been categorized into at least two broad categories based on their association with acute inflammation and cytotoxic antitumor responses (type 1) or with chronic inflammation and predominantly suppressive effects in the tumor context (type 2). T cell subsets are characterized by the predominant cytokines that they produce and are also characterized by immune gene signatures that reflect the downstream regulation of gene expression by cell type-associated transcription factors. For example, T helper 1 CD4+ (Th1) cells, a subset of CD4+ T cells, responding in large part to the action of IL-12 from mature antigen-presenting cells (APCs), produce IL-2, IFNγ, and tumor necrosis factor (TNF) and depend on the transcription factor T-bet,

while Th2 cells produce IL-4, IL-5, IL-10, and IL-13; are characterized by the transcription factor GATA-3; and are facilitated by exogenous IL-10. A third subset, Th17 cells, characterized by the production of IL-17, participate in autoimmune disease processes as well as potentially in some aspects of tumor immunity. These cells respond to IL-6 and IL-23 signals, and use the transcription factor RORγT in the control of their lineage fate.[6-10] Although these categories of helper T cells are not perfectly fixed but are subject to a degree of plasticity, they do provide a foundation for phenotypic and functional groupings that need to be considered in the understanding of antitumor immune responses and the design of immunotherapeutic interventions.

CD8+ T cells can also be polarized toward Th1-like, Th2-like, and Th17-like phenotypes, but type 1 CD8+ T cells are considered the most critical for immune-mediated tumor control. These effector cells are typically lytic and are also called cytotoxic T lymphocytes (CTLs). They contain cytotoxic granules (the content of which includes perforin and granzymes) that are released on encounter of antigen-expressing target cells. In addition to cytotoxic T cells (CTC), NK cells recognize a tumor through a number of alternative ligand–receptor interactions and are highly responsive to some of the same γ_c cytokines that activate or promote the proliferation of T cells, such as IL-2 and IL-15. Considering that T cell recognition of target cells requires antigen presentation through the major histocompatibility complex (MHC)–peptide–TCR complex while NK recognition of target cells is predominantly inhibited by class I MHC molecules, it is theoretically possible that close collaboration of NK cells and CTL, representing innate and adaptive immune responses, could cooperate to eradicate tumors that escape control through mutations in the class I antigen processing and presentation machinery. However, even in the presence of brisk innate and adaptive immune responses, multiple negative regulatory mechanisms limit the efficiency of immune control of malignant disease and must be taken into consideration in the design of effective immunotherapies.

IL-2, The Prototypical γ_c Cytokine—From T Cell Growth Factor to Cancer Immunotherapy

Recombinant Human IL-2, Aldesleukin

IL-2 is produced mainly by CD4+ T cells and acts on CD4+ T cells, CD8+ T cells, NK cells, T_{reg} cells, and B cells. The net effects of physiologic IL-2 production as well as the response to pharmacologic doses and schedules depend on factors that are not fully understood but probably include germline polymorphisms of selected immunomodulatory genes, the dose administered, the absolute and relative numbers of T cells and their subsets infiltrating primary and metastatic tumors, and the pre- and on-therapy expression of different co-stimulatory and activation/exhaustion markers (such as the programmed-death receptor 1 [PD-1]). The relative expression of activating and inhibitory receptors on NK cells, the activity of which is determined in part by the host HLA determinants and multiple other cellular and circulating ligands, also contribute to the overall balance of IL-2 effects in cancer.[11] The critical role of IL-2 in maintaining the function of CTC is evidenced by the loss of IL-2 production as one of the first functional deficits occurring during the process of T cell exhaustion, followed by other functional deficits such as proliferation and secretion of molecules required for cytotoxicity.[12]

The discovery and cloning of recombinant IL-2 provided for the study of animal models in which escalating doses of this cytokine, especially with the addition of ex vivo, IL-2-exposed PBMCs, demonstrated dose-dependent tumor regression and a substantial rate of cure, even in the "nonimmunogenic" tumor models that most closely approximate human spontaneously arising tumors. While the cellular components and characteristics of the blood, tumor microenvironment (TME), vasculature, and tumor biology required for IL-2–mediated antitumor effects remain to this day inadequately understood, an important result of these studies was the definition of lymphokine-activated killer cells (LAKs), derived from the action of IL-2 on NK cells, as a predominant mediator of antitumor cytotoxicity. These studies also led to extensive characterization of IL-2 receptor forms on various subsets of T cells (including, importantly, the high-affinity α receptor, IL-2RA, on T_{reg} cells) and NK cells, which can be subsetted by their differential expression of the neural cell adhesion receptor (NCAM) CD56 and functionally by their response to IL-2 (predominant cytokine secretion [CD56^{bright}] vs activation/cytotoxic granule production [CD56^{dim}]).[13]

IL-2 is a 15-kD single-chain cytokine that signals predominantly through a heterotrimeric receptor that includes the α chain, β chain, and the common γ chain ($γ_c$; Figure 24.3).[14]

On ligand binding, the IL-2R conveys signal transduction mainly via JAK1/JAK3 and signal transducers and activators of transcription 5 (STAT5). Additional signaling has been observed involving STAT1 and STAT3 transcription factors, and the PI3K, Ras, and NF-κβ signaling pathways. The predominant functional effect of IL-2 signaling in lymphocyte responses to this cytokine is promotion of cell cycle progression/proliferation, although IL-2 additionally can influence cell death pathways (in its promotion of activation-induced T cell death, AICD), acquisition of cytolytic activity, and development of T cell memory.[10]

The β subunit of the receptor (CD122), common to IL-2 and IL-15, narrows the specificity of these $γ_c$ receptor cytokines but has no intrinsic signaling function. Each of the $γ_c$ receptor cytokines has its own specific α-receptor that determines the circulating, tissue and tumor concentrations of the active cytokine, its structural characteristics (such as the presentation of IL-15 by its α receptor in cell-bound form on APCs that produce both the receptor subunit and the cytokine in tandem), and its target cell features—sites of action, target cell specificity, receptor structure and affinity, kinetics, and interactions with other cell functions.[15] While the $γ_c$ receptor is responsible for the signaling functions of cytokines in this family, the signaling cascades triggered by the non-$γ_c$ components of their receptors confer their distinct features and functions.

T_{reg} cells have been shown to have a distinct IL-2R signaling pattern compared to activated CTC. Engagement of the IL-2R on T_{reg} cells results in the activation of the JAK/STAT signaling pathway but does not appear to activate downstream targets of the PI3K signaling pathway due to the inhibitory effects of phosphatase and tensin homolog (PTEN) on the latter.[16] The net effects of IL-2 on T_{reg} cells include antiapoptosis and enhanced cellular survival, while its effect on CTL includes AICD, the mechanisms of which involve upregulation of FasL expression and the suppression of FLICE-inhibitory protein (FLIP) expression, an inhibitor of Fas signaling. Thus, IL-2-induced AICD may be related to the engagement of Fas–FasL interaction in T cells. In addition, AICD has been implicated as a major mechanism by which IL-2 controls autoreactive T cells and thus host protection against autoimmunity as well as curbing potentially harmful effector T cell responses to pathogens.[17]

The entry of recombinant human IL-2 in its commercially approved form was based on encouraging preclinical studies in a variety of tumor models that showed the dose-response effect and the apparent benefit of adding autologous (or, in animals, syngeneic) LAK cells in conjunction with high-dose IL-2. Melanoma and renal cancer (RCC), being highly resistant to cytotoxic chemotherapy, minimally responsive to IFN-α, and in many models responsive to immunomodulation, were chosen for initial clinical development. In these trials, which long predated immune checkpoint blockade (ICB) for melanoma and the vascular endothelial growth factor-directed therapies for RCC, the level of antitumor activity—as well as the lack of additional benefit from LAK cells and thus a reduction in the complexity, risks and costs of the regimen—was sufficient to support the approval of Aldesleukin, a single amino acid-substituted form of recombinant human IL-2. This drug, given in high doses with ICU-level support, provided objective responses in the 15%-20% range for advanced melanoma and in the 25% range for advanced clear-cell RCC, with 5–8% of treated patients (about 1/3 of all responders) experiencing durable responses that are considered

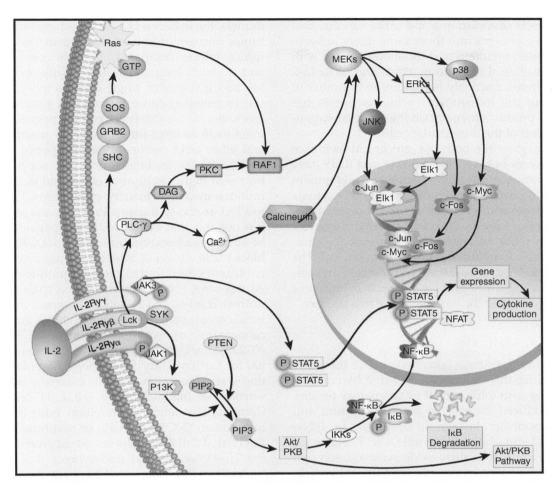

Figure 24.3 **Detailed schematic of IL-2 signaling in cells expressing the high affinity trimeric IL-2 receptor.** IL-2 signaling is mediated by the high affinity IL-2Rαβγ, a multichain receptor complex consisting of an α (CD25), β (CD122), and γ (CD132) chain. IL-2Rα primarily increases the affinity of ligand binding without signaling; β and γ subunits participate in both ligand binding and signal transduction. Phosphorylation of the cytoplasmic domains of the β- and γ-subunits of the IL-2R provides docking sites for JAK1/3, resulting in docking and phosphorylation STAT3 and STAT5. Phosphorylation induces dimerization and nuclear translocation of STAT3 and STAT5 complexes, where they promote specific target gene transcription. The IL-2R signals through at least three different pathways, which mediate proliferation and survival: Ras/MAPK and Syk lead to expression of the protooncogenes c-Fos, c-Jun, and Elk, and the protein tyrosine pathway results in BCL2 expression and antiapoptosis. IL-2 also activates Lck, which is involved in T cell receptor signaling.[14]

BCL2, B-cell leukemia-2; IL, interleukin; JAK, Janus kinase; Lck, lymphocyte-specific protein tyrosine kinase; MAPK, mitogen-activated protein kinase; STAT, signal transducer and activator of transcription.

immune-mediated cure. High-dose IL-2 (HD-IL-2) was the mainstay of first-line treatment for advanced melanoma and RCC for at least a decade, until the first trials of angiogenesis-directed kinase inhibitors (TKI) for RCC demonstrated high regression rates and tolerability for long-term exposure, which moved the TKIs into frontline therapy for RCC, increased the fraction of patients who could be treated safely, and opened the field to investigations of so-called personalized therapy approaches based on predictive biomarkers for benefit from specific therapies and the ideal sequencing of therapies in RCC.[18] Analogous events in advanced melanoma—the advent

of ICB, first with CTLA-4 and then PD-1 blockade followed by their combination—also rendered high-dose IL-2 nearly obsolete, as the safety and activity of the ICBs far exceeded those of high-dose IL-2 (although those of IL-2 are more acute and reversible, while the toxicities of ICB can begin at any time and may be permanent). Although there are now data supporting the use of high-dose IL-2 after failure of ICB, the patient numbers are small, patients highly-selected, and therapeutic index still unsatisfactory.[19–24] Current efforts are directed at defining the role of molecular characteristics of the tumor, particularly the driver and passenger mutations in various subsets of melanoma and other cancers, that would segregate patients into those more likely to benefit from IL-2-based regimens and those best treated with ICBs. The main clinical scenario in which high-dose IL-2 is still administered routinely is as a limited number of doses following cell infusion of various adoptive cell transfer (ACT) products to maintain the survival, expansion and function of the therapeutic cells.

The rapidly growing body of preclinical evidence suggesting synergy between γ_c cytokines and ICB[25] have provided the rationale for new studies in development that combine these two classes of agents and evaluate less intensive doses and schedules of IL-2 administration. Also in development are a series of engineered γ_c receptor cytokines with more favorable characteristics for clinical administration than aldesleukin or native IL-15. The engineered IL-2/IL-15 cytokines, characterized by predominant signaling through their common $\beta\gamma_c$ receptor complex, are detailed in the next section of this chapter.

Engineered IL-2 Molecules

Other approaches have been taken to enhance the activity and/or reduce the toxicities of HD-IL-2 by combining the cytokine with inhibitors of inflammatory toxicity mediators (produced by cells of the endothelium and monocyte-macrophage lineage in response to IFN-γ secreted by IL-2-stimulated CD4+ and CD8+ T cells) such as TNF-α, IL-1, inducible nitric oxide synthase, selected fatty acid intermediates, or vascular endothelial growth factor, but these efforts have so far failed to improve the therapeutic index;[26–30] other combinations designed to synergize with IL-2 and thus potentially lower the need for high doses of the cytokine or otherwise bias the effect towards antigen-specific effector CD8+ cells were also disappointing.[31–33]

Molecular engineering has been used to create bempegaldesleukin, a polyethylene glycol (PEG)-modified aldesleukin featuring enhanced binding to the $\beta\gamma_c$ receptor complex and thus to decrease T_{reg} cell activation and AICD that retains its potent stimulation of effector CD8+ and NK cell cytotoxicity at lower concentrations than required for native aldesleukin in HD-IL-2 regimens. Bempegaldesleukin was designed to be active and less toxic than therapeutic doses of aldesleukin when given as a single agent or in combinations with other immunomodulatory therapies.[34] These strategies parallel other engineering approaches to enhance the other $\beta\gamma_c$ receptor binder, IL-15, detailed in the following section. The PEGylation of bempegaldesleukin occurs at 6 non-random lysine residues within the α receptor-binding domain that are slowly hydrolyzed *in vivo* to yield a mono-or di-PEGylated IL-2 that preferentially binds to the $\beta\gamma_c$ receptor while the α receptor binding site remains partially blocked by remaining PEG. In preclinical

models, the enhanced CD8+:T_{reg} ratio within the immune tumor microenvironment (TME) provided superior antitumor effects compared with the parent aldesleukin and a much longer half-life.[35] While bempegaldesleukin had insufficient single-agent activity to warrant its use in patients whose tumors had progressed on PD-1 blockade, a combination of bempegaldesleukin with nivolumab as front-line therapy for melanoma and several other solid tumors appears superior to the activity of PD-1 blockade alone[36,37] and may support a combination with higher antitumor effects but lacking the added immune-mediated toxicity of adding CTLA-1 blockade to PD-1 antibody therapy. Pursuing the same reasoning, it is possible that safe doses of bempegaldesleukin could be added to a backbone of lower-dose CTLA-4 and PD-1 blockade in a regimen with maximum immune-mediated antitumor effects and minimum immune-related toxicity. At this time, Phase III combination trials are ongoing in untreated advanced melanoma (versus nivolumab) and renal cancer (versus investigator choice among sunitinib, cabozantinib or nivolumab) patients (NCT 03635983 and 03729245), and Phase II trials to test its activity and potential for further study of bempegaldesleukin in combination with nivolumab are also underway in patients with sarcoma or bladder cancer (NCT 03729245 03282344). Combination bempegaldesleukin with nivolumab and ipilimumab (NCT 02983045) or nivolumab plus a novel PEGylated Toll 7/8-receptor agonist given intratumorally (NCT03435640) are also underway.

Another PEGylated IL-2 has been designed that contains an amino acid substitution in the α receptor-binding domain and a single PEG molecule at this site that interferes with binding to the α receptor, resulting in a "not alpha" IL-2 with strong bias toward the desired binding of $\beta\gamma_c$ on target CD8+ and NK cells,[38] and this agent has recently entered clinical trials.

Several other IL-2 structures have been designed that retain the desirable features of the native molecule while reducing or eliminating the undesirable effects of binding to the IL-2 receptor α chain, and some of these structures incorporate elements that direct the active IL-2 moiety to a specific site where its function is sequestered or enhanced: for example, Alks 4230 contains a fusion of circularly-permuted IL-2 with the extracellular domain of the IL-2 α receptor that blocks binding of the molecule to the cellular high-affinity IL-2 receptor and thus biases the cytokine towards $\beta\gamma_c$ functions;[39] this molecule is currently being evaluated in combination with the PD-1 antibody pembrolizumab (NCT 02799095 and 03861793). The L19IL-2 molecule is a human fusion protein consisting of the L19 antibody against fibronectin fused to human interleukin-2;[40] FAP:IL-2 is a mutein IL-2 (3 residues altered) fused to fibroblast-activating protein (FAP) that was designed to concentrate the activity of IL-2 in the TME of FAP-expressing tumors (many carcinomas plus sarcomas and melanoma) as well as cells of the TME such as mesenchymal stem cells and cancer-associated fibroblasts.[41] The FAP-IL-2 bifunctional molecule is currently in trials with ICB (PD-1 or PD-L1 antibody) for several solid tumors as well as with disease-directed antibodies trastuzumab and cetuximab for Her2+ breast and squamous cancer of the head and neck, respectively (NCT 03386721, 03193190, 03424005, 03875079, 02627274, and 03063762).

Structure and Function of Other T Cell Immunomodulatory Cytokines

Interleukin-15 and Its Engineered Derivatives

Recombinant IL-15, rhIL-15

IL-15 along with its α receptor (IL-15R) is synthesized by APCs, which chaperones the IL-15RA to the cell surface,

where it is presented in cell-bound form to cells expressing the common $\beta\gamma_c$ used by IL-2.[42] These differences in the structure and presentation of their α receptors account for major differences in how the two cytokines function distinctly. In contrast with the predominant physiologic T cell growth factor function of IL-2, IL-15 functions in homeostatic fashion as a growth factor for NK cells and memory CD8+ T cells. IL-15 also lacks two of the suppressive or regulatory functions of IL-2 that are therapeutic disadvantages in cancer—the stimulation of T_{reg} cell expansion (through the high-affinity $\alpha\beta\gamma_c$ receptor specific for IL-2, which is expressed constitutively on T_{reg} cells but only transiently on activated CD8+ T cells) and the promotion of AICD.[43]

Figure 24.4[44] illustrates the action of IL-15, which is critical to the generation of durable, high avidity, memory CD8+ T cells.

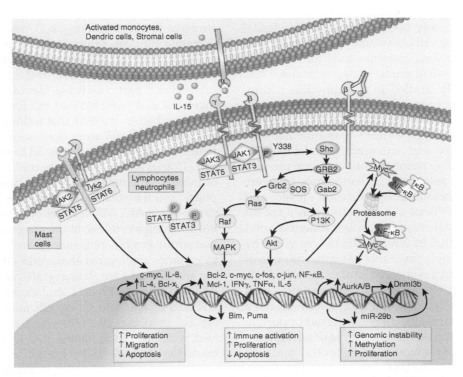

Figure 24.4 **Schematic illustration of IL-15 signaling and resulting downstream transcriptional products.** In one scenario (right), IL-15 binds to its high affinity IL-15Rα expressed on an APC and in turn is presented *in trans* to the IL-2/15Rβγ heterodimer. Effector cell activation can then proceed via three distinct pathways: JAK-STAT activation with the phosphorylated STAT proteins forming a heterodimer and trafficking to the nucleus for transcriptional activation; a second recruits Shc to a phosphorylated site on the IL-2/15Rβ chain followed by activation of Grb2. Grb2 can activate PI3K, phosphorylate AKT, or can bind the guanine nucleotide exchange factor SOS to activate RAS-RAF and MAPK. Each leads to effector cell survival and activation. In mast cells (left), IL-15 signals through a unique receptor chain, IL-15RX, to activate the JAK2/STAT5 pathway. IL-15 can also bind to the common γ chain to transmit its signals via Tyk2/STAT6 for initiation of a survival (BCL-X$_L$) and a Th2 immune response.

DC, dendritic cell; IFNγ, interferon γ; IL, interleukin; JAK, Janus kinase; NF-κB, nuclear factor-κB; NK, natural killer; NKT, natural killer T cells; STAT, signal transducers and activators of transcription; TNF-α, tumor necrosis factor-α; TSLP, thymic stromal lymphopoietin; TSLPR, TSLP receptor.

Source: Adapted from Mishra A, Sullivan L, Caligiuri MA. Molecular pathways: interleukin-15 signaling in health and in cancer. *Clin Cancer Res.* 2014;20(8):2044–2050. doi:10.1158/1078-0432.CCR-12-3603

When used in large doses and altered patterns of exposure such as in cancer therapy regimens, IL-15, which lacks the T_{reg} cell and AICD functions of IL-2, could potentially stimulate T cell clones cytotoxic for self-antigen-expressing cells and thus result in immune toxicities similar to those of the immune checkpoint blocking antibodies, particularly CTLA-4 blockade.[45] Indeed, "disordered" IL-15 activity has been associated with promotion of malignancy and of autoimmune diseases and may be a therapeutic target for immunomodulatory strategies to suppress IL-15 signaling.[46–48] To date, preliminary study results with various IL-15-based agents (summarized in the text that follows) have not confirmed this concern, possibly because the main focus of current approaches is to use IL-15 in support of antigen-directed regimens, taking advantage of CD8+ cell epitope-specificity as well as the powerful ADCC functions mediated by NK cells expanded and stimulated by IL-15, particularly the engineered IL-15 agonists that also contain an IgG Fc fragment. Synergy between IL-15 and ICB antibodies has already been observed in preclinical models,[49] and it will be critical to analyze the short- and long-term toxicities of these combinations for the emergence of new or excessive immune-related toxicities.

IL-15 was originally studied in its unmodified form, using the recombinant human molecule (rhIL-15) grown in *Esherichia coli* cells and administered intravenously on a daily schedule because of its short ~40-minute half-life. At doses that expanded and activated NK cells from 10 to 50 times their baseline numbers and cytokine production, the cytokine was associated with moderate to severe IL-2-like toxicities, including hypotension, fever, and thrombocytopenia[50] without clinical activity in a cohort of heavily pretreated patients with an assortment of solid tumors. A follow-on trial in which rhIL-15 was given by daily s.c. injection to more favorable patients with one of four different malignancies showed similar immunologic effects and no objective responses,[51] suggesting again that IL-15, like other T cell modulatory cytokines, is not a stand-alone therapy but is most likely to play a supportive role in other combinatorial regimens, some of which were already detailed in the previous section on IL-2 and will be further mentioned in the text that follows. The observation of an association between remissions and high serum levels of IL-15 among patients with B cell lymphomas achieving remission in response to CD19-chimeric antigen receptor (CAR) T cells suggests that an important role of IL-15 in cancer therapy is also as a growth factor for cytotoxic effector cells with antigen-specificity.[52]

Engineered Derivatives of IL-15

Several forms of IL-15 that exploit the unique physiologic features of its trans-presentation on APCs and its signaling via the $\beta\gamma_c$ receptor common to IL-2 and IL-15 have been engineered and demonstrated proof of concept for

their superiority over native IL-15—superior antitumor activity, longer half-life, synergy with other immunomodulators, and lack of immunogenicity. The IL-15-binding domain of IL-15RA has been named the "sushi" domain, and IL-15 structures containing the entire α receptor or its sushi domain are termed "superagonists" or IL-15SAs.[53] The enhanced IL-15SA that has been tested in the largest number of patients and combination strategies is the ALT-803/N-803 molecule (hereafter called by its original name, ALT-803), a complex of two molecules of IL-15 with enhanced $\beta\gamma_c$ receptor binding conferred by the N72D substitution, associated to two molecules of IL-15Rα sushi fused with one human IgG1Fc fragment that contributes the most to prolonging the half-life to ~25 hours in the circulation and may also contribute to the immunotherapeutic potential of the complex by activating NK cells through Fc receptor binding.[54] Initial studies of ALT-803 were designed in part based on the experience of rhIL-15 and the desire to create a molecule with a longer half-life, stronger IL-15RA binding, and unimpaired binding and signaling function through the $\beta\gamma_c$ receptor. The preclinical experience of ALT-803 was remarkably favorable in showing its superiority over rhIL-15 in multiple preclinical models,[55] particularly bladder cancer, colon cancer, and myeloma, that provided the basis for the ongoing trials that are described in the text that follows. The Phase I safety studies of ALT-803 were done in one trial of pretreated patients with the same four solid tumors treated in the s.c. rhIL-15 trial and in a separate trial for patients in relapse of hematologic malignancy following allogeneic hematopoietic cell transplant. While there was little activity with single-agent ALT-803 in either of these settings, the potential for using a cytokine in the allogeneic transplant setting that stimulates NK cells more than T cells may be optimal to enhance graft-versus-leukemia effects while minimizing the risk of stimulating graft-versus-host syndromes. ALT-803 in these Phase I studies, like rhIL-15, expanded NK cells several-fold, CD8+ cells modestly, and stimulated NK cell cytokines like IFN-γ when given at doses associated with mild to moderate IL-2-like effects.[50] In patients treated with ALT-803 by the s.c. route, a local injection reaction characterized as large, tender wheals with histologic evidence of lymphocytic and monocytic infiltrates suggested the ability of IL-15 to induce the influx of T cells and mononuclear cells with therapeutic activity in sites of tumor metastases.[56,57] ALT-803 also showed synergy in preclinical models with immune checkpoint blockade[49,58] and provided the rationale for current Phase II studies of this cytokine in combination with PD-1 blockade, which preliminarily showed activity in lung cancer[59] and is now in Phase III with pembrolizumab versus pembrolizumab alone (NCT 03520686).

Uniquely, ALT-803 has also been studied as intravesical therapy in non-muscle-invasive bladder cancer (NMIBC), where it had potent activity in preclinical models and can be given safely in combination with intravesical bacillus Calmette-Guerin (BCG), the standard therapy for early bladder cancer.[60] It is possible that the first setting in which ALT-803 will demonstrate sufficient activity to fill an unmet need and thus qualify for FDA approval will be in patients with NMIBC in combination with BCG.

Interleukin-7

IL-7, a single-chain 20 kD protein, is a homeostatic growth factor for naïve and memory T cells that promotes proliferation and supports antigen responses, in part by preventing and reversing anergy and modulating expression of exhaustion molecules, including PD-1.[42,43] IL-7 also plays a key role in lymph node organogenesis, T cell homing to lymph nodes, and development of secondary lymphoid organs in nonlymphoid tissues.[61] The IL-7 receptor has no β chain, and its cytokine-specific α-receptor (CD127) interacts directly with the γ_c receptor to stimulate signaling through JAK1/3 and STAT5 as well as the PI3K/AKT pathways, with the resulting upregulation of cell cycle molecules, metabolic enhancers like glucose transporter 1 (GLUT-1), and the antiapoptotic molecules BCL-2 and Mcl-1.

IL-7 is produced mainly by thymic and lymph node stromal cells, and it promotes the survival of naïve and memory T cells. IL-7, along with IL-15, is a "homeostatic cytokine" that tightly regulates the number and function of circulating T lymphocytes—mainly CD8+ T cells—in normal and pathologic states and modulates the effector-to-memory transition.[62] IL-7 also increases TCR diversity and stimulates antigen-specific vaccine responses, and it promotes the expansion of conventional over regulatory T cells.[63] The production of both of the homeostatic cytokines, IL-7 and IL-15, is elevated during lymphopenia and suppressed during lymphocytosis. Animal models have shown enhancement of the activity of tumor antigen-specific CTL used for ACT by in vitro culture with IL-7 and IL-15, and IL-7 has also shown activity in animal models and limited human subject studies, given by a variety of routes, schedules, and vectors.[61]

The clinical development of IL-7 is ongoing. The early trials of recombinant IL-7 in cancer patients showed that the cytokine was safe without dose-limiting toxicities and expanded T cell repertoire and circulating CD8+ and CD4+ T cells, while reducing T_{reg} cell percentage and suppressive function.[64,65] IL-7 is now undergoing further investigation in combination with an approved DC-based prostate cancer vaccine comprised of a prostatic acid phosphatase:GM-CSF fusion protein that triggers antigen-specific T cell responses and B cell epitope spread that has been associated with improved outcomes.[66,67] The trial (clinicaltrials.gov NCT01881867) was designed to test whether IL-7 mediates broadening and deepening of the T cell response and improves the modest antitumor

activity of the vaccine as well as other immune responses while avoiding the nonspecific or off target immune-related toxicities of other immunomodulatory agents. Results from this completed trial are currently undergoing analysis (Fong L., personal communication).

Until IL-7 and IL-15 become commercially available, an alternative strategy to achieve T cell repertoire enhancement as well as the other desired activities of these cytokines is to use lymphodepleting chemotherapy, generally consisting of high-dose cyclophosphamide and fludarabine, to dramatically reduce the circulating lymphocyte count and thus trigger a reactive increase in the levels of homeostatic cytokines IL-7 and IL-15 until lymphoid reconstitution is achieved. The latter approach has been used extensively in ACT regimens, based on preclinical evidence that lymphodepletion/homeostatic reconstitution of antigen-specific effector T cells is a critical element of these multicomponent regimens.[68]

Interleukin-21

IL-21, another well-studied γ_c receptor cytokine with therapeutic potential in human cancer, is a pleiotropic molecule produced predominantly by CD4+ T cells (particularly the TFH, or follicular helper cells, and Th17, or IL-17-secreting subsets) and natural killer T (NKT) cells. IL-21 regulates effector functions of T cells, NK cells, and B cells. IL-21 actions include co-stimulation of B cell differentiation and immunoglobulin (Ig) production, cooperating as a T cell mitogen, and stimulation of NK and CD8+ T cell cytotoxic function. Like IL-15, IL-21 can promote antitumor cytotoxic CD8+ T cell functions without stimulating T_{reg} cells or AICD, likely due to differences in signal transduction by the γ_c receptor that are impacted by its binding to the cytokine-specific α-receptor:cytokine complex.[69]

IL-21 is a single-chain molecule with a unique α receptor that signals through γ_c to activate JAK1/JAK3 and STATs 1, 5a, 5b, and, most potently, STAT3 (see Figure 24.5).[69] IL-21 also signals through PI3K/AKT, which leads to mTOR activation. Although IL-21, along with IL-4, has a critical role in support of normal B cell differentiation and production of Ig, IL-21 also exerts a regulatory effect on B cells, inducing their apoptosis, a process that may be analogous to IL-2 in stimulating effector cells but also contributing to their physiologic regulation to avoid host damage associated with an excessive or autoreactive action. The other unique effects of IL-21 include its stimulation of B cell antitumor cytotoxicity (presumably nonantigen-specific, analogous to NK cell cytotoxicity and similarly mediated by cytotoxic granules such as granzyme B) and a paradoxical inhibition of GM-CSF-induced DC activation and maturation—again possibly in a cross counterregulatory fashion with GM-CSF. The net effect of exogenous IL-21 on antitumor immune responses is difficult to predict, because of the multiple

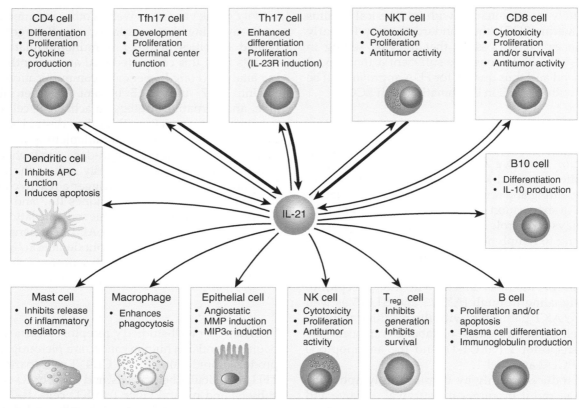

Figure 24.5 Sources of IL-21 and its cellular targets. IL-21 is produced by CD4+ T cell populations, with the highest production by TFH cells and Th17 cells, and slightly lower levels produced by NKT cells (bold arrows). CD8+ T cells can also produce IL-21. IL-21 exerts actions on multiple lymphoid and myeloid populations as well as on epithelial cells. The consequences of IL-21 signaling in each cell type are listed.

APC, antigen-presenting cell; IL-23R, interleukin-23 receptor; MIP3α, macrophage inflammatory protein 3α; MMP, matrix metalloproteinase; NKT, natural killer T; TFH, T follicular helper; T_reg, regulatory T.

Source: Adapted from Spolski R, Leonard WJ. Interleukin-21: a double-edged sword with therapeutic potential. *Nat Rev Drug Discov*. 2014;13(5):379–395. doi:10.1038/nrd4296

and potentially opposing effects detailed previously and also to its support of CD4+ subsets that contribute to the regulation of B cell biology (follicular helper, TFH, cells) and inflammatory Th17 cells. The effects of IL-21 on conventional CD8+ T cells include its support of an earlier, less differentiated memory CD8+ T cell subset with enhanced in vivo persistence, and the induction of CD8+ T cell expression of granzyme B. IL-21 also promotes NK cell ADCC and NKT cell function and showed synergy with the other important γ_c cytokines IL-2 and IL-15 in animal models of transplantable tumors.[70,71]

IL-21 has undergone extensive early testing in patients with malignancy and has shown modest clinical activity (5%–22% objective response rates) in pretreated patients with renal cancer and melanoma,[72–74] but its evaluation as an in vivo therapeutic was superseded by the advent of immune checkpoint blocking antibodies and other highly active immunotherapy strategies in these patients. Initial trials of combination IL-21 with CTLA-4 blockade showed hepatotoxicity that did not permit dose escalation to levels

likely to be needed for anticancer activity (Thompson, J.A., unpublished observations). Nevertheless, important in vitro synergy with other γ_c cytokines and the unique characteristics of IL-21 support its further exploration in preparation of the effector cell product for ACT.[75]

Interleukin-4

IL-4, while highly pleiotropic like IL-21, has important effects on B cell function as well as on T cells, and it is the only well-characterized cytokine in the γ_c receptor family with predominantly immunomodulatory effects that support type 2-polarized immune responses. While IL-4 shares the γ_c chain with the other members of this family, all of which support cytotoxic and/or homeostatic T cell responses, the α receptor of IL-4 is the same as that of IL-13, a type 2 cytokine that signals through a second, unique α1 receptor and mainly supports allergic inflammatory responses.[76] Unexpectedly, IL-4 was one cytokine that showed antitumor effects when expressed transgenically in tumor cells as a form of autologous cancer vaccine[77]—an approach that eventually led to the broader use of GM-CSF transduction of tumor cells, which is still showing promise in selected tumors. On the basis of additional preclinical activity of IL-4 as a single agent and in combination with IL-2, IL-4 was taken into the clinic soon after the discovery of IL-2's remarkable properties and antitumor activity. However, IL-4 failed to demonstrate sufficient activity in the settings in which it was tested; in view of its polarization toward type 2 responses as well as the presence of IL-4 receptors in a wide variety of tumor cells, it is unlikely that this cytokine has a place in in vivo therapy of cancer but continues to be used in vitro in combination with GM-CSF in the preparation of DC from peripheral blood-derived mononuclear cells[78] to use as APCs for tumor vaccines.

Interleukin-9

IL-9, initially purified and characterized as a T cell and mast cell growth factor, is a pleiotropic cytokine that has documented effects on lymphocytes, mast cells, and resident lung macrophages. It has been mostly associated with allergic inflammation and immunity to extracellular parasites, although developing literature has demonstrated a role for IL-9 or IL-9–responsive cells in Th1/Th17-mediated inflammation and in T_{reg} cell responses. The factors required for IL-9 production in T cells are only beginning to be elucidated and require the integration of signals from multiple cytokines. IL-9 is produced by long-term T cell lines, antigen-specific T cell lines, and naïve murine T cells,[79] IL-9 production was initially associated with the Th2 phenotype, and many of the preliminary functions of IL-9 were tested in models of Th2-associated immunity.[80] It is unclear, however, if there are specialized cells programmed for IL-9 production as has been established for other cytokines such as IL-4 and IFNγ in Th2 and Th1 cells, respectively.[81] Naïve CD4+ T cells primed in vitro in the presence of TGF-β and IL-4 or Th2 cells in the presence of TGF-β secreted high levels of IL-9 and displayed low expression of other transcription factors and lineage-specific cytokines.[82] The ability of IL-4 to inhibit expression of Foxp3 in cultures containing TGF-β, which mediated the generation of inducible T_{reg} cells, and to promote an IL-9-secreting phenotype was dependent on STAT6. Likewise, the transcription factor GATA3 was required for the generation of IL-9-secreting cells, suggesting that Th2 cells, and the IL-9-secreting population termed Th9 cells, have shared factors in their development. In addition, human T cells cultured in the presence of TGF-β and IL-4 acquire IL-9-secreting capacity. The stability of the IL-9-secreting phenotype is still not well described, although several studies suggest that Th9 cells can be maintained, but remain highly plastic and able to acquire additional cytokine-secreting capacity.[83–85]

Thymic Stromal Lymphopoietin

Originally shown to promote the growth and activation of B cells, TSLP is an epithelial cell-derived cytokine that exerts its biological function through TSLP receptor (TSLPR). TSLP is known to have wide-ranging effects on both hematopoietic and nonhematopoietic cell lineages, including DCs, basophils, eosinophils, mast cells, CD4+ and CD8+ T cells, NKT cells, B cells, and epithelial cells. While TSLP's role in the promotion of Th2 responses has been extensively studied in the context of lung- and skin-specific allergic disorders, it has become increasingly clear that it may be involved in multiple disease states within multiple organ systems, including the blockade of Th1/Th17 responses and the regulation of cancer and autoimmunity. TSLP genetic variants and its dysregulated expression have been linked to atopic diseases such as atopic dermatitis and asthma.[86] In a breast cancer model, the inflammatory properties of TSLP have been associated with oncogenic capacity.[87] In addition, independent studies showed that TSLP-mediated inflammation can be tumor suppressive in two mouse models of skin cancer.[88,89] To study skin carcinogenesis in these mouse models, skin-specific expression of Cre recombinase to inactivate genes involved in NOTCH signaling was used. In the skin, NOTCH signaling is typically tumor suppressive. Deletion of NOTCH signaling led to the development of noncancerous skin lesions, which were inflammatory owing to the expression of TSLP by the keratinocytes. Surprisingly, the subsequent inactivation of TSLP signaling led to malignant skin lesions, suggesting that it can suppress the tumorigenic effects of NOTCH signaling disruption in the skin. The reconstitution of TSLPR-deficient mice with wild-type bone marrow restored the tumor-suppressive effects, indicating that the hematopoietic cells responding to TSLP were responsible for its antitumor activity. These observations highlight the context-dependent activity of TSLP signaling in cancer and suggest caution in the current development of TSLP-based therapeutics.

IL-12

This immunomodulatory cytokine entered the clinic early in the era of recombinant cytokine-based therapies based on its powerful induction of IFN-γ and type 1 polarized immune responses mediated by effector NK and T cells.[2] It was anticipated that the systemic administration of pure IL-12 could provide the type of stimulus to immune effector cells that normally depends on the interaction between APC stimulated by a variety of ligands—such as tumor cell-derived damage-associated molecules interacting with pattern-recognition receptors—and tumor and effector cells. These events lead to potent stimulation of IFN-γ, which, along with effector cell-derived perforin and granzyme, is one of the most critical molecules in antitumor cytotoxicity. However, recombinant human IL-12 in its unmodified form proved to have a very unfavorable therapeutic index, characterized by toxic inflammatory effects, especially fevers and hepatotoxicity,[90] which led investigators to seek alternative ways to exploit IL-12 via innovative delivery methods. Thus, IL-12 was the first cytokine to be investigated using a form of molecular engineering that involves the insertion of its gene into a bacterial plasmid that is administered intratumorally by injection followed by local electroporation, using a small electrical current that transiently permeabilizes the tumor cells and promotes the expression of the IL-12 gene in tumor cells. Initial studies of the IL-12/plasmid/electroporation strategy provided evidence of antitumor activity and proof of principle for the proposed mechanism of action, including the ability to induce an abscopal response at distant, uninjected tumor sites.[91,92] This agent, now called Tavokinogene telseplasmid, is now being investigated in combination with PD-1 blockade for melanoma after progression on PD-1 blockade alone (NCT 03132675). Another form of IL-12 intratumoral administration is via IL-12 gene delivery in a novel Newcastle disease virus vector,[93] which will enter clinical trials soon. All of these methods for intratumoral delivery of IL-12 are designed to create a locoregional lymphoid follicle in which antigen taken up and presented by APC along with the appropriate co-stimulatory signals can prime and stimulate effector cell cytotoxicity, mediated by both CD8+ and NK cell subsets.

CONCLUSION

The γ_c cytokines are a family of proteins that control the activities of lymphocytes of the innate and adaptive immune system, predominantly acting on T cells. While the physiologic roles of these cytokines relate to the development of immunologic memory and to immunosurveillance and cytotoxic activity against invading pathogens, including the emergence of immunologic memory, they also contribute to host protection against malignancy. Paradoxically, however, selected γ_c cytokines also contribute to chronic inflammation that supports malignant transformation and the propagation of tumors, related in part to their promotion of suppressive cells and their secretory products. However, selected γ_c cytokines have been used successfully in cancer immunotherapy and have been employed in a variety of routes, including systemic administration, intratumoral injection, and in vitro expansion of therapeutic cell products. The first and foremost of these therapeutically valuable γ_c cytokines is IL-2, used in many doses and schedules to support effector cells both in vivo and as part of ACTs. While high-dose IL-2 alone is approved in advanced melanoma and renal cancer, its therapeutic index is unfavorable and its use has been replaced in a large part by the more active and less toxic immune checkpoint blocking antibodies. However, IL-2 may find a role in combination regimens with these

antibodies or other immunomodulators. IL-7 may have clinical potential in the expansion of T cells and immune reconstitution, while IL-4 appears to be valuable in the production of therapeutic DC products for cancer vaccines. IL-15 has recently demonstrated a high potential to stimulate the expansion and cytotoxicity of NK and CD8+ T cells. When administered in one of its optimized forms of delivery—bound to its cytokine-specific α receptor—IL-15 may have potential similar to IL-2 with fewer undesirable effects such as activation-induced T cell death and stimulation of T_{reg} cells. One form of IL-15, bound to its α-receptor and an IgG1 Fc receptor, has a long half-life in vivo, expands NK and CD8+ T cells, and has demonstrated a favorable safety profile when given intravenously, subcutaneously, or intravesically and has shown early evidence of antitumor activity in patients with several malignancies. This and other γ_c cytokines are now being studied in combinations with other immunomodulatory agents that are likely to have powerful antitumor effects in the future management of a wide variety of malignancies.

KEY REFERENCES

Only key references appear in the print edition. The full reference list appears in the digital product on Springer Publishing Connect: connect.springerpub.com/content/book/978-0-8261-3743-2/part/part02/chapter/ch24

19. Atkins MB, Lotze MT, Dutcher JP, et al. High-dose recombinant interleukin 2 therapy for patients with metastatic melanoma: analysis of 270 patients treated between 1985 and 1993. *J Clin Oncol.* 1999;17(7):2105–2116. doi:10.1200/JCO.1999.17.7.2105

35. Charych DH, Hoch U, Langowski JL, et al. NKTR-214, an engineered cytokine with biased IL-2 receptor binding, increased tumor exposure, and marked efficacy in mouse tumor models. *Clin Cancer Res.* 2016;22(3):680–690. doi:10.1158/1078-0432.CCR-15-1631

37. Bentebibel SE, Hurwitz ME, Bernatchez C, et al. A first-in-human study and biomarker analysis of NKTR-214, a Novel IL2Rβγ-biased cytokine, in patients with advanced or metastatic solid tumors. *Cancer Discov.* 2019;9(6):711–721. doi:10.1158/2159-8290.CD-18-1495

51. Miller JS, Morishima C, Mcneel DG, et al. A first-in-human Phase I study of subcutaneous outpatient recombinant human IL-15 (rhIL15) in adults with advanced solid tumors. *Clin Cancer Res.* 2018;24(7):1525–1535. doi:10.1158/1078-0432.CCR-17-2451

65. Sportès C, Babb RR, Krumlauf MC, et al. Phase I study of recombinant human interleukin-7 administration in subjects with refractory malignancy. *Clin Cancer Res.* 2010;16(2):727–735. doi:10.1158/1078-0432.CCR-09-1303

73. Thompson JA, Curti BD, Redman BG, et al. Phase I study of recombinant interleukin-21 in patients with metastatic melanoma and renal cell carcinoma. *J Clin Oncol.* 2008;26(12):2034–2039. doi:10.1200/JCO.2007.14.5193

75. Chapuis AG, Roberts IM, Thompson JA, et al. T-cell therapy using interleukin-21-primed cytotoxic T-cell lymphocytes combined with cytotoxic T-cell lymphocyte antigen-4 blockade results in long-term cell persistence and durable tumor regression. *J Clin Oncol.* 2016;34(31):3787–3795. doi:10.1200/JCO.2015.65.5142

76. May RD, Fung M. Strategies targeting the IL-4/IL-13 axes in disease. *Cytokine.* 2015;75(1):89–116. doi:10.1016/j.cyto.2015.05.018

Non-Engineered Adoptive T Cell Therapy

Farah Hasan and Cassian Yee

KEY POINTS

- Non-engineered adoptive cell transfer (ACT) is a cancer immunotherapy modality rooted in the premise that there are endogenous/existing tumor-reactive T cells that can be isolated and expanded in sufficient quantity and quality for infusion into patients, with the expectation that they will kill tumor cells and provide long-term immunoprotection.

- When combined with a lymphodepleting preconditioning regimen and a rapid expansion protocol, tumor-infiltrating lymphocyte (TIL) therapy has achieved durable responses in a subset of patients with advanced cancers, in particular metastatic melanoma.

- Endogenous T cell (ETC) therapy sources tumor antigen-specific T cells from the peripheral blood and can achieve durable responses without the use of high-dose lymphodepleting preconditioning regimens or post-infusion high-dose Interleukin-2 (IL-2).

- Challenges to application of ACT to broader patient populations include the identification of immunogenic target antigens while minimizing off-tumor toxicity, poor trafficking to and infiltration of tumor sites, and an immune-evasive, hostile tumor microenvironment.

- Combination of ACT with therapies such as checkpoint blockade, oncolytic viruses, or low-dose radiotherapy, as well as intrinsic strategies that influence T cell phenotype and function, may be used to increase the efficacy of ACT by promoting antigen spreading, improved trafficking, function, and *in vivo* persistence.

- γδ T cells have potential for antitumor activity against a broad range of tumor types, and their major histocompatibility complex (MHC)-independence reduces requirements for human leukocyte antigen (HLA)-matching while enabling them to treat tumors that escape the conventional T cell response via MHC downregulation.

INTRODUCTION

Adoptive cell transfer (ACT) is a form of cellular immunotherapy whereby tumor-reactive T cells are enriched and expanded ex vivo for the treatment of patients with cancer. This approach has become an increasingly attractive treatment modality due to its potential for high specificity, combination with other therapies, and promise of long-term immunoprotection against disease recurrence. The effector cells used for ACT may be derived from peripheral blood T cells (endogenous T cell therapy) or tumor-infiltrating lymphocytes (TIL therapy), or genetically engineered to express receptors that recognize tumor antigens (TCR-engineered T cell therapy and chimeric antigen receptor T cell [CAR T] therapy). This chapter will focus on non-engineered ACT modalities whereby the structures and signaling involved in antigen recognition and T cell activation are unadulterated; in contrast to engineered T cell approaches, non-engineered T cell therapies can offer greater flexibility in tumor targeting and opportunity for combination strategies that can lead to functional enhancement, antigen spreading, and increased T cell persistence. A variety of non-engineered ACT approaches are under clinical investigation and these are summarized in Figure 25.1.

THE BEGINNINGS OF ADOPTIVE T CELL THERAPY

Adoptive cellular immunotherapy for cancer is arguably rooted in early studies on stem cell transplantation, perhaps the crudest form of ACT, to treat leukemia in a murine model.[1] The original intent behind this therapy was to ablate the abnormal, cancerous bone marrow (leukemia) and reconstitute it with normal donor marrow. In human (allogeneic) studies, it was observed that transplant recipients who developed graft-versus-host disease trended to lower rates of relapse, and that this phenomenon was dependent on the presence of donor T cells, suggesting their role in this antileukemia effect.[2-5] In the 1970s, studies at the University of Washington showed that splenocytes from mice whose tumors had regressed could be used in conjunction with cyclophosphamide to treat tumors in recipient mice.[6,7] Simultaneously, studies on a T cell growth factor present in conditioned media of stimulated lymphocytes

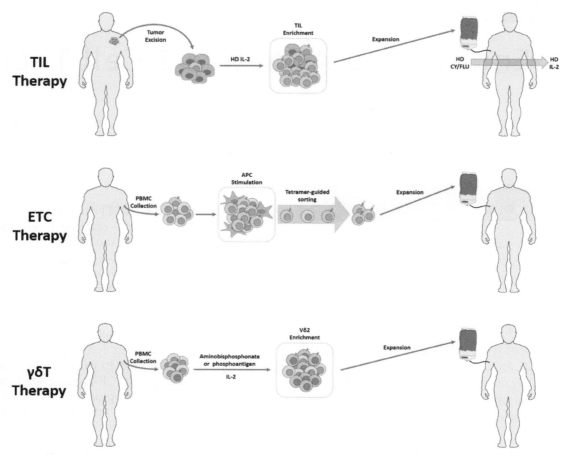

Figure 25.1 Non-engineered adoptive T cell therapy approaches. Tumor-reactive T cells used for non-engineered adoptive T cell therapy are derived from peripheral blood mononuclear cells (endogenous T cell and γδT therapies) or tumor-infiltrating lymphocytes (tumor-infiltrating lymphocyte therapy), enriched and expanded ex vivo, and infused to treat patients with cancer.

APC, antigen-presenting cell; ETC, endogenous T cell; IL-2, interleukin-2; PBMC, peripheral blood mononuclear cell; TIL, tumor-infiltrating lymphocyte.

(later characterized as interleukin-2; IL-2) enabled in vitro expansion of antitumor lymphocytes for adoptive transfer, laying the foundation for current adoptive T cell therapy paradigms, and defining three requirements operative in the elimination of cancer: lymphodepletion, a source of effector cells, and helper function.[8–14] In the 1980s, Rosenberg and colleagues at the National Cancer Institute (NCI) demonstrated that systemic administration of recombinant IL-2 could cause durable responses in some patients with metastatic cancer, providing empiric evidence for the existence of endogenous tumor-reactive T cells that can be expanded to mediate tumor regression.[15,16] Since these seminal studies, methods have been developed to isolate and expand antitumor T cells for clinical use and ACT has been actively pursued as a cancer treatment modality.

ADOPTIVE TRANSFER OF TUMOR-INFILTRATING LYMPHOCYTES

Early attempts to generate large numbers of tumor-reactive immune cells for adoptive transfer led to the development of lymphokine-activated killer cells (LAK): peripheral blood lymphocytes endowed with the ability to lyse tumor cells after exposure to IL-2.[17] However, treatment with LAK required very large numbers of cells and administration of toxicity-inducing doses of systemic IL-2 to effectively mediate regression; thus, in order to reduce these requirements, TILs were investigated as a source of more concentrated, potent tumor-reactive lymphocytes.[18,19] The initial murine studies demonstrated that TILs were 50 to 100 times more effective than LAK cells in eliminating established tumors, providing rationale for further development of TILs for the treatment of patients with cancer.[19] The standard approach to TIL expansion for adoptive therapy, pioneered by Rosenberg and colleagues at the Surgery Branch of the NCI, involves resection of tumor tissue dissected into small tumor fragments or enzymatically digested into single-cell suspensions and culture in media containing high-dose IL-2 to enable outgrowth of TILs.[20–22] The TILs can then be harvested and further expanded to numbers sufficient for infusion using a Rapid Expansion

Protocol (REP) of soluble anti-CD3, irradiated feeder cells, and IL-2—a method first established by Riddell and Greenberg and modified by the NCI Surgery Branch for TIL expansion.[22,23]

Tumor-Infiltrating Lymphocyte Therapy: Clinical Experience and Optimization

In a 1988 pilot study treating 12 patients with various advanced cancers with 0, 25, or 50 mg/kg cyclophosphamide, escalating doses of IL-2, and infusion of autologous TIL, two partial responses were observed among the patients who had received cyclophosphamide, mirroring the prior murine studies indicating that enhanced efficacy required pretreatment with cyclophosphamide and co-administration of IL-2.[19,24] Subsequent trials in metastatic melanoma patients produced encouraging results with partial responses in some patients; however, toxic side effects due to the high-dose IL-2 were common, although manageable.[20,25,26] In an effort to increase efficacy and promote engraftment and persistence of the infused TILs, a nonmyeloablative lymphodepleting preconditioning regimen of cyclophosphamide and fludarabine (adapted from stem cell transplant practices) was incorporated into clinical protocol, yielding overall response rates of 38% to 51% and durable responses of 10% to 15%.[27,28] Responses were often accompanied by vitiligo and anterior uveitis—autoimmune destruction of melanocytes in the skin and uvea, which was largely reversible. As desired, these studies provided evidence of in vivo expansion and persistence of the transferred cells; however, in some cases, the endogenous T cell repertoire was replaced almost completely with the transferred TIL population. Addition of total body irradiation (TBI) to this preconditioning regimen in a small cohort of patients reported in 2008 achieved overall response rates of 72% and dramatic and durable complete responses of up to 40%, but the additional benefit of TBI was not confirmed in a follow-up randomized trial in 2016.[29,30] Among major institutions conducting TIL therapy using a "standard" nonmyeloablative regimen of fludarabine and cyclophosphamide (Sheba Medical Center, Moffitt Cancer Center, and MD Anderson Cancer Center), the overall response rate achieved is 40% to 49% with a complete response rate of 6% to 15%.[31–36] Although temporary lymphodepletion prior to infusion seems to benefit TIL therapy, further studies are necessary to determine the optimal regimen to increase efficacy while minimizing toxicity.

The initially established procedure for TIL product generation involved culture in IL-2, selection of tumor-reactive cultures based on reactivity to autologous tumor or HLA-matched tumor cell lines, followed by further expansion, resulting in a lengthy process that could not always successfully generate an infusion product. Thus, many patients ultimately did not receive the therapy because their TIL failed testing for tumor reactivity, there was no tumor material to conduct such tests, or their disease progressed during the TIL production process.[37] To address these limitations, selection based on tumor reactivity was discontinued and a "minimal culture" method was adopted.[38,39] This simplified process reduced production time, increased the success rate for product generation (up to 94% in some series), and produced "young" TIL associated with improved efficacy.[33,37,39,40] Alternatively, the infusion of unselected TIL expanded from tumor fragments in 74 metastatic melanoma patients generated similar response rates (42%), further supporting the absence of benefit from selection based on tumor reactivity for TIL derived from melanoma.[41] Even with these improvements, requirements of tumor fragment excision, specialized production, and optimal management of adverse reactions currently limits TIL therapy to a handful of large medical centers.

Tumor-Infiltrating Lymphocyte Therapy: The Next Stage

TIL products are heterogeneous, containing CD4+ and CD8+ T cells with varying antigen specificity and tumor reactivity, and the composition is unique to each patient, the tumor site, and even intratumoral localization of biopsy sampling.[42] Specificity and efficacy may be improved by enriching for TIL that express markers associated with tumor reactivity. At the NCI, PD-1, which is upregulated following TCR triggering, was used as a selection marker for melanoma-reactive TILs: following PD-1 expression-based sorting and expansion, CD8+ PD-1+ TILs from fresh tumors displayed increased IFN-γ production and cytotoxicity after co-culture with autologous tumor cell lines.[43] Similarly, other groups have shown that expression of CD137 (4-1BB), another T cell-associated activation marker, designates tumor-specific TIL that are more reactive in vitro and more effective at controlling tumors in an NSG model.[44,45] In a related approach, the addition of agonistic anti-4-1BB antibody during the initial tumor fragment culture phase of TIL production seems to favor outgrowth of tumor-reactive CD8+ TIL.[46–49] Whether the results of these preclinical studies translate to increased clinical efficacy will be determined in clinical trials.

Advances in optimization of growth conditions, such as the use of 4-1BB-agonistic antibodies, have overcome the limitation of low infiltrate and enabled successful expansion of TIL from multiple nonmelanoma solid tumors including ovarian cancer, cervical cancer, breast cancer, bladder cancer, pancreatic cancer, and even very poorly infiltrated GI cancers.[49–54] Various case reports and pilot studies have shown objective responses and clinical benefit from TIL therapy in patients with metastatic colorectal cancer, metastatic breast cancer, cervical cancer, and metastatic ovarian cancer, but to date there have been few larger-scale studies employing current TIL therapy protocols in solid tumors, aside from advanced cutaneous melanoma.[55–59] A single-arm, Phase II trial of TIL therapy to treat metastatic uveal melanoma reported objective responses in 35% of evaluable patients, including one complete response.[60] Strategies to expand the application of TIL therapy to other solid tumors are discussed in a later section.

Defining the antigen specificity of antitumor response in TIL products can provide a rich source of potential tumor-rejection antigens but has been challenging due to the diversity of lymphocyte repertoires and the labor-intense antigen screening process. Profiling of melanoma TIL against a panel of all known HLA-A2-restricted melanoma-associated epitopes revealed reactivity to melanocyte differentiation antigens (e.g., MART-1), germline antigens (also known as cancer-testis antigens, CTAs; e.g., NY-ESO-1 and MAGE family), and overexpressed antigens (e.g., Survivin); however, these cells comprised a small proportion of the total CD8$^+$ T cell pool.[61] Reactivity was mostly observed against MART-1, diverse germline antigens, and overexpressed antigen epitopes derived from cryptic open reading frames or alternative splicing events, suggesting a relationship to T cell escape of central tolerance.[62] Attention has increasingly shifted to neoantigens arising from tumor-specific mutations, which are postulated to be immunogenic to T cells. New prediction and screening approaches have identified melanoma neoantigens that elicit antitumor T cell reactivity, and these studies also suggest that neoantigen-specific T cells are important mediators of tumor regression.[43,63,64] Encouragingly, the NCI has reported durable complete responses in four patients who received infusions of TIL products enriched for melanoma neoantigen reactivity.[65–67] The promise of enrichment for neoantigen-specific TIL as a strategy to increase therapeutic efficacy is counterbalanced by the additional time and resources necessary to identify these cells for each patient; however, this process may be streamlined by preselection based on PD-1 or CD137 expression.[43,68]

ENDOGENOUS T CELL THERAPY

Endogenous T cell (ETC) therapy uses peripheral blood as a source of T cells for ACT and is based on the premise that there exists a population of tumor-reactive T cells that can be identified, isolated, and expanded in sufficient quantity and of desired quality for infusion into patients, with the expectation that they will kill tumor cells and provide long-term immunoprotection. The low frequencies at which circulating tumor-reactive T cells are found in patients required the development of enabling technologies to facilitate the isolation and expansion of antigen-specific T cells from peripheral blood using various in vitro strategies.

Development of Engogenous T Cell Therapy

The direct demonstration that a circulating population of potentially tumor-reactive antigen-specific T cells exists in patients with cancer first became possible following the development of peptide-MHC (pMHC) multimers.[69,70] Direct labeling of T cells recognizing tumor-associated melanocyte differentiation antigens (gp100, tyrosinase, MART-1) revealed measurable populations of circulating T cells in melanoma patients, at frequencies as high as 2%; typically, the prevalence of tumor-associated antigen-specific cytotoxic T lymphocytes (CTLs) in the peripheral circulation is <0.2% and often at the lower limits of detection (0.01%).[70,71] Tetramer-guided cell sorting enabled in vitro expansion of this population to near uniform specificity (80–100%) but would not be translated into clinical practice until more than a decade later and has since transformed the feasibility of ETC therapy.[72,73]

Initial ETC therapy studies involved a lengthy protocol of in vivo stimulation, limiting dilution cloning, screening, and expansion requiring upwards of 12–14 weeks.[74] To expedite this process, a clinical-grade cell sorter and protocol was developed.[75] On this basis, subsequent studies began using tetramer-guided cell sorting for the generation of a usable T cell product resulting in a 50% reduction in time from leukapheresis to infusion and enabling routine generation of tumor antigen-specific T cells present at very low frequencies. Although the initial sorter was a stream-in-air device, current strategies incorporate a Micro-Electro-Mechanical Systems-based microfluidics device that allows for turnkey operation and closed-path manipulation of intake and output of antigen-specific T cells.

Strategies to isolate or enrich for tumor antigen-specific T cells involve an in vitro recapitulation of in vivo priming events, namely, TCR triggering by the peptide-MHC complex presenting tumor antigenic epitopes, engagement of co-stimulatory molecules, and cytokine-induced expansion. Multiple rounds of stimulation may be necessary to expand tumor antigen-specific populations to levels that can be sorted and further expanded via Rapid Expansion Protocol (REP).[23] Autologous dendritic cells (DCs) present antigen in a relatively "physiologic" manner in vitro and can be used in various ways. Immature DCs can be loaded with tumor lysate, tumor antigen protein, or opsonized tumor particles, and then matured (using cytokine cocktails and Toll-like receptor agonists) to facilitate antigen presentation and upregulation of co-stimulatory ligands.[76] DCs may also be engineered to express the antigen of interest after introduction of RNA encoding the antigen, or, in some cases, total tumor RNA.[77–79] These approaches may provide a more comprehensive antitumor T cell response as they would present multiple epitopes on MHC class I and II to stimulate CD8$^+$ and CD4$^+$ T cells, respectively. The most widely used approach, due to its relative facility, is to pulse mature DCs with known antigenic class I– or class II–restricted peptides. This method underlies the majority of ETC therapy clinical trials to date. Efforts are also being made in pursuit of more "universal" artificial antigen-presenting cells (APCs) based on genetically engineered insect cell lines and K562 cells, as well as artificial beads coated with anti-CD3/CD28+/– HLA-immunoglobulin domains.[80–82] Finally, addition of IL-21 during in vitro priming can significantly augment the frequency of high-affinity tumor antigen-specific CTL, as exposure to IL-21 resulted in a 10- to 100-fold increase in the frequency and absolute numbers of MART-1-specific CTLs generated in cultures.[83,84]

Endogenous T Cell Therapy in the Clinic

Initial trials of ETC therapy in the clinic generally involved infusion of monoclonal T cell products, were conducted without lymphodepleting preconditioning, and showed that in vitro generation of tumor antigen-specific T cells for adoptive therapy is feasible, infused T cells trafficked to sites of disease, and the treatment is relatively well-tolerated and safe.[74,85–87] Although not overwhelming, clinical benefit was observed in some patients as partial and mixed responses, with a complete regression that could be attributed to CD8+ T cells alone. Infused T cells persisted for up to 14 days in vivo and persistence correlated with response. ETC therapy utilizing CD4+ T cells has also been used to treat refractory, bulky metastatic melanoma and, impressively, a single infusion of NY-ESO-1-specific CD4+ T cells resulted in a durable complete response, accompanied by T cell product persistence of greater than 80 days post-infusion with evidence of antigen-spreading.[88]

ETC therapy has also been used with some success to treat Epstein-Barr virus (EBV)-associated lymphomas and nasopharyngeal carcinomas, which express the less immunogenic EBV antigens LMP1, LMP2, and EBNA1.[89] Generation of EBV-specific T cells for infusion typically employs repeated stimulation with EBV-LCLs or APCs in the presence of IL-2, without a rapid expansion phase.[90–94] A study testing the use of EBV-specific ETC therapy in the adjuvant setting for high-risk or multiple-relapse lymphoma patients and as treatment for patients with active disease observed that 28 of 29 patients receiving adjuvant therapy remained in remission 3.1 years (median) after infusion, and there were 13 clinical responses (two partial, 11 complete) out of 21 patients with active disease.[93] There was also evidence of epitope spreading in a subset of responders. Trials of EBV-specific ETC therapy to treat nasopharyngeal carcinoma have achieved modest success with some complete responses and partial responses in those with local disease, but limited control of disease progression

in patients with advanced refractory and metastatic disease.[90,92,94] Results may be improved by combination with chemotherapy, as a Phase II trial treating nasopharyngeal carcinoma with cycles of gemcitabine and carboplatin followed by infusion of EBV-specific T cells had an overall response rate of 71%.[95]

Efforts to increase the efficacy of ETC therapy focused on combination with lymphodepleting preconditioning regimens and enhancing persistence of infused T cells. As discussed earlier, nonmyeloablative but lymphodepleting chemotherapy conditioning regimens (high-dose cyclophosphamide and fludarabine) prior to TIL therapy had been shown to facilitate the in vivo engraftment and expansion of adoptively transferred cells.[35] Wallen et al. evaluated the use of fludarabine preconditioning in an intrapatient study and found a modest increase in T cell persistence without an increase in response rate.[96] Similarly, a small study of EBV-specific CTL infusion to treat nasopharyngeal carcinoma found that addition of a cyclophosphamide and fludarabine preconditioning regimen did not enhance clinical benefit.[97] Chapuis et al. evaluated the use of high-dose cyclophosphamide followed by low-dose IL-2 post-ETC infusion and found one out of 10 patients had a complete response and five patients experienced clinical benefit of stable disease up to at least week 8.[98] Plasma IL-15 levels were increased post-infusion and the infused T cells appeared to enter the cell cycle (Ki67+) within 1 week of transfer, but this did not translate to in vivo persistence. Importantly, the complete response was associated with long-term persistence of the infused T cell clone and in vivo conversion to a central memory phenotype.

While most of the focus on generation of persistent memory T cells centered on IL-15 on the basis of murine studies, in 2005 a unique role was discovered for IL-21 for human CD8+ T cells: exposure to IL-21 during in vitro priming led to the development of a central memory pool of tumor antigen-specific CD28+, CD127+, CD8 T cells with high replicative potential.[83,84] These tumor-reactive helper-independent CTLs produced antigen-driven autocrine IL-2. The clinical significance of these findings was confirmed when WT1-specific T cells generated in the presence or absence of IL-21 were administered to high-risk of relapse acute myeloid leukemia (AML) patients following stem cell transplant: only IL-21–primed T cells demonstrated long-term in vivo persistence and maintained or acquired phenotypic and functional characteristics associated with long-lived memory CD8+ T cells.[99] The transcriptional and epigenetic mechanisms underlying the effects of IL-21 in human CD8+ T cell priming were recently described.[100] Subsequent studies utilizing IL-21-primed ETC therapy approaches have confirmed persistence of the cells after transfer and in some cases have achieved durable responses.[101–103] Although clinical trials of ETC therapy have thus far been small in scale and achieved varying degrees of success, current ETC therapy offers several advantages as a therapeutic modality: it requires only access to peripheral blood, sourcing a wider, unbiased TCR repertoire, and does not require high-dose IL-2 or high-dose lymphodepletion, avoiding toxicities associated with those treatments and allowing for potential outpatient therapy. In addition, ETC therapy has shown efficacy with minimal, self-limited toxicities, and the neurotoxicity and cytokine release syndrome sometimes observed with CAR T therapy do not occur with ETC therapy, though there may be a mild, transient, lymphopenia. As with other ACT modalities, greater ETC therapy efficacy will likely be achieved through further enhancing the persistence of adoptively transferred cells and incorporating combination therapies to mitigate the impact of a hostile tumor microenvironment and augment T cell function (discussed in later sections). Table 25.1 summarizes the key differences between TIL and ETC adoptive therapy.

ADOPTIVE T CELL THERAPY FOR SOLID TUMORS BEYOND MELANOMA

To date, most successes observed for TIL and ETC therapies have been observed in patients with metastatic melanoma; this section will briefly discuss some of the major challenges to their application in other solid tumor types.

Target Antigen Identification and Selection

Identification and selection of target tumor antigens is of central importance to effective ACT. Being that cancerous cells are originally derived from normal cells of "self" tissue origin, the preponderance of antigens that may be targeted are weakly immunogenic (i.e., poorly recognized by T cells). The consequence of this is illustrated by the observations that cancers with higher mutational burden like melanoma, non-small cell lung cancers, and mismatch repair deficient colorectal cancers are more likely to be successfully treated with immune checkpoint therapy than less "immunogenic" tumors.[104–108] For antigen-specific ACT, the number of TCR targets are few, limited to a handful of tumor types such as melanoma and sarcoma, for which immunogenic epitopes to differentiation antigens (e.g., MART-1, gp100) or CTAs (e.g., NY-ESO-1, MAGE-A4) have been identified. Chapters 4 and 37 on human tumor antigens and tumor antigen profiling provide a more comprehensive discussion; for the purposes of TIL and ETC therapy, we focus on mutated and non-mutated tumor-associated antigens.

Neoantigens as TCR Targets for Adoptive T Cell Therapy

Mutations resulting in neoantigens that are processed and presented are postulated to be more amenable to T cell recognition. TIL targeting neoantigens may improve efficacy in solid tumors, and as more neoantigen epitopes are identified they may also be used in other T cell-based modalities.[109] Neoantigens have been identified in a variety of solid tumors such as gastrointestinal and ovarian cancers, and the screening of TIL for neoantigen reactivity has shown that mutations are very frequently recognized by CD8+ and/or CD4+ TIL.[63,110,111] Preliminary studies have shown adoptive transfer of TIL enriched for reactivity to neoantigens can result in objective responses in patients with solid tumor malignancies including colorectal cancer and breast cancer.[53,55,57,112,113] It is important to note that mutations may be found in all tumor cells (clonal), or a fraction of the tumor mass (subclonal). A complete response to TIL therapy was achieved in a metastatic breast cancer patient using TIL enriched for recognition of four distinct private mutations, including two clonal mutations.[57] This result suggests that even for mutated antigens, attention should be given to select antigens that are uniformly expressed across the whole tumor mass to maximize the odds of response. In addition to intratumoral heterogeneity of expression, neoantigens resulting from somatic mutations are rarely shared across patients, restricting this approach to highly personalized therapy requiring ad hoc identification and screening for neoantigen expression on patient tumor before generating a T cell product—a process that can have significant constraints on sample acquisition, manufacturing, and patient selection.[111] Ideally, antigens derived from more ubiquitous gene mutations, such as those that support oncogenesis, would be identified and targeted, and for this purpose TIL serve as a valuable resource, exemplified by studies targeting neoantigens of mutant KRAS and TP53, some of the most common mutations in epithelial cancers.[55,110,114]

Nonmutated Cancer-Testis Antigens as TCR Targets for Adoptive T Cell Therapy

Germline antigens (more commonly known as cancer-testis antigens, CTA), which have expression restricted to germ cells and placental cells but can be reexpressed by tumor cells of various tissues, are another promising class of antigens. The most recognizable CTA are probably NY-ESO-1 and the MAGE family antigens. Recent studies have identified additional families of CT and CT-like antigens whose derived immunogenic epitopes can be presented by a broader array of HLA alleles.[115] Due to the restriction of their expression among adult somatic tissues to immune-privileged sites such as testis, fetal ovary, and placenta, CTA are expected to be immunogenic, and this is supported by the presence of CTA-reactive T cells among endogenous TIL from melanoma patients.[61] CTA have the advantage of being more widely expressed across patients and tumor types, but their expression may be low or heterogeneous within tumors; however, demethylating

Table 25.1 Comparison of Tumor-Infiltrating Lymphocyte Therapy Versus Endogenous T Cell Therapy

	TIL THERAPY	ETC THERAPY
Source	Tumor biopsy (T cell infiltrated)	Peripheral blood mononuclear cells
Target antigen	Undefined, mixed, or neoantigen	Defined antigen (known immunogenic epitopes)
In vitro processing	Tumor disaggregation	Stimulation with antigen-presenting cells (autologous or artificial)
	Culture with high dose IL-2	Low dose IL-2
		Low dose IL-21 (in some protocols)
Production time (*current standard)	Standard TIL: 7–8 weeks	Monoclonal product: 8–12 weeks
	Young TIL*: 4–5 weeks	Polyclonal cultures*: 4–6 weeks
Cell therapy product	Heterogeneous, CD4+ and CD8+ T cells, varying antigen specificity and tumor reactivity	Generally uniform, tumor-reactive CD8+ T cells; central memory phenotype (IL-21 protocols)
Pre-infusion conditioning	High dose cyclophosphamide	Low dose cyclophosphamide (optional)
	Fludarabine	
Post-infusion cytokine administration	High dose IL-2	Low dose IL-2 (optional)
Tumor types treated (to date)	Melanoma	Melanoma
	HPV-associated carcinomas	EBV-associated lymphomas and carcinomas
	Uveal melanoma	Uveal melanoma
	Ovarian cancer	Ovarian cancer
	Gastrointestinal cancers	Pancreatic and gastrointestinal cancers
	Breast cancer	Merkel cell carcinoma
		NSCLC
Toxicities		
Cytokine-induced	Pulmonary failure	Fever
	Renal failure	
	Hypotension	
	Fever	
On-target	Vitiligo (melanoma)	Vitiligo and rash (melanoma)
	Uveitis (melanoma)	

EBV, Epstein-Barr virus; ETC, endogenous T cell; HPV, human papillomavirus; NSCLC, non-small cell lung cancer; TIL, tumor-infiltrating lymphocyte.

Source: Adapted with permission from Yee C. The use of endogenous T cells for adoptive transfer. *Immunol Rev.* 2014;257(1):250–263. doi:10.1111/imr.12134

agents and other epigenetic modifiers may be used to enhance their expression in tumor cells.[116,117] Furthermore, emerging evidence indicates that CTA have functional roles in tumor cells and may contribute to oncogenic processes.[116] Several clinical trials are evaluating CTA-specific ETC therapies, alone or in combination with the demethylating agent decitabine. Immune escape by tumor antigen loss should be less of an issue for polyclonal TIL and ETC therapies, compared to more homogenous TCR-T and CAR T approaches; however, they could be further improved by discovery of target antigens which confer some oncogenic advantage to tumor cells and survival dependency, as well as combination therapies that encourage antigen spreading. It must be noted that tumors may still escape recognition by T cells via diminished antigen presentation, such as by downregulation of MHC.[118,119]

Nonmutated Tumor-Associated Differentiation Antigens as Targets for Adoptive T Cell Therapy

Toxicities to normal tissues are a serious concern in target antigen selection, as many shared tumor-associated differentiation antigens are expressed by both malignant and normal cells. An example of this is the autoimmune vitiligo that often accompanies response to immunotherapies in melanoma patients, which is due to T cell-mediated destruction of normal melanocytes.[120] Such "on-target/off-tumor" toxicity is further illustrated by studies using TCR-engineered T cells (TCR-T). Administration of autologous T cells engineered to express a TCR recognizing CEA, an antigen which is also present in normal colonic epithelia, resulted in transient but severe colitis.[121] Treatment of melanoma using autologous PBMCs transfected with a nonmutated MART-1 TCR led to uveitis and decreased hearing, presumably due to MART-1 expression among pigmented cells in the uvea and stria vascularis of the inner ear.[122,123] No such toxicity was observed in responding patients receiving non-engineered MART-1-specific endogenous T cells, suggesting that overexpression of even a nonmutated TCR can lead to unwanted on-target/off-tumor toxicities. That ETC therapy can effect tumor regression without inducing toxicity to tissues expressing nominal levels of antigen demonstrates that a "goldilocks" window of therapeutic efficacy can be achieved without undue autoimmune toxicity using peripheral blood-derived, naturally occurring MART-1-specific T cells. When targeting differentiation antigens, shared expression with normal tissues may not be prohibitive if such tissues do not represent critical organ sites such as the CNS, heart, lungs, and so on. For example, tumor-associated antigens shared by breast cancer or prostate cancer and their normal tissue counterpart may be targetable especially if patients have already undergone a mastectomy or prostatectomy.[124,125] Finally, a shared tissue antigen selectively overexpressed

in uveal melanoma, but not mature melanocytes, may offer a wider therapeutic window than differentiation antigens, which are expressed at high levels in both melanoma and melanocytes (such as gp100 and MART-1).[126]

Trafficking and Infiltration

After infusion, adoptively transferred T cells must find and enter tumors to exert their antitumor response; however, poor trafficking to and infiltration of tumors is currently a significant barrier in solid tumors. T cells navigate to tissues in response to chemokine gradients and extravasate via interactions with adhesion molecules on endothelial cells; however, tumors can subvert this process. By decreasing T cell-homing chemokines and increasing chemokines for which T cells have low cognate receptor expression and/or that attract immunosuppressive cells, tumors can render an unfavorable tumor microenvironment.[127–129] Preclinical studies indicate that engineering ACT products to express receptors for tumor-produced chemokines could improve trafficking, but this approach would be tailored to the varying chemokine milieus of different tumor types.[130–133] Tumors may also inhibit T cell infiltration via aberrant vasculature and downregulation of endothelial adhesion molecules.[134] Anti-angiogenic therapies may normalize tumor vasculature, and use of VEGF-neutralizing antibody reportedly increased lymphocyte infiltration in a murine melanoma model.[135] The enhanced efficacy of adoptively transferred T cells in this study may also have been due in part to mitigation of various immunosuppressive effects of VEGF.

The tumor control provided by TIL therapy in metastatic melanoma patients strongly suggests that TIL have the ability to home back to the tumor tissue. Additionally, the fact that TIL grown from one tumor lesion can eliminate not only the lesion that they were grown from but also other lesions throughout the body, including brain metastasis, demonstrates their ability to traffic to various tumor sites and suggests that the breadth of antigens targeted by TIL is sufficient to circumvent tumor heterogeneity, at least in the subset of patients deriving long-term benefit. Recent work has demonstrated a correlation between the presence of tissue-resident memory (T_{RM}) phenotype T cells in tumor tissue and survival in several solid tumor types, suggesting that there may be a distinct, tissue homing, population of TIL that is most desirable to select for expansion.[136,137] The potential of tissue-resident lymphocytes to expand ex vivo has not yet been thoroughly investigated owing to a variety of technical challenges: the propensity for T_{RM} cell death due to tissue processing, a lack of T_{RM} markers that are maintained during conventional expansion protocols, and/or a paucity of in vitro culture methods suitable for T_{RM}; as a result, it is unclear if T_{RM} comprise a substantial portion of the expanded TIL infused to patients and whether they retain their tissue imprinting.[138–140] The elucidation of the molecular underpinning of tissue-resident programming also offers the possibility of engineering T cells with qualities that facilitate tissue homing.

The Immunosuppressive Tumor Microenvironment

Once T cells enter the tumor they must contend with an immunologically hostile microenvironment. Soluble mediators such as IL-10, TGF-β, and VEGF can inhibit the antitumor effector response and upregulate inhibitory checkpoint molecules on T cells. These factors may be countered through the use of neutralizing antibodies, receptor blocking antibodies, or genetic approaches involving expression of dominant-negative receptors that can act as cytokine sinks without signaling, or chimeric cytokine receptors that combine the exodomain of the suppressive factor's receptor with stimulatory or pro-survival endodomains, thereby redirecting an inhibitory ligand to trigger positive signals.[141–143] Metabolites produced by tumor cells and other cells in the tumor microenvironment can also inhibit T cell function. The ectonucleotidases CD39 and CD73 contribute to immunosuppression by reducing pro-inflammatory extracellular ATP and producing adenosine, which can directly inhibit T cells through the adenosine A2A receptor.[144] These effects may be mitigated using CD39/CD73 blocking antibodies, small-molecule inhibitors targeting A2AR, or gene editing of A2AR in T cells.[145,146] Indoleamine 2,3-dioxygenase (IDO) depletes the T cell-essential amino acid tryptophan and produces regulatory T cell (T_{reg} cell)-promoting kynurenine.[147] To address this, IDO inhibitors are currently in clinical development, but results have not yet fulfilled expectations.[148] Suppressive immune cells such as myeloid-derived suppressor cells (MDSCs) and T_{reg} cells are responsible for production of the inhibitory factors detailed previously, are sources of ligands for inhibitory checkpoint receptors, and interventions to modulate their function or eliminate such cells would be expected to improve antitumor T cell response.[149] Finally, T cell competition with tumor cells for glucose, which constrains effector functions in the glucose-deficient tumor microenvironment, might be overcome by augmenting metabolic fitness via checkpoint blockade, genetic strategies such as expression of phosphoenolpyruvate carboxykinase 1 (PCK1), and other innovative approaches.[150,151]

ADOPTIVE T CELL THERAPY IN COMBINATION STRATEGIES

To disable many of these immunoevasive mechanisms, combination strategies that target suppression must be implemented so that transferred T cells can achieve their full effector potential. Given the ever-increasing number of targetable pathways, the ability to track and rigorously analyze a highly uniform T cell population with defined specificity and phenotype, while exposed to immunologic countermeasures in vivo, would be invaluable in understanding the reasons for success or failure of a given combination strategy. In this way, the role of adoptively transferred T cells as a "transferrable cellular biomarker" becomes experimentally and empirically important in immune-based therapies not only as a therapeutic modality, but an analytical one as well.

Lymphodepleting Preconditioning Regimens

ACT combination strategies were first evaluated more than 20 years ago, beginning with studies by North et al. demonstrating the requirement for lymphodepleting preconditioning regimens to augment ACT efficacy in tumor-bearing murine models.[13] These regimens are thought to improve ACT by multiple mechanisms, including lymphopenia-induced elevation of homeostatic cytokines such as IL-15, removal of cytokine sinks (endogenous effectors), depletion of suppressive cells such as T_{reg} cells, bacterial translocation across GI barriers leading to Toll-like receptor activation, and increased tumor antigen availability and presentation as a result of tumor cell death.[152–156] These conditioning regimens continue to be practiced today (see the previous text), but rationale for their use should be contextualized for any given cell therapy approach. For example, while host immune suppression for gene-modified T cells may contribute to extended in vivo persistence by reducing the probability of endogenous immune rejection of the transgene, a finding that was noted even before CAR T cell-based therapies, it is less clear if such an immunosuppressive regimen is necessary for non-engineered T cell therapy.[157]

Clearing not only suppressive T cells, but also endogenous effector cells, with high dose cyclophosphamide and fludarabine also eliminates any possibility of antigen spreading. Antigen spreading, whereby targeting a specific antigen (in this case, with a tumor antigen-specific T cell), can elicit T cell responses to nontargeted antigens by tumor destruction, cross-presentation of immunogenic proteins and induction of a broad effector response in the presence of a favorable milieu is associated with a durable clinical response in the absence of antigen immune escape, even when the antigen targeted is dispensable for tumor survival or metastasis.[88,102,103] The absence of antigen spreading may be one reason for the high rates of relapse seen in patients receiving T cell therapy preceded by high-dose immunosuppressive conditioning.

Checkpoint Blockade Therapy

Immune checkpoint blockade and ACT have achieved some early successes in melanoma when checkpoint inhibitor therapy fails, and their combination holds promise in extending effective immunotherapy to more cancer types. Underpinning this strategy is the concept that in cancers where endogenous tumor-reactive T cells are sparse, infusing a bolus of tumor antigen-specific T cells would provide effectors that can respond more vigorously in vivo following the reduced inhibition and increased metabolic fitness afforded by checkpoint blockade. In a small, recent trial testing the combination of anti-CTLA-4 and standard TIL therapy in patients with metastatic melanoma, of the 12 patients who received both therapies five had objective responses, four of which were durable, and one of which later became a complete response.[158] Importantly, this trial began anti-CTLA-4 administration weeks before TIL infusion and had a reduced rate of attrition due to progression during the ACT production process (7% compared to 32%).

In a first-in-human, prospectively designed study evaluating the combination of memory MART-1-specific ETC therapy and CTLA-4 blockade in 10 patients with refractory metastatic melanoma, three of whom had failed prior anti-CTLA-4 monotherapy, seven out of 10 patients received clinical benefit.[103] Two patients achieved a durable complete response, one of them despite failing prior anti-CTLA-4 monotherapy. T cell persistence was observed for all patients for as long as samples could be collected (>500 days), accompanied by upregulation of central memory markers (CD28, CD127, CD62L, and CCR7) among all seven responders. In addition, all responders showed increased reactivity to nontargeted melanoma-associated antigens, indicating antigen spreading. In this study, upregulation of central memory markers and the emergence of antigen spreading was positively associated with clinical response.

PD-1 blockade represents an attractive option for combination ACT, as PD-1 expression can mark tumor-reactive T cells, and its antagonism may be used to relieve T cell exhaustion in the tumor microenvironment.[43,159,160] Indeed, at the NCI, treatment of a single metastatic breast cancer patient with neoantigen-specific TIL therapy and anti-PD-1 resulted in a complete durable regression.[57] Multiple larger studies are planned or underway to evaluate the combination of PD-1 pathway blockade and ACT.

Effects of Prior Checkpoint Blockade Therapy on Adoptive T Cell Therapy

As immune checkpoint blockade therapy becomes more commonly used, it is important to consider its effects on later adoptive cellular therapy treatment. Although earlier studies seemed to suggest that prior treatment with anti-CTLA-4 therapy had no effect on later TIL therapy, a larger, more recent study of 43 checkpoint-naïve metastatic melanoma patients and 31 patients who had received prior checkpoint blockade therapy reported reduced survival, overall response, and duration of

response, and less expansion of TIL during product generation in patients who had received prior checkpoint blockade.[33,41,161] It is unclear whether these results were a function of an inherent patient population refractory to anti-CTLA-4, effects of anti-CTLA-4 treatment on endogenous lymphocytes and/or tumor stroma, or both. One study of patients with regionally advanced melanoma receiving neoadjuvant anti-CTLA-4 therapy reported increases in circulating tumor antigen-specific T cells and increased tumor infiltration by activated T cells.[162] Interestingly, another study of TIL grown from patients with metastatic melanoma reported higher CTLA-4 expression but also broader, more frequent tumor antigen responses in T cells from patients who had received anti-CTLA-4 therapy.[163] Perhaps one advantage to pre-TIL harvest PD-1 therapy may be the infiltration and replacement of TILs with T cell clones that are more likely to be functionally tumor-reactive.[164] Further studies will be important in helping to determine treatment sequences and patient populations amenable to the combination of checkpoint inhibitor therapy and ACT.

Genetic Inhibition of Checkpoint Molecules

To avoid possible unwanted systemic effects of immune checkpoint blockade, intrinsic modification of transferred T cells ex vivo may be achieved by gene editing. The advent of CRISPR-Cas9 gene editing technology has stirred great interest in genetic approaches to checkpoint inhibition, in particular deletion of (PD-1), with a number of recent clinical trials testing this approach in ACT.[165] In preclinical studies, genetic disruption of PD-1 improved antitumor function in both CAR T cells and ETC; however, this may be at the expense of generating memory cells from the infused T cells.[166–169] A study in a chronic viral infection model showed PD-1 knockout in virus-specific T cells resulted in accumulation of terminally differentiated cells and greater contraction due to decreased survival, indicating an inability to establish memory, which may be due to a deficiency in upregulation of fatty acid oxidation.[170,171] These results were mirrored in a recent Phase I clinical trial testing the safety of PD-1-edited TCR-T cells (also edited for endogenous TCR alpha and beta chains).[172] Infusion of a mixed product containing PD-1 knockout and PD-1 sufficient cells could allow for enhanced antitumor function without sacrificing memory formation. Use of self-delivering small interfering RNA to knock down PD-1, rather than knock out, is an interesting alternative that has been successfully applied to TIL in a preclinical in vitro study.[173]

Oncolytic Viruses

Oncolytic viruses are designed to selectively replicate in cancer cells and induce immunogenic cell death that can act as an in situ vaccine and, more importantly for combination ACT strategy, as a means to enhance trafficking and in situ T cell activation.[174] Being viruses, they provide ligands for pattern recognition receptors and can promote a pro-inflammatory environment via induction of the antiviral response, resulting in the production of cytokines and chemokines that improve T cell infiltration and tumor antigen presentation, among other effects. They may also be used as vectors for gene delivery to tumor cells, modifying them to express desired cytokines, chemokines, co-stimulatory ligands, antigens, or other molecules.[174,175] Currently, there is one U.S. Food and Drug Administration (FDA)-approved oncolytic virus therapy: talimogene laherparepvec (T-VEC), an attenuated herpes simplex virus type 1 (HSV-1) encoding granulocyte-macrophage colony-stimulating factor (GM-CSF), approved for the treatment of some melanomas.[176] The successes of combined checkpoint blockade therapy and T-VEC suggests that combination of ACT with oncolytic viruses may also be effective.[177,178] A preclinical study identified adenovirus as the most effective virus when combined with TIL transfer; an oncolytic adenovirus encoding IL-2 and TNF-α (TILT-123) is currently being evaluated in combination with TIL therapy for melanoma in an ongoing clinical trial.[179]

Radiation Therapy

Early evidence supporting the combination of radiation therapy and ACT was the observation of synergy between TIL therapy and localized radiotherapy in a murine model of colon adenocarcinoma.[180] In similar manner to oncolytic viruses, radiation causes DNA damage-induced immunogenic tumor cell death that releases tumor antigens and promotes pro-inflammatory cytokines and the interferon (IFN) response, and may also enhance T cell infiltration by inducing the production of chemokines and tumor vasculature remodeling.[181,182] More recent preclinical studies in models of glioblastoma and pancreatic adenocarcinoma have shown that low-dose (subtherapeutic), local radiotherapy can increase the efficacy of adoptively transferred CAR T cells by improved trafficking to the tumor and sensitization of the tumor cells to T cell-mediated cytotoxicity.[183,184] Although the combination strategy of ACT and radiation therapy has yet to be evaluated in clinical trials, a case report of durable response in a single myeloma patient who was treated with localized radiotherapy for spinal cord compression shortly after infusion of CAR T cells shows promise.[185] Increases in inflammatory cytokines and TCR diversity were also observed post-radiation therapy.

DESIRABLE T CELL PHENOTYPES FOR ADOPTIVE T CELL THERAPY

Selection of Functional Cells

In contrast to vaccine-based or immune checkpoint therapies, ACT allows for ex vivo selection and enrichment of a desired effector phenotype for adoptive transfer. As T cells can develop a progressive state of dysfunction known as "exhaustion" following chronic in vivo or ex vivo stimulation, a means to evaluate and mitigate this phenotype would be desirable. Exhausted T cells are characterized by expression of several immune checkpoint molecules and a gradual loss of effector functions: proliferative capacity and production of IL-2, TNF-α, and IFN-γ.[186] Exhaustion was originally studied in models of chronic viral infection, but it has also been found that T cells isolated from tumor models and cancer patients exhibit many of the characteristics of T cells exhausted from chronic infection. In the context of tumors, in addition to persistent antigen and inflammation, causes of T cell dysfunction may be attributable to poor antigen presentation and/or priming, deficient co-stimulation, and immunosuppressive soluble mediators, which can lead to upregulation of inhibitory receptors including checkpoint molecules.[159,186] Multiple studies have shown that tumor antigen-specific T cells isolated from the peripheral blood, tumor, and lymph-node metastases of melanoma patients express checkpoint molecules, in particular PD-1 and TIM-3, and are deficient in cytokine production.[187–189] Interestingly, it has been reported that expression of PD-1, TIM-3, and LAG-3 designate tumor-reactive TIL, as measured by IFN-γ production and cytotoxicity in response to autologous tumor cell lines.[43,190] In this latter case, the cells were tested after a two-week period of in vitro expansion, suggesting that expression of checkpoint molecules indicated activation of these cells in vivo by tumor antigens and possible restoration of some effector function during in vitro culture.

Studies in chronic viral infection and tumor models have shown that exhausted T cells are a heterogeneous population consisting of a spectrum of different cell states, and significant efforts have been made to characterize these various states based on marker expression. A study comparing single-cell RNA sequencing profiles of T cells from chronic LCMV infection and melanoma models found both conditions produced T cells that were enriched for the canonical exhaustion signature defined by Wherry et al.[191,192] Several groups have identified that within TIL there are "progenitor" and "terminal" exhausted T cells which can be distinguished by their expression of PD-1, TIM-3, and TCF1, and determined that progenitor exhausted T cells (PD-1$^+$ TIM-3- TCF1$^+$) mediate tumor control and response to PD-1 checkpoint blockade.[192–194] As TCF1 is a transcription factor and therefore an intracellular marker, SLAMF6 has been identified as a surrogate cell-surface marker, based on high co-expression of SLAMF6 and TCF1, enabling the selection of live progenitor exhausted T cells.[192] Strategies to enhance ACT by sorting progenitor exhausted TIL based on these markers are being developed.[195] Even more recently, Beltra, Wherry, and colleagues have further defined four subsets of exhausted T cells based on their expression of SLAMF6 and CD69, with SLAMF6 marking the progenitor subsets.[196] Selection of tumor antigen-specific T cells that are not terminally exhausted could prove to be a fundamental requisite for ACT efficacy, especially in combination with PD-1 pathway blockade therapies.

Enhancing Persistence of Transferred Cells

Commensurate with these research studies are clinical studies demonstrating that in vivo persistence of adoptively transferred T cells correlates with patient response to ACT.[88,98,102,103,197–199] As discussed earlier, one of the original goals of lymphodepleting preconditioning regimens was to enhance persistence of transferred cells; however, this may also be achieved by selection of less differentiated T cells or manipulation of T cells in vitro to enrich for less differentiated or memory phenotypes. Preclinical studies have shown that less differentiated T cells, such as stem cell memory T cells (T_{scm}) or effectors derived from naïve or central memory precursors, have increased proliferative capacity, persistence, and antitumor function.[200–204] These cells are typically identified by their expression of CD62L, CCR7, CD95 (Fas), CD127, CD28, and/or CD27. Stem-like T cells may also be identified based on their mitochondrial membrane potential.[205]

Most current ACT production protocols involve (sometimes repeated) stimulation and extended culture in IL-2 in order to produce a sufficient number of cells for infusion; however, this can drive differentiation of effector T cells in vitro resulting in suboptimal performance in vivo.[203] The first demonstration, in 2005, that it was possible to modulate the phenotype of human CD8+ T cells was achieved by IL-21 exposure during priming and led to expansion of helper-independent central memory type T cells, which were later demonstrated to be critical for in vivo persistence of these cells at high frequencies in patients for more than nine months after adoptive transfer.[83,99] Since then, several studies using a combination of gamma-chain receptor cytokines (IL-7, IL-15, and IL-2) with IL-21 have reportedly resulted in T cells with a less differentiated phenotype, combinations which were later revealed to be counterproductive once an understanding of the signaling mechanisms leading to central memory development were elucidated.[100,206–208] Limitation of differentiation and preservation of "stemness" may also be achieved by inhibition of Akt signaling, limiting ROS metabolism with antioxidants such as N-acetylcysteine, or exposure to extracellular potassium-inducing autophagy.[209–211] Lastly, alteration of T cell mitochondrial dynamics by culturing with fusion promoting and fission inhibiting chemicals or enforced expression of the mitochondrial inner membrane fusion protein Opa1 can promote a memory phenotype.[212]

The in vitro priming used in ETC therapy offers an opportunity to influence T cell phenotype. A pilot study using artificial APCs expressing co-stimulatory ligands and IL-2/IL-15 to generate infusion products resulted in a mixture of effector memory and central memory phenotype T cells that persisted post-infusion, reminiscent of the phenotypic and functional attributes of memory T cells.[81,213] As discussed in an earlier section, exposure to IL-21 during priming promotes CD28+ central memory phenotype with high replicative potential and enhanced persistence without negatively affecting cytolytic activity.[83,84,99] Additionally, the effects of IL-21 are exerted predominantly through enhancement of tumor antigen-specific CTL derived from naïve CD8+ T cells, resulting in a younger, less differentiated ACT product.[83] It has also recently been shown that IL-21 can be combined with epigenetic remodeling via histone deacetylase inhibition to reprogram effector CTL to central memory phenotype cells.[100] Enhancing persistence of ACT cells should not only increase antitumor efficacy, but also provide a long-lived population of tumor-reactive T cells to protect against metastasis and recurrence.

ADOPTIVE TRANSFER OF GD T CELLS

Most adoptive T cell therapy approaches focus on "conventional" αβ T cells; however, "unconventional' γδ T cells are also being actively pursued for antitumor therapy. As their name indicates, γδ T cells are defined by their T cell receptors (TCRs), which are composed of a gamma (γ) chain and delta (δ) chain associated with CD3 complexes. γδ T cells generally do not express CD4 or CD8 coreceptors and recognize antigens independent of MHCs. While the antigen and antigen-presenting molecule for most γδ T cells are unknown, a subset of γδ T cells directly bind to an antigen's superstructure, whereas other minor subsets recognize lipid presented by CD1d and possibly metabolites presented by MR1.[214] γδ T cells comprise 1% to 5% of T cells circulating in human peripheral blood and are also found in peripheral tissues.[214] These unconventional T cells are typically distinguished by the variable (V) domain of their TCRδ chains, with Vδ2 (preferentially paired with Vγ9) cells predominating in the blood and Vδ1 cells commonly found in tissues.[214] γδ T cell antigens have not yet been comprehensively characterized but it is known that Vγ9Vδ2 T cells recognize nonpeptide phosphoantigens, such as isopentenyl pyrophosphate (IPP), that are metabolites derived from the mevalonate pathway.[215] Tumor cells with increased HMG-CoA reductase activity have increased endogenous phosphoantigens; this can also be achieved by exposure to aminobisphosphonate drugs such as Zoledronate, which trigger accumulation of phosphoantigens via disruption of the mevalonate pathway, rendering tumor cells susceptible to γδ T cell recognition.[215]

Conformational changes in CD277 (BTN3A1) appear to be involved in γδ T cell detection of phosphoantigens. Vγ9Vδ2 T cells also reportedly recognize stress-induced cell surface proteins on tumor cells such as heat shock protein 60 and FI-ATPase.[216]

In addition, some γδ T cells can express DNAM-1, NKG2D, CD244 (2B4), KIRs, NKp30, and/or NKp44 markers more commonly associated with natural killer (NK) cells, and recognize their ligands Nectin-2 and PVR, MIC A/B, and ULBPs. Hence, γδ T cell recognition of tumor cells likely involves more than one ligand and possibly concurrent detection of conformational changes. Following activation, the γδ T cell response is similar to that of conventional T cells by initiating cytotoxic pathways that produce IFN-γ, TNF-α, perforin, and granzymes to directly kill tumor targets. It has been suggested that they may form memory cells.[217] Thus, γδ T cells may be potentially effective against a variety of cancers and are especially attractive effector populations for treating tumors that escape the conventional T cell response by MHC downregulation.

In an early study of leukemia, patients who received allogeneic partially HLA-mismatched bone marrow transplants depleted of αβ T cells (to reduce graft-versus-host reactions) there was an association between high levels of circulating γδ T cells and improved disease-free and overall survival rates, suggesting that transferred γδ T cells can mediate an antitumor effect.[218,219] Most γδ T cell ACT studies to date have focused on Vγ9Vδ2 T cells, as they are the most common and accessible subtype in peripheral blood and can be expanded in vitro using cytokines and aminobisphosphonate drugs (e.g., Zoledronate) or synthetic phosphoantigens.[214] No studies used lymphodepleting preconditioning; however, most employed in vivo Zoledronate to sensitize tumor cells to the transferred γδ T cells.[217] Unfortunately, these trials had very limited success. While the trials have shown that γδ T cell ACT is generally well-tolerated, transferred cells can traffic to tumor sites and can achieve partial responses; complete responses were rare—although the few observed have been in varied tumor types (RCC, CRC, and breast cancer).[220-222]

Improving the Efficacy of γδ T Cell Adoptive T Cell Therapy

In vitro studies suggest the possibility of combination γδ T cell ACT with approved treatments. For example, when exposed to the chemotherapeutic temozolamide, GBM cells can upregulate cell-surface NKG2D ligands, enabling γδ T cell-mediated lysis.[223] Similarly, treatment of colon cancer cells with 5-fluorouracil or doxorubicin sensitizes them to γδ T cell cytotoxicity via a mechanism dependent on NKG2D.[224] Combining tumor-targeting antibodies such as rituximab (anti-CD20) or trastuzumab (anti-HER2) with γδ T cell therapy could increase efficacy by promoting tumor cell killing via antibody-dependent cellular cytotoxicity (ADCC) and allowing γδ T cells to present tumor antigens to conventional αβ T cells.[225-227] Furthermore, γδ T cells from tumor sites can express PD-1 and reportedly increase degranulation (CD107 expression) in vitro in response to anti-PD-1, suggesting γδ T cell ACT may also benefit from combination with PD-1 blockade therapy.[228]

Efforts to improve the efficacy of γδ T cell ACT are generally hampered by the dearth of knowledge regarding γδ T cell antigens, target cell recognition, activation, and regulation, as well as the considerable diversity among γδ T cells.[217] As with conventional T cells, γδ T cells are functionally diverse; in some tumor types, they can play important immunosuppressive and/or pro-tumorigenic roles, though the data regarding this has been contentious.[229,230] The endogenous suppressive or IL-17-producing γδ TIL in these reports were primarily of the Vδ1 subtype, but in vitro studies have shown that particular cytokine milieus can direct Vγ9Vδ2 T cells toward regulatory or IL-17+ phenotypes, and it is unknown whether adoptively transferred Vγ9Vδ2 T cells might undergo phenotypic alterations in the tumor microenvironment.[231,232] Although the expansion approach used in most γδ T cell ACT trials to date results in a bulk product that contains primarily Vγ9Vδ2 T cells, the individual clones can vary widely in TCR affinity as well as their expression of activating and inhibitory NK receptors; thus, identification and enrichment of a population with high antitumor reactivity might lead to improved efficacy.[233,234] An interesting alternative approach is to introduce high-affinity γδTCRs into αβ T cells, creating T cells engineered with defined γδTCRs (TEGs).[217,233] Transgenic expression of γδTCRs leads to downregulation of endogenous αβTCR expression on the cell surface, and this phenomenon, combined with γδTCR MHC-independence, opens the possibility for use in a broad patient population with reduced requirements for HLA-matching.[234] A Phase I trial using this approach in patients with AML or multiple myeloma is currently underway (NTR6541). Finally, methods have recently been developed for clinical-grade expansion of Vδ1 T cells, which are characterized favorably for tissue localization properties and enhanced cytotoxicity, and may have some advantages for ACT such as greater persistence and resistance to activation-induced cell death.[235-237] Overall, the lack of MHC-restriction and potential for antitumor activity against a broad range of tumor types will continue to fuel interest in γδ T cells (and their TCRs) for cancer immunotherapy, and a greater understanding of their biology should inform and improve future γδ T cell ACT approaches.

CONCLUSION

Over the last 30 years, ACT has developed from a boutique-type therapy, limited to selected patients with anecdotal clinical responses, to an established treatment modality. The reinvigoration of cancer immunotherapy by the advent of checkpoint blockade therapy has set the stage for a new era of ACT, aided by scientific advances, enabling technologies, and judicious application of combination strategies to enhance trafficking, function, and persistence of adoptively transferred antitumor T cells. Successes of ACT will be extended to broader patient populations through improvements in target antigen selection and strategies to overcome T cell dysfunction and the immunosuppressive tumor microenvironment.

KEY REFERENCES

Only key references appear in the print edition. The full reference list appears in the digital product on Springer Publishing Connect: connect.springerpub.com/content/book/978-0-8261-3743-2/part/part02/chapter/ch25

35. Dudley ME, Wunderlich JR, Yang JC, et al. Adoptive cell transfer therapy following non-myeloablative but lymphodepleting chemotherapy for the treatment of patients with refractory metastatic melanoma. *J Clin Oncol.* 2005;23(10):2346–2357. doi:10.1200/JCO.2005.00.240

74. Yee C, Thompson JA, Byrd D, et al. Adoptive T cell therapy using antigen-specific CD8+ T cell clones for the treatment of patients with metastatic melanoma: in vivo persistence, migration, and antitumor effect of transferred T cells. *Proc Natl Acad Sci U S A.* 2002;99(25):16168–16173. doi:10.1073/pnas.242600099

88. Hunder NN, Wallen H, Cao J, et al. Treatment of metastatic melanoma with autologous CD4+ T cells against NY-ESO-1. *N Engl J Med.* 2008;358(25):2698–2703. doi:10.1056/NEJMoa0800251

103. Chapuis AG, Roberts IM, Thompson JA, et al. T-cell therapy using interleukin-21-primed cytotoxic T-cell lymphocytes combined with cytotoxic T-cell lymphocyte antigen-4 blockade results in long-term cell persistence and durable tumor regression. *J Clin Oncol.* 2016;34(31):3787–3795. doi:10.1200/JCO.2015.65.5142

109. Gros A, Parkhurst MR, Tran E, et al. Prospective identification of neoantigen-specific lymphocytes in the peripheral blood of melanoma patients. *Nat Med.* 2016;22(4):433–438. doi:10.1038/nm.4051

197. Robbins PF, Dudley ME, Wunderlich J, et al. Cutting edge: persistence of transferred lymphocyte clonotypes correlates with cancer regression in patients receiving cell transfer therapy. *J Immunol.* 2004;173(12):7125–7130. doi:10.4049/jimmunol.173.12.7125

199. Chapuis AG, Desmarais C, Emerson R, et al. Tracking the fate and origin of clinically relevant adoptively transferred CD8+ T cells in vivo. *Sci Immunol.* 2017;2(8):eaal2568. doi:10.1126/sciimmunol.aal2568

26

CAR T Cell Therapy

Shivani Srivastava, Alexander I. Salter, and Stanley R. Riddell

KEY POINTS

- Adoptive cell transfer (ACT) of genetically modified T cells is a personalized cancer therapy that involves selection, modification, expansion, and reinfusion of tumor-reactive T cells.

- Tumor-associated antigens that are selectively or preferentially expressed on tumor cells but not normal tissues have been identified and represent ideal targets for ACT.

- Genetic modification with engineered receptors (T cell receptor [TCR] or chimeric antigen receptor [CAR]) can redirect T cell specificity to tumor-associated determinants.

- T cells modified with major histocompatibility complex (MHC)–restricted TCRs display antitumor activity in some patients with melanoma and synovial cell sarcoma.

- CAR T cells targeting lineage molecules and incorporating co-stimulatory signaling domains have demonstrated significant efficacy in patients with relapsed or refractory B cell malignancies.

- Using defined phenotypic T cell subsets with intrinsic capacity for self-renewal and proliferation may enhance persistence of transferred cells *in vivo* and therapeutic efficacy.

- New strategies for genetic manipulation can improve safety and enhance the efficacy of transferred T cells in the immunosuppressive microenvironment of solid tumors.

INTRODUCTION

Adoptive cell transfer (ACT) is a personalized cancer therapy that involves the administration of tumor-reactive T lymphocytes that are derived from the patient's blood or tumor infiltrate or are engineered by gene transfer to express receptors that recognize tumor antigens. ACT was shown to mediate antitumor activity against transplanted tumors in murine models even before the molecular nature of tumor antigens, and the fundamentals of antigen processing and presentation were understood.[1,2] ACT with endogenous, nongenetically modified T cells derived from the blood or tumor infiltrates established the principle that T cell immunotherapy could be effective in human cancers, and this approach is covered in detail in Chapter 25. However, it is challenging to isolate and expand highly functional tumor-reactive T cells from blood or tumor infiltrates in most cancer patients. Overcoming this barrier has been facilitated by better characterization of antigens expressed on tumor cells and advances in our ability to efficiently deliver, express, and edit genes in T cells. Genetically modified T cells are now providing curative therapy for a subset of patients with hematologic malignancies (Figure 26.1).[3,4] This chapter focus on ACT with genetically modified T cells.

GENETIC MODIFICATION OF T CELLS WITH T CELL RECEPTORS

An initial focus in the field of T cell engineering was to identify, clone, and engineer T cell receptors (TCRs) specific for tumor-associated antigens (TAAs) presented by major histocompatibility complex (MHC) molecules. Such TCRs, if specific for C/T or viral antigens or public neoantigens that are shared by many patients' tumors, could provide off-the-shelf reagents for endowing autologous T cells with tumor reactivity. Several TCRs have been isolated, characterized, and made their way into clinical trials, but it should be noted that most antigens recognized by tumor-specific T cells are specific for nonshared, patient-specific neoantigens. Isolating TCRs to engineer T cells for the therapy of each individual patient is logistically challenging, particularly if viral vectors are used to deliver the TCR gene to T cells. Viral or nonviral gene insertion can efficiently express the TCR in autologous T cells to confer antigen specificity; however, as discussed in the text that follows, unless the endogenous

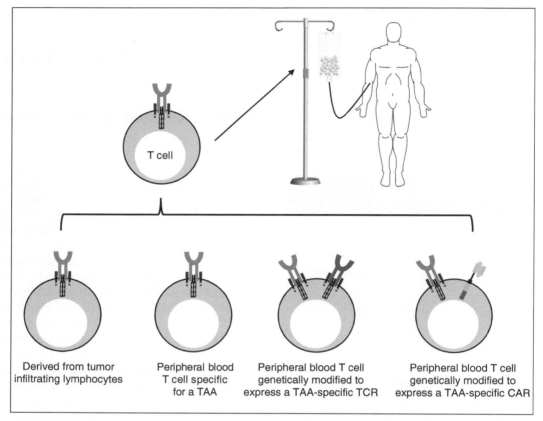

Figure 26.1 Genetic modifications of T cells for adoptive T cell transfer. T cells can be modified by gene transfer to express a T cell receptor (TCR) or chimeric antigen receptor (CAR) that is specific for a TAA (tumor-associated antigen) and edited to enhance efficacy.

TCR chains are silenced, the introduced TCR chains must compete with endogenous chains for cell surface expression. After in vitro expansion of TCR gene-modified T cells, preferably under conditions that limit T cell differentiation during culture, the reprogrammed T cells can be reinfused back into the patients.

Optimal Antigen Targets for T Cell Receptor–Targeted Therapy

The utility of T cells for cancer therapy is predicated on identifying antigens that are selectively or preferentially expressed on tumor cells and has limited or absent expression on vital normal tissues. Numerous antigens that are selectively or preferentially expressed on cancer cells have been identified and prioritized for clinical translation.[5] When performing ACT using TCR-modified T cells, it is critical that expression of the target antigen be restricted to transformed or dispensable normal cells. Ideally, the peptide antigen should be a "driver" mutation critical for the oncogenic process or for cell survival so that tumor cells cannot easily down-regulate the protein product during T cell therapy.

Emerging data from analysis of T cell responses to tumors suggests that tumor-reactive T cells are often specific for peptides that result from mutations that are only present in that patient's tumor but not necessarily responsible for oncogenesis.[6] In this circumstance, the antigen should be encoded by a truncal mutation that is uniformly expressed in all tumor cells to minimize the outgrowth of antigen-negative tumor cells, or multiple antigens should be targeted. It would also be ideal for shared antigen(s) to be presented by common HLA class I molecules so that a maximum number of patients could benefit and a sufficient number of individuals can be treated to obtain robust data on safety and efficacy. The peptide must be generated by the proteasome subunits expressed in the tumor cells and bind to the MHC molecule with high affinity.[7,8] Finally, the TCRs that target the antigen should be of sufficiently high avidity to efficiently recognize the level of peptide-MHC (pMHC) expressed on tumor cells.[9]

Several categories of antigens have been identified and are actively being pursued for ACT. A major category is self-proteins that are overexpressed in transformed cells compared with normal cells or expressed in differentiated normal tissues and tumors originating from those lineages. Examples include Melan-A (MART-1), glycoprotein 100 (gp100), carcinoembryonic antigen (CEA), Wilms tumor antigen 1 (WT-1), and survivin.[10–16] Cancer-testes (C/T) antigens such as NY-ESO-1 and melanoma-associated antigen (MAGE) family members represent another class of self-antigens that are expressed only in normal testes and aberrantly expressed in many tumors.[17] Tumors that result from oncogenic transformation caused by viruses, such as human papillomavirus (HPV), Epstein–Barr virus (EBV), and Merkel cell polyomavirus, express viral antigens that can be targets for ACT.[18–27] Finally, coding mutations, frameshift mutations, gene fusions, or splice variants of expressed genes can give rise to public or private neoantigens that are presented by MHC molecules on tumor cells (Table 26.1).[28,29]

Isolating T Cell Receptors and Engineering T Cells for Adoptive T Cell Transfer

Generating TCR-modified T cells requires the isolation of TCR alpha and beta gene sequences that, when introduced into T cells, reliably and safely redirect T cell specificity to tumor antigens. Exogenous TCRs specific for self-antigen and mutated antigen have been isolated from tumor-infiltrating lymphocyte (TIL) products that mediated clinically effective antitumor responses, from the endogenous TCR repertoire in the blood of autologous and allogeneic donors, and from TCR and/or HLA-humanized mice that were immunized with peptide antigens.[30–32] Recent studies have shown that a subset of T cells in tumor infiltrates and blood that express the programmed cell death protein 1 (PD-1) molecule, which is normally upregulated by activation and serves to inhibit T cell signaling, are enriched for tumor reactivity.[33–35] This observation facilitates a new strategy for isolating tumor-reactive T cells and cloning their TCRs.

High-affinity TCRs that bind strongly to pMHCs are believed to be optimal for ACT. However, the affinity of TCRs that can be isolated to self-antigens is limited by thymic negative selection, which deletes T cells with TCRs that bind too strongly to MHCs presenting self-peptides.[36] To circumvent the effects of central tolerance on TCR affinity, many groups have sought to enhance the avidity of naturally isolated TCRs. This can be accomplished by mutating complementarity determining regions in TCR alpha and beta chain genes that define peptide specificity. Simple amino acid substitution and selection using phage display or T cell display have been harnessed for affinity enhancement.[37,38] The TCRs produced by these methods can have significantly increased avidity compared with their natural counterparts but, as discussed later, come with the potential risk of new undesired and unpredicted reactivities.

Table 26.1 Representative Examples of Tumor-Associated Antigens That May Serve as Targets for Major Histocompatibility Complex–Restricted T Cells

CLASS OF TUMOR ANTIGEN	EXAMPLES	EXAMPLES OF TUMOR TYPE(S)
Self-differentiation antigens	MART-1, gp100	Melanoma
	Proteinase 3	Leukemia
Self-overexpressed antigens	WT-1	Leukemia, epithelial cancers
	Mesothelin	Mesothelioma, lung, ovarian, pancreatic, and cervical cancers
	Her2	Breast, ovarian
Self-C/T antigens	NY-ESO-1	Melanoma, sarcoma, myeloma, and other tumor types
	MAGE A3	Melanoma, many tumors
	Other C/T members	Many tumors
Viral antigens	EBV (LMP-1, 2)	Lymphoma
	HPV (E6, E7)	Cervical cancer, head and neck cancer
	Merkel cell polyomavirus	Merkel cell cancer
Neoantigens from oncogenic mutations	KRAS	Lung, pancreas, colorectal
	BRAF	Melanoma, hairy cell leukemia
Neoantigens from random somatic mutations	Patient-specific	Common in melanoma, lung cancer, and bladder cancer

C/T, cancer-testes; EBV, Epstein–Barr virus; gp100, glycoprotein 100; Her2, receptor tyrosine-protein kinase ErbB-2; HPV, human papillomavirus; LMP, latent membrane protein; MAGE-A3, melanoma-associated antigen 3; MART-1, melan-A; NY-ESO-1, cancer/testis antigen 1; WT-1, Wilms tumor antigen 1.

Techniques for Genetic Modification of Primary Human T Cells

The most well-studied methods for modifying human T cells use retroviral or lentiviral vectors to deliver a transgene that becomes stably integrated into the host cell genome. Early work focused on optimizing the tropism, structure, promoter, and packaging of retroviruses and lentiviruses for obtaining high expression of exogenous

TCRs in viable primary T cells.[39-41] As the TCR is composed of two independent chains (α and β), these studies also sought to determine how best to express two proteins from a single transgene cassette—whether to use two open-reading frames with distinct promoters or an internal ribosomal entry site or one open-reading frame separated by a 2A ribosomal skip element that mediates cotranslational polypeptide cleavage.[42] A disadvantage of two open-reading frames is that the transgene includes a second promoter, which increases the size of the DNA insert and can result in lower viral titer and transduction efficiency. In addition, because promoters vary in strength, the TCR chains encoded in each open-reading frame may not be produced in equimolar amounts, thereby reducing the absolute number of appropriately paired alpha and beta chains on the cell surface. At present, the field has coalesced around the use of 2A ribosomal skip elements to provide for equimolar production of both TCR chains. Several retrovirus and lentivirus vectors have been developed that provide a stable expression of exogenous TCRs and other transgenes, and thus far, there has been no evidence that gene insertion results in transforming mutations in human T cells.[43,44] This was a relevant issue because clinical studies of retroviral gene transfer into hematopoietic stem cells to correct immunodeficiency syndromes resulted in insertional mutagenesis and leukemia development in a fraction of patients.[45,46] Although this remains a concern, the improved design of viral vectors and apparent intrinsic resistance of T cells to insertional mutagenesis have reassured investigators and regulators alike, and clinical applications of viral gene transfer into T cells have proceeded rapidly.[44]

The production of retrovirus and lentivirus vectors for clinical use poses several challenges for investigators outside of industry or major academic centers.[47,48] First, clinical-grade production of lentiviral or retroviral vectors can take several weeks and is expensive. Second, viral stocks must be tested for safety, including the absence of a replication-competent virus that could be generated by sporadic recombination events during manufacturing. Third, the size of the transgene payload is constrained by the size of the retroviral and lentiviral capsids. These limitations have made it difficult thus far to test different TCR designs, multiple TCRs targeting different tumor antigens in a single trial, or TCRs targeting private neoantigens that would be relevant only for an individual patient.

Because of the limitations of viral gene delivery, there has been significant interest in using nonviral techniques for modifying T cells. The Sleeping Beauty (SB) transposon system for genetic modification uses an engineered transposase to integrate a co-transfected transgene carrying transposon into the genome of human cells.[49,50] Inverted repeat sequences flanking a genetic payload are recognized by the coexpressed transposase, which then catalyzes the integration of the transgene–transposon cassette into the genome. Two studies demonstrated the ability of the SB system to transfer an exogenous TCR into primary human T cells.[51,52] In one report, SB yielded a slightly lower gene transfer efficiency compared with a lentiviral vector, but the T cells exhibited similar functions in preclinical testing.[51] SB delivery also integrated the transgene into the genome in similar genomic loci as a lentiviral vector. Because plasmid DNA can be produced for clinical use more rapidly and inexpensively, there is considerable interest in SB and other nonviral delivery systems, and Phase 1 clinical applications are now being reported.[53] A limitation of the SB transposon system is the risk of genome instability because of uncontrolled transposase gene activity when the transposase is introduced by a DNA vector. Rational protein design based on knowledge from the crystal structure of the hyperactive SB100X variant has been used to create an SB transposase with enhanced solubility and stability.[54,55] This novel transposase spontaneously penetrates cells, including T cells, and can be delivered with transposon DNA to genetically modify cells without the risk of uncontrolled transposase activity.

Modifications of T Cell Receptors to Improve Expression and Prevent Mispairing With Endogenous Chains

The initial studies transferring exogenous TCRs into T cells uncovered issues that required further modifications of the transgene. First, there were substantial variations in the cell surface expression levels of different TCRs, which impaired the function of engineered T cells. Exhaustive mapping of the framework sequences of TCR variable regions identified that substitution of three amino acid residues consistently increased TCR expression on the surface of engineered T cells and improved the in vitro and in vivo functions.[56] Second, because the TCR is an alpha beta heterodimer and both chains are required for recognition of pMHC, the introduction of exogenous alpha and beta chains into a T cell by gene transfer could lead to mispairing of these chains with the endogenous TCR alpha and beta chains.[57] Mispaired TCR chains diminish the absolute number of correctly paired species on the cell surface and, if expressed in post-thymic T cells, can confer new specificities including self-reactivity. Indeed, when a TCR was transferred into polyclonal murine T cells, mispairing led to systemic autoimmunity resulting in bone marrow failure, pancreatitis, and colitis.[58] Mispairing was also reported in primary human T cells and led to undesired reactivity against lymphoblastoid cell lines and hematopoietic cell lineages in vitro, raising concern that mispairing could lead to toxicity in patients.[59]

Several strategies have been developed to prevent or minimize TCR mispairing and promote strong TCR expression. One relies on "murinization" or swapping of sequences in the human TCR constant regions not involved in pMHC recognition with those of the murine TCR alpha and beta chains. These efforts began with the observation that a mouse TCR could be expressed in human T cells at higher levels than the endogenous human TCR counterpart.[60,61] However, when murine TCRs specific for human TAAs were transduced into human T cells and used for ACT in a clinical trial, a subset of patients developed anti-TCR antibody responses.[61] This led to the creation of human–mouse hybrid TCRs containing human variable regions and murine alpha and beta constant regions that preferentially pair with each other and not with human constant regions.[62–64] Careful analysis of the murine constant region showed that only nine murine amino acid residues needed to be incorporated into the human constant region to abrogate mispairing.[65] More recently, it was found that interchanging the constant regions between human TCR alpha and beta chains, so that the alpha chain contains the beta constant region and vice versa, could prevent mispairing.[66] Other methods to prevent mispairing have been described. In near simultaneous publications, two groups showed that incorporation of cysteine residues at defined positions in the TCR alpha and beta chains led to preferential pairing and increased expression of the exogenous TCR.[67,68] These effects were likely mediated by disulfide bonds formed between the cysteine residues.

The problem of mispairing might be eliminated completely using genome-editing techniques including RNA interference, zinc-finger nucleases (ZFNs), transcription activator-like effector nucleases, and clustered regularly interspaced short palindromic repeats (CRISPR)/Cas9 to silence, delete, or replace endogenous TCR chains. Silencing of endogenous TCR expression using transgene-encoded endogenous TCR loci-specific inhibitory RNA sequences increased expression of the introduced TCR, improved T cell cytotoxic responses against cells presenting the antigen targeted by the exogenous TCR, and reduced mispairing toxicity in mice.[69–72] ZFNs have been targeted to DNA sequences in the endogenous TCR alpha and beta loci to create DNA double-strand breaks that, when repaired by error-prone nonhomologous end joining (NHEJ), disrupt the coding sequence, resulting in a knockout of endogenous TCR expression.[73] This approach is cumbersome as it requires sequential delivery of ZFNs targeting each TCR chain, with the introduction of the corresponding tumor-specific TCR chain.

A logical next step was to employ CRISPR/Cas9 gene editing with homologous recombination of an insert encoding exogenous TCR alpha and beta chains into the native TCR alpha and beta loci.[74,75] This has the advantage of both preventing mispairing and placing the introduced TCR chains under natural regulatory control to provide for regulated expression of only the exogenous TCR at normal levels. A limitation of CRISPR/Cas9 is low-editing efficiency in primary cells, particularly when homologous recombination is required.[76] Recent studies showing that homologous recombination can be favored over NHEJ for repairing nuclease-induced strand breaks suggest the utility of this approach for clinical applications, such as TCR gene transfer, will be improved and provide for physiologic TCR regulation.[77,78]

T Cell Receptor Gene Transfer Into CD8+ and CD4+ T Cells

Studies to determine the optimal T cell subsets to engineer for ACT are ongoing. It is established that CD4+ T cells synergize with CD8+ T cells in ACT,[79,80] suggesting it would be advantageous to engineer both tumor-reactive CD8+ and CD4+ T cells with MHC class I- and class II-restricted TCRs, respectively. However, bioinformatics techniques for predicting and immunological reagents for detecting MHC class I antigens are significantly more robust than for MHC class II antigens. As a result, most TCRs that have been isolated for use in ACT are MHC class I-restricted and selected for function in CD8+ T cells.

The CD8 or CD4 coreceptors bind to a conserved region on MHC class I or class II, respectively, and coreceptor binding is important for stabilizing the TCR–pMHC interaction and recruiting Lck, a critical kinase that phosphorylates the TCR-associated CD3 chains and initiates TCR signaling after pMHC engagement.[81] Thus, placing a class I-restricted TCR into CD4+ T cells disrupts the natural format of TCR recognition because CD4 does not strongly interact with MHC class I molecules. To this end, investigators assessed the function of MHC class I-restricted TCRs in CD4+ T cells and found that transducing CD4+ T cells with CD8 alpha and beta chains allows for antigen recognition, but altered effector responses.[82–84] An alternative approach is to use avidity-enhanced TCRs that are not dependent on coreceptor binding for peptide recognition.[85,86]

Modulation of T Cell Differentiation in Culture

There is substantial data demonstrating that the differentiation state of T cells used for ACT can affect their in vivo potency. Previous studies with T cell clones or polyclonal T cells used prolonged culture in interleukin 2 (IL-2) to obtain the numbers of T cells that were perceived to be necessary for efficacy. After culture, the T cells expressed a highly differentiated phenotype, with absent or low expression of CD62L, CD28, and CD27, which, based on our current understanding of T cell differentiation, would be suboptimal for ACT.[87–90] Fate mapping of T cells after ACT in preclinical models have provided evidence for a model of progressive T cell differentiation whereby naïve CD45RA⁺CD62L⁺ T cells differentiate into long-lived memory stem (CD45RA⁺CD62L⁺CD95⁺) and central memory cells (CD45RO⁺CD62L⁺CD95⁺) that, in turn, give rise to short-lived effector memory (CD45RO⁺CD62L⁻CD95⁺) and effector (CD45RO⁺CD62L⁻CD95⁺) T cell subsets.[89,91–94] Advances in cell selection technologies have made it feasible to isolate naïve or central memory T cells from patient blood prior to genetic modification to confer tumor specificity.[95] This has the advantage of starting with less differentiated cells and also prevents the "quorum sensing" that occurs when more differentiated cells present in cultures confer more rapid acquisition of effector differentiation.[96] In other systems, clinical trials of CD19-specific chimeric antigen receptor (CAR) T cells have demonstrated that isolating central memory CD8⁺ T cells and CD4⁺ T cells for cell manufacturing and combining the resulting CD8⁺ and CD4⁺ CAR T cells in a 1:1 ratio in the final cell product leads to remissions of refractory leukemia and lymphoma and a predictable dose–effect relationship.[97,98]

Investigation of alternative culture conditions for propagating antigen-specific gene-modified CD8⁺ T cells has also identified a variety of methods for limiting T cell differentiation during in vitro expansion, including the use of media containing high levels of K⁺ or 2-hydroxycitrate, which alter T cell metabolism, and the use of alternative cytokine cocktails such as IL-7, IL-15, or IL-21, which favor the maintenance or outgrowth of specific T cells from the naïve pool that retains CD28 expression.[99–102] Based on these findings, IL-21 was used during isolation of T cell clones targeting WT-1, which is expressed at high levels in acute myeloid leukemia (AML). Patients with AML who received WT-1-specific T cell clones cultured with IL-21 demonstrated improved persistence compared with those cultured with IL-2, although antitumor efficacy in both groups of patients was limited, perhaps reflecting the low affinity of T cells specific for the self-antigen WT-1.[103]

Clinical Trials of T Cell Receptor–Modified T Cells Demonstrate Antitumor Activity

In 2006, Rosenberg et al. at the National Cancer Institute (NCI) reported the results of a trial in HLA-A*02:01 individuals with progressive metastatic melanoma who received T cells genetically modified to express a MART-1-specific TCR previously isolated from a melanoma patient with a near-complete regression after TIL therapy.[104,105] Two of 15 (13%) patients obtained transient partial responses, demonstrating that TCR-modified T cells could produce therapeutic responses in a subset of individuals with melanoma. None of the patients in this trial experienced off-target or on-target, off-tumor toxicity to normal melanocytes.

The same group later reported that higher avidity TCRs targeting MART-1 and gp100 had antitumor activity in individuals with melanoma.[106] Objective antitumor responses were achieved in six of 20 (30%) patients receiving the anti-MART-1 T cells and three of 16 (19%) patients receiving anti-gp100 T cells. Both types of TCR-modified T cells persisted in the blood of all patients for more than 1 month, but a substantial fraction of patients suffered from eye and ear toxicities. Biopsies of affected tissues showed a CD3⁺ infiltrate, suggesting that the toxicities resulted from on-target off-tumor T cell recognition and destruction of nontransformed melanocytes in these sites. These findings advise caution when using a high-avidity TCR targeting a self-antigen that is also expressed on normal tissues.

Findings from trials evaluating TCR-modified T cells specific for the C/T antigen NY-ESO-1 (aa157-165) in HLA-A*02:01 individuals have also been reported. Individuals with metastatic synovial cell sarcoma and melanoma were treated with a TCR containing two amino acid substitutions in the CDR3 region that enhanced T cell function.[37,107,108] Objective responses were observed in 11 of 18 (61%) patients with synovial cell sarcoma and 11 of 20 (55%) patients with melanoma. In a second study, multiple myeloma patients were given an autologous stem cell transplant and infused two days later with TCR-modified T cells expressing an affinity-enhanced NY-ESO-1-specific TCR.[109] The TCR-modified T cells expanded in vivo, trafficked to the bone marrow, and persisted for up to two years in some patients. The fact that the T cells were infused immediately after transplant complicates the evaluation of their antitumor efficacy, but the expression level of NY-ESO-1 on tumor cells decreased after treatment and relapses were NY-ESO-1-negative, suggesting that the TCR-modified T cells recognized antigen in vivo. Thus, T cells modified to express this NY-ESO-1-specific TCR are safe and can produce antitumor responses in some patients. Collectively, these studies establish the principle that TCR-modified T cells can have therapeutic utility.

Numerous groups are now attempting to target neoantigens with TCR-engineered T cells, which may overcome the problem that many self-reactive T cells are of low avidity. Whether this will be sufficient to improve responses or whether additional modifications to T cells to overcome barriers in the tumor microenvironment (TME) are needed remains to be determined.

Combining Adoptive T Cell Transfer With Checkpoint Inhibitors

Multiple immunotherapeutic modalities have antitumor efficacy, and it is logical to investigate combining these approaches to improve outcomes. Upon antigen recognition, adoptively transferred T cells upregulate inhibitory receptors, such as cytotoxic T-lymphocyte–associated protein 4 (CTLA-4), PD-1, Lag3, TIM3, and TIGIT in vivo, and administering antibodies that target one or more of these immune checkpoints with ACT can enhance efficacy in murine tumor models.[110–112] A small clinical study in melanoma patients combined the infusion of polyclonal CD8+ MART-1-specific T cells with CTLA-4 blockade. Two of 10 patients achieved a complete remission and T cell responses to additional tumor antigens were evident after therapy, suggesting both improved activity of the transferred T cells and recruitment of new responses.[113] These results provide encouragement that efficacy of ACT with TCR-engineered T cells can be improved with combination therapy.

An alternative strategy is to use gene knockout technology to genetically engineer the T cell to be resistant to immune checkpoints. Results from a first-in-human Phase 1 clinical trial of CRISPR/Cas9-edited and lentivirus-transduced T cells in three patients with refractory cancer were recently published.[114] The trial built upon prior studies demonstrating that editing of human T cells with CRISPR/Cas9 was feasible in vitro, and PD-1-edited cells could improve antitumor responses in preclinical mouse models.[115–117] The trial enrolled six patients with refractory cancer expressing NY-ESO-1 and the authors attempted to manufacture autologous T cell products containing CRISPR/Cas9 knockouts of TCR alpha and beta loci (TCRA, TCRB) as well as PD-1. During manufacturing, T cells were also transduced with a TCR transgene specific for NY-ESO-1 to confer tumor specificity. However, T cell products could only be made for four patients (66%) and the characteristics of these products were unimpressive as fewer than 1% of infused cells were transduced and edited appropriately. Although this was a technical tour de force, the vast majority of the infused T cell product was unmodified T cells, making it impossible to draw conclusions with regard to feasibility, efficacy, or safety.

On-Target and Off-Target Toxicities of T Cell Receptor–Modified T Cells

In addition to clinical responses, reports of severe toxicities caused by TCR-modified T cells have emerged and are instructive for future applications of this approach. One study evaluated a TCR specific for CEA, which is often not only overexpressed on tumors of the digestive tract but also expressed by normal colonic epithelial cells.[118] Dose-limiting transient colitis developed in all three treated individuals soon after infusion of TCR-modified T cells. The colitis was traced to T cell–mediated attack of normal gastrointestinal tract tissues expressing the target antigen, indicating that certain overexpressed antigens may not be viable targets for TCR-modified T cells.[119] It remains unknown whether CEA might be

safely targeted with T cells modified with a lower affinity CEA-specific TCR.

Toxicity has also been observed with TCR-modified T cells targeting the C/T antigen MAGE-A3, which is a member of the MAGE family of antigens expressed by many tumors.[120,121] In this study, an avidity-enhanced TCR was derived from HLA-A2 transgenic mice by immunizing the mice with two MAGE-A3 peptides and introducing a single amino acid mutation in the CDR3 region of the TCR.[122] After infusion into nine patients with metastatic melanoma, synovial sarcoma, or esophageal cancer, the T cells persisted for at least 1 month in each patient and five of nine (56%) patients achieved an objective response. However, three patients developed severe neurologic toxicities without major changes in serum cytokine levels after T cell infusion.[123] In subsequent analyses, the authors failed to find off-target reactivity of their TCR using in vitro immunological assays, but discovered that MAGE-A12, which contains a highly homologous peptide sequence to the MAGE-A3 epitope, is expressed in the normal human brain. The authors concluded that the neurologic toxicity likely resulted from recognition of MAGE-A12 expressed on a subset of neurons. Their findings speak to the challenges of targeting epitopes that are similar or shared among proteins from the same family and of screening avidity-enhanced TCRs for off-target toxicity.

In 2013, another trial targeting a distinct HLA-A*01:01 restricted epitope of MAGE-A3 with an affinity-enhanced TCR had to be halted after two patients died from cardiogenic shock.[124] In preclinical testing, the authors enhanced the affinity of the TCR by mutating four residues in the CDR2 region of the alpha chain. They did not detect cross-reactivity with other known MAGE family members and infused autologous T cells modified to express the affinity-enhanced TCR into individuals with melanoma and multiple myeloma. The first two treated patients developed severe cardiac abnormalities within days of the T cell infusion. Further analysis revealed that the TCR cross-reacted with a peptide derived from titin, which is expressed by cardiomyocytes.[125,126] Although TCR affinity enhancement remains an intriguing strategy for improving the antitumor efficacy of TCR-modified T cells, a more sophisticated understanding of TCR cross-reactivity as well as improved strategies for characterizing affinity-enhanced TCRs and screening for peptides that are cross-reactive are necessary to reduce the likelihood of unanticipated off-target toxicity to normal tissues.[127,128]

More recently, two cases of transient acute inflammatory demyelinating polyneuropathy were reported in patients with synovial cell sarcoma who received T cells expressing a high-affinity NY-ESO-1-reactive TCR.[129] The TCR in question was previously shown to mediate sustained activity in patients with myeloma and synovial cell carcinoma.[109] While the underlying pathogenesis of the polyneuropathy is incompletely understood, mispairing of exogenous and endogenous TCR chains could have introduced new specificities to gene-modified T cells. Thus, caution is warranted when utilizing TCR-modified T cells without endogenous TCR alpha and beta gene disruption or other strategies to prevent TCR chain mispairing.

Unresolved Questions and Future Directions of T Cell Receptor–Modified T Cells

Marked progress has been made in the characterization of TCRs specific for peptide antigens, the optimization of these TCRs in vitro, and their testing in clinical trials. Preclinical and clinical data have demonstrated that T cells modified with exogenous TCRs can mediate anti-tumor responses for some antigens in certain clinical settings. However, a number of questions remain to be addressed in future work. Clinical trials of TCR-modified T cells showed that the antitumor responses were highly variable, despite the similarity between the transduction levels and numbers of transduced T cells administered to individual patients. One plausible source of variability is the level of expression of the exogenous TCR in the final cell product. Retroviral, lentiviral, and SB techniques mediate transgene integration into actively transcribed areas of the genome. However, this process is relatively nonspecific and, in contrast to the tightly regulated TCR locus, each integration site will possess a unique chromatin architecture that is subject to differential enhancer regulation. Thus, transgene expression can be highly variable from cell to cell. This can affect the functional avidity of the introduced TCR because the avidity of the TCR–pMHC interaction depends not only on the binding affinity but also on the number of TCR molecules that can be engaged. Future studies using ZFNs or CRISPR/Cas9 to insert exogenous TCR alpha and beta chains into the endogenous TCR loci may improve therapeutic efficacy.

Several factors in the TME have been identified to inhibit the local function of T cells, including deficiencies in metabolites critical for T cell function, low levels of class I or II MHC molecules on tumor cells, expression of programmed death ligand 1 (PD-L1) on tumor and/or infiltrating immune cells, and infiltration with immunosuppressive CD4+Foxp3+ regulatory T cells (T_{reg} cells) and/or myeloid cells.[130,131] Antibodies that target CTLA-4, PD-1, or PD-L1 can overcome suppression mediated through these immune checkpoints and are effective in many cancers, particularly those with high mutational burden.[132–134] However, it is important to note that in melanoma, ACT with TILs can be effective in patients who have failed prior treatment with checkpoint-blocking antibodies, suggesting unique benefits in combining lymphodepleting chemotherapy, ACT, and IL-2 for overcoming resistance to immune-mediated tumor eradication. Future combinations of antibodies and/or small molecules that target the immunosuppressive mechanisms operative in the TME may be effective without TIL infusion and narrow the therapeutic applications of TILs. However, the analysis of location, phenotype, specificity, transcriptional, and epigenetic properties of TILs has enriched our understanding of interactions between the tumor and the immune system and identified opportunities for intervention.

Chronic stimulation of tumor-specific T cells can drive a progressive loss in T cell effector function and "exhaustion" that limits antitumor activity. During productive T cell activation, TCR and co-stimulatory receptor signaling induce activation of the transcription factors nuclear factor of activated T cells (NFAT) and activator protein 1 (AP-1), respectively, which together drive the expression of genes involved in proliferation and effector function. By contrast, TCR stimulation in the absence of sufficient co-stimulation results in insufficient AP-1 activation and drives expression of Tox and Nr4a, which have been identified as master regulators of the "exhausted" state.[135–141] Reversing T cell exhaustion with immune checkpoint blockade is only partly effective because many exhausted T cells adopt a fixed epigenetic state that is difficult to reverse. Advances in our understanding of T cell exhaustion suggest that T cells might be rendered resistant to exhaustion before infusion. Deletion of Tox or Nr4a,[137,138,140] or overexpression of the AP-1 subunit c-Jun,[142] improves the function and antitumor activity of tumor-specific T cells in preclinical models, suggesting that adoptively transferred T cells can be engineered to resist the development of exhaustion.

Finally, as will be discussed in subsequent sections, it is now possible to engineer additional functions into T cells using synthetic receptors. Fully synthetic proteins that provide additional co-stimulation or cytokine support as well as resistance to transforming growth factor beta (TGF-β) signaling and PD-1 signaling have recently been described and tested in T cells.[143–146] Combining them with an exogenous TCR could lead to improved antitumor efficacy.

GENETIC MODIFICATION OF T CELLS WITH SYNTHETIC RECEPTORS

Advantages of Synthetic Receptors

Advances in synthetic biology and genetic modification have led to novel approaches for retargeting T cells to tumor antigens using synthetic CARs. In its most basic designs, a CAR links a tumor-specific extracellular recognition domain to an intracellular signaling domain that induces T cell activation upon antigen binding (Figure 26.2).[147–149] An advantage of CARs over TCRs is that they confer HLA-independent recognition of tumor

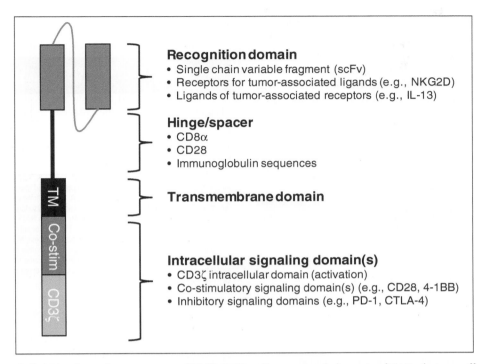

Figure 26.2 Elements of chimeric antigen receptor (CAR) design. Key structural elements of CARs that can affect the sensitivity of antigen recognition and T cell function after ligand engagement.

4-1BB, tumor necrosis factor receptor superfamily member 9; CTLA-4, cytotoxic T-lymphocyte–associated protein 4; Ig, immunoglobulin; IL-13, interleukin 13; NKG2D, NKG2-D type II integral membrane protein; PD-1, programmed cell death protein 1.

cells, allowing one receptor to be used regardless of the patient's HLA haplotype. For this reason, CARs recognize tumor cells that have downregulated expression of HLA or antigen-processing molecules, which are common mechanisms of tumor immune evasion.[150,151] Moreover, because of their modular structure, CAR components can be differentially configured to maximize T cell function in various settings. From the recognition domain to the intracellular signaling domain(s), optimization of each CAR component can improve recognition of tumor cells and T cell effector function.

Principles of Chimeric Antigen Receptor Design: The Recognition Domain

The recognition domain of CARs can be composed of virtually any molecule that has sufficient binding affinity for a tumor cell surface molecule (Figure 26.2). Most CARs that have advanced to clinical testing have been built using single-chain variable fragments (scFvs) as recognition domains because monoclonal antibodies (mAbs) to several TAAs are readily available, and new mAbs can be obtained by conventional technologies and by screening antibody phage display libraries; however, natural ligand-binding domains are also being tested in clinical trials.[152–154] CARs have been developed from mAbs specific for mutated receptors (e.g., epidermal growth factor receptor variant III [EGFRvIII]), cell lineage molecules (e.g., CD19, CD20, CD22, and CD7), developmental molecules (e.g., receptor tyrosine kinase–like orphan receptor 1 [ROR1], disialoganglioside [GD2], and glypican-3 [GPC3]) that are expressed on some tumors, and molecules overexpressed in tumors relative to normal tissues (e.g., receptor tyrosine-protein kinase ErbB-2 [Her2], mesothelin, Mucin 1 [MUC1], and MUC16; Table 26.2).[155–163] CARs can also be designed using the ectodomain of natural molecules, such as the NKG2-D type II integral membrane protein (NKG2D) receptor that binds to stress-induced ligands upregulated on tumor cells or the TNF superfamily protein APRIL (TNFSF13) that binds to B cell maturation antigen (BCMA) and transmembrane activator and calcium-modulator and cytophilin ligand interactor (TACI).[154,164–167] Other groups have exploited the selective expression of the cytokine receptor IL-13Rα2 on glioblastoma by designing CARs using the receptor's natural ligand, the cytokine IL-13, as an ectodomain.[168,169] IL-13 "zetakine" CAR T cells have shown partial efficacy and safety in a Phase 1 clinical trial for glioblastoma.[170]

Because designing and optimizing a new CAR for each TAA is time-consuming and labor-intensive, another strategy is to develop a "universal" CAR that can theoretically target any tumor antigen. One group tested this idea by constructing a CAR specific for the fluorochrome fluorescein isothiocyanate (FITC) molecule. By infusing FITC-labeled antibodies specific for TAAs in vivo, they could label the tumor with FITC and mark it for killing by FITC-specific CAR T cells.[171] Similar approaches have

Table 26.2 Representative Examples of Tumor-Associated Antigens That May Serve as Targets for CAR T Cells

CLASS OF TUMOR ANTIGEN	EXAMPLES	EXAMPLES OF TUMOR TYPE(S)
Cell lineage molecules expressed on tumors and normal cell lineage	CD19	ALL, NHL, CLL
	CD20	ALL, NHL, CLL
	CD22	ALL, NHL, CLL
	BCMA	Multiple myeloma
	Ig light chain	NHL, CLL, myeloma
	CD123	AML
Self-antigen with overexpression on tumors	Her2	Breast, ovarian
	CEA	Colorectal, breast
Self-antigen with limited normal tissue expression	L1CAM	Neuroblastoma
	GD2	Neuroblastoma, Ewing sarcoma
	ROR1	CLL, mantle cell lymphoma, ALL, NSCLC, triple-negative breast, pancreatic, ovarian, and cancer
	Mesothelin	Mesothelioma, ovarian cancer, pancreatic cancer
	MUC1	Ovarian, breast, and pancreatic cancer
	MUC16	Ovarian cancer
	Folate receptor alpha	Ovarian, breast, and lung cancer
	IL-13Rα2	Glioblastoma
Viral antigens	EBV (LMP-1)	Nasopharyngeal carcinoma, lymphoma
Peptide/MHC	HA-1/HLA-A2	Leukemia (allogeneic stem cell transplant)

(continued)

Table 26.2 Representative Examples of Tumor-Associated Antigens That May Serve as Targets for CAR T Cells (continued)

CLASS OF TUMOR ANTIGEN	EXAMPLES	EXAMPLES OF TUMOR TYPE(S)
Peptide/MHC (cont'd)	PR-1/HLA-A2	AML, CML
	WT-1/HLA-A2	AML, epithelial cancers
	AFP/HLA-A2	Hepatocellular carcinoma

ALL, acute lymphoblastic leukemia; AML, acute myeloid leukemia; BCMA, B cell maturation antigen; CAR, chimeric antigen receptor; CEA, carcinoembryonic antigen; CLL, chronic lymphocytic leukemia; EBV, Epstein–Barr virus; GD2, disialoganglioside; HA-1, immunogenic peptide derived from minor histocompatibility antigen HA-1; Her2, receptor tyrosine-protein kinase erbB-2; IL-13Rα2, interleukin 13 receptor subunit alpha-2; L1CAM, neural cell adhesion molecule L1; LMP, latent membrane protein; MHC, major histocompatibility complex; MUC16, Mucin 16; NHL, non-Hodgkin lymphoma; MUC1, Mucin 1; NSCLC, non-small cell lung cancer; PR-1, immunogenic peptide derived from proteinase 3 and neutrophil elastase; ROR1, receptor tyrosine kinase–like orphan receptor 1; WT-1, immunogenic peptide derived from Wilms tumor antigen 1.

been taken using biotinylated antibodies and biotin-specific CAR T cells, or using CARs with a CD16 recognition domain that binds the Fc portion of human immunoglobulins (Igs).[172,173] Although "universal" CARs have been effective against multiple tumors in preclinical models, clinical trials are necessary to determine whether they remain effective in patients without binding endogenous biotin or free Ig and eliciting off-tumor toxicity.

Despite the versatility and plethora of recognition domains, a limitation of current CARs is that they primarily recognize tumor cell surface molecules that are also expressed on normal tissues (Table 26.2). Because transcription factors and intracellular signaling molecules are often mutated in tumor cells and represent potential tumor-specific targets, several groups have attempted to develop "TCR-like" antibodies that recognize specific pMHCs and could be used as recognition domains for CARs. Investigators are now using phage display and hybridoma strategies to isolate scFvs specific for pMHC, and CARs built from such "TCR-like" antibodies have shown efficacy in preclinical models. For example, T cells expressing TCR-like CARs specific for gp100/HLA-A2, PR1/HLA-A2, WT1/HLA-A2, and AFP/HLA-A2 mediate antitumor activity in vitro and in xenograft mouse models.[153,174–176] Thus, in principle CARs can be designed to target intracellular antigens, although additional study of the biophysical interactions of TCR-like CAR T cells with tumor cells is necessary to optimize specificity, antitumor activity, and safety, and to determine whether there are potential advantages over TCRs.

Several properties of CAR recognition domains are amenable to manipulations that can influence antitumor activity. Receptor affinity for tumor antigens can significantly affect downstream CAR signaling and functionality, and the optimal affinity may be different depending on ligand density and epitope location. A lower affinity CD19 CAR showed enhanced proliferation and cytotoxicity in preclinical studies and improved CAR T cell expansion in patients with B cell ALL compared with published results with a higher affinity CD19 CAR.[177] Likewise, lower affinity CARs have shown equivalent or superior activity against human epidermal growth factor receptor 2 (Her2) and intercellular adhesion molecule 1 (ICAM-1).[178,179] Faster off-rates may enable CARs to be serially triggered, resulting in enhanced signaling and proliferation. By contrast, studies evaluating CARs specific for ROR1 or folate receptor beta found that scFvs with higher affinity exhibited superior antitumor activity against antigen-positive tumor cells in vitro and in vivo.[180,181] Other studies show that there may be an affinity threshold that provides for selective recognition of tumor cells when targeting molecules, such as Her2 or epidermal growth factor receptor (EGFR), that are expressed at low levels on some normal tissues.[178] Even the framework regions of an scFv, which do not participate in antigen binding, can influence CAR signaling and function. When comparing CD19 and GD2 CARs, the framework regions of a GD2 scFv contributed to antigen-independent clustering of the scFvs on the T cell surface, resulting in tonic signaling, early exhaustion, and poor antitumor function both in vitro and in vivo.[182] Thus, scFvs may need to be screened for both antigen-binding and antigen-independent expression properties.

Principles of Chimeric Antigen Receptor Design: Hinge/Spacer and Transmembrane Sequences

CARs often contain a hinge or spacer region derived from CD8α, CD28, or Ig sequences inserted between the scFv and the transmembrane domain. Notably, the spatial properties of the TCR–pMHC interaction are conserved and have evolved to elicit optimal T cell activation; however, the distance between a CAR and its antigen will vary based on the location of the target epitope and the protrusion of the scFv from the T cell membrane.[183,184] Tailoring the length of the spacer region is one way to modify this distance and maximize T cell activity, and several studies have demonstrated that lengthening the spacer can improve the function of scFvs targeting membrane–proximal epitopes, presumably by adding the flexibility and length needed to access these epitopes.[185,186] It is interesting to note that lengthening the spacer diminishes the function of CARs targeting tumor cell membrane–distal epitopes, suggesting that too much space between the T cell and the target cell is suboptimal.[185,186] Thus, the location of the target epitope may dictate the length of the spacer required for optimal CAR T cell function.

The amino acid sequences of the spacer can also affect CAR T cell function in vivo. Spacer regions derived from the Ig Fc region and CARs designed with IgG1- or IgG4-based spacers can inadvertently bind to and activate Fc receptor (FcR)–expressing innate immune cells in vivo.[187] Binding of the CARs to FcR+ cells in vivo can also activate CAR T cells and induce activation-induced T cell death, thereby compromising antitumor activity.[186] Mutating five amino acids to abrogate FcR binding in the spacer region improves CAR T cell persistence and antitumor activity for applications that require long spacers.

Additionally, the identity of the hinge/transmembrane region can affect the functionality and sensitivity of CARs to different antigen levels. As previously noted, a CD8α hinge and transmembrane sequence can be used in CAR structures.[188] One group added 15 amino acids from the native CD8α molecule to the most frequently used CD8α hinge and transmembrane variant.[189] The additional amino acids reduced CAR T cell cytokine and proliferation in vitro without reductions in efficacy in both preclinical mouse models and human patients. The authors suggest that the modified CAR might reduce the risk of CAR T cell–related toxicities because of the lessened production of proinflammatory cytokines, but further clinical studies are necessary to evaluate this possibility. Replacing the CD8α hinge/transmembrane domain with a CD28 hinge/transmembrane can also lower the threshold for CAR activation, alter the immunological synapse, and enhance CAR activity against antigen-low tumors, indicating that modulating the hinge/transmembrane region can tune CAR sensitivity independent of the scFv and signaling domains.[190]

Principles of Chimeric Antigen Receptor Design: Intracellular Signaling Domains

Initial CAR designs linked recognition domains to a single signaling module from FcRγ or CD3ζ to induce T cell activation.[147-149] Expression of these "first-generation" CARs in T cells redirected lytic activity in vitro but provided limited persistence and antitumor activity in vivo.[191,192] T cells require two signals for full activation: signal 1 provided by the TCR via CD3ζ and signal 2 provided by co-stimulatory receptors like CD28.[193] In an effort to recapitulate both signals, "second-generation" CARs were designed to carry the signaling endodomains of CD3ζ and CD28 linked in cis. A clinical trial directly comparing first-generation (CD3ζ alone) and second-generation (CD28–CD3ζ) versions of the same CAR demonstrated that CD28 co-stimulation improved CAR T cell persistence and expansion in vivo.[194] It is interesting to note that although second-generation CAR T cells are generally superior to first-generation CAR T cells, the converse was observed in tumors infiltrated by T_{reg} cells, and this was linked to greater IL-2 production from second-generation CAR T cells that supported T_{reg} cell activity.[195]

Co-stimulatory domains other than CD28 have also been tested for their ability to support T cell survival and long-term persistence. Most notably, incorporating the 4-1BB (CD137) signaling domain improved CAR T cell persistence, tumor localization, and antitumor activity in some preclinical models compared with CD28/CD3ζ and CD3ζ only CARs,[188] as well as ameliorated tonic signaling and T cell exhaustion in certain CAR constructs.[182] Initial work comparing CAR T cells possessing CD28 or 4-1BB co-stimulatory domains revealed that the CAR designs imparted distinct metabolic phenotypes and that CD28/CD3ζ CAR T cells may be less likely to promote memory T cell development.[144,196] Based on these findings, it was assumed that the differential T cell phenotypes resulted from co-stimulatory signaling through unique pathways. However, in-depth analysis of phosphoprotein signaling demonstrated that CD28/CD3ζ and 4-1BB/CD3ζ CAR T cells signaled through nearly identical pathways.[197] Instead, signaling from the two CARs differed in kinetics and strength whereby CD28/CD3ζ CAR stimulation promoted more rapid and stronger intracellular phosphorylation and signaling.

A major finding from comparisons of CD28/CD3ζ and 4-1BB/CD3ζ CAR T cells was that CD28/CD3ζ CAR T cells were more likely to exhaust in preclinical models of leukemia and lymphoma.[144,197] This phenomenon heralded back to early studies of TCR signaling demonstrating that progressively stronger TCR signals promote T cell dysfunction.[198,199] Based on this framework, researchers tested ways to alter CAR signal strength. CD28/CD3ζ CAR signaling could be partly abrogated by mutating the Lck-binding site in the CD28 co-stimulatory domain[197] and systematic mutation of the three immuno-tyrosine activating motifs in the CD3ζ domain demonstrated that CD28/CD3ζ CAR T cells with mutated tyrosine residues in the CD3ζ domain possessed improved tumor control and were less likely to exhaust.[200]

Despite intensive research of CD28/CD3ζ and 4-1BB/CD3ζ CAR designs, alternative co-stimulatory domains, including OX40, CD27, and ICOS, alone, or in tandem, can be included with CD3ζ in CARs.[201] CARs have also been designed to encode both CD28 and 4-1BB co-stimulatory domains alongside CD3ζ, although there is limited evidence that including additional co-stimulatory domains on the CAR molecule improves antitumor functions in patients.[202,203] In summary, an emerging principle is that CAR signal strength can drive disparate T cell phenotypes and fates. While the rules for tuning CAR signaling characteristics are not well defined, efforts are already underway to tune CAR signaling for a variety of clinical applications. Optimal signaling parameters are, however, likely to differ by clinical setting based on varying target ligand densities, targeting domain affinities, and T cell subsets. Thus, further study of how CAR signaling impacts therapeutic efficacy is needed. The application of innovative technologies that probe CAR signaling quality and kinetics and evaluate synapse composition could guide the development of new CAR designs with enhanced signaling qualities.[204,205]

Considerations for Selecting Targets for Chimeric Antigen Receptor T Cell Therapy

CARs can be developed to target almost any surface-expressed molecule, and it is important to define which targets will safely elicit antitumor activity. A major consideration when choosing candidate target antigens is the selectivity of their expression on tumors to avoid off-tumor toxicity to vital normal tissues. The most advanced clinical applications of CAR T cells target B cell lineage molecules (CD19, CD20, and CD22) expressed on B cell malignancies such as acute lymphoblastic leukemia (ALL), non-Hodgkin lymphoma (NHL), and chronic lymphocytic leukemia (CLL). BCMA is another validated CAR target that is expressed by multiple myeloma. As discussed in the following section, CAR T cells targeting these antigens can not only induce complete remissions but also eliminate healthy B cell lineages that express the target molecules. This on-target off-tumor toxicity is manageable transiently, but persistent B cell deficiency reduces Ig titers and increases susceptibility to infections.

Other targets such as neural cell adhesion molecule L1 (L1CAM), GD2, Her2, mesothelin, MUC16, and ROR1 are being pursued as targets for CAR T cells, but have the limitation of being expressed in some normal tissues (Table 26.2).[206–211] There is some evidence that GD2-specific CAR T cells can have antitumor activity without on-target toxicity[212]; however, CAR T cells specific for Her2 caused serious pulmonary toxicity in one patient, although high-dose IL-2 administered after the CAR T cells may have contributed.[160] Cell surface molecules that are mutated in cancer cells, such as EGFRvIII, which is deleted in exons 2 through 7 and signals constitutively, would provide a true tumor-specific CAR target, but its heterogeneous tumor expression may limit efficacy.[213] A recent study demonstrated that a cancer-associated glycoform of MUC1 could be targeted with CAR T cells with no recognition of the alternative glycoform in normal cells, suggesting this may be a safe and effective target.[162] It remains to be determined whether CARs can be designed to discriminate between high and low levels of antigen expression as a means of sparing normal tissues, and trials currently in progress should delineate the risks for individual target molecules.

In addition to the selective expression on tumor cells, antigen density and homogeneity of expression on the tumor are important factors. Studies suggest that the threshold for CAR T cell signaling is higher than that for TCRs, which require only one to 10 pMHCs for activation. For a CD20 CAR, ~200 molecules per target cell were required to induce lytic activity, and the requirement for cytokine production by CAR T cells was 10-fold higher.[214] Target antigens for CARs should ideally be expressed homogeneously throughout the tumor to minimize the escape of antigen-negative variants. In the case of B cell malignancies, CD19 is expressed homogeneously on tumor cells, and CAR T cells mediate complete remissions in many patients. Similarly, BCMA is expressed uniformly in at least 60% to 70% of myeloma cases. Identifying homogeneously expressed antigens is more difficult for solid tumors, which do not express a common lineage marker like CD19 on all tumor cells. ROR1 is an attractive target because it is highly and homogeneously expressed on many different types of solid tumors, but this molecule is expressed on a restricted subset of normal tissues and on-target off-tumor toxicity remains a concern despite the safety of ROR1-specific CAR T cells in animal models.[206,215]

First-Generation Chimeric Antigen Receptor T Cells Fail to Mediate Antitumor Responses in Patients

Clinical trials testing ACT with T cells modified with first-generation CARs demonstrated feasibility but failed to show objective antitumor responses. In two early studies, patients with NHL, mantle cell, or follicular lymphoma were treated with autologous T cells expressing a CD20- or CD19-specific CAR.[216,217] Both studies used plasmid electroporation for transduction and antibiotic selection to enrich CAR T cells, which required long in vitro culture and resulted in highly differentiated "effector" phenotype T cells. CAR T cells were only detectable in the blood by polymerase chain reaction for a short time after transfer and antitumor activity was not observed. Another clinical trial evaluated carbonic anhydrase IX (CAIX)-specific CAR T cells to treat renal cell carcinoma.[218] CAR T cell persistence was short and significant off-tumor toxicity occurred because CAIX+ epithelial cells in the liver bile ducts were targeted. No antitumor responses were observed and immune responses to the murine scFv used to construct the CAR were detected in patients after therapy,[219] which was not surprising given prior studies demonstrating immune responses to foreign transgene products in patients receiving ACT.[220,221] Thus, studies with first-generation CAR T cells highlighted the need to modify the signaling domain, improve gene transfer efficiency, and attenuate immunogenicity.[148,222,223]

CD19 Chimeric Antigen Receptors Incorporating Co-Stimulatory Domains Mediate Antitumor Responses

T cells transduced to express a CD19-specific CAR with one or more co-stimulatory domains in addition to CD3ζ

exhibited more potent antitumor activity in preclinical models.[188,223] In the only clinical trial to directly compare first- and second-generation CAR T cells, superior proliferation and persistence in vivo was observed for T cells expressing a CD28/CD3ζ CAR compared with those with a CAR containing only CD3ζ.[194] Results of large Phase 1 and 2 clinical trials using autologous T cells expressing CD19-specific CARs containing either 4-1BB/CD3ζ or CD28/CD3ζ signaling domains are described subsequently for the treatment of relapsed or refractory B cell malignancies and provide insight into the efficacy, toxicities, and current limitations.[224–233] However, comparing efficacy and toxicity across trials is challenging because of differences in scFvs, construct design, method of gene transfer, T cell culture conditions, composition of T cell products, lymphodepleting chemotherapy regimens, cell dose, and patient heterogeneity.

Acute Lymphoblastic Leukemia

ACT with CD19-specific 4-1BB/CD3ζ or CD28/CD3ζ CAR T cells after lymphodepleting chemotherapy induced complete remission in 80% to more than 90% of pediatric and adult patients with relapsed or refractory ALL.[97,226,228,231,234,235] CAR T cell activation and proliferation occurred in a majority of patients and, in those individuals, CD19+ leukemia cells were cleared rapidly from bone marrow, cerebrospinal fluid, and extramedullary sites. Studies in which CAR T cells were formulated with a uniform CD4:CD8 ratio revealed correlations between cell dose, antitumor response, and toxicity, and allowed better definition of the therapeutic window compared with heterogeneous products in other trials.[97] The degree of CAR T cell proliferation depended on tumor burden, and prolonged CAR T cell persistence of at least three to six months was associated with superior relapse-free survival.[97,228] Loss of detectable CAR T cells from peripheral blood was shown in some patients to be caused by T cell immune responses directed against epitopes in the murine scFv and other CAR components.[97,231] Many ALL patients who achieved a remission after CAR T cells had a subsequent stem cell transplantation, and long-term follow-up of patients who did not receive transplant are ongoing to determine whether this approach can cure a subset of patients. Notably, relapses with CD19− leukemia cells caused by mutations, alternative splicing of CD19 messenger RNA (mRNA), or a lineage switch to a myeloid phenotype do occur, suggesting that targeting more than one antigen may be important to achieve a higher cure rate and prevent relapse.[228,232,233,236]

Non-Hodgkin Lymphoma

CD19-specific CAR T cells were also shown to have antitumor activity in relapsed refractory NHL.[229,237] The largest reported single-center series used a 4-1BB/CD3ζ CAR, and a CAR T cell product prepared with a defined CD4:CD8 formulation.[98] This study showed that lympho-depletion with both cyclophosphamide and fludarabine (Cy/Flu) resulted in increased CAR T cell expansion and persistence, and higher response rates compared with Cy alone. The complete response (CR) rate in patients treated with Cy/Flu at the maximally tolerated CAR T cell dose was 64% in this study and all histologic lymphoma classifications responded.[98] CD28/CD3ζ and 4-1BB/CD3ζ CAR T cell products achieve complete remission rates of 54% and 40% and objective response rates of 82% and 52%, respectively, in relapsed refractory diffuse large B cell lymphoma and have been approved for this indication.[238–240] Studies are ongoing to investigate the mechanisms of nonresponse to determine whether resistance is at the level of the tumor cell and/or TME or reflects properties of CAR T cells in individual patients.

Chronic Lymphocytic Leukemia

Despite advances in targeted therapies for CLL, patients who become refractory to these agents have a poor prognosis. The initial studies of refractory CLL patients treated with CD19-specific CAR T cells reported objective response rates of 57% to 74% and CR rates of 21% to 29%.[241,242] CLL patients often have defects in T cell function, and some groups have reported difficulty transducing and expanding CAR T cell products in a significant fraction of patients. It has since been reported that the quality of the leukapheresis product used to generate CAR T cells, particularly the frequency of CD27⁺CD45RO⁻ memory-like T cells, correlates with clinical responses.[243] The ability to expand CAR T cells is improved in patients receiving the Bruton's tyrosine kinase inhibitor ibrutinib, and ibrutinib has been shown to improve CAR T cell function in preclinical animal models.[244,245] A subsequent clinical trial showed that CD19-specific CAR T cells with concurrent ibrutinib were well tolerated with an overall response rate of 83% (using 2018 International Workshop on CLL criteria), and a minimal residual disease (MRD)–negative marrow response by immunoglobulin heavy (IGH) sequencing of 61%.[246] Thus, combination therapies and other advances may improve the feasibility and efficacy of CAR T cells in CLL.

CD19-Specific Chimeric Antigen Receptor T Cells Can Cause Serious Toxicity

Toxicities of CD19-specific CAR T cells include cytokine release syndrome (CRS), neurologic sequelae, and persistent B cell aplasia. CRS typically occurs one to 10 days after the T cell infusion and is associated with elevated levels of cytokines including interferon gamma (IFNγ), tumor necrosis factor alpha (TNFα), IL-6, and IL-1, as well as acute phase reactants such as C-reactive protein and ferritin.[234,247,248] The clinical and biochemical manifestations of CRS may include fever, hypotension, tachypnea and hypoxemia, disseminated intravascular coagulation, azotemia, transaminitis, and neurologic alterations. A study of CRS in mice showed that the production of catecholamines by immune cells may play a key role in pathogenesis and suggested that interfering with catecholamine production might mitigate CRS.[249] The timing and type of interventions to manage CRS in patients continue to evolve; however, ICU management and administration of tocilizumab (antihuman IL-6R monoclonal antibody) are indicated in patients with significant hypotension and/or organ toxicity,[247] and has been shown to mitigate CRS without impacting antitumor efficacy.[250] Most groups are now using corticosteroids (dexamethasone or methylprednisolone) simultaneously with tocilizumab in patients with serious CRS.[247,251] Other agents that target cytokines or cytokine receptors may have utility in treating CRS. Ongoing studies are likely to elucidate the pathophysiology of CRS and determine whether early intervention with corticosteroids might compromise antitumor activity as suggested by one study.[234] An important issue is to identify patients at highest risk for CRS, where altering the CAR T cell dose or intervening early with immunosuppression may be necessary to avoid life-threatening toxicity. The heterogeneity in the design of CARs and in the composition of the CAR T cell products administered in various trials makes this task more difficult.

Neurologic complications including headache, mental status changes, focal neurologic deficits, seizures, and coma have been observed in all trials of CD19-specific CAR T cells. Neurotoxicity may occur concurrently with CRS or be delayed and is not as rapidly responsive to tocilizumab or corticosteroids as CRS.[252] Neurologic abnormalities fully resolve in most patients, but a small subset develops permanent impairments or rapid-onset cerebral edema. Severe neurotoxicity was associated with increased blood–brain barrier permeability and increased concentrations of systemic cytokines like IFNγ in the CSF, which induced vascular pericyte stress and secretion of endothelium-activating cytokines.[253] Preclinical studies suggest that monocyte/macrophage-derived IL-1 may promote both CRS and neurotoxicity, and that the IL-1R antagonist Anakinra can protect against both complications.[254,255] Nevertheless, the pathologic basis for neurologic abnormalities remains incompletely understood, making it difficult to intervene prophylactically or with specific therapy.

B cell aplasia occurs in patients with persisting CAR T cells that recognize CD19 on normal B cells. Nearly, all patients initially become B cell–deficient; however, many patients do not have long-term persistence of CAR T cells and recover B cells from hematopoietic progenitors.

In some patients, a T cell response to foreign components of the CAR can be detected, providing an explanation for the loss of detectable CAR T cells.[97,98,231] Patients in whom CAR T cells do persist long-term have B cell aplasia that could compromise immune responses to infection. However, a recent study demonstrated that virus-specific IgG levels were maintained in B cell aplastic patients for up to one year post treatment, presumably because long-lived plasma B cells are CD19[-], indicating that preexisting humoral immunity may be preserved.[256]

Several strategies for the conditional elimination of adoptively transferred T cells have been developed including expression of the herpes simplex virus thymidine kinase (HSV-TK) that renders T cells susceptible to ganciclovir, expression of an inducible caspase 9 that is activated by a dimerizer drug, and cell surface expression of molecules, such as CD20, or a truncated epidermal growth factor receptor (EGFRt) that may render cells susceptible to antibody-dependent cell-mediated cytotoxicity on infusion of a U.S. Food and Drug Administration (FDA)–approved mAb.[257] HSV-TK is immunogenic in humans, making it less attractive as a conditional suicide gene.[221] The inducible caspase is effective in the clinic for eliminating transduced polyclonal T cells that cause graft-versus-host disease (GVHD) in allogeneic stem cell transplant recipients,[258] and targeting EGFRt is effective in reversing B cell aplasia induced by CD19-specific CAR T cells in preclinical models.[259] Dasatinib, an FDA-approved tyrosine kinase inhibitor that interferes with Lck and thus inhibits CD3ζ/Zap70 phosphorylation, is an attractive alternative drug that can rapidly and reversibly ablate CAR signaling without affecting T cell viability.[260,261] Administering dasatinib early after infusion of CAR T cells was shown to protect mice from lethal CRS, although how transient inhibition of CAR T cells affects subsequent tumor control has not been demonstrated.[260] More refined strategies for regulating CAR expression and T cell survival are the subject of ongoing research.[160,170,212,218,262–266]

B Cell Maturation Antigen–Specific Chimeric Antigen Receptor T Cells Mediate Activity Against Multiple Myeloma

Building on the success of CD19-specific CAR T cells in B cell leukemia and lymphoma, CAR T cells have also been developed to treat resistant/refractory multiple myeloma. Multiple myeloma develops from clonal plasma cells that highly express BCMA, and, as such, BCMA-specific CAR T cells have shown impressive responses in initial clinical trials. In a first-in-human study, T cells expressing a murine anti-BCMA scFv linked to CD28/CD3ζ signaling domains induced an objective response rate of 81% at the highest dose level, with 13% of patients achieving a

complete response.[267,268] Subsequent clinical trials using a BCMA CAR-expressing 4-1BB/CD3ζ signaling domains resulted in objective response rates of 64% to 88% at the highest dose levels, with up to 74% to 76% achieving complete responses.[269–272] A high frequency of CRS was observed in all studies, with some cases of neurotoxicity, similar to that observed with CD19-specific CAR T cells in B cell leukemia and lymphoma. However, median progression-free survival lasted for only 11 to 15 months in most trials,[270,272] calling the durability of responses into question. Relapse and/or progressive disease was associated, in part, with anti-CAR immune responses, with more durable responses demonstrated in patients who had previously received autologous hematopoietic stem cell transplantation.[272] As such, several trials are ongoing using fully human scFvs.

Escape of BCMA-low or BCMA-negative myeloma cells is also a mechanism of relapse,[268,269] and BCMA can be shed from the surface of plasma cells by γ-secretase.[273] A recent study demonstrated that inhibition of γ-secretase could increase surface BCMA levels on myeloma cells and improve CAR T cell antitumor activity in vitro and in vivo in preclinical models.[274] Other strategies to combat antigen loss or downregulation include co-infusion with CD19 CAR T cells[275] and use of an APRIL-based CAR which enables targeting of both BCMA and TACI.[154,276] Combination therapy with lenalidomide, an immunomodulatory drug already approved for the treatment of myeloma, was also shown to enhance CAR T cell activity against antigen-low tumors and in the presence of inhibitory ligands like PD-L1.[277,278]

Chimeric Antigen Receptor T Cells Targeting Solid Tumors Mediate Incomplete Antitumor Activity

In contrast to the robust clinical efficacy achieved by targeting CD19 with CAR T cells, the treatment of solid tumors has produced less-striking results. The efficacy of a first-generation CAR specific for the TAA GD2 was evaluated in 11 neuroblastoma patients, and four of eight (50%) patients with evaluable tumors had evidence of tumor necrosis or regression and no evidence of on-target off-tumor toxicity.[212,262] Mesothelin was targeted in two patients with mesothelioma and pancreatic cancer, respectively, with autologous T cells that expressed a mesothelin-specific CAR after mRNA transfection. The CAR T cells migrated to sites of disease and transient shrinkage of one lesion was detected by MRI. Despite previous toxicity targeting Her2 with CAR T cells,[160] different Her2-specific CARs were tested in 19 patients with sarcoma. The Her2-specific CAR T cells persisted in some patients for six weeks and there were no dose-limiting toxicities and no evidence of antitumor efficacy.[264] More recently, an interleukin 13 receptor subunit alpha 2 (IL-13Rα2)–specific CAR produced modest antitumor activity in three glioblastoma patients.[170] In this study, subjects received up to 12 intracranial infusions in the tumor resection cavity, and two of the patients had evidence of transient antitumor activity with clinically manageable temporary brain inflammation as the only toxicity. Collectively, these results indicate that targeting certain overexpressed surface antigens on solid tumors with CAR T cells can lead to transient antitumor activity without off-tumor toxicity. Numerous clinical trials aimed at improving responses through additional genetic engineering and/or T cell culture techniques are currently in progress but have not yet reported the results.

BARRIERS TO EFFECTIVE ADOPTIVE T CELL TRANSFER AND POTENTIAL SOLUTIONS

Tumor Escape by Antigen Loss

CAR T cells are MHC-independent and tumors with low MHC expression remain susceptible to recognition. However, loss, downregulation, or differential splicing of the target antigen or epitope, as observed in some patients who received CD19-specific CAR T cells, are now established mechanisms of tumor escape.[97,233,279] Likewise, BCMA loss is associated with treatment failure in multiple myeloma.[268,269] This problem may be circumvented by targeting multiple antigens at once with multiple cell products or bispecific CARs targeting CD19 and CD20, or CD19 and CD22 for example, to reduce the probability of selecting for escape variants that lack expression of multiple antigens.[280–283] This is an attractive strategy for B cell malignancies and multiple myeloma where multiple targets have been identified, but finding pairs of TAAs that are coexpressed on the same tumor cell and can be safely targeted may prove challenging for other malignancies.

Toxicity to Normal Host Tissues

CAR T cells can result in toxicity because of off-tumor expression of the antigen on normal tissues. Because few truly tumor-specific antigens exist, developing new methods that enable CAR T cells to discriminate between tumor and normal cells expressing the same antigen would vastly improve both the efficacy and the safety of CAR T cell therapy (Figure 26.3). Recent studies have demonstrated that tuning the affinity of the scFv for Her2 or EGFR might allow selective recognition of tumor cells that express high levels of these molecules and not normal cells that express lower levels.[264,284,285] Whether this ability to discriminate target cells based on the level of antigen expression is maintained in vivo in relevant settings remains to be determined.

Another strategy to increase tumor specificity is to use "AND" logic gates that require recognition of two distinct TAAs on the same target cell to elicit full CAR T cell activation. Such a split-receptor system was designed in which a Her2-specific scFv was linked to the CD3ζ signaling domain and a second MUC1-specific scFv was linked to the CD28 signaling domain.[286] Both Her2 and MUC1 are commonly overexpressed in many tumors but have limited overlap in expression in normal tissues. The dual-specific CAR T cells only proliferated in response to Her2/MUC1 double-positive tumor cells that delivered both CD3ζ and CD28 signals, but not in response to Her2 or MUC1 single-positive "normal" cells. These dual-signaling CAR T cells, however, would fail to function against antigen-loss variants, and CD3ζ signaling alone is sufficient to induce some T cell activity against single-positive cells, suggesting that toxicity to single-positive normal tissues may still occur. The latter problem may be addressed by screening low-affinity scFvs that, when linked to a CD3ζ signaling domain, are incapable of inducing T cell activation without co-stimulation.[287] Thus, development of dual-signaling CAR T cells is likely to require further optimization for individual scFvs as well as identification of antigen pairs that are selectively coexpressed in tumor tissues, but not in normal tissues.

Tumor specificity can also be increased by using a split-receptor system to provide negative signaling in the presence of normal, but not tumor tissues, tissues. This principle is used naturally by the immune system, in which T cells upregulate the inhibitory receptor PD-1 on activation that engages ligands on normal cells to dampen T cell activity.[288] In principle, this mechanism can be exploited by coexpressing a second inhibitory synthetic receptor that activates PD-1 signaling after engaging an antigen expressed on normal tissues, but not on tumor tissues.[289] Here again, the utility of this approach will depend on identifying appropriate antigen pairs that are coexpressed on normal cells but where only the activating ligand is on tumor cells.

Sophisticated applications are emerging from the field of synthetic biology to regulate the activity of CAR T cells to minimize toxicity in vivo. Constructs have been designed in which CAR expression is regulated by a drug-inducible promoter or in which the recognition domain and signaling domain only associate together in the presence of a small molecule dimerizer.[265,290,291] Because CAR expression and/or signaling depend on the presence of an externally supplied drug, their activity can theoretically be halted if toxicity occurs simply by withdrawal of the drug.

Rather than using a drug to induce CAR expression, an inducible dual-receptor system has been described in which engagement of a receptor specific for one TAA is used to induce expression of a CAR specific for a second TAA.[292] The advantage of this approach is that expression of the CAR is restricted to sites where the first receptor is engaged; in order for a target cell to be lysed, it must also express the CAR ligand. Therefore, this approach can improve tumor selectivity by requiring

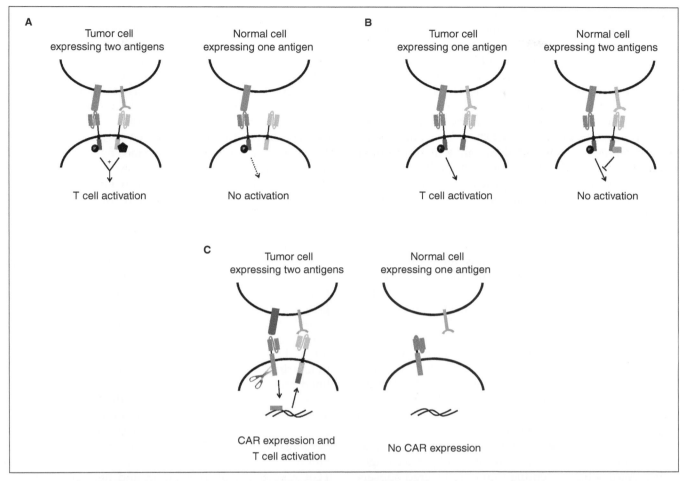

Figure 26.3 Strategies to improve tumor selectivity of CAR T cells. (A) T cells may be engineered to express a CAR and a chimeric costimulatory receptor specific for two different tumor-associated antigens (TAAs). The CAR contains the CD3ζ endodomain, whereas the CCR contains a co-stimulatory (e.g., CD28 or 4-1BB) endodomain. Dual-receptor T cells are only activated when both receptors are simultaneously engaged. Normal cells expressing only one antigen do not induce T cell activation and are spared from toxicity (right); only tumor cells expressing both antigens are capable of fully activating CAR T cells (left). **(B)** T cells may be engineered to coexpress a CAR capable of fully activating T cells and a chimeric receptor that delivers an inhibitory signal (e.g., via the programmed cell death protein 1 [PD-1] endodomain). Engagement of both targets on normal cells suppresses T cell activation (right), whereas recognition of only the activating ligand on tumor cells results in T cell activation (left). **(C)** CAR expression can be linked to an inducible system, such as a synthetic Notch receptor. Engagement of the Notch receptor specific for one TAA activates a transcription factor that induces transcription and expression of a CAR specific for a second tumor antigen. Tumor cells that express both antigens are capable of activating CAR T cells and are killed (left); normal tissues expressing either antigen alone cannot activate CAR T cells and are protected from killing (right).

recognition of two TAAs to elicit CAR T cell activity. This approach has several drawbacks: first, it takes ~8 hours for CAR expression to degrade after the first receptor is disengaged, creating a window during which the T cell expressing CAR can migrate and potentially engage normal tissues that express the ligand; second, the normal tissue cells that express the CAR target must be spatially segregated from the tumor or they will be susceptible to recognition and killing.[293] Nevertheless, this approach illustrates an important new principle that, if refined to

relevant CAR targets on solid tumors, might improve the therapeutic index of CAR T cells.

Overcoming the Immunosuppressive Tumor Microenvironment

Although CAR T cells are highly effective for hematologic malignancies, targeting epithelial cancers, which account for 80% to 90% of all cancers, has proven more challenging due, in part, to the immunosuppressive TME. Genetic engineering strategies have been used to generate CAR T cells intrinsically capable of resisting or overcoming particular immunosuppressive pathways. For example, several groups have attempted to block inhibitory PD-1 signaling by engineering CAR T cells to secrete anti-PD-L1 or anti-PD-1 antibodies,[294,295] to block endogenous expression of PD-1 via CRISPR/Cas9 or short hairpin RNAs,[144,296] or to coexpress "switch receptors" linking the PD-1 ectodomain to the CD28 endodomain such that engagement of PD-L1 delivers an activating rather than inhibitory signal to the T cell.[145,146] CAR T cells that were rendered resistant to suppressive TGF-β or Fas-mediated death signaling via genetic engineering have also shown improved activity in preclinical models of solid tumors.[297,298] Other strategies to genetically enhance CAR T cells include enabling them to secrete extracellular matrix-degrading enzymes that allow them to infiltrate solid tumors better[299,300] or engineering them to secrete the proinflammatory cytokine IL-12, which modulates many different immune cells, such as monocytes and macrophages, to promote antitumor immunity.[299,301–303] While each of these approaches has shown some degree of efficacy in preclinical models, none has yet been documented to improve CAR T cell activity in the native human TME.

A recent focus has been improving CAR T cell antitumor activity by altering their metabolic profiles to enhance their overall fitness. Memory T cells exhibit distinct metabolic profiles from effector T cells, such as a reliance on oxidative phosphorylation over glycolysis, that endow them with the ability to survive and persist longer in vivo. Studies have identified and engineered subsets of T cells with better metabolic profiles that enable them to resist immunosuppressive mechanisms in the TME. For example, T cells with low mitochondrial membrane potentials demonstrated superior persistence, metabolic fitness, and enhanced antitumor activity when engineered and adoptively transferred into tumor-bearing mice.[304] Another study identified a master regulator of mitochondrial membrane fusion, Opa1, that when transduced into T cells remodeled their mitochondria and endowed them with superior antitumor activity and memory-like characteristics such as elevated CD62L, chimeric costimulatory receptor 7 (CCR7), and CD127 expression; increased mitochondrial mass; and reliance on oxidative phosphorylation over glycolysis.[305] These studies suggest that new engineering, culturing, or selection methods that enhance the metabolic fitness of CAR T cells may improve efficacy in the immunosuppressive TME of solid tumors.

CELL MANUFACTURING AND ALLOGENEIC APPROACHES

A limitation for broader application of ACT as a therapeutic modality for cancer is the need to manufacture T cells under current good manufacturing practice (cGMP) conditions. The manufacturing of tumor-specific T cells selected from blood or engineered with TCRs has been facilitated by improved clinical cell-sorting capabilities, but cell doses of 10^9 to 10^{10} are routinely employed.[103,113,306,307] CAR T cells have been shown to be effective in doses of 10^7 to 10^8, which are relatively easy to manufacture, and potency may be further enhanced by engineering naïve and central memory T cell subsets that have superior capacity to proliferate and persist in vivo, culturing the T cells under cytokine or pharmacologic conditions that limit differentiation in vitro, and/or formulating cell products to contain both tumor-specific CD8+ and CD4+ T cell subsets.[80,89,90,93,97,98] Further genetic manipulation to confer superior function in immunosuppressive TMEs and combining T cells with checkpoint inhibitors or small molecules that target specific mechanisms that inhibit T cells should further reduce the cell doses needed for efficacy.

Separately, researchers and companies are developing technologies to enable the adoptive transfer of allogeneic T cells that are prepared in large quantities and stored until use.[308] Potential advantages of allogeneic CAR T cells include their availability for immediate use, the ability to re-treat patients without additional manufacturing, and cost reductions stemming from streamlined manufacturing operations. However, allogeneic T cells may be rapidly eliminated by the host immune system, which would limit treatment efficacy. Allogeneic T cells may also cause life-threatening GVHD, as has been demonstrated after hematopoietic stem cell transplantation.[309,310] Virus-specific memory T cells with limited TCR repertoires or TCR alpha and beta gene-edited T cells can be used for CAR T applications; they have the potential to mitigate GVHD, but further studies are necessary to assess the efficacy and limitations of these strategies.[311–313] Until further research demonstrates the ability of allogeneic T cells to safely mediate tumor regressions in patients, autologous T cells will continue to be used as the primary source of CAR T cell therapies.

CONCLUSION

ACT with genetically modified T cells has emerged as a curative modality for a subset of patients with refractory cancers. Recent advances in synthetic biology, genome engineering, and cell manufacturing have made it possible to develop highly specific and potent tumor-reactive T cells and offer many opportunities for experimentation and broader clinical translation. Extending the success of ACT to additional patient populations will require new strategies to overcome immunosuppression and toxicity to normal tissues. Recent proof-of-principle studies have demonstrated that synthetic signaling systems allow for physician-controllable and/or inducible T cell activity in preclinical models.[265,292,314] Advances in genome and cell engineering technologies could also further improve ACT.

For example, targeted insertion of a CAR into the TCR alpha constant locus using CRISPR/Cas9 improved CAR T cell antitumor function compared with CAR T cells conventionally generated using retroviral-based gene transfer methods.[315] Additionally, improvements to cell isolation, culture, and manufacturing are being pursued to improve the phenotype, composition, and potency of infused T cells. With these and other advances, the field is poised for increasingly more effective applications of ACT.

KEY REFERENCES

Only key references appear in the print edition. The full reference list appears in the digital product on Springer Publishing Connect: connect.springerpub.com/content/book/978-0-8261-3743-2/part/part02/chapter/ch26

32. Stronen E, Toebes M, Kelderman S, et al. Targeting of cancer neoantigens with donor-derived T cell receptor repertoires. *Science.* 2016;352:1337–1341. doi:10.1126/science.aaf2288

89. Gattinoni L, Klebanoff CA, Restifo NP. Paths to stemness: building the ultimate antitumour T cell. *Nat Rev Cancer.* 2012;12:671–684. doi:10.1038/nrc3322

135. Khan O, Giles JR, McDonald S, et al. TOX transcriptionally and epigenetically programs CD8+ T cell exhaustion. *Nature.* 2019;571:211–218. doi:10.1038/s41586-019-1325-x

225. Kalos M, Levine BL, Porter DL, et al. T cells with chimeric antigen receptors have potent antitumor effects and can establish memory in patients with advanced leukemia. *Sci Transl Med.* 2011;3:95ra73. doi:10.1126/scitranslmed.3002842

228. Maude SL, Frey N, Shaw PA, et al. Chimeric antigen receptor T cells for sustained remissions in leukemia. *N Engl J Med.* 2014;371:1507–1517. doi:10.1056/NEJMoa1407222

238. Neelapu SS, Locke FL, Bartlett NL, et al. Axicabtagene ciloleucel CAR T-cell therapy in refractory large B-cell lymphoma. *N Engl J Med.* 2017;377:2531–2544. doi:10.1056/NEJMoa1707447

292. Roybal KT, Rupp LJ, Morsut L, et al. Precision tumor recognition by T cells with combinatorial antigen-sensing circuits. *Cell.* 2016;164:770–779. doi:10.1016/j.cell.2016.01.011

Immunotherapy Based on Blocking T Cell Inhibitory Pathways

Randy F. Sweis and Jason J. Luke

KEY POINTS

- Many naturally existing counterregulatory pathways can inhibit immune responses. This negative regulation is physiologically advantageous under many circumstances, such as the prevention of uncontrolled autoimmunity or in maternal–fetal tolerance, but unfavorable in the context of cancer.

- Negative immune regulation occurs through surface receptor–ligand interactions including cytotoxic T lymphocyte-associated protein 4 (CTLA-4), programmed cell death protein 1 (PD-1), lymphocyte activation gene 3 (LAG-3), T cell immunoglobulin 3 (TIM-3), and T cell immunoreceptor with immunoglobulin and ITIM domain (TIGIT). Negative immune regulation can also occur through metabolic pathways including adenosine A_{2A} and indoleamine 2,3-dioxygenase 1 (IDO).

- Given the presence of neoantigens generated from tumor mutations, an antitumor immune response often occurs in patients with cancer. However, tumors exploit negative regulatory pathways to evade antitumor immunity.

- Blocking negative regulation through small molecules or antibodies has proven to be the most successful cancer immunotherapy strategy to date. Specifically, anti-PD-1/programmed death ligand 1 (PD-L1) antibodies have clinical activity in numerous cancer types.

- Key clinical advantages to blocking negative immune regulation include durability of responses and tolerability with manageable toxicities.

- There are challenges to blocking negative regulation, including the lack of response in tumors with more than one active negative regulatory pathway and tumors that are "non-T cell-inflamed," which lack preexisting immune priming. Combination strategies such as targeting multiple immune checkpoints simultaneously or adding chemotherapy, vaccines, or radiation therapy to overcome resistance are now being investigated.

INTRODUCTION

Negative regulation of the immune system is a critical evolutionary process necessary to prevent unrestrained immune activation and autoimmunity. This regulation occurs through a variety of mechanisms including expression of cell surface proteins that regulate intracellular pathways in immune cells, alteration of cytokines and chemokines, and modulation of metabolic states. Discoveries in recent years have indicated that immune inhibitory pathways often dominate in the setting of malignancy, thwarting the ability of the endogenous immune response to eliminate cancer cells. This concept has been critical to the development of modern cancer immunotherapies, as numerous therapeutic agents now target negative immune regulatory pathways. This therapeutic approach has led to a surge in effective immunotherapies available to patients, with dramatic responses observed in some patients with previously refractory metastatic cancers.

BASIC BIOLOGY OF NEGATIVE REGULATORY PATHWAYS

Effective antitumor immunity requires complex processes involving antigen presentation, lymphocyte activation, and proliferation in peripheral lymphoid tissue, trafficking to the tumor microenvironment, and execution of effector function to eliminate malignant cells. Priming and activation of tumor antigen-specific T cells are dependent on both the engagement of the T cell receptor (TCR) with the antigen/major histocompatibility complex (MHC) and a co-stimulatory signal from CD28 binding with B7-1 (CD80) or B7-2 (CD86) on antigen-presenting cells (APCs). This second signal results in the production of stimulatory cytokines, enhanced cell survival and differentiation, increased metabolism, and T cell proliferation. Additional co-stimulatory molecules with similar effects have been identified during the past decades, and concurrently, inhibitory molecules have been discovered that can be expressed on the cell surface of T lymphocytes and other immune cells (Table 27.1). Negative regulatory pathways are commonly engaged within the tumor microenvironment of cancers. In general, negative regulation can occur during each of the steps involved in antitumor immune responses including processing and presentation of antigens, priming and activation of T cells, recruitment of cytotoxic lymphocytes to the tumor microenvironment, and effector T cell engagement of tumor cells. Currently, the agents with proven efficacy block engagement of inhibitory receptors expressed by tumor-specific T cells within the tumor microenvironment. The most therapeutically successful targets have been cytotoxic T-lymphocyte-associated protein 4 (CTLA-4) and programmed cell death protein 1/programmed death ligand 1 (PD-1/PD-L1), with U.S.

Food and Drug Administration (FDA) approvals now achieved in multiple cancer types. Additional antibodies or small molecules in clinical testing are targeting lymphocyte-activation gene 3 (LAG-3) protein and hepatitis A virus cellular receptor 2 (HAVCR2), also known as T cell immunoglobulin 3 (TIM-3), and indoleamine 2,3-dioxygenase 1 (IDO). Finally, the presence of adenosine in the tumor microenvironment has been shown to suppress the immune response, and thus inhibitors of the adenosine A_{2A} receptor/CD39/CD73 pathway are currently in clinical development.

Cytotoxic T-Lymphocyte-Associated Antigen 4
Structure and Discovery

CTLA-4, also known as CD152, was initially identified in 1987 as a member of the immunoglobulin superfamily.[1] Its expression was noted to be restricted to lymphoid lineage cells, mainly on activated T cells. The molecule CTLA-4 was noted to be homologous with CD28, which has been identified as a co-stimulatory molecule[2] as both CTLA-4 and

Table 27.1 Negative Regulatory Pathways Being Targeted for Cancer Immunotherapy

TARGET	GENE SYMBOL	ALIASES	GENOMIC LOCATION	EXONS	PROTEIN	BINDING PARTNERS
CTLA-4	CTLA-4	CD152	2q33	4	Cytotoxic T-lymphocyte-associated protein 4	B7-1 (CD80) B7-2 (CD86)
PD-1	PD-1	CD279	2q37.3	6	Programmed cell death protein 1	PD-L1 (CD274) PD-L2 (CD273)
PD-L1	CD274	B7-H1 PDCD1L1	9p24	8	Programmed cell death 1 ligand 1	PD-1 (CD279) CD80
PD-L2	PDCD1LG2	CD273 B7-DC	9p24.2	7	Programmed cell death 1 ligand 2	PD-1 (CD279)
LAG-3	*LAG-3*	CD223	12p13.32	8	Lymphocyte-activation gene-3 protein	MHC class II Lectin FGL1
TIM-3	HAVCR2	CD366 KIM-3	5q33.3	7	Hepatitis A virus cellular receptor 2	Galectin-9 Ceacam1 HMGB1 PtdSer
TIGIT	TIGIT	WUCAM VSIG9 VSTM3	3q13.31	6	T cell immunoreceptor with Ig and ITIM domains	CD155 CD112
IDO	IDO1	INDO	8p11.21	10	Indoleamine 2,3-dioxygenase 1	n/a
A2AR	ADORA2A	RDC8	22q11.23	6	Adenosine A_{2A} receptor	Adenosine (via CD39 or CD73)

A2AR, adenosine A_{2A} receptor; CTLA-4, cytotoxic T-lymphocyte-associated protein 4; FGL1, fibrinogen-like protein 1; IDO, indoleamine 2,3-dioxygenase 1; ITIM, immunoreceptor tyrosine-based inhibitory motif; *LAG-3*, lymphocyte-activation gene 3; MHC, major histocompatibility complex; HAVCR2, Hepatitis A virus cellular receptor 2; PD-1, programmed cell death protein 1; PD-L1, programmed death ligand 1; PD-L2, programmed death ligand 2; TIGIT, T cell immunoreceptor with immunoglobulin and ITIM domain; TIM-3, T cell immunoglobin 3.

CD28 share common protein elements including a single extracellular IgV domain. The sequence of these proteins is highly conserved across several species with greater than 70% homology between humans and mouse including complete conservation of the cytoplasmic domain.[3] The *CTLA-4* gene contains four exons, encoding a signal peptide sequence, an IgV-like ligand-binding domain, a transmembrane region, and a cytoplasmic domain. There are four known splice variants with the first being a full-length transcript including all four exons. Other variants include a soluble CTLA-4 lacking the transmembrane exon 3, a variant lacking exons 2 and 3, and a ligand-independent variant lacking exon 2. CTLA-4 binds the same ligands as CD28, namely B7-1 and B7-2. CTLA-4 forms covalent homodimers that bind two B7 molecules at the cell surface, which differs from the monovalent binding of CD28 homodimers. Thus, CTLA-4 binds B7 molecules with greater affinity than CD28, with the following K_D values[4,5]: CD28:B7-1: $K_D = 4$ μM, CD28:B7-2: $K_D = 20$ μM; CTLA-4:B7-1: site 1 $K_D = 0.2$ μM, site 2 $K_D = 1.4$ μM; CTLA-4:B7-2: site 1 $K_D = 2.6$ μM, site 2 $K_D = 22.4$ μM. Thus, when CTLA-4 becomes expressed, the dominant functional effect of B7 ligands on T cells is favored to be inhibitory.[6]

Expression and Function

In resting T cells, CTLA-4 is present mainly in the intracellular compartment in perinuclear Golgi vesicles, endosomes, and lysosomes. A small fraction is present on the cell surface, and in the absence of phosphorylation, it is continually internalized by clathrin-mediated endocytosis via AP-2. Intracellular calcium influx from TCR activation enhances localization to the cell surface, and phosphorylation of its cytoplasmic domain inhibits internalization. In this manner, the expression of surface CTLA-4 is mainly restricted to activated T cells. The expression after activation is also regulated transcriptionally.

Given its similarity to CD28, CTLA-4 was initially believed to be a co-stimulatory molecule.[7,8] Early reports suggested that CTLA-4 and CD28 synergistically increased CD4[+] T cell proliferation.[9] However, even at that time, qualitative differences were noted between the effects of the two molecules, such as the lack of intracellular calcium mobilization or interleukin-2 (IL-2) production induced by CTLA-4 antibody binding. Subsequent work demonstrated that CTLA-4 is actually an inhibitor of T cell function and plays a critical role in regulating immune priming.[10–14] Evidence for an inhibitory effect of CTLA-4 was noted in CTLA-4 knockout mice, which develop a lymphoproliferative disease and tissue destruction due to infiltration of activated polyclonal T lymphocytes.[15] These mice die within 4 weeks of life, primarily due to severe myocarditis and pancreatitis. They also develop mononuclear infiltrates in the liver, lungs, and salivary glands, while some organs such as the kidney and thyroid gland appear to be spared.

Once on the surface of CD4[+] or CD8[+] T cells, CTLA-4 can bind B7-1 and B7-2 on APCs (Figure 27.1). Furthermore, CD28-mediated co-stimulation of the T cell is inhibited partially not only through competition for B7-1 and B7-2 binding but also through other mechanisms. CTLA-4 can remove ligands from APC through transendocytosis, and binding and activation of CTLA-4 inhibits the production of IL-2 and limits cellular proliferation through interactions with tyrosine phosphatases Src homology region 2 domain-containing phosphatase-1 (SHP-1), Src homology region 2 domain-containing phosphatase-2 (SHP-2), and protein phosphatase 2 (PP2A). In addition, ligation of B7 on APCs by CTLA-4 has been reported to induce reverse signaling and induction of inhibitory factors such as IDO.[16] Binding of CTLA-4, therefore, results in blunting of TCR signal transduction and CD8[+] lymphocyte inhibition through multiple mechanisms.

An inhibitory impact on CD4[+] T cells has also been ascribed to CTLA-4. The X-linked transcription factor forkhead box P3 (Foxp3) is a hallmark of immunosuppressive regulatory T cells (T$_{reg}$ cells) and leads to constitutive expression of CTLA-4 on this CD4[+] T cell subset.[17] It has been demonstrated that the effects of CTLA-4 blockade in a preclinical model increased antitumor immunity through the effects on both CD8[+] and CD4[+] T$_{reg}$ cell subsets.[18] Evidence for the T$_{reg}$-dependent effect of CTLA-4 blockade has been demonstrated by the restoration of polyclonal activation of T cells with CTLA-4 antibody treatment, even when the conventional T cells lacked CTLA-4 and could not be affected by the treatment.[19] The relationship between CTLA-4 and T$_{reg}$ cells, however, is not straightforward and has been the subject of much debate with conflicting data in preclinical models. Some data suggest that the inhibitory function of T$_{reg}$ cells from CTLA-4$^{-/-}$ mice is not lost in vitro.[20] In sum, extensive bodies of work indicate at least a partial role for T$_{reg}$-dependent effects of CLTA-4 blockade.[21]

Despite the existence of some uncertainty around its precise mechanism of action, numerous studies confirmed that CTLA-4 inhibits antitumor immunity, and the development of therapeutic antibodies soon followed. Preclinical studies confirmed that anti-CTLA-4 monoclonal antibodies augmented the proliferation of stimulated T lymphocytes.[10] This eventually led to the clinical development of anti-CTLA-4 antibodies such as ipilimumab, which was approved in 2011 for the treatment of metastatic melanoma and ushered in a new era of modern immunotherapy.

Programmed Cell Death Protein 1 and its Ligands

Structure and Discovery

Programmed Cell Death Protein 1

Shortly after the discovery of CTLA-4, the PD-1/PD-L1 axis was also characterized and found to have inhibitory

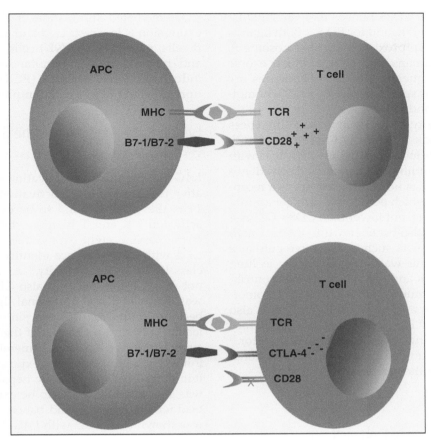

Figure 27.1 T cell activation requires both binding of the MHC-presented antigen from the APCs to the TCR and a co-stimulatory signal from CD28 binding B7-1/B7-2 molecules (top). CTLA-4 surface expression becomes upregulated, and binding of B7 results in inhibition of T cell activation both through competitive binding to B7 ligands and through inhibition of downstream TCR/CD28 signaling.

APC, antigen-presenting cells; CTLA-4, cytotoxic T-lymphocyte-associated protein 4; MHC, major histocompatibility complex; TCR, T cell receptor.

effects on antitumor immunity. PD-1, also known as CD279, is a member of the immunoglobulin superfamily. It is part of the CD28/CTLA-4 subfamily, and its sequence is conserved across human and mouse species.[22] It lacks a cysteine present in CTLA-4 that leads to homodimerization, and fluorescence resonance energy transfer (FRET) experiments have indicated that PD-1 exists as a monomer on the cell surface.[23] The gene contains five exons, encoding: a signal peptide sequence, an IgV-like ligand-binding domain, a stalk and transmembrane region, a cytoplasmic domain encoding an immunoreceptor tyrosine-based inhibitory motif (ITIM), and a cytoplasmic domain encoding an immunoreceptor tyrosine-based switch motif (ITSM).

There have been five splice variants described for PD-1. In addition to the full-length transcript, variants lacking exon 2, exon 3, exons 2 and 3, and exons 2 to 4 have been described.[24] The splice variant lacking the transmembrane exon 3 is similar to the analogous splice variant of CTLA-4 in that it results in a soluble form of PD-1. This form has been detected in the serum of patients with autoimmune diseases such as rheumatoid arthritis.[25] PD-1 lacks the amino acid sequence MYPPPY responsible for CD28 and CTLA-4 binding of B7-1 and B7-2. However, two novel PD-1-binding ligands, PD-L1 (CD274) and PD-L2 (PDCD1LG2), were subsequently identified.

Programmed Death Ligand 1 and Programmed Death Ligand 2

It was noted that, unlike CTLA-4 and CD28, PD-1 did not bind B7-1 and B7-2. A search to identify PD-1 ligands resulted in the discovery of two B7 homologs: PD-L1 and PD-L2. Human and murine cDNAs for PD-L1 were identified in 1999 by a B7 homology-based search of expressed sequence tag databases.[26,27] PD-L1 is a 290 amino acid type I transmembrane protein. It was noted that PD-L1 bound exclusively to PD-1 and demonstrated no binding to CTLA-4 or CD28. Shortly thereafter, PD-L2 was identified as a second ligand for PD-1.[28] Both ligands are genomically in close proximity on chromosome 9, only 42 kb apart in humans, and have a similar exonic structure with 34% sequence identity.[29] Sequences are highly conserved across species with 69% to 70% homology between humans and mouse.

Despite their similarity, there are important differences between the two ligands. First, the PD-1 binding affinity with PD-L2 is twofold to sixfold higher than that with PD-L1.[30] Additional binding partners have been identified. For instance, CD80 is now known to act as a receptor for PD-L1 binding, which occurs with greater affinity than CD80-CD28 binding, but lower than CD80–CTLA-4 binding.[31,32] PD-L2 has also been shown to interact with additional binding partners such as repulsive guidance molecule B (RGMb). This was shown to occur in lung interstitial macrophages and alveolar cells and contributed to respiratory, immune tolerance through promoting the initial clonal expansion of T cells.[33] There is also evidence that PD-L1 and PD-L2 may have co-stimulatory function through binding to an unidentified receptor.[34] Lastly, each ligand has unique expression and functional patterns, as outlined in the next section.

Expression and Function

PD-1 is inducibly expressed on activated T cells in response to TCR signaling, similar to CTLA-4. The expression of PD-1 on T cells also is upregulated by γ-chain cytokines, such as IL-2, IL-7, IL-15, IL-21, and also with type I interferons.[35] Prolonged antigen stimulation results in T cell effector dysfunction, as evidenced by studies showing reduced cytokine production in PD1[+] compared with PD1[−] tumor-infiltrating lymphocytes (TILs).[36]

The PD-1 ligands, both PD-L1 and PD-L2, are expressed in response to γ-chain cytokines as well as type I and type II interferons. PD-L2 expression is also strongly increased in response to granulocyte-macrophage colony-stimulating factor (GM-CSF) and IL-4. The expression of both ligands is context-dependent and highly dynamic. PD-L1 is generally more widely expressed but is not restricted to hematopoietic cells. In fact, its expression has been found extensively on tumor cells of numerous cancer types. PD-L1 binding to PD-1 was shown to inhibit CD3-mediated T-lymphocyte proliferation.[27] PD-1-mediated inhibition is more potent in the context where CD28 co-stimulation is inadequate.

Inhibition of T cell activation has been demonstrated by the binding of PD-1 to each of its ligands. While the PD-1 pathway bears some resemblance to CTLA-4, in that it serves to inhibit the activity of T cells, there are several distinctions between these two pathways. Expression of PD-1, similar to CTLA-4, is upregulated following CD3/ CD28-mediated stimulation of T cells. However, PD-1 expression is less restricted and also occurs on activated B cells, natural killer (NK) cells, dendritic cell subsets, and myeloid cells.[37,38] Similar to TCR-mediated PD-1 induction, B cell receptor (BCR) activation results in upregulation of PD-1 on B lymphocytes.[38]

Lymphocyte-Activation Gene 3

Structure and Discovery

LAG-3, or lymphocyte-activation gene 3, is another negative regulator of T cell activation. It was discovered in 1990 after it was found to be expressed selectively in activated NK and T lymphocytes.[39] The gene is 6.6 kb encompassing eight exons. It is structurally similar to CD4 with 20% sequence identity and also binds MHC class II with higher affinity.[40] As it is known to impact not only CD4[+] T cells but also CD8[+] T and NK cells, it was postulated that additional ligands exist for LAG-3 besides MHC class II. Liver sinusoidal endothelial cell lectin (LSECtin), a member of the C-type lectin receptor superfamily, is a type II transmembrane protein that was initially found to be highly expressed in the liver where it impairs T cell immunity to hepatitis B virus.[41] LSECtin was subsequently found to be expressed in melanoma, bladder, endometrial, and pancreatic cancer tissues and was shown to interact with LAG-3.[42]

Expression and Function

The expression of LAG-3 is found on CD4[+] and CD8[+] T lymphocytes. Early evidence of LAG-3 as a negative regulator of T cell proliferation was first published in the 1990s. It was reported that LAG-3 binding to MHC class II results in a decreased proliferative response in CD4[+] T cells and cross-linking of LAG-3 with CD3 inhibits TCR function.[43,44] The downstream signaling mechanism of LAG-3 is not fully understood, but it appears that the cytoplasmic tail contains a KIEELE motif that is essential for its inhibitory function.[45] It has been found to be highly expressed by Foxp3[+]CD4[+] T_{reg} cells relative to effector CD4[+] T cells, and antibodies to LAG-3 were shown to inhibit T_{reg}-mediated immunosuppression in both in vitro and in vivo model systems.[46] Additionally, ectopic expression of LAG-3 in those studies resulted in potent suppression of T cell stimulation relative to control T cells, even with a mutant of LAG-3 without affinity to MHC class II. LAG-3 is also commonly co-expressed on dysfunctional CD8[+] T cells along with PD-1, and inhibition of both synergistically reverses T cell anergy.[47–49] Additional ligands independent of MHC class II may also play a key role in LAG-3 signaling. Preclinical data have implicated fibrinogen-like protein 1 (FGL1) as a major inhibitory ligand that is expressed by cancer cells and binds to LAG-3.[50] In sum, the breadth of data supporting *LAG-3* as a negative immune regulator supported the development of neutralizing antibodies for clinical testing.

T Cell Immunoreceptor With Immunoglobulin and Immunoreceptor Tyrosine-Based Inhibitory Motif Domain

Structure and Discovery

T cell immunoreceptor with immunoglobulin and ITIM domain (TIGIT) is a cell surface protein, which is a member of the immunoglobulin family. It was discovered in 2009 through a genomic search for structural analogs for immunomodulatory receptors specifically expressed on T cells.[51] Through this search, a gene was identified that contained an immunoglobulin variable (IgV) domain, a transmembrane domain, and an ITIM domain. Hence, it was named TIGIT. TIGIT has six exons and its protein product has 244 amino acids. It is also known as WUCAM, Vstm3, or VSIG9. In the original report on the discovery of TIGIT, a screen for binding receptors was performed. A single high-affinity receptor was identified, poliovirus receptor (PVR), which is also known as NECL5 or CD155.

Expression and Function

TIGIT is expressed in activated CD4$^+$ T cells, CD8$^+$ T cells, and NK cells. Unstimulated CD4$^+$CD45RA cells did not express TIGIT, suggesting that it is inducibly expressed after activation. It is not expressed in either activated or naïve B cells. Knockdown of TIGIT had no effect on T cell proliferation or cytokine production, indicating that TIGIT has no T cell-intrinsic function. In contrast, its binding partner PVR is expressed on dendritic cells, and binding of TIGIT led to an alteration in cytokine production. The ratio of IL-10 to IL-12 in dendritic cells was increased after TIGIT-PVR binding, and T cell activation in co-culture studies was reduced by half. Additional reports found that binding of TIGIT to PVR and PVRL2 leads to inhibition of NK cell cytotoxicity.[52] Taken together, these data indicated that TIGIT is an important negative regulator of the antitumor immune response and a potential target for cancer immunotherapy.

T Cell Immunoglobulin 3 (Hepatitis A Virus Cellular Receptor 2)

Structure and Discovery

The T cell immunoglobulin (TIM) family of surface proteins was discovered in 2001, and TIM-3 was identified in 2002.[53,54] In that study, antibodies generated through immunization of rats with T helper type 1 (Th1) T cell mouse clones were used to identify Th1-specific cell surface proteins by expression cloning. This screen identified a 281 amino acid type I membrane protein, designated TIM-3, and the human homolog was subsequently characterized by a database search. Human and murine proteins have 63% sequence identity with 77% identity in the cytoplasmic domain. Human TIM-3 was noted to be structurally similar to kidney injury molecule 1 (KIM-1), also known as HAVCR1, the receptor for hepatitis A virus cellular receptor 1. Both were found to be located on chromosome 5 in humans. The extracellular domain contains four sites for N-linked glycosylation and five sites for O-linked glycosylation, whereas the cytoplasmic domain contains five tyrosine residues, and two—Y256 and Y263—can be phosphorylated by Src kinases or IL-2-inducible T cell kinase (ITK).[55,56]

Expression and Function

TIM-3 was identified initially as a cell surface protein selectively expressed on the surface of Th1 cells. Flow cytometric analyses showed the absence of expression on naïve T and B cells, or macrophages and dendritic cells. Its expression has now been well characterized and noted to be also found on T$_{reg}$ cells, dendritic cells, NK cells, and monocytes. TIM-3 has been extensively studied in models of autoimmunity, and reduced expression is thought to play an important role in diseases such as multiple sclerosis, rheumatoid arthritis, and psoriasis.[57] Treatment of mice with an antibody to TIM-3 resulted in the development of hyperacute allergic encephalomyelitis and uncontrolled macrophage activation, which first indicated that it played a role in inhibiting effecter Th1 immune responses.[58] It has also been studied in models of chronic viral infections where its role likely parallels that in cancer. In the lymphocytic choriomeningitis virus (LCMV) chronic viral infection model, TIM-3 was found to mark dysfunctional virus-specific T cells.[59–61] Similar TIM-3$^+$ virus-specific T cells have been found in patients with chronic viral infections such as hepatitis B, hepatitis C, and HIV.[62–64]

TIM-3 expression has also been studied in the cancer context, where it is found on the surface of dysfunctional CD8$^+$ T cells in the tumor microenvironment, similar to PD-1. In fact, the expression of both is found on the most severely dysfunctional TILs, and it has now been observed in preclinical models that blockade of both is synergistic in promoting antitumor immune responses.[65]

METABOLIC NEGATIVE REGULATORS OF T CELLS

Adenosine A$_{2A}$ Receptor

Structure and Discovery

In the early 1970s, it was noted that adenosine can lead to increases in intracellular cyclic adenosine monophosphate (cAMP) in vitro,[66] prompting investigation to identify a cell surface receptor. Both the A_1 and A_{2A} receptors were first characterized in the 1970s and found to have opposing effects on the concentration of intracellular cAMP.[66-68] A total of four adenosine receptors (AdoRA$_1$, AdoRA$_{2A}$, AdoRA$_{2B}$, and AdoRA$_3$) were ultimately identified.[69] Binding of adenosine to AdoRA$_1$ and AdoRA$_3$ leads to inhibition of adenyl cyclase reducing intracellular cAMP. Binding of adenosine to AdoRA$_{2A}$ and AdoRA$_{2B}$ has the opposite effect, activating adenyl cyclase and increasing intracellular cAMP. The adenosine A$_{2A}$ receptor is encoded by the gene *ADORA2A*. ADORA2 is located on chromosome 22q11.23 and encodes the seven transmembrane, 410 amino acid AdoRA$_{2A}$ G protein-coupled receptor AdoRA$_{2A}$.[70-73] This receptor has a higher affinity for adenosine than AdoRA$_{2B}$ and has become a key therapeutic target in cancer immunotherapy.

Expression and Function

Adenosine receptors are expressed in numerous cell and tissue types including the brain and immune compartments such as the thymus, lymph nodes, and bone marrow. Adenosine is a nucleoside generated from adenosine triphosphate (ATP) that is found in intracellular or extracellular spaces including the tumor microenvironment. Adenosine is generated in the tumor microenvironment from ectonucleosides CD39 and CD73. Adenosine is converted to adenosine monophosphate (AMP) by adenosine kinase. However, hypoxia inhibits adenosine kinase, leading to increases in the concentration of adenosine in the extracellular space under hypoxic conditions.[74] Adenosine in the extracellular space can bind adenosine receptors. When bound to the adenosine A$_{2A}$ receptor, it results in abrogation of the antitumor immune response, thus making it an attractive target for cancer immunotherapeutics. Of note, A$_1$ and A$_3$ receptors are not expressed in peripheral T and B lymphocytes. In preclinical models, A$_{2A}$ receptor inhibition through both knockout experiments or exogenous antagonists resulted in activation of cytotoxic T cell response.[75,76] These findings have now led to the clinical exploration of A$_{2A}$ inhibitors to restore an antitumor immune response.

Indoleamine-2,3-Dioxygenase

Structure and Discovery

The description of an enzyme pathway that converted tryptophan to kynurenine was suggested initially in the 1950s from biochemical studies in bacteria and mammalian systems. An enzyme found in the rabbit intestine was shown to oxidize tryptophan to yield kynurenine and was tentatively called D-tryptophan pyrrolase.[77] This intracellular enzyme acted as a dioxygenase that incorporates an oxygen molecule into a substrate ($R + O_2 \rightarrow R[O]_2$). Through oxidation, this intracellular enzyme

cleaves the double bond of the indole moiety of tryptophan. It has subsequently been extensively characterized and is now known as IDO.[78] Its structure was confirmed by x-ray crystallography and is characterized by a heme molecule between two domains.[79] The large domain contains 13 alpha-helices and two 3$_{10}$ helices, while the smaller domain includes six alpha-helices, two betasheets, and three 3$_{10}$ helices.

Expression and Function

IDO has been found to be expressed in endothelial cells of various tissues including the lung and placenta, and also in dendritic cells. It was originally found to facilitate maternal tolerance to the fetus[80,81] and is now known to inhibit antitumor immunity. It catalyzes the oxidative cleavage of the pyrrole ring of tryptophan, which is the first and rate-limiting step of tryptophan degradation through the kynurenine pathway. In the tumor microenvironment, this leads to the reduction of free tryptophan, which cannot be synthesized de novo in mammalian systems. The depletion of this essential amino acid, in turn, restricts the clonal expansion of T cells and results in their dysfunction and can also facilitate differentiation to T$_{reg}$ cells by activation of the stress response kinase GCN2.[82,83] Preclinical mechanistic data have indicated that IFNγ produced by activated T cells is responsible for inducing IDO expression in the tumor microenvironment.[84] The resulting accumulation of kynurenine and its downstream metabolites also result in immunosuppressive activity by activating the aryl hydrocarbon receptor (AHR). Activation of AHR promotes T$_{reg}$ cell differentiation.[85] Both AHR and GCN2 can also impact dendritic cells and macrophages to promote an immunosuppressive environment by the production of IL-10 and transforming growth factor-beta (TGF-β).[86] Together with several other studies, IDO has been demonstrated to negatively impact antitumor immunity, and inhibition of the enzyme has shown promise in reactivating antitumor immunity in vivo.[87,88]

The Tumor Microenvironment and Negative Immune Regulation

The negative immune regulatory molecules described thus far have been noted to occur as an adaptive inhibitory response to the presence of tumor antigen-specific T cells present in the tumor microenvironment. The emergence of adaptive immune inhibition is dependent on the occurrence of spontaneous immune priming that involves the presence of APCs, T cells, type I interferons, and an appropriate milieu of chemokines and cytokines (Figure 27.2). In human tissue samples from several cancers, this phenotype has been identifiable through gene expression profiling as well as

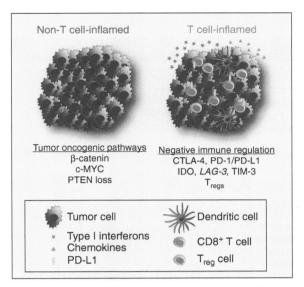

Figure 27.2 **Schema depicting T cell-inflamed versus non-T cell-inflamed tumor microenvironments.** T cell-inflamed tumors are associated with upregulation of various negative immune regulatory pathways that suppress the antitumor immune response. In contrast, non-T cell-inflamed tumors lack infiltrating T cells; thus, they generally do not develop adaptive immune resistance. Several oncogene pathways have been reported to contribute to a non-T cell-inflamed tumor microenvironment and likely contribute to immunotherapy resistance.

CTLA-4, cytotoxic T-lymphocyte-associated protein 4; IDO, indoleamine 2,3-dioxygenase 1; LAG-3, lymphocyte-activation gene 3; PD-1/PD-L1, programmed cell death protein 1/programmed death ligand 1; PTEN, phosphatase and tensin homolog; TIM, T cell immunoglobulin; T_reg, regulatory T.

immunohistochemistry for immune cell populations and has been referred to as a T cell–inflamed tumor microenvironment.[89,90] It has been shown that negative immune regulators such as PD-1, LAG-3, TIM-3, and IDO correlate strongly together with the presence of T cells.[91] Thus, it is important to note that targeting these negative regulatory elements may be limited to a subset of patients unless strategies are pursued to overcome the lack of immune priming and T cell infiltration observed in the non-T cell-inflamed tumors.[92] Preclinical mechanistic data have shown that immune checkpoint blockade approaches largely rely on T cells already within the tumor microenvironment for efficacy,[93] consistent with the notion that these therapies are refunctionalizing T cells already present within the tumor site. Recent work has identified several tumor-intrinsic oncogenic pathways that may play a role in preventing immune infiltration, including beta-catenin and c-myc activation, or phosphatase and tensin homolog (PTEN) loss,[94–96] which may lead to new predictive biomarkers for resistance and also indicate potential drug targets for improving immunotherapy efficacy.

THERAPEUTIC TARGETING OF IMMUNE CHECKPOINTS

With the increasing understanding of negative regulatory pathways in cancer immunity, monoclonal antibodies and, in some cases, small molecules have been developed for exploration in human clinical trials. The first approved checkpoint therapy, ipilimumab, is an anti-CTLA-4 mAb that began a sea change in the treatment of advanced cancers. Since that time, anti-PD-1/PD-L1 targeted therapies have also been approved, and combination therapy targeting CTLA-4 and PD-1 has also become a standard of care option for many cancer patients. Targeting other negative regulatory pathways such as LAG-3, TIGIT, and IDO has also shown promise in clinical trials, although the clinical development of those agents is ongoing and has not yet resulted in regulatory approval.

Therapeutically targeting immune negative regulatory pathways has transformed the ability to treat cancers such as melanoma, for which the 2-year survival rate has increased from 10% to nearly 50% with the recent combination immunotherapeutic approaches. Some responses have been found durable beyond 10 years, potentially raising the possibility of long-term survival and even possibly a cure in a subset of patients. Since 2011, when the anti-CTLA-4 mAb ipilimumab was approved for metastatic melanoma by regulatory agencies, clinical exploration of this therapeutic class has been occurring in virtually every malignancy and disease state. In most cases, cancers at advanced stages have been studied first; however, trials have also progressed toward studying the postsurgical adjuvant stage, the neoadjuvant setting, and in multiple combination regimens.

Success in targeting negative regulatory pathways has been shown to be broadly applicable across numerous cancer types in an unprecedented manner (Table 27.2). Therapeutic efficacy by type of malignancy is summarized separately in this text, but specific agents and their clinical development are reviewed in Table 27.2.

Anti-Cytotoxic T Lymphocyte-Associated Protein 4 Antibodies

Once it became apparent that CTLA-4 was a negative regulator of immune responses, it was postulated that inhibition of this pathway with monoclonal antibodies could be used to facilitate rejection of cancers through activation of endogenous antitumor T cells. The first preclinical studies were published in 1996 and indicated that this might be a viable therapeutic strategy to bring to the clinic.[11]

Ipilimumab

The first approved checkpoint therapy, ipilimumab, is a fully human monoclonal IgG1 antibody that targets

Table 27.2 Summary of U.S. Food and Drug Administration–Approved Therapies Targeting Immune Negative Regulation

DRUG	APPROVAL YEAR	CANCER TYPE	REFERENCES
Ipilimumab	2011	Melanoma	(97–99)
Pembrolizumab	2014	Metastatic melanoma	(100)
	2015	Non-small cell lung cancer	(101)
	2016	Head and neck cancer	(102)
	2017	Urothelial cancer	(103)
	2017	MSI-H or dMMR solid tumors	(104)
		Gastric cancer	
	2017	Cervical cancer	(105)
	2018	Primary mediastinal large B cell lymphoma	(106)
	2018	Hepatocellular cancer	(107)
	2018	Merkel cell cancer	(108)
	2018	Renal cancer (with axitinib)	(109)
	2019	Esophageal squamous cancer	(110)
	2019	Endometrial cancer (with lenvatinib)	(111)
	2019	Small cell lung cancer	(112)
	2019	TMB-H solid tumors	(113)
	2020	Cutaneous squamous cell cancer	(114)
	2020	MSI-H or dMMR colorectal cancer	(115)
	2020	Classical Hodgkin lymphoma	(116)
		Triple-negative breast cancer	
	2020		(117)
	2020		(118)
Nivolumab	2014	Metastatic melanoma	(119, 120)
	2015	Non-small cell lung cancer	(121)
	2015	Renal cancer	(122)
	2016	Urothelial cancer	(123)
		Classical Hodgkin lymphoma	(124)
	2016	Head and neck cancer	(125)
	2017	MSI-H or dMMR colorectal cancer	(126)
		Hepatocellular cancer	
	2017	Small cell lung cancer	(127)
	2018	Esophageal squamous cancer	(128)
	2020		(129)
Atezolizumab	2016	Urothelial cancer	(130)
	2016	Non-small cell lung cancer	(131)
	2019	Triple-negative breast cancer (with nab-paclitaxel)	(132)
	2019	Small cell lung cancer (with carboplatin and etoposide)	(133)
	2020	Hepatocellular cancer (with bevacizumab)	(134)
	2020	Metastatic melanoma (BRAF V600 mutation-positive, with cobimetinib and vemurafenib)	(135)
Durvalumab	2017	Urothelial cancer	(136)
	2018	Non-small cell lung cancer	(137)
	2020	Small cell lung cancer (with cisplatin or carboplatin and etoposide)	(138)
Avelumab	2017	Urothelial cancer	(139, 140)
	2017	Merkel cell cancer	(141)
	2019	Renal cancer (with axitinib)	(142)
Cemiplimab	2018	Cutaneous squamous cell cancer	(143)
Ipilimuimab + Nivolumab	2015	Metastatic melanoma	(144)
	2017	Renal cancer (intermediate/poor risk)	(145)
	2018	MSI-H or dMMR colorectal cancer	(126)
		Non-small cell lung cancer	
	2020	Malignant pleural mesothelioma	(146)
	2020	Hepatocellular cancer	(147)
	2020		(127)

dMMR, mismatch repair–deficient; MSI-H, microsatellite instability-high; TMB-H, tumor mutational burden-high.

CTLA-4 and was approved by regulatory agencies in 2011.[97] Two large, international randomized Phase 3 studies were performed. The first included 676 patients who had progression on prior treatment. Ipilimumab was given as an intravenous infusion at a dose of 3 mg/kg every 3 weeks for four cycles. A gp100 vaccine was given as a series of two modified HLA-A*0201-restricted peptides, gp100:209–217(210M) and gp100:280–288(288V). Each peptide was injected subcutaneously into opposite thighs at a dose of 1 mg, as an emulsion with Montanide ISA-51. This study included three treatment arms randomly assigned in a 3:1:1. The first group received ipilimumab plus the gp100 peptide vaccine, the second group received ipilimumab plus vaccine placebo, and the third group received gp100 plus ipilimumab placebo. The median overall survival in the ipilimumab group was 10.0 months (95% confidence interval (CI): 8.5–11.5) compared with 6.4 months (95% CI: 5.5–8.7) for the gp100 group, with a hazard ratio for death of 0.66 with a p value of .0003. There was no difference detected between the ipilimumab groups.

In a separate large Phase 3 randomized trial, ipilimumab was compared with dacarbazine in patients with previously untreated metastatic melanoma.[148] In this study, 502 patients were randomized 1:1 to ipilimumab at 10 mg/kg plus dacarbazine at 850 mg/m² versus dacarbazine plus placebo. Dacarbazine was given every 3 weeks for a total of eight cycles, and ipilimumab or placebo was given along with dacarbazine every 3 weeks for the first four cycles. Overall survival was significantly longer in the ipilimumab group at 3 years (20.8% vs. 12.2%), with a hazard ratio for death of 0.72 (p <.001). Percent survival was also significantly higher in the ipilimumab group at 1- and 2-year time points. This trial used a higher dose of ipilimumab when compared with the other Phase 3 trial (10 mg/kg vs. 3 mg/kg), and the combination of 10 mg/kg ipilimumab and dacarbazine had a higher incidence of grade 3 to 4 adverse events than ipilimumab 3 mg/kg plus gp100 vaccine (56.3% vs. 45.5%). Nonetheless, this trial importantly demonstrated efficacy in a previously untreated population.

The dosing of ipilimumab has been explored in a randomized Phase 2 study that compared 0.3 mg/kg, 3 mg/kg, and 10 mg/kg given every 3 weeks for four cycles followed by maintenance dosing in previously treated melanoma patients.[149] Ipilimumab demonstrated dose-dependent efficacy and dose-dependent toxicity. In order of increasing dosing, the best overall response rates were 0%, 4.2%, and 11.2%, whereas immune-related grade 3 to 4 adverse events were 26%, 65%, and 70%. Dosing of 3 and 10 mg/kg has been compared in a large Phase 3 study (NCT01515189), which has not yet been reported.

Long-term follow-up from a pooled analysis of 1,861 patients from 12 clinical trials reporting survival data from ipilimumab-treated melanoma patients indicated that responses have been durable with a plateau in the survival curve at 3 years.[150] The median overall survival was 9.5 months, and the 3-year overall survival rate was 26% for treatment-naïve patients and 20% for previously treated patients. Survival in some patients extended to 10 years after treatment with ipilimumab, thus raising the possibility of cure and generating further excitement in the strategy of targeting immune negative regulatory pathways.

Ipilimumab has also been evaluated and FDA approved in the adjuvant setting in melanoma. Historically, interferon alpha was demonstrated to prolong disease-free survival, and possibly overall survival, in multiple trials published since 1990. Typically, high-dose interferon alpha has been tested in stage IIB or III melanoma patients and involves the intravenous infusion of 20 million units/m² 5 days per week for 4 weeks followed by 10 million units/m² three times weekly for 11 months. This regimen is associated with significant adverse events including, but not limited to, fatigue, granulocytopenia, liver toxicity, and depression. Nonetheless, a meta-analysis of 14 randomized controlled trials involving 8,122 patients indicated a statistically significant improvement in disease-free and overall survival with a hazard ratio for disease recurrence of 0.82 (p <.001), and 0.89 (p = .002) for death.[151] With these data as a foundation, ipilimumab was explored in the adjuvant setting. In a trial of 951 patients randomly assigned to either placebo or ipilimumab 10 mg/kg every 3 weeks for four doses followed by every 3 months for 3 years, median relapse-free survival was improved from 17 to 26 months.[98] Given that a high dose of ipilimumab was used, there were significant adverse events including five treatment-related deaths. The 5-year overall survival rate improved from 54.4% with placebo to 65.4% with ipilimumab.[99] On the basis of this trial, ipilimumab was approved for adjuvant treatment of melanoma. A second Phase 3 trial evaluating both 10 and 3 mg/kg versus high-dose interferon in the adjuvant setting showed that 3 mg/kg, but not the 10 mg/kg, dose resulted in a survival benefit. This finding was likely a result of the high discontinuation rate of ipilimumab at the high dose. Thus, the 3 mg/kg dosing is recommended when using in the adjuvant setting.

Tremelimumab

Ipilimumab was the first approved therapy to target an immune checkpoint; however, another CTLA-4-targeting agent, tremelimumab, has also demonstrated activity in cancer patients. Tremelimumab is a fully human monoclonal antibody against CTLA-4. A clinical trial including 655 patients was completed and compared tremelimumab 15 mg/kg every 90 days versus physician choice standard-of-care chemotherapy (temozolomide or dacarbazine). Overall survival for tremelimumab was 12.6 months versus 10.7 months for chemotherapy, which was not statistically significantly different (p = .88). However, the duration of response was longer for tremelimumab (35.8 vs. 13.7 months, p = .0011). It is widely assumed that post-treatment crossover to ipilimumab compromised the survival analysis in the Phase 3 trials of tremelimumab; however, regulatory approval was never obtained. This drug is again being studied clinically and is currently being investigated in combination clinical trials.

Anti-Programmed Cell Death Protein 1/ Programmed Death Ligand 1 Antibodies

Therapeutic targeting of the anti-PD-1 pathway has been the most broadly successful therapeutic approach in cancer immunotherapy to date. Signs of early success in melanoma spawned the development of numerous antibodies targeting this pathway, which has resulted in regulatory approval for multiple drugs for the treatment of over a dozen cancer types to date (see Table 27.2). It is anticipated that targeting this pathway will be successful in more tumor types and in newer combinations based on current clinical trial data.

Pembrolizumab

Pembrolizumab is a highly selective humanized, monoclonal IgG4-κ antibody against PD-1. The approval was based on results from a randomized clinical trial with 135 advanced melanoma patients, including some who received prior ipilimumab. Results showed a confirmed response rate of 38%, with no difference in patients who received prior ipilimumab.[152] The durability of responses was also demonstrated with 81% of patients still responding at the time of publication. Subsequent data expanded from this series of studies included 655 patients (581 with measurable disease) and showed a similar objective response rate of 33%.[153] Median overall survival was 23 months, and 74% of responses were durable (defined as lasting more than 1 year). Pembrolizumab subsequently gained approval for non-small cell lung cancer and advanced head and neck squamous cancer.

Over the next years, pembrolizumab gained 19 distinct cancer approvals (Table 27.2). The activity of this drug has been confirmed in cancers with few to no prior approved therapies, such as Merkel cell cancer and hepatocellular cancer.[154] Importantly, pembrolizumab initiated a new paradigm in drug development when it became the first tumor histology-agnostic drug ever approved by the FDA. In 2017, it was approved for microsatellite instability-high (MSI-H) or mismatch repair–deficient (dMMR) solid tumors, regardless of the origin of cancer. Pembrolizumab has been studied in earlier stages of

various cancers. For example, it gained approval in early-stage, nonmuscle–invasive bladder cancer making it the first systemic therapy used in cancer that is typically only treated with intravesical agents. Pembrolizumab is also effective in combinations with chemotherapy in lung cancer and targeted therapies such as lenvatinib and axitinib in renal cell carcinoma (RCC). New combinations are currently being explored in hundreds of clinical trials. Pembrolizumab has also been combined with stereotactic body radiation therapy (SBRT) in a Phase 1 trial including 79 patients.[155] The response rate was 13.1% in a patient population with highly refractory disease with a median number of five prior therapies.

From the early development of pembrolizumab, potential biomarkers predictive of response were evaluated with a major goal of selecting the optimal patient population for treatment. The most widely explored predictive biomarker for pembrolizumab efficacy has been PD-L1 immunohistochemistry. In clinical trials with pembrolizumab, the 22C3 antibody was used to measure the proportion of cells that were positive in a histologic tumor sample. Tumors were given a score called the tumor proportion score (TPS), and exploration into response rates at various TPS cutoffs was explored in the original Phase 1 study. In non-small cell lung cancer (NSCLC), for example, the response rate in patients with PD-L1 expression 50% or higher was 45.2%.[101] This compared favorably versus patients who had tumors with TPS between 1% and 49% or <1%, which had response rates of 16.5% and 10.7%, respectively. Similar patterns have been observed in other tumor types, and TPS is now validated for lung, gastric, esophageal, head and neck, cervical, urothelial, and triple-negative breast cancers. In some cancer settings, regulatory approvals are restricted to a population based on PD-L1 testing.

Nivolumab

Nivolumab is a fully human IgG4 antibody that blocks PD-1. In an early Phase 1 study, an objective response rate of 28% was observed in 94 melanoma patients.[119] In that study, responses were also noted in non-small cell lung cancer (18%) and renal cancer (27%). The length of response of more than 6 months was noted in 20 of 31 patients with a follow-up of 1 year or more. This study also highlighted the PD-L1 expression by immunohistochemistry as a potential biomarker. In 42 patients with staining performed, all nine responders were noted to be PD-L1-positive. In a follow-up study in melanoma patients, the median overall survival was 16.8 months and the objective response was noted in 31% of patients, with a median response duration of 2 years.[120] In the years after, nivolumab was also approved for renal cancer, non-small cell lung cancer, and relapsed Hodgkin lymphoma.[121–123] The latter was the first hematologic malignancy to gain immune checkpoint therapy approval.[156] Nivolumab ultimately has received approval in 10 cancer types (Table 27.2), including diseases with high unmet needs such as small cell lung cancer and hepatocellular carcinoma. It has been successfully evaluated in combination with CTLA-4 inhibitor ipilimumab, which is reviewed in the section on combination immunotherapy. Newer combination studies are ongoing with hundreds of trials actively accruing.

Atezolizumab

Atezolizumab is an engineered, high-affinity human IgG1 antibody that blocks PD-L1 and inhibits its interaction with PD-1. In a Phase 1 study in refractory bladder cancer patients, the objective response rate was 43% in patients with PD-L1-positive tumors (defined by positive PD-L1 immunohistochemistry on tumor-infiltrating immune cells) including a 7% complete response rate, and 11% in PD-L1-negative tumors.[157] As with the anti-PD-1 antibodies, extended clinical benefit was noted with responses of more than 6 months ongoing in 16 of 17 patients at the time of publication and a maximum duration of response over 30 weeks. Follow-up publications noted an overall objective response rate of 15% (including PD-L1-positive and PD-L1-negative patients) with 84% of responses ongoing with a median follow-up of 11.7 months.[130] This drug is being evaluated in several other cancer types and has now also gained approval in non-small cell lung cancer based on significantly improved overall survival versus docetaxel chemotherapy (12.6 vs. 9.7 months), small cell lung cancer, triple-negative breast cancer, and hepatocellular carcinoma (in combination with bevacizumab).[131]

Durvalumab

Durvalumab is a selective, high-affinity, engineered human IgG1 monoclonal antibody targeting PD-L1. The constant domain of the antibody was engineered to reduce antibody-dependent cellular cytotoxicity (ADCC) and complement-dependent cytotoxicity (CDC) by the introduction of three-point mutations that reduce binding to C1q and the Fc gamma receptors.[158] An objective response rate of 31% was reported in 42 patients with advanced urothelial bladder cancer from a Phase 1/2 study expansion cohort.[136] When enriched for patients with PD-L1-positive tumors, the response rate was 46.4%. In lung cancer, durvalumab was evaluated in patients treated with at least two prior therapies, including one platinum-based chemo regimen. Data from 444 patients from two cohorts of this Phase 2 study indicated objective response rates of 12.2% to 30.9%, with the highest response rate observed in patients with 90% or more of tumor cells staining positive for PD-L1.[159] Durvalumab was also successfully developed in combination with chemotherapy for small cell lung cancer and for non-small cell lung cancer as consolidation after chemoradiotherapy for stage III disease.

Avelumab

Avelumab is a fully human IgG1 anti-PD-L1 monoclonal antibody. It inhibits the interaction between PD-1 and PD-L1, and preclinical models suggest that ADCC may contribute to the activity of avelumab.[160,161] An objective response rate of 31.8% was reported in an 88-patient Phase 2 study in chemotherapy-refractory metastatic Merkel cell carcinoma.[141] Eight complete responses were observed. Responses were durable, with the majority (82%) ongoing at the time of reporting and the longest ongoing response being 17.5 months. Based on this significant activity in a disease with few available effective therapies, avelumab received regulatory approval. In 2020, it received approval as maintenance therapy for urothelial carcinoma treated with platinum chemotherapy with stable disease or an objective response. This approval was based on a substantial overall survival benefit in the randomized Phase 3 Javelin Bladder 100 trial.[140] Median overall survival for maintenance avelumab was 21.4 months versus 14.3 months for best supportive care (HR: 0.69, 95% CI: 0.56–0.86, $p = .001$). The combination of avelumab plus axitinib in frontline renal cancer significantly prolonged progression-free survival compared with sunitinib (13.8 months vs. 7.2 months; HR: 0.61, 95% CI: 0.47–0.69, $p < .001$).[142] Avelumab is also currently under investigation in several other tumor types and in combinations.

Cemiplimab

Cemiplimab is a fully human IgG4 anti-PD1 monoclonal antibody that was developed for advanced cutaneous squamous cell carcinoma. In 2018, it became the first ever drug approved by the FDA specifically in this indication. Approval was based on a Phase 1 open-label study that evaluated cemiplimab in multiple solid tumors.[143] An expansion cohort for cutaneous squamous-cell carcinoma was carried out in 26 patients and the objective response rate was 50%. A Phase 2 study was then performed that showed a response rate of 47% in 59 patients, with four patients achieving a complete response (CR). Six of the 10 locally advanced patients, nonmetastatic patients included, had an objective response.

Anti-T Cell Immunoreceptor With Immunoglobulin Immunoreceptor Tyrosine-Based Inhibitory Motif Domain Therapy

After the recognition that TIGIT may impair T cell activation, antibodies targeting this protein soon entered clinical development. Tiragolumab is a fully human IgG1/kappa antibody designed to block the interaction between TIGIT and PVR. This drug was combined with the anti-PD-L1 antibody in a randomized, Phase 2 study in patients with NSCLC.[162] Initial data indicated that tiragolumab plus atezolizumab versus placebo plus atezolizumab resulted in an improved objective response rate (37% vs. 21%) and progression-free survival (PFS; 5.55 months vs. 3.88 months; HR: 0.58, 95% CI: 0.38–0.89). The benefit appeared to be restricted to patients with PD-L1 tumor expression of 50% or greater. This study led to a randomized Phase 3 study that is ongoing. Vibostolimab is another anti-TIGIT antibody that has been studied as monotherapy and in combination with the anti-PD-1 inhibitor pembrolizumab.[163] In a Phase 1 study expansion cohort in 79 patients with anti-PD-1/PD-L1 refractory NSCLC, the objective response rate was 7% with vibostolimab monotherapy and 5% with combination therapy including pembrolizumab.

Anti-Lymphocyte–Activation Gene 3 and Anti-T Cell Immunoglobulin 3 Therapy

The first therapy involving the *LAG-3* pathway that entered clinical trials was IMP321, a soluble *LAG-3*Ig fusion protein. The safety and tolerability of this drug were established in clinical trials from 2009 to 2014. In two Phase 1 studies, IMP321 was found to be tolerated and with no treatment-related adverse events. In one study of 18 pancreatic cancer patients, IMP321 at doses from 0.5 to 2.0 mg was evaluated in combination with gemcitabine (1,000 mg/m²).[164] No significant treatment-related events were noted. Similarly, it was shown to be generally well-tolerated in patients with renal cancer. However, no clinical activity was reported in either of these trials. In another trial where it was combined with a melanoma antigen recognized by T cells 1 (MART-1) peptide vaccine, an increase in antigen-specific T cells and a reduction in T_{reg} cells were reported, although with no associated objective responses. A potential for efficacy was shown in metastatic breast cancer when combined with paclitaxel, where the response rate reached 50% compared with a reported historical control rate of 25%.[165] A monoclonal antibody, relatlimab (BMS-986016), is another drug in clinical development that targets *LAG-3*. This drug has been explored as monotherapy and in combination with anti-PD-1 therapy (NCT 01968109). A Phase 3 study is now ongoing comparing the combination of relatlimab plus nivolumab to nivolumab alone in melanoma (NCT03470922).

An antibody targeting TIM-3 is a recent addition to the clinical development pipeline targeting negative immune regulators. Several TIM-3 inhibitors including TSR-022, LY3321367, Sym023, and INCAGN02390 have entered clinical trials as monotherapy and in combination with anti-PD-1 therapy.

Indoleamine 2,3-Dioxygenase 1-Targeting Therapy

Several IDO inhibitors were developed based on strong preclinical rationale including epacadostat (INCB 024360), indoximod (NLG2101), and NLG919. Epacadostat is an oral hydroxyamidine small molecule that inhibits IDO1. This drug was investigated in several clinical trials both as monotherapy and in combination with other immune checkpoints (ipilimumab, pembrolizumab, and durvalumab), cancer vaccines, or molecularly targeted therapies. In 2015, data from 54 patients treated with the combination of epacadostat and pembrolizumab were presented. Patients had advanced refractory solid tumors including melanoma, renal cancer, urothelial bladder cancer, non-small cell lung cancer, endometrial adenocarcinoma, and head and neck squamous cancer. Objective response rate was 53% in the melanoma cohort, and clinical development advanced to a Phase 3 trial.[166] Subsequent reporting of the Phase 3 randomized, placebo-controlled trial was negative and subsequent development was not pursued.[167] This negative trial dampened enthusiasm for this class of therapy. Nonetheless, some ongoing studies remain with other drugs. Indoximod is a selective IDO inhibitor with reported Phase 1 data and is being pursued for malignant glioma in pediatric patients.[168] Finally, linrodostat (BMS-986205) is an orally available inhibitor of IDO1 that is currently under development for urothelial carcinoma. It is being investigated in combination with nivolumab both in the BCG-unresponsive nonmuscle invasive bladder cancer setting (NCT 3519256) and for muscle-invasive bladder cancer in the perioperative setting (NCT03661320). Newer approaches targeting the tryptophan–kynurenine–AHR pathway are now being explored.[169] Promising methods include targeting Kyn-degrading enzymes, inhibiting the AHR, and tryptophan mimetics.

Adenosine A$_{2A}$ Receptor Pathway Inhibition

Therapeutics targeting this pathway have advanced through Phase 1 studies now and early results have been promising. Ciforadenant, an A$_{2A}$ receptor antagonist, has shown activity in several cancer types such as prostate cancer, renal cancer, and NSCLC.[170] Other A$_{2A}$ receptor antagonists in clinical development are taminadenant, AZD4635, PBF-999, EOS100850, and CS3005. AB928 is another adenosine receptor antagonist that is under development that blocks both A$_{2A}$ and A$_{2B}$. A second strategy to target the A$_{2A}$ pathway is to inhibit the production of adenosine through targeting ectonucleotidases that produce adenosine, namely CD39 and CD73. CPI-006 is a human IgG1 Fcγ receptor-deficient antibody that binds to CD73, blocking the ectoenzyme's catalysis of AMP to adenosine and also has agonist intracellular activity. CPI-006 has shown tumor regression with monotherapy and in combination with A_{2A} receptor blockade.[171] Patient selection for A_{2A} pathway–targeted therapy may play a role, as an adenosine gene signature has shown to be associated with response to therapy.

Combination Therapy

Given the successes of monotherapy with drugs targeting CTLA-4 and PD-1/PD-L1, and the fact that each target regulates different aspects of antitumor immunity, combination therapeutic approaches were then rapidly pursued. Preclinical data have indicated that certain combination immunotherapies are synergistic in mouse models, providing a mechanistic basis for clinical development.[93,172] In 2016, the FDA approved the combination of ipilimumab and nivolumab based on improvement in outcome compared with ipilimumab monotherapy in a randomized, double-blind study of 142 patients with metastatic melanoma.[173] Objective response rate for the combination was 61% versus 11% for ipilimumab alone. Median progression-free survival was not reached for the combination group and was 4.4 months in the ipilimumab group. A separate study also demonstrated similar improvement in outcomes for combination versus monotherapy with either agent.[144] The combination was subsequently approved for intermediate and poor-risk advanced RCC based on a randomized Phase 3 study versus sunitinib.[145] The potency of this combination has proven successful now in a variety of cancers. Between 2018 and 2020, the ipilimumab/nivolumab combination received approvals for MSI-H or dMMR colorectal cancer, NSCLC, malignant pleural mesothelioma, and hepatocellular cancer. Innumerable combination studies with anti-PD-1/PD-L1 mAbs are currently underway with many other agents, and it is expected that additional combination therapies will be high priorities for clinical investigation in the near future.

Dual-Targeted Therapies

Given the expected synergies of combining therapies that block negative immune regulation, the clinical development of dual-targeted single agents has grown. MGD013 is an IgG4κ bispecific protein using dual-affinity re-targeting (DART) technology by MacroGenics. This approach employs variable regions of heavy and light chains of an antibody that each recognize a different antigen. Regions are linked together with a spacer, then two polypeptides are joined through disulfide bonds. MGD013 is engineered to bind LAG-3 and PD-1. This drug has advanced through Phase 1 clinical trials and has shown preliminary activity in several tumor types.[174] Xencor has advanced multiple IgG bispecific antibodies into Phase 1 development including therapies with dual targeting of PD-1/CTLA-4 (XmAb20717) and CTLA-4/LAG-3 (XmAb22841). Bintrafusp alpha (M784)

is a bifunctional fusion protein that both blocks PD-L1 and traps transforming growth factor beta (TGF-β). Bintrafusp alpha is a fully human IgG1 monoclonal antibody that binds PD-L1 fused to the extracellular domain of the receptor. The latter portion functions as a trap for TGF-β.[175] This drug has now shown activity with durable responses observed in solid tumors including lung cancer and head and neck cancer.[176,177] Many other dual-targeting agents are in development and ongoing clinical trials will determine whether this approach to blocking multiple negative regulation pathways will emerge as a new standard of care in cancer immunotherapy.

IMMUNE-RELATED TOXICITIES ASSOCIATED WITH IMMUNE CHECKPOINT INHIBITORS

One of the most important challenges with cancer immunotherapy is the unintended consequence of immune activation resulting in immune-related adverse events. Blocking negative regulation not only results in activation of a tumor antigen-specific T cell response but also may activate self-reactive T cells, resulting in toxicity. As demonstrated in preclinical models, this can result in infiltration of activated polyclonal T cells into normal tissues, resulting in organ dysfunction and clinical toxicity (Exhibit 27.1). While immune checkpoint therapy is generally well-tolerated compared with other types of cancer therapy, such as chemotherapy or even molecularly targeted therapy, clinicians and patients must be aware of the unique toxicity profile of these drugs.

The time of onset is variable depending on the specific type of toxicity. Generally, the timing of most immune-related adverse events occurs in the first 6 months of treatment but is widely variable.[120,178–180] Some patients may experience toxicities as early as the first 2 weeks of therapy, while others may develop toxicities much later, even after discontinuation of the drug. The rate of certain toxicities may be differently observed between different drugs targeting negative immune regulation. For example, complications, such as colitis and hypophysitis, are more common with anti-CTLA-4 therapy compared with PD-1/PD-L1-targeted therapy. Even among the same class of drugs, there may be subtle differences. Avelumab, an anti-PD-L1 inhibitor, is linked with a higher incidence of infusion-related reactions compared with other PD-1/PD-L1-targeted agents. In general, combination therapy with anti-CTLA-4 and anti-PD-1 antibodies carries the highest risk for immune-related adverse events.

Prior to starting treatment, consensus guidelines recommend baseline testing with a complete blood count, comprehensive metabolic panel, thyrotropin, hemoglobin A1C, free T4, total CK, and fasting lipid profile.[181] Additionally, an EKG, troponin, and an infectious disease screen are recommended including

EXHIBIT 27.1

SELECTED COMMON TOXICITIES WITH IMMUNOTHERAPY TARGETING NEGATIVE REGULATION

Manifestations of immune-mediated adverse events by organ system

Pulmonary

- Pneumonitis

Endocrine

- Hypothyroidism and hyperthyroidism
- Adrenal insufficiency
- Hypophysitis and panhypopituitarism

Gastrointestinal

- Autoimmune hepatitis (elevated AST, ALT)
- Diarrhea
- Colitis

Dermatologic

- Dermatitis
- Vitiligo
- Pruritis
- Bullous dermatoses

Renal

- Nephritis

Musculoskeletal

- Arthritis
- Myositis

Ocular

- Conjunctivitis
- Scleritis
- Uveitis
- Graves' ophthalmopathy

Neurologic

- Myopathy
- Guillain–Barré syndrome
- Myasthenia gravis
- Encephalitis

Hematologic

- Thrombotic thrombocytopenic purpura
- Aplastic anemia

Cardiovascular

- Myocarditis

ALT, alanine transaminase; AST, aspartate transaminase.

hepatitis B surface antigen, hepatitis B surface antibody, hepatitis B core antibody, hepatitis C antibody, cytomegalovirus (CMV) antibody, T-spot test, HIV antibody, and HIV antigen (p24). After initiation of any immune checkpoint inhibitor therapy, patients should be monitored frequently for the development of toxicities. Monitoring typically involves a clinical evaluation initially every 2 weeks with laboratory tests including a complete blood count, comprehensive metabolic panel, thyroid function tests, and troponin (every 6 weeks). Additional laboratory tests, EKGs, and imaging tests should be obtained based on specific reported new symptoms.

Treatment of immune-related adverse events can be summarized based on grade and there are now multiple consensus guideline publications available to aid in management.[181,182]

- Grade 1: Close monitoring and symptomatic treatment as needed. Continue therapy with some exceptions.
- Grade 2: Close monitoring and symptomatic treatment that may include systemic corticosteroids, discontinue therapy, and resume after improvement to Grade 1 or less. If recurrent or persistent, manage as grade 3.
- Grade 3: Close monitoring, symptomatic treatment, including administration of systemic corticosteroids. Consult appropriate specialists. Permanently discontinue drug therapy, except for certain toxicities (i.e., asymptomatic laboratory abnormalities) that may allow for rechallenge according to guidelines.
- Grade 4: Close monitoring, symptomatic treatment, including administration of systemic corticosteroids and additional immunosuppressive medications according to guidelines (mycophenolate, infliximab, etc.). Consult appropriate specialists. Permanently discontinue drug therapy.

Grade 3 to 4 events typically require systemic steroids that should be tapered over a minimum of 4 weeks. A rapid taper early can lead to recurrences of immune-related adverse events. Most drugs blocking negative immune regulation are antibodies with half-lives measured in weeks. When managing immune toxicities, one must consider the prolonged on-target effects of the drug that can persist even after cessation of treatment. During tapering, patients should be monitored closely for recurrences of immune toxicities. For grade 4 or relapsing grade 3 events, additional therapies such as mycophenolate mofetil, azathioprine, tacrolimus, methotrexate, or infliximab are typically indicated and consultation with appropriate disease specialist is warranted (gastroenterology, rheumatology, etc.).

Other treatments for immune-related adverse events are organ-specific. For instance, endocrine disorders can be managed with hormone replacement therapy. Most events are manageable and will resolve with treatment and cessation of the drug. However, as combination therapies are much more commonly becoming the standard of care, the incidence of toxicities, including those that are severe, is expected to increase. Although rare, serious or even fatal immune-related toxicities, such as myocarditis, may occur. Serious toxicities may even develop rapidly within the first 2 weeks. Thus, early recognition of immune-related adverse events is critical. Patients starting on therapies that block negative immune regulation should be educated to expeditiously report any new symptoms they experience, even those perceived to be minor.

CONCLUSION

Targeting negative immune regulation has led to the uptake of clinical cancer immunotherapy in multiple tumor types. The rapid and dramatic responses observed in patients with refractory advanced cancers have proven the concept that harnessing the immune system can be effectively used to control or even eradicate cancer on a significant scale. There are at least three aspects of this approach that have had a "disruptive" technological impact on clinical practice. First, the broad applicability across cancer types is almost unique in the history of oncology drug development. Clinical activity has been shown in over a dozen cancer types, many of which previously had very limited therapeutic options available. Second, therapies targeting negative regulatory pathways have generally been more tolerable than conventional chemotherapies or even molecularly targeted

therapies. While the associated toxicities are not insignificant, most patients are able to tolerate therapy, and if side effects do occur, they are generally very manageable when recognized and treated early. Finally, the durability of responses in some patients has been long enough to entertain the concept of cure, at least in a fraction of patients. Given results reported to date, immunotherapy directed toward negative immune regulation is likely to remain the backbone of modern cancer treatments for many years.

KEY REFERENCES

Only key references appear in the print edition. The full reference list appears in the digital product on Springer Publishing Connect: connect.springerpub.com/content/book/978-0-8261-3743-2/part/part02/chapter/ch27

11. Leach DR, Krummel MF, Allison JP. Enhancement of antitumor immunity by CTLA-4 blockade. *Science*. 1996;271(5256):1734–1736. doi:10.1126/science.271.5256.1734

27. Freeman GJ, Long AJ, Iwai Y, et al. Engagement of the PD-1 immunoinhibitory receptor by a novel B7 family member leads to negative regulation of lymphocyte activation. *J Exp Med*. 2000;192(7):1027–1034. doi:10.1084/jem.192.7.1027

97. Hodi FS, O'Day SJ, McDermott DF, et al. Improved survival with ipilimumab in patients with metastatic melanoma. *N Engl J Med*. 2010;363(8):711–723. doi:10.1056/NEJMoa1003466

100. Ribas A, Puzanov I, Dummer R, et al. Pembrolizumab versus investigator-choice chemotherapy for ipilimumab-refractory melanoma (KEYNOTE-002): a randomised, controlled, Phase 2 trial. *Lancet Oncol*. 2015;16(8):908–918. doi:10.1016/S1470-2045(15)00083-2

119. Topalian SL, Hodi FS, Brahmer JR, et al. Safety, activity, and immune correlates of anti-PD-1 antibody in cancer. *N Engl J Med*. 2012;366(26):2443–2454. doi:10.1056/NEJMoa1200690

181. Puzanov I, Diab A, Abdallah K, et al. Managing toxicities associated with immune checkpoint inhibitors: consensus recommendations from the Society for Immunotherapy of Cancer (SITC) Toxicity Management Working Group. *J Immunother Cancer*. 2017;5(1):95. doi:10.1186/s40425-017-0300-z

28

Agonistic Antibodies to Co-Stimulatory Molecules

Rebekka Duhen, Alexandra K. Frye, and Andrew D. Weinberg

KEY POINTS

- Several T cell co-stimulatory pathways are currently being targeted for cancer immunotherapy.

- Both preclinical and clinical trial data show that antibodies targeting the co-stimulatory pathways can increase immune cell activation.

- Human agonist antibodies to co-stimulatory pathways can target CD4+, CD8+, and regulatory T cells.

- The majority of co-stimulatory proteins that have been targeted belong to the CD28 superfamily (ICOS, CD28) or tumor necrosis factor receptor superfamily (TNFRSF), such as 4-1BB, OX40, glucocorticoid-induced TNFR-related protein (GITR), CD27, and CD40.

- While single-agent co-stimulatory treatments have shown limited success in clinical trials, co-stimulatory antibodies are currently being evaluated in combination with checkpoint blockade, adoptive T cell therapy, and vaccination to boost immune responses.

INTRODUCTION

Treatment of cancer with immunotherapeutic agents has advanced tremendously throughout the last decade. Not only has our understanding of basic T cell function grown but also the ways to manipulate their function for clinical benefit in tumor-bearing hosts. The immune response against viruses, bacteria, and other pathogens is under tight regulation because resolving infections involves tissue inflammation, followed by clearance of the pathogenic microorganism. Several mechanisms involved with downregulation of T cell function following infections to limit tissue damage are unfortunately used within the tumor microenvironment to quell ongoing T cell responses. This chapter summarizes the use of several therapeutic agonist antibodies (Abs) that target T

cells in an attempt to overcome suppression and increase T cell function within tumor-bearing hosts, leading to immune-mediated cancer destruction.

CD4+ and CD8+ T cells are composed of a vast naïve T cell repertoire capable of responding to the large number of antigens that are encountered during a lifetime—with each naïve T cell clone being present at very low frequency.[1-3] Positive selection takes place in the thymus via antigen-presenting cells (APCs), which helps to ensure that T cells entering the periphery will recognize and respond to foreign peptides bound on self-major histocompatibility complex (MHC) molecules. Concomitantly, negative selection depletes the majority of T cells that would be self-reactive or bind with high affinity to self-MHC.[4,5] T cells, encountering their cognate Ag in the periphery, can undergo different fates depending on the activation status of the APCs they encounter. If the T cell receptor (TCR) is triggered in the absence of co-stimulatory signals, the T cells can be deleted through apoptosis or become refractory to restimulation and are termed "anergic." If, however, the T cell recognizes its cognate peptide in the context of an activated APC expressing a variety of co-stimulatory signals, it proliferates and acquires proinflammatory/cytotoxic functions. Co-stimulatory signals between an APC and a T cell usually occur within the immunologic synapse, allowing for clustering of signals via a distinct spatial organization, which fosters positive molecular interactions.[6] Furthermore, co-stimulation of T cells leads to the production of a variety of secreted proteins (cytokines and chemokines) that can influence the outcome of an immune response (e.g., T cell lineage and/or migratory pattern).[7] The classic co-stimulatory signal, otherwise known as signal 2, is provided via the interaction of CD80/CD86 (or B7-1, a bivalent dimer and B7-2, a bivalent monomer), two molecules expressed on activated APCs, with CD28, a protein that is expressed on the surface of naïve and most memory T cells.

CD28 is the founding member of a subfamily of molecules characterized by an extracellular variable immunoglobulin-like domain, which includes the inducible T cell co-stimulator (ICOS), and both molecules act as positive regulators of T cell function. Other co-stimulatory proteins are 4-1BB (CD137), OX40 (CD134), glucocorticoid-induced tumor necrosis factor receptor–related protein (GITR), and CD40L, which are all members of the tumor necrosis factor receptor (TNFR) superfamily (TNFRSF). As opposed to T cell co-stimulatory proteins, there are several proteins responsible for limiting T cell responses, which are termed "co-inhibitory proteins." These co-inhibitory proteins, also known as checkpoints, help reduce tissue damage by limiting excessive T cell proliferation, cytokine production, and cytotoxicity. These molecules include programmed cell death protein 1 (PD-1), T cell immunoglobulin (Ig), mucin-domain containing 3 (TIM-3), cytotoxic T-lymphocyte-associated protein 4 (CTLA-4), B- and T-lymphocyte attenuator (BTLA), lymphocyte-activation gene 3 (LAG-3), and T cell immunoreceptor with Ig and ITIM domains (TIGIT) among others. Blocking these checkpoint molecules with Abs has a profound therapeutic impact on cancer progression, and their role and function were covered Chapter 27.

Cancer initiation occurs when cells undergo neoplastic transformation and begin to proliferate abnormally, most often as a result of genetic alterations. Selection then results in the expansion of rapidly growing cells, leading to an outgrowth of a clonal population of tumor cells. The tumors then increase in size; the malignant cells constantly undergo clonal selection during this expansion phase and acquire properties that increase their survival, metabolism, and metastatic potential. In the past, it was hypothesized that tumors were not recognized by the immune system; however, more recent evidence has shown that the immune system can recognize and destroy tumor cells.[8] There is proof that tumor-specific T cells can recognize mutated proteins/peptides within the tumor and hence mount a high-affinity T cell response against the tumor.[9–11] However, when tumors enter into a progressive cycle of coevolution with the immune system, they can drive T cells into a refractory or anergic state through several immune suppressive mechanisms, leading to T cells that cannot respond to tumor antigens. One way to overcome this unresponsive state is through the administration of "agonist Abs" that target molecules expressed on CD4+, CD8+, and regulatory T cells (T$_{reg}$ cells).

CO-STIMULATORY MOLECULES AND THEIR EFFECTS IN CANCER DEVELOPMENT

CD28 Superfamily Members

CD28

CD28 is a glycoprotein well known for its role in co-stimulation of naïve T lymphocytes. While TCR ligation alone is not sufficient for complete T cell activation, co-stimulation provided by activated APCs, such as monocytes, dendritic cells (DCs), and B cells, increases T cell activation and prevents unresponsiveness.[12,13] These observations led to the discovery of CD28 (then named Tp44) in 1986.[14,15] and its function on tumor-infiltrating lymphocytes (TILs) was first described in 1992.[16] CD28 engagement results in protection from cell death, enhanced cytokine production, stronger and sustained proliferation, and increased cytotoxic capabilities. After engagement of CD80/CD86 with CD28 during T cell activation, a negative feedback loop occurs, resulting in the expression of the checkpoint protein CTLA-4, which binds CD80 with higher affinity and decreases CD28 signaling. CTLA-4 signaling leads to a dampening of T cell activation and self-limits the T cell response.[17,18] To modulate the function of effector T cells, a soluble CTLA-4-binding domain linked to an Ig constant region was developed and found to be effective at blocking CD28 interactions with CD80/86. In animals, CTLA-4:Ig can induce tolerance to allografts and decrease symptoms of autoimmune diseases. Two CTLA-4:Ig drugs (abatacept and belatacept) are approved by the U.S. Food and Drug Administration (FDA) in autoimmune settings and have ameliorated symptoms in a subset of autoimmune diseases, while their effect is still being investigated in many other autoimmune diseases.[19]

Several attempts have been made to exploit the CD28 co-stimulatory pathway to enhance tumor immunity in preclinical cancer models. Initially, engagement of CD28 was attempted through CD80/CD86 transfection of tumor cells and it was found that these transfected tumors were more easily rejected by the immune system.[20–22] The transfected tumor lines were then used as vaccines to elicit tumor-specific T cell responses; however, this technique had limited success because CD80/86 expression by the host cells (APCs) was shown to be critically important to stimulate CD8+ T cells.[23,24] CD28 co-stimulation has also been used to activate T cells for adoptive T cell therapies and its intracellular signaling domain, coupled with CD3ζ, has been used in chimeric antigen receptor (CAR) T cell constructs. The CD28 signaling domain enhances CAR T cell activation and proliferation, as well as differentiation into an effector memory phenotype. Preclinical models have also tested the use of systemic CD28 Abs to enhance in vivo immune responses. These studies demonstrated preferential activation of type 2 T helper cells (Th2) and of CD4+ CD25+ regulatory T cells with increased lymphocyte counts but no detectable toxic effects.[25,26] A human antibody developed by TeGenero (TGN1412) was found to be a superagonist monoclonal antibody (mAb), targeting and activating all cell types expressing CD28, and this co-stimulation was found to be independent of TCR ligation.[27] Although preclinical data in nonhuman primates lacked any evidence of toxic side effects, six subjects treated simultaneously with a low dose of the Ab developed severe and life-threatening toxicity (due to a cytokine storm followed by systemic inflammation) during a Phase 1 trial.[28,29] The adverse events observed during this trial led to a reluctance to further develop CD28 mAbs for cancer immunotherapy. It is now understood that in cynomolgus macaques, CD4[+] effector cells selectively downregulate CD28, alleviating the source of proinflammatory cytokines and allowing for high tolerance of the CD28 superagonists.[27] After additional preclinical work, the same superagonist antibody (renamed TAB08) is now under evaluation in clinical trials led by TheraMAB in autoimmune diseases and advanced solid neoplasms to determine safety and optimal dose.[30] A Phase I study beginning at a dose 1,000-fold lower than applied in 2006 proved safe in healthy volunteers and showed selective activation of T_{reg} cells. Subsequently, a Phase 1b trial (NCT01990157) initiated in patients with rheumatoid arthritis (RA) showed favorable responses and few adverse events.[19,27] TheraMAB is currently recruiting for a Phase 1b clinical trial to determine the maximum-tolerated dose (MTD) in patients with metastatic or unresectable advanced solid malignancies (NCT03006029).

More recently, the anti-CD28 Ab has been incorporated into bispecific and trispecific antibodies, which engage both tumor-specific antigens (TSAs) and co-stimulatory molecules (CD3, CD28) to mimic signal 1 and/or signal 2 of T cell activation. Wu et al. designed a CD38/CD3xCD28 trispecific antibody, aiming to direct stimulated T cells to several hematologic malignancies.[31] Compared to daratumumab (an approved anti-CD38 mAb for the treatment of multiple myeloma), the trispecific antibody was more potent at killing CD38[+] multiple myeloma cells. In vivo modeling with the trispecific led to reduced myeloma growth in a humanized mouse model and increased CD8[+] T cell proliferation in cynomolgus macaques.[31] Waite et al. have described a new class of bispecifics with co-stimulatory properties that crosslinks the TSA with either CD3 or CD28. Unlike CD28 superagonists, TSA x CD28 bispecifics display a safe toxicity profile and can synergize therapeutically with PD-1 blockade. The TSA x CD3 bispecifics promote T cell activation, decrease tumor growth, and increase survival in murine tumor models.[32] Bispecifics and trispecifics represent a similar approach to CAR T cells, in that multiple proteins are used to artificially trigger both signal 1 and signal 2 to induce T cell activation. The distinct advantage of antibody therapy over CAR T cells lies in the ability to provide therapy without individual customization and the lack of preemptive lymphodepletion as a requisite.[32]

Recently, Hui et al. have found that the expression of co-stimulatory proteins in CD8[+] T cells is an important factor for responsiveness to anti-PD-1 and that PD-1 suppresses T cell function primarily by inactivating CD28 signaling.[33] In line with these findings, it was shown that loss of CD28 expression on CD8[+] TIL can serve as a

biomarker for resistance to anti-PD-1 treatment, casting some doubt on the efficacy of anti-CD28 Abs on tumor-reactive TIL in the clinic.[34,35] Moreover, studies using an MC38 mouse tumor model have revealed that antitumor efficacy of PD-1 blockade could be rescued by co-administration of interleukin 15 (IL-15), and did so in a CD8[+] T cell-dependent manner. Further interrogation using human CD8[+] TIL indicated that IL-15 increased the cytotoxic capacity and effector function of the CD28[-] progeny of CD28[+]PD-1[+] TIL.[35] Concomitantly, our laboratory has found that tumor-reactive T cells (characterized by surface expression of CD39 and CD103) express low levels of CD28, as revealed by protein and gene set enrichment analysis.[10] Although the use of anti-CD28 in the context of tumor immunology has been met with some challenges, the co-stimulatory pathway will likely have enduring contributions to the field.

Inducible T Cell Co-Stimulator (CD278)

Another member of the CD28 superfamily is ICOS, which has 36% homology to CD28 and was first described in 1999.[36,37] ICOS is expressed on activated T cells and mediates its function by signaling as a homodimer. Its ligand is expressed on the surface of B cells, APCs, and somatic cells.[38] ICOS co-stimulation is important to generate effective T cell-mediated immune responses.[39] Stimulation through ICOS has garnered significant attention for its role in promoting differentiation of follicular T helper cells (Tfh) as well as Th2 and T helper 17 (Th17) lymphocytes.[40–43] In peripheral blood, T_{reg} cells express the highest level of ICOS[44] and, when triggered by ICOS agonist antibodies, can promote tumor growth. Thus, both agonistic antibodies (enhancing CD4[+] T cell activation and effector function) and antagonistic antibodies (reducing T_{reg} cell-mediated suppression and interaction with ICOSL[+] cells) are being developed for cancer immunotherapy.[45] Interest in ICOS as a target has grown, as increased expression was observed on peripheral blood T cells in patients treated with ipilimumab (anti-CTLA-4).[46,47] Consequently, upregulation of ICOS on T cells was proposed as a pharmacodynamic biomarker for CTLA-4 inhibition, but whether clinical response to CTLA-4 can be correlated to its expression is still under investigation.[48,49] Preclinical studies using tumor models for melanoma and pancreatic cancer demonstrated synergistic effects when combining ICOS stimulation with CTLA-4 blockade.[50,51] More recently, James Allison showed that intratumoral administration of Newcastle disease virus expressing ICOSL led to the rejection of the virus-injected and distant B16 tumors when combined with CTLA-4 blockade.[52] Synergism with anti-CTLA-4 was also observed using intratumoral ICOS bispecific aptamers.[53] Several biotechnology and pharmaceutical companies now have an interest in Abs or fusion proteins targeting the ICOS pathway. GlaxoSmithKline (GSK), MedImmune (now AstraZeneca), Kymab Limited, and Jounce Therapeutics have ongoing clinical trials with agonist and antagonist ICOS Abs. The first agonist anti-ICOS antibody (IgG1 isotype; termed JTX-2011 or vopratelimab, Jounce Therapeutics) entered the clinic in August 2016. However, the Phase 1/2 trial was disappointing, as the data showed one partial response out of 67 patients treated and in combination with PD-1 blockade, eight partial responses out of 106 patients (NCT02904226). Jounce Therapeutics is refining this approach and is now testing vopratelimab in combination with CTLA-4 blockade in lung and urothelial cancers (NCT03989362).

Anti-CTLA-4 treatment has been shown to increase ICOS expression on CD4+ T cells, which, in combination with anti-ICOS, would be more efficient.[54] GSK also has an anti-ICOS Ab with an IgG4 Fc-tail (GSK3359609), which was tested in patients with advanced or recurrent solid tumors. While only one patient of 16 achieved an objective clinical response to monotherapy, eight of 34 responded to the antibody combined with pembrolizumab (anti-PD-1; NCT02723955). GSK has now entered a randomized Phase 3 combination trial in head and neck cancer, enrolling up to 600 patients. In contrast, AstraZeneca and more recently Kymab have produced an ICOS antagonist IgG1 antibody, which is thought to promote antibody-dependent cellular cytotoxicity

Table 28.1 Summary of Clinical Trials With Anti-ICOS Antibodies (Since 2016)

STUDY AGENT	CANCER TYPE	IN COMBINATION WITH	SPONSOR	NCT NUMBER + PHASE
MEDI-570 (anti-ICOS afucosylated mAb) ANTAGONIST	Recurrent or refractory peripheral T cell lymphoma follicular variant Angioimmunoblastic T cell lymphoma	None	NCI	NCT02520791 Phase 1
KY1044 (anti-ICOS IgG1 mAb) ANTAGONIST	Advanced cancer	Atezolizumab (anti-PD-L1)	Kymab Limited	NCT03829501 Phase 1/2
GSK3359609 (humanized anti-ICOS IgG4 mAb) AGONIST	Neoplasms Head and neck cancer	Pembrolizumab (anti-PD-1)	GSK	NCT04128696 Phase 3
	Neoplasms	Tremelimumab (anti-CTLA-4) Cetuximab (anti-EGFR) Docetaxel Paclitaxel	GSK	NCT03693612 Phase 2
	Neoplasms	GSK3174998, Pembrolizumab (anti-PD-1) Docetaxel Pemetrexed Paclitaxel Gemcitabine Fluorouracil Carboplatin Cisplatin	GSK	NCT02723955 Phase 1
	Neoplasms	Docetaxel	GSK	NCT03739710 Phase 2
JTX-2011 (anti-ICOS IgG1 mAb) Vopratelimab AGONIST	Cancer	Ipilimumab (anti-CTLA-4) Nivolumab (anti-PD-1)	Jounce Therapeutics	NCT04319224 Phase 1/2
	Cancer	Ipilimumab (anti-CTLA-4) Nivolumab (anti-PD-1) Pembrolizumab (anti-PD-1)	Jounce Therapeutics	NCT02904226 Phase 1/2
	NSCLC Urothelial cancer	Ipilimumab (anti-CTLA-4)	Jounce Therapeutics	NCT03989362 Phase 2

CTLA-4, cytotoxic T-lymphocyte-associated protein 4; EGFR, epidermal growth factor receptor; GSK, GlaxoSmithKline; ICOS, inducible T cell co-stimulator; IgG, immunoglobulin G; mAb, monoclonal antibody; NCI, National Cancer Institute; NSCLC, non-small cell lung cancer; PD-1, programmed cell death protein 1; PD-L1, programmed death ligand 1.

(ADCC) against ICOS+ cells, targeting T_{reg} cells for depletion. Overall, the data suggest that targeting ICOS is safe and in combination with immune checkpoint inhibitors could have therapeutic benefits in future clinical trials. Ongoing trials are summarized in Table 28.1.

Tumor Necrosis Factor Receptor Family Members

At the same time that CD28 family members were being targeted for immunotherapy, members of the TNF family of proteins were being explored in the context of cancer immunotherapy. TNF has been a target in the field of autoimmunity for many years, and TNF inhibitors have been successfully applied and approved for the treatment of inflammatory bowel disease (IBD), RA, and psoriasis.

The TNF superfamily is composed of 19 related proteins that bind to one or more TNFRSF member (29 related) molecules.[55] TNF receptors (TNFR) are widely expressed throughout the body, most notably on the cell surface of leukocytes. When TNFRs are engaged by their ligand, they form trimeric complexes within the plasma membrane and signal through adaptor proteins. In the immune system, this family of receptors can promote cell activation, survival, and inflammation, which includes CD40, lymphotoxin alpha (LT-α), OX40, CD27, 4-1BB, TNFRSF1B, and BAFF. Other members can induce cell death via death domains found in some of these proteins, including FAS, TNF-related apoptosis-inducing ligand (TRAIL), DR3 and DR5. They can also act as decoy receptors (e.g., OPG and DcR3), which are devoid of signal transduction capabilities and negatively regulate signals from their ligands.

As alluded to earlier, these receptors do not contain enzymatic or direct signaling activity, which is provided by adaptor proteins, such as TRADD, TRAF, RIP, and FADD. These proteins interact with the cytoplasmic tail of the receptor and transmit downstream signaling via nuclear factor κB (NF-κB), activation of mitogen-activated protein kinases, and PI3-kinase signaling to promote leukocyte activation.[56]

Figure 28.1 highlights the principle of signal transduction in the TNFRF member OX40.

The original TNF family member, tumor necrosis factor alpha (TNFα), was discovered in 1975 and cloned 9 years later.[57,58] Initial excitement regarding this protein involved inducing necrosis in tumors of bacillus Calmette–Guérin–primed and endotoxin-treated mice. However, the enthusiasm subsided as several Phase 1 and 2 clinical trials showed little therapeutic efficacy and induced toxic side effects.[59] Preclinical models also showed antitumor efficacy by injecting LT-α in melanoma tumor models.[60] However, similar to TNFα, there was limited efficacy, and toxicity concerns in clinical trials prevented its pursuit as an anticancer agent.[61] A new

era of Ab development started when certain members of the TNFR family such as 4-1BB (CD137) were recognized for expanding as well as limiting T cell-based immune responses.[62] Seven members of the TNFR family are currently being targeted with Abs to treat cancer patients, five of which are discussed in detail subsequently. Figure 28.2 highlights those interactions.[63]

Contrary to anti-PD-1 and anti-CTLA-4, which release T cell inhibition, these Abs stimulate their ligands to enhance the immune response and have been termed "agonist Abs." A plethora of clinical trials are combining T cell stimulation using agonist co-stimulatory Abs with checkpoint blockade to achieve maximum T cell activation, expansion, cytotoxic capabilities, and survival. These therapeutic combinations have worked extremely well in preclinical cancer models and are further discussed later in this chapter.

4-1BB (CD137 or TNFRS9)

4-1BB is a co-stimulatory receptor expressed on the surface of activated T cells, natural killer (NK) cells, and monocytes, and is constitutively present on the surface of T_{reg} cells. It is also expressed, at least transiently, on the surface of B cells, γδ T cells, DC, mast cells, and thymocytes. It was first cloned in 1989[64] and further characterized in 1993 as induced lymphocyte activation (ILA) protein.[65,66] The 4-1BB ligand (4-1BBL) is mainly expressed by activated APCs, which include DCs, macrophages, and B cells.[67] Due to 4-1BB's widespread pattern of expression, treatment with agonistic Abs can have side effects such as neutropenia, transaminitis, and liver toxicity, which has been frequently observed in clinical trials.[68,69] Liver toxicity has also been observed in preclinical studies, where toxicity was attributed to activation of liver myeloid cells, resulting in inflammatory cytokine production.[70,71]

4-1BB appears to have a dual role—on one hand, when engaged with its ligand it potentiates effector immune responses and can boost antigen-specific CD8+ T cell immunity to viruses such as influenza and cytomegalovirus. On the other hand, it has also been shown to dampen autoimmune pathologies. Engaging 4-1BB with an agonist antibody has led to decreased signs of autoimmunity in experimental autoimmune encephalomyelitis (EAE), systemic lupus erythematosus (SLE), IBD, and RA.[72] The stimulatory effects of agonist 4-1BB Abs on CD8+ T cells include promoting survival, enhanced T cell memory formation via Bcl-2, Bcl-xl, and Bfl-1,[73] as well as increased CD8+ T cell proliferation and effector function.[74] The enhancement of effector T cell activity is mediated through increased cytokine production, including the Th1 cytokines interferon gamma (IFNγ), TNFα, and IL-2.[75,76] The unique ability of 4-1BB agonist Abs to enhance immune responses in cancer and infectious diseases while limiting autoimmune pathologies

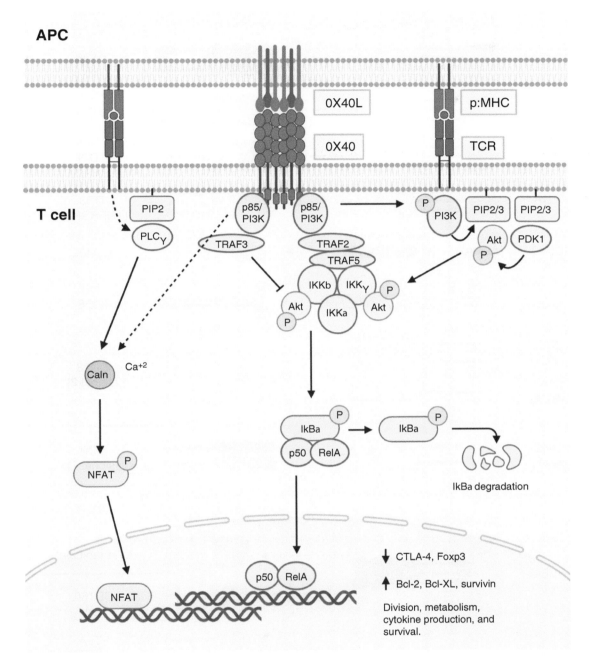

Figure 28.1 **OX40 signaling pathway.** The binding of OX40L to OX40 results in trimerization of OX40 monomers and the recruitment of TRAF2, TRAF3, and TRAF5. This leads to the formation of a signaling complex, formed by IKKα, IKKβ, IKKγ, the p85 subunit of PI3K, and Akt. The signalosome then leads to phosphorylation and degradation of IkBα, leading to the activation of NF-kB (p50+RelA subunits) and its translocation to the nucleus. Upon TCR–pMHC interaction, OX40 synergizes with the TCR to promote strong Akt phosphorylation. TCR-initiated Ca2+ influx leads to NFAT dephosphorylation and entry into the nucleus, a process that is also enhanced by OX40. This combination of antigen-mediated and OX40-mediated signals leads to transcription of prosurvival/antiapoptotic genes, cytokines, and chemokines, as well as changes in the metabolic state of the T cell.

Akt/PKB, protein kinase B; APC, antigen-presenting cell; Bcl-2, B cell lymphoma 2; Bcl-XL, B cell lymphoma-extra large; Caln, calcineurin; CTLA-4, cytotoxic T-lymphocyte-associated protein 4; Foxp3, forkhead box p3; IKKs, inhibitor of nuclear factor kappa-B kinase; NFAT, nuclear factor of activated T cell; PDK1, phosphoinositide-dependent protein kinase-1; PI3K, phosphatidylinositol-4,5-bisphosphate 3-kinase; PIP2, phosphatidylinositol 4,5-bisphosphate; PIP3, phosphatidylinositol 4,5-triphosphate; PLCγ, phospholipase Cγ; p:MHC, peptide-major histocompatibility complex; TCR, T cell receptor; TRAF, TNFR- associated factor.

Source: Created with BioRender.com

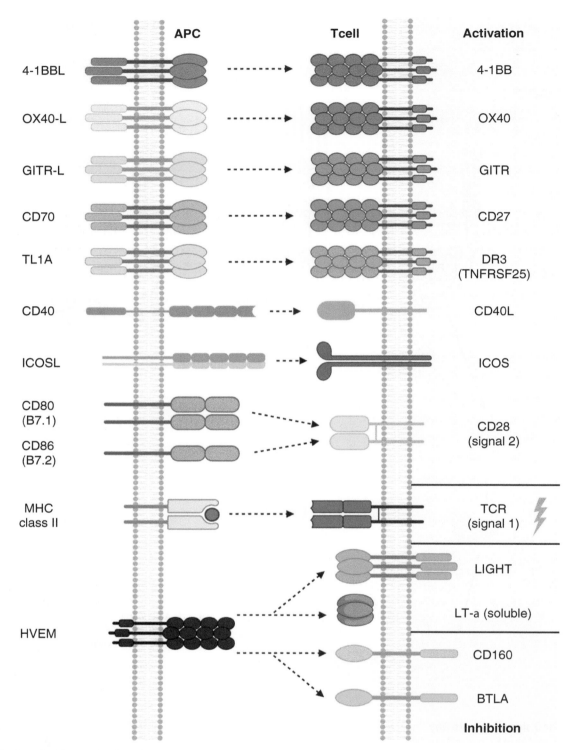

Figure 28.2 Co-stimulatory molecules. Signal 1 is delivered when a TCR on a T cell recognizes its cognate antigen/peptide presented by the MHC. Optimal and functional activation of T cells requires signal 2, which is provided by the interaction of CD28 on the T cell with CD80/CD86 on the APC. More interactions occur between co-stimulatory (green shaded area) and coinhibitory (yellow shaded area) proteins to foster T cell activation and differentiation. Antibodies to those molecules are in various stages of clinical development for the treatment of cancer as discussed in this chapter.

APC, antigen-presenting cell; BTLA, B- and T-lymphocyte attenuator; DR3, death receptor 3; GITR, glucocorticoid-induced TNFR-related protein; HVEM, herpes virus entry mediator; ICOS, inducible T cell co-stimulator; LIGHT, homologous to lymphotoxins, exhibits inducible expression, and competes with HSV glycoprotein D for HVEM, a receptor expressed by T lymphocytes; LT-α, lymphotoxin alpha; MHC, major histocompatibility complex; TCR, T cell receptor; TL1A, TNF-like ligand 1A; TNFRSF25, TNF receptor superfamily member 25.

Source: Adapted from Mahoney KM, Rennert PD, Freeman GJ. Combination cancer immunotherapy and new immunomodulatory targets. *Nat Rev Drug Discov.* 2015;14(8):561–584. doi:10.1038/nrd4591; Created with BioRender.com

makes this treatment modality an interesting target for cancer immunotherapy.

4-1BB was the first member of the TNFRSF identified as an immunotherapy target in tumor-bearing hosts. Melero et al. spearheaded the work showing that agonist 4-1BB Abs were therapeutic in murine tumor models.[77] His work was followed by many preclinical studies with anti-4-1BB mAbs that demonstrated efficacy alone or in combination with anti-CTLA-4,[78,79] PD-1 or programmed death ligand 1 (PD-L1),[80–82] CD40 activation,[83] and cellular vaccines.[78,84] IFNγ plays a vital role in 4-1BB-mediated immunotherapy and this was demonstrated in IFNγ-deficient animals that were treated with anti-4-1BB, in which antigen-specific cytotoxic T lymphocytes (CTLs) were unable to traffic to the tumor site and cause tumor regression.[85] 4-1BB expression also allows for accurate identification of antigen-specific CD8[+] T cells independent of precursor frequency and knowledge of the immunogenic antigen in acute infections.[86] Several cancer immunotherapy groups have found that upregulation of 4-1BB and PD-1 on CD8[+] TIL could potentially serve as a biomarker for 4-1BB-specific therapeutics.[87,88] 4-1BB can also be used as a surrogate marker for TCR activation when T cells are co-cultured with autologous tumor or tumor peptides. These in vitro assays have helped to identify tumor-specific mutated peptides that are recognized by the immune system.[89]

Preclinical studies targeting 4-1BB with agonist Abs as monotherapy in the P815 mastocytoma tumor model as well as in combination with anti-CD40 or CTLA-4 were promising and led to clinical trials.[68,83,90] Early trials showed limited success, but there has been a resurgence of using this Ab in recent years. Two agonist 4-1BB Abs have largely been investigated in clinical trials: urelumab (Bristol Myers Squibb [BMS]), an IgG4 antibody, which does not block interaction with 4-1BBL, and utomilumab (Pfizer), which inhibits binding to endogenous 4-1BBL.[89] Urelumab entered the clinic in 2005; however, its study was halted in 2009 due to substantial liver toxicity (NCT00612664).[68] The results led to the termination of that trial and other ongoing Phase 1 trials. Preclinical studies of combination therapies, as well as the finding that in humans much lower doses of urelumab could have beneficial effects, have revived some interest in the drug. Urelumab continues to be studied in clinical trials in combination with other therapeutics, including nivolumab (anti-PD-1), anti-LAG-3, anti–colony-stimulating factor 1 receptor (CSF1R), TIL infusion, and chemotherapy. In October of 2018, BMS closed their urelumab development program, leading to the subsequent termination of treatment arms and new clinical trials. One of the most promising combination trials evaluating urelumab alone or in combination with rituximab (anti-CD20) initially showed potential. Three of 60 patients with B cell non-Hodgkin lymphoma achieved a complete response and three more achieved a partial response on monotherapy alone. In combination with rituximab, four of 46 patients achieved complete remission and five achieved partial remission.[91] Despite several durable remissions, many were achieved at doses exceeding the determined MTD in the study, indicating less than optimal potency for safe and reliable clinical effect.

In 2011, Pfizer launched a Phase 1 trial with their mAb, utomilumab (PF-05082566, IgG2), in advanced cancer after showing in vitro bioactivity and safety in nonhuman primates.[92] Results from the initial trial showed no dose-limiting toxicity, limited side effects, and evidence of disease stabilization in multiple patients (NCT01307267). These results have led to multiple Phase 1/2 trials in combination with checkpoint inhibitors, agonist Abs, CAR T cells, CD8+ TIL, peptide vaccines, and others, which are summarized in Table 28.2. Data from a Phase 1 combination trial with utomilumab and rituximab showed promising results in patients with rituximab refractory follicular lymphoma (FL). The overall response rate (ORR) was 33% (8/24), with four complete and four partial responses. Increases in circulating CD8[+] T cells were observed in these patients and led to an expansion cohort in rituximab refractory FL patients.[93] A Phase 1b trial combining utomilumab and pembrolizumab in various solid tumors achieved an ORR of 26% (6/23), including two CRs and four PRs. Biomarker analyses from both trials indicated increased levels of circulating memory CD8[+] T cells and supported the continuation of further studies.[89,94]

Despite efficacy in preclinical models, moving urelumab and utomilumab beyond early-stage clinical development has been hindered by severe liver toxicity or low efficacy, respectively.[71] Qi et al. feel that urelumab is a strong agonist based on its ability to co-stimulate T cells via 4-1BB activation without FcγR crosslinking, and classify utomilumab as a weaker agonist, based on its reliance on FcγRIIA or FcγRIIB expressing cells for activity. To circumvent the efficacy and safety concerns of both Abs, the authors proposed engineering an Fc with selective FcγRIIB binding and a Fab that has weaker agonist activity, giving rise to LVGN6051 (Lyvgen Biopharma), an Ab that is currently in a Phase 1 trial as a single agent and in combination with pembrolizumab (NCT04130542). Compass Therapeutics pursued the development of a fully human IgG4 4-1BB agonist, termed CTX-471, which binds CD137 at a nonligand competitive epitope, but does require FcγR binding to induce IFNγ production. Most interestingly, CTX-471 was able to eradicate very large established tumors as monotherapy in the CT26 tumor model.[95]

Table 28.2 Summary of Clinical Trials With Anti-4-1BB Antibodies (Since 2015)

STUDY AGENT	CANCER TYPE	IN COMBINATION WITH	SPONSOR	NCT NUMBER + PHASE
MSB0010718C (anti-PD-L1 mAb) Avelumab	Advanced cancer	Utomilumab (anti-4-1BB) PF-04518600 (anti-OX40) PD-0360324 (anti-M-CSF) CMP-001 (TLR9 agonist)	Pfizer	NCT02554812 Phase 2
AGEN2373 (anti-CD137 IgG1 mAb)	Advanced cancer	None	Agenus	NCT04121676 Phase 1
ADG106 (anti-CD137 IgG4 mAb)	Solid tumors Non-Hodgkin lymphoma	None	Adagene	NCT03707093 Phase 1
	Solid tumors Non-Hodgkin lymphoma	None	Adagene	NCT03802955 Phase 1
LVGN6051 (humanized IgG1 mAb)	Cancer	Pembrolizumab (anti-PD-1)	Lyvgen Biopharma Holdings Limited	NCT04130542 Phase 1
ATOR-1017 (anti-CD137 mAb)	Solid tumors Neoplasms	None	Alligator Bioscience AB	NCT04144842 Phase 1
MCLA-145 (IgG1 bispecific PD-L1xCD137)	Advanced solid tumors B-cell lymphoma	None	Merus N.V.	NCT03922204 Phase 1
PRS-343 (bivalent bispecific 4-1BBxHER2)	HER2-positive solid tumors	Atezolizumab (anti-PD-L1)	Pieris Pharmaceuticals	NCT03650348 Phase 1
	HER2-positive solid tumors	None	Pieris Pharmaceuticals	NCT03330561 Phase 1
PF-05082566 (humanized anti-4-1BB IgG2 mAb) Utomilumab	Advanced HER2-positive breast cancer	Trastuzumab (anti-HER2) Trastuzumab Emtansine (anti-HER2-DM1)	George W. Sledge Jr., Stanford University	NCT03364348 Phase 1
	Breast cancer	Vinorelbine Trastuzumab (anti-HER2) Avelumab (anti-PD-L1)	Ian E. Krop, MD, PhD, Dana-Farber Cancer Institute	NCT03414658 Phase 2
	HPV-16-positive oropharyngeal cancer	ISA101b (HPV16 E6/E7 peptide vaccine)	MD Anderson Cancer Center	NCT03258008 Phase 2
	Refractory large B-cell lymphoma	Cyclophosphamide Fludarabine Axicabtagene Ciloleucel	Kite Pharma	NCT03704298 Phase 1/2
	Recurrent or refractory diffuse large B cell lymphoma Recurrent or refractory mantle cell lymphoma	Avelumab (anti-PD-L1) Carboplatin Etoposide Phosphate Ibrutinib Ifosfamide Rituximab	City of Hope Medical Center	NCT03440567 Phase 1
	Colorectal cancer	Cetuximab (anti-EGFR) Irinotecan Irinotecan hydrochloride	MD Anderson Cancer Center	NCT03290937 Phase 1

(continued)

Table 28.2 Summary of Clinical Trials With Anti-4-1BB Antibodies (Since 2015) (*continued*)

STUDY AGENT	CANCER TYPE	IN COMBINATION WITH	SPONSOR	NCT NUMBER + PHASE
PF-05082566 (humanized anti-4-1BB IgG2 mAb) Utomilumab	Recurrent ovarian cancer	Aldesleukin (interleukin-2) CD8+ T cell infusion	MD Anderson Cancer Center	NCT03318900 Phase 1
BMS-663513 (human anti-4-1BB IgG4 mAb) Urelumab	Urothelial carcinoma Bladder cancer	Nivolumab (anti-PD-1)	Sidney Kimmel Comprehensive Cancer Center at Johns Hopkins	NCT02845323 Phase 2
	Neoplasms	Nivolumab (anti-PD-1)	Clinica Universidad de Navarra	NCT03792724 Phase 1/2
	Cancer	Nivolumab (anti-PD-1) Cabiralizumab (anti-CSF1R)	University of Chicago	NCT03431948 Phase 1
	Glioblastoma	BMS 986016 (anti-LAG-3) Nivolumab (anti-PD-1)	Sidney Kimmel Comprehensive Cancer Center at Johns Hopkins	NCT02658981 Phase 1
	Melanoma	Nivolumab (anti-PD-1) Cyclophosphamide Fludarabine TIL infusion Interleukin-2	H. Lee Moffitt Cancer Center and Research Institute	NCT02652455 Phase 1
	Pancreatic cancer	Cyclophosphamide GVAX Nivolumab (anti-PD-1)	Sidney Kimmel Comprehensive Cancer Center at Johns Hopkins	NCT02451982 Phase 1/2

CSF1R, colony-stimulating factor 1 receptor; EGFR, epidermal growth factor receptor; HER2, human epidermal growth factor receptor 2; HPV, human papillomavirus; ICOS, inducible T cell co-stimulator; IgG, immunoglobulin G; LAG-3, lymphocyte-activation gene 3; mAb, monoclonal antibody; M-CSF, macrophage colony-stimulating factor; PD-1, programmed cell death protein 1; PD-L1, programmed death ligand 1; TIL, tumor-infiltrating lymphocytes; TLR, Toll-like receptor.

Future efforts are focused on minimizing systemic exposure while maximizing safe clinically active levels. Next-generation Ab trials may include bispecifics (engaging both a TSA and 4-1BB), "masked" antibodies, and intratumoral administration.[96] Further clarifying the role of 4-1BB in T_{reg} cells and APCs will also be important to inform the ways in which this pathway can be further exploited to enhance the development of current and next-generation 4-1BB therapies.[89]

OX40 (CD134 or TNFRS4)

OX40 was first discovered in 1987 as a cell surface protein that was upregulated upon activation of rat CD4+ T cells[97] and the human homologue was characterized in 1994.[98] OX40 is a type 1 transmembrane protein, transiently expressed on the cell surface of activated CD4+ and CD8+ T lymphocytes. When T cells are stimulated by their cognate antigen or anti-CD3, OX40 expression is induced within 12 hours and maintained for 48 to 72

hours on the cell surface. The expression is transient and declines rapidly on CD8+ T cells and decays with slower kinetics on cells of the memory lineage.[99] OX40 is also expressed on NK cells, NK T cells, and neutrophils, whereas its ligand OX40L is predominantly expressed by DCs, B cells, and macrophages and can be upregulated on NK cells and mast cells. T cells can also express the OX40L and it is thought that T cell expression can act in a paracrine fashion to enhance T cell function during activation.[100] In addition to TCR stimulation, common gamma chain cytokines (IL-2, IL-7, and IL-15) are critical for inducing maximal OX40 expression on murine and human T cells through a STAT5-dependent mechanism[101] and provide a rationale for combining anti-OX40 therapy with IL-2. Engagement of OX40 during antigen presentation to T cells promotes proliferation and increases release of proinflammatory cytokines of both Th1 and Th2 lineages.[102,103] Furthermore, OX40 ligation promotes survival and generation of long-lived memory

T cells.[103] Constitutive expression of OX40L in transgenic mice increases T cell activation and enhances Ag-specific T cell responses to immunization; however, these transgenic mice are susceptible to autoimmune disease as the mice age.[104,105] In human TIL, OX40 expression on T cells has been identified in breast cancer, melanoma, and head and neck cancer, and its expression in the tumor microenvironment is one of the rationales for using OX40 agonistic Abs in tumor immunotherapy studies.[106,107]

Of note, murine CD4$^+$ T$_{reg}$ cells express OX40 constitutively, whereas in humans, T$_{reg}$ cells upregulate OX40 upon activation.[108,109] T$_{reg}$ cells isolated from human tumors express very high levels of OX40, suggesting they are highly activated within the tumor.[110] However, the effect of OX40 agonists on T$_{reg}$ cells is controversial. Initially, it was published that OX40 stimulation inhibited the induction of T$_{reg}$ cells.[108,109] This OX40-mediated inhibition to TGF-β1-induced T$_{reg}$ cell conversion was later explained by increased IFNγ produced by activated effector T cells in these cultures.[111,112] A subsequent study showed that OX40-induced T$_{reg}$ cell expansion was attributed to the cytokine milieu present within the local microenvironment.[113] At the same time, other studies observed depletion of intratumoral T$_{reg}$ cells and inhibition of their function after administration of OX40 agonists.[109,114–117] Following these reports, we observed that depletion of T$_{reg}$ cells within the tumor (and periphery) was accentuated when using a depleting Fc-isotype (murine IgG2a) OX40 agonist Ab.[118] Data from our laboratory demonstrated that T effector cells generated with an OX40 co-stimulatory Ab instead can become resistant to T$_{reg}$ cell-mediated suppression and exhibit increased effector function, as has been determined for GITR agonist Ab stimulation.[119–121]

Several preclinical studies have been investigating the effects of OX40 stimulation (as monotherapy via agonist Abs or OX40L:Ig fusion proteins) to enhance T cell function in tumor-bearing hosts.[115,122–126] OX40 agonist monotherapy was therapeutically effective in many tumor models, including MCA-induced sarcoma lines, CT26 colon carcinoma, SM1 breast cancer, E.G7 thymoma, and B16 melanoma.[126] Due to positive preclinical results either as monotherapy or in combination with other immune modulatory Abs, radiation, chemotherapy, vaccines, cytokines, or immune adjuvants,[126] OX40 agonists entered the clinic.

Clinical studies began with a murine monoclonal antihuman OX40 agonist Ab (9B12, MEDI6469) developed by the Providence Cancer Center and was tested in a dose-escalation study in 30 patients. Immune monitoring revealed enhanced immune activation with a significant increase in proliferation of peripheral blood CD4$^+$ and CD8$^+$ T cells, as well as NK cells.[127] The study also showed antitumor activity as tumor regression occurred in at least one metastatic lesion in 12 of 30 patients treated. Following these findings, trials in breast, prostate, and metastatic colon cancers were initiated, with fewer positive results. More recently, a neoadjuvant trial in head and neck cancer showed encouraging results, where patients, treated 2 weeks prior to surgery, demonstrated a substantial increase in activation of TIL after OX40 administration, and long-term survival of human papillomavirus (HPV)–negative patients (*Nat Comm*, submitted). In parallel, AstraZeneca humanized the 9B12 murine Ab (termed MEDI-0562) and launched clinical trials in 2015 (NCT02318394 and NCT02705482). Due to lack of responses and toxicity in the combination study, AstraZeneca dropped the development of MEDI-0562 in 2019. Similarly, Genentech (now Roche) discontinued the OX40 program (MOXR0916) in the same year, when the Phase 1b combination study with anti-PD-L1 only showed partial responses in two of 51 (4%) patients.

Other companies and investigators are still pursuing the development and optimization of OX40 agonists. Pfizer's OX40 agonist Ab (PF-04518600) was first tested as a monotherapy to determine safety (NCT02315066) and was then tested in a clinical trial with the aforementioned 4-1BB Ab, utomilumab. GSK has recently completed their anti-OX40 (GSK3174998) Phase 1 clinical trial in combination with pembrolizumab (NCT02528357), and results are pending. While expectations were high for combination studies with checkpoint proteins (PD-1, PD-L1, and CTLA-4) based on data in preclinical models,[128,129] the dosing and biological mechanisms have yet to be further elucidated before mono- and combination therapies show sufficient antitumor activity.

BMS has also developed an OX40 agonist IgG1 Ab, which is being studied in combination with a TLR9 agonist (SD-101; NCT03410901 and NCT03831295) or anti-PD-1 and anti-CTLA-4 (NCT02737475). Novel monoclonal antibodies were developed by Innovent Biologics, BeiGene, Incyte/Agenus, and Inhibrx (developing a hexavalent OX40 agonist). Moderna is examining the use of intratumoral delivered OX40L mRNA encapsulated in lipid nanoparticles, together with IL-23 and IL-36γ mRNA in patients based on preclinical observations.[130] Alligator Biosciences has also tested a bispecific OX40xCTLA-4 antibody, which was superior compared with each treatment alone in preclinical settings (MB49 and MC38 tumor models).[131]

Table 28.3 summarizes all clinical trials with OX40 agonist Abs currently being tested either as monotherapy or in combination with checkpoint inhibitors and other standard-of-care treatments.

Glucocorticoid-Induced TNFR-Related Protein (CD357 or TNFRSF18)

The glucocorticoid-induced TNFR-related protein (GITR, also known as CD357 or TNFRSF18) was discovered in 1997 on the surface of murine T cell hybridomas.[132] The

Table 28.3 Summary of Clinical Trials With Anti-OX40 Antibodies (Since 2015)

STUDY AGENT	CANCER TYPE	IN COMBINATION WITH	SPONSOR	NCT NUMBER + PHASE
BMS-986178 (anti-OX40 IgG2 mAb)	Low-grade B cell non-Hodgkin lymphoma	TLR9 agonist SD-101	Ronald Levy, Stanford University	NCT03410901 Phase 1
	Advanced metastatic solid neoplasms	TLR9 agonist SD-101	Ronald Levy, Stanford University	NCT03831295 Phase 1
	Advanced cancer	Nivolumab (anti-PD-1) Ipilimumab (anti-CTLA-4) Tetanus vaccine DPV-001 vaccine Cyclophosphamide	BMS	NCT02737475 Phase 1/2
INCAGN01949 (anti-OX40 IgG1 mAb)	Locally advanced solid neoplasms Metastatic pancreatic adenocarcinoma Stage IV pancreatic cancer	CMP-001 (VLP-encapsulated TLR9 agonist)	University of Southern California	NCT04387071 Phase 1/2
BGB-A445 (anti-OX40 mAb)	Advanced solid tumors	Tislelizumab (anti-PD-1)	BeiGene	NCT04215978 Phase 1
mRNA-2416 (lipid nanoparticle encapsulated OX40L mRNA)	Relapsed or refractory solid tumors Lymphoma Ovarian cancer	Durvalumab (anti-PD-L1)	ModernaTX, Inc.	NCT03323398 Phase 1/2
INBRX-106 (hexavalent OX40 agonist Ab)	Advanced or metastatic solid tumors	Pembrolizumab (anti-PD-1)	Inhibrx, Inc.	NCT04198766 Phase 1
IBI101 (anti-OX40 IgG1 mAb)	Advanced solid tumors	Sintilimab (anti-PD-1, IgG4)	Innovent Biologics (Suzhou) Co. Ltd.	NCT03758001 Phase 1
PF-04518600 (anti-OX40 IgG2 mAb)	Neoplasms	PF-05082566 (anti-4-1BB)	Pfizer	NCT02315066 Phase 1
	Recurrent or refractory acute myeloid leukemia	Avelumab (anti-PD-L1) Azacitidine Gemtuzumab Ozogamicin Glasdegib Venetoclax	MD Anderson Cancer Center	NCT03390296 Phase 1/2
	Renal cell carcinoma	Axitinib (tyrosine kinase inhibitor)	University of Southern California	NCT03092856 Phase 2
	Breast cancer	Avelumab (anti-PD-L1) Binimetinib Utomilumab (anti-4-1BB)	University of California, San Francisco	NCT03971409 Phase 2
	Malignant neoplasms Prostate cancer	Avelumab (anti-PD-L1) Utomilumab (anti-4-1BB)	MD Anderson Cancer Center	NCT03217747 Phase 1/2
	Follicular lymphoma	Rituximab (anti-CD20) Avelumab (anti-PD-L1) Utomilumab (anti-4-1BB)	Dana-Farber Cancer Institute	NCT03636503 Phase 1

(continued)

Table 28.3 Summary of Clinical Trials With Anti-OX40 Antibodies (Since 2015) (*continued*)

STUDY AGENT	CANCER TYPE	IN COMBINATION WITH	SPONSOR	NCT NUMBER + PHASE
MEDI0562 (humanized IgG4 anti-OX40 mAb) Tavolimab	Head and neck cancer Melanoma	None	Providence Health & Services	NCT03336606 Phase 1
	Ovarian cancer	Durvalumab (anti-PD-L1) Tremelilumab (anti-CTLA-4) Oleclumab (anti-CD73)	Nordic Society for Gynaecological Oncology	NCT03267589 Phase 2
GSK3174998 (anti-OX40 IgG1 mAb)	Neoplasms	Pembrolizumab (anti-PD-1)	GSK	NCT02528357 Phase 1
ATOR-1015 (bispecific CTLA-4xOX40)	Solid tumors Neoplasms	None	Alligator Bioscience AB	NCT03782467 Phase 1

BMS, Bristol Myers Squibb; CTLA-4, cytotoxic T-lymphocyte-associated protein 4; GSK, GlaxoSmithKline; HER2, human epidermal growth factor receptor 2; IgG, immunoglobulin G; mAb, monoclonal antibody; PD-1, programmed cell death protein 1; PD-L1, programmed death ligand 1; TLR, Toll-like receptor.

human homolog, which shares 55% amino acid homology with the mouse protein, was characterized shortly thereafter.[133,134] Similar to OX40 and 4-1BB, GITR is a T cell activation marker that is upregulated 24 to 72 hours after initial TCR stimulation of $CD4^+$ and $CD8^+$ T cells and maintained on the cell surface for several days. The delayed pattern of expression on T cells suggests that signaling may be required at the effector stage to establish and maintain T cell memory. Interestingly, GITR is expressed constitutively on both human and murine T_{reg} cells.[119,120] Other cell types expressing GITR include DCs, monocytes, granulocytes, and NK cells. The ligand, GITR-L, is expressed at low levels on the surface of APCs in immunologically naïve hosts, but rapidly upregulated at sites of inflammation on the surface of epithelial cells and activated APCs.[76,99,135]

Interest in GITR as cancer immunotherapy was sparked when experiments showed that triggering GITR signaling could overcome self-tolerance and rendered T cells resistant to T_{reg}-mediated suppression.[119,120] The first preclinical evidence of antitumor efficacy with a GITR agonist was published in 2004 when the rat mAb DTA-1 protected mice from the B16 melanoma tumor challenge, presumably by blocking T_{reg} cell suppression.[136,137] This was further characterized by the Wolchok group when they showed that the DTA-1 Ab could cure small established primary tumors.[138] Agonist Abs to GITR also cured established sarcomas leading to the induction of long-lasting memory in these mice.[139] Beneficial effects of GITR ligation were also demonstrated in colon carcinoma CT26 and A20 lymphoma models.[140,141] A GITR agonist showed impressive antitumor efficacy when combined with anti-PD-1 in the poorly immunogenic ID8 ovarian cancer model and 4T1 breast tumor model.[128] GITR ligation combined with stereotactic radiation increased survival in a glioblastoma model.[142]

Based on the previously noted preclinical studies, several mechanisms appear to be involved with the GITR Ab-mediated antitumor activity. Initially, it was shown that both $CD4^+$ and $CD8^+$ T cells play an essential role in GITR-based therapy, as the efficacy was decreased when either $CD4^+$ or $CD8^+$ T cells were depleted.[140,143] Functionally, anti-GITR stimulation increases T cell activation, which leads to increased IFNγ release.[143] Additionally, anti-GITR seems to decrease T_{reg} cell function. Whether this is a direct effect on T_{reg} cells or T effector cells are more resistant to their suppression is still under investigation.[138,139] Depletion of T_{reg} cells with anti-GITR Abs can also contribute to the therapeutic outcome.[144,145]

These findings led to several clinical trials; currently, six different GITR agonist Abs are being tested in safety and efficacy trials, summarized in Table 28.4. Most notably, the first trial utilized a humanized GITR-targeting mAb (TRX518) developed by Leap Therapeutics. This mAb was evaluated in a Phase 1 dose escalation study in patients with refractory solid tumors (NCT01239134). While T_{reg} cells were reduced in tumors and the periphery of patients, no clinical responses were observed. The study is being followed up in combination with PD-1 blockade to increase responsiveness to GITR therapy (NCT02628574).[146] Merck has investigated the effects of MK-4166, an anti-GITR IgG1 mAb, and demonstrated increased proliferation of TIL and inhibition of T_{reg} cells in vitro.[147] The safety is currently being evaluated in patients with advanced solid tumors in a Phase 1 study (NCT02132754). Amgen has investigated the effects of their GITR antibody, AMG 228, in a Phase 1 dose-escalation study, but terminated enrollment prior to the expansion phase due to the lack of immune modulatory effects and objective responses.[148] Incyte Corporation and BMS are also characterizing the use of their GITR agonists in

Table 28.4 Summary of Clinical Trials With Anti-GITR Antibodies (Since 2015)

STUDY AGENT	CANCER TYPE	IN COMBINATION WITH	SPONSOR	NCT NUMBER + PHASE
INCAGN01876 (humanized IgG1 anti-GITR mAb)	Glioblastoma	INCMGA00012 (anti-PD-1)	University of Pennsylvania	NCT04225039 Phase 2
	Advanced or metastatic cancer	Nivolumab (anti-PD-1) Ipilimumab (anti-CTLA-4)	Incyte Corp	NCT03126110 Phase 1/2
	Advanced or metastatic cancer	Epacadostat (IDO inhibitor) Pembrolizumab (anti-PD-1)	Incyte Corp	NCT03277352 Phase 1/2
BMS-986156 (anti-GITR IgG1 mAb)	Advanced or metastatic lung/ chest or liver cancers	Ipilimumab (anti-CTLA-4) Nivolumab (anti-PD-1)	MD Anderson Cancer Center, NCI	NCT04021043 Phase 1/2
	Solid tumors	Nivolumab (anti-PD-1)	BMS	NCT02598960 Phase 1/2
TRX518 (humanized aglycosyl IgG1 anti-GITR mAb)	Advanced solid tumors	Cyclophosphamide Avelumab (anti-PD-L1)	Leap Therapeutics	NCT03861403 Phase 1/2
	Solid tumors	Gemcitabine Pembrolizumab (anti-PD-1) Nivolumab (anti-PD-1)	Leap Therapeutics	NCT02628574 Phase 1
MK-4166 (humanized IgG1 anti-GITR mAb)	Advanced solid tumors	Pembrolizumab (anti-PD-1)	Merck Sharp & Dohme Corp.	NCT02132754 Phase 1
AMG 228 (anti-GITR IgG1 mAb)	Advanced solid tumors	None	Amgen	NCT02437916 Phase 1

BMS, Bristol Myers Squibb; CTLA-4, cytotoxic T-x lymphocyte-associated protein 4; GITR, glucocorticoid-induced tumor necrosis factor; IDO, indoleamine 2,3-dioxygenase; IgG, immunoglobulin G; mAb, monoclonal antibody; PD-1, programmed cell death protein 1; PD-L1, programmed death ligand 1.

advanced solid tumors. In conclusion, while the preclinical data were encouraging, GITR agonists have not been effective as single agents and AstraZeneca as well as Novartis abandoned their GITR programs in 2019.

CD27 (TNFRSF7)

CD27 (or TNFRSF7), initially discovered in 1987 as Tp55, is constitutively expressed on lymphoid cells, primarily on the surface of T cells, memory B cells, and NK cells, and can be further upregulated upon activation.[149–151] On terminally differentiated memory CD4[+] and CD8[+] T cells, CD27 (and CD28) expression is decreased, whereas KLRG-1 is increased.[152]

The CD27 ligand, CD70, is transiently expressed on the surface of APCs, NK cells, and T cells, and ligation of CD27 enhances T cell proliferation, expansion, and survival, similar to the function of the aforementioned TNFRSF members. Membrane-bound CD70 strongly stimulates CD27-associated signaling pathways, while soluble CD70 molecules are less able to trigger those pathways.[153] Interestingly, CD27 is expressed as a homodimer, which is surprising, considering most

TNFR ligand–receptor interactions occur as trimers.[151,154] However, this phenomenon can be explained by clustering of CD27 and CD70 oligomers; hence, three dimers of CD27 may bind two trimeric CD70 ligands. This may explain why soluble CD70 does not induce a potent transduction signal, which is greatly enhanced in supramolecular clusters.[153]

CD70 is absent on cells of nonhematopoietic origin, and expression is low in lymphoid tissues. In contrast, CD70 is highly expressed on B cell and T cell lymphomas and is also present on a majority of human solid tumors.[155] This suggests that CD70 may have immunosuppressive activity, potentially through the induction of T cell exhaustion, apoptosis, and/or expansion of T_{reg} cells.[153] These immune suppressive effects do not seem to override the strong CTL response triggered by anti-CD27, potentially because of the transient nature of agonist Abs.

In the context of T cell priming, CD27 co-stimulation promotes effector CD8[+] T cell differentiation and generates Th1-skewed CD4[+] T helper cells in both mice and humans.[156] The skewing of Th1 cells leads to a decrease in the development of Th17 cells in both species.[157,158] CD27 signaling also influences CD8[+] T cell memory formation via direct stimulation of CD27 on the cell surface and indirectly through CD4[+] T cell help.[159,160] CD27 co-stimulation is necessary to enhance CD4[+] and CD8[+] T cell survival,[161] as well as IL-2 production, which enhances CTL survival in nonlymphoid tissues.[162] Similar to other TNFR members (e.g., 4-1BB and OX40), combined blockade of co-inhibitory signals (e.g., anti-PD-L1) can reprogram exhausted CD8[+] T cells to increase their proliferation and effector function.[161,163]

Owing to constitutive expression of CD27 on the T cell surface as well as its strong co-stimulatory capacity, the CD27–CD70 axis is a promising target for immunotherapy. In mice, transgenic expression of CD70 in B cells, DCs, or tumor cells greatly increased antitumor immunity leading to therapeutic benefit.[164,165] Likewise, in preclinical studies, French et al. showed that an agonistic anti-CD27 Ab has antitumor activity in the Bcl1 lymphoma model.[166] CD27 agonists are also effective in the B16 melanoma model, which was dependent on activation of CD8[+] T cells and NK cells.[167]

A fully human IgG1 monoclonal CD27 agonist Ab (clone 1F5, also known as CDX-1127 or varlilumab), developed by Celldex Therapeutics, is the only anti-CD27 Ab currently in several Phase 1 and 2 trials evaluating therapeutic efficacy in cancer patients. Early trials targeting CD27 as monotherapy have indicated feasibility as well as safety, with the most common side effects being nausea, fatigue, and thrombocytopenia. CDX-1127 (varlilumab) has shown modest efficacy, leading to a durable complete response in one patient with stage 4 Hodgkin lymphoma and a partial response (78% tumor shrinkage) in one of 15 patients with metastatic renal cell carcinoma (RCC; NCT01460134).[168–170] Combination approaches using CD27 agonist Abs and PD-1 blockade have achieved the most promising preclinical efficacy, leading to tumor eradication in murine models.[171,172] In the TC-1 tumor model, administration of anti-CD27 together with PD-1 blockade was able to recapitulate the effects of CD4[+] T cell helper epitopes during therapeutic vaccination, with 100% cure rates. In addition, generation of tumor-specific effector CD8[+] T cells was further improved when tumor-unrelated CD4[+] T cell epitopes were administered with anti-CD27.[171] Growing preclinical evidence suggests that the agonist effect of anti-CD27 can be enhanced in combination with Abs to OX40 or CD40, as well as in combination with CTLA-4 blockade.[170] Preliminary results presented at the 2018 ASCO Annual Meeting from a Phase 1/2 study combining varlilumab and nivolumab were particularly noteworthy in ovarian cancer. The combination was able to turn immune cold tumors into hot ones, increasing CD8[+] T cell tumor infiltration (n = 14 of 24; 58%) and tumor PD-L1 expression (n = 14 of 23; 61%), and further correlated with improved clinical outcomes. Recent preclinical models

have also shown that anti-CD27 combined with PD-1/PD-L1 blockade synergize to increase CD8[+] T cell effector function and expansion, as evidenced by transcriptome analyses.[172]

Current trials include combination studies of varlilumab (anti-CD27) with nivolumab or rituximab (anti-CD20) in B cell lymphomas (NCT03038672; NCT03307746), and atezolizumab (anti-PD-L1) in patients with lung cancer. Additional Phase 1 and 2 trials are being pursued in melanoma and glioma in combination with multiantigen vaccines and DC vaccines, with and without the addition of varlilumab. Furthermore, a number of agents targeting CD70 tumor cell expression, including anti-CD70 mAbs (cusatuzumab, SEA-CD70) and CAR T cells, are in clinical trials (e.g., NCT02830724 and NCT03030612).[170] Most recent trials are summarized in Table 28.5.

CD40 (TNFRSF5)

In contrast to the aforementioned TNFRSF members, CD40 is expressed on APCs (B cells, DCs, macrophages, and monocytes) and activated CD8[+] T cells, whereas the ligand, CD40L (or CD154), is induced on T cells after activation. CD40 was first discovered in 1985 as the p50 surface antigen[173] CD40L is upregulated on CD4[+] T cells after TCR engagement, and upon interaction of CD40 with CD40L on the APC they license DCs via increased MHC expression, cytokine production, adhesion molecules, and increased co-stimulatory proteins to enhance priming of CD4[+] and CD8[+] T cells.[174,175]

In the late 1990s, several studies examined the effect of CD40 to stimulate tolerized CD4[+] T cells and increase the cytotoxic function of CD8[+] T cells in various tumor models. It was shown that CD4[+] T cell tolerance could be overcome by administering anti-CD40 with a vaccine in a renal cell carcinoma model.[176] Similar results were obtained in B cell and T cell lymphoma models with CD40 agonist stimulation.[177,178] Interestingly, CD40 is also present on the surface of several tumors and therefore the mechanism of action could be twofold. Anti-CD40 could enhance Ab-dependent phagocytosis of tumor cells via FcγR binding, and second, could induce the activation of APCs and thus help prime a vigorous T cell response to the tumor.[179] In addition to combining anti-CD40 with vaccination, its antitumor efficacy can be enhanced in combination with irradiation or chemotherapy. These treatments cause breakdown of the tumor, which increases immune priming. Anti-CD40 can boost this autovaccination strategy.[180,181]

There have been several clinical trials targeting CD40 in cancer patients during the past 20 years. The first trial was completed in early 2000 and reported encouraging antitumor results in lymphoma and advanced solid malignancies.[182] Seven Abs are currently under

Table 28.5 Summary of Clinical Trials With Anti-CD27 Antibodies (Since 2017)

STUDY AGENT	CANCER TYPE	IN COMBINATION WITH	SPONSOR	NCT NUMBER + PHASE
CDX-1127 (human IgG1kappa anti-CD27 mAb) Varlilumab	B cell lymphoma	Rituximab (anti-CD20)	University Hospital Southampton NHS Foundation Trust	NCT03307746 Phase 1/2
	Low-grade glioma	IMA950 vaccine Poly-ICLC	Nicholas Butowski, University of California, San Francisco	NCT02924038 Phase 1
	Glioblastoma	pp65-LAMP pulsed and control autologous DCs Temozolomide Tetanus–diphtheria 111 In-labeled DCs HIV-Gag pulsed autologous DCs	Gary Archer PhD, Duke University	NCT03688178 Phase 2
	Melanoma	6MHP Montanide ISA-51 Poly-ICLC	Craig L Slingluff, Jr, University of Virginia	NCT03617328 Phase 1/2
	Relapsed or refractory B cell lymphomas	Nivolumab (anti-PD-1)	NCI	NCT03038672 Phase 2
	NSCLC	Atezolizumab (anti-PD-L1) SBRT	Rutgers, The State University of New Jersey	NCT04081688 Phase 1

DC, dendritic cell; HIV, human immunodeficiency virus; IgG, immunoglobulin G; mAb, monoclonal antibody; NCI, National Cancer Institute; NSCLC, non-small cell lung cancer; PD-1, programmed cell death protein 1; PD-L1, programmed death ligand 1, Poly-ICLC, complex of carboxymethylcellulose, polyinosinic-polycytidylic acid, and poly-L-lysine double-stranded RNA; SBRT, stereotactic body radiation therapy.

investigation in clinical trials for the treatment of cancer, and three of them have been extensively studied in the clinic and are currently being assessed in Phase 2 trials: (a) selicrelumab (RG-7876; RO-7009789) from Roche, (b) CDX-1140 from Celldex Therapeutics, and (c) APX005M from Apexigen.

Selicrelumab was the first anti-CD40 Ab tested in humans and the agent was well tolerated, displaying promising single-dose results in patients with advanced melanoma (partial responses in four of 15 patients), but no efficacy in other solid tumors.[183] Interestingly, a follow-up trial with weekly dosing that included 11 advanced melanoma patients had no efficacy. Subsequently, the CD40 Ab was combined with gemcitabine (NCT01456585, in pancreatic adenocarcinoma) or carboplatin and paclitaxel chemotherapy (NCT00607048, in metastatic solid tumors) and led to partial responses in both trials.[184,185] Interestingly, the antitumor effect appeared to be DC and T cell-independent and mediated by CD40-expressing macrophages.[184] Current trials have combined selicrelumab with atezolizumab (anti-PD-L1), small molecule antagonists and inhibitors, anti-CD38, chemotherapy, and more. Like selicrelumab, CDX-1140 is also an IgG2 CD40 Ab that does not block the CD40L binding site.

Additive access to the CD40L binding motif enables enhanced APC activation, while also limiting side effects like cytokine release syndrome.[183,186] Neither CDX-1140 nor selicrelumab Abs require FcR crosslinking, which may decrease the therapeutic efficacy of these Abs.[183]

APX005M is currently under investigation in 10 clinical trials, targeting solid cancers including those found in the lung, pancreas, central nervous system (CNS), skin, rectum, esophagus, and other soft tissues (see Table 28.6). APX005M is a humanized rabbit IgG1 CD40 Ab that blocks the CD40L binding site and maintains a very high activation potency. In line with preclinical studies, APX005M requires FcR crosslinking in vivo, reflecting the pharmacodynamics and molecular features of anti-mouse agonist CD40 Abs.[183] The first-in-human study of APX005M was safe and showed increased activation of T cells and APCs, as well as augmented systemic levels of IL-12. Unfortunately, the study yielded no clinical responses. Current clinical trials are combining APX005M with nivolumab, pembrolizumab, ipilimumab, and personalized cancer vaccines. The Cancer Research UK Institute developed a fourth anti-CD40 Ab, termed Chi Lob 7/4, for use in cancer patients. A Phase 1 trial with the Ab in patients with advanced malignancies reported

Table 28.6 Summary of Clinical Trials With Anti-CD40 Antibodies (Since 2015)

STUDY AGENT	CANCER TYPE	IN COMBINATION WITH	SPONSOR	NCT NUMBER + PHASE
ABBV-927 (anti-CD40 mAb)	Cancer	ABBV-181 (anti-PD-1)	AbbVie	NCT02988960 Phase 1
	Locally advanced or metastatic solid tumors	ABBV-368 (anti-OX40) ABBV-181 (anti-PD-1) Carboplatin Nab-paclitaxel	AbbVie	NCT03893955 Phase 1
	Head and neck cancer	ABBV-368 (anti-OX40) ABBV-181 (anti-PD-1)	AbbVie	NCT03818542 Phase 1
RO7009789 (anti-CD40 mAb) Selicrelumab	Refractory or relapsed B cell lymphoma	Atezolizumab (anti-PD-L1)	The Lymphoma Academic Research Organization	NCT03892525 Phase 1
	Metastatic or locally advanced triple-negative breast cancer	Capecitabine Atezolizumab (anti-PD-L1) Ipatasertib SGN-LIV1A Bevacizumab (anti-VEGF) Tocilizumab (anti-IL-6R) Nab-paclitaxel Sacituzumab govitecan chemotherapy	Hoffmann-La Roche	NCT03424005 Phase 1/2
	Colorectal cancer	Regorafenib Atezolizumab (anti-PD-L1) Imprime PGG Bevacizumab (anti-VEGF) Isatuximab (anti-CD38) Idasanutlin AB928 (A2aR/A2bR antagonist)	Hoffmann-La Roche	NCT03555149 Phase 1/2
CDX-1140 (anti-CD40 mAb)	Advanced cancer	CDX-301 (Flt3L) Pembrolizumab (anti-PD-1)	Celldex Therapeutics	NCT03329950 Phase 1
	Melanoma	6MHP NeoAg-mBRAF Poly-ICLC	Craig L Slingluff, Jr, University of Virginia	NCT04364230 Phase 1/2
SEA-CD40 (nonfucosylated, humanized IgG1 anti-CD40 mAb)	Advanced cancer	Pembrolizumab (anti-PD-1) Gemcitabine Nab-paclitaxel	Seattle Genetics, Inc.	NCT02376699 Phase 1
JNJ-64457107 (anti-CD40 IgG1 mAb) ADC1013	Advanced solid neoplasms	None	Janssen Research & Development, LLC	NCT02829099 Phase 1
APX005M (humanized anti-CD40 mAb)	Soft tissue sarcoma	Doxorubicin	Columbia University	NCT03719430 Phase 2
	NSCLC Metastatic melanoma	Nivolumab (anti-PD-1)	Apexigen, Inc.	NCT03123783 Phase 1/2
	Melanoma	Pembrolizumab (anti-PD-1)	MD Anderson Cancer Center	NCT02706353 Phase 1/2

(continued)

Table 28.6 Summary of Clinical Trials With Anti-CD40 Antibodies (Since 2015) (*continued*)

STUDY AGENT	CANCER TYPE	IN COMBINATION WITH	SPONSOR	NCT NUMBER + PHASE
	Pediatric CNS tumors	None	Pediatric Brain Tumor Consortium	NCT03389802 Phase 1
	Resectable esophageal cancer Gastroesophageal junction cancers	Paclitaxel Carboplatin Radiation	Apexigen, Inc.	NCT03165994 Phase 2
	Unresectable or metastatic melanoma	None	Apexigen, Inc.	NCT04337931 Phase 2
	Locally advanced rectal adenocarcinoma	None	University of Texas Southwestern Medical Center	NCT04130854 Phase 2
	Metastatic pancreatic adenocarcinoma	Nivolumab (anti-PD-1) Nab-paclitaxel Gemcitabine	Parker Institute for Cancer Immunotherapy	NCT03214250 Phase 1/2
	Advanced melanoma NSCLC Renal cell carcinoma	Cabiralizumab (anti-CSF1R) Nivolumab (anti-PD-1)	Yale University	NCT03502330 Phase 1
	Metastatic melanoma	NEO-PV-01 Nivolumab (anti-PD-1) Ipilimumab (anti-CTLA-4) Poly-ICLC	Neon Therapeutics, Inc.	NCT03597282 Phase 1
2141-V11 (Fc-engineered anti-CD40 mAb)	Solid tumors	None	Rockefeller University	NCT04059588 Phase 1
NG-350A (oncolytic adeno-vector expressing anti-CD40 Ab)	Metastatic cancer Epithelial tumors	None	PsiOxus Therapeutics Ltd	NCT03852511 Phase 1

CNS, central nervous system; CSF1R, colony-stimulating factor 1 receptor; CTLA-4, cytotoxic T-lymphocyte-associated protein 4; IgG, immunoglobulin G; IL, interleukin; mAb, monoclonal antibody; NSCLC, non-small cell lung cancer; PD-1, programmed cell death protein 1; PD-L1, programmed death ligand 1, Poly-ICLC, complex of carboxymethylcellulose, polyinosinic-polycytidylic acid, and poly-L-lysine double-stranded RNA; VEGF, vascular endothelial growth factor.

low levels of toxicity and sustained B cell depletion as well as peripheral T cell activation. Stable disease was observed in 15 of 29 patients treated.[187] Taken together, selicrelumab, APX005M, and ChiLob7/4 have been able to elicit stable disease in patients with highly refractory solid tumors at a rate of 24% to 50%. Immune monitoring has revealed the ability of CD40 Abs to augment antigen presentation (increased expression of MHC class 1/2, CD54, CD80, CD86), deplete circulating B cells, and in some cases cause a significant increase in circulating IL-12.[183]

Seattle Genetics had performed nine clinical trials in hematologic malignancies with a first-generation CD40 Ab (SGN-40 or dacetuzumab) and has now developed a second-generation Ab, SEA-CD40, which is a nonfucosylated humanized IgG1 anti-CD40 Ab derived from dacetuzumab with higher binding capabilities. This second-generation CD40 Ab has improved agonist activity due to enhanced binding to FcγRIIIa and is currently being tested in a Phase 1 trial (NCT02376699). Other CD40 agonist Abs currently under investigation include ADC-1013, developed by Alligator Bioscience AB; 2141-V11, designed by The Rockefeller University; and ABBV-927, developed by AbbVie. Additionally, researchers have been investigating CD40 activation by intratumoral injections with an adenoviral vector encoding CD40L. Injection of the adenovirus (ISF35) in a B16 melanoma model resulted in an increase in tumor-specific CD8+ T cells that expressed PD-1 and produced significantly higher levels of cytokines including IFNγ, TNFα, IL-13, IL-6, and granulocyte-macrophage colony-stimulating factor (GM-CSF).[188] The addition of anti-CTLA-4 and anti-PD-1 resulted in complete eradication of 40% to 45% of melanoma tumors, even in brain metastases, and led to a higher ratio of CD8[+] T cells to T$_{reg}$ cells in the TIL. In summary, anti-CD40 agonists are being tested extensively and there are several ongoing clinical trials studying anti-CD40 stimulation in combination with other immune therapies, all of which are listed in Table 28.6.

Other Tumor Necrosis Factor Receptor Superfamily Targets

Other members of the TNFRSF that are presently under investigation by biotechnology and pharmaceutical companies as potential immunotherapy targets are as follows: herpes virus entry mediator (HVEM; TNFRSF14), death receptor 3 (DR3; TNFRSF25), CD30 (TNFRSF8), and TRAIL receptors 1 and 2 (TNFRSF10A and B). The therapeutic mode of action for the last two targets is via direct tumor cell killing and will not be covered in this chapter. In the remaining paragraphs, we have chosen to focus on the other TNFRSF that enhance T cell function in the tumor immunology setting.

Herpes Virus Entry Mediator (CD270 or TNFRSF14)

HVEM was initially described as herpes virus entry mediator and has some interesting characteristics not typically found in other TNFRSF members. First discovered in 1996 and characterized for its function on T cells,[189,190] HVEM interacts with multiple binding partners. Upon engagement, it induces variable downstream signals that can both positively and negatively affect T cell activation.[191] In contrast to other TNFRSF members, HVEM is highly expressed on resting or naïve T and B cells and is down-regulated upon activation. It is also expressed on APCs, NK cells, and endothelial cells. Besides the ligand for which it is named (the glycoprotein gD expressed on the HSV envelope), four other ligands for HVEM have been identified thus far: the TNF family members LIGHT and LT-α, as well as the immunoglobulin superfamily members BTLA and CD160.[191] The former ligands (LIGHT and LT-α) are expressed by lymphocytes, monocytes, and DCs, and have stimulatory effects on T cells as observed by increased proliferation, survival, and Th1 differentiation.[192] Stimulation through these ligands can also enhance CD40–CD40L interaction on B cells to increase their activation and Ig secretion.[193] In contrast, both BTLA and CD160 have been reported to have inhibitory effects on T cell and B cell stimulation. Expression of BTLA is inversely correlated with HVEM expression, presumably to reduce T cell activation. Recent work by Mintz et al. determined engagement of HVEM on B cells with BTLA on T cells reduced TCR signaling and subsequent expression of CD40L on T cells. HVEM functions to restrain B cell selection, differentiation, and proliferation by reduction of T cell help in the germinal center.[194] These negative regulatory proteins have also been found to decrease T

cell function in tumor-bearing hosts.[195,196] Drugs designed to block BTLA/CD160–HVEM interactions could prove to be potent immune activators and will hopefully be explored in the near future as therapeutics (patents by BMS and INSERM). One drawback of directly targeting HVEM to enhance T cell activation is its systemic expression on naïve T cells. Therefore, several preclinical studies have investigated the effect of targeting HVEM in antitumor settings, mainly by increasing LIGHT expressed within the tumor microenvironment.[197,198] However, LIGHT can also bind DR3 or LTβR, both of which have numerous biologic activities that can impact T cell function and activation. One study assessed the effect of a single-chain variable fragment (scFv) of an anti-HVEM agonistic Ab in the P815 mouse model of mastocytoma. On treatment with this agent, they observed tumor rejection and an increase in long-term T cell memory.[199] This positive antitumor effect was even more pronounced when the anti-HVEM Ab was combined with anti-4-1BB.[199] In 2018, a patent published by Daniel Olive's group (Marseille, INSERM) proposed to exploit the BTLA/HVEM pathway for therapeutic use to increase the proliferation of Vγ9Vδ2-specific γδ-T cells and induce antitumor responses in hematologic and solid malignancies. Due to the complex interactions of HVEM with several ligands, as well as its immunostimulatory versus immunosuppressive effects, manipulating the HVEM pathway may be a promising route in the future, but necessitates further preclinical development to understand its potential in cancer immunotherapy.

Death Receptor 3 (TNFRSF25)

DR3 or TNFRSF25 was first described in the late 1990s[200,201] and has the greatest homology (63%) with TNFR1. Expression of TNRSF25 is high on CD4[+] and CD8[+] T cells, especially following activation,[202] and is constitutive on T$_{reg}$ cells.[203] Its ligand is the TNF-like ligand 1A (TL1A) present on epithelial cells. The ligand is also expressed on APCs and is increased upon Toll-like receptor (TLR) stimulation.[204] In addition to TNFRSF25, TL1A can bind to DcR3, a decoy receptor that also binds LIGHT and Fas ligand.[205] The proposed function of this decoy receptor is as a negative regulator of the TL1A--DR3 signaling pathway.[206] Induction of apoptosis through a classic TNFR death domain was one of the first functions associated with TNFRSF25. However, it was later determined that downstream signaling after receptor engagement can also lead to cell activation and survival. Like TNFR1, it can recruit the adapter protein TRADD, which in turn signals via TRAF2 to deliver activating signals through NFκB and MAPK pathways.[207] If NF-κB is blocked in cells signaled through DR3 then FADD and caspase-8 are recruited, leading to cell death. The DR3 stimulatory functions described in immune cells mainly include increased effector functions in both CD4[+] and CD8[+] T cells, and these immune stimulatory effects would be

Table 28.7 Summary of Clinical Trials With an Anti-DR3 Antibody (Since 2020)

STUDY AGENT	CANCER TYPE	IN COMBINATION WITH	SPONSOR	NCT NUMBER +PHASE
PTX-35 (anti-TNFRSF25 IgG2 mAb)	Advanced solid tumors	None	Pelican Therapeutics	NCT04430348 Phase 1

IgG, immunoglobulin G; mAb, monoclonal antibody; TNFRSF, tumor necrosis factor receptor superfamily.

beneficial in tumor immunity.[208,209] Interestingly, one study compared anti-OX40 with DR3-agonist Abs and anti-DR3 was more potent at enhancing CD8$^+$ T cell responses, whereas OX40 agonists had greater activity on CD4$^+$ T cells.[210] More research is underway to analyze DR3 agonists in tumor immunology, but it is likely that its function might be unique and/or complementary to other TNFRSF members such as OX40, 4-1BB, GITR, and CD27. Pelican Therapeutics (a subsidiary of Heat Biologics) recently began a Phase 1 first-in-human clinical trial evaluating the safety and efficacy of PTX-35, a humanized agonistic mAb to TNFRSF25 (NCT04430348; see also Table 28.7). The study aims to enroll 30 patients with refractory advanced solid tumors and determine the optimal or MTD dose of the Ab. Pelican Therapeutics describes the Ab as a selective and potent stimulator of memory CD8$^+$ T cells, which is particularly useful to enhance the activity of T cells that have already seen their cognate antigen.

CONCLUSION

In summary, targeting T cell co-stimulatory proteins with agonist Abs is a promising approach to enhance immunity to a wide variety of malignancies. However, as demonstrated from the multitude of cancer clinical trials chronicled in this review, agonist co-stimulatory Abs may have the most therapeutic potential when combined with other immune-stimulating pathways. As illustrated with the CD28 co-stimulatory agonist, caution has to be taken when preclinical findings from mice and nonhuman primates are taken to the clinic. This requires careful characterization of the drug and its effect on the immune system, as well as titration, dosing, and timing. To comprehend the therapeutic potential of the TNFR pathways, it is crucial to improve our understanding of the expression (both spatial and temporal) of TNFRSF members on TIL, healthy tissue, and in peripheral blood. Furthermore, each cancer-bearing host may have a distinct set of immune evasion mechanisms, so that treatments with co-stimulatory agonist Abs may need to be tailored not only by tumor type but also to each individual patient.

Combining agonist Abs together with other treatment modalities, such as radiation/chemotherapy, targeted small molecule inhibitors, or with checkpoint blockade, will increase the clinical efficacy of these agents. Many ongoing preclinical studies and clinical trials are currently investigating these questions, and understanding the principles that drive immune-mediated tumor regression via agonist Abs will help guide their use in the future.

KEY REFERENCES

Only key references appear in the print edition. The full reference list appears in the digital product on Springer Publishing Connect: connect.springerpub.com/content/book/978-0-8261-3743-2/part/part02/chapter/ch28

19. Esensten JH, Helou YA, Chopra G, et al. CD28 costimulation: from mechanism to therapy. *Immunity*. 2016;44(5):973–988. doi:10.1016/j.immuni.2016.04.020
30. Jeong S, Park SH. Co-stimulatory receptors in cancers and their implications for cancer immunotherapy. *Immune Netw*. 2020;20(1):e3. doi:10.4110/in.2020.20.e3
32. Waite JC, Wang B, Haber L, et al. Tumor-targeted CD28 bispecific antibodies enhance the antitumor efficacy of PD-1 immunotherapy. *Sci Transl Med*. 2020;12(549):eaba2325. doi:10.1126/scitranslmed.aba2325
45. Amatore F, Gorvel L, Olive D. Inducible Co-Stimulator (ICOS) as a potential therapeutic target for anti-cancer therapy. *Expert Opin Ther Targets*. 2018;22(4):343–351. doi:10.1080/14728222.2018.1444753
71. Qi X, Li F, Wu Y, et al. Optimization of 4-1BB antibody for cancer immunotherapy by balancing agonistic strength with FcγR affinity. *Nat Commun*. 2019;10(1):2141. doi:10.1038/s41467-019-10088-1
89. Chester C, Sanmamed MF, Wang J, Melero I. Immunotherapy targeting 4-1BB: mechanistic rationale, clinical results, and future strategies. *Blood*. 2018;131(1):49–57. doi:10.1182/blood-2017-06-741041
99. Croft M. Control of immunity by the TNFR-related molecule OX40 (CD134). *Annu Rev Immunol*. 2010;28:57–78. doi:10.1146/annurev-immunol-030409-101243
146. Zappasodi R, Sirard C, Li Y, et al. Rational design of anti-GITR-based combination immunotherapy. *Nat Med*. 2019;25(5):759–766. doi:10.1038/s41591-019-0420-8
170. Starzer AM, Berghoff AS. New emerging targets in cancer immunotherapy: CD27 (TNFRSF7). *ESMO Open*. 2020;4:e000629. doi:10.1136/esmoopen-2019-000629
186. Piechutta M, Berghoff AS. New emerging targets in cancer immunotherapy: the role of cluster of differentiation 40 (CD40/TNFR5). *ESMO Open*. 2019;4:e000510. doi:10.1136/esmoopen-2019-000510

Immune Effects of Conventional Cancer Therapeutics

Sandra Demaria, Giulia Petroni, and Lorenzo Galluzzi

KEY POINTS

- Conventional chemotherapy, targeted anticancer agents, and radiotherapy have immunological effects that contribute to their activity *in vivo*.

- Immunological effects can be "on-target" (affecting cancer cells directly) or "off-target" (affecting immune cells).

- "On-target" immunostimulatory effects enhance immunogenicity of the cancer cells by improving antigenicity (increased expression of antigens or major histocompatibility complex [MHC] molecules) and/or adjuvanticity (generation of danger signals or damage-associated molecular patterns [DAMPs]).

- "Off-target" immunostimulatory effects are direct when the drug activates antitumor immune effectors or indirect when the drug eliminates or inhibits immunosuppressive cells.

- Cancer therapy can also mediate immunosuppressive effects as it promotes the accumulation or activation of regulatory and suppressor cells or factors.

- Treatments able to induce an immunogenic form of cancer cell death are often synergistic with immune checkpoint inhibitors.

- Rational combinations of conventional chemotherapy and/or radiotherapy with immunotherapy are undergoing clinical testing.

INTRODUCTION

Conventional cancer therapeutics, which include cytotoxic chemotherapy and radiotherapy, were developed with the goal of killing transformed cells while sparing normal cells as much as possible. An improved understanding of the molecular alterations that drive a specific cancer type has fostered the development of targeted therapeutics with increased selectivity and limited toxicity.[1] Technological advances in imaging and radiation dose delivery have also improved tumor targeting by radiotherapy.[2] At the same time, unequivocal demonstration that the malignant potential of transformed cells is regulated by the immune system fostered the development of anticancer therapeutics that target immune cells.[3] The success of the latter approach urges revisiting long-held assumptions about the mechanisms through which conventional cancer therapeutics work and assessing their effects on cells of the immune system and on tumor–host interactions.[4,5] This information becomes essential in the new era of immuno-oncology, in which several immune checkpoint inhibitors are approved for treatment of a growing list of cancer types and many more immunotherapies are likely to enter routine clinical care in the coming years.[6] In this new landscape, the immunological effects of conventional and targeted therapeutics used to treat patients before, during, or after immunotherapy need to be clearly understood as they can profoundly influence disease outcome.

Conventional chemotherapy and radiation preferentially affect proliferating cells, a feature not only of cancer but also of cells of the adaptive immune system, and have been considered uniformly immunosuppressive. While this is true for some agents, especially when used

Authors' Disclosure: SD has received compensation for consultant/advisory services from Lytix Biopharma, Mersana Therapeutics, Genentech, and EMD Serono, and research support from Lytix Biopharma and Nanobiotix. GP has no relevant conflicts of interest to disclose. LG has received consulting fees from OmniSEQ, Astra Zeneca, Inzen, and the Luke Heller TECPR2 Foundation, and he is a member of the Scientific Advisory Committee of Boehringer Ingelheim, The Longevity Labs, Onxeo, and OmniSEQ.

at high doses, experimental and clinical evidence accumulating over the past 15 years shows that many cytotoxic cancer treatments can stimulate antitumor immune responses and that the latter contribute significantly to their therapeutic activity.[7–14] Immunostimulatory effects of chemotherapy can be categorized as "on-target" when they result directly from the interaction of the drug with cancer cells or "off-target" when they result from effects of the drug on immune cells (Figure 29.1). A similar definition applies to targeted therapeutics, at least in part to focal radiotherapy, since radiation affects all compartments of the tumor stroma including immune cells. For

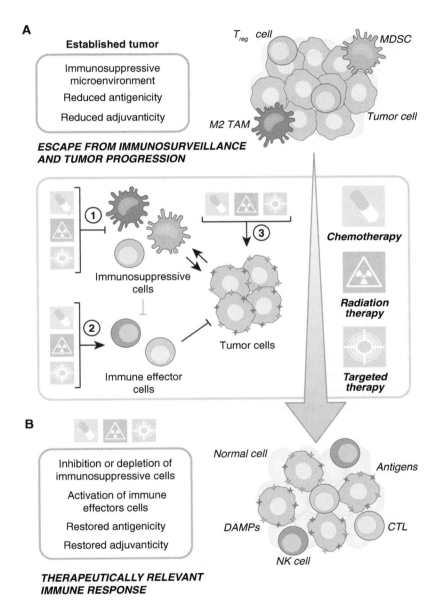

Figure 29.1 Immunostimulatory effects of conventional chemotherapeutics, targeted anticancer agents, and radiation therapy. According to current models, malignant precursors only form clinically manifest tumors as they escape immunosurveillance. Such an escape generally involves the selection of cancer cell variants with reduced immunogenicity (i.e., reduced antigenicity or reduced adjuvanticity) and/or the establishment of robust immunosuppressive mechanisms that operate locally (i.e., within the tumor microenvironment) and systemically (**A**). Multiple chemotherapeutics, targeted anticancer agents, and radiation therapy support the (re-)activation of tumor-targeting immune responses by (1) inhibiting or depleting immunosuppressive cell populations, (2) boosting the activity of immune effectors cells, and/or (3) restoring the antigenicity or adjuvanticity of neoplastic cells (**B**).

CTL, CD8+ cytotoxic lymphocyte; DAMPs, damage-associated molecular patterns; MDSC, myeloid-derived suppressor cell; NK, natural killer; TAM, tumor-associated macrophage; T_reg, CD4+CD25+Foxp3+ regulatory T.

the purpose of discussion in this chapter we will categorize on-target and off-target effects as outlined next and refer the reader to Section I of this book for a more detailed description of the key components and mechanisms of antitumor immune responses.

ON-TARGET IMMUNE EFFECTS

Tumors that become clinically evident have escaped immunological elimination by becoming less immunogenic or by suppressing antitumor immune effectors[15,16] (Figure 29.1A). Some cytotoxic agents can trigger a number of molecular responses in cancer cells that restore (at least part of) their immunogenicity. The immunogenicity of cancer cells is determined by their antigenicity and adjuvanticity. "Antigenicity" involves the expression of proteins that are not covered by central or peripheral tolerance.[16] Somatic mutations that accumulate in cancer cells are a major (but not the sole) source of the so-called tumor neoantigens.[17,18] Alternative tumor-specific antigens can also originate from nonmutated proteins that are overexpressed and/or ectopically expressed,[19] splice variants or lipids derived from noncanonical posttranscriptional or posttranslational events,[20] re-expression of latent proteins that are normally silenced by DNA methylation during development (e.g., the so-called "oncofetal antigens"),[21] as well as proteins aberrantly expressed from normally noncoding genomic regions[22] or endogenous retroelements.[20] Such antigens must be presented to CD8+ cytotoxic T lymphocytes (CTLs) in association with major histocompatibility complex class I (MHC-I) molecules. Thus, both the number of antigenic epitopes and MHC-I expression affect cancer cell antigenicity. "Adjuvanticity" refers to the expression or release of danger signals collectively known as "damage-associated molecular patterns" (DAMPs).[23,24] For the purpose of the present discussion, DAMPs can be broadly subdivided into two (partially overlapping) groups: (a) cell death–associated DAMPs and (b) cell stress–associated DAMPs.[24] A stressful cell death, as occurs when cells are infected or exposed to some cytotoxic agents that trigger the premortem activation of the DNA damage response (DDR), endoplasmic reticulum (ER) stress response, and autophagy, results in release of DAMPs that promote the recruitment and activation of dendritic cells (DCs) by binding to pattern recognition receptors (PRRs), and thus initiate the presentation of tumor-derived antigens to T cells.[24,25] An instance of cell death associated with elevated antigenicity and considerable DAMP emission is therefore defined as immunogenic cell death (ICD).[26] Molecules that are expressed by cells coping with (but surviving) therapy include ligands for natural killer (NK) cell-activating receptors like killer cell lectin-like receptor K1 (KLRK1, best known as NKG2D),[27] as well as the death receptor FAS/CD95, and adhesion molecules that improve recognition and

killing of the cancer cells by CTLs.[28] Although these molecules do not interact with PRRs as bona fide DAMPs do,[29] they contribute to the activation of the antitumor immune effectors and are therefore considered here as cell stress–associated DAMPs.

OFF-TARGET IMMUNE EFFECTS

Multiple immunosuppressive mechanisms operate locally (i.e., within the tumor microenvironment) and systemically to hinder tumor rejection by the immune system.[15] Inhibition of DCs, CTLs, and NK cells is mediated by suppressive cytokines, such as transforming growth factor beta 1 (TGF-β1), and co-inhibitory receptors, like cytotoxic T lymphocyte associated protein 4 (CTLA-4), programmed cell death 1 (PD-1),[3] and hepatitis A virus cellular receptor 2 (HAVCR2, best known as TIM-3),[30] within a network of interactions with immune cells mediating tolerogenic and suppressive function such as regulatory T (T_{reg}) cells, myeloid-derived suppressor cells (MDSCs), or M2-polarized macrophages.[31,32] Conventional and targeted anticancer treatments have been shown to mediate immunostimulatory effects by *direct* interaction with immune effector cells or *indirectly* by eliminating or reprogramming immunosuppressive cells (Figure 29.1B).

Conventional Chemotherapy

Increased Antigenicity

Multiple chemotherapeutic agents currently employed in clinical practice have been found to boost the antigenicity of cancer cells by upregulating the levels of surface-expressed MHC-I molecules, an "on-target" immunostimulatory activity that likely contributes to the efficacy of these drugs.[9] In combination with type I interferon (IFN-I), 5-fluorouracil (an irreversible inhibitor of thymidylate synthase used for the treatment of several solid tumors) as well as doxorubicin (an anthracycline frequently employed in women with breast carcinoma) restored MHC-I expression on murine Panc02 pancreatic cancer cells, and this regimen had prominent therapeutic activity against Panc02 cells growing orthotopically in immunocompetent syngeneic mice.[33,34] Gemcitabine (a nucleoside analogue mainly used for therapy of pancreatic carcinoma) had similar effects on human non–small cell lung carcinoma (NSCLC) A549 cells, human colorectal carcinoma HCT-116 cells, and human breast carcinoma MCF-7 cells.[35] The upregulation of MHC-I molecules induced by gemcitabine was associated with (a) increased tumor-specific T cell cytotoxicity in vitro, and this could be inhibited by an MHC-I-targeting monoclonal antibody[35]; and (b) with increased beta 2 microglobulin expression (which is required for MHC-I exposure), upregulation of immune-proteasomal subunits, and altered antigenic epitopes exposed by tumor cells.[36] Along similar lines, cisplatin (a DNA-damaging agent platinum derivative approved for use in patients with a wide variety of solid tumors) employed at low doses efficiently upregulated surface-exposed MHC-I molecules in cultured mouse lung adenocarcinoma TC-1 cells and in human head and neck squamous cell carcinoma (HNSCC) UMSCC-46 and UMSCC-74A cell lines,[37,38] as did oxaliplatin (another platinum-based DNA-damaging agent commonly used in combinatorial regimens for the treatment of colorectal cancer).[38] Moreover, MHC-I expression was upregulated by two topoisomerase inhibitors employed against different solid cancers, topotecan and irinotecan, in human breast carcinoma ZR-75-1 cells and murine mammary FM3A carcinoma cells, respectively, most likely as a consequence of autocrine/paracrine IFN-I signaling.[39,40] At least theoretically, a wide panel of DNA-damaging agents, including radiation therapy (RT) employed at suboptimal doses (i.e., doses that are unable to promote cell death),[41] could increase the antigenicity of cancer cells by favoring the generation of mutational neoantigens.[17] These agents include cisplatin and other platinum derivatives (like carboplatin, which is frequently employed against ovarian carcinoma, and oxaliplatin, which is approved for the treatment of colorectal carcinoma),[42] doxorubicin and other anthracyclines (such as idarubicin, which is also part of the chemotherapeutic options for acute myeloid leukemia [AML]),[43] topotecan and other topoisomerase inhibitors (like etoposide, which is employed against multiple hematological and solid neoplasms),[44] and alkylating agents (such as temozolomide, which is approved for use in glioblastoma and astrocytoma patients).[45] However, a recent study of gliomas recurring after temozolomide-based chemotherapy demonstrates that hypermutated tumor cells do not necessarily become more sensitive to immunotherapy,[46] lending further support to the emerging notion that neoantigen quality may be critical for immunogenicity.[47–49]

Increased Adjuvanticity

Multiple conventional chemotherapeutic agents mediate "on-target" immunostimulatory effects by increasing the capacity of malignant cells to emit danger signals as they respond to stress.[9,50] Cell stress–associated DAMPs are emitted by malignant cells that successfully cope with the potentially lethal effects of chemotherapy, and hence survive treatment.[51] Prototypic DAMPs of this class include various ligands for the activating NK-cell receptor NKG2D, including MHC-I polypeptide-related sequence A (MICA), MHC-I polypeptide-related sequence B (MICB), and retinoic acid early transcript 1E (RAET1E), which are upregulated on the membrane of cancer cells experiencing DNA damage.[27] On the other hand, cell death–associated DAMPs are emitted by neoplastic cells that are unable to cope with the

damaging effect of chemotherapy and eventually die as they attempt to do so (i.e., they activate adaptive stress responses that are insufficient for the recovery of homeostasis).[23] DAMPs liberated following chemotherapy-induced cancer cell death trigger signaling cascades that ultimately result in the induction of adaptive immune responses.[24,26,52] The optimal perception of ICD has been reported to involve the following cascade of events: (a) the exposure of calreticulin (CALR) and other ER chaperones on the cell surface, where they facilitate the phagocytosis of dead cells and corpses by antigen-presenting cells (APCs);[53,54] (b) the secretion of ATP, which functions both as a chemotactic cue for myeloid cells and as a pro-inflammatory signal;[55,56] (c) the release of annexin A1 (ANXA1), which guides the final approach of myeloid cells toward dying cells;[57] (d) the liberation of high-mobility group box 1 (HMGB1), a nuclear protein with multipronged immunostimulatory activity;[58] (e) the activation of an autocrine/paracrine type I IFN signaling pathway, via cyclic GMP-AMP synthase (CGAS), culminating with the release of chemotactic cytokines, including C-X-C motif chemokine ligand 10 (CXCL10, a chemoattractant for T cells);[59,60] and (f) passive release of nucleic acids which can engage Toll-like receptor 3 (TLR3), TLR7/8, and/or TLR9.[60]

Several chemotherapeutics have been shown to upregulate NKG2D ligands on the surface of cancer cells.[9,24] 5-Fluorouracil as well as doxorubicin (both in combination with type I IFN) efficiently stimulated the exposure of RAET1E and UL16 binding protein 1 (ULBP1, which also activates NKG2D) on the surface of murine Panc02 cells maintained in vitro.[33,34] Treatment with doxorubicin plus interleukin-12 (IL-12) also restored expression of the NKGD2 ligands MICA, MICB, RAET1E, and ULBP2 in vivo, in multiple murine tumors encompassing 4T1 breast carcinomas, CT26 colorectal carcinomas, Lewis lung carcinomas (LLCs), and K7M3 osteosarcomas, as well as in a genetically engineered model of mammary carcinoma, which was coupled to CD8[+] CTL-dependent tumor regression.[61] Gemcitabine at doses not affecting cell proliferation upregulated surface-exposed MICA and MICB in two out of six human pancreatic cancer cell lines tested in vitro (i.e., PANC-1 and HPAF-II cells), but this failed to correlate with increased T cell cytotoxicity, possibly as a result of the concomitant release of soluble MICA and/or MICB.[62] Gemcitabine also upregulated the expression of ULBP2, ULBP5, and ULBP6, as well as other NKG2D ligands, and of death receptor FAS/CD95 in human HCT-116 colorectal carcinoma cells and A549 NSCLC cells, and weakly increased the expression of FAS/CD95 on the surface of MCF7 breast carcinoma cells.[63] Docetaxel (a taxane employed for the treatment of various carcinomas) promoted the exposure of MICA, MICB, ULBP1, and/or ULBP2 on cultured human breast carcinoma BT474 and MDAMB361 cells, as well as in MDAMB361 cells grown in SCID mice, which was accompanied by a 15% to 40% increase in NK cell-dependent antibody-mediated cellular cytotoxicity.[64] Along similar lines, dacarbazine (a mainstay in the treatment of melanoma) robustly upregulated multiple NKG2D ligands including MICA, MICB, RAET1E, and/or ULBP1 in cultured mouse melanoma B16F10 cells and human melanoma Mel-C cells (at both the mRNA and protein level), correlating with the ability of dacarbazine to improve the efficacy of checkpoint blockers in immunocompetent mice bearing B16F10 melanomas.[65]

In addition, multiple chemotherapeutics commonly employed in clinical practice have been shown to promote bona fide ICD, as monitored in gold-standard vaccination experiments involving immunocompetent mice and syngeneic tumors.[66] These agents include (but may not be limited to) doxorubicin, idarubicin, and epirubicin (yet another anthracycline used for the treatment of breast carcinoma, most often in the context of combinatorial chemotherapeutic regimens)[67–69]; oxaliplatin[70–74]; cyclophosphamide (an alkylating agent approved for the therapy of hematological and solid neoplasms)[75–77]; bortezomib (a proteasome inhibitor used for the treatment of multiple myeloma)[78]; and pemetrexed (an antimetabolite approved for use against pleural mesothelioma and NSCLC).[79] Recently, other chemotherapeutic agents that are under clinical development for cancer therapy, such as lurbinectedin (a synthetic alkaloid analogue) and PT-112 (a platinum-pyrophosphate conjugate), have been shown to induce several markers of ICD in different tumor models.[80,81] Of note, ICD is accompanied by such an adjuvanticity that chemotherapeutic ICD inducers appear to synergize with checkpoint blockers to induce potent therapeutic responses even in tumors that are normally insensitive to checkpoint blockade.[73,79–85] A considerable number of clinical trials is currently focusing on the safety and efficacy of ICD-inducing chemotherapeutics plus immune checkpoint blockers (ICBs) in patients affected by a variety of solid and hematological tumors.[86,87]

Direct Immunostimulation

Although it may seem counterintuitive, some conventional chemotherapeutics mediate "off-target" immunostimulatory effects by delivering activating signals to the myeloid cell populations that initiate anticancer immune responses and/or to lymphoid immune effectors.[9] Thus, while dose-intensive cyclophosphamide has been employed for decades as part of myelo- and lymphoablative preconditioning (to prepare patients for hematopoietic stem cell transplantation),[88] metronomic cyclophosphamide has multipronged immunostimulatory effects. Low-dose cyclophosphamide has been shown to support therapeutically relevant Th1 and Th17 responses in immunocompetent mice

developing KRAS^{G12D}-driven lung cancer in the absence of functional p53 through a gut microbiota–dependent mechanism.[89] This regimen promoted CTL activity and the expansion of circulating NK cells in C57BL/6 mice implanted with syngeneic GL261 gliomas, an effect that contributed to the efficacy of treatment.[76] Along similar lines, metronomic cyclophosphamide synergized with a tumor lysate–based vaccine in the eradication of aggressive mouse AgN2a neuroblastomas growing in syngeneic hosts, an activity that also depended on CD8$^+$ CTL expansion.[90] In combination with radiotherapy, 5-fluorouracil promoted tumor infiltration by CD8$^+$ CTLs in a cohort of 52 locally advanced rectal cancer patients,[91] and an increased number of CD8$^+$ tumor-infiltrating lymphocytes (TILs) expression have also been found in a cohort of 69 patients with esophageal squamous cell carcinoma treated with 5-fluorouracil and cisplatin. This effect has been linked to compensatory upregulation of the immunosuppressive ligand CD274 (best known as PD-L1).[92] Of note, other chemotherapeutic agents can upregulate the expression of PD-L1 on cancer cells or tumor-infiltrating myeloid cells in preclinical[85] and clinical settings,[93–96] most likely reflecting increased tumor infiltration by CD8$^+$ CTLs. Moreover, low-dose 5-fluorouracil enabled a peptide-based anticancer vaccine to mediate therapeutic effects in immunocompetent mice bearing syngeneic E.G7 lymphoma cells, an effect that was linked to enhanced CD8$^+$ CTL activity.[97]

In a cohort of 28 pancreatic cancer patients, gemcitabine administration was associated with considerably increased numbers of circulating CD11c$^+$ DCs and CD14$^+$ monocytes (both of which are known to contribute to natural and therapy-elicited anticancer immunosurveillance).[98,99] Similarly, gemcitabine restored defective cross-presentation by tumor-infiltrating DCs in a model of mouse AB1 mesothelioma engineered to express an exogenous immunoreactive antigen,[100,101] as did paclitaxel (a taxane used for the treatment of multiple solid tumors) in mice bearing transgenic breast carcinomas.[102] Oxaliplatin potently boosted the anticancer activity of neutrophils and macrophages in immunocompetent mice bearing syngeneic EL4 lymphomas via a microbiota-dependent circuitry, thus resembling metronomic cyclophosphamide.[103] Moreover, oxaliplatin also favored the activation of DCs by increasing IL-12 production and concomitantly decreasing PD-L1 expression by DCs themselves.[104] Neoadjuvant paclitaxel favored the accumulation of TILs in a cohort of 25 breast carcinoma patients, correlating with clinical responses to treatment.[105] Finally, pemetrexed stimulated IFN-γ production by circulating NK cells from pancreatic cancer patients, an immunostimulatory effect that was abrogated by concurrent gemcitabine treatment and associated with the depletion of CD45RO$^+$ memory T cells.[106] Pemetrexed also increased T cell activation in vitro and in preclinical models of colorectal carcinoma by simultaneously inducing ICD and mediating direct "on-target" effects on T cells.[79] Taken together, these observations suggest that the direct immunostimulatory effects of specific chemotherapeutics may be sensitive to contextual variables including the presence of additional drugs.

Indirect Immunostimulation

Arguably the most common mechanism through which conventional chemotherapeutics employed at metronomic doses promote therapeutically relevant immunostimulation is by inhibiting or depleting immunosuppressive cell populations.[9] Thus, it appears possible to find doses and/or schedules of chemotherapeutic agents that preferentially deplete immunosuppressive cells over immune effector cells in vivo. Molecular mechanisms are understood in only a subset of cases. Human $CD4^+CD25^+Foxp3^+$ T_{reg} cells have been shown to be particularly sensitive to cyclophosphamide-driven cell death as they do not express ATP-binding cassette, subfamily B (MDR/TAP), member 1 (ABCB1), which normally extrudes the active metabolite of the drug.[107] On the contrary, why other immunosuppressive cells succumb so easily in response to a wide panel of chemotherapeutic agents employed at low doses remains unknown.[9]

Metronomic cyclophosphamide has been reported to preferentially deplete $CD4^+CD25^+Foxp3^+$ T_{reg} cells in nine end-stage cancer patients, correlating with the restoration of NK-cell and $CD8^+$ CTL activity.[108] A similar effect has been seen in C57BL/6 mice bearing syngeneic GL261 gliomas[76] and in rats bearing syngeneic colorectal carcinomas.[109] Conversely, in mice bearing syngeneic 4T1 breast carcinoma cells and A20 B-cell lymphoma cells, low-dose metronomic cyclophosphamide slightly increased circulating T_{reg} cells as it decreased circulating B and effector T cells.[110] Despite these latter observations, cyclophosphamide and an anti-PD-L1 antibody synergized in the control of 4T1 and A20 tumors.[110] A T_{reg} cell-depleting activity has also been ascribed to docetaxel, in a cohort of 40 NSCLC patients;[111] gemcitabine, in 53 subjects with pancreatic cancer[112] and in 40 NSCLC patients (receiving gemcitabine plus cisplatin);[113] and vinorelbine (a vinca alkaloid employed for the treatment of solid tumors), in 14 NSCLC patients treated with this agent in combination with cisplatin.[114] 5-Fluorouracil was reported to deplete circulating MDSCs from immunocompetent mice bearing carcinogen-driven colorectal cancer[115] or syngeneic EL4 lymphomas,[116] as well as from 23 patients with stage IV colorectal carcinoma,[116] an indirect immunostimulatory effect that was abolished by the concomitant administration of irinotecan but not oxaliplatin.[115] In mice bearing FM3A breast carcinomas, irinotecan depleted T_{reg} cells when used as monotherapy, but an increase in $CD8^+$ T cells in tumors or lymph nodes was

only observed when used in combination with an anti-PD-L1 antibody.[40] Finally, doxorubicin could increase the percentage of CTLs secreting IFN-γ through reducing the accumulation of T_{reg} cells in LLC and 4T1 breast carcinomas only when coadministered with IL-12, while the administration of doxorubicin alone resulted in T_{reg} cell accumulation in the same models.[117]

Gemcitabine caused a decrease in the percentage of circulating MDSCs in a variety of syngeneic tumor models, including CT26 colorectal carcinomas,[118] A20 lymphomas,[119] WEHI-164 fibrosarcomas,[120] AB12 mesotheliomas,[121] L1C2 bronchoalveolar carcinomas,[121] and K7M2 osteosarcomas[120] established in BALB/c mice, as well as LLC or TC-1 lung adenocarcinomas,[121,122] L1C2 bronchoalveolar carcinomas,[121] AE-17 mesothelioma,[121] and EL4 lymphoma[116] established in C57BL/6 mice. Along similar lines, paclitaxel was capable of depleting circulating MDSCs from mice bearing transgene-driven melanoma, accounting for most of the therapeutic efficacy of the drug in this setting.[123] Moreover, low levels of MDSCs have been found in the peripheral blood of patients with gastric cancer treated with paclitaxel.[124]

Finally, the experimental platinum-pyrophosphate conjugate PT-112 has been linked to a reduction in immunosuppressive cells (i.e., MDSCs, tumor-associated macrophages, and T_{reg} cells) and a concomitant increase in $CD8^+$ CTLs in the tumor microenvironment of CT26 colon carcinomas.[81] A similar indirect immunostimulatory effect has been ascribed to oxaliplatin, which reduced peritoneal metastasis by decreasing the number of tumor-associated macrophages and MDCSs in the spleen of BALB/c mice bearing syngeneic CT26 colon carcinomas,[125] and to a nanoparticle formulation of doxorubicin that causes the repolarization of murine M2-polarized immunosuppressive tumor-associated macrophages into their M1-polarized tumoricidal counterparts in 4T1 mammary carcinoma established in BALB/c mice.[126] Interestingly, gemcitabine and paclitaxel have also been shown to cause the M2-to-M1 repolarization of human and murine macrophages in vitro and in tumor samples from ovarian cancer patients.[127,128] However, it remains unclear to which extent such a conversion occurs in pancreatic cancer patients treated with gemcitabine-based chemotherapy in vivo, and whether such indirect immunostimulatory effects are therapeutically relevant in the clinic. Irrespectively, these observations corroborate the notion that a wide panel of chemotherapeutics currently employed in clinical practice can inhibit immunosuppressive cell populations, especially when employed according to metronomic regimens.

Overall, these data highlight the multiple effects of conventional chemotherapeutics on the antitumor host response (Table 29.1). While it remains to be established to which degree the therapeutic response to chemotherapy in patients is the result of direct tumor cytotoxicity

Table 29.1 Immunological Effects of Conventional Chemotherapy (Examples)

EFFECT	AGENT	SETTING	NOTES	REF.
"On-target" effects				
Increased antigenicity	5-Fluorouracil (plus type I IFN)	Orthotopic Panc02 mouse pancreatic carcinoma	Restored MHC class I expression	[33]
	Cisplatin	Mouse lung adenocarcinoma TC-1 cells	Restored MHC class I expression	[37]
		Human HNSCC UMSCC-46 and UMSCC-74A cells	Restored MHC class I expression	[38]
	Doxorubicin (plus type I IFN)	Mouse pancreatic carcinoma Panc02 cells	Restored MHC class I expression	[34]
	Gemcitabine	Human breast carcinoma MCF-7 cells	Restored MHC class I expression	[35, 36]
		Human NSCLC A549 cells	Restored MHC class I expression	[35, 36]
		Human colorectal cancer HCT-116 cells	Restored MHC class I expression	[35, 36]
	Irinotecan	Transplantable FM3A mouse breast carcinoma	Restored MHC class I expression	[40]
	Oxaliplatin	Human HNSCC UMSCC-46 and UMSCC-74A cells	Restored MHC class I expression	[38]
	Topotecan	Human breast carcinoma ZR-75-1 cells	Restored MHC class I expression	[39]
Increased adjuvanticity	5-Fluorouracil (plus type I IFN)	Mouse pancreatic carcinoma Panc02 cells	Restored RAET1E and ULBP1 expression	[33]
	Bortezomib	Human multiple myeloma U266 cells	ICD induction	[78]
	Cyclophosphamide	Transplantable EL4 mouse lymphoma and GL261 mouse glioma	ICD induction	[75, 76]
		Mouse glioma GL261 and CT-2A cells	ICD induction	[77]
	Dacarbazine	Human melanoma Mel-C cells and mouse melanoma B16F10 cells	Restored MICA, MICB, RAET1E, and/or ULBP1 expression	[65]
	Docetaxel	Human breast carcinoma BT474 and MDAMB361 cells	Restored MICA, MICB, ULBP1, and/or ULBP2 expression	[64]
	Doxorubicin	Various human and mouse cancer cells	ICD induction	[67, 68]
	Doxorubicin (liposome-microbubble)	Mouse lung carcinoma LL/2 cells	ICD induction	[69]
		Mouse colon carcinoma CT26 cells	ICD induction	[69]
	Doxorubicin (plus type I IFN)	Mouse pancreatic carcinoma Panc02 cells	Restored RAET1E and ULBP1 expression	[34]
	Doxorubicin (plus IL-12)	Various transgenic and transplantable mouse tumors	Restored RAET1E, MICA/B, and ULBP2 expression	[61]
	Gemcitabine	Human pancreatic carcinoma PANC-1 and HPAF-II cells	Restored MICA and MICB expression	[62]

(continued)

Table 29.1 Immunological Effects of Conventional Chemotherapy (Examples) (*continued*)

EFFECT	AGENT	SETTING	NOTES	REF.
	Lurbinectedin	Various human and mouse cancer cells	ICD induction	[80]
	Gemcitabine	Human breast carcinoma MCF-7 cells	Restored CD95 expression	[63]
		Human NSCLC A549 cells	Restored ULBP2/5/6 and CD95 expression	[63]
		Human colorectal cancer HCT-116 cells	Restored ULBP2/5/6 and CD95 expression	[63]
	Oxaliplatin	Various human and mouse cancer cells	ICD induction	[70–73]
	Pemetrexed	Mouse colorectal carcinoma Colon26 and MC38 cells	ICD induction	[79]
	PT-112	Mouse breast carcinoma TSA cells	ICD induction	[81]
"Off-target" effects				
Direct immunostimulation	5-Fluorouracil	Rectal cancer patients	Tumor infiltration by CD8+ CTLs	[91]
		Transplantable E.G7 mouse lymphoma	Enhanced CD8+ CTL activity	[97]
	5-Fluorouracil plus cisplatin	Esophageal squamous cell cancer patients	Tumor infiltration by CD8+ CTLs	[92]
	5-Fluorouracil plus oxaliplatin	Transplantable Colon26 and MC38 mouse colorectal carcinomas	Enhanced CD8+ CTL activity	[85]
	5-Fluorouracil plus docetaxel plus a platinum-based agent	HNSCC patients	Tumor infiltration by CD8+ CTLs	[93]
	Cyclophosphamide	Endogenous KRAS^{G12D}-driven lung cancer	Improved T_H1 and T_H17 responses, dependent on the gut microbiota	[89]
		Transplantable AgN2a mouse neuroblastomas	CD8+ CTL expansion	[90]
		Transplantable GL261 mouse gliomas	Enhanced CD8+ CTL activity and peripheral NK cell expansion	[76]
	Gemcitabine	Pancreatic cancer patients	Increased circulating CD11C+DCs and CD14+ monocytes	[98]
		Transplantable AB1 mouse mesothelioma	Restored cross-presentation by tumor-infiltrating DCs	[100, 101]
	Oxaliplatin	Transplantable MC38 mouse colon carcinoma	Induced DCs phenotypic maturation	[104]

(*continued*)

Table 29.1 Immunological Effects of Conventional Chemotherapy (Examples) (*continued*)

EFFECT	AGENT	SETTING	NOTES	REF.
	Paclitaxel	Breast carcinoma patients	Increased levels of TILs, correlating with clinical responses	[105]
		Transgenic mouse breast carcinoma	Restored cross-presentation by tumor-infiltrating DCs	[102]
	Pemetrexed	Pancreatic cancer patients	Enhanced IFN-γ-secretory activity in circulating NK cells	[106]
		Primary T cells and transplantable Colon26 and MC38 mouse colon carcinomas	Activated T cells and enhanced CD8$^+$ CTL activity	[79]
Indirect immunostimulation	5-Fluorouracil	Colorectal carcinoma patients	Depletion of circulating MDSCs	[115]
		Mouse carcinogen-driven colorectal cancer	Depletion of MDSCs, abolished by irinotecan coadministration	[115]
		Transplantable EL4 mouse lymphoma	Depletion of circulating MDSCs	[116]
	Cyclophosphamide	Advanced cancer patients	Depletion of T_{reg} cells, linked to NK cell and CD8$^+$ CTL activity	[108]
		Transgenic rat colorectal carcinoma	Depletion of T_{reg} cells	[109]
		Transplantable GL261 mouse glioma	Depletion of T_{reg} cells	[76]
	Docetaxel	NSCLC patients	Depletion of T_{reg} cells	[111]
	Doxorubicin (plus IL-12)	Transplantable LLC lung and 4T1 breast carcinomas	Depletion of T_{reg} cells linked to CD8$^+$ CTL activity	[117]
	Doxorubicin (nanoparticles)	Transplantable 4T1 breast carcinoma	M2-to-M1 repolarization linked to CD8$^+$ CTL activity	[126]
	Gemcitabine	Pancreatic cancer patients	Depletion of T_{reg} cells	[112]
		Human M2-polarized macrophages	M2-to-M1 repolarization	[127]
		Transplantable K7M2 mouse osteosarcomas and WEHI-164 mouse fibrosarcomas	Depletion of T_{reg} cells	[120]
		Various transplantable mouse tumors	Depletion of circulating MDSCs	[116, 118–122]
	Gemcitabine (plus cisplatin)	NSCLC patients	Depletion of T_{reg} cells	[113]
	Irinotecan	Transplantable FM3A mouse breast carcinoma	Depletion of T_{reg} cells	[40]
	Oxaliplatin	Transplantable CT26 mouse colon carcinoma	Depletion of TAMs and of MDCSs in the spleen, linked to CD8$^+$ CTL activity	[125]

(continued)

Table 29.1 Immunological Effects of Conventional Chemotherapy (Examples) (*continued*)

EFFECT	AGENT	SETTING	NOTES	REF.
	Paclitaxel	Transgenic mouse melanoma	Depletion of circulating MDSCs	[123]
		Gastric cancer patients	Depletion of circulating MDSCs	[124]
		Ovarian cancer patients	M2-to-M1 repolarization	[128]
		Murine M2-polarized macrophages	M2-to-M1 repolarization	[128]
	PT-112	Transplantable CT26 and MC38 mouse colon carcinomas	Depletion of MDSCs, TAMs, and T_{reg} cells, linked to CD8$^+$ CTL activity	[81]
	Vinorelbine (plus cisplatin)	NSCLC patients	Depletion of T_{reg} cells	[114]

CTL, cytotoxic T lymphocyte; DC, dendritic cell; HNSCC, head and neck squamous cell carcinoma; ICD, immunogenic cell death; IFN, interferon; LCC, Lewis lung carcinoma; MDSC, myeloid-derived suppressor cell; MHC, major histocompatibility complex; MICA, MHC class I polypeptide-related sequence A; MICB, MHC class I polypeptide-related sequence B; NK, natural killer; NSCLC, non–small-cell lung carcinoma; RAET1E, retinoic acid early transcript 1E; TAM, tumor-associated macrophages; T_H, helper T; TIL, tumor-infiltrating lymphocyte; T_{reg}, CD4$^+$CD25$^+$Foxp3$^+$ regulatory T; ULBP1, UL16 binding protein 1; ULBP2, UL16 binding protein 2.

Source: Modified with permission from Galluzzi L, Buqué A, Kepp O, et al. Immunological effects of conventional chemotherapy and targeted anticancer agents. *Cancer Cell.* 2015;28(6):690–714. doi:10.1016/j.ccell.2015.10.012

versus the induction of antitumor immunity, it is clear that the immunomodulatory effects of a given chemotherapy can influence its interaction with immunotherapeutic agents, either positively or negatively.

Targeted Therapy

Similar to conventional chemotherapy, targeted anticancer agents can have unintended immunomodulatory effects that are the result of their on-target action (inhibition of a mutated or overexpressed oncogene product) or may result from the interaction of the drug with other targets expressed by immune cells. These effects can have positive or negative influences on antitumor immune responses and are important yet incompletely understood determinants of clinical efficacy. In support of this notion, in a mouse model of oncogene addiction, durable responses to specific targeting of an oncogene were shown to require the contribution of T cells.[129]

The tyrosine kinase inhibitor (TKI) imatinib mesylate developed against the oncogenic fusion protein BCR-ABL is the prototype-targeted anticancer therapeutic and one of the most successful clinically. Initially developed for BCR-ABL$^+$ chronic myelogenous leukemia (CML),[130] imatinib was later shown to also have activity against the oncogenic kinase KIT, which is expressed by gastrointestinal stromal tumors (GISTs),[131] and platelet-growth factor receptor beta (PDGFRB), which is expressed by several solid tumors.[132] Induction of antileukemia T cell responses was reported in nine of 14 CML patients in remission after imatinib treatment.[133] In another study, BCR-ABL–specific T cells were detected in 10 of 10 CML

patients in maintenance with imatinib, more frequently in the bone marrow than in the peripheral blood. There was a correlation between BCR-ABL–specific T cells and lower minimal residual disease, and absence at leukemia relapse.[134] Moreover, ibrutinib, which targets Bruton tyrosine kinase, has been reported to increase diversification of the T cell compartment by increasing the TCR repertoire diversity in patients with chronic lymphocytic leukemia.[135]

An impact of kinase targeting on host immune responses has also been observed in the context of GIST. In a mouse model of GIST driven by an activated *KIT* mutation, the therapeutic activity of imatinib was shown to be partially dependent on antitumor CD8$^+$ T cells. The activation of antitumor immunity was due to downregulation of the immunosuppressive enzyme indoleamine 2,3-dioxygenase 1 (IDO1) in cancer cells, resulting in reduced T_{reg} cells and increased effector CTL infiltration into the tumor, a change that correlated with imatinib sensitivity in human GISTs.[136] Thus, activation of antitumor immunity is an *on-target* effect of imatinib in GISTs, which can be categorized as enhancing their *adjuvanticity*. In contrast, an *off-target* inhibitory activity of this drug against colony-stimulating factor 1 receptor (CSF1R) was likely responsible for decreased tumor-associated macrophage (TAM) recruitment to imatinib-treated GISTs. Despite such reduction, TAM interaction with apoptotic cancer cells in treated tumors was shown to promote M2 polarization, resulting in increased immunosuppression.[137] Consistent with this data, coadministration of imatinib and an anti-CD40 antibody activated TAMs and resulted in superior antitumor activity.[138] In other studies, the ability of imatinib to inhibit KIT on DCs was shown to promote DC-mediated NK-cell activation, culminating in antitumor effects against imatinib-resistant GISTs.[139,140] Imatinib also induced the M2-to-M1 repolarization of macrophages by TLR engagement and the M1-mediated NK-cell activation in neuroblastoma and CML samples, as did the imatinib-like drug nilotinib.[141] Recent findings also demonstrate that imatinib can augment antitumor immunity by inducing selective depletion of T_{reg} cells and increasing the number of effector CD8+ T cells in patients with CML or melanoma. Mechanistically, imatinib appears to inhibit the lymphocyte-specific protein tyrosine kinase LCK proto-oncogene, Src family tyrosine kinase (LCK), which is highly expressed by T cells other than T_{reg} cells, rendering the latter more sensitive to apoptosis upon TCR inhibition in the presence of imatinib.[142] The analysis of samples from dermatofibrosarcoma patients after treatment with imatinib also demonstrated that PDGFRB inhibition favors antigen presentation, linked to enhanced infiltration of the tumor by T cells and strong PD-L1 expression on the malignant cells themselves.[143] Consistent with this, coadministration of PD-1/PD-L1 blockers correlated with superior therapeutic activity in a model of GISTs.[144] ICBs also synergized with crizotinib, a TKI used to treat NSCLC, which acted as a potent ICD stimulator when combined with non-ICD–inducing chemotherapeutics like cisplatin, and induced off-target effects by promoting immune infiltration in NSCLC tumors established in immunocompetent mice.[145] These data highlight the complex and unsuspected effects of a molecularly targeted drug on the intended and unintended targets, which contribute to, and in some circumstances could hinder, the therapeutic response via immunological mechanisms.[132]

Many other TKIs used in the clinical practice for the treatment of different malignancies have been found to mediate direct and indirect effects on the immune system.[9] For example, dasatinib, a second-generation TKI active against BCR-ABL, SRC, KIT, PDGFR, and ephrin tyrosine kinases, reduced the levels of MDSCs and T_{reg} cells in a mouse melanoma model, leading to improved T cell responses to a tumor vaccine, an off-target indirect immunostimulatory effect.[146] A similar reduction of MDSCs and T_{reg} cells was reported for sorafenib, another broad-spectrum TKI, in mice and patients with renal cell carcinoma,[147,148] and sunitinib, which also upregulated CXCL10 and CXCL11 on the tumor endothelium, improving the recruitment of T cells in mouse melanoma and hepatocellular models, effects that are at least in part the consequence of the antiangiogenic activity of these drugs.[149,150] Erlotinib and gefitinib, which target epidermal growth factor receptor (EGFR), were shown to increase the expression of NKG2D ligands on lung cancer cells, increasing their susceptibility to NK

cell-mediated lysis, an example of an *on-target* increase in *adjuvanticity*.[151] *Off-target immunostimulatory* effects have also been reported for lenvatinib, which showed potent antitumor activity in the tumor microenvironment of murine colorectal and hepatocellular tumors, characterized by reduced TAMs and increased percentage of CTLs secreting IFN-γ and granzyme B. Moreover, combination treatment of lenvatinib plus anti-PD-1 further increased these effects resulting in greater antitumor activity.[152,153]

Activating mutations in B-Raf proto-oncogene (*BRAF*), encoding a serine/threonine kinase of the mitogen-activated protein kinase (MAPK) pathway, are frequent in melanoma and can be successfully targeted by specific BRAF inhibitors vemurafenib, encorafenib, and dabrafenib, alone or in combination with inhibitors of downstream mitogen-activated protein kinase kinase 7 (MAP2K7, best known as MEK, such as trametinib, cobimetinib, and binimetinib), but responses are generally short-lived.[154,155] Treatment of melanoma cells with BRAF and MEK inhibitors was shown to increase expression of melanocyte differentiation antigens, resulting in improved recognition by T cells, an *on-target* increase in cancer cell *immunogenicity*. In a recent study, combined inhibition of BRAF and MEK also led to DC activation following the release of HMGB1 by melanoma cells.[156] Although a previous study demonstrated that MEK inhibitor can impair T cell function,[157] MEK inhibition has recently been linked to a blockage of naïve CD8+ T cell expansion and priming but an increased number of antigen-specific effector CD8+ T cells in the tumor microenvironment (TME), and limited T cell exhaustion in vitro upon TCR stimulation.[158] These findings have been confirmed in mouse models of AML as well as in primary samples of AML patients sensitive to trametinib.[159] Moreover, the MEK inhibitor selumetinib combined with the PD-L1 blocker atezolizumab augmented antitumor immunity by upregulating MHC-I expression, boosting the production of several cytokines (i.e., IFN-γ, IL-6, IL-1β, and TNF), and reducing PD-L1 expression in a panel of NSCLC cell lines.[160] Other studies also suggest that T cell impairment may not be significant in vivo since patients co-treated with BRAF and MEK inhibitors showed increased infiltration of the tumor by T cells, which was associated with increased expression of PD-L1 (which is reflective of local IFN-γ secretion).[161,162] Importantly, responses to BRAF inhibitors correlated with the presence of an oligoclonal CD8+ T cell infiltrate in pretreatment biopsies, suggesting a contribution of the immune system to clinical responses, while reduced levels of intratumoral CD8+ T cells were seen at progression.[163,164] Interestingly, BRAF inhibition has also been shown to have *off-target direct immunostimulatory* effects on mouse and human NK cells, leading to increased phosphorylation of ERK1/2, CD69 upregulation, and improved effector functions. In a mouse model of BRAF^V600E-driven melanoma, NK cells and perforin

1 (PRF1) were required for therapeutic effects of BRAF inhibitors.[165] Moreover, BRAF and MEK inhibitors combined with a PD-1 blocker decreased TAM and T$_{reg}$ cell accumulation, improved IFN-γ release, and enhanced antigen presentation in a preclinical melanoma model, and increased the frequency of long-lasting antitumor responses in patients with BRAF-mutated melanoma.[166]

Improved antitumor immunity and synergy with ICBs has been described for MEK inhibitors in different preclinical models of tumors driven by mutant KRAS proto-oncogene, GTPase (KRAS).[167,168] Activating mutations of KRAS, which impact several signaling pathways including BRAF-MEK signaling and sustain carcinogenesis as well as treatment resistance in multiple oncological settings,[169] have recently been considered as novel targets to impair tumor growth and enhance antitumor immunity. Interestingly, pharmacological inhibition of KRAS^{G12C} with AMG510 resulted in tumor regression linked to the activation of ICD in several KRAS^{G12C}-driven tumor models. In addition, AMG510 improved the therapeutic efficacy of MEK inhibitors and a PD-1 blocker in KRAS^{G12C}-expressing mouse colorectal tumors growing in immunocompetent syngeneic mice.[170,171]

Some of the therapeutics targeting growth factor receptors that are overexpressed by cancer cells, including HER2/ERBB2 and EGFR, are monoclonal antibodies (e.g., trastuzumab, cetuximab). Not surprisingly, these agents not only mediate direct cytostatic or cytotoxic effects on cancer cells, but also engage immunological mechanisms such as antibody-dependent cellular cytotoxicity (ADCC), which likely contributes to their efficacy.[172] Interestingly, EGFR-targeting antibodies were shown to induce ICD and facilitate the elicitation of antitumor T cells in mouse models,[173,174] and the clinically relevant antibodies cetuximab and panitumumab induced ICD via a mechanism dependent on the mutational status of the EGFR signaling pathway and involving inhibition of the unfolded protein response, leading to ER stress, CALR translocation to the cell surface, and phagocytosis of the cancer cells by DCs.[173] Trastuzumab in combination with chemotherapy induced humoral responses to the intracellular domain of HER2 and other tumor-associated antigens, including carcinoembryonic antigen (CEA) and p53, in breast cancer patients, an effect that was associated with improved survival.[175] Trastuzumab-mediated ADCC was enhanced when conjugated to an anthracycline derivative, an effect that was linked to off-target immunostimulatory effects and synergy with an anti-PD-1 antibody in a murine orthotopic breast cancer model resistant to other HER2-targeted therapies.[176] Cetuximab has also been attributed off-target immunostimulatory effects by activating human CD8$^+$ T and NK cells in patients with colorectal cancer, correlating with T$_{reg}$ cell inhibition,[177] as well as systemic effects linked to improved infiltration of liver metastases in colorectal cancer patients.[178]

Epigenetic modifiers are another group of therapeutics with potentially important effects on antitumor immunity. For instance, decitabine, an inhibitor of DNA methyltransferases, has been reported to upregulate interferon signaling, antigen processing and presentation, and cytokine/chemokine-dependent signal transduction, as well as cancer-testis antigen expression in breast, colorectal, and ovarian cancer cells.[111] These data were confirmed in human samples from patients with colorectal and ovarian cancer responding to low-dose decitabine.[179] Such a response was attributed to the upregulation of hypermethylated endogenous retroviruses coupled to cytosolic sensing of double-stranded (ds) RNA by TLR3 and mitochondrial antiviral signaling protein.[180] The antitumor activity of histone deacetylase (HDAC) inhibitor trichostatin A, which is similar to the U.S. Food and Drug Administration (FDA)-approved HDAC inhibitor vorinostat, was shown to depend (at least in part) on the inhibition of intratumoral CD4$^+$ T cell apoptosis via downregulation of FAS ligand.[181]

DDR targeting can also mediate immunostimulatory effects and several reports are evaluating the therapeutic efficacy of combining these agents with immunotherapy.[87] For example, the FDA-approved poly(ADP-ribose) polymerase 1 inhibitors olaparib and rucaparib showed on-target immunostimulatory effects by inducing the accumulation of single-stranded (ss) DNA and micronuclei into the cytosol of NSCLC and triple-negative breast cancer cells.[182,183] In turn, this activated CGAS and consequent type I IFN secretion (linked to increased PD-L1 expression) and recruitment of CD8$^+$ T cells into the tumor.[182,183] Moreover, coadministration of ICBs led to superior disease control in tumors with DDR deficiency (including tumors with BRCA1 or BRCA2 mutations).[184]

Cyclin-dependent kinase 4 (CDK4) and CDK6 are frequently upregulated in human malignant cells.[185] These proteins are involved in cell-cycle regulation and can be specifically targeted with CDK4/6 inhibitors, including palbociclib, ribociclib, and abemaciclib, all of which have recently been approved for the treatment of patients with hormone receptor (HR)-positive breast cancer.[186] Their therapeutic activity has been largely attributed to their ability to induce cell-cycle arrest in malignant cells, but accumulating reports also highlighted a role for cell-cycle inhibitors in promoting on-target and off-target immunostimulatory effects.[187] In particular, CDK4/6 inhibition can induce on-target effects by enhancing antigen presentation via MHC-I on breast and colorectal cells.[188,189] Malignant cells treated with CDK4/6 inhibitors can also secrete type III IFN plus multiple inflammatory cytokines as a part of the senescence-associated secretory phenotype (SASP),[188,189] resulting in the modulation of anticancer immune responses.[190] Moreover, CDK4/6 inhibitors can induce *off-target immunostimulatory* effects by promoting effector T cell proliferation upon nuclear factor of activated T cell 1 activation and downregulating T_{reg} cell proliferation.[188,189,191] Recent findings also demonstrated that the combination of palbociclib with a MEK inhibitor (trametinib) favors a SASP that recruits NK cells with anticancer activity or favors a vascular remodeling that enables CD8+ CTL infiltration in preclinical models of KRAS-driven lung or pancreatic adenocarcinomas, respectively.[192,193] Enhanced T cell activation downstream of genome destabilization has been recently documented for pharmacological CDK7 inhibitors.[194] Moreover, targeting CDK8 resulted in NK cell-dependent antitumor responses in mice bearing B16F10 melanoma.[195] Finally, superior tumor eradication has been observed in different mouse tumor models following coadministration of cell-cycle inhibitors with ICBs.[188,189,191,193,194,196,197]

Radiation Therapy

Radiation has been known for a long time to have dose-dependent pro-inflammatory effects.[198] In fact, the multifraction radiation regimens traditionally used in clinical practice, which consist of small daily doses given for several weeks (1.5–2.2 Gy/day to a total dose of 50–80 Gy depending on the tumor type), were developed to minimize inflammatory reactions in normal tissue incorporated in the radiation field to account for differences in the daily reproducibility of the patient position. Technological advances have dramatically expanded the range of doses that can be safely delivered to the tumor with each fraction by improving the precision of tumor targeting with stereotactic body radiotherapy (SBRT).[2,199] One or a few high radiation doses (above 8 Gy and up to 30 Gy) are used to "ablate" the tumor by increasing the amount of cancer cell death. However, experimental evidence shows that the ability of radiation to activate antitumor immunity is an important determinant of radiation response,[200,201] and hence that the quality of cancer cell death, namely the induction of ICD, may be more important than its quantity.[10,202] In some preclinical studies, the local response to radiation given at doses in the SBRT range (single dose of 20–30 Gy) was largely dependent on T cells and a single large dose was more effective at inducing antitumor T cells than several small doses,[11,203] but other studies reported activation of antitumor T cells with a few comparatively lower dose fractions (e.g., 2 Gy X 5, 3 Gy X 5, or 8 Gy X 3),[204–206] suggesting some degree of model-dependency in this regard.[207]

Overall, the influence of the dose and fractionation regimen on the immunogenic effects of radiation therapy remains incompletely understood. The direct comparison of different radiation doses and fractionation schedules in a few mouse tumor models showed that hypofractionated regimens of 8 Gy X 3 or 6 Gy X 5 (but not single-dose radiation of 20 or 30 Gy) were able to induce a potent immune response leading to systemic tumor regression when combined with ICBs.[206,208] However, when the immunogenicity of radiation is assessed by the immunological control of the tumor in experimental models, several factors (many of which are model-specific) may contribute to outcome, including intrinsic radiosensitivity, immune contexture, and the type of immunotherapy combined with radiation.[209]

Besides contributing to the control of the irradiated lesion, radiation-induced antitumor T cells can reject metastases outside of the radiation field, a phenomenon known as abscopal effect.[207,210–212] Tumor responses in non-irradiated metastases have been reported in patients receiving radiation alone but are very rare.[213,214] However, when radiation was used in patients treated with immunotherapy, either to palliate progressing tumors or in the setting of clinical trials testing combinations of radiation and immune modulators, abscopal responses were detected at increased frequency.[215–222] The ability of focal tumor radiotherapy in combination with ICBs to induce abscopal responses in patients with NSCLC has been tested prospectively in various studies. In patients with chemorefractory metastatic NSCLC, which is poorly sensitive to ICBs targeting CTLA-4 used alone or combined with chemotherapy,[223] fractionated radiation (6 Gy X 5 and 9.5 Gy X 5) combined with the anti-CTLA-4 agent ipilimumab induced objective abscopal responses in 18% of individuals, accompanied by evidence of tumor-specific CD8+ T cell responses.[219] In another study, metastatic NSCLC patients were randomized to receive the anti-PD1 agent pembrolizumab alone or combined with focal radiation (8 Gy X 3), and the latter treatment was associated with superior overall response rate and median overall survival,[224] supporting the hypothesis that local radiotherapy can play a role in metastatic disease by sensitizing tumors to immunotherapy.[8] However, results have not been conclusive across different clinical studies,[225–228] highlighting the need to improve the current understanding of the immunological effects of radiotherapy.

Overall, radiation seems to mediate both on-target and off-target immunomodulatory effects that influence its therapeutic activity and identify novel targets for the development of combinatorial treatment regimens with superior clinical efficacy (Figure 29.2).

Immunostimulatory Effects of Radiation

Increased Antigenicity

Multiple studies have shown that radiation enhances the expression of MHC-I molecules as well as some tumor antigens in mouse and human cancer cells maintained in vitro.[229,230] In one study analyzing the

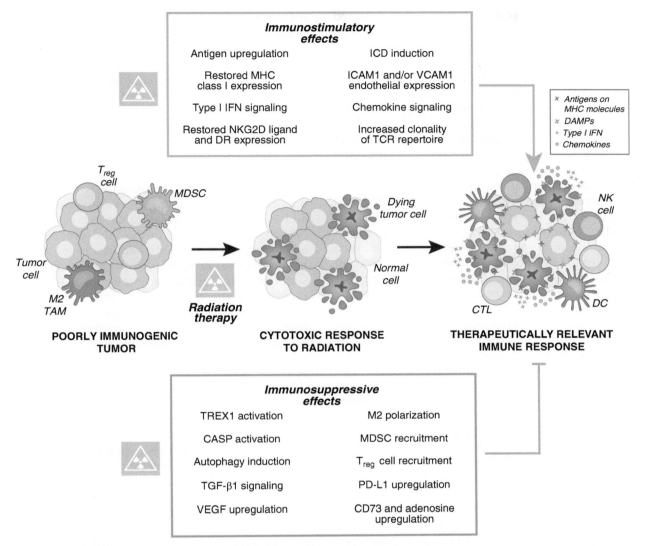

Figure 29.2 Immunostimulation and immunosuppression by radiation therapy. Malignant cells can die in response to radiation therapy as a consequence of irreparable damage to macromolecules and organelles. Importantly, such a cytotoxic response only affects a fraction of the tumor, implying that it is not sufficient to eradicate established neoplasms. Alongside, radiation therapy also mediates immunostimulatory (**A**) and immunosuppressive (**B**) effects, originating not only within cancer cells, but also within the stromal, endothelial, and immunological tumor compartments. The balance between such immunostimulatory and immunosuppressive effects determines whether radiation therapy can ultimately stimulate a therapeutically relevant anticancer immune response resulting in tumor eradication.

CD73 (official name: NT5E), 5'-nucleotidase ecto; CTL, CD8+ cytotoxic lymphocyte; DAMP, damage-associated molecular pattern; DC, dendritic cell; DR, death receptor; ICAM1, intercellular adhesion molecule 1; ICD, immunogenic cell death; IFN, interferon; MDSC, myeloid-derived suppressor cell; NK, natural killer; NKG2D (official name KLRK1), killer cell lectin-like receptor K1; PD-L1 (official name, CD274); TAA, tumor-associated antigen; TAM, tumor-associated macrophage; TGFβ1, transforming growth factor β1; T_{reg}, CD4+CD25+Foxp3+ regulatory T; TREX1, three prime repair exonuclease 1; VCAM1, vascular cell adhesion molecule 1; VEGF, vascular endothelial growth factor.

effects of radiation on expression of MHC-I and two tumor antigens, that is, CEA and mucin-1 (MUC-1), exposure to a single radiation dose of 10 or 20 Gy induced the upregulation of MHC-I and MUC-1 in eight of 23 human colon, lung, and prostate carcinoma cell lines tested, and CEA in 16 of them.[28] In mouse colorectal carcinoma MC38 cells growing in syngeneic immunocompetent mice, MHC-I upregulation was shown to occur in vivo after a single 10 Gy radiation dose, improving tumor rejection by adoptively transferred tumor-specific CTLs.[231] Similar findings have been obtained in human NSCLC A549 and H1975 cell lines maintained in vitro, with a plateau effect at 20 Gy single-dose radiation.[232]

In another study, the mechanisms of radiation-induced MHC-I upregulation were investigated using human melanoma cells.[231] Upregulation was detected at doses of 4 Gy or above and plateaued between 10 and 25 Gy. In the first few hours postradiation (clean-up phase), increased expression of surface MHC-I was supported by degradation of cellular proteins damaged by reactive oxygen species (ROS) generated by radiation, resulting in a larger pool of peptides available for loading onto MHC-I molecules. In a second phase (repair phase), activation of mechanistic target of rapamycin was required to sustain the increased availability of antigenic peptides, which largely originated from overall enhanced protein synthesis resulting in enhanced generation of defective ribosomal products. Importantly, some peptides displayed on surface MHC-I molecules by irradiated cells were not detected in the immunopeptidome of non-irradiated cells, and originated from proteins synthesized in response to DNA damage.[231] These data suggest that radiation modulates cancer cell antigenicity by altering the repertoire of epitopes displayed by MHC-I. This may result in increased expression of genes that encode immunogenic mutations, thus exposing neoantigens to the immune system.[230] Evidence in support of this hypothesis comes from the identification of CD8+ T cell clones specific for an immunogenic mutation encoded in karyopherin subunit alpha 2 (KPNA2), a gene upregulated by radiation, in an NSCLC patient with complete response to radiation and ipilimumab.[219]

The upregulation of MHC-I in vivo is not always the result of an on-target effect of radiation. For instance, in the B16 mouse melanoma model, host-produced IFN-γ was required for MHC-I upregulation in tumors treated with a single dose of 15 Gy.[233] This effect has also been observed in an orthotopic HNSCC murine model in which a single radiation dose of 10 Gy promoted IFN-γ secretion by CD4+ and CD8+ T cells, ultimately increasing tumor immunogenicity.[234]

Regardless of the mechanisms involved, which include a stable increase in expression of MHC-I heavy chain mRNA in mouse melanoma cells after prolonged exposure to 2 Gy daily radiation doses,[235] the increased antigenicity of irradiated cancer cells can contribute to their ability to serve as vaccines, especially when doses that are not ablative but may sensitize tumor cells to CTLs are used. In fact, in a mouse intracranial GL261 glioma model, peripheral vaccination with irradiated GM-CSF-transduced GL261 tumor cells had little effect, and whole brain radiotherapy with two doses of 4 Gy only minimally extended survival. However, when combined, the two treatments cured 40% to 80% of the mice.[236] Interestingly, restored MHC-I expression was seen in invading glioma cells at the edge of the tumor growing in the irradiated brain, suggesting that it may have contributed to complete tumor elimination by vaccine-elicited T cells.

Increased Adjuvanticity

Similar to chemotherapy, radiation has been shown to increase the capacity of malignant cells to emit danger signals. Cell stress–associated danger signals expressed on cells that survive irradiation include several NKG2D ligands, death receptors, adhesion molecules, and co-stimulatory molecules.[237] Ionizing radiation induced the expression of NKG2D ligands ULBP1 and RAET1E in mouse ovarian cancer cells,[238] and MICB, ULBP1, and ULBP2 in several human cancer cells, increasing their sensitivity to NK cell-mediated lysis.[239] Radiation also promoted the immunogenicity of different glioma cell lines, including glioma stem-like cells, in vitro and in vivo, by upregulating the expression of several NKG2D ligands at the mRNA and protein levels and enhancing DDR.[240] Consistently, decreased NKG2D ligand expression coupled to increased PD-L1 expression has been found in radioresistant NSCLC cell lines, protecting these cells from the cytotoxic action of NK cells.[241] Sensitivity of cancer cells to NK cell-mediated lysis was also increased by radiation-induced release of diablo IAP-binding mitochondrial protein (DIABLO) from mitochondria, which increases granzyme-induced cytotoxicity by blocking X-linked inhibitor of apoptosis (XIAP).[242] Moreover, inhibition of XIAP has been related to enhanced radiation-induced antigen presentation, induction of ICD, and recruitment of T cells in mouse models of HNSCC.[243] In the 4T1 mouse breast cancer model, in vivo irradiation increased the expression of intercellular adhesion molecule 1 (ICAM1) and induced the exposure of RAET1E on the surface of cancer cells. The interaction of RAET1E with NKG2D expressed on CD8+ T cells was critical for formation of stable immune synapses between these immune effectors and cancer cells in mice treated with an anti-CTLA-4 antibody.[244] Expression of death receptor FAS/CD95 was induced in MC38 colorectal mouse tumor cells after in vivo irradiation with a single 8 Gy radiation dose and increased tumor rejection by CD8+ T cells.[245] Similar findings have been obtained in models of pancreatic adenocarcinoma treated with CAR T cells.[246] In this setting, low-dose (1–2 Gy) irradiation caused the upregulation of TNF receptor superfamily member 10b (TNFRSF10B, best known as DR5) on the surface of malignant cells, ultimately resulting in some degree of antigen-independent cytotoxicity by CAR T cells.[246] Finally, irradiation of human colorectal cancer cells in vitro resulted in the upregulation of OX40L and 41BBL through epigenetic modulation, resulting in improved CTL survival, activation, and effector functions.[247]

Radiation has also been shown to induce the expression and release of many pro-inflammatory cytokines and chemokines by cancer cells. In vitro, a single radiation dose of 20 Gy induced IL-1β release by leukemia cells.[248] Human sarcoma cells produce TNF in response to a single radiation dose of 5 Gy.[249] CXCL16 was induced in vitro in human breast cancer cells and murine mammary, prostate, and colon carcinoma cells by a single dose of 12 Gy.[250,251] Moreover, radiation-induced CXCL16 was required for optimal infiltration of 4T1 mouse breast tumors by activated CD8+ T cells in mice treated with anti-CTLA-4 antibody.[250] Other than CXCL16, CXCL10, CCL2, and CCL5 also increased in B16 melanoma tumors after 30 Gy of radiation given in two fractions, resulting in increased CD8+ T cells and decreased CD11b+Gr1+ MDSCs tumor infiltration.[252]

Importantly, radiation-induced cancer cell death is associated with the generation of at least some of the DAMPs that characterize ICD induced by chemotherapy: CALR translocation to the cell surface, ATP secretion, and HMGB1 release, all of which have been shown to manifest in a radiation dose-dependent manner.[53,58,218,253,254] In addition, DNA released by cancer cells succumbing to radiation in vivo can be taken up by tumor-infiltrating DCs and provide a critical signal by activating IFN-I production via CGAS and stimulator of interferon response cGAMP interactor 1 (STING1),[255] an effect that may depend, at least in part, on tumor-derived exosomes.[256] At least in some settings, STING1 activation and consequent IFN-I production also occurs in irradiated cancer cells downstream of the accumulation of double-stranded (ds) DNA in the cytosol.[257] The ability of cancer cells to produce IFN-I is dependent on multiple factors, including expression levels of CGAS and STING1, the status of the cofactors and posttranslational modifications that modulate their functions, and the radiation dose and fractionation schedule.[258] One of the regulatory mechanisms limiting the secretion of IFN-I by irradiated cells is mediated by three prime repair exonuclease 1 (TREX1), which degrades cytosolic dsDNA and is upregulated at least in some cancer cells by radiation doses above 12 Gy. Conversely, production of IFN-I following CGAS-STING1 activation appears to be optimal when radiation is given in hypofractionated doses (8 Gy X 3). Upregulation of IFN-inducible chemokines (i.e., CXCL9, CXCL10, CXCL11, and CXCL16) and consequent recruitment of conventional type 1 DCs (cDC1s) and effector CD8+ T cells to the irradiated tumor were also seen in mouse tumors following fractionated radiation doses that optimally induce IFN-I.[206] Thus, in vivo radiation amplifies a pathway responsible for priming of spontaneous antitumor immunity to immunogenic tumors.[10,259]

Off-Target Immunostimulatory Effects

Some of the stromal cells present within the irradiated tumor have been shown to respond to radiation with phenotypic changes that improve tumor infiltration of effector T cells. Most of the studies have analyzed changes in tumor endothelium, showing upregulation of vascular cell adhesion molecule (VCAM1), which was associated with increased tumor-specific CD8+ T cell infiltration into irradiated mouse B16 melanomas.[204] Ionizing radiation also induced ICAM1 and VCAM1 expression on lymphatic endothelial cells in MC38 and B16 tumors grown in mice, an effect that was partially mediated by TGF-β1.[260] In another study based on a mouse model of spontaneous pancreatic islet carcinogenesis, radiation used at a low dose of 0.5 to 2 Gy normalized the aberrant vasculature by re-programming macrophages into a M1 phenotype, resulting in endothelial activation and recruitment of adoptively transferred T cells.[261] Interestingly, a recent study using longitudinal in vivo imaging of mouse tumors demonstrated that a significant fraction of tumor-infiltrating T cells survives therapeutic doses of radiation and exhibits increased motility and cytokine secretion as compared to T cells from unirradiated tumors.[13] These data indicate that, unlike circulating naïve T cells, tumor-resident T cells respond to radiation with increased effector functions rather than apoptosis.

Overall, the previously described multiple immune activating signals elicited by radiation explain the ability of radiation to convert the tumor into an "in situ vaccine" and induce antitumor immune responses that have been shown to contribute to control of the irradiated tumor in experimental studies.[200,262] However, the immune activation is usually insufficient to overcome negative regulatory networks that can also be upregulated by radiation, precluding the development of systemic responses capable of mediating abscopal effects. This could also be because radiation dose and fractionation schedules for inducing the optimal antitumor immune response and for reducing toxicity are not well defined and may vary between tumors with different genomic alterations and immune contextures.[199] Clearly, evidence for development of systemically detectable antitumor T cells in radiotherapy-treated patients is tenuous,[263] and abscopal responses are rarely seen in patients, as well as in tumor-bearing mice treated with radiation alone,[209] suggesting that the immunostimulatory effects of radiation are often insufficient to generate robust antitumor immune responses that overcome existing and radiation-driven immunosuppressive barriers.

Immunosuppressive Effects of Radiation

Radiation causes DNA damage that activates several stress responses including a cytoprotective DDR.[264] As previously described, the removal of cytosolic DNA fragments by TREX1 can limit the secretion of type I IFN by cancer cells.[206] In this context, ATR serine/threonine kinase (ATR), a regulator of the DDR, has shown to decrease IFN-I secretion by cancer cells, PD-L1 upregulation on tumor cells, and CD8+ T cell exhaustion. Enhancing DNA damage and accumulation of micronuclei by ATR pharmacological inhibition in combination with radiation significantly increased radiation-mediated IFN-I responses and MHC-I antigen presentation in lung cancer cells, and potentiated CD8[+] T cell activity in mouse models of KRAS-mutant cancer.[265-267] Another DNA damage regulator, ATM serine/threonine kinase (ATM), has been shown to activate NF-κB signaling pathway in radioresistant cancer cells,[268] resulting in the secretion of pro-inflammatory cytokines but limited STING-mediated type I IFN production.[269,270] As a consequence of DDR or ROS generation by damaged mitochondria, cancer cells can also activate autophagy as a mechanism of defense in response to radiation,[202,264] and radiation-induced autophagy can act as an immunosuppressive mechanism by removing the cytosolic sources of dsDNA including micronuclei[271,272] and limiting CGAS-STING pathway activation.[273] Moreover, CGAS-STING–dependent type I IFN production can be prevented by caspase 9 (CASP9) and CASP3, both of which are activated in cells succumbing to radiation-driven ICD.[5,264,274,275] In particular, both Casp9[-/-] and Casp3[-/-] cells growing in immunocompetent mice are more sensitive to radiation and generated a superior abscopal response in combination with ICBs.[212,275,276] In addition, CASP3 mediated prostaglandin E2 release by irradiated cancer cells, which is known to favor the establishment of an immunosuppressive tumor microenvironment.[277]

Radiation has been shown to upregulate expression of a number of growth factors and chemokines that promote the influx of myeloid cells into the tumor and foster their differentiation into immunosuppressive and tumor-promoting MDSCs and/or M2-polarized TAMs.[32] In the MycCaP mouse model of prostate carcinoma, radiation increased CSF1 release by cancer cells, leading to a systemic increase in circulating MDSCs, which were recruited to the tumor. Response of the irradiated tumor was improved by administration of an inhibitor of CSF1R. Increased levels of CSF1 were also found in the serum of prostate cancer patients after radiotherapy.[278] In a model of pancreatic ductal adenocarcinoma, radiation upregulated the chemokine CCL2, which increased the recruitment of Ly6C[+]CCR2[+] monocytes and their differentiation into pro-tumorigenic and pro-angiogenic TAMs.[279] Induction of TAMs in irradiated pancreatic tumors in mice also correlated to fewer CD8[+] T cells and increased numbers of effector CD4[+] T cells and T_{reg} cells.[280] Genetic or antibody-mediated CCL2 blockade, neutralization of macrophage colony-stimulating factor, and treatment with anti-CCR2 antibody alleviated immunosuppression, improving tumor response to radiation.[279-281] Interestingly, CCL2 was not induced by radiation in MycCaP prostate carcinomas, indicating that different tumors rely on different pathways to recruit myeloid cells in response to radiation.[278] Another radiation-induced pathway that promotes immunosuppression involves the upregulation of hypoxia-inducible factor 1 and consequently vascular endothelial growth factor A (VEGFA),[282] which promotes tumor infiltration by MDSCs and T_{reg} cells.[283] In vivo treatment with an aptamer platform that targets radiation-induced VEGFA and 4-1BB (an immune-stimulatory receptor expressed on activated CD8[+] T cells) potentiated both local tumor control and abscopal responses and reduced tumor-infiltrating T_{reg} cells.[284] T_{reg} cells have also been shown to be more radioresistant than conventional T cells, resulting in a relative increase postradiation,[285,286] although tumor-infiltrating effector T cells also appear to be more radioresistant than their circulating counterparts.[13] Moreover, radiation promotes the expansion and enhances the suppressive function of suppressive tumor-infiltrating T_{reg} cells, characterized by higher expression of CTLA-4, CD137, and Helios, in several murine tumor models (B16/F10, RENCA, and MC38).[287] T_{reg} cell depletion improved tumor control achieved by radiation in different cancer models.[288,289] Finally, STAT3 inhibition decreased T_{reg} cells, MDSCs, and M2 macrophages in response to radiotherapy, but enhanced effector T cells and M1 macrophages, improving tumor growth delay in preclinical models of HNSCC.[289]

Many tumors are rich in TGF-β1 but the vast majority is bound to latency-associated peptide (LAP) and inactive. Radiation-induced ROS causes TGF-β1 dissociation from LAP and its activation,[290] an event that plays a major role in inhibiting DC activation and priming of tumor-specific T cells. When TGF-β1 was neutralized by an antibody, radiation elicited T cell responses to multiple tumor antigens and abscopal effects in mouse models of metastatic breast cancer.[291] Abscopal responses were not documented in a prospective randomized clinical study testing systemic TGF-β blockade (fresolimumab) in two doses in the context of local hypofractionated radiation in a cohort of 23 patients with metastatic breast cancer. However, patients receiving the higher dose of fresolimumab showed changes consistent with decreased immunosuppression and improved CD8[+] T cell memory and experienced longer median overall survival compared to the patients treated with the lower fresolimumab dose.[292]

In vivo upregulation of PD-L1 by radiation has been reported in cancer cells and infiltrating myeloid cells in murine tumors.[205,234,241,291,293] In most cases, PD-L1 upregulation was driven by IFN-γ produced by radiation-induced antitumor T cells and acted as a barrier to tumor rejection.[205,234] However, CASP9 activation in irradiated cells has also been mechanistically linked to PD-L1 upregulation.[275] Other than PD-L1, the adenosine-generating enzyme CD73 and adenosine are upregulated in irradiated mouse and human breast cancer cells.[294] The CD73-adenosine axis on tumor cells is well known to impair antitumor T cell responses[295] and CD73 blockade with radiotherapy was able to restore DC infiltration in settings in which induction of IFN-I by radiotherapy alone was suboptimal.[294]

Other factors that may exert an immunosuppressive effect in the context of some tumors include the complement system, which was activated in a mouse model of lymphoma and mediated fast clearance of apoptotic cells reducing the generation of inflammatory signals,[296] as well as galectin-1 (as demonstrated in a mouse lung carcinoma model).[297] In summary, radiation can elicit a variety of immunosuppressive mechanisms that, at least potentially, limit its therapeutic efficacy and thus offer valuable targets for the development of combinatorial therapeutic regimens (Figure 29.2).

POTENTIAL ROLE OF THE GENETIC BACKGROUND OF THE HOST

Accumulating clinical data indicate that the genetic background of cancer patients can influence disease outcome as it influences the ability of malignant cells to elicit an immune response following chemotherapy, targeted therapy, or radiation therapy.[298] Loss-of-function single nucleotide polymorphisms (SNPs) affecting *TLR3* (encoding the receptor for cancer cell-derived ssRNA), *TLR4* (encoding the receptor for extracellular HMGB1), *P2RX7* (encoding the immunostimulatory receptor for extracellular ATP), and *FRP1* (encoding the receptor for extracellular ANXA1) have all been associated with reduced disease-free or overall survival in cohorts of breast carcinoma patients treated with neoadjuvant anthracycline-based chemotherapy.[55,57,58,299] Along similar lines, SNPs in *FPR1* and *TLR4* have been linked to poor disease outcome in two independent cohorts of colorectal carcinoma patients.[299,300] Moreover, a genetic variant of advanced glycosylation end-product specific receptor (*AGER*; another HMGB1 receptor best known as RAGE) has been associated with poor response to chemotherapy among NSCLC patients.[301] Finally, SNPs in *IDO1* and *CD24* (encoding an adhesion molecule involved in the interaction between DCs and T cells) have been linked to decreased 5-year survival rate in patients with resected colorectal liver metastases.[302] Altogether, these observations exemplify the potential effect of the genetic background of the host on the elicitation of anticancer immune responses by different treatment modalities.

CONCLUSION

Growing evidence indicates that the therapeutic effect of cytotoxic treatments is mediated by the interaction of stressed and dying cancer cells with the host immune system. Success likely depends on the balance between activating and suppressive signals generated by treatment, which is determined by the interaction of at least three factors: (1) the effects of therapy on cancer cells and immune cells; (2) the intrinsic immunogenicity of the cancer cells; and (3) germline polymorphisms in key immune players. Moreover, accumulating evidence supports a key role for the gut microbiota and a number of environmental and metabolic factors in the immunological fitness of the host and hence its capacity to mount

robust anticancer responses to treatment.[303–306] Finally, some neoplasms (the so-called "cold tumors") are able to prevent infiltration by immune cells compromising the immunostimulatory effects of chemotherapy, radiotherapy, and targeted therapy, and the efficacy of immunotherapy.[5,307] To which degree cancer cell death and the disruption of the tumor microenvironment imposed by chemotherapy and/or radiotherapy can turn cold tumors into hot ones remains to be determined.

As previously mentioned, the immunogenicity of a tumor is determined by antigenicity and adjuvanticity. Some tumors are more antigenic due to the presence of large numbers of mutations, some of which will encode neoantigens.[16,17] Others have mutations in MHC-I genes resulting in irreversible loss of expression.[308–312] Oncogenic pathways activated in different tumors are emerging as important regulators of tumor adjuvanticity,[313,314] and polymorphisms in genes encoding DAMP receptors such as TLR4 and P2RX7 affect immune cell activation.[7,55,58] Each of these factors provides opportunities to improve treatment outcome by devising personalized combinations of agents and ultimately induces a robust and persistent antitumor T cell memory response that not only contributes to cancer control but provides life-long protection from recurrence in the patient.[315] Multiple clinical trials testing combinations of immune checkpoint inhibitors and other immunotherapies with chemotherapy,[86] targeted anticancer agents,[316–319] or radiotherapy[320,321] are ongoing. Research to improve our understanding of the immune effects of currently used drugs, agents that are still under development, and the various radiation doses and fractionation regimens employed is urgently needed to accelerate progress and achieve therapeutic success in ever more, and eventually all, cancer patients.

KEY REFERENCES

Only key references appear in the print edition. The full reference list appears in the digital product on Springer Publishing Connect: connect.springerpub.com/content/book/978-0-8261-3743-2/part/part02/chapter/ch29

5. Galluzzi L, Chan TA, Kroemer G, et al. The hallmarks of successful anticancer immunotherapy. *Sci Transl Med.* 2018;10(459):eaat7807. doi:10.1126/scitranslmed.aat7807
14. Rodriguez-Ruiz ME, Vanpouille-Box C, Melero I, et al. Immunological mechanisms responsible for radiation-induced abscopal effect. *Trends Immunol.* 2018;39(8):644–655. doi:10.1016/j.it.2018.06.001
26. Galluzzi L, Vitale I, Warren S, et al. Consensus guidelines for the definition, detection and interpretation of immunogenic cell death. *J Immunother Cancer.* 2020;8(1):e000337. doi:10.1136/jitc-2019-000337
219. Formenti SC, Rudqvist NP, Golden E, et al. Radiotherapy induces responses of lung cancer to CTLA-4 blockade. *Nat Med.* 2018;24(12):1845–1851. doi:10.1038/s41591-018-0232-2
258. McLaughlin M, Patin EC, Pedersen M, et al. Inflammatory microenvironment remodelling by tumour cells after radiotherapy. *Nat Rev Cancer.* 2020;20(4):203–217. doi:10.1038/s41568-020-0246-1

Oncolytic Viruses

Ragunath Singaravelu, Larissa Pikor, John Bell, and Howard L. Kaufman

KEY POINTS

- Oncolytic viruses (OVs) are an emerging class of cancer biotherapeutics.

- Tumor evolution (acquisition of the hallmarks of cancer) favor viral infection and replication specifically in cancer cells.

- OVs have an excellent safety record and can be genetically manipulated to minimize off-target replication and maximize therapeutic efficacy.

- Oncolytic viruses kill cancer cells through multiple mechanisms.

- Viral infection of tumors enhances antitumor immune responses and can generate durable responses.

- OVs can be combined with chemotherapy, radiation, targeted therapy, and immunotherapy to improve the efficacy of both drugs with minimal additional toxicity.

- Systemic and physical barriers within the tumor microenvironment remain major obstacles in the successful delivery of therapeutically relevant doses of virus into the tumor.

HISTORY OF ONCOLYTIC VIRUSES

Oncolytic viruses (OVs) are a class of cancer biotherapeutics that utilizes replication-competent viruses designed or selected to specifically infect and destroy tumor cells without harming normal tissues. The use of viruses for the treatment of cancer originated from anecdotal evidence in multiple case reports dating back to the early 1900s in which tumor regression coincided with natural viral infections, such as measles,[1–3] influenza,[4,5] rabies,[6] and chicken pox[7] (Figure 30.1). While these remissions were generally short lived, lasting only a month or two, and observed mostly in patients with hematologic malignancies (acute leukemia, Hodgkin lymphoma, and Burkitt's lymphoma), they suggested that under the

right conditions some viruses are capable of destroying tumor cells while causing minimal harm to the patient.

Interest in the field of oncolytic viruses has varied significantly over the past 60 years. In the 1950s and 1960s, excitement about the potential of OVs for cancer treatment was at its peak, with numerous in vitro and in vivo studies, as well as clinical trials, conducted in an attempt to identify a lead candidate.[8] Flaviviruses, such as the West Nile, dengue, and yellow fever viruses (all transmitted by mosquitoes) were exceedingly common in the population at this time and among some of the first used for virotherapy.[9–12] Despite viremia and intratumoral virus replication, tumor responses were rare. While immunosuppressed patients were more likely to respond to treatment, they were also at a higher risk of fatal neurotoxicity.[8] Attempts at reducing neurotoxicity were met with limited success, leading to the search for viruses that display efficacy as well as an acceptable safety profile.

The use of animal cancer models to test OVs conclusively demonstrated the ability of viruses to infect and destroy cancer cells in an immune competent host. Importantly, the extensive and pioneering work of Alice Moore showed that in some cases, if the viral dose was high enough, it was possible to induce complete regressions.[13] As a result, a number of human pathogens were tested in rodent models to search for oncolytic activity. Evidence of responses in these models became a necessary step in establishing "proof of principle" data for oncolytic activity before moving into clinical testing of new potential OVs. From these studies, adenovirus, poxviruses, herpes viruses, picornaviruses, and paramyxoviruses emerged as leading candidates.[8] One of the most promising candidates identified through preclinical models was the adenoidal-pharyngeal-conjunctival virus (APC, now known as adenovirus). As an oncolytic agent with relatively modest side effects, APC moved quickly into clinical trials.[14] Administered either by intravenous, intravascular, or intra-arterial routes to 30 patients with advanced epidermoid carcinoma of the cervix, APC produced striking effects in two-thirds of cases, causing severe hemorrhage, necrosis, and shedding of neoplastic tissue.[15] However, infection was quickly eradicated by the host immune response, with

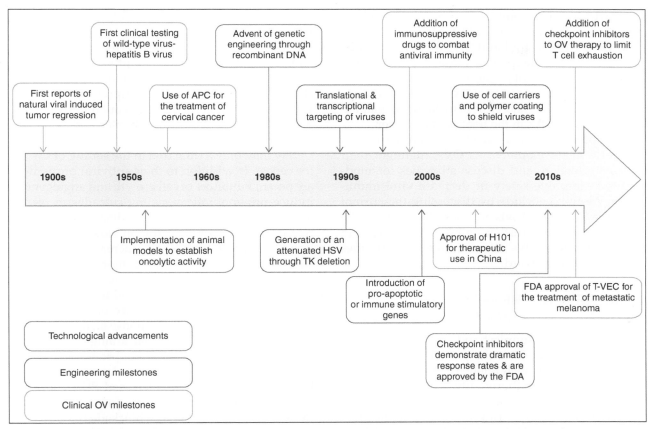

Figure 30.1 Milestones in the clinical development of oncolytic virotherapy. Technological advances are highlighted in blue, engineering milestones in purple, and notable clinical advances in orange. The milestones highlighted in this figure include the first case reports describing remissions upon viral infection (early 1900s); the first clinical testing of a wild-type virus (hepatitis B, 1949); the use of animal models to demonstrate efficacy (early 1950s); clinical testing of the first virus identified to have efficacy in preclinical models (APC, 1956); the advent of recombinant DNA technologies enabling genetic engineering of viral backbones, leading to the resurgence of OV therapy (1980s); translational and transcriptional targeting of replication-competent HSV to improve safety (1991 and 1997); attenuation of HSV in normal tissues through the deletion of thymidine kinase (early 1990s); the addition of immunosuppressive drugs such as cyclophosphamide to inhibit innate and adaptive antiviral immunity, leading to enhanced spread on HSV (1999); the introduction of pro-apoptotic (adenovirus death protein, ADP) or immune-stimulating genes (IL-12 and GM-CSF) into viral backbones to enhance cytotoxicity and recruit T lymphocytes to improve antitumor immune responses, respectively (2001); approval of the first OV for clinical use in China (H101, 2005); the application of cell carriers and polymer coating to shield the virus and improve delivery of oncolytic viruses into tumor beds (2006,2008); FDA approval of the CTLA-4 checkpoint inhibitor (ipilimumab) following the demonstration of a 20% survival benefit in advanced melanoma; the first drug ever shown to extend survival in this deadly disease (2011); FDA approval of the first OV, TVEC (talimogene laherparepvec) for use in metastatic melanoma (2015); addition of immune checkpoint inhibitors to OV therapy, which limits T cell exhaustion and improves efficacy of both treatment regimes (2014).

APC, adenoidal-pharyngeal-conjunctival virus; FDA, U.S. Food and Drug Administration; HSV, herpes simplex virus; OV, oncolytic virus; TK, thymidine kinase; T-VEC, talimogene laherparepvec.

no significant survival benefit reported. Importantly, patients with preexisting anti-adenovirus antibodies displayed diminished responses, emphasizing the issue of premature immune-mediated elimination of virus. Despite the undeniable efficacy in animal cancer models, it quickly became clear that clinical development was going to be more complicated.[11,15,16]

Due to the safety concerns associated with the use of live replication, nonattenuated viruses, coupled with the disappointing results of several clinical trials, by the 1970s oncolytic virotherapy was virtually all but abandoned.[8] It wasn't until the advent of recombinant DNA technologies in the 1980s, which enabled the modification of viruses to increase attenuation and decrease immunogenicity, that there was renewed interest in OVs. Within the past two decades the OV field has made a dramatic resurgence following the demonstration of therapeutic efficacy in a number of tumor types, an improved understanding of the multiple mechanisms through which OVs induce cell death, and the advent of immune checkpoint inhibitors, which can be combined with OVs to enhance systemic antitumor immunity. In October 2015, the U.S. Food and Drug Administration (FDA) approved the first OV (Talimogene Laherparepvec, commonly referred to as T-VEC) for the treatment of advanced melanoma, quickly followed by regulatory approvals in Australia and Europe (for treatment of stage III and IV M1a melanoma), validating a clinical role for OVs in the treatment of cancer.

In this chapter, we summarize the different virus families currently in development as OVs, highlight their mechanisms of action, and discuss strategies for modifying OVs to improve safety or decrease viral immunogenicity. We will conclude by discussing the current status of OVs in clinical trials and describe some of the emerging strategies to further improve delivery and therapeutic efficacy of OVs. We also highlight priorities for moving the field forward.

VIRUS BIOLOGY AND THE PRINCIPLES OF ONCOLYTIC VIROTHERAPY

Viruses are among the simplest and smallest infectious agents known to man.[17] Over the past 50 years, viruses have been studied with such intensity that their biology is now understood more thoroughly.[8] Largely regarded as nonliving, viruses are incapable of growing or multiplying on their own, requiring a host for replication. Viruses exist as independent particles known as virions, all of which are comprised of two components: a genetic element composed of DNA or RNA, and a protein coat known as the capsid which protects the nucleic acid. In addition, some viruses also possess a lipid envelope that surrounds the capsid and aids in cellular attachment through the presentation of glycoproteins. For entry into a host cell, viruses must attach to cell surface receptors and fuse with or penetrate the cell membrane. Each virus uses a specific mechanism for cell entry, which is often mediated by a host cell surface receptor. The distribution of these receptors often dictates the cell preference of a particular virus. For example, HIV binds both CD4 and its co-receptor CCR5, which are expressed exclusively on T cells, and thus, HIV enters and replicates preferentially in T cells.[18] Similarly, the neurotoxicity associated with several OVs (discussed in the text that follows) is due to the high expression of viral receptors on neurons.

In humans and animals, the detection, neutralization, and subsequent immune response to viral infections is mediated through the highly sophisticated interferon (IFN) signaling pathway. Type I and III IFNs and antiviral effector genes are induced upon the recognition of (a) viral elements by Toll-like receptors (TLRs),[19] (b) viral RNA by retinoic acid-induced gene I (RIG-I) and melanoma differentiation-associated protein 5 (MDA5),[20] and (c) viral DNA by the cytosolic DNA sensor protein cGAS, which activates the Stimulator of Interferon Genes

(STING) protein.[21,22] IFNs act in both an autocrine and paracrine manner to induce broadly antiviral gene programs, which inhibit viral entry, replication, and spread, and stimulate innate and adaptive immune responses through production of pro-inflammatory cytokines and chemokines.[23] A detailed description of the IFN pathway and its role in mediating cellular antiviral response is beyond the scope of this chapter and is reviewed in detail elsewhere.[23,24]

IFN may play a dual role in the setting of OV therapy for cancer. In addition to their antiviral properties, IFNs are potent inhibitors of cell growth and angiogenesis, and induce pro-apoptotic signaling cascades in response to infection. In this sense, local production of IFNs induced by OVs may also play a role in slowing tumor growth upon viral infection. IFNs also increase tumor cell expression of MHC class I and some tumor-associated antigens, which supports a role for OVs in promoting systemic antitumor immune responses and fostering T cell recognition of tumor cells. The release of IFN, however, can also promote an immune response against the virus limiting infection and tumor cell killing. In addition, IFN signaling activates expression of programmed cell death ligand 1 (PD-L1) as a counterregulatory response to limit immune responses. Also, increased PD-L1 levels resulting from OV infection may serve to increase tumor sensitivity to immune checkpoint blockade.[25]

As neoplastic cells undergo malignant transformation, they may activate oncogenic signaling pathways such as the Wnt-β-catenin, epidermal growth factor (EGF)/EGF receptor (EGFR), Ras/mitogen activated protein kinase (MAPK), phosphatidylinositol-4,5-bisphosphate 3-kinase (PI3K)/protein kinase B (AKT)/mechanistic target of rapamycin (mTOR), and vascular endothelial growth factor (VEGF) pathways, or repress tumor suppressor genes, such as P53 and RB, to acquire the hallmarks of cancer and overcome normal cellular restraints.[26] While disruption of these pathways provides growth and survival advantages for tumor cells, they come at the expense of the cell's antiviral response as they also inhibit IFN signaling. Defective IFN signaling is one of the most common genetic changes in tumors, estimated to occur in 65% to 70% of tumors. This defective antiviral response results in tumor cells being hypersensitive to viral infection and replication, and creates a clear distinction between normal and tumor cells, and this difference can be exploited by OVs. Some viruses, such as Newcastle disease virus (NDV), reovirus, herpes simplex virus (HSV), and mumps virus have a natural, albeit nonexclusive, tropism for cancer cells regardless of the state of antiviral signaling due to the overexpression of their receptors on cancer cells. These viruses were among some of the first to be used as OVs.[27–30] In general, OVs derive their specificity for tumor cells by exploiting dysfunctional intracellular signaling pathways and cell surface receptor expression patterns that arise during malignancy to promote cell growth and survival.

The ability of OVs to use abnormal IFN and oncogenic signaling defects in cancer cells explains how they can promote antitumor activity. Thus, it is likely that certain tumors may be more or less responsive to individual OVs that take advantage of individual signaling defects. Further investigation is needed to optimize OV therapy to the most appropriate cancer setting.

METHODS FOR IMPROVING OV SAFETY AND EFFICACY

While viruses possess tremendous potential as cancer therapeutics, the optimal OV needs to selectively infect and/or replicate in tumor cells, promote tumor cell death while not killing normal cells or promoting viral pathogenicity, and induce antitumor immune responses while avoiding antiviral immune elimination. Although some native viruses do share many of these properties, most viruses require manipulation in order to enhance specificity and subsequently improve efficacy, while also limiting toxicities and avoiding rapid viral clearance. The pathogenicity of a virus depends on its ability to replicate and/or induce latency, the presence of attenuation factors (natural or engineered), and the interaction between the virus and the host immune response (refer to Table 30.2).[31] Attenuation of viral pathogenesis (first generation OVs) can be achieved by using naturally occurring less virulent strains or vaccine strains, or through genetic engineering to delete specific viral pathogenesis genes or restrict their expression to cancer cells. Specific examples of attenuation are discussed in the following section that describes the different families of viruses currently in use as OVs.

While attenuation of pathogenesis successfully mitigates undesired toxicities, it may also produce less effective therapeutic OVs. Second generation OVs, therefore, focused on tumor-specific targeting to enhance efficacy while maintaining desirable safety profiles. Tumor targeting of OVs can be achieved through a variety of mechanisms, occurring either during viral infection or replication. For example, cell surface receptors overexpressed specifically on cancer cells such as EGFR, folate receptor, and prostate-specific membrane antigen (PSMA) can be targeted for use as receptors to facilitate virus entry[32,33] or essential viral genes can be placed under the regulation of tumor-specific promoters, such as prostate specific antigen (PSA), nestin, or human telomerase reverse transcriptase (hTERT) such that viral growth is restricted to those cells that can support transcription via the specific promoter.[33,34] However, the later approach is limited to nuclear DNA viruses (not including poxviruses).[35] Alternatively, viruses can be engineered to exploit the defective apoptotic, metabolic, and antiviral responses that distinguish tumor cells from normal cells, creating viruses that are attenuated/nonpathogenic in normal cells but still able to propagate in tumor cells. Examples include the E1 protein of adenovirus, the matrix (M) protein of vesicular stomatitis virus (VSV), γ34.5 of herpes simplex virus (HSV), and the vaccinia virus (VV) thymidine kinase gene. Specific details of viral manipulation to improve safety and efficacy are discussed in the following section.

FAMILIES OF ONCOLYTIC VIRUSES IN CLINICAL DEVELOPMENT

Viruses are classified according to their mechanism of viral mRNA synthesis (Baltimore Classification), and are currently classified into seven classes (I–VII). With each of the over 6,000 different mammalian species, each to be infected by an average of 58 unique viruses,[36,37] there exists a virtually endless possibility of potential OV candidates for clinical development. Ideally, clinically relevant OVs should be amenable to manufacturing at high titers, be easily manipulated in vitro while being genetically stable, exhibit selective tumor cell lysis, be safe, and be capable of simple patient delivery. The advent of viral genome modification to mediate tumor selectivity and enhance oncolytic activity while also limiting toxicity dramatically increased the number of viruses that could be used as OVs. Targeted OVs have demonstrated an excellent safety record in the clinic, with adenovirus and herpes virus being the most extensively studied. To date, one oncolytic HSV, talimogene laherparepvec (T-VEC), has been approved for the treatment of advanced melanoma in the United States, Europe, Australia, and Israel, while two other OVs have received limited approvals. This includes an oncolytic adenovirus, H101, approved in China for the treatment of refractory nasopharyngeal cancer in combination with chemotherapy, respectively; and an oncolytic reovirus, Rigvir, approved for advanced melanoma in Poland, Estonia, Belarus, and Latvia. Many other oncolytic viruses are currently in clinical development as monotherapies and in combination strategies for a variety of cancer indications. In the following section we describe the features of viruses currently in use as OVs and highlight the leading clinical candidates within each family. Table 30.1 highlights the properties of all virus families currently in use as OVs.

Adenoviruses

Adenoviruses (Ad) are non-enveloped viruses with a double-stranded 36 kb DNA genome that infects both dividing and nondividing cells across a wide range of species. The compact Ad genome has been well characterized and shown to be permissive to insertion of large transgenes without risk of integration into the host genome due to episomal viral replication. Human Ads are

Table 30.1 General Properties of Common Oncolytic Viruses

VIRUS FAMILY	STRAINS	GENOME	GENOME ORGANIZATION	GENOME SIZE	ENVELOP	CAPSID SYMMETRY	NATURAL HOST	SITE OF REPLICATION	MECHANISM OF ENTRY	RECEPTOR
Poxviridae	Vaccinia virus (VV)	dsDNA	Linear, nonsegmented	190 kb (250 genes)	Yes	Complex	Humans	Cytoplasm	Plasma membrane fusion	N/A
Rhabdoviridae	Vesicular stomatitis virus (VSV)	ssRNA (-)	Linear, nonsegmented	11.1 kb (5 genes)	Yes	Helical	Animals & insects	Cytoplasm	Receptor mediated	Low-density lipoprotein receptor (LDLR)
	Maraba virus	ssRNA (-)	Linear, nonsegmented	11 kb (5 genes)	Yes	Helical	Animals & insects	Cytoplasm	Receptor mediated	LDLR
Herpesviridae	Herpes simplex virus (HSV-1)	dsDNA	Linear, nonsegmented	154 Kb (74 genes)	Yes	Icosahedral	Humans & animals	Nucleus & Cytoplasm	Receptor mediated	Glycoprotein D (epithelial cells) herpes virus entry mediator (HVEM, immune cells), nectin-1 and nectin-2 (neurons)
Adenoviridae	Adenovirus (Ad)	dsDNA	Linear, nonsegmented	26–48 Kb	No	Icosahedral	Humans & animals	Nucleus & Cytoplasm	Receptor mediated	Human coxsackie and adenovirus receptor (hCAR) for species A, C-G, CD46 and Desmoglein 2(DSG-2) for B viruses
Paramyxoviridae	Newcastle disease virus (NDV)	ssRNA (-)	Linear, nonsegmented	15 kb	Yes	Helical	Birds	Cytoplasm	Plasma membrane fusion	N/A
	Measles virus (MeV)	ssRNA (-)	Linear, nonsegmented	16 kb	Yes	Icosahedral	Humans	Cytoplasm	Receptor mediated	CD46, signaling lymphocyte activation molecule (SLAM) and nectin-4
Picornaviridae	Coxsackievirus	ssRNA (+)	Linear, nonsegmented	28 Kb	No	Icosahedral	Humans & animals	Cytoplasm	Receptor mediated	Coxsackie- adenovirus receptor (CAR), intracellular adhesion molecule 1 (ICAM-1) decay accelerating factor (DAF)
	Poliovirus	ssRNA (+)	Linear, nonsegmented	7.5 Kb	No	Icosahedral	Humans	Cytoplasm	Receptor mediated	CD155
Parvoviridae	Parvovirus	ssDNA	Linear, nonsegmented	5 kb	No	Icosahedral	Humans & animals	Nucleus & cytoplasm	Receptor mediated	Erythrocyte P antigen, sialic acid residues
Reoviridae	Reovirus	dsDNA	Linear, segmented	10–48 kb	No	Icosahedral	Humans & animals	Cytoplasm	Receptor mediated	Sialic acid residues and junctional adhesion molecule-a (JAM-A)

classified into seven species (A–G, based on their DNA homology, hemagglutination status, and oncogenic/neutralization properties) and are commonly associated with mild human disease including upper respiratory tract infections (B and C), conjunctivitis (B and D), or gastroenteritis (F and G).[38,39] Due to the mild nature of Ad-related disease, substantial clinical experience, and ability to recombine and express heterologous genes, Ad has been developed as both an oncolytic virus and as a vector for gene therapy/vaccine delivery. Details regarding non-oncolytic vectors are reviewed elsewhere.[40]

Serotype 5 of species C (Ad5) is the most commonly used Ad delivery vector and has undergone multiple generations of development as an OV. First generation vectors harbored mutations of the E1/E3 genes responsible for viral replication and modulation of immune responses, respectively, creating conditionally replicating (crAdV) viruses with specific and enhanced replication in cancer cells and an improved safety profile. Second generation Ads encompassed an E4 deletion in addition to E1/E3 mutations to further improve both safety and efficacy.[41] The first oncolytic Ad5-based vectors used in cancer clinical trials was ONYX-015, later licensed as H101, which was approved in China for the treatment of head and neck cancer and nasopharyngeal cancer, respectively.[42] These viruses harbor complete deletion of E1B, rendering viral particles capable of selectively infecting cells with defective p53 signaling and, thus, improving safety. In a Phase 3 trial of H101, the combination of chemotherapy with virus led to a significant increase in response rate versus chemotherapy alone and led to the approval of H101 by the Chinese regulatory agency in 2005.[43] Early trial data of ONYX-015 identified a number of issues that may have limited efficacy and led to the development of third generation Ad vectors expressing suicide genes, immunostimulatory molecules, drug converting enzymes, or immunotherapeutic molecules.[41,44,45]

Despite the high transduction efficiency and ability to achieve tumor infection in both human and animal trials, high levels of preexisting humoral immunity against Ad in the general population (30%–100%) results in the formation of neutralizing antibodies that rapidly target systemically administered Ad vectors for elimination and severely limit its therapeutic efficacy. Attempts to improve efficacy have included creating non-Ad5-based species, such as ColoAd1 (a chimeric Ad3/Ad11p virus with ΔE1A/E1B), exploiting defects in the Rb pathway by deleting the Rb-binding region (E1A-CR2, known as Delta24), and circumventing liver sequestration and retargeting to limit humoral immunity.[38,40,41] While these manipulations have generated viruses that appear to be more potent than parental vectors, the efficacy of Ad as a monotherapy remains low. Nonetheless, the potent immunogenicity of Ad vectors has been successfully employed in prime-boost regimens.[46,47] Moreover, the combination of Ad vectors with existing therapies such as chemotherapy and radiotherapy have shown greater efficacy compared to virus alone, likely due to multi-mechanistic cell killing and stimulation of durable immune responses.[48,49] Therefore, it seems likely that the future of Ad as an oncolytic will be in combination with other treatment modalities.

More than half a dozen Ad vectors are currently under clinical investigation and their clinical characteristics are summarized in Table 30.2. Among the vectors currently in use, CG0070, an Ad5 encoding granulocyte-macrophage colony-stimulating factor (GM-CSF) (CG Oncology, Inc.), is the most advanced.[48] Data from a Phase 1/2 trial of CG0070 showed response rates of 48% to 77% in cancer patients depending on the dose schedule used, warranting further exploration.[50] An interim analysis of a Phase 2 clinical trial of CG0070 in 45 patients with BCG-unresponsive non-muscle-invasive bladder cancer demonstrated a 6-month complete response rate of 47% with most adverse events being low grade bladder spasm, hematuria, dysuria, and urgency.[51] These results have prompted a trial of CG0070 in combination with pembrolizumab for the treatment of bladder cancer.

Herpes Simplex Virus-1

Herpes simplex virus-1 (HSV-1) is an enveloped, dsDNA virus that causes cold sores in humans. A member of the alphaherpesvirus family, HSV-1 infects and replicates in the majority of tumor types, has a large genome (152 kb, of which 30 kb encodes nonessential genes for viral infection), and is easy to manipulate, allowing for the insertion of multiple transgenes. Importantly, while HSV-1 replicates in the nucleus, it does not cause insertional mutagenesis and, as such, was one of the first recombinant viruses to be developed. As HSV-1 is a minor human pathogen causing cold sores and is neurotropic resulting in latent infections, much work has been directed to mitigating these potential safety issues. Importantly, HSV-1 is sensitive to antiviral agents and in the case of severe toxicity, clinically approved antivirals can be used to limit viral replication.

To increase safety, HSV-1 oncolytics were engineered to harbor deletions of genes that: (a) are essential for replication in nondividing cells (e.g., UL39), (b) counteract the IFN response (e.g., $\gamma_1 34.5$), or (c) promote immune evasion (e.g., $\alpha 47$). HSV-1-based OVs were also armed with immune stimulatory transgenes to boost antitumor cytotoxic immune responses within the tumor microenvironment (e.g., GM-CSF).[38,52] Despite an improved safety profile, the deletion of multiple viral genes can also attenuate the virus in some tumor cells. Attempts to improve cytotoxicity of these viruses have focused on changing the tropism or transcriptional specificity of these viruses.

Table 30.2 General Considerations in Oncolytic Virus Development

VIRAL SPECIES	MODIFICATIONS	ARMING	COMBINATIONS	ROUTES	INDICATIONS
DNA viruses • Adenovirus • Herpes virus • Parvovirus • Vaccinia virus (and modified Vaccinia Ankara)	• Native viral gene deletions (e.g., to enhance tumor cell selective replication, decrease pathogenicity, alter immunogenicity) • Insertion of transgenes (e.g., to arm virus for better antitumor therapeutic activity—see arming column or provide imaging capability) • Cell specific promoters (helps promote tumor-specific replication and safety) • Alteration of capsid proteins (enhances efficiency and specificity of tumor cell targeting)	Cytokines • GM-CSF • IL-2 • IL-12 • IL-15 • IL-18 • IL-21 • IFN • TGF-β trap • FLT3	Chemotherapy • Standard of care regimens • Myeloablative • Metronomic • Chemoradiation	Intratumoral	Cutaneous malignancies • Melanoma • Cutaneous squamous cell carcinoma • Merkel cell carcinoma • Mycosis fungoides
RNA viruses • Coxsackievirus • Maraba virus • Measles virus • Newcastle disease virus • Poliovirus • Reovirus • VSV		Chemokines • CCL5 • CCL19 • CCL20 • CCL21 • CXCL10	Immunotherapy • Checkpoint blockade (e.g., anti-CTLA-4, anti-PD-1) • Cytokine (e.g., IL-2) • CAR T cells • TLR agonists • STING agonists • Tumor vaccines • Other oncolytic viruses (prime-boost)	Intravenous	Solid tumors • Glioblastoma • Non-small cell lung cancer • Colorectal cancer • Cholangiocarcinoma • Pancreatic cancer • Esophageal cancer • Hepatocellular carcinoma • Prostate cancer • Ovarian cancer • Endometrial cancer • Head and neck cancer • Breast cancer • Soft tissue sarcoma • Renal cell carcinoma • Pediatric tumors
		Co-stimulatory molecules • CD28 • B7.1 • ICAM-1 • LFA-3 • ICOS • 4-1BBL • CD40 • OX40 • CD30	Radiation • External beam • Stereotactic • Proton	Intrapleural	Hematologic tumors • Lymphoma • Multiple myeloma • Leukemia
		Co-inhibitory molecule inhibitors • Anti-CTLA-4 • Anti-PD-1 • Anti-PD-L1 • Anti-TIM-3 • Anti-LAG-3	Targeted therapy • Sorafenib • BRAF inhibitors • MEK inhibitors • Bevacizumab	Intraperitoneal	

(continued)

Table 30.2 General Considerations in Oncolytic Virus Development (*continued*)

VIRAL SPECIES	MODIFICATIONS	ARMING	COMBINATIONS	ROUTES	INDICATIONS
		Suicide genes • HSV-TK • Cytochrome P450 • Nitroreductase • GALV	Surgery • Neoadjuvant	Intra-arterial	
		Tumor suppressors • P53 • PTEN • P16 • RB • MnSOD		Convection-enhanced delivery	
		Anti-angiogenesis • VEGF • Vasculostatin • Canstatin • FGF receptor		Cell carriers	
		Tumor-associated antigens • CEA • PSA • MAG-A3 • Mesothelin • hDCT • CLND6		Nanoparticles	

CAR, chimeric antigen receptor; CCL, CC chemokine ligand; CD, cluster of differentiation; CEA, carcinoembryonic antigen; CLND6, claudin 6; CTLA-4, cytotoxic T lymphocyte antigen 4; CXCL, C-X-C chemokine ligand; FGF, fibroblast growth factor; GALV, Gibbon ape leukemia virus; GM-CSF, granulocyte-macrophage colony-stimulating factor; hDCT, human dopachrome tautomerase; HSV-TK, herpes simplex virus thymidine kinase; ICAM, intercellular adhesion molecule; ICOS, inducible T cell co-stimulator; IFN, interferon; IL, interleukin; LAG, lymphocyte activation gene; LFA, lymphocyte function-associated antigen; MAGE, melanoma-associated antigen gene; MnSOD, manganese superoxide dismutase; PD-1, programmed cell death 1; PD-L1, programmed cell death ligand 1; PSA, prostate specific antigen; PTEN, phosphatase and tensin homolog; RB, retinoblastoma; TGF, transforming growth factor; TIM, T cell immunoglobulin and mucin domain; VEGF, vascular endothelial growth factor; VSV, vesicular stomatitis virus.

For example, by fusing the receptor binding protein of HSV (Glycoprotein D) with a heterologous ligand, it is possible to retarget the virus to a tumor-specific receptor of choice (e.g., include EGFR, HER2, and IL-13Rα2), simultaneously de-targeting the normal receptor.[53–56]

Several early HSV oncolytics have been evaluated in clinical trials, with the majority demonstrating a good safety profile and some degree of therapeutic benefit. To date, T-VEC is the only OV to be approved by the FDA, and further information on the development of T-VEC is discussed in detail later in this chapter. Other promising HSV-1 candidates currently under clinical investigation include: (a) HF10 for the treatment of melanoma, administered in combination with the checkpoint inhibitor nivolumab (NCT03259425), and (b) G207 for the treatment of brain cancer.

Paramyxoviruses

Paramyxoviruses are enveloped, negative-sense single-stranded RNA viruses that cause a number of different diseases in humans and animals. Paramyxoviruses can accommodate large amounts of foreign genetic material and maintain good genetic stability both in vitro and in vivo due to their cytoplasmic replication, making them attractive viral vectors. The most well-known viruses in this family include mumps virus, measles virus (MeV) (both human viruses), Sendai virus (rodent virus), and Newcastle disease virus (NDV), an avian virus. Paramyxoviruses possess a natural selectivity for cancer cells due to the overexpression of viral receptors on their cell surface (sialic acid glycoproteins for Sendai and mumps viruses, and CD46 and SLAM for MeV), promoting preferential association of the virus with malignant cells over normal cells. NDV and mumps virus were among some of the earliest viruses used in virotherapy; however, today, most of the work on paramyxoviruses is focused on NDV and measles.

NDV strains are classified into three groups according to disease severity in birds: lentogenic (low), mesogenic (moderate), and velogenic (highly virulent).[57,58] However, as oncolytic agents, NDV strains are categorized as lytic or non-lytic based on their ability to infect tumor cell monolayers. Lytic strains produce infectious particles that can infect other cells and amplify the viral load whereas non-lytic strains produce non-infectious particles.[59] NDV strains that have been evaluated as oncolytic agents include the lytic mesogenic strains MTH68/H, PV-701, and 73-T and the non-lytic lentogenic strains Ulster and HUJ.[57,59] NDV causes no serious illness in humans because it is highly sensitive to type I IFNs and has been shown to be safe even at high doses administered intravenously.[60] Despite a wealth of preclinical data suggesting antitumor activity of recombinant NDV in a variety of cancers, clinical trials using these viruses are limited, and there are currently no active trials using NDV.

Measles virus is highly contagious and causes serious illness in humans, requiring population-wide vaccination using live, attenuated derivatives of the wild-type strain to prevent disease. The majority of oncolytic MeV research has used the Edmonston B strain, shown to preferentially lyse cancer cells expressing CD46 and considered to be safe.[61] While this strain displays potent antitumor activity in vitro and in animal tumor models, the prevalence of preexisting immunity and neutralizing antibodies greatly limits its therapeutic efficacy in humans. Difficulty in bringing effective MeV oncolytics into the clinic is further hampered by the fact that mice don't express the MeV receptors, requiring the use of other animal models for preclinical studies. Efforts to enhance oncolytic activity and evade neutralization while maintaining safety are underway and have the potential to improve the therapeutic efficacy of oncolytic MeV. Currently, there are multiple active clinical trials (Phase 1 and 2) using MeV. Studies out of the Mayo Clinic are testing the safety and toxicity of a recombinant MeV expressing the carcinoembryonic antigen (CEA) or the thyroidal sodium iodide symporter (NIS).[57,59] The use of an attenuated MeV encoding NIS (MV-NIS) enables imaging following the administration of radioiodine. Another clinical study is investigating a combination approach consisting of 5-fluorocytosine, a prodrug, and MeV encoding a prodrug converting enzyme (NCT04195373).

Parvovirus

Parvoviruses are small, non-enveloped viruses with a single-strand DNA genome of roughly 5 kb that infect a broad range of hosts and are capable of crossing the blood-brain barrier. The Parvoviridae family contains two subfamilies: Parvovirinae, which infect vertebrates, and Densovirinae, which infect invertebrates. Parvoviruses replicate only in dividing cells or in the presence of a helper virus (e.g., adeno-associated viruses, AAV). Recently, it has been shown that rodent protoparvoviruses, specifically H-1PV, the minute virus of mice (MVM), and the LuIII virus, possess natural anticancer

activity, activating multiple cell death pathways while being nonpathogenic to humans.[62] With a lack of preexisting antiviral immunity in the human population and the ability of these viruses to elicit robust anticancer immune responses upon tumor cell lysis, parvoviruses have emerged as attractive oncolytic viral candidates. Parvovirus selectivity is due to the dependence of the viral life cycle upon cellular factors involved in the control of cell proliferation and differentiation, such as Cyclin A and E2F, which are frequently dysregulated in tumor cells, rather than a disparity in virus uptake between transformed and normal cells.[62]

H-1PV has been extensively evaluated in the preclinical setting. Upon infection of tumor cells, H-1PV stimulates expression of danger- and pathogen-associated molecular patterns (DAMPs and PAMPs) and the release of tumor-associated antigens, promoting cross-presentation of tumor antigens on dendritic cells and facilitating recognition by the host's immune system.[63] The importance of this immune effect on tumor regression was confirmed in vivo through adoptive cell transfer,[64] providing a strong rationale for the use of H-1PV as cancer virotherapy. Given the strong antiviral immune response elicited by these viruses, neutralizing antibodies are expected to limit efficacy. However, the lack of exposure to these viruses in the human population is thought to provide a window in which treatment may be effective. In late 2011, the first clinical trial using H-1PV (ParvOryx) for the treatment of grade IV glioblastoma multiforme (GBM) was initiated (NCT01301430). Current efforts to increase anticancer efficacy of H-1PV through genetic engineering are underway and include capsid modification, generation of chimeric vectors to increase viral titers, and arming with specific PAMPs, namely CpG motifs.[63,65] In vitro and in vivo combinations of H-1PV with other cancer therapies including ionizing radiation, gemcitabine, and HDAC inhibitors resulted in significant synergy and could prove to be critical in maximizing the anticancer effects of these therapies.[66,67] As the use of parvoviruses as oncolytics is still relatively new, a better understanding of the parvovirus/host factors that govern infection, replication, and oncolytic properties could elucidate novel, rationally derived targets for therapeutic intervention.

Picornavirus

Picornaviruses are small, non-enveloped single-stranded RNA viruses. The two family members used as OVs are coxsackievirus and poliovirus, both human enteroviruses. Coxsackievirus is categorized into two subgroups, A and B, which differ in their pathogenesis in murine models. In humans, coxsackievirus infections are typically asymptomatic, and as such the viral genome does not require manipulation for safety. Coxsackievirus has a natural tropism for cancer cells, due to the overexpression of viral receptors, ICAM-1 and decay accelerating factor (DAF), in melanoma, breast cancer, and multiple myeloma.[68,69] These viruses have also been shown to induce strong immune responses upon infection due to the release of DAMPs, which promote the infiltration of CD8$^+$ T cells and NK cells, and enhance antigen presentation through the activation of dendritic cells.[70] Cavatak® (coxsackievirus A21, Merck Inc.) is the leading clinical oncolytic coxsackievirus candidate and early phase clinical trials have demonstrated safety while also suggesting therapeutic efficacy in patients with advanced melanoma.[71] Additional clinical studies are evaluating Cavatak® in combination with ipilimumab and pembrolizumab in advanced cutaneous melanoma, as well as expansion to other cancers, including bladder cancer, non-small cell lung carcinoma, and uveal melanoma.[72] In addition, Cavatak® is being evaluated using intravenous delivery.[72] Previous exposure to coxsackievirus can cause immunity to infection; however, antibodies against serotypes do not appear to be cross-reactive, indicating that the use of different serotypes could be useful in overcoming neutralization and clearance in exposed individuals.

Poliovirus is highly pathogenic in humans, and while asymptomatic or mildly symptomatic in the vast majority of cases, 1% of infections result in paralytic poliomyelitis due to viral replication and selective destruction of motor neurons. Major outbreaks of polio in the early 20th century led to population-wide vaccination programs in the mid-1950s, which have dramatically reduced the number of cases. For use as an OV, poliovirus must be attenuated, which has been achieved by replacing the viral internal ribosome entry site (IRES) of the Sabin vaccine strain (PV1) with an IRES from the related human rhinovirus type 2.[73] This recombinant, attenuated poliovirus known as PVS-RIPO displays tropism for glioma cells ,which upregulate CD155, the poliovirus receptor,[74] and is currently in early phase trials assessing intratumoral infusion in GBM (NCT01491893). Preliminary results in 61 patients with recurrent, supratentorial WHO grade IV malignant gliomas evaluated safety in a dose escalation cohort of PVS-RIPO (range, 10^7 to 10^{10} TCID$_{50}$) and identified 5.0 x 10^7 TCID$_{50}$ as the recommended Phase 2 dose.[75] In this study, an expansion cohort at the Phase 2 dose demonstrated a 21% overall survival at 24 months with 19% of patients experiencing a grade 3 or greater adverse event.[75]

Poxviruses

The Poxviridae family is comprised of large, complex, enveloped dsDNA viruses that replicate in the cytoplasm of vertebrates and invertebrates. This family includes, among its most notable members, variola virus, the cause of smallpox, cowpox, myxoma, fowlpox, and ALVAC (avian poxviruses), and vaccinia virus (VV), the agent used in smallpox eradication programs worldwide. Advantages of VV as an oncolytic include: wide host range, rapid replication (first particles are produced and secreted within 8 hours and infected cells are destroyed 48 to 72 hours post-infection), cytoplasmic restriction of the life cycle, induction of cell lysis in a wide range of tumor cell types due to the absence of a defined surface receptor for entry, a lack of genomic integration, and a genome capable of accommodating large transgenes.

Deletion of several nonessential viral genes has been used to successfully enhance tumor-specific replication and improve safety. These include the vaccinia virus growth factor (VGF) gene, which results in VV targeted to cells with EGFR pathway activation; viral thymidine kinase (TK) gene, which creates a virus dependent on overexpressed cellular TK for replication; and the viral B18R gene, which encodes a soluble decoy IFN receptor and inhibits cellular antiviral innate immune responses and promotes selective lysis in IFN-deficient cells.[76–78] Poxviruses are highly immunogenic, producing strong cytotoxic T lymphocyte responses and circulating antiviral neutralizing antibodies.[79] In an attempt to improve the innate immune response induced upon viral infection and replication, VV harboring deletions have also been armed with immune stimulators (e.g., GM-CSF, IL-2, IL-12, etc.), co-stimulatory molecules (e.g., B7.1, ICAM-1, LFA-3, etc.), apoptotic proteins, prodrug-converting enzymes, and anti-angiogenic antibodies/proteins.[78,80–83]

To date, clinical trials with oncolytic VV have demonstrated minor side effects and preliminary evidence of tumor responses.[84,85] The leading VV clinical candidate, Pexa-Vec (previously known as JX-594), is a TK-deleted, GM-CSF-encoding Wyeth strain of VV and was tested in a randomized Phase 3 trial in combination with the kinase inhibitor sorafenib in hepatocellular carcinoma (HCC) patients without previous systemic therapy, but failed to meet the primary study endpoints (NCT02562755). In this study, no safety issues were noted. GL-ONC1 (GLV-1h68) is a triple-modified Lister strain VV expressing Renilla luciferase fused to green fluorescent protein, β-galactosidase, and β-glucuronidase in place of F14.5L, TK, and A56R (hemagglutinin), respectively, and is another poxvirus under clinical investigation.[86,87] The safety of GL-ONC1 has been assessed in a variety of solid tumor types, both alone and in combination with chemotherapy. This OV has also been evaluated through both intratumoral and intravenous delivery routes. To date, GL-ONC1 has been well tolerated, with minimal toxicity with preliminary evidence of antitumor activity. Another series of Phase 1 studies utilized Wyeth strain VV encoding the B7.1 co-stimulatory molecule or three co-stimulatory molecules (B7.1, ICAM-1, and LFA-3) in patients with metastatic melanoma.[88,89] In these studies, clinical responses were detected and correlated with the emergence of melanoma-specific CD8⁺ T cells and autoimmune vitiligo while patients experienced low-grade constitutional type adverse events. Lastly, a double deleted Western Reserve strain Vaccinia bearing two deletions in the VGF and TK genes (JX-929) has also been tested in Phase 1 clinical trials for advanced solid cancers with intravenous delivery,[90] with high tolerance rates reported.

Rhabdoviruses

Over 250 different viruses make up the Rhabdoviridae family.[91] These enveloped viruses are characterized by a single-stranded, negative-sense RNA genome, a distinct bullet-like shape, and are capable of infecting and replicating in plants, invertebrates, or vertebrates. The best-known virus of this family is the rabies virus. While treatment with a live attenuated rabies virus was anecdotally associated with tumor necrosis,[6] today two rhabdoviruses currently under clinical investigation are Maraba virus and vesicular stomatitis virus (VSV), both of the *vesiculovirus* genus. VSV has been widely studied as the prototypical negative stranded RNA virus and, as such, there exists an extensive body of knowledge about its genome, replication, and safety. In humans, VSV can cause acute febrile disease, although laboratory-adapted strains are rarely pathogenic. Maraba virus is an insect virus that was recently identified in a screen of rhabdoviruses as having potent oncolytic properties without causing disease in humans.[92]

Rhabdoviruses possess a number of properties that make them attractive oncolytic agents. They replicate very rapidly; produce high titers in a wide range of mammalian cells; harbor a small, easy-to-manipulate genome (five genes); their life cycle is independent of cell cycle regulation and occurs exclusively in the cytoplasm, eliminating the risk of genomic integration; and antibodies to these viruses are rare, limiting preexisting humoral immunity.[93] The oncoselectivity of these viruses is predominantly based on impaired type I IFN responses,[94,95] which is common among tumor cells. However, these viruses are also highly neurotropic, limiting the dose at which they can be safely delivered. Improved safety and selectivity have been achieved by mutating the M (delta51 in VSV and L123W in Maraba) and G (Q242R in Maraba) proteins to abolish inhibition of IFN such that normal cells are able to sense and prevent viral replication, significantly reducing associated neurotoxicity and also improving efficacy.[92,95] These attenuated strains are referred to as VSVΔ51 and MG1, respectively. Other attempts at improving efficacy of rhabdoviruses have used approaches that have been previously described, which include arming with immune stimulatory molecules or tumor antigens, tumor-specific targeting, and combination with other therapeutics.

While there exists a wealth of preclinical data on VSV and to a lesser extent Maraba, these agents are still in the early stages of clinical development. VSV expressing human IFN-β (VSV-hIFN-β) was shown to induce tumor regression in vivo, and this regression was enhanced in the presence of CD8⁺ T cells. The expression of IFN-β also increased safety, protecting immune-deficient mice and nonhuman primates from lethal neurotoxicity.[96,97] Early phase clinical trials of VSV-hIFN-β in patients with various cancers, such as hepatocellular carcinoma, endometrial cancer, and others, are in progress.

Maraba virus displays broad oncotropism and the attenuated MG1 strain demonstrates potent antitumor activity in vivo, superior to that observed with VSVd51.[92] In an attempt to improve antitumor immunity, MG1 was engineered to express the human melanoma-associated tumor antigen, dopachrome tautomerase (hdCT). While MG1-hdCT alone was unable to generate adaptive immunity against the tumor, when used as a boosting vector in a heterologous prime-boost regimen with an adenovirus expressing hDCT, MG1 generated a powerful T cell-specific immune response leading to complete remissions in >20% of animals.[98] A Phase 1/2 trial testing MG1 encoding the melanoma-associated antigen 3 (MAGEA3), with or without an Ad-MA3 prime, was initiated in 2015 in patients with advanced or metastatic solid tumors expressing MAGEA3 and is being further evaluated with pembrolizumab in patients with previously treated melanoma and cutaneous squamous cell carcinoma (NCT03773744).

Reovirus

Members of the *Reoviridae* family form non-enveloped virions containing a segmented double-stranded RNA (dsRNA) genome with 9 to 12 discrete segments. Reovirus infection in humans usually involves the respiratory and gastrointestinal tracts, with mild signs and symptoms, although some family members, such as rotaviruses, are more pathogenic. Three serotypes of reovirus are ubiquitous within the environment, and it is estimated that 50% to 70% of adults have been exposed to reovirus and harbor antibodies against the virus, potentially complicating the widespread use of reovirus as a therapeutic agent.[99]

The ability of reoviruses to specifically infect and replicate in transformed cells was first observed in the late 1970s.[29] It was later shown that cells overexpressing the native or truncated form of EGFR or with activated Ras signaling are more susceptible to reovirus infection than cells lacking these alterations, making reoviruses inherently oncolytic.[28,100,101] Reoviruses induce cell lysis by activating both intrinsic and extrinsic apoptotic pathways. The lead clinical reovirus candidate is Reolysin, a mammalian orthoreovirus of the T3D strain developed by

Oncolytics Biotech Inc. Reolysin has been evaluated in a number of clinical trials for different cancer types.[102,103] It is well tolerated at high doses without dose-limiting toxicities when delivered intravenously, with some appreciable antitumor effects. Importantly, reovirus activity has been shown to increase when combined with chemotherapy or radiation and many of the ongoing trials are examining the combination of Reolysin with various chemotherapies.[104] In addition to the many Reolysin trials, the combination of wild-type reovirus with chemotherapy (paclitaxel or bortezomib, for the treatment of ovarian cancer and multiple myeloma, respectively) is also under clinical investigation.

THE CLINICAL DEVELOPMENT OF TALIMOGENE LAHERPAREPVEC (T-VEC)

The first oncolytic virus to achieve regulatory approval was talimogene laherparepvec (T-VEC; Imlygic™), originally termed Oncovex^GM-CSF. T-VEC is a first-in-class OV based on an attenuated HSV-1 strain (JS-1) designed to selectively replicate in tumor cells and stimulate tumor-specific immunity. The pathway to approval provides important insights into the clinical development of oncolytic viruses and will be briefly reviewed. While T-VEC is now being evaluated in several different types of cancer, the initial clinical development focused on advanced melanoma, since these tumors are known to be immunogenic and, in many patients, are accessible for intralesional injection.[105] The use of a live, replicating virus, the multiple mechanisms of action associated with oncolytic viruses and the adoption of local administration into established tumors required additional considerations with respect to biosafety, drug storage, dosing and delivery mechanisms, and clinical trial design and study endpoints.

Characteristics of Talimogene Laherparepvec

In T-VEC, both copies of the HSV-infected cell protein (ICP) gene ICP34.5, which encodes the neurovirulence factor, are deleted, resulting in reduced pathogenicity and selective tumor cell replication.[95] In addition, the ICP47 gene, which encodes a protein that blocks peptide entry into the major histocompatibility complex (MHC) pathway and hence blocks antigen presentation, is also deleted and this allows peptide presentation promoting antitumor immunity.[106] Deletion of ICP47 also results in the earlier transcription of the herpes US11 gene product that further promotes preferential replication of the virus in tumor cells. T-VEC also harbors two recombinant genes encoding human GM-CSF under the control of the cytomegalovirus promoter, providing high levels of expression. Local production of GM-CSF helps recruit and mature regional dendritic cells which are thought to foster the induction of T cell immunity against

tumor-associated antigens released during viral lysis of the tumor cells in association with local viral DNA and cellular danger signals.[31] Importantly, T-VEC retains susceptibility to standard antiviral agents (e.g., acyclovir, valacyclovir, ganciclovir) that can prevent viral replication in the event of overdose or inadvertent infection.[107]

The initial preclinical studies with TVEC confirmed lytic activity in vitro against a variety of human tumor cell lines, and therapeutic activity in vivo was confirmed in murine tumor models using comparable doses to those now in clinical use.[107–109] The preclinical studies further supported the role of GM-CSF in promoting host antitumor immunity as an important part of the mechanism of action. In the A20 B cell lymphoma tumor model, for example, established bilateral flank tumors treated with JS-1 or HSV-1 vectors induced similar dose-related antitumor effects in injected ipsilateral tumors but uninjected contralateral tumors experienced therapeutic responses only when GM-CSF was expressed by the vector.[107] Tumor rejection in this model was also associated with higher levels of IFN-γ produced by A20-exposed murine splenocytes in the presence of treatment with the GM-CSF-containing virus.[107] These data were used to support the final version of T-VEC as ICP34.5⁻, ICP47⁻, GM-CSF⁺ for clinical development.

Pivotal Talimogene Laherparepvec Melanoma Clinical Trials

The first-in-human study of T-VEC was designed primarily to evaluate the safety profile and biological activity, as well as to define an appropriate dose and treatment schedule for further development.[110] In the initial studies, local intratumoral injection was chosen as the mode of administration since this mirrored the murine studies; it was anticipated to be associated with enhanced therapeutic efficacy and tolerability compared with systemic delivery since over 50% of the melanoma population has likely been exposed to HSV-1 and was expected to have preexisting (i.e., circulating) anti-HSV antibody titers. The Phase 1 trial enrolled 30 patients with cutaneous or subcutaneous tumor lesions accessible for injection who had previously failed standard treatment. The final study population consisted of patients with breast cancer ($n = 14$), head and neck cancer ($n = 5$), colorectal cancer ($n = 2$), and melanoma ($n = 9$). The trial also utilized several treatment designs to better assess safety and allow induction of antibodies in seronegative subjects. The study included a single-dose cohort in which doses of 10^6, 10^7, or 10^8 plaque-forming units (PFU)/mL were tested ($n = 13$) and a multidose group in which various dose-escalation regimens were evaluated ($n = 17$). The maximum volume of virus to be used was 4 mL based on prior murine studies. This volume was divided between lesions based on the largest diameter of injectable tumor using the measurements shown in Table 30.3.

Table 30.3 Talimogene Laherparepvec Recommended Dosing Volume

TUMOR SIZE (LONGEST DIMENSION)	INJECTION VOLUME
5.0 cm	≤4.0 mL
>2.5 cm to 5.0 cm	≤2.0 mL
>1.5 cm to 2.5 cm	≤1.0 mL
>0.5 cm to 1.5 cm	≤0.5 mL
≤0.5 cm	≤0.1 mL

Note: At each patient visit, accessible tumors are measured by longest diameter (left column) and injected with the volume shown (right column). The first visit uses a dose of 10^6 PFU/mL and 3 weeks later the dose is 10^8 PFU/mL, and this dose is repeated every 2 weeks until complete response, confirmed disease progression, or unacceptable toxicity.

This Phase 1 trial demonstrated that T-VEC was well tolerated with the most frequently reported adverse events being low-grade systemic constitutional symptoms (fever, chills, and nausea) and local injection site reactions (erythema and pain).[110] The injection site reactions were more pronounced and took longer to resolve in HSV-seronegative subjects when compared to those patients who were herpesvirus seropositive at baseline. These side effects were considered dose limiting at the 10^7 PFU/mL dose in the seronegative cohort. Thus, an initial priming dose of 10^6 PFU/mL and a 3-week interval between the first and second injection was selected as the initial dose schedule in the multidose cohort to allow for seroconversion in patients not previously exposed to herpesvirus, and after 3 weeks all patients received higher doses at 2-week intervals.

The study revealed evidence of viral replication at the injection site and local GM-CSF expression was confirmed in vivo.[110] Careful histologic review of postinjection biopsy material showed that treatment was associated with inflammation and tumor necrosis in 14 of 19 available specimens and necrotic tumor cells strongly expressed viral proteins. In contrast, nonmalignant cells within the tumor microenvironment did not contain significant HSV-1 protein expression or undergo necrosis, suggesting preferential infection and lysis of tumor cells. Three subjects had stable disease and six patients had flattening of injected and regionally uninjected lesions. In four patients, there was evidence of distant metastatic disease regression. There was no difference in response between HSVseronegative and seropositive subjects. Based on the results of the Phase 1 trial, the recommended dosing regimen was to use a priming dose of 10^6 PFU/mL followed, 3 weeks later, by multiple 10^8 PFU/mL doses every 2 weeks in seronegative and seropositive patients.

Following the Phase 1 trial, a decision to focus on melanoma was made and a single-arm, open-label, multi-institutional clinical trial was conducted in which 50 patients with unresectable, stage IIIC-IV melanoma were treated at the dosing regimen recommended by the Phase 1 trial (NCT00289016; EudraCT 2006-003841-17).[111] In this study, the primary endpoint was overall response rate and additional safety outcomes were collected. The majority of subjects (74%) had received prior therapy with most being cytotoxic chemotherapy (dacarbazine or temozolomide) or high-dose IL-2, a reflection of the precheckpoint blockade era. A similar adverse event profile as reported in Phase 1 was seen with most patients reporting low grade, transient constitutional symptoms or local injection site reactions. After a median of six T-VEC injections, the overall response rate, as determined by standard RECIST criteria and incorporating all lesions (injected or not), was 26%.[111] This included 10 patients with complete responses and three additional patients with partial responses rendered disease-free through resection of remaining disease. The clinical responses appeared to be durable, with ongoing responses lasting 16 to 40 months from the time of first T-VEC dosing. In this trial, urine samples and injection site swabs were taken within 48 hours for urine and 24 to 72 hours for injection sites after receiving the first injection. Of 78 urine and 102 injection site samples from 13 and 19 subjects, respectively, only one injection site swab tested positive for viral DNA by polymerase chain reaction (PCR) assay albeit at very low titers (<10 PFU), supporting the notion that viral shedding was rare.

The impact of T-VEC treatment on local and distant antitumor immunity was assessed in a single institution subset of subjects from the Phase 2 clinical trial using matched peripheral blood and tumor samples.[112] In this analysis, T-VEC injection was associated with lower frequency of CD4$^+$Foxp3$^+$ regulatory T (T_{reg}) cells, CD8$^+$Foxp3$^+$ suppressor T cells, and myeloid-derived suppressor cells (MDSC) when compared to established tumors collected from 20 nonstudy metastatic melanoma patients. Interestingly, analysis of regressing lesions identified a high level of MART-1-specific CD8+ T cells capable of IFN-γ-production. A similar pattern of MART-1-specific CD8$^+$ effector T cells and a decrease in T_{reg} cells and MDSC cells were also seen in uninjected lesions, but the change in frequency was less pronounced than in the injected lesions. These findings support the induction of host antitumor immunity with T-VEC but suggest that this effect is greater in injected lesions and may require additional immune stimulation to enhance rejection of distant disease.

Based on the early phase study results suggesting that T-VEC had both a direct oncolytic effect in injected tumors and a secondary induction of host antitumor immunity, a prospective randomized Phase 3 clinical trial was proposed (termed Oncovex^{GM-CSF} Pivotal Trial in Melanoma; OPTiM; NCT00769704, EudraCT 2008-006140-20).[113] Given the novel mechanisms of action and local delivery of the agent, the study was designed as an open-label study and used recombinant GM-CSF as the control arm. By the time this study was designed it was also evident that some patients in the Phase 2 clinical trial demonstrated tumor growth or developed new lesions prior to entering an objective response, suggesting that T-VEC might be associated with "pseudo-progression" as has been reported for other types of immunotherapy, such as ipilimumab. Thus, in order to incorporate both response rate and a time element into the study, a primary endpoint of durable response rate (DRR) was selected for the Phase 3 trial. DRR was defined as an objective response as measured by modified World Health Organization (WHO) criteria starting within 12 months of beginning T-VEC treatment and lasting for at least 6 months or longer. A 6-month duration was selected based on the natural history of melanoma in which nearly all patients experienced disease progression within 6 months. The trial also required confirmation of objective response or disease progression prior to removing subjects from therapy. Any patients with investigator-reported objective response and all subjects on trial for ≥9 months were evaluated by an independent, blinded endpoint assessment committee (EAC). Secondary endpoints included overall response rate, duration of response, time to treatment failure, and overall survival.

The OPTiM trial accrued 436 patients with unresectable stage IIIB/C-IV melanoma and subjects were allowed prior therapy but this was not required since stage IIIB/C patients had few other established options. Patients were stratified based on disease stage, prior therapy, and location of metastatic disease. The subjects were randomized 2:1 to receive T-VEC (10^6 PFU/mL up to 4 mL, followed 3 weeks later by 10^8 PFU/mL up to 4 mL every 2 weeks for up to 24 total doses; $n = 295$) or recombinant GM-CSF (125 µg/m^2 subcutaneously daily for 14 days on and 14 days off for up to 1 year; $n = 141$). In this trial, all melanoma lesions could be injected as well as any new lesions appearing after regression of established disease. After 12 months, T-VEC treatment was able to continue for another 6 months in subjects with clinically stable or responding disease. Those patients who received the maximum allowable T-VEC doses and who were not progressing, or patients with new lesions within 12 months after achieving a complete response, as well as those experiencing a CR in OPTiM but who then developed new lesions within 12 months, were eligible for participation in an extension study (NCT02173171; EudraCT 2010-021070-11).

At the time of initial OPTiM reporting, patients treated with T-VEC demonstrated a significantly higher DRR versus patients treated with GM-CSF (16.3% vs. 2.1%; odds ratio: 8.9 [95% confidence intervals (CI): 2.7–29.2], p <.001). Further, T-VEC treatment was also associated with an improvement in objective response rate (ORR) (26.4% vs. 5.7%) with 11% of patients treated with T-VEC achieving an objective complete response (including injected and uninjected disease) compared with <1% complete response rate in patients receiving GM-CSF.[113] In addition, upon primary analysis, T-VEC was associated with an improvement in overall survival compared to GM-CSF therapy (23.3 vs. 18.9 months; HR 0.79 {95% CI: 0.62-1.00}; p = .051). In a preplanned final descriptive analysis of overall survival scheduled to occur 3 years after the last patient was randomized, T-VEC treatment continued to demonstrate an improvement in overall survival with a 21% reduction in the risk of dying from melanoma (HR 0.79 {95% CI: 0.62–1.00}; p = .049 [descriptive]).[114] The majority of T-VEC responses were ongoing at a median follow-up of 2.8 months with 88% of patients who initially responded and 78% of patients who had initial disease progression followed by an objective response still responding. The median time to treatment failure was longer in patients treated with T-VEC compared to GM-CSF (8.2 vs. 2.9 months; HR 0.42 [95% CI: 0.32–0.54]). These data resulted in initial approval of T-VEC for the treatment of melanoma in the United States and Australia in late 2015, and subsequently, it was also approved in Europe and Israel.

The OPTiM trial results further highlighted several key features of T-VEC. First, 42 of 78 objective responders (54%) had evidence of disease progression, as defined by 25% or greater increase in lesion size or appearance of new lesions, prior to achieving an objective response. This finding is consistent with delayed response kinetics observed with other forms of immunotherapy and reiterates the need to continue treatment in patients who are clinically stable despite growth in preexisting tumors or the presence of new lesions.[115] A second lesson was revealed from a preplanned subset analysis in which pronounced responses and improved overall survival were noted in those patients with stage III or IVM1a disease compared to those with more advanced visceral metastases, and in patients receiving T-VEC as first-line treatment compared to treatment after failing other therapeutic options.[113] For example, in the stage III cohort DRR was 33% for T-VEC compared to 0% for GM-CSF treatment, and in stage IVM1a, T-VEC was associated with a 16% DRR versus 2.3% for GM-CSF. The overall survival for the combined stage III and IVM1a population was significantly improved in patients who received T-VEC (41.1 vs. 21.5 months, HR 0.57, p <.001). This data was used to obtain regulatory approval of T-VEC for patients with stage III and IVM1a disease in Europe. Patients who received T-VEC as first-line treatment had a DRR of 23.9% compared to 0% for GM-CSF treatment and improved overall survival (33.1 vs. 17.0 months; HR 0.50, p <.001). Collectively, this data suggests that T-VEC was especially useful when given early in the course of the disease and in patients with locally and regionally advanced disease. Nonetheless, it was also noted that 15% of measurable visceral metastases responded with a 50% or greater regression in size even when the lesions were not injected with virus.

There were 30 patients from the OPTiM study that met criteria for the extension trial, which included 27 subjects treated with T-VEC and three with GM-CSF.[116] These patients continued on treatment for a median duration of 91 weeks in the T-VEC arm and five new complete responses were noted, although none were seen in the GM-CSF cohort. This observation supports the potential for achieving responses late in the course of treatment with T-VEC.

The OPTiM trial also contributed important safety information with very few patients discontinuing treatment due to adverse events (4% vs. 2% for patients treated with T-VEC and GM-CSF, respectively).[113] In line with the early phase clinical trials, the most common side effects observed included systemic constitutional-like symptoms (e.g., fatigue, fever, chills, nausea) and local injection-site reactions. T-VEC treatment was associated with an overall grade 3 or greater adverse event rate of 36% but the only grade ≥3/4 adverse event occurring in more than six patients was cellulitis. There was no treatment-related mortality. Thus, the safety profile of T-VEC appears quite tolerable and supports the use of the agent in patients with other comorbid conditions and makes it attractive for use in combination immunotherapy regimens.

Clinical experience with T-VEC has now been reported confirming initial clinical trial data defining a tolerable safety profile and validating monotherapy response rates. In a multi-institutional retrospective observational study, 76 patients with unresectable melanoma were treated with T-VEC.[117] The median age of the patients was 73%, and 55% had stage IIIB-IVM1a disease, 40% had stage IVM1b-c, and 5% were unknown. After a median follow-up of 9.4 months, 15 patients (20%) completed T-VEC and had no evidence of residual melanoma. Overall survival at 1 year was 77% in patients with stage IIIB-IVM1a disease and 65% in those with stage IVM1b-c disease. The median number of T-VEC doses given was six and median duration of treatment was 3 months. In another single institution study in Germany, 27 melanoma patients were treated with T-VEC as part of standard care and followed for outcomes.[118] In this study, the median age was 68 and the median duration of treatment was 22 weeks for all patients and 28 weeks in those with stage IIIB-C only disease. All patients had received definitive excision

of the primary melanoma and overall patients had a median of three recurrences treated by re-excision with a median of 10 months from time of re-excision to T-VEC initiation. No new safety signals were noted but patient outcomes were not reported. In another multi-institutional retrospective study, 121 patients received T-VEC and 80 were evaluable for response with follow-up of 3 months or greater.[119] In this trial, adverse events were collected and found to be similar to those reported in the OPTiM trial. At a median follow-up of 9 months, 31 (39%) patients had a complete response and 14 (18%) had a partial response. The median number of T-VEC doses was six. Collectively, these real-world data with T-VEC confirm the safety profile with no evidence of herpetic skin outbreaks in patients or evidence of household contact transmission. In addition, monotherapy T-VEC responses are similar to those reported in clinical trials and may be especially useful when given first-line in older melanoma patients, and for those with stage IIIB-IVM1a disease. Most patients can be expected to respond within 3 to 6 months.

Talimogene Laherparepvec Clinical Trials for Other Cancers

The success of T-VEC in melanoma and the lytic effects on other cell lines in vitro support the clinical development of T-VEC for other types of cancer. This includes studies in pediatric cancers, bladder cancer, malignant pleural effusions, cutaneous squamous cell carcinoma, Merkel cell carcinoma, Kaposi's sarcoma, mycosis fungoides, peritoneal malignancies, triple negative breast cancer, sarcoma, pancreatic cancer, rectal cancer, hepatic metastases from colorectal and breast cancers, and head and neck cancer. T-VEC was evaluated in a Phase 1/2 dose-finding clinical trial with concurrent cisplatin-based chemotherapy and radiation therapy.[120] This trial was designed to evaluate the safety of T-VEC in head and neck cancer patients in combination with chemotherapy and radiation, while also determining response rates using standard RECIST criteria. Seventeen patients with untreated stage III/IV squamous cell cancer of the head and neck (SCCHN; EudraCT 2005-000777-21) were treated with cisplatin (100 mg/m² every 3 weeks for three doses and radiation (70 Gy over 35 fractions). The patients also received T-VEC every 3 weeks with an initial 10^6 PFU/mL dose, followed by further doses at 10^6, 10^7, or 10^8 PFU/mL. A neck dissection was completed 6 to 10 weeks after the fourth dose of T-VEC.

In this trial, T-VEC was safely delivered with both chemotherapy and radiation. All patients experienced treatment-emergent adverse events with most (86%) classified as grade 2 or less, including two injection site reactions.[120] There was at least one grade 3 or 4 adverse event observed in each patient but only two treatment-emergent adverse events related to T-VEC (pyrexia and fatigue). There were also two injection-site reactions reported as related to T-VEC. The study investigators also measured viral shedding from the injection site, and virus could be detected for up to 6 days after treatment in three patients. The trial established a dosing regimen of 10^6 PFU/mL initially followed by three doses of 10^8 PFU/mL, as optimal. The objective clinical response rate was 82% with four complete and 10 partial responses. Of note, the pathologic complete response rate in the resected surgical specimens was 93%. With median follow-up of 29 months, the patients had a disease-specific survival of 82% and relapse-free survival of 76%. The data support further exploration of T-VEC in head and neck cancer while confirming the safety profile of combination T-VEC with chemoradiation.

Another Phase 1 pilot study was conducted to evaluate the optimal dose and safety profile of T-VEC in advanced pancreatic cancer patients. Seventeen subjects who had previously failed therapy or were unable to receive standard therapy for pancreatic cancer were enrolled (NCT00402025).[121] T-VEC was injected into visceral lesions using ultrasound-guided endoscopy and fine-needle injection. The initial study design planned to enroll three patients in sequential cohorts starting at an initial dose of 10^4 PFU/mL followed by two doses of 10^5 PFU/mL, and progressing to a group starting at 10^6 PFU/mL dose followed by two 10^8 PFU/mL doses.

The study proceeded to the third cohort in which T-VEC was given as a priming dose at 10^6 PFU/mL followed by two doses of 10^7 PFU/Ml.[121] While 41% of the subjects received all three planned doses and 47% underwent posttreatment imaging, most patients (59%) needed to discontinue therapy due to rapid disease progression. At the highest doses administered to four patients, two subjects had evidence of tumor regression. Although this trial demonstrated the feasibility of visceral injections, it also suggested that T-VEC may not be ideal for very advanced and rapidly progressing cancers. Further trials of visceral injection into hepatic metastases and pancreatic cancers are in progress. As detailed in the text that follows, several clinical studies have been focused on using T-VEC in combination with immune checkpoint blockade, and these are especially interesting as early results appear promising for improving therapeutic responses without increasing toxicity.[122]

Priorities in Talimogene Laherparepvec Clinical Development

T-VEC is the first-in-class oncolytic virus approved for the treatment of cancer based on clinical benefit and an acceptable safety profile as confirmed through a prospective, randomized Phase 3 clinical trial in melanoma. The agent is distinguished by a highly tolerable safety profile,

making it clinically useful in patients with extensive comorbid conditions where more toxic systemic agents may be more challenging to administer. The results of the Phase 3 trial highlight the pronounced effects of treatment in patients with advanced locoregional disease and support the evaluation of combination approaches in those patients with more extensive visceral metastases, and studies of T-VEC and other OVs may be appropriate for neoadjuvant consideration. Major clinical priorities for T-VEC will be to determine the impact on both clinical activity and safety of various combination strategies and extending trials of T-VEC to other cancers.[123] The need for direct intratumoral injection may limit such studies to cancers with easily accessible tumors, but further study of visceral injection as through interventional CT-guided delivery, endoscopic ultrasound administration, or application at the time of surgical resection are all interesting avenues of clinical investigation.

In addition to the high priority clinical studies, a better understanding of the molecular and cellular mechanisms through which T-VEC mediates antitumor activity is needed. Much of the currently accepted thinking on the mechanism of action is hypothetical and requires confirmation in well-designed translational research laboratories. These studies may also identify predictive biomarkers, which could help identify eligible patients likely to respond to T-VEC and suggest more rational combination strategies for further clinical development. As a live, replicating virus, T-VEC requires careful attention to storage, preparation, and administration.[124] The biosafety issues and need to determine dosing volume at each clinic visit mandates that clinicians receive training in the proper administration of T-VEC and become comfortable with incorporating T-VEC into their clinical practice.

ONCOLYTIC VIRUSES EXERT THEIR ANTITUMOR EFFECTS THROUGH MULTIPLE MECHANISMS OF ACTION

Inherent or acquired resistance to first-line therapeutics is a major limitation in the successful treatment of cancer and is attributed in large part to the highly heterogeneous nature of the majority of tumors. Although originally conceived as tumor lysing agents, OVs are multimechanistic agents that elicit their effect through both direct and indirect tumor cell lysis, as well as induction of innate and adaptive immune responses (Figure 30.2). The lytic potential of an OV is dependent on the type of virus, cell tropism, the efficiency of cell receptor targeting, and viral replication, as well as the susceptibility of the cancer cells to cell death and the strength of the host cell antiviral response.[31] Rhabdoviruses, such as Maraba and VSV, are among the most lytic OVs currently in use. More in-depth studies of how OVs induce cell death are a high priority for future investigation in the field.

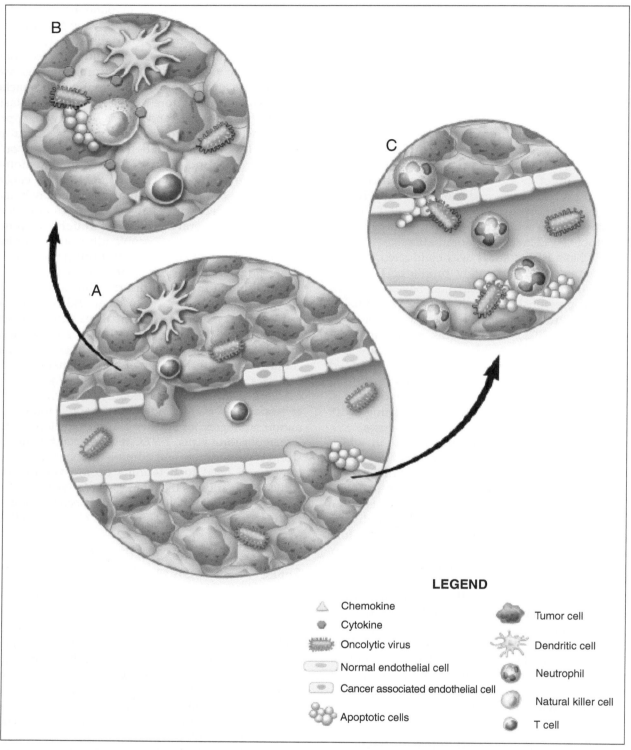

LEGEND

△ Chemokine

● Cytokine

▨ Oncolytic virus

▭ Normal endothelial cell

▭ Cancer associated endothelial cell

⬡ Apoptotic cells

⬢ Tumor cell

☆ Dendritic cell

◉ Neutrophil

◐ Natural killer cell

● T cell

Figure 30.2 Oncolytic viruses kill tumor cells through multiple mechanisms of action. (A) Following delivery to the tumor, oncolytic viruses infect, replicate, and lyse tumor cells, resulting in the release of viral progeny, inflammatory cytokines, growth factors, and tumor-associated antigens, which spread through the tumor microenvironment acting on neighboring cells within the tumor microenvironment. **(B)** The release of immune stimulatory cytokines attracts immune cells into the tumor and stimulates the innate and adaptive immune responses, which can lead to long-lasting antitumor responses. **(C)** Upregulation and secretion of growth factors such as vascular endothelial growth factor upon viral infection by some oncolytic viruses sensitize endothelial cells to infection. Apoptosis of endothelial cells leads to a massive infiltration of neutrophils and subsequent vascular collapse.

Immune-Mediated Cell Death

While the precise mechanisms that underlie viral-mediated cell death following direct infection depends on the type of virus, they all display variable features of apoptosis and necrosis, which results in the release of tumor-associated antigens, DAMPs, and PAMPs into the tumor microenvironment. These danger signals and antigens can then activate antigen-presenting cells (APCs), such as dendritic cells and macrophages, to stimulate immune responses. In addition to antiviral responses, it is also likely that cross presentation of tumor antigens results in adaptive antitumor immunity. In murine models, durable immune responses have been shown to lead to an in situ vaccine effect, protecting against tumor re-challenge. This protection is specific to the tumor cell line used in the original model as challenge with different syngeneic cell lines results in tumor growth, highlighting the specificity of the immune response generated by OV treatment. Importantly, targeted infection of tumor beds can also serve to perturb immune tolerance created by the cancer, re-activating tumor immune surveillance and facilitating tumor elimination.[125] The stimulation of long-lasting antitumor immune response likely plays a pivotal role in the duration and extent of clinical responses. With this increased appreciation for the role of immune stimulation in OV efficacy, many OVs are now being designed to express transgenes encoding immune stimulatory cytokines to enhance OV immunogenicity (refer to Table 30.1). In contrast to the beneficial effects of antitumor immune responses and tumor rejection, a hyperactive immune response can also lead to premature viral clearance, diminishing the lytic capacity of the virus (discussed in greater detail in the following section). At present, there is little data on the balance between antiviral and antitumor immunity with OVs.

Tumor Vasculature Effects

In addition to the indirect cell lysis mediated by immune cell killing, some OVs such as VV and VSV have demonstrated the ability to induce substantial cell death of non-infected tumor cells through infection and destruction of tumor-associated endothelial cells. This leads to the recruitment of neutrophils into the tumor microenvironment and subsequent vascular collapse.[126,127] This phenomenon was shown to be mediated through the expression of vascular endothelial growth factor A (VEGF-A), which sensitizes endothelial cells to infection by attenuating type I IFN signaling through induction of the transcriptional repressor positive regulatory domain 1-binding factor 1 (PRD1-BF1).[128] From preclinical and clinical data, it is clear that while cell lysis alone can be sufficient to induce tumor regression in tumors lacking immune suppression, the most effective OVs will combine potent oncolysis with a durable antitumor immune response. This is perhaps best exemplified by T-VEC although the exact mechanism(s) of T-VEC antitumor activity are incompletely understood.

BARRIERS TO ONCOLYTIC VIRUSES DELIVERY AND ALTERNATIVE STRATEGIES TO OVERCOME THEM

Many OVs show promising results in preclinical models; however, achieving therapeutically relevant doses of virus within established human tumors has proven significantly more complicated. A number of factors can significantly limit viral delivery and spread, tumor uptake, and therapeutic effectiveness. These include neutralizing antibodies, complement inactivation, and physical barriers within the tumor, such as poor vascularization (hypoxia), necrosis, high interstitial fluid pressure, acidosis, and a dense extracellular matrix.[129–131] As such, one of the major unresolved questions in the field is whether systemic/intravenous (IV) or intratumoral (IT) delivery of OVs is better. While systemic administration doesn't require an accessible tumor and can, in theory, target metastases throughout the body, the virus must reach the tumors at therapeutic concentrations to elicit a response and avoid premature immune-mediated clearance. Conversely, IT injections bypass architectural barriers within the tumor, but are limited to tumors that are palpable or accessible by imaging. The potential route of delivery may also depend on unique features of the virus, tumor location (e.g., within the CNS), and preexisting immunity to the virus selected (through both infection and vaccination).

Presence of Antiviral Neutralizing Antibodies

As mentioned, there exists a fine balance between induction of effective antitumor responses and the rapid clearance of the virus by the host's natural antiviral immune response. To date, the majority of OVs have been administered by direct injection into the tumor bed, due in large part to concerns about being able to overcome natural barriers within the blood such as preexisting antibodies and complement. These latter factors can also preclude repeated IV dosing. The virus selected is important as it dictates if and when neutralizing antibodies develop, how likely preexisting immunity will exist in the patient population, and the potential for the virus to be delivered systemically. Viruses such as HSV-1 that are widely prevalent in humans have often evolved techniques to evade immunosurveillance, while viruses that do not typically infect humans are unlikely to encounter preexisting immunity. For viruses such as measles, adenovirus, and polio where vaccination or previous exposure significantly reduces efficacy, strategies to limit neutralization and clearance such as serotype switching, polymer coating, and covalent conjugation of viral particles to prevent antibody binding are being applied.[132–134] In addition to virus modification, suppression of the host immune system by pretreatment with cyclophosphamide has been shown to improve efficacy of HSV-1 virotherapy.[135]

Inactivation by Complement

Even in the absence of neutralizing antibodies, IV delivery of OVs, such as HSV-1 and VV, has been shown to be inhibited by antiviral activity present in serum due to the activation of the complement system.[136–138] The complement system acts as a first line of innate immune defense, opsonizing and neutralizing foreign pathogens, targeting them for phagocytosis and clearance from the circulatory system.[139] Antibody-mediated complement activation enhances the neutralizing capacity of antibodies, making complement of particular relevance for OVs in which preexisting immunity may be prevalent. In the absence of complement, residual protective immunity provides weak to no neutralizing activity in vitro, suggesting that inactivation of complement could enhance OV stability and subsequently delivery to the tumor tissue.[79,140] Evgin et al. showed that the use of a complement inhibitor CP40, which targets complement C3, the key molecule common to all three complement activation pathways, inhibited VV neutralization in the blood of immunized individuals.[138] In immunized animals, inhibition of complement prolonged the length of time in which infectious virus was detectable, eliciting a 10-fold increase in infectious titers within the blood and improving virus delivery into the tumor.[138] Importantly, it was also demonstrated that IT delivery of OVs was improved following complement inhibition, suggesting that complement plays a role not only in the circulation but also within the tumor microenvironment. These findings suggest that short-term complement inhibition prior to OV therapy could dramatically improve therapeutic efficacy of viral vectors that generate complement-fixing antibodies.

Tumor Heterogeneity

Tumorigenesis is a multi-step evolutionary process that results in the accumulation of tens to thousands of genetic alterations. Next generation sequencing of tumors by The Cancer Genome Atlas (TCGA) has revealed dramatic and somewhat unexpected inter- and intratumoral heterogeneity in human cancers. Acquired resistance to cancer therapeutics, especially targeted therapy, is often attributed to intratumoral heterogeneity and represents a major obstacle in the successful treatment of cancer. Tumor heterogeneity also presents a problem for OVs as residual antiviral activity enables tumor cells to resist OV

infection. In an attempt to facilitate OV growth in heterogeneous tumors where partial responsiveness to IFN exists, the use of small molecule viral sensitizers (VSe) that mimic the activity of viral virulence gene products, sensitizing cells to infection, have been used.[141,142] Various sensitizers have been shown to synergize with OVs to increase replication and subsequently enhance efficacy both in vitro and in vivo. Elucidation of the mechanisms underlying these sensitizers will provide a better understanding as to the cellular signaling pathways that impact OV growth and spread.

Tumor heterogeneity with respect to mutation burden may potentiate immunotherapy with checkpoint blockade.[143] This relationship, as well as data supporting improved responses to checkpoint blockade when a high number of tumor-infiltrating lymphocytes are present, suggests that the presence of multiple tumor neoantigens may promote antigen-specific T cell responses and improved response to immunotherapy.[144] Since OVs express numerous viral-specific antigens it has been hypothesized that OVs may be able to substitute for high mutation burden and could help promote immunotherapy, especially with immune checkpoint inhibitors.[145] Further studies are needed to understand how OVs may be limited and may overcome the innate heterogeneity in cancers.

Tumor Microenvironment Suppression

The tumor microenvironment (TME) is a complex milieu in which tumor cells interact with stromal cells, including endothelial cells, adipocytes, cancer associated fibroblasts (CAFs), and infiltrating immune cells. These stromal cells are known to play an important role in the response to immunotherapy and OV therapy (the role of endothelial cells and immune infiltrating have been previously discussed). For example, Ilkow et al. demonstrated that CAFs have an increased sensitivity to OV infection compared to normal fibroblasts. They also secrete high levels of fibroblast growth factor 2 (FGF2), which impedes antiviral responses in tumor cells through the inhibition of RIG-I expression.[146] FGF2 was found to promote viral infection of endothelial cells and a Maraba virus encoding FGF2 was more effective than the parental virus at controlling tumor burden.[146] However, these cells are also responsible for creating physical barriers such as dense fibrotic capsules, necrosis, and acidosis, which can impede viral delivery into the tumor. Moreover, the IFN responsiveness of a tumor is determined by both its malignant and stromal compartments; therefore, while tumor cells may harbor defects in the IFN pathway, the tumor as a whole may still possess some antiviral activity. It has become clear that reciprocal crosstalk between cells within the TME dramatically influences OV replication and subsequent therapeutic efficacy; however, much work remains to be done before a comprehensive understanding of these complex interactions between all the cells within the TME are fully understood.

ALTERNATIVE STRATEGIES TO ENHANCE ONCOLYTIC VIRUS EFFICACY

Combination Therapy

OV-mediated cell death (through both direct and indirect lysis) occurs through distinct mechanisms from those induced by chemotherapy, targeted therapy, and radiotherapy, suggesting that combinations may portend additive or even synergistic effects. The combination of OVs with these standard treatment modalities has been shown to potentiate the therapeutic effect of both approaches, significantly enhancing tumor response rates as well as overcoming resistance to conventional therapy (Figure 30.3). There has been considerable attention to the role of radiation therapy potentiating immunotherapy by promoting an abscopal effect through induction of immune responses, and combining radiation with immunotherapy may be a logical therapeutic approach.[147–149] Several trials of T-VEC and other OVs in combination with radiation therapy are currently in clinical development for a variety of cancers including melanoma, head and neck cancer, and soft tissue sarcoma. While targeted therapies often result in rapid clinical responses, the emergence of drug resistance is inevitable and limits long-term efficacy of these agents. There are data to suggest that targeted agents such as BRAF inhibitors may promote the accumulation of lymphocytes in the tumor microenvironment, allowing for better responses to immunotherapy.[150] Moreover, given the safety profiles of OVs, overlapping toxicities with such targeted therapies are not expected. JX-594 was well tolerated in combination with the VEGFR inhibitor sorafenib, and the combination of T-VEC and BRAF inhibitors for the treatment of melanoma is anticipated in the near future (NCT03088176).

One class of therapeutics garnering substantial attention as a promising candidate for combination therapy is the checkpoint inhibitors (CKIs). CKIs are a relatively new class of immunotherapies that aim to overcome tumor-induced immune suppression and evasion caused by the expression of immune checkpoints. Monoclonal antibodies that inhibit programmed cell death protein 1 (PD-1), its ligand (PD-L1), and cytotoxic T lymphocyte antigen 4 (CTLA-4) have demonstrated remarkable responses in melanoma, non-small cell lung cancer (NSCLC), renal cell carcinoma, bladder cancer, head and neck cancer, Hodgkin's lymphoma, Merkel cell carcinoma, and likely other cancers as well.[151] Although responses with CKIs can be durable, some patients do not respond and some will eventually develop drug resistance.[152] Further, CKI

therapy is predicated on the presence of tumor-reactive T cells within the TME, and some tumors may not contain such cells. Thus, an emerging combination strategy is to combine agents that generate T cell responses with CKIs.

Given their tolerable safety profile as well as their ability to induce innate immune responses and promote IFN production, OVs are attractive agents for use in combination immunotherapy regimens. In particular, oncolytic viruses may be able to convert tumors that are lymphocyte-poor into "hot" lesions characterized by the influx of T and NK cells. The direct lysis of tumor cells also results in the release of soluble tumor antigens, cellular danger signals, viral DNA, and necrotic cell material, which can all help generate an adaptive immune response against the cancer. CKIs and OVs are thought to act synergistically to potentiate and improve each other's efficacy as OVs enhance immune cell recruitment into the tumor and local IFN production results in increased expression of immune checkpoints. CKIs can then activate the immune cells within the tumor microenvironment, producing more robust T cell responses against the tumor.

Preclinical studies have validated this concept demonstrating durable remissions with combination OV and CKI treatment.[153] These initial findings, however, have also highlighted the importance in timing of administration for both agents. CTLA-4 expression peaks 24 to 48 hours after T cell activation and the benefit of inhibition decreases as the length of time after OV treatment increases.[154,155] Optimization of treatment schedules will therefore be essential in order to maximize therapeutic efficacy. In addition to systemic coadministration of CKIs and OVs, proof-of-concept studies have demonstrated the feasibility of encoding OVs with antibodies against specific checkpoints. This strategy is attractive as it restricts the expression of CKIs to within the TME, possibly alleviating systemic immune-related adverse events.

The clinical translation of checkpoint inhibitors with OVs is well underway. In a Phase 1b cohort of 19 metastatic melanoma patients treated with T-VEC and ipilimumab, an encouraging objective response rate of 50% was reported and 44% of the subjects demonstrated durable responses persisting for 6 months or more.[156] These response rates are higher than those observed with either monotherapy, suggesting improved efficacy with the combination. Importantly, there were no unexpected adverse events or drug reactions noted during these trials. A larger randomized Phase 2 cohort comparing combination T-VEC and ipilimumab to ipilimumab alone in patients with metastatic melanoma was conducted.[157] In this study, 198 patients were randomized and the primary study endpoint was ORR. There was a 39% ORR in the combination arm compared to 18% in the ipilimumab alone arm (odds ratio 2.9; 95% CI, 1.5 to 5.5; $p = .002$). In this trial, regression of visceral, uninjected lesions occurred in 52% in the combination arm versus 23% with

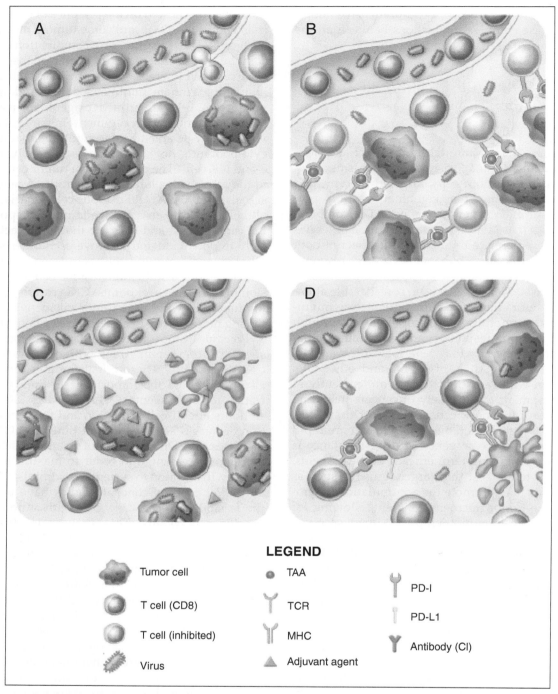

Figure 30.3 Combination therapies improve OV efficacy. (A) OV infection of tumor cells results in lysis and the release of viral progeny and tumor antigens, leading to immune cell recruitment. However, neutralizing antibodies, physical barriers within the tumor microenvironment, and tumor heterogeneity often limit infection and immune cell infiltration and thus efficacy. **(B)** OV infection results in the upregulation of PD-L1 on tumor cells leading to exhaustion of T cells and limiting effective innate antitumor immunity. **(C)** The addition of adjuvant agents such as chemotherapy, radiotherapy, or targeted therapy whose mechanisms of action are distinct from OVs act synergistically to improve infection and cell lysis, leading to improved responses. **(D)** The combination of checkpoint inhibitors (CKIs) with OVs prevents the binding of PD-L1 to PD-1, maintaining an active CD8+ T cell compartment capable of killing tumor cells and generating long-lasting antitumor immunity.

MHC, major histocompatibility complex; OV, oncolytic viruses; PD-1, programmed cell death protein 1; PD-L1, programmed death ligand 1; TAA, tumor-associated antigen; TCR, T cell receptor.

ipilimumab alone, suggesting an improved systemic response with combination treatment. The incidence of grade 3 or greater adverse events was 45% and 35% in the combination and ipilimumab alone arm, respectively.

In a Phase 1b clinical trial, T-VEC was combined with pembrolizumab in patients with advanced melanoma.[145] Although the study was small, 21 patients were treated and no new toxicity signals were noted. ORR were reported in 62% of the patients with 33% achieving a complete response by immune-related response criteria. Biomarker analysis in this study demonstrated an increase in CD8[+] T cell recruitment to OV-injected tumor sites, increased PD-L1 expression, and reported complete responses in patients with T cell excluded tumors and in those with a low inflammatory gene signature score at baseline, suggesting that T-VEC could promote responses to pembrolizumab in tumors typically not responsive to anti-PD-1 therapy.[145] These data led to a larger randomized Phase 3 clinical trial comparing T-VEC and pembrolizumab to pembrolizumab alone in advanced melanoma (NCT 02965716).

T-VEC and pembrolizumab was also investigated in an open-label, single-institution Phase 2 trial in patients with locally advanced or metastatic sarcoma who had failed at least one prior treatment (PMID:31971541). In this study, 20 patients were treated, and the trial met its primary endpoint of best ORR at 24 weeks determined by RECISTv1.1 criteria. The best ORR was 30%, with overall ORR 35%; only four patients reported grade 3 or worse treatment-related adverse events. Other viruses being investigated in combination with CKIs include adenovirus, poxviruses, and reovirus.

Heterologous Prime-Boost

In recent years, it has become apparent that there are patients who respond mostly to the oncolytic properties of a virus, while other responses are driven by the in situ vaccine effect following tumor cell lysis. To confer protective immunity, vaccination usually requires multiple immunizations in the form of a prime-boost. Traditionally, the same vaccine is given multiple times (homologous boost); however, heterologous prime boost strategies that use different delivery methods (recombinant DNA and a viral vector or different viral vectors expressing the same antigens) have been shown to be more immunogenic than homologous prime boosts.[158] This approach is designed to educate or "prime" the immune system to recognize the specified antigen and then locally boost the response through virus-directed expression of the antigen at high levels within the tumor. Importantly, heterologous prime boost is thought to prevent development of antivector immunity resulting from repeated administrations of the same vector, as well as overcome preexisting vector immunity.[159,160]

Multiple variations of the prime-boost strategy have been used with OVs. A common approach has been the use of two distinct OV strains expressing a common tumor-associated antigen.[161,162] Preclinical studies of antigens that have been used in the OV prime-boost setting include ovalbumin (OVA) and dopachrome tautomerase (DCT). While individual Ad or VSV vectors encoding DCT provided minimal improvements in survival, successful antigen-specific immune responses and viral replication within the tumor leading to lysis were observed when a prime-boost approach was employed using both vectors.[98,163] The use of an Ad-DCT prime followed by VSV-DCT boost in the murine B16 melanoma model led to 40% of circulating T cells being directed against DCT and immunity against additional tumor antigens, suggestive of epitope spreading, a dampened immune response against VSV, breaking of tolerance against endogenous cellular antigens, and the generation of durable tumor responses.[163]

Cell Carriers

The use of combination therapy and prime boosting to potentiate the effect of OVs has improved therapeutic effectiveness in several tumor models, although a remaining weakness of all OVs is their vulnerability to antiviral host defenses. Viruses that enter the circulation as free-floating particles can be neutralized or sequestered within half an hour. Thus, the ability to shield virus from the host immune response and delay elimination has potential to improve OV delivery and efficacy. One of the most popular methods to protect OVs such as adenovirus, VSV, and measles from preexisting circulating antibodies is the use of cell-based carriers.[164,165] For best results, in addition to protecting the virus from host immunity, carriers should be able to effectively take up the virus ex vivo, respond to tumor-secreted soluble factors, and traffic to established tumors to unload unaltered virus into the TME.[166] This approach has led to tumor-infiltrating immune cells such as macrophages, dendritic cells, MDSCs, and mesenchymal stem cells emerging as the cell-carriers of choice. Several preclinical studies have shown that viruses can be loaded into or onto these different cells without affecting activity of the virus or cell carrier, and that these carriers provide significant protection against neutralization and antiviral responses. Not only are these cells usually increased in tumors due to the secretion of immunosuppressive cytokines, but both chemotherapy and radiation are known to induce hypoxia and necrosis, leading to a marked increase in macrophage and MDSC recruitment into tumors, facilitating delivery of these carriers.[167] The use of cell carriers has led to improvements in tumor control of both primary tumor and metastases as well as survival in murine models.[164,168] In vivo human work using cell-based carriers has yet to be performed, so the true potential of this strategy as a legitimate therapeutic approach remains unknown.

Convection-Enhanced Delivery

Intratumoral delivery of OVs is one of the best means by which to bypass viral neutralization and sequestration; however, few tumor types are amenable to IT injection. The brain, while highly accessible for nutrients, is an extremely challenging location in which to deliver therapeutics (including OVs) due to the blood-brain barrier (BBB). In attempts to circumvent the BBB, convection-enhanced delivery (CED) has been designed for the administration of pharmacological agents that wouldn't normally cross the BBB. CED uses several catheters placed stereotactically within or around the tumor to continuously and homogenously deliver drugs directly into the brain parenchyma.[169] This approach allows enhanced delivery to the site of interest, limiting systemic side effects and possibly increasing efficacy, making it a promising new treatment strategy for the treatment of brain cancers. CED has been used to deliver standard chemotherapy as well as targeted drugs and resulted in improved outcomes. The use of CED for oncolytic virus delivery has been examined by several groups.[170–173] While these studies have met with variable success, evidence of safety and antitumor efficacy in preclinical and early phase clinical studies has warranted further investigation. CED is being used to deliver PVS-RIPO in GBM trials and has produced some impressive results.[75] Not all viral vectors may be amenable to CED due to virion size; however, the early results with PVS-RIPO suggest that CED may be a valuable delivery strategy in the treatment of brain tumors.

SAFETY CONCERNS WITH ONCOLYTIC VIRUS CLINICAL DEVELOPMENT

Within the past decade there have been significant advances in oncolytic virotherapy that have revolutionized the field. While OVs have proven to have an excellent safety record in the clinic, there remain a number of unique challenges in the clinical development of OVs. The live replicating nature of oncolytic viruses poses unique biosafety concerns and regulatory issues compared to standard cancer therapeutics. Chief among them is environmental shedding of infectious particles, which refers to shedding of viral products from the patient's body through one or all of the following routes: blood, fecal, urine, saliva, or wounds/sores on the skin. Shedding is a considerable biosafety concern as it raises the possibility of transmission of OV products from treated to untreated individuals. As such, the FDA has established guidelines as to how and when data regarding shedding should be

collected during preclinical and clinical development and how it is to be used to assess the potential for transmission to untreated individuals.[174] Some viruses such as HSV, VSV, and reovirus, display minimal shedding, whereas other viruses including Ad and VV are known to be more problematic. Shedding of Ad from injection sites and excretions has been reported in several trials and found to increase with higher viral doses and following systemic administration. Shedding of Ad vectors can result in homologous recombination with wild type Ad, leading to new strains; however, to date recombination has yet to be detected following clinical administration. Live VV is known to shed from skin injection sites following vaccination and it is not recommended for use in immunocompromised individuals, patients with eczema, or pregnant women. Conversely, shedding of animal viruses such as NDV pose an environmental risk since shedding could result in the infection of animals. While viral shedding has yet to be associated with any documented outbreaks, it is imperative that bioshedding studies are carried out for all newly developed OVs, especially as more OVs enter the clinic and are being administered on a greater scale.

The emerging real-world data with T-VEC suggests that treatment is safe, and no evidence of household or healthcare provider transmission has been reported. There are now several consensus guidelines with recommendations for how to establish a safe and standardized approach to integrating T-VEC into ambulatory clinical practices.[175,176] Provider education and coordination with local pharmacy and infection control experts is useful in developing local protocols for OV delivery and establishing mechanisms for viral transmission surveillance.

CONCLUSION

Oncolytic viruses represent a new class of drugs for the treatment of cancer. OVs are composed of native or genetically modified live, typically replication competent viral particles. Most OVs are selected for preferential infection and replication in tumor cells and mediate antitumor activity through a multimodal mechanism of action. This includes direct lysis of infected tumor cells, which is often enhanced by aberrant oncogenic and interferon signaling pathways within cancer cells, and indirect lysis through induction of innate and adaptive antitumor immunity. The ability to manipulate the viral genome and capsid have provided a variety of strategies for improving therapeutic efficacy, limiting pathogenicity and enhancing antitumor immunogenicity. A large number of potential viruses can be considered for development as oncolytic agents but the most clinical progress has been seen with adenovirus, herpes virus, paramyxovirus, parvovirus, picornavirus, poxvirus, rhabdovirus, and reovirus families. An attenuated HSV-1 virus encoding GM-CSF, termed talimogene laherparepvec (T-VEC), has demonstrated clinical benefit and an acceptable safety profile in a prospective, multi-institutional, global clinical trial for patients with advanced melanoma leading to the first regulatory approval of an OV in the United States, Europe, Israel, and Australia.

Despite the success of T-VEC and emerging early phase clinical trials with other OVs, there continue to be challenges with optimizing the therapeutic window. The induction of neutralizing antibodies and complement inactivation of viral particles can limit viral replication and spread, and, hence, impact efficacy. The heterogeneous nature of neoplastic cells and suppressive mechanisms inherent in the tumor microenvironment can also limit the induction of effective antitumor immune responses. The clinical development of OVs is also complicated by concerns over viral shedding and biosafety issues related to drug storage, preparation, and administration. As is true with any new class of pharmacologic agents, these issues are being addressed through increased research in the laboratory and clinic. Further discussion with regulatory agencies on appropriate study populations, eligibility, endpoints, and biomarker priorities for OV clinical studies should provide guidance for further clinical development.

In addition to addressing some of the inherent challenges in OV clinical development, there are other priorities that have emerged for the field. The recognition that tumor-infiltrating T cells are associated with improved outcomes in patients with cancer and in those treated with immunotherapy, and the inherent ability of most OVs to induce lymphocyte trafficking into tumors, suggests a rational strategy of combination treatment with OVs and other immunotherapy or conventional cancer treatments. Of particular interest is the emerging therapeutic data observed with OV and immune checkpoint blockade, suggesting significant improvements in the therapeutic window with combination treatment. Although validation will require completion of prospectively randomized clinical trials, the acceptable safety profile observed with most OV therapies further support combination studies. Another important development may be the concept of using OVs in a prime-boost strategy by combining different vectors to avoid rapid viral clearance. Further investigation is needed to determine what the best viruses and sequences will be in specific cancers. Optimizing delivery of viruses to established tumors is another high priority, and while clinical studies using various routes of clinical administration are already underway, novel delivery vehicles, such as synthetic nanodelivery particles, will also be of further interest for OV drug development. Finally, as a new form of treatment, some attention to educating the healthcare providers on the safe management of patients on oncolytic virotherapy will be important to ensure that eligible patients receive the highest quality care and achieve the most benefit from oncolytic virus therapy.

KEY REFERENCES

Only key references appear in the print edition. The full reference list appears in the digital product on Springer Publishing Connect: connect.springerpub.com/content/book/978-0-8261-3743-2/part/part02/chapter/ch30

31. Kaufman HL, Kohlhapp FJ, Zloza A. Oncolytic viruses: a new class of immunotherapy drugs. *Nat Rev Drug Discov*. 2015;14(9):642–662. doi:10.1038/nrd4663

61. Russell SJ, Peng KW. Measles virus for cancer therapy. *Curr Top Microbiol Immunol*. 2009;330:213–241. doi:10.1007/978-3-540-70617-5_11

113. Andtbacka RH, Kaufman HL, Collichio F, et al. Talimogene laherparepvec improves durable response rate in patients with advanced melanoma. *J Clin Oncol*. 2015;33(25):2780–2788. doi:10.1200/JCO.2014.58.3377

145. Ribas A, Dummer R, Puzanov I, et al. Oncolytic virotherapy promotes intratumoral T cell infiltration and improves anti-PD-1 immunotherapy. *Cell*. 2017;170(6):1109–1119. doi:10.1016/j.cell.2017.08.027

157. Chesney J, Puzanov I, Collichio F, et al. Randomized, open-label Phase II study evaluating the efficacy and safety of talimogene laherparepvec in combination with ipilimumab versus ipilimumab alone in patients with advanced, unresectable melanoma. *J Clin Oncol*. 2018;36(17):1658–1667. doi:10.1200/JCO.2017.73.7379

Metabolism of Tumor Immunity

Robert D. Leone and Jonathan D. Powell

INTRODUCTION

Reprogrammed cellular metabolism is a critical aspect of both cancer and cells of the immune system. The manner in which metabolic pathways intersect between cancer and immune cells, as well as how cells adapt to establish viable metabolic phenotypes within the tumor microenvironment (TME), is a critical determinant of the nature and success of the antitumor immune response. Recent work has demonstrated that the metabolic activity of cancer cells can create a potent checkpoint to the antitumor immune response. As such, a nuanced understanding of the metabolism of the native immune response to cancer has the potential to identify biomarkers as well as therapeutic targets to induce, enhance, and sustain a meaningful and long-lived antitumor response.

THE METABOLISM OF HIGHLY PROLIFERATIVE CELLS

Metabolism is the manner in which cells transform nutrients and biomolecules to support functional, proliferative, or growth requirements. Metabolic programs function in a network to meet the energy, biomolecular synthesis, and redox demands of the cell. The differential activity of pathways within this network can allow a cell to be exquisitely responsive to signaling events, cellular stress, and nutrient conditions. As such, the specific pathways and mechanisms enacted to support metabolic activity are highly reflective of cellular differentiation states or physiologic roles within a tissue or organism.

The cellular metabolism of glucose is among the most well studied metabolic pathways in eukaryotic cells. During glycolysis, glucose can be enzymatically broken down to generate pyruvate and a modest yield of ATP (Figure 31.1). In the presence of sufficient oxygen, pyruvate can enter the mitochondria where it can be metabolized through the tricarboxylic acid (TCA) cycle. TCA cycle activity generates NADH and FADH2 which, along with molecular oxygen, are used in the electron transport chain to produce high yields of ATP in a process called oxidative phosphorylation (OXPHOS). Alternatively, pyruvate can be metabolized to lactate in the cytosol by lactate dehydrogenase (LDH), which does not produce additional ATP, but regenerates NAD^+, which is a critical cofactor for GAPDH, a key enzyme of glycolysis. Regeneration of NAD^+ is especially critical during conditions of low oxygen tensions, during which OXPHOS is curtailed and mitochondrial generation of NAD^+ is suppressed. Thus, NAD$^+$ generation through pyruvate conversion to lactate can be a critical mechanism to support glucose metabolism during limited oxygen conditions. Because it is the primary source of energy production during hypoxic conditions, this lactate-generating glycolysis pathway is referred to as "anaerobic glycolysis." OXPHOS and anaerobic glycolysis are the two main energy-generating pathways in eukaryotic cells.

Interestingly, through the pioneering work of Otto Warburg, it was found that cancer cells and malignant tissues grown in culture employ high levels of lactate-generating glycolysis even in the presence of sufficient oxygen levels.[1,2] This phenomenon is known as "aerobic glycolysis," or the "Warburg effect." While the basis of the cellular advantage of engaging in aerobic glycolysis is still a matter of debate, it is important to appreciate that it renders cells highly glucose avid and can generate significant quantities of lactate and acid. Importantly, over the past few decades aerobic glycolysis has been observed not only in malignant cells and tissues, but as a common feature in highly proliferative cells, including highly activated immune cells such as T cells.[3–8] That said, the fact that both immune activation and malignant transformation have been

consistently observed to engage high levels of aerobic glycolysis (requiring high levels of glucose uptake) suggests that a fundamental competition for nutrients exists during the antitumor immune response. Furthermore, despite the Warburg effect having been identified as a hallmark of cancer cell metabolism, malignant cells upregulate a broad range of metabolic pathways which are critical for survival and proliferation. In fact, in addition to aerobic respiration, mitochondrial respiration (OXPHOS) is now understood to make a significant contribution to the energetics of cancer cell metabolism.[9–12]

In addition to the energy-producing pathways of aerobic glycolysis and OXPHOS, metabolic pathways emanating from intermediates in both glycolysis and the TCA cycle (i.e., "central carbon metabolism") are fundamental to biomolecule synthesis and homeostatic control in both cancer and highly proliferative cells such as activated T cells (Figure 31.1).[13] The pentose phosphate pathway (PPP) uses glycolysis-derived glucose-6-phosphate (G6P) to generate NADPH and ribose sugars, to maintain REDOX balance and support nucleic acid synthesis, respectively. The serine glycine one-carbon pathway (SGOC) branches from the glycolysis intermediate

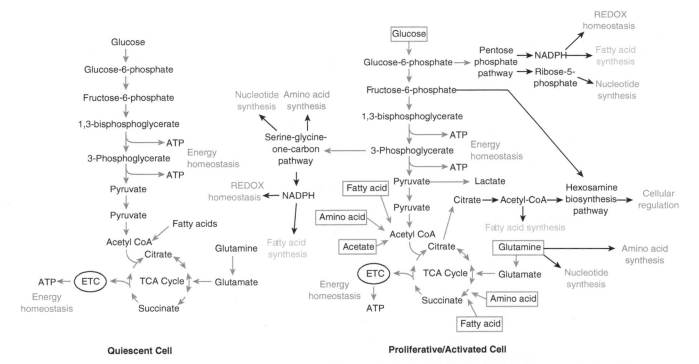

Figure 31.1 Metabolic reprogramming of immune activation and cancer transformation. Metabolic reprogramming is an integral aspect of the transition from a quiescent cell to a highly proliferative one. This requires marked upregulation of aerobic glycolysis as well as other pathways integral to anabolic metabolism. Proximal glycolytic pathways, such as the pentose phosphate pathway, the serine-glycine-one carbon pathway, and the hexosamine biosynthetic pathway, are critical metabolic programs to support cellular processes, such as REDOX homeostasis, fatty acid synthesis, nucleotide synthesis, cellular regulation, and amino acid synthesis. Although the TCA cycle and oxidative metabolism can also be upregulated to support energy homeostasis, anaplerotic processes, such as glutaminolysis, are particularly critical to support biomolecule syntheses. Metabolic flexibility is determined by the ability of a cell to utilize distinct nutrient sources (outlined in green) to fuel these anabolic processes.

3-phosphogluconate for de novo synthesis of serine, glycine, and one-carbon units that are critical in nucleic acid synthesis and posttranslational protein modifications. Intermediates in the TCA cycle are also crucial starting points for biomolecular synthesis. Citrate, for example, is actively exported from the mitochondria to the cytosol wherein it can be metabolized to acetyl CoA to support massive demands for fatty acids and cholesterol to support plasma membrane synthesis, which is crucial in highly proliferative cells such as cancer and many activated immune cells. Other TCA intermediates such as oxaloacetate and a-ketoglutarate (aKG) are used to support amino acid synthesis and an array of other diverse cellular processes. As intermediates are siphoned away for these critical roles, the amino acid glutamine becomes a critical nutrient to replenish the TCA cycle. Glutamine is the most highly abundant amino acid in plasma and can be imported into highly proliferative cells at elevated rates. Through a process called "glutaminolysis," glutamine can be metabolized to glutamate and aKG, which can enter the TCA cycle to replenish intermediates and support the previously outlined functions. Alternatively, glutamine can undergo a process known as "reductive carboxylation," leading to cytosolic citrate synthesis as fuel for de novo lipogenesis. Lastly, uptake of essential amino acids from the extracellular space is also a critical determinant of metabolic viability in these cells.

METABOLISM, THE TUMOR MICROENVIRONMENT, AND IMMUNITY

While the metabolic pathways described are highly characteristic of malignant cells, they are also highly upregulated in several activated immune cell subsets during an inflammatory response. In fact, most of the immune cell subtypes which comprise an inflammatory or antitumor response rely on similar metabolic pathways as malignant cells.[3–8] As mentioned, this convergence of highly active metabolic phenotypes within the TME creates a fundamental competition for nutrients and oxygen between cancer cells and inflammatory antitumor immune cells.[14–17] A highly dysregulated vasculature in the TME further exacerbates nutrient depletion and hypoxia. Another important consequence of cancer cell metabolism is the generation of toxic (i.e., immunosuppressive) metabolites such as lactate, acid, adenosine, and kynurenine. Lastly, in addition to the metabolic derangements created by cancer cell metabolism, other cells within the TME, such as myeloid suppressive cells, macrophages, and regulatory T cells, employ metabolic mechanisms that deplete key nutrients and generate toxic metabolites. We will discuss the specific metabolic programs, nutrient dependencies, and vulnerabilities of the major immune subsets within the TME.

The Metabolism of Energy Production

Immune Cell Catabolism

Catabolism is the means by which nutrient fuels such as glucose are degraded in a manner to produce cellular energy in the form of ATP. The specific metabolic pathways that a particular immune cell type engages to produce ATP is a reflection of their function and proliferative state (Figure 31.2). Effector CD4+ and CD8+ T cells (Teff) are antigen-specific immune cells which orchestrate and execute cytotoxic antitumor responses. Upon activation, naïve T cells undergo dramatic signaling events

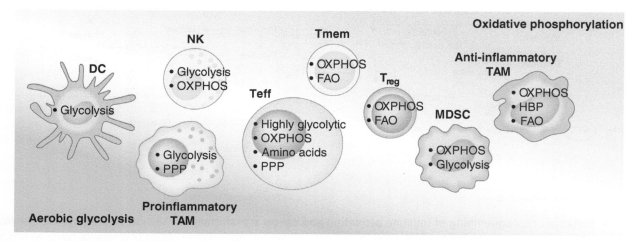

Figure 31.2 Predominant metabolic programming of tumor-associated immune cells. Effector (green and orange) and suppressive (yellow and purple) immune cells arise as part of innate and adaptive immune response to cancer. Each cellular type and subtype is metabolically programmed in this manner to support specific functional activities.

DC, dendritic cell; FAO, fatty acid oxidation; HBP, hexosamine biosynthesis pathway; MDSC, myeloid-derived suppressor cell; NK, natural killer; OXPHOS, oxidative phosphorylation; PPP, pentose phosphate pathway; TAM, tumor-associated macrophage; Teff, effector T cell; Tmem, memory T cell; T$_{reg}$, regulatory T cell.

and metabolic reprogramming to support immense proliferation and effector functions. Driven primarily by the transcription factors MYC and hypoxia-inducible factor 1 (HIF-1), T cells undergoing activation dramatically upregulate their reliance on aerobic glycolysis through upregulation of key glycolytic enzymes, pyruvate kinase (PKM), hexokinase 2 (HK2), glucose transporter 1 (GLUT1), and LDH.[8,18-20] It is important to note that TCA cycle metabolism and OXPHOS are also upregulated during Teff activation.[3-8] However, like many cancer cells, a comparatively greater increase in aerobic glycolysis is characteristic of this immune cell subtype (at least in in vitro studies). It is important to remember that, aside from its role in supplying the electron transport chain with reducing equivalents for ATP synthesis, TCA cycle intermediates are in high demand in activated T cells, supplying building blocks for lipid and cholesterol synthesis, nucleic acid synthesis and amino acid synthesis. Like cancer cells, activated T cells upregulate glucose shuttling into the PPP, generating NADPH and ribose sugars that are critical for fatty acid synthesis for membranes and nucleic acid synthesis, respectively. Glycolytic intermediates also supply the hexosamine biosynthetic pathway (HBP) in activated T cells. The HBP generates UDP-GlcNAc, the key cellular substrate for posttranslational glycosylation reactions, which are critical for broad cellular regulation of protein function and essential for activated T cell proliferation and effector function (Figure 31.1). Lastly, the serine-glycine synthesis pathway, as well as the one-carbon pathway, are required for optimal T cell proliferation.

Another critical CD4+ T cell subtype that plays an important role in the antitumor response is the regulatory T cell (T_{reg} cell) compartment. While T_{reg} cells are crucial to maintenance of self-tolerance and microbiome homeostasis, their robust suppressive effect on Teff cells is maladaptive in the setting of the antitumor immune response. Quite distinct from Teff cells, T_{reg} cells generally rely primarily on mitochondrial respiration and TCA cycle metabolism.[21,22] In contrast to Teff cells, T_{reg} cells express lower levels of GLUT1 and show decreased levels of glucose uptake.[22] Furthermore, catabolism of fatty acids plays a prominent role in T_{reg} cell metabolism, fueling the TCA cycle and OXPHOS through fatty acid oxidation (FAO; Figures 31.1 and 31.2). While this metabolic profile is most commonly associated with T_{reg} cells, it has become clear that similar to effector CD4+ T cells, effector T_{reg} cells, which are highly active, also rely on the upregulation of glycolysis.[23] The metabolic flexibility of T_{reg} cells is likely a critical aspect of their ability to sustain viability and function within the tumor metabolic environment.

An important facet of the successful T cell response to tumors is the generation of immunologic memory through the formation of T memory cells.[24,25] While several subtypes comprise these cells (reviewed elsewhere), it is clear that the generation of Tmem cells as a whole are critical in producing long-lived responses to immunotherapy, both checkpoint blockade and CAR T cell therapy.[24,26] Similar to T_{reg} cells, Tmem cells preferentially rely on TCA cycle activity and OXPHOS, rather than aerobic glycolysis.[27-30] That said, the most characteristic metabolic feature of Tmem cells is the capacity to dramatically upregulate OXPHOS from baseline.[29] This is referred to as spare respiratory capacity (SRC) and allows a metabolic reserve which is in concert with the ability of Tmem cells to respond especially rapidly to antigen rechallenge. While initial reports had shown that oxidation of long chain fatty acids using the carnitine palmitoyl transferase (CPT1) transporter was the primary fuel for OXPHOS in Tmem cells, this pathway has subsequently been shown not to be uniquely contributing to the metabolic phenotype of these cells.[29,31] Indeed, in addition to glucose, glutamine, and long chain fatty acids, amino acids and short- and medium-chain fatty acids can also fuel the TCA cycle and OXPHOS. Acetate is the smallest short chain fatty acid and, through the activity of Acyl-CoA Synthetase Short-Chain Family Member 1 (ACSS1), has recently been shown in several studies to be an important contributor to the TCA cycle in Tmem cells.[32,33,34] Also, recent data has shown that a Tmem subset known as resident memory T cells (Trm), which are noncirculating and reside long-term in peripheral tissues, are specifically reliant on uptake of exogenous fatty acids through fatty acid binding proteins (FABP4/5) to support FAO. Trm cells are emerging as playing important roles in effective antitumor immune responses.[35,36]

Natural killer (NK) cells form a critical part of the antitumor immune response. In vitro activation of NK cells by IL-12 and IL-15 led to upregulation of both aerobic glycolysis as well as OXPHOS in NK cells.[37] These metabolic changes are broadly dependent on SREBP, the inhibition of which not only curtails metabolic reprogramming, but also suppresses cytokine production, cytotoxicity, and antitumor response.[38] Though both glycolytic and mitochondrial pathways have been shown to be active in stimulated NK cells, a number of studies have found that these cells, like Teff cells, are particularly dependent on aerobic glycolysis for viability and function.[39] To this end, inhibition of FBP1, which is induced by TGF-β and curtails glycolytic activity as well as NK cell function and viability, rescues metabolic reprogramming, cytotoxic capacity, and antitumor cytotoxicity of NK cells. Notably, these findings were dependent on rescue of the glycolytic pathway, as inhibition of glycolysis by the hexokinase inhibitor 2-deoxyglucose (2DG) blocked NK cell rescue from FBP1 inhibition.

Some myeloid immune cells within the TME also rely on aerobic glycolysis, which is an important determinant of phenotype and function in these cells. Although there is clearly a spectrum of macrophage phenotypes, pro-inflammatory macrophages, or M1-like macrophages, are critical innate effector cells in the antitumor response.[40,41,42] Similar to activated T cells, inflammatory macrophages stimulated through Toll-like receptor (TLR) signaling dramatically increase glucose uptake and lactic acid production.[43] Interestingly, these metabolic changes directly impact effector function of these cells. Upon stimulation, HIF-1alpha is stabilized by increased succinate generated through TCA cycle activity, leading to expression of the pro-inflammatory IL-1-beta.[44] Other metabolic pathways emanating from glycolysis are also direct and critical determinants of effector function of these cells. The generation of reactive oxygen species (ROS) is an important aspect of effector function in antitumor inflammatory macrophages. Generation of high levels of ROS to fuel the oxidative burst characteristic of these macrophages requires dramatic upregulation of the PPP as a primary source of NADPH, which is critical for ROS synthesis.[44-46]

Anti-inflammatory macrophages, so-called "M2-like" macrophages, generally form the largest intratumoral macrophage subpopulation. Contrasting with M1-like macrophages, these cells can be highly suppressive of the antitumor response and adopt a distinct metabolic phenotype. Like Tmem and T_{reg} cells, M2-like macrophages rely primarily on OXPHOS, with considerable contribution of FAO in this regard.[47-49] Strikingly, forced induction of mitochondrial biogenesis and FAO through PGC1 overexpression in macrophages led to suppression of inflammatory cytokines and promoted the immunosuppressive, M2-like phenotype.

Another group of intratumoral myeloid cells, called myeloid-derived suppressive cells (MDSCs), appear to engage both aerobic glycolysis and OXPHOS to a significant degree within the TME.[50] Although more work is needed to more completely understand the metabolic phenotype of MDSCs, present evidence suggests that, like T_{reg} cells, this highly immunosuppressive subset is metabolically flexible, which may likewise impart an inherent ability to adapt to the nutrient stress and metabolic derangement within the TME. That said, MDSC expansion and intratumoral accumulation are attenuated through blocking one of the rate determining enzymes of the glycolytic pathway, hexokinase 2 (HK2), with 2-deoxyglucose (2DG).[51]

Dendritic cells (DCs) function as the primary antigen-presenting cell (APC) in antitumor T cell activation. Activation of DCs triggers maturation and antigen processing, leading to antigen presentation to T cells within the major histocompatibility complex (MHC). Metabolic reprogramming is an integral process during DC activation. Studies have demonstrated that DC activation through either LPS stimulation (via HIF1-alpha) or TLR agonism (via PI3K/AKT pathway) leads to metabolic reprogramming away from OXPHOS and toward increased aerobic glycolysis.[52,53] Interestingly, forced OXPHOS through AMPK activation has been shown to block DC maturation, and inhibition of glycolysis suppressed DC survival, maturation, and ability to activate T cells.[54]

Catabolic Metabolism in the Tumor Microenvironment

As discussed, most cancer cells are highly metabolically active. This, along with a compromised supply of nutrients and oxygen due to disorganized and dysregulated vasculature, create a fundamental competition for nutrients within the TME (Figure 31.3).[15-17] Given the similarly high catabolic requirements of many antitumor immune cells, nutrient restrictions within the TME present a significant challenge or "checkpoint" to immune cell function. This is particularly true regarding glucose and oxygen, which are fundamental to glycolysis and OXPHOS. Importantly, curtailing catabolic metabolic processes of a given immune cell phenotype can not only suppress function and viability, but may also induce dramatic changes in cell subtype by impacting cellular differentiation.

Glucose Limitation in the Tumor Microenvironment

Several recent studies have defined the effect of glucose limitations within the TME on the antitumor Teff cell response. As such, the degree of glucose availability within the TME is inversely related to CD8+ T cell cytokine expression.[15,16] And more specifically, both T cell glucose uptake as well as effector function are progressively limited with increased glycolytic activity of cancer cells within the TME. This inverse relationship between cancer cell glycolysis and Teff response was corroborated by a study of TCGA data from melanoma patients, showing that the expression of key Teff genes, CD40lg and IFN-γ, was inversely proportional with the rate-limiting step in glycolysis, HK2.[16] Similarly, overexpression of key glycolytic genes in tumor cells led to marked decreases in CD8+ T cell infiltration and function in mouse tumor models compared to empty vector transfected control tumors.[15]

Further observations on the effect of glucose limitations on T cell biology have been reported from extensive in vitro studies. Limiting glucose concentration in media suppressed both aerobic glycolysis as well as OXPHOS in both CD4+ and CD8+ Teff cells.[55-57] This metabolic suppression was coupled to attenuated effector cytokine production, including IL-17, IFN-γ, and granzyme B, as well as marked suppression of mTOR signaling.[56-59] The suppression of mTOR signaling is of particular significance as studies have demonstrated that mTOR blockade with rapamycin can skew CD4+ T cell differentiation from effector phenotype to that of protumorigenic T_{reg} cells, underlining the idea that suppression of antitumor responses as well as augmentation of protumorigenic responses are closely tied to the metabolic programming

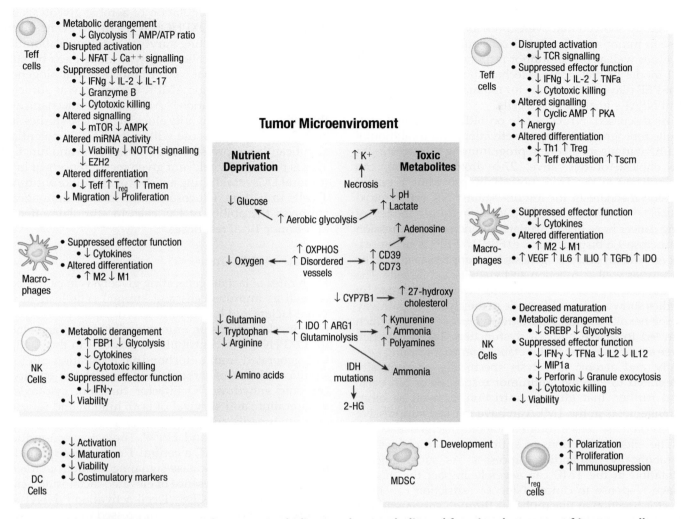

Figure 31.3 **Potential consequences of cancer metabolism on the metabolic and functional response of immune cell populations within the TME.** The metabolic milieu of the TME is a reflection of cancer metabolic programs. Nutrient deprivation, hypoxia, toxic metabolites, and intercellular metabolic reprogramming, or "cross-talk," are conditions within the TME that confront and influence immune cell metabolism and function. The consequences of TME conditions on specific immune cell responses can be predicted based on a growing literature of preclinical, translational, and clinical studies.

DC, dendritic cell; IDO, indoleamine 2,3-dioxygenase; IFN, interferon; MDSC, myeloid-derived suppressor cell; NK, natural killer; OXPHOS, oxidative phosphorylation; SREBP, sterol regulatory element-binding protein; Teff, effector T cell; TME, tumor microenvironment; Tmem, memory T cell; T$_{reg}$, regulatory T; VEGF, vascular endothelial growth factor.

and nutrient exposure of Teff cells.[60] That said, it is also true that rapamycin treatment induces Tmem cell differentiation in CD8+ T cells, which are an important cell type for sustained antitumor responses.[60–62] Interestingly, both transcription and translation of the IFN-γ locus in T cells has been molecularly linked to glycolytic activity in these cells. Chang et al. showed that suppressed lactate-forming glycolysis (i.e., Warburg physiology) led to suppressed activity of the NAD+-dependent glycolytic enzyme, GAPDH, which consequently binds to upstream regions of IFN-γ mRNA, blocking translation.[3] Interestingly, Peng et al. have shown that direct blockade of lactate dehydrogenase A (LDHA) in T cells alters

acetyl-CoA metabolism and triggers epigenetic remodeling of the IFN-γ locus, suppressing transcription.[3] Glucose depletion in ovarian cancer cell conditioned media was found to suppress Teff cell function and viability through downregulation of the key epigenetic remodeling enzyme EZH2 through miRNA-mediated decay.[63]

It is notable that, while increased cancer cell glycolytic activity can have profound suppressive effects on the T cell response, Ho et al. demonstrated, conversely, that augmentation of glycolysis in antitumor Teff cells can improve antitumor response.[16] Initially demonstrating that generation of the glycolysis intermediate phosphoenolpyruvate

(PEP) was curtailed in Teff cells during glucose restriction, this group showed that overexpression of PEP carboxykinase in tumor-specific CD4+ T cells augmented both PEP levels as well as the antitumor response in an adoptive T cell model of melanoma. Mechanistically, it was shown that PEP plays a critical role for maintaining Ca++- dependent NFAT signaling in Teff cells.

As discussed, NK cells rely on SREBP-mediated metabolic reprogramming upon activation, and inhibition of SREBP curtails metabolic reprogramming.[38] Interestingly, the cholesterol derivative, 27-hydroxycholesterol, can be enriched in the TME, potentially providing a potent evasion mechanism for tumors against NK cell cytotoxicity.[37,64–68] Furthermore, TGF-β levels in mouse models of lung cancer have been correlated to increased expression of fructose-1,6-bisphosphatase (FBP1).[39] FBP1 is an important enzyme in gluconeogenesis but suppresses glycolytic activity, as well as function and viability in NK cells. The central role of glycolysis in this effect was corroborated by studies showing direct blockade of the glycolytic pathway by the hexokinase inhibitor 2-deoxyglucose (2DG), which also led to severe NK cell dysfunction. Taken together, these studies suggest that metabolic reprogramming generally, and aerobic glycolysis specifically, are critically integrated to effective antitumor responses of NK cells. And further, that glucose restriction, as well as other derangements in the TME, can have marked suppressive effects on these cells through metabolic mechanisms.

The effector functions of antitumor macrophages are metabolically demanding processes. As such, glucose limitation in the TME can severely impact the macrophage response to cancer. Glucose restriction can limit effector function in macrophages through suppression of glycolysis and related pathways such as the PPP and the glucose entry into the TCA cycle, curtailing generation of NADPH, which is required for ROS elaboration for oxidative burst, as well as succinate, which is critical for stabilization of HIF1 and HIF1-mediated effector functions.[48,44,69] Studies have demonstrated that pro-inflammatory cytokines are markedly reduced in macrophages during glycolytic blockade with 2-DG, and conversely, overexpression of the glucose transporter GLUT1 induces a hyperinflammatory state in macrophages. Lastly, elevated AMP-activated protein kinase (AMPK) activity in response to diminished cellular energy reserves has been found to diminish pro-inflammatory macrophage responses and promote polarization to antiinflammatory, M2-like, phenotypes.[70] Cancer cell intrinsic metabolism can also impact the MDSC response. In a recent study, MDSC response to triple-negative breast cancer was a direct function of the intrinsic glycolytic rates in the cancer cells.[71] Restricting glycolysis in the cancer cells inhibited expression of granulocyte–macrophage colony-stimulating factor (GM-CSF) and granulocyte colony-stimulating factor (G-CSF) and limited MDSC development.

As discussed, upregulation of aerobic glycolysis and downregulation of OXPHOS is a critical event during DC activation, impacting survival, cytokine elaboration, and activation of T cells. This was made clear by studies demonstrating that forced mitochondrial biogenesis through pharmacologic AMPK activation was sufficient to inhibit DC maturation.[53] Although the mechanism of this effect has not been fully elucidated, these studies suggest that limiting glucose within the TME is potentially significantly suppressive of DC maturation and function. This is particularly relevant given recent reports of intratumoral DCs establishing a niche for stem-like antitumor T cells to mature. Glucose limitation may dramatically suppress the ability of DC cells to stimulate effective anti-tumor T cell responses.[72]

Lactate and Acidosis

High rates of lactate-generating glycolysis in cancer cells as well as immune cells and stromal cells lead to elevated lactate and low pH in the TME, both of which can have marked effects on immune cell function and stability. OXPHOS also contributes to acidosis in the TME, as CO_2 generated from mitochondrial respiration can form significant levels of carbonic acid through the activity of carbonic anhydrase.[73,74] Effector function, cytotoxicity, proliferation, and survival of both human and mouse T cells are broadly suppressed in the presence of elevated extracellular lactate and H+.[75,76] The activation-induced upregulation of NFAT, a central T cell transcription factor, as well as MAP kinase signaling are both markedly suppressed in the presence of elevated lactate and acidosis in media during CD8+ T cell activation.[75] NFAT signaling was also found to be suppressed in NK cells with associated decreased cytotoxicity and effector function in the presence of elevated lactate and acidosis during in vitro studies.[75,77,78] Interestingly, Treg cells are much more well adapted to these conditions. By suppressing MYC and downstream metabolic programming toward aerobic glycolysis, Foxp3, the defining transcription factor in Treg cells, maintains OXPHOS. Because OXPHOS activity is independent of lactate transport, Treg cells are relatively resistant to extracellular lactate-induced metabolic, functional, and proliferative constraints.[79] Lactate and acidosis are also suppressive factors for myeloid cells within the TME, modulating DC cell activation and antigen expression.[80] and suppressing inflammatory cytokine production and inducing anti-inflammatory polarization in tumor-associated macrophages.[81,82]

Hypoxia in the Tumor Microenvironment

Hypoxia can present a significant additional hurdle for immune cell energetics within the TME. Despite many effector cell programs (e.g., Teff, M1-like macrophages, DCs) relying primarily on aerobic glycolysis, OXPHOS still plays a significant role in many of these cell subtypes. This is particularly true in effector T cells, wherein, despite engaging proportionally higher levels of aerobic glycolysis upon activation, OXPHOS is also upregulated compared with the naïve state.[11] Oxygenation in tumors due to cancer cell metabolic activity and dysfunctional vasculature can reach as low as 0.3%, compared with 5% on average in normal tissues.[83,84] It must also be stated that, while commonly observed in tumors, hypoxic areas can be chronic or acute and heterogeneously distributed.[73] That said, the precise consequences of hypoxia on T cell phenotype and function has not been clearly established. While early work had demonstrated that hypoxic CD8+ Teff cells were suppressed in proliferative potential as well as IL-2 and IFN-γ production, they simultaneously displayed improved lytic capacity, activation markers, and longevity. Subsequent in vitro studies showed that T cells exposed to hypoxic conditions had markedly diminished cytokine production, cytotoxicity, and activation but, unexpectedly underwent increased proliferation and survival, and mounted an improved antitumor response upon in vivo transfer.[85] Many of these effects were found to be mediated by altered cellular metabolism leading to the generation of the metabolite (S)-2-hydroxyglutarate (S-2-HG). 2-S-HG can inhibit a broad range of demethylating enzymes, and thus can dramatically influence cellular processes through modulating posttranslational modifications and epigenetic remodeling.[86] Subsequent studies confirmed improved in vivo antitumor cytotoxicity of adoptively transferred CD8+ Teff cells cultured in 1% (vs. 20%) oxygenation, further showing that increased granzyme B was the primary mechanism of improved in vivo performance.[87] Later in vivo studies exposing mice to hypoxic conditions have generally demonstrated suppressed T cell activation, proliferation, and effector function.[88,89]

Present understanding of the effects of hypoxia on T_{reg} cells is equally muddled. While separate studies have reported that hypoxia mediates T_{reg} cell migration, stabilization of the T_{reg} cell defining transcription factor Foxp3, and increased proliferation and immunoregulatory function,[90–96] others have reported hypoxia stabilization of HIF1-alpha destabilizes T_{reg} cells and promotes alternative differentiation programs favoring IL-17-producing CD4+ effector T cells (Th17 cells).[58,59,97]

Innate immune cells are also impacted by hypoxia in the TME. Hypoxia suppresses NK cell cytolytic activity, downregulating the expression of activating receptors NKp46 and NKp30.[98,99] Hypoxia has also been shown to induce M2-like anti-inflammatory polarization in macrophages, which accumulate in hypoxic regions of the tumor.[100–102] These macrophages are particularly adept at aiding tissues in hypoxic stress as they are programmed to elaborate angiogenic factors and mitogenic factors, all of which are maladaptive in the setting of

malignancy. Hypoxia-induced adenosine signaling suppresses inflammatory macrophages and augments the function and differentiation of M2-like protumorigenic macrophages.[103,104] Interestingly, hypoxia also modulates MDSCs toward a potently immunosuppressive, M2-like phenotype in in vitro studies—an effect that was HIF1-alpha dependent. Tumor growth was significantly suppressed in mouse models with bone marrow reconstituted with knockout of HIF1-alpha during anti-tumor adoptive cell therapy with wild type T cells.[103,104]

An important consequence of hypoxia in the TME is the upregulation of pathways that generate supraphysiological levels of adenosine, which is broadly immunosuppressive. Hypoxia induces upregulation of two ectonucleotidases, CD39 and CD73, which metabolize extracellular ATP to adenosine.[105,106] The activation of adenosine A2a and A2b receptors, which are highly expressed on a range of immune cells, widely suppresses antitumor effector cells (e.g., Teff cells, NK cells, inflammatory macrophages) and, at the same time, enhances the generation, stability, and function of immune suppressive populations such as T_{reg} cells and M2 macrophages.[104,107–111] In a study by Hatfield et al., supplemental oxygen promoted the antitumor immune response of NK cells and Teff cells through downregulation of the adenosine signaling pathway.[88] While a complete discussion of the effects of hypoxia on the tumor immune response is beyond the scope of this review, future study would benefit this important subject area.

Induced Mitochondrial Dysfunction

Mitochondrial function is emerging as a critical determinant of antitumor immune response, particularly regarding T cell dynamics. As mentioned, although aerobic glycolysis is a prominent feature of activated T cells, mitochondrial respiration is also fundamentally involved in T cell activation and effector function. Interestingly, recent reports have demonstrated that decreased mitochondrial mass and dysfunction in T cells is a common phenomenon in some cancer patients and mouse tumor models.[112–114] In one study, the clinical response of patients receiving CAR T cell therapy for chronic lymphocytic leukemia was correlated to the fitness of the mitochondria of the infused CAR T cells.[114] Another study of renal cell cancer patients demonstrated high levels of reactive oxygen species and hyperpolarization in infiltrating T cells.[113] Recently, a study by the Thompson Group was able to define a causal connection between persistent antigenic stimulation, such as that which occurs in a tumor, and uncoupling of mitochondrial functions, such as that for which high levels of ROS are generated, triggering severe dysfunction or T cell exhaustion.[115] In these latter two studies, T cell function could be rescued with the use of pharmacologic antioxidants.

The Metabolism of Biomolecule Synthesis

In addition to generating energy through glycolysis and OXPHOS, highly proliferative and active cells, including cancer and activated immune cells, require large amounts of biomolecular building blocks to fuel extensive synthetic requirements for proteins, nucleic acids, and lipids (Figure 31.1). While some of these can be synthesized from *de novo* pathways, many biomolecular building blocks must be directly imported from the extracellular environment. In either case, the high demand for essential nutrients or nutrients required to drive de novo pathways (e.g., glucose or glutamine) can form the basis for a metabolic battleground within the TME.

Immune Cell Anabolism

Amino Acids

Amino acids are vital for cellular synthesis of proteins and nucleic acids. Upon activation, Teff cells become highly amino-acid avid, markedly upregulating several key amino acid transporters, including SLC7A5 (transporter for large neutral amino acids, such as leucine and tryptophan), SLC38A1/2 (sodium-dependent cotransporter for glutamine and neutral amino acids), and SLC1A5 (sodium-dependent cotransporter for glutamine, asparagine, and neutral amino acids).[116–118] Interestingly, while deletion of SLC7a5 led to failure during in vitro Teff cell activation, T_{reg} cell differentiation was unaffected.[119,120] Arginine is highly metabolized by activated T cells, with increased extracellular arginine especially important for generation of long-lived T memory cells.[121] Arginine is also important for NK cell function, with low arginine levels suppressing NK cell proliferation and cytokine production.[98,122,123] Additionally, through the expression of high levels of inducible nitric oxide synthase (iNOS), inflammatory macrophages are critically reliant on sufficient arginine to fuel generation of cytotoxic nitric oxide, a potent antitumor effector molecule.[124,125,126] Glutamine, tryptophan, serine, and cysteine are also well established as critical nutrients for activated T cell function.[116,127–130]

Glutamine is in particularly high demand for many cancer cell types, as well as for activated T cells and inflammatory macrophages. Glutamine contributes to biosynthetic processes in two fundamental ways. It is both the primary source of nitrogen for biosynthesis of amino acids and nucleic acids, as well as the critical source of carbon skeletons for replenishing TCA cycle intermediates, a process called anaplerosis. Anaplerosis is a vital facet of highly active cells in that TCA intermediates are themselves critical raw materials for biosynthetic processes such as production of amino acids, nucleic acids, and lipids. For example, the TCA cycle metabolite citrate can be exported to the cytoplasm where it is converted to acetyl COA to fuel cholesterol and phospholipid biosynthesis, which is critical for plasma membrane generation. As these intermediates are taken away from the TCA cycle to fuel biosynthesis, glutamine, through its proximal metabolite a-ketoglutarate, allows continued function of the cycle. As such, glutamine also supports energetics through fueling the TCA cycle and OXPHOS. Because glutamine is involved in fueling a broad array of metabolic processes, the effect of glutamine restriction on dynamic cell populations such as activated T cells can be multifaceted as well as highly specific to a particular cell state. For instance, while glutamine deprivation can profoundly hamper the function and proliferation of differentiated Teff cells,[116] it can also alter differentiation during activation of naïve T cell priming, leading to the development of long-lived memory T cells.[131] While the former is antithetical to optimal antitumor response, the latter may aid in supporting long-term responses. To this end, combining glutamine blockade with anti-PD-1 checkpoint blockade in mouse models is able to generate a high proportion of long-lived antitumor T cells that markedly improve the efficacy of checkpoint blockade.[34]

Lipids

Lipid synthesis is a vital aspect of immune cell function, especially for inflammatory macrophages and highly proliferative post-activation T cells.[132] As such, antiviral activity of Teff cells is critically dependent on activation-induced metabolic reprogramming by sterol regulatory element-binding protein 1 (SREBP1) and SREBP2 activity. SREBP1 and SREBP2 induce de novo lipid synthesis and cholesterol uptake, respectively.[133,134] The importance of cholesterol metabolism to activated Teff cells is also demonstrated by the role of acetyl-CoA acetyltransferase (ACAT1). ACAT1 typically catalyzes the esterification and storage of cholesterol ester in neutral lipid droplets. In ACAT1 knockout T cells, absence of this enzyme causes redirection of cholesterol metabolism and favors increased membrane cholesterol.[134] Increased membrane cholesterol facilitated clustering of the T cell receptor, enhancing signaling and improving effector function and proliferation of antitumor Teff cells in mouse models. A significant improvement in tumor control in mouse models of melanoma was noted when mice were treated with the pharmacologic ACAT1 inhibitor, avasimibe.[134]

Challenges to Immune Cell Anabolic Metabolism in the Tumor Microenvironment

The TME can present clear hurdles to anabolic metabolic programs that are crucial for effective immune response (Figure 31.3). This mechanism of immune evasion is perhaps most clearly demonstrated in studies of amino acid metabolism within the TME. Tryptophan and arginine, which are critical for Teff function, are actively depleted in the TME by a variety of cells. Cancer cells, MDSCs, cancer-associated fibroblasts, and anti-inflammatory macrophages can each express high levels of the tryptophan-depleting enzyme indoleamine 2,3-dioxygenase (IDO).[135] Distinct from inflammatory macrophages, anti-inflammatory macrophages and MDSCs upregulate arginase 1 (ARG1), which leads to significant depletion of arginine within the TME.[136–139] While depletion of tryptophan and arginine can starve immune effector cells of critical nutrients, the products of these enzymatic processes are, in and of themselves, immunosuppressive. Specifically, polyamines and the amino acid kynurenine, products of ARG1 and IDO activity, respectively, have been shown to be highly immunosuppressive in preclinical studies.[136–140] IDO blockade has shown significant impact in rescuing immune responses in mouse studies, though clinical studies have thus far failed to demonstrate significant benefit. ARG1 inhibitors are presently being investigated as a single agent and in combination with checkpoint blockade in clinical trials.

Until recently, the contribution of lipid biology to immune cell function in the TME was not well studied. However, several recent reports have begun to uncover the notable impact of lipid biology in this regard. Despite the beneficial effect of ACAT1 blockade in upregulating cholesterol content in T cell plasma membrane and associated enhancement of TCR signaling, Ma et al. have demonstrated that high cholesterol content in tumors can induce a robust endoplasmic stress response leading to T cell dysfunction.[141] Similarly, Manzo et al. have recently reported that accumulation of specific long-chain fatty acids in the TME impaired mitochondrial function of infiltrating T cells. T cell metabolism, function, and survival could be augmented by forced expression of the very-long-chain acyl-CoA dehydrogenase (VLCAD) enzyme as a means to catabolize toxic fatty acids.[142] Interestingly, a recent study by Wang et al. demonstrated that intratumoral T_{reg} cells can adapt to lipid conditions in the TME by expression of the lipid transporter CD36.[143] CD36 inhibition led to T_{reg} cell instability, enhanced Teff cell function, and significantly improved antitumor responses. Notably, CD36-mediated fatty acid uptake is also a critical mechanism of activation for immune suppressive M2-like macrophages.[144] Lastly, in a study of ovarian cancer, it was found that high expression of fatty acid synthase (FAS) led to marked fatty acid accumulation in mouse tumor models, which subsequently led to DC cell functional defects and blunted T cell activation.[81]

THERAPEUTIC IMPLICATIONS OF CANCER IMMUNOMETABOLISM

As better tools for studying cellular metabolism emerge, a progressively clarified understanding of immune cell metabolism in the context of cancer will uncover novel targets to enhance immunotherapy. Although there is significant overlap in metabolic pathways in cancer and many immune cell subtypes, cell types may often have heretofore unsuspected vulnerabilities which can be differentially targeted to great effect. For example, marked improvements in antitumor immune responses in the setting of glutamine blockade have been observed in mouse tumor models.[34] In these studies, alternative metabolic pathways (upregulation of acetate metabolism with concomitant increased glucose anaplerosis through the pyruvate carboxylase pathway)—pathways that were not accessible to the cancer cells— were identified in antitumor Teff cells that allowed these cells to thrive during glutamine blockade. Exploiting this differential metabolic flexibility effectively reset the metabolic balance of power in the TME and produced significant improvement in cure rates. In addition, other studies have demonstrated that glutamine blockade simultaneously induces immunogenic cell death in cancer cells, as well as remodels the myeloid compartment in the TME from a highly immunosuppressive population to an inflammatory one.[145] Recent studies using the folate pathway inhibitor, pemetrexed, in combination with PD-1 blockade has similarly shown a dramatic enhancement of mitochondrial function and T cell activation, while simultaneously inducing immunogenic cell death in cancer cells, allowing significant improvement in antitumor responses in clinical trials.[146]

This proposed paradigm of inducing differential metabolic programs in cancer and antitumor immune cells to tip the scales in favor of antitumor immune response is further underlined by the metabolic effects of checkpoint blockade. Several studies have emerged detailing the effect of checkpoint pathways on metabolic pathways. Notably, cell intrinsic signaling of the PD-1/PD-L1 pathway on cancer cells and T cells trigger divergent metabolic programming in each of these cell types.[15,147] Chang et al.[15] demonstrated that PD-L1 signaling can drive AKT-mediated glycolysis and glucose uptake. In another study, PD-1 and CTLA-4 signaling suppressed glucose metabolism as a mechanism of T cell suppression. Because of the overlap between checkpoint signaling and metabolic reprogramming, the combination of metabolic approaches within current anti-PD-1 regimens is particularly attractive as a therapeutic approach.

Adoptive cell transfer (ACT) offers a particularly attractive platform for metabolic control of immunotherapeutic responses. As discussed, metabolic interventions, such as blockade of glycolysis or glutamine metabolism, may induce phenotypic changes in active immune cells that could be beneficial for T cell function and/or longevity. As such, genetic editing of metabolic pathways during ex vivo CAR T cell reprogramming, for example, presents a feasible approach to induce precisely defined metabolic interventions. A recent study demonstrated this approach through forced expression of mitochondrial-inducing peroxisome proliferator-activated receptor-γ co-activator 1α (PGC1α) in adoptively transferred CD8$^+$ T cells.[122] By enforcing mitochondrial biogenesis in this way, the authors reported enhanced intratumoral T cell function and tumor control in mouse models. As our understanding of the full range of metabolic pathways accessible to antitumor immune cells grows, this synthetic biologic approach can broaden our ability to produce highly defined T cell phenotypes with predictable metabolic capabilities tailored for long-lived activity and tumor control.

CONCLUSION

The TME presents significant hurdles to mounting an effective immune response. Tumors are highly active, heterogeneous, and complex metabolic tissues. As such, the large range of cell types and array of metabolic phenotypes require careful examination to infer specific vulnerabilities and capacities. That said, studies are beginning to reveal the remarkable therapeutic potential attainable through metabolic intervention of cancer immunity. Future studies enlisting systems biology approaches will undoubtedly be critical in elucidating metabolic patterns and opportunities. While the inherent complexities of the system pose a formidable challenge, the breadth of metabolic pathways and phenotypes at play also offers significant promise for reconfiguring the metabolic balance of power from immune evasion to immune response.

KEY REFERENCES

Only key references appear in the print edition. The full reference list appears in the digital product on Springer Publishing Connect: connect.springerpub.com/content/book/978-0-8261-3743-2/part/part02/chapter/ch31

4. Frauwirth KA, Riley JL, Harris MH, et al. The CD28 signaling pathway regulates glucose metabolism. *Immunity*. 2002;16(6):769–777. doi:10.1016/s1074-7613(02)00323-0

14. Cascone T, Mckenzie JA, Mbofung RM, et al. Increased tumor glycolysis characterizes immune resistance to adoptive T cell therapy. *Cell Metab*. 2018;27(5):977–987. doi:10.1016/j.cmet.2018.02.024

15. Chang CH, Qiu J, O'Sullivan D, et al. Metabolic competition in the tumor microenvironment is a driver of cancer progression. *Cell*. 2015;162(6):1229–1241. doi:10.1016/j.cell.2015.08.016

16. Ho PC, Bihuniak JD, Macintyre AN, et al. Phosphoenolpyruvate is a metabolic checkpoint of anti-tumor T cell responses. *Cell*. 2015;162(6):1217–1228. doi:10.1016/j.cell.2015.08.012

34. Leone RD, Zhao L, Englert JM, et al. Glutamine blockade induces divergent metabolic programs to overcome tumor immune evasion. *Science*. 2019;366(6468):1013–1021. doi:10.1126/science.aav2588

112. Scharping NE, Menk AV, Moreci RS, et al. The tumor microenvironment represses T cell mitochondrial biogenesis to drive intratumoral T cell metabolic insufficiency and dysfunction. *Immunity*. 2016;45(2):374–388. doi:10.1016/j.immuni.2016.07.009

32

Principles of Combination Immunotherapies

Inderjit Mehmi, Raphael Brandao, Omid Hamid, and Patrick A. Ott

KEY POINTS

- The clinical efficacy of single-agent programmed cell death 1 (PD-1) pathway inhibition across subsets of patients with solid and hematologic malignancies coupled with low toxicity provides a rationale for combination immunotherapy with PD-1 or programmed cell death ligand 1 (PD-L1) directed agents as the backbone. Additive or even synergistic effects can be achieved using agents that target tumor growth and immune regulatory pathways.

- Combining immunotherapy with standard-of-care approaches, such as chemotherapy and radiation therapy, may enhance immune responses through neoantigen release and inducing interferon-gamma (IFN-γ) signatures; counteracting immunosuppressive mechanisms in the tumor by targeting T cell immunoglobulin and mucin domain-containing 3 (TIM-3), lymphocyte activation gene 3 protein (LAG-3), T cell immunoreceptor with Ig and ITIM domains (TIGIT), and B- and T-lymphocyte attenuator (BTLA) are also potentially attractive combination approaches.

- The tumor microenvironment (TME), macrophage-associated colony-stimulating factor 1 receptor (CSF-1R), myeloid-derived stem cells, and T cell suppressive indoleamine 2,3-dioxygenase (IDO) and vascular endothelial growth factor (VEGF) are novel targets for combination immunotherapy.

- Current combination trials highlight the challenges and risks in using immuno-oncology agents at standard doses and schedules. It is reasonable to anticipate that adjustments in standard dosing and schedules will be necessary to appropriately balance clinical benefit against acceptable safety and tolerability.

- Despite numerous advances, overall response rates (ORRs) across clinical trials still average less than 50%, and unusual response patterns including delayed or mixed tumor regression pose a further clinical dilemma. These challenges underscore the need for biomarker development to help identify patients who will derive the most clinical benefit, and also provide early recognition of nonresponders.

INTRODUCTION

The striking antitumor activity of immune checkpoint blocking antibodies in a wide spectrum of solid and hematologic malignancies has substantially increased the scope of immunotherapy for cancer. Only recently considered a niche treatment for select cancers, such as renal cancer and melanoma, cancer immunotherapy has become an increasingly important treatment tool for oncologists, even moving into the first-line systemic treatment setting for melanoma, non-small cell lung cancer (NSCLC), renal cell carcinoma (RCC), and potentially a number of other malignancies. Programmed cell death 1 (PD-1) inhibitors are already approved in several solid and hematologic malignancies including melanoma, Merkel cell carcinoma, cutaneous squamous cell carcinoma, hepatocellular carcinoma, NSCLC, RCC, bladder cancer, Hodgkin lymphoma, and head and neck cancer, along with a broad category of tumors with microsatellite instability high phenotype (MSI-H). A turning point was the recognition that these antibodies could be effective in cancers, such as NSCLC, long-considered nonresponsive to immune interventions.[1]

Fast-paced clinical development testing the safety and antitumor activity of anti-PD-1 and programmed cell death ligand 1 (PD-L1) antibodies in the entire spectrum of solid and hematologic malignancies has proven that these agents are safe across tumors and are effective in a subset of patients in almost every tumor type tested. However, while response rates (RRs) with monotherapy have been high in some tumors, such as melanoma, Hodgkin lymphoma, and Merkel cell cancer, single-agent PD-1/PD-L1 inhibition typically achieves relatively low RRs in unselected patient cohorts (an average of 10%–30% across trials). These RRs can be increased by enriching study populations with the use of predictive biomarkers, including assessment of PD-L1 expression by tumor and/or immune cells, CD8$^+$ T cell infiltrates in the tumor microenvironment (TME), interferon-gamma (IFN-γ)-centric gene expression profiles, and high tumor cell mutational load. However, patient selection using predictive biomarkers effectively eliminates some patients from consideration for potential benefit from these agents. An alternative or complementary strategy is combination therapy, such that the proportion of responding patients can be increased by combining other agents or interventions with PD-1 blockade.

In principle, the efficacy of PD-1-blocking therapies might be improved with the following interventions: (a) expansion of the peripheral tumor-specific T cell repertoire (through checkpoint inhibition, engaging co-stimulatory receptors, vaccines, cytolytic viral therapy, and cytokines); (b) induction of an innate immune response to tumor (through radiation, cytolytic viral therapy, IFN, and Toll-like receptor [TLR]/stimulator of interferon gene [STING] pathways); or (c) counteracting other immunosuppressive mechanisms in the tumor and its microenvironment (depletion of regulatory T cells [T$_{reg}$ cells], blockade of inhibitory receptors [T cell immunoglobulin and mucin domain-containing 3 (TIM-3) and lymphocyte

activation gene 3 protein (LAG-3)], T cell immunoreceptor with Ig and ITIM domains (TIGIT), B- and T-lymphocyte attenuator (BTLA), blockade of macrophage-associated CSF-1R, depletion of myeloid-derived suppressor cells [MDSCs], adenosine, and vascular endothelial growth factor [VEGF]). A summary of these varying mechanisms may be found in Table 32.1 and is described in further detail in this chapter.

Given the heterogeneity of patient populations and tumor types, predictive and prognostic biomarkers of response are an intense area of clinical investigation. Identifying subgroups of patients with higher likelihood of response therefore not only helps profile future populations of eligible patients, but also identifies patient subgroups for whom combination therapy may be more effective and appropriate. Considering the host of resistance mechanisms that can be in the way of a successful antitumor immune response, the observation of durable antitumor activity with single receptor–ligand inhibition with anti-PD-1 agents is in fact rather surprising. Indeed, it has already become clear from a number of trials investigating monotherapy with antibodies against other immune checkpoints and agonistic antibodies (i.e., LAG-3, CD137, OX-40, ICOS, GITR, and CD40) that these agents have modest (if any) single-agent activity. Thus, PD-1 blockade may be rather exceptional in terms of its single-agent activity and relatively benign toxicity profile.

Stimulated largely by clinical activity of immune checkpoint inhibitors, which provided a proof of principle that immunotherapy can be effective for cancer patients beyond cancers known to be "immune responsive," a

Table 32.1 Mechanisms of Inducing an Antitumor Response

EXPANSION OF PERIPHERAL TUMOR-SPECIFIC T CELL REPERTOIRE	INDUCTION OF INNATE IMMUNE RESPONSE IN TUMOR OR LYMPHATIC ORGANS	COUNTERACT IMMUNE SUPPRESSIVE MECHANISMS IN THE TUMOR			
		INHIBITORY RECEPTORS	SUPPRESSIVE IMMUNE CELLS	INHIBITORY METABOLIC PATHWAYS	ANGIOGENESIS/ INHIBITORY SOLUBLE FACTORS
CTLA-4 inhibition	TLR agonist	Anti-PD-1/PD-L1	T$_{reg}$ cell depletion	Arginase inhibitors	Anti-VEGF
Enhancement of co-stimulation (CD28, CD40, OX-40, 4-1BB)	STING agonist	Anti-LAG-3	TAM polarization (CSF-1R—blockade)	A2aR inhibition	Anti-Ang-2
Vaccines	Radiation	Anti-TIM-3	MDSC depletion		
Cytolytic viral therapy	Cytolytic viral therapy	Anti-KIR TIGIT inhibition			
IL-2	IFNα, GM-CSF	BTLA inhibition			

A2ar, adenosine receptor 2a; BTLA, B- and T-lymphocyte attenuator; CSF-1R, colony-stimulating factor 1 receptor; CTLA-4, cytotoxic T lymphocytic antigen 4; GM-CSF, granulocyte-macrophage colony-stimulating factor; IFN, interferon; KIR, killer cell immunoglobulin-like receptor; LAG-3, lymphocyte-activation gene 3; MDSC, myeloid-derived suppressor cells; PD-1, programmed cell death-ligand 1; STING, stimulator of interferon genes; TAM, tumor-associated macrophage; TIGIT, T cell immunoreceptor with Ig and ITIM domains; TIM, T cell immunoglobulin and mucin-domain containing-3; TLR, Toll-like receptor; T$_{reg}$, regulatory T; VEGF, vascular endothelial growth factor;

large number of immunotherapeutic agents are currently in preclinical and clinical testing. Although this expanded development platform provides a tremendous opportunity, it also harbors considerable challenges for the field. The number of combinations that can theoretically be tested is substantially higher than the available resources (e.g., financial, patients, infrastructure), and there are already more than 1,000 cancer immunotherapy trials ongoing, many of which are exclusively combinatorial or include combinatorial regimens. Judicious trial design must acknowledge not only these limitations but also must incorporate better understanding of the complexities of an antitumor immune response. As this chapter later aims to illustrate, this response consists of several components that are regulated on multiple levels in a coordinated temporal–spatial fashion and is dependent on both host and tumor immune dynamics.

BUILDING COMBINATION THERAPIES ON THE BACKBONE OF THE PROGRAMMED CELL DEATH 1 PATHWAY INHIBITION

General Concepts

The clinical efficacy of a single-agent PD-1 pathway inhibition across subsets of patients with solid and hematologic malignancies coupled with low toxicity provides a rationale for combination immunotherapy with PD-1 or PD-L1-directed agents as the backbone. Preclinical mouse studies and early clinical trial data have indicated that additive or even synergistic effects can be achieved using agents that target distinct immune regulatory pathways. The correlation between baseline CD8+ T cell infiltration and IFN-γ gene signatures in the tumor and response to PD-1 inhibition in melanoma and other tumors indicate that T cell inflammation of a tumor is a prerequisite for maximal efficacy of PD-1 inhibition. The absence of T cell infiltration in a tumor may be due to (a) lack of an innate immune response, (b) lack of chemokine secretion, or (c) activation of tumor cell intrinsic oncogenic pathways that actively undermine an antitumor immune response as has been shown for the β-catenin pathway.[2] There are many therapeutic strategies that can increase frequencies of tumor-specific T cells and potentially mediate increased trafficking of T cells into the tumor. They include cancer vaccines, oncolytic viral therapy, co-stimulatory molecule stimulation, targeted therapy, radiation, chemotherapy, and adoptive cell transfer (ACT; T cells, chimeric antigen receptors [CARs]). These interventions may therefore be particularly useful in tumor types with low or absent RRs with PD-1/PD-L1-directed monotherapy. Combination approaches built on the backbone of PD-1 pathway inhibition that counteract additional inhibitory mechanisms in the TME, such as IDO inhibition, transforming growth factor beta (TGF-β) blockade, regulatory T cell (T_reg cell)

depletion, and angiogenesis inhibition, may be particularly appropriate for T cell inflamed tumors to enhance or rescue tumor responses achieved with anti-PD-1/PD-L1 monotherapy. The myriad of potential therapeutic approaches built on an anti-PD-1/PD-L1 "backbone" is illustrated in Figure 32.1.

Looking ahead to the future of precision therapy and personalized medicine, selection of appropriate patients for specific combinations may be guided by predictive biomarkers, although valuable biomarkers for combinations may be distinct from monotherapies as the experience of tumor PD-L1 expression with PD-1 inhibition versus combined PD-1 and cytotoxic T lymphocytic antigen 4 (CTLA-4) inhibition in advanced melanoma has shown.

"IMMUNO PLUS IMMUNO" COMBINATION THERAPIES

Blockade of Inhibitory Receptors

The U.S. Food and Drug Administration (FDA) approval of the anti-CTLA-4 antibody ipilimumab for metastatic melanoma heralded the arrival of modern immunotherapy in solid tumor oncology, the success of which was further bolstered by later FDA approvals of the anti-PD-1 drugs nivolumab and pembrolizumab. Acting through different mechanisms of T cell stimulation, it was postulated that combined inhibition of both pathways would have an enhanced effect.[3-5] The synergy of combined PD-1/PD-L1 and CTLA-4 inhibition was shown in the B16 melanoma model and other preclinical models.[3] Based on this evidence, a remarkably successful clinical trial program combining the α-PD-1 antibody nivolumab and the α-CTLA-4 antibody ipilimumab demonstrated an initial RR of more than 50% in metastatic melanoma; the majority of responses were rapid (evident at the time of the first radiographic assessment at 12 weeks) and durable.[5] Consistent RRs of nearly 60% and superior progression-free survival (PFS), and updated data showing 5-year OS of 50% for patients treated with combination compared to 26% for patients treated with monotherapy ipilimumab was shown in Phase 2 and 3 trials, leading to FDA approval of this combination for advanced melanoma in the United States in 2015.[3-5] This impressive antitumor activity of combined PD-1 and CTLA-4 inhibition in melanoma has triggered the initiation of clinical trials testing combined with CTLA-4 pathway inhibition with either anti-PD-1 or anti-PD-L1 antibodies in a number of cancers, including lung cancer (small cell and non-small cell), renal cell cancer, hepatocellular carcinoma, colorectal cancer, bladder cancer, and a number of other malignancies. A summary of key combination immunotherapy trials are listed in Table 32.2, and trial data are discussed in further detail in this chapter. Initial assessments of clinical efficacy appear superior compared with

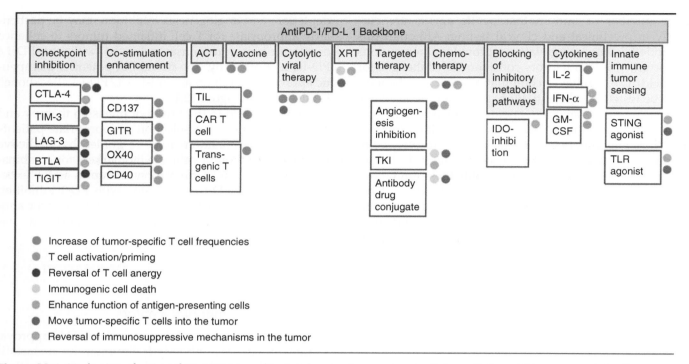

Figure 32.1 Mechanism of action of PD-1/PD-L1 combinatorial partnering agents potentially mediating additive or synergistic effects.

ACT, adoptive cell transfer; BTLA, B- and T-lymphocyte attenuator; CAR, chimeric antigen receptor; CTLA-4, cytotoxic T lymphocytic antigen 4; GITR, glucocorticoid-induced TNFR-related protein; GM-CSF, granulocyte macrophage-colony stimulating factor; GITR, glucocorticoid induced tumor necrosis factor receptor; IDO, indoleamine 2,3-dioxygenase; IFN, interferon; IL-2, interleukin 2; LAG-3, lymphocyte activation gene 3 protein; PD-1, programmed cell death 1; STING, stimulator of IFN genes; TIGIT, T cell immunoreceptor with Ig and ITIM domains; TIL, tumor-infiltrating lymphocyte; TIM, T cell immunoglobulin and mucin domain-containing 3; TKI, tyrosine kinase inhibitor; TLR, Toll-like receptor; XRT, radiotherapy.

Table 32.2 Combination Immunotherapy Trials With Additive/Synergistic Activity

COMBINATION	CANCER TYPE	DEVELOPMENT STAGE WITH DOCUMENTED EFFICACY	OBJECTIVE RESPONSE RATE	CURRENT DEVELOPMENT STAGE
α-CTLA-4 plus α-PD-1/PD-L1	Melanoma	Phase 1–3	55%–61%	FDA approved
α-CTLA-4 plus α-PD-1/PD-L1	Other solid tumors	Phase 1–2	38%–40% (RCC) 39% (NSCLC) 26%–38% (TCC) 33% (HCC) 46% (MSI-H/dMMR mCRC)	FDA approved in RCC Under priority review in NSCLC FDA approved in HCC FDA approved in mCRC with MSI-H/dMMR
α-CTLA-4 plus GM-CSF	Melanoma	Phase 1	21%	Phase 2
α-CTLA-4 plus TVEC	Melanoma	Phase 1	50%	Phase 2
α-PD-1 plus IDO inhibitor	Melanoma, NSCLC, RCC	Phase 1	57% (melanoma) 40% (RCC)	Studies halted due to lack of efficacy
α-PD-1 plus TVEC	Melanoma	Phase 1	48%	Phase 3
α-PD-L1 plus bevacizumab	Melanoma	Phase 1	DCR 67%	Phase 2
α-PD-L1 plus BRAF and MEK inhibitors	Melanoma	Phase 1	RR 70%	Phase 2

CTLA-4, cytotoxic T lymphocytic antigen 4; DCR, disease control rate; FDA, U.S. Food and Drug Administration; GM-CSF, granulocyte-macrophage colony-stimulating factor; HCC, hepatocellular carcinoma; IDO, indoleamine 2,3-dioxygenase; mCRC, metastatic colorectal cancer; NSCLC, non-small cell lung cancer; PD-L1, programmed cell death-ligand 1; RCC, renal cell carcinoma; SCLC, small cell lung cancer; TCC, transitional cell carcinoma; TVEC, talimogene laherepavec.

anti-PD-1/PD-L1 monotherapy previously reported in several tumor types. There is a preclinical rationale for the combination of PD-1 inhibition with a blockade of other inhibitory receptors, such as TIM-3 and LAG-3, that has been further supported by clinical studies that are ongoing either as single agents or in combination with PD-1/PD-L1. Preclinical evidence for synergy between PD-1 pathway blockade and LAG-3 inhibition as well as TIM-3 inhibition, respectively, has been reported.[6,7] A number of early phase trials are ongoing that evaluate safety and efficacy of these targets in combination with PD-1/PD-L1 inhibition. Harding et al. reported a Phase 1/1a study testing an anti-TIM-3 antibody as monotherapy or in combination with anti PD-L1.[8] Data reported in 23 patients that the combination was well tolerated (most AEs were less than grade 2, with one grade 3 event of anemia). Although limited efficacy data was reported, clinical activity in relapsed/refractory patients was demonstrated. Blockade of another inhibitory receptor, LAG-3, has been pursued in multiple clinical trials. Eastgate et al. reported Eftilagimod alpha LAG-3-fusion protein's activity in combination with anti-PD-1, pembrolizumab, in unresectable/metastatic melanoma.[9] In this Phase 1 dose escalation study, 18 patients who had previously been treated with pembrolizumab and showed refractory disease, no dose limiting toxicities were observed. Eight of 16 patients who were eligible for response evaluation had tumor regression.[9] However, in a larger Phase 1/2 study of LAG525 (LAG-3 humanized IgG4 mab) +/- spartalizumab (anti-PD mAb), clinical efficacy was modest.[10] The combination arm of this study showed dose limiting toxicity in four patients (grade 3 hyperglycemia, pneumonitis, brain tumor edema, fatigue, and grade 4 autoimmune hepatitis). There were 12 responses (11 PRs, one CR) in patients with solid tumors, whereas therapy was discontinued in 99/121 due to disease progression. Phase 2 evaluation in selected cohorts is ongoing (NCT02460224). A number of additional clinical trials targeting TIGIT are in early phases (NCT04150965 and NCT02913313).

Stimulation of Co-Stimulatory Receptors With Agonistic Antibodies

Co-stimulatory receptors including CD137 (also known as 4-1BB), glucocorticoid-induced tumor necrosis factor receptor (GITR; CD357), CD40, OX40, and CD27 are expressed predominantly by activated T cells but can also be upregulated by activated natural killer (NK) cells, T_{reg} cells, and other immune cells.[11] Agonistic antibodies may promote NK cell-mediated antibody-dependent cellular cytotoxicity (ADCC).[12] Stimulation of co-stimulatory receptors can increase T cell frequencies in the periphery, modulate T effector (Teff) functions, reverse T cell anergy in the tumor, counteract the suppressive

activity of T_{reg} cells, and enhance cytokine secretion by NK cells. Synergy between PD-1 and CD137 inhibition has been demonstrated preclinically.[12,13] Urelumab, an agonistic CD137 antibody, has been in clinical development for several years. Initial clinical trials were stopped due to hepatotoxicity, leading to substantial dose reduction in later trials. Furthermore, aggregated analysis of three studies showed that dose of 0.1 mg/kg every 3 weeks carried the immune stimulation function and had a safety profile that was acceptable.[14] In particular, doses greater than 1 mg/kg showed significant incidence of hepatotoxicity. The combination of urelumab with the α-PD-1 antibody nivolumab was studied in NSCLC, squamous cell head and neck cancer, and lymphoma.[15] Initially reported RRs in these four cancers were modest and not higher compared with historical controls of PD-1 monotherapy. A second CD137 agonist, utomilumab, has also been evaluated in a Phase 1 study as a single agent.[16] In this study, 55 patients were evaluated for safety, tolerability, pharmokinetics, preliminary clinical activity, and pharmacodynamics. The ORR was found to be only 3.8%; the incidence of hepatotoxicity was much lower at the doses tested. From these two studies, it seems that CD137 is a suboptimal target for a single agent approach; perhaps a combination with anti-PD-1/PD-L1 will yield desired responses in a first-line setting or in refractory setting. GITR is a co-stimulatory molecule expressed primarily by T_{reg} cells, effector T cells, and NK cells that inhibit the suppressive activity of T_{reg} cells. AMG 228, an agonistic human IgG1 monoclonal antibody that binds to GITR, was studied in a Phase 1 setting involving heavily pretreated solid malignancies.[17] This 30-patient study included mCRC, HNSCC, TCC, NSCLC, and melanoma. Overall, ANG 228 was well tolerated with most adverse events being low grade.[1-2] However, 12 patients (40%) had serious adverse events that were considered treatment related and included one death due to pneumonitis related to AMG 228. Additionally, there was modest anti-tumor activity with single agent therapy. Combination strategies with anti-PD-1/PD-L1 are currently being evaluated in multiple clinical trials. Another co-stimulatory molecule of interest, OX-40, which is primarily expressed on activated T cells, has been in clinical development as a single agent or in combination with PD-1/PD-L1 backbone. Hamid et al. presented data on a first-in-human study of PF-8600 as a single agent, an OX40 agonist fully human IgG2 mAB. The reported data in a small number of patients demonstrated tolerability and some clinical activity. The most common adverse event reported was fatigue (33%). Four patients of nine had the best ORR of stable disease.[18] Follow-up combination studies with anti-PD-1/PD-L1 are ongoing. Lastly, CD27, another co-stimulatory molecule, has entered the clinical picture with early data showing clinical activity as a single agent and in combination with anti-PD-1/PD-L1.[19]

However, caution is encouraged, since most of the trials are in their early phase and reports available, if any, are on a small number of patients with select cohorts.

Vaccines and Toll-Like Receptor Agonists

The antitumor activity of PD-1/PD-L1-directed therapy may be compromised by a limited preexisting pool of both naïve and primed tumor-specific T cells. An effective cancer vaccine has the potential to expand preexisting tumor-reactive T cells and to stimulate naïve tumor-reactive T cells, thereby broadening the tumor-specific T cell repertoire. A therapeutic vaccine is composed of a target antigen and an immunological adjuvant; tumor antigens used for cancer vaccines have included differentiation antigens, cancer-testis antigens, tumor-associated viral antigens, and overexpressed antigens. Antigens can be delivered in the form of protein, peptide, RNA, recombinant DNA transfected into viral vectors, or whole tumor cell lysates engineered to secrete cytokines, such as granulocyte-macrophage colony-stimulating factor (GM-CSF) or fms-like tyrosine kinase 3 (FLT-3) ligand. The immune adjuvant is designed to provide the necessary inflammatory context leading to activation of antigen-presenting cells (APCs), most importantly dendritic cells (DCs); examples of effective adjuvants are TLR agonists, cytokines, and agonists for co-stimulatory molecules. There is now compelling evidence supporting neoantigens as the targets of effective tumor-specific T cell responses, and multiple studies in a number of cancers have shown a correlation between effectiveness of checkpoint therapy and neoantigen load.[20] Expansion of neoantigen-specific T cells has also been demonstrated in various effective treatment settings including ACT,[21] checkpoint blockade,[22] and stem cell transplantation.[23] Neoantigen-reactive T cells were found to effectively kill cancer in both mice and humans. These data provide a strong rationale for vaccination targeting neoantigens as a personalized cancer therapy approach, and portends synergistic combination with immune checkpoint inhibition, particularly the PD-1 pathway inhibition. Evidence for vaccine and anti PD-1 combination has been observed in several small early phase trials. Ott et al. reported a Phase 1b study testing NEO-PV-01 (a personalized neoantigen vaccine) in combination with nivolumab.[24] In an interim report, encouraging antitumor activity was seen in 34 patients (16 with melanoma, 11 with NSCLC, and seven with bladder cancer). The combination was well tolerated with adverse events including injection site reaction and flu-like symptoms.[24] Other personalized neoantigen vaccines are being tested in clinical trials (NCT03639714, NCT03289962).

Toll-like receptor 9 agonism has revealed promising activity in metastatic melanoma patients. Two studies testing TLR9 agonists SD-101 and CMP-001, both in combination with pembrolizumab, are ongoing. Early phase data presented by Milhem et al. of combination approach with CMP-001 (CpG-A oligodeoxynucleotide packaged in viral -ike particle, TLR-9 agonist) and pembrolizumab in 68 patients (44 in dose escalation and 24 in dose expansion) showed an ORR 23% in patients with anti-PD-1 resistant advanced melanoma.[25] Safety data was reported in 63 patients, and combination was tolerable with adverse events of greater than grade 3 to 4 of hypotension (7), anemia (2), chills (2), hypertension (2), and fever (2). SD-101, a synthetic CpG oligonucleotide in combination with pembrolizumab, was evaluated in treatment-naïve advanced melanoma patients.[26] In 86 patients, ORR was 71% with responses in both injected and noninjected lesions. The combination was well tolerated; adverse events ≥ grade 3 included headache (7%), fatigue (7%), malaise (5%), myalgia (4%), and chills (4%).

Adoptive T Cell Therapy

A direct method to increase frequencies of tumor-specific T cells is the adoptive transfer of large numbers of T cells after in vitro expansion. This approach has been effective in advanced melanoma patients using tumor-infiltrating lymphocytes (TILs) harvested from surgically resected tumor. For maximal efficacy (and to deplete non-TIL lymphocytes in bone marrow and circulation) patients are treated with myeloablative chemotherapy and whole-body irradiation followed by high-dose interleukin-2 (IL-2) following the TIL transfer. To date, this therapy has only been available at a few select, highly experienced centers with RRs of more than 50% consistently reported; however, RRs are presumably lower in an intention-to-treat population. The reasons for dilution of the therapeutic effect are multifactorial, as not all tumors generate sufficient TILs for transfer, patients drop out due to decreasing performance status while TILs are prepared, and myeloablative therapy followed by IL-2 is clinically very challenging. Despite these challenges, recent progress has been reported in patients with melanoma. Sarnaik et al. demonstrated that treatment with cryopreserved autologous TIL in advanced metastatic melanoma patients is feasible, safe, and effective.[27] In 55 patients, the ORR was 38% (21 patients with 2 CR, 18 PR, 1 uPR), with a disease control rate of 76%. Most of these patients had received three or more lines of therapy before enrolling on the study. Additionally, data from Jazaeri et al. showed the safety and efficacy of this approach beyond melanoma.[28] In 27 cervical cancer patients who had progressed on an average of 2.6 lines of therapy, an ORR of 44% and disease control rate of 89% was observed. Novel approaches to adoptive T cell therapy that have shown clinical efficacy in melanoma and other tumors include the use of T cells with transgenic T cell receptors (TCRs) that recognize tumor antigens, CAR T cells, or clonal tumor-derived T cells that are expanded ex vivo after the selection for (neo)antigens are identified in the respective tumors.[29–31]

Given that ACT regimens include cytokine therapy with IL-2 as well as conditioning chemotherapy—interventions that are aimed at sustaining the survival and function of the transferred T cells in vivo and preventing a cytokine sink—ACT arguably by itself is a rationally designed combination immunotherapeutic approach. Numerous clinical studies partnering ACT (TIL, CAR T), or TCR modulation with additional strategies to inhibit suppressive mechanisms or engage T cells in the TME—including anti-PD-1, anti-CTLA-4, and others—are currently underway.

Bispecific Molecules

Bispecific antibodies or molecules are proteins engineered to target multiple antigens and have generated significant interest in cancer immunotherapy. Blinatumomab (Amgen, Thousand Oaks, Ca) is the trailblazing bispecific antibody for B-cell precursor acute lymphoblastic leukemia. It is designed with two specificities: (a) against CD3; (b) against CD19; and allows T cell engagement against leukemia cells.[32] Unfortunately, similar approaches in solid malignancies have not reached the success found in hematologic malignancies. One of the more promising bispecific agents belonging to the ImmTAC (immune-mobilizing monoclonal T cell receptor against cancer) platform has recently demonstrated encouraging clinical activity in patients with metastatic uveal melanoma. Tebentafusp, a first-in-class, bispecific fusion protein that redirects $CD3^+$ T cells to gp100-expressing melanoma cells, has shown promising activity in controlling tumors.[33] IMCgp100-01 evaluated tebentafusp as a single agent in 15 patients with uveal melanoma and resulted in 73% 1-year overall survival. It is well-established that uveal melanoma is a very immune-infiltrate-deprived tumor, with limited treatment options and poor prognosis. The treatment was overall well tolerated, and combination approaches with anti-PD-1/PD-L1 are now ongoing in uveal melanoma, cutaneous melanoma, and other solid malignancies (NCT04262466, NCT03973333).

Cytokines

IL-2 can boost the differentiation of naïve T cells into effector T cells and sustain survival of T cells. In advanced melanoma patients, high-dose IL-2 induced an RR of 10% to 15% with many of these responses being durable, resulting in long-term survival for a small subset of patients.[34] GM-CSF and IFN-α can promote the maturation of DCs, leading to improved priming and activation of T cells. Other cytokines found to expand T cells include IL-7, IL-15, and IL-21. IL-7 and IL-15 have also

been shown to reverse T cell anergy,[35] potentially rescuing the function of T cells that have become anergic in the tumor environment. IL-10 stimulates expansion and cytotoxicity of tumor-infiltrating $CD8^+$ T cells and also inhibits inflammatory $CD4^+$ T cells, thereby suppressing chronic inflammation. In a Phase 1 trial using PEGylated IL-10, safety and single-agent activity in solid tumors was shown, leading to its exploration in combination with PD-1 inhibition and different chemotherapeutic regimens in multiple tumor types.[36]

The use of GM-CSF as an immune-stimulating agent in the treatment of melanoma first emerged in preclinical models in the late 1990s, when Allison et al. demonstrated the synergistic effect of GM-CSF and anti-CTLA-4 therapy in poorly immunogenic murine tumors.[37] Investigators examined the effectiveness of CTLA-4 blockade, alone or in combination with a GM-CSF-expressing tumor cell vaccine, on rejection of a highly tumorigenic, poorly immunogenic murine melanoma. Recently established tumors could be eradicated in 80% (68/85) of the cases using combination treatment, whereas each treatment by itself showed little or no effect. The same treatment regimen was found to be therapeutically effective against the outgrowth of lung metastases, inducing long-term survival. Of all mice surviving after combination treatment, 56% (38/68) developed depigmentation, including CD4-depleted mice, strongly suggesting that the effect was mediated by cytotoxic T lymphocytes (CTLs).

The combination of GM-CSF and anti-CTLA-4 also has important effects on the TME. Investigators examined the impact of an anti-CTLA-4 and a GM-CSF–transduced tumor cell vaccine on the balance of Teffs and T_{reg} cells in an in vivo model of B16/BL6 melanoma.[38] Although anti-CTLA-4 did not deplete T_{reg} cells or permanently impair their function, GM-CSF primed the tumor-reactive Teff compartment, inducing activation, tumor infiltration, and a delay in tumor growth. The combination with CTLA-4 blockade induced greater infiltration and a striking change in the intratumor balance of T_{reg} cells and Teffs that directly correlated with tumor rejection.

A series of Phase 1 studies were carried out to examine whether intralesional GM-CSF could induce regression of subcutaneous melanoma metastases.[39] Thirteen patients had 15–50 doses of GM-CSF injected into two subcutaneous metastases, with one metastasis treated with five injections before excision, whereas the other received weekly injections for up to 6 months. Metastases from the responding patients had marked increases and high absolute numbers of T cell infiltrates into the tumor, particularly of the $CD4^+$ subset.

Systemic GM-CSF has been studied in clinical trials in combination with both high-dose ipilimumab (10 mg/kg) and standard-dose ipilimumab (3 mg/kg). The Eastern Cooperative Oncology Group (ECOG) 1608 trial randomly assigned patients to ipilimumab 10 mg/kg every 3 weeks for four cycles, then maintenance every 12 weeks, or the same schedule plus sargramostim at 250 μg subcutaneously (self-administered) daily for days 1 to 14 of a 21-day cycle, for four cycles.[40] The addition of GM-CSF to ipilimumab significantly improved overall survival (OS), from a median of 12.7 months with ipilimumab alone to 17.5 months ($p = 0.014$), and 1-year OS rates were 52.9% with ipilimumab alone versus 68.9% with the combination. The combination also appeared to reduce the severity of immune-related adverse events (irAEs), as grade 3 to 5 adverse events (AEs) occurred in 45% of the combination arm and 58% of the single-agent arm ($p = 0.038$). At a lower dose of ipilimumab (3 mg/kg) in 32 patients treated at a single institution,[41] combination with GM-CSF yielded similar toxicity and preliminary patient outcomes. The best ORR by Response Evaluation Criteria In Solid Tumors (RECIST) was found to be 21%, and a more favorable toxicity profile was again seen with grade 3 or higher events reported in 9.4% of patients ($n = 3$), in particular colitis, which was lower than the rate of high-grade toxicity seen with administration of ipilimumab 3 mg/kg alone. A clinical trial investigating the combination of ipilimumab and nivolumab with or without GM-CSF (NCT02339571) was halted due to increased toxicity. The combination of tremelimumab, another anti-CTLA-4 antibody, and IFN-α also showed potential synergy in patients with advanced melanoma.[42] Davar et al. evaluated interferon alpha-2b in combination with pembrolizumab in advanced melanoma patients.[43] In this Phase 1b/2 study, 43 patients with cutaneous (76.7%), mucosal (7%), and unknown primary 16.3%) patients were enrolled. The majority of the patients had elevated lactate dehydrogenase (LDH), prior treatment with adjuvant IFN (48.8%), adjuvant ipilimumab (2.3%), or systemic ipilimumab (23.3%). The overall response rate was 60.5%; 46.5% of patients had ongoing responses at a median duration of 25 months. Similarly, PEGylated IL-2 and nivolumab combination has been evaluated in the PIVOT-12 Phase 1/2 study.[44] A proposed advantage of PEGylated IL-2 over IL-2 is that it activates CD122-prefrential IL-2 pathway and increases TIL, T cell clonality, and PD-1 expression.[44] In this study, 41 patients with untreated advanced melanoma were treated with PEGylated IL-2 at 0.006 mg/kg and nivolumab at 360 mg/kg given IV every 3 weeks. This combination was well tolerated, with the most common adverse events being grade 1-2 flu-like symptoms. At a follow-up period of 18.6 months, ORR was 53%, CR 34%, and a median time to achieve CR was 7 months. Lastly, 90% of the patients had 75% reduction in their target lesion(s), considered to be a marker for good outcome. Additionally, clinical trials testing the combination of IL-7, IL-12 in combination with anti PD-1 are ongoing, as is IL-12 in combination with anti-PD-L1. These strategies are attempting to increase the ORR and also capturing more patients who can benefit from immunotherapies for various malignancies.

"IMMUNO PLUS STANDARD OF CARE" COMBINATION THERAPIES

Chemotherapy

Chemotherapy has various effects on the immune response, including modification of the immune microenvironment and potential neoantigen generation by direct tumor mechanisms, including induction of "immunogenic cell death" and possibly accumulation of mutations. Cyclophosphamide, an alkylating chemotherapeutic agent, leads to a reduction in the number and the function of T_{reg} cells in the peripheral blood of cancer patients and may improve the effective induction of $CD4^+$ and $CD8^+$ effector T cells by a tumor vaccine.[45,46] $CD4^+CD25^+$forkhead box p3 (Foxp3$^+$) T_{reg} cells play a key role in the maintenance of peripheral immune tolerance including the prevention of organ-specific autoimmune diseases,[47–49] and T_{reg} cell depletion enhances antitumor T cell responses in melanoma and other cancers.[50,51] In preclinical tumor models, T_{reg} cell depletion has shown synergy with various different immunotherapies.[50,52]

Gemcitabine, a nucleoside analog, has been reported to lead to decreased numbers of MDSCs in tumor-bearing mice while frequencies of $CD4^+$ and $CD8^+$ T cells, NK cells, macrophages, and B cells were unaffected.[53] The combination of carboplatin and paclitaxel was also shown to lower myeloid cells in the peripheral blood of patients with advanced cervical cancer,[54] indicating that chemotherapy may generate a more favorable immune milieu than earlier thought. Chemotherapy can also increase tumor antigen presentation as cancer cell death may lead to neoantigen release, potentially leading to improved priming of tumor-specific T cells in addition to its capacity to directly stimulate immune effectors and inhibit immune suppressive factors.[55] Some chemotherapy agents, including cyclophosphamide, doxorubicin, mitoxantrone, and oxaliplatin, induce immunogenic cell death,[56] which generates an immune response distinct from necrosis and apoptosis. Immunogenic cell death has numerous beneficial effects on the antitumor immune response, including increased uptake of cancer cell-derived antigens by DCs, activation of DCs and T cells, and increased infiltration of the tumor by immune cells. Based on the hypothesis that chemotherapy could be partnered with immunotherapies, a number of trials are ongoing and several have been reported. In the age when data from Phase 2 trials have led to approval by the FDA, large randomized trials when available and carry positive results are very reassuring. IMpower130, KEYNOTE-189, and KEYNOTE-407 are examples of such trials.[57–59] IMpower 130 enrolled 724 patients with metastatic nonsquamous NSCLC, previously untreated, to evaluate chemotherapy with or without atezolizumab (anti-PD-L1 mAb) in a randomized Phase 3 clinical trial. This trial demonstrated clinically significant improvement in median overall survival of 18.6 months for atezolizumab + chemotherapy group versus 13.9 months for the chemotherapy alone group; median progression free survival was 7 months for atezolizumab + chemotherapy versus 5 months for chemotherapy group. A modest increase in treatment-related adverse events was seen in the atezolizumab + chemotherapy arm of the study. Similarly, both KEYNOTE-189 and KEYNOTE-407 evaluated pembrolizumab + chemotherapy and met their endpoints in untreated metastatic NSCLC by showing improvement of median overall survival and progression free survival. Chemoimmunotherapy activity has also been shown in breast cancer: nab-paclitaxel + atezolizumab in metastatic breast cancer;[60] and pembrolizumab + chemotherapy in neoadjuvant setting in early stage breast cancer.[61] Neoadjuvant chemotherapy is a common approach for locally advanced breast cancer, especially high-risk tumors (e.g., triple negative and Her-2 positive breast cancers). Post neoadjuvant chemotherapy, pathological complete response (pCR) has been a surrogate marker for outcomes in breast cancer. To evaluate if addition of pembrolizumab to standard of care chemotherapy will lead to improvement in pCR along with improved event-free survival, KEYNOTE-522 evaluated 602 patients with untreated stage II or III triple-negative breast cancer in a randomized (2:1) Phase 3 trial. Patients were randomized to pembrolizumab + paclitaxel and carboplatin every 3 weeks for four cycles versus placebo + paclitaxel and carboplatin every 3 weeks for four cycles, followed by four cycles of doxorubicin/epirubicin-cyclophosphamide followed by definitive surgery. Up to nine cycles of pembrolizumab or placebo were given in the adjuvant setting. Pembrolizumab addition to the neoadjuvant setting led to 13.6% improvement in pCR, and this addition was well tolerated. Ongoing neoadjuvant trials are evaluating addition of immune checkpoint blockers to other subtypes of breast cancers as well.

Radiation Therapy

Radiation therapy (RT), in addition to its effect on local tumor control, may also increase tumor immunogenicity by inducing tumor cell death.[62] In animal models, radiation has shown synergy with CTLA-4 blockade.[63–65] Irradiation of tumors can induce danger signals (damage-associated molecular patterns [DAMPs]; e.g., heat shock proteins or high-mobility group protein B1 [HMGB1] alarmin protein) that lead to DC activation. In particular, the STING pathway, induced by cyclic guanosine monophosphate-adenosine monophosphate (cGAMP) or DNA released from irradiated cells, is a critical component of the type I IFN-dependent antitumor effects of radiation, including DC activation and radiation-induced adaptive immune responses.[56,62] RT can thus act similar to an immune adjuvant, providing the inflammatory context that activates and promotes immune responses,[66] leading to recruitment of T cells and the production of Th1 cytokines.[67,68] Radiation therapy also facilitates recruitment of effector T cells into tumors through induction of chemokines.[69] Furthermore, RT increases cell adhesion molecules (e.g., intercellular adhesion molecule 1 [ICAM-1]) promoting the extravasation of immune cells.[70] RT when administered with anti CTLA-4-induced diversification of the TCR repertoire of TILs and shaped the repertoire of expanded T cell clones in the B16 melanoma model.[71] Resistance to radiation and CTLA-4 blockade was found to be mediated by upregulation of PD-L1, leading to subsequent inhibition of T cell functionality.

Clinical evidence supporting an abscopal effect was demonstrated in a patient with metastatic melanoma who had developed secondary resistance to maintenance therapy with ipilimumab.[72] Palliative RT to a spinal mass induced regression of nonirradiated splenic and lymph node metastases. A temporal association between a decrease in tumor burden and NY-ESO-1 antibody response, as well as changes in frequencies of peripheral blood immune cells (increase in CD4+ICOS^{high} cells with reciprocal decrease of MDSCs), were seen.[72] Abscopal responses were also demonstrated in about a quarter of patients (11/41) with NSCLC, breast cancer, and thymic cancer who received fractionated irradiation (3.5 Gy × 10 daily fractions) in combination with GM-CSF in addition to single-agent chemotherapy or hormonal therapy on a Phase 2 trial.[73] Nonirradiated lesions were evaluated by physical examination or by CT scans. Abscopal response was interpreted as at least 30% reduction in size from baseline. The patients with abscopal responses had better OS (21 vs. 8 months) compared with patients without abscopal responses.

The preclinical and initial clinical evidence for the potential synergistic effect of RT with immunotherapy has led to a number of clinical trials assessing various combinations.[74] Resistance to radiation and CTLA-4 blockade was found to be mediated in part by upregulation of PD-L1, thus providing rationale for future trials combining anti-PD-1 and RT. This hypothesis was tested by Luke et al. in a 79-patient Phase 2 study with multisite stereotactic body radiotherapy (SBRT) in combination with pembrolizumab in advanced solid malignancies.[75] A total of 73 patients who received SBRT (given to two to four sites) and at least one cycle of pembrolizumab were included in the analysis. At a median follow up of 5.5 months, 68 patients had follow-up imaging and were evaluated for response. In these heavily pretreated patients (median number of prior therapies 5), overall ORR was 13.2%, median OS 9.6 months, and median PFS

3.1 months. Biomarker analysis found that expression of IFN-γ associated genes in post-SBRT tumor had a significant correlation with distant tumor response.

Targeted Therapy

Immune checkpoint blockade and BRAF (proto-oncogene B-Raf)/MEK (mitogen-activated protein kinase)-directed targeted therapy have drastically changed the treatment of advanced melanoma—as it happened, these two fundamentally different treatment approaches reached the patient's bedside almost in parallel. The substantial clinical activity of both treatment approaches and their nonredundant mechanisms of action provide a rationale for their use in combination. Activation of signaling pathways in tumor cells has long been implicated in promoting suppressive immune networks in the TME.[76,77] Years before the successes of immune checkpoint inhibition and mitogen-activated protein kinase (MAPK)-directed therapy in melanoma, it had become evident that MEK inhibition with the specific inhibitor U0126, or via RNA interference targeting BRAF, could result in decreased production of the immunosuppressive cytokines IL-6, IL-10, and VEGF. Additional experiments showed that constitutive activation of the MAPK pathway in melanoma cells could lead to compromised function of DCs, and this immune evasion could be reversed by MAPK inhibition. There are extensive data supporting a link between the MAPK pathway and the antitumor immune response in melanoma, indicating that BRAF/MEK inhibition affects the immune response on multiple levels, including T cells, DCs, tumor cells, stromal cells, and soluble factors.[78,79] These effects include:

1. *Increased expression of tumor antigens:*[80] Both BRAF and MEK inhibition result in upregulation of melanoma differentiation antigens, which is associated with improved antigen recognition by T cells.
2. *Migration of T effector cells into the tumor and expansion of TILs.*[81] In melanoma patients treated with BRAF inhibitors, increased numbers and clonality of CD8+ T cells infiltrating metastatic tumors were found.
3. *Increased functionality of TILs alone:* In transgenic mouse models, adoptive T cell therapy in combination with BRAF inhibition demonstrated improved antitumor immune responses compared with monotherapy with either of the treatments.

Taken together, these data provide a strong rationale for combined MAPK pathway inhibition and immune checkpoint blockade. Of note, MEK inhibition had been associated with decreased T cell function in vitro, but a recent study in a transgenic mouse model demonstrated that the addition of MEK inhibition to BRAF inhibition and either ACT or PD-1 inhibition did not impair T cell function in vivo and provided superior tumor control.[74] These data support the investigation of combined BRAF/MEK inhibition with immunotherapy in patients with advanced melanoma, with multiple studies in advanced melanoma ongoing, testing BRAF and/or MEK inhibition in sequence or concurrent combination with PD-1/PD-L1 and CTLA-4 inhibitors. IMspire170 tested the hypothesis that improved clinical benefit would be possible by adding the MEK inhibitor cobimetinib to atezolizumab (anti-PD-L1 mAb) versus pembrolizumab in untreated advanced BRAF^{V600} WT melanoma. This trial was built on data from a Phase 1b dose-escalation and dose-expansion study testing atezolizumab + cobimetinib. An ORR of 45% and disease control rate of 75% were demonstrated in the combination, and toxicities included diarrhea and dermatitis acneiform, which were manageable.[82] However, in Phase 3, IMspire failed to meet its endpoints, both in colorectal cancer and advanced BRAF^{V600} WT melanoma. Patients with BRAF^{V600}-mutated advanced melanoma treatment with atezolizumab in combination with cobimetinib and vemurafenib demonstrated an ORR of 71.8% with median duration of response at 17.4 months and 39.3% patients with ongoing response at median follow-up of 29.9 months.[83] In an update published recently by Gutzmer et al., detailed findings were reported in 514 randomized patients to two arms: vemurafenib/cobimetinib/atezolizumab versus atezolizumab, with a primary endpoint of PFS. At a median follow-up of 18.4 months, PFS was 15.1 months versus 10.6 months in favor of triplicate therapy. Overall, the therapy was well tolerated.[84]

Intratumoral Oncolytic Viral Therapy

The oncolytic virus talimogene laherparepvec (T-VEC) received regulatory approval in the United States and other countries for the treatment of advanced or unresectable cutaneous melanoma after promising results from the OPTiM trial were reported.[85] In OPTiM, 436 patients with advanced stage accessible unresectable melanoma received either intralesional T-VEC or subcutaneous GM-CSF; T-VEC demonstrated a superior ORR compared with GM-CSF (26.4% vs. 5.7%; p <0.001) and prolonged OS (median 23.3 months vs. 18.9 months; p = 0.051). In addition to effects in injected lesions, 34% of uninjected nonvisceral lesions and 15% of visceral lesions also showed reduction in tumor size. Given its dual mechanism of action as a directly cytolytic agent and an in situ vaccine, T-VEC results in killing of cancer cells and priming of tumor-specific T cells in the directly injected lesions, leading to trafficking of these T cells into distant metastatic sites. Consequently, similar to vaccination, oncolytic virus therapy has the potential to induce priming of T cells, leading to T cell-mediated cytolysis of directly injected and distant tumor metastases through a presumed abscopal effect. This mechanism of action argues strongly for combination with checkpoint blocking antibodies, and a Phase 1b trial of T-VEC in combination with ipilimumab in 18 patients showed an ORR of 50% (CR [complete response] = 4, PR [partial response] = 5); all but one patient were still responding at 6 months.[86] The combination therapy did not add to the toxicity expected with each regimen alone. T-VEC showed similar efficacy when combined with pembrolizumab in a Phase 1b study of 21 patients with advanced melanoma; the confirmed ORR was 48%, with a CR rate of 14% and a median time to respond of 17 weeks.[87] Update of MASTERKEY-265 Phase 1b data showed objective response of 62% and complete response of 33%.[88] These responses included patients whose pretreatment biopsies showed a low CD8+ T cell count or negative IFN-γ gene signature. On treatment, biopsy demonstrated increased infiltration of CD8+ T cell and elevation of IFN-γ gene signature. Based on this experience, the benefit of adding T-VEC to ipilimumab was evaluated in Phase 2 randomized study in patients with stage IIIB-IV melanoma. Addition of T-VEC to ipilimumab led to improved ORR of 38.8% compared to 18% with ipilimumab alone.[89] Combination led to increased toxicity with the most common symptoms being fatigue, chills, and diarrhea. Grade 3 or higher AEs were also observed in combination (28% vs. 18%).

Antibody Drug Conjugates

Striking synergy between combined CTLA-4 and PD-1 blockade and the antibody drug conjugate trastuzumab emtansine (T-DM1) was reported in an orthotopic human epidermal growth factor receptor (HER-2) breast cancer mouse model.[90] Although CTLA-4 plus PD-1 inhibition without T-DM1 was ineffective in this model, T-DM-1 led to upregulation of CTLA-4 on T cells and the combination resulted in durable survival. Substantial increases in the expression of inhibitory receptors including CTLA-4, PD-1, and TIM-3 (consistent with T cell activation) were observed. Additionally, IFN-γ and granzyme B were markedly increased in TIL from orthotopic tumors, highlighting the immune-enhancing properties of T-DM-1 therapy, and provides a rationale for the combination of immune checkpoint blockade and T-DM-1 in patients with HER-2+ breast cancer. A clinical trial using T-DM-1 in combination with pembrolizumab is ongoing.

Glembatumumab vedotin links a fully human immunoglobulin G2 monoclonal antibody against the melanoma-related glycoprotein NMB (gpNMB) to the potent cytotoxin monomethyl auristatin E and has shown single-agent activity in advanced melanoma and breast cancer.[91,92] Based on preclinical evidence of potential synergy, it is currently being tested in combination with the anti-CD27 antibody varlilumab in metastatic melanoma.

TARGETING THE MICROENVIRONMENT

Inhibition of Indoleamine 2,3-Dioxygenase

IDO1 is an enzyme that converts the amino acid tryptophan, an essential amino acid for T cell function, into kynurenine, a metabolite that has a direct toxic effect on T cells. Physiologically, IDO activity thus leads to decreased T cell and NK cell activation,[93,94] and is exploited by tumors as a component of immune resistance. IDO is also expressed by macrophages and DCs and can be induced by IFN-γ and other cytokines that are secreted by tumor-specific T cells, counteracting their antitumor activity.[95,96] Combined inhibition of IDO and immune checkpoint blockade (CTLA-4, PD-1, and PD-L1) was found to be synergistic in melanoma and breast cancer mouse models[97] and is currently being tested in combination with anti-CTLA-4 and anti-PD-1 antibodies in a number of solid tumor trials. Initial efficacy data from a Phase 1 study using the IDO-inhibitor epacadostat in combination with pembrolizumab demonstrated encouraging antitumor activity and a remarkably benign toxicity profile in multiple tumor types.[98] Initial safety data on 28 patients (melanoma [n = 11], RCC [n = 5], NSCLC [n = 5], transitional cell carcinoma [TCC] [n = 3], EA (esophageal adenocarcinoma), and SCCHN (squamous cell carcinoma of the head and neck) [n = 2 each]) showed the combination of epacadostat 50 mg orally BID plus pembrolizumab 2 mg/kg intravenously every 3 weeks was well tolerated with no dose limiting toxicity (DLT). Reductions in tumor burden were observed in 15 of 19 evaluable patients, in all tumor types, and all were ongoing. Based on these encouraging data, a Phase 3 trial (ECHO-301/KEYNOTE-252) was conducted in patients with metastatic melanoma.[99] In the trial, 706 patients were randomized to receive either epacadostat + pembrolizumab or placebo + pembrolizumab. At median follow-up at 12.4 months, there were no significant differences in progression-free survival or overall survival between the two study arms. These unexpected findings have led to a halt of most trials evaluating this approach in several other solid malignancies.

Arginase 1 (ARG1), expressed in hepatocytes and myeloid-derived suppressor cells, is an isomer of arginase involved in L-arginine metabolism. The developing picture of ARG1 indicates that it mediates immune function suppression via MDSC's interaction with effector T cells.[44] A number of ARG1 inhibitors in preclinical settings show their ability to retard tumor growth when used as a single agent or in combination with immune checkpoint blockers.[100]

Adenosine, which causes an immunosuppressive TME, is an endogenous purine nucleoside that is produced both intracellularly and extracellularly. It is mainly generated extracellularly by the sequential enzymatic cleavage of adenosine triphosphate (ATP) to adenosine monophosphate (AMP) by CD39 ectonucleotidase and AMP (to adenosine) by CD73 ectonucleotidase. Therefore, targeting adenosine receptors has emerged as a novel approach to stimulate antitumor immunity. CPI-006 (anti-CD73 mAb) and CPI-444 (ciforadenant) are two molecules that are currently in clinical development as single agents or in combination with immune checkpoint blockers. Phase 1 data reported at the Society for Immunotherapy of Cancer's 2019 meeting showed that these agents are safe with very few grade 3 to 4 adverse events, and demonstrated antitumor activity in renal and prostate cancer patients.[101]

Angiogenesis Inhibition

Another mechanism of tumor survival and immune evasion is angiogenesis, as tumor vasculature mediates tumor growth and angiogenic factors, such as VEGF, have a direct impact on the immune response against the tumor. VEGF has various effects on the antitumor response,[102–104] including the following:

1. Promotion and expansion of inhibitory immune cell subsets (T_{reg} cells and MDSCs)
2. Inhibition of DC maturation
3. Suppression of T cell responses
4. Inhibition of immune cell trafficking across tumor endothelia.

In the B16 melanoma model, enhanced antitumor activity was seen when mice bearing established melanoma tumors were treated with anti-VEGF antibody in addition to adoptive transfer of gp-100-specific Pmel-1 TCR transgenic T cells compared with the adoptive T cell therapy alone. A single treatment with anti-VEGF antibody leads to significantly enhanced antitumor activity, as measured by infiltration of Pmel-1 T cells into treated tumors.[105] In an independent study (also in the B16 melanoma model), the combination of a GM-CSF-secreting tumor cell vaccine and a VEGF inhibition with a chimeric adeno-associated virus vector expressing soluble VEGF receptor (sVEGFR1/R2) resulted in significantly increased frequencies of activated DCs and effector T cells and decreased T_{reg} cell numbers. Mice treated with the combination had prolonged survival compared with the vaccine by itself, suggesting synergy.[106]

Single-institution experience of combining ipilimumab and bevacizumab in patients with metastatic melanoma showed favorable results. Forty-six patients were treated in four dosing cohorts of ipilimumab (3 or 10 mg/kg) with four doses at 3-week intervals and then every 12 weeks, and bevacizumab (7.5 or 15 mg/kg) every 3 weeks. Clinical responses included a disease control rate (DCR) of 67.4% and a median OS of 25.1 months. Combination therapy had a manageable safety profile with grade 3 and 4 toxicities observed in 11 of 46 patients

(23.9%). AEs included colitis, hepatitis, uveitis, and one case of giant cell arteritis and were consistent with toxicities that are expected with either of the two drugs alone. On-treatment tumor biopsies revealed activated vessel endothelium with extensive CD8$^+$ and macrophage cell infiltration, alterations of the tumor vasculature reminiscent of high endothelial venules in secondary lymphoid organs associated with lymphocyte trafficking into the tumor site. Increased numbers of memory CD4$^+$ and CD8$^+$ T cells (C–C chemokine receptor type 7 [CCR7]$^{+/-}$ CD45RO$^+$) in the peripheral blood were also observed.[107]

The encouraging clinical activity in melanoma patients and the earlier described observations in posttreatment biopsies and peripheral blood suggesting mechanisms that support synergy between CTLA-4 and VEGF inhibition have led to a randomized Phase 2 trial testing the combination of ipilimumab plus bevacizumab versus ipilimumab alone (NCT01950390). Furthermore, several trials using the anti-PD-1 antibodies nivolumab and pembrolizumab as combination partners with bevacizumab are ongoing in melanoma, RCC, NSCLC, and glioblastoma multiforme, among other tumor types. Given the VEGF suppressive effects of tyrosine kinase inhibitors (TKIs), synergy based on this mechanism may be achieved in clinical trials exploring combinations of TKI and checkpoint inhibition in patients with hepatocellular carcinoma, gastrointestinal stromal tumors, and other malignancies. A Phase 3 trial of pembrolizumab + axitinib (TKI) versus sunitinib (TKI) in advanced RCC (KEYNOTE-426) led to FDA approval of this combination approach.[108] In the study, 861 RCC patients were evaluated in randomized fashion with primary endpoints of overall survival and progression-free survival, along with a key secondary endpoint of objective response rate. At a median follow-up of 12.8 months, 89.9% patients were alive in combination arm versus 78.3% in sunitinib arm. Progression-free survival was noted to be 15.1 months for combination arm and 11.1 months for sunitinib arm. Adverse events were slightly increased in combination arm (75.8% vs. 70.6%). This approach is also being pursued in HCC and several other solid malignancies.

STRATEGIES TO MINIMIZE COMBINATION-ASSOCIATED TOXICITY: DOSING, SEQUENCING, AND LESSONS FROM INITIAL EXPERIENCE

Ipilimumab Plus Nivolumab in Advanced Melanoma

As described earlier, the first Phase 1 study of ipilimumab plus nivolumab in advanced melanoma showed impressive antitumor activity, leading to a rapid succession of Phase 2 and 3 programs and the eventual FDA approval of this regimen for the first-line treatment of metastatic melanoma. The landmark trial comparing ipilimumab versus nivolumab versus the combination showed an investigator-assessed ORR of 19% in the ipilimumab group, 43.7% in the nivolumab group, and 57.6% in the group treated with combination therapy.[109] Nevertheless, the increased efficacy came at the cost of substantial toxicity, with a grade 3/4 AE rate of more than 53% across doses in the Phase 1 study and greater than or equal to 50% grade 3/4 toxicity in both the Phase 2 and 3 trials, leading to the discontinuation of therapy in almost half of the patients treated. Notably, the combination of ipilimumab plus nivolumab at their single-agent doses (3 mg/kg) exceeded the maximum tolerated dose in the Phase 1 study and was not further tested. Importantly, the increase in immune-related toxicities compared with anti-CTLA-4 and PD-1 monotherapy was purely quantitative and could be managed with the employment of toxicity treatment algorithms. No deaths in the ipilimumab plus nivolumab combination group were reported in the multi-institutional international Phase 3 study. Furthermore, no qualitatively different, previously unknown toxicities were observed with the combination regimen.[110]

Of note, the combination of pembrolizumab with ipilimumab at a lower dose (1 mg/kg) showed similar efficacy but improved tolerability in 153 patients with advanced, treatment-naïve melanoma.[111] Patients were treated with pembrolizumab 2 mg/kg and ipilimumab 1 mg/kg every 3 weeks for four doses, then pembrolizumab 2 mg/kg every 3 weeks until intolerable toxicity, progression, or the 24-month endpoint. Safety analysis showed 41 patients (38%) had more than or equal to one grade 3 to 4 drug-related AE (DRAE); 68% of these DRAEs resolved by data cutoff. DRAEs led to the discontinuation of combination therapy in 8% of patients, ipilimumab alone in 10%, and pembrolizumab alone in 4%; there were no treatment-related deaths. Immune-mediated AEs of any grade and grade 3 to 4 severity occurred in 57 (53%) and 21 (20%) patients, respectively. ORR by central review was 51%, with 9% CR and 42% PR. Although data from this ongoing trial of ipilimumab at a lower dose in combination with pembrolizumab have yet to mature, similar RRs with a more favorable safety profile may inform future decisions regarding combination strategies for melanoma and other advanced cancers.

Ipilimumab Plus BRAF/MEK in Advanced Melanoma

The flexibility that may be required for testing of novel immunotherapy is also highlighted by the early experience in combining CTLA-4 inhibition with BRAF/MEK-targeted agents. A Phase 1 trial combining ipilimumab and vemurafenib (based on emerging preclinical and clinical rationale for this combination as discussed earlier in this chapter) revealed unexpected toxicity associated with this novel combination. In a Phase 1 dose safety study, melanoma patients with advanced BRAF^{V600E} mutant melanoma received standard doses of vemurafenib (960 mg PO daily) concurrently with ipilimumab at the standard dose of 3 mg/kg every 3 weeks for four doses.[112] Six of the initial 10 patients developed grade 3 transaminitis leading to early termination of the study. Another Phase 1 trial included an arm in which ipilimumab was administered concurrently with dabrafenib and trametinib at below standard doses (100 mg PO BID and 1 mg PO daily, respectively) to patients with BRAF^{V600} mutant melanoma.[113] Two of seven patients developed immune-related colitis, which was complicated by bowel perforation, leading to the discontinuation of this "triple combination" arm of the trial. These experiences suggest that dose escalation, run-in, or sequenced schemas should be considered in the early phase of clinical development of combination regimens.

A recent follow-up study evaluated the combination of vemurafenib and ipilimumab using a sequential schedule of administration.[114] This regimen demonstrated a substantially improved safety profile, with marked reduction in hepatotoxicity compared with the earlier study that administered ipilimumab and vemurafenib concurrently. Similar experience was gained with the combination of a PD-L1 inhibitor, atezolizumab, with vemurafenib and the MEK inhibitor cobimetinib.[115] Patients with untreated BRAF^{V600} mutant unresectable or metastatic melanoma received triplet therapy after a 28-day run-in period with BRAF and MEK inhibition alone. Atezolizumab was given at 800 mg IV every 2 weeks, cobimetinib was given at 60 mg PO daily for the first 21 days of each 28-day cycle, and vemurafenib was given 960 mg PO BID during the run-in, then reduced to 720 mg PO BID thereafter. In 14 evaluable patients, 13 (93%) showed responses by RECIST, including 1 CR and 12 PRs (one patient with PR had a 100% reduction in target lesions). Responses were unconfirmed, and median duration of response (DOR) and PFS were not estimable due to limited follow-up at the time of data cutoff. All-grade AEs that occurred in more than 20% of patients were nausea, fatigue, flu-like symptoms, photosensitivity, maculopapular rash, elevated ALT/AST and bilirubin, mucosal inflammation, and arthralgia. Six patients had drug-related grade 3 to 4 AEs during the run-in period, and five patients had drug-related AEs during the triple combination period; all were manageable and reversible. As discussed elsewhere in this chapter, the triple combination was found to mediate high rates of objective responses, many of which were durable, in advanced BRAF^{V600} mutant melanoma.

These studies highlight the clinical development challenges and risks in combining immuno-oncology agents at standard doses and schedules. Attempts to combine standard doses of drugs in doublet and triplet combination strategies resulted in substantial incremental toxicity. Although demonstrable improvements in clinical benefit were seen in a highly selected clinical trial population, when immunotherapy agents are used in combination or with conventional antineoplastic agents, it is reasonable to anticipate that adjustments in standard dosing and schedules will be necessary to appropriately balance clinical benefit against acceptable safety and tolerability.

Ipilimumab Plus Nivolumab in Other Solid Tumors

The toxicity with combined ipilimumab and nivolumab also appear to differ between tumor types. In patients with advanced NSCLC, the combination of ipilimumab 3 mg/kg and nivolumab 1 mg/kg every 3 weeks was compared with ipilimumab 1 mg/kg and nivolumab 3 mg/kg every 3 weeks. Significant toxicities were noted in both cohorts, with any grade treatment-related AEs reported in 39 of 46 patients (85%). Grade 3/4 AEs were seen in 22 patients (48%) and led to treatment discontinuation in 16 patients. Treatment-related deaths ($n = 3$) were due to respiratory failure, bronchopulmonary hemorrhage, and toxic epidermal necrolysis.[116] This experience led to the development of different dosing schedules with a focus on lengthening the dosing intervals of ipilimumab given at 1 mg/kg from every 3 weeks to every 6 and every 12 weeks.[117] Remarkably, this change of dosing intervals resulted in a decrease of the grade 3/4 AE rate from 48% in the original trial to 29% in the subsequent trial. ORR ranged from 13% to 39% across dosing groups, with the maximal ORR seen in patients treated with nivolumab 3 mg/kg every 2 weeks and ipilimumab 1 mg/kg every 12 weeks ($n = 38$). These data suggest that lower dose intensity of the ipilimumab plus nivolumab combination regimen can result in substantially lower toxicity and, perhaps surprisingly, increased antitumor activity. A subsequent Phase 3 study in advanced NSCLC (CheckMate 227) confirmed the benefit of nivolumab 3 mg/kg every 2 weeks + ipilimumab 1 mg/kg every 6 weeks.[118] In comparison to chemotherapy (platinum doublet), in patients with PD L-1 expression ≥1%, the median overall survival and 2-year overall survival for the immunotherapy combination versus chemotherapy were 17.1 months versus 14.9 months and 40% versus 32.8%, respectively. There was also a significant difference in the duration of responses in favor of immunotherapy combination (23.2 months) versus chemotherapy (6.2 months).

Furthermore, switching the dosing of ipilimumab at 3 mg/kg and nivolumab at 1 mg/kg (the FDA-approved dosing regimen for advanced melanoma) to ipilimumab at 1 mg/kg and nivolumab at 3 mg/kg was found to be better tolerated in tumor types, such as RCC and small cell lung cancer. In RCC, the rate of grade 3/4 immune-related toxicities was 34% with ipi 1/nivo 3 versus 64% with ipi 3/nivo 1, while the ORR was nearly identical at 40% in both groups ($n = 47$ each).[119] Lower toxicity, albeit to a lesser degree, was also reported in patients with small cell lung cancer who received ipi 1/nivo 3 compared with ipi 3/nivo 1, while the RR was also similar in the two groups (19% vs. 23%, respectively).[120] Nivolumab and ipilimumab have been approved for advanced hepatocellular patients based on data from CheckMate 040.[121] In this study, 148 patients previously treated with sorafenib were randomized to three arms: nivolumab 1 mg/kg + ipilimumab 3 mg/kg (every 3 weeks x 4), nivolumab 3 mg/kg + ipilimumab 1 mg/kg (every 3 week x 4), or nivolumab 3 mg/kg every 2 weeks + ipilimumab 1 mg/kg every 6 weeks and followed by nivolumab 240 mg every 2 weeks for each of the arms. Primary endpoints were safety and tolerability, whereas secondary endpoints were ORR, disease control rate, duration of response, and overall survival. At a minimum follow-up of 24 months, ORR was 31%, disease control rate was 49%, duration of response was 17 months, and 24-month overall survival was 40%. Disease control rate, median overall survival, 12-month overall survival rate, and 24-month overall survival rate were all improved in the higher dose ipilimumab arm. Adverse events were similar as in other studies involving this combination. Similarly, the CheckMate 032 study in extensive stage small cell lung cancer showed 1-year overall survival of 42% and 2-year survival of 30%, disease control rate of 49% with the combination of nivolumab 1 mg/kg and ipilimumab 3 mg/kg in 61 patients evaluated.[122] These findings illustrate the importance of flexibility with regards to the dosing, scheduling, and sequencing of combination regimens. The observations also indicate that there may be no "one regimen fits all" approach and that optimal dosing and scheduling may need to be carefully tested for each tumor type individually.

BIOMARKERS FOR COMBINATION IMMUNOTHERAPIES

As described earlier, recent clinical developments with immune checkpoint blockade have entered the therapeutic mainstream in oncology. Although anti-CTLA-4 therapy has shown reproducible antitumor activity only in patients with advanced melanoma, anti-PD-1 and anti-PD-L1 antibodies seem to have a broad range of activity for an expanding list of cancers. Notable exceptions, such as microsatellite stable (nonmicrosatellite-instability [MSI] high) colorectal cancer and prostate cancer, have proved much more resistant to anti-PD-1 therapies and present a therapeutic challenge. Moreover, despite numerous advances, ORRs across trials still average below 50%, and unusual response patterns including delayed or mixed tumor regression pose a further clinical dilemma. These challenges underscore the need for biomarker development to help identify patients who will derive the most clinical benefit, and also provide early recognition of nonresponders.

This chapter has previously detailed how the immune system is just one half of the equation in immunotherapy, as the tumor and its stromal microenvironment play critical roles in immune tolerance, cancer metabolism, and propagation of malignant cells. Improved understanding of immune-tumor interaction has led to a dichotomous, yet complex, approach to the biology of cancer and its host. Derivation of biomarkers, then, may depend on profiling of activated T cells and their target, as well as host factors that impact antitumor immunity, as illustrated in Figure 32.2, and detailed subsequently.

Tumor Profiling

The predominant impact of the PD-1 pathway suggests that the tumor site itself contains the most important clues for the identification of biomarkers, including PD-L1 expression, oncogenic driver mutations, mutational burden, and cancer-associated viruses.

Considering the mechanism of PD-1/PD-L1 interaction, high expression of PD-L1 in tumors suggests early recognition of cancer and subsequently induced PD-L1 overexpression as a means of immune evasion. PD-L1 as a means of adaptive immune resistance was first described in human melanoma samples,[123] where immune infiltrates in PD-L1+ versus PD-L1− melanomas were compared by mRNA expression profiling. A CD8+ T cell cytokine signature characterized by IFN-γ expression was identified in PD-L1+ melanomas, and T cell-derived IFN-γ was shown to be required for induction of both PD-L1 and IDO expression in tumors.[120] As the initial description of adaptive immune resistance in melanoma, PD-L1 expression has been described in other tumor types, including NSCLC and breast cancer,[124–126] and in each instance, PD-L1 expression was found to be a positive prognostic feature. Correlations with driver mutations have not been as clear: KRAS mutant lung adenocarcinomas may demonstrate heightened PD-L1 expression compared with wild-type tumors; however, in melanoma, BRAF^{V600E} mutation does not seem to correlate with PD-L1 expression.[127,128] PD-L1 expression also varies across cancer types, as it has also been observed that certain cancers (SCCHN, melanoma, breast, RCC) express PD-L1 on both tumor cells and TIL,[129,130] while colon and gastric cancers almost exclusively have PD-L1 on TIL.[124,131] The role of PD-L2 and its predictive importance is unknown. Analysis of a limited number of solid tumors demonstrated the expression of PD-L2 in approximately 20% of the cases, but its expression did not enhance the predictive power of PD-L1 expression for responsiveness to anti-PD-1 therapy.[130]

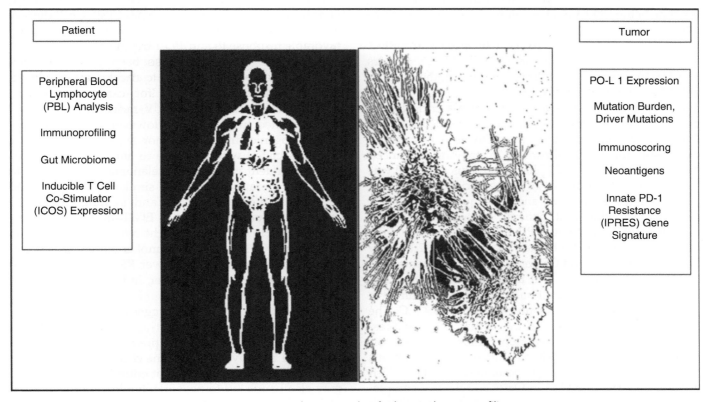

Figure 32.2 Biomarker approaches for host and tumor profiling.

The initial evidence that PD-L1 expression could predict anti-PD-1 therapy response was provided in the first-in-human study of nivolumab in 39 patients with several solid tumor types.[132] PD-L1-positive patients, defined as having at least 5% of tumor cells with cell surface PD-L1 protein expression, were twice as likely to respond to treatment compared with the overall study population.[1] However, variable expression levels of PD-L1 were observed in multiple tumor biopsies collected over time and from different anatomical sites in individual patients, illuminating a potential pitfall of developing PD-L1 immunohistochemistry (IHC) as an unequivocal biomarker based on a single biopsy specimen. Since these initial reports, expanded investigations in several solid tumor types, including NSCLC, melanoma, SCCHN, RCC, and bladder cancer, using several different PD-L1 IHC assays and cut-off criteria for positivity, have validated the general conclusion that PD-L1 expression in pretreatment tumor specimens portends a greater likelihood of response to anti-PD-1 and anti-PD-L1 drugs.[133,134] It is worth noting that patients with PD-L1 negative tumors will obtain a lower, but still detectable, RR, calling into question the use of this marker as an absolute selection criterion for therapy.[132] In a recent analysis of multiple reports, ORR in patients with PD-L1+ tumors was 48% compared with 15% in patients with PD-L1− tumors.[134] Although the relationship between PD-L1 expression and long-term outcomes, such as PFS and OS, has yet to be firmly established, for the time being PD-L1 expression might be used to prioritize treatment sequencing. As an example, patients with PD-L1+ tumors might be advised to receive anti-PD-1 as first-line therapy, while patients with PD-L1− tumors may be considered for combination immunotherapies or anti-PD-1 in the second line.

The type of PD-L1 assay used is also a critical component of biomarker selection. In October 2015, a PD-L1 IHC test was approved by the FDA as a companion diagnostic for pembrolizumab in treating advanced NSCLC (PD-L1 IHC 22C3 pharmDx). This approval was based on results from a large Phase 2 trial that included patients with squamous and nonsquamous NSCLC subtypes, showing that patients whose tumors were more than or equal to 50% PD-L1+ (approximately 20% of NSCLC cases) had a higher RR to anti-PD-1 therapy and prolonged PFS and OS compared with patients with lower PD-L1 expression.[135] A different companion diagnostic was used in the two Phase 3 trials of nivolumab in patients with squamous or nonsquamous NSCLC. The PD-L1 IHC 28-8 pharmDx showed that PD-L1 expression on tumor cells in pretreatment tumor specimens correlated with improved OS in patients with nonsquamous NSCLC, but not in those with squamous NSCLC.[136,137] It was approved by the FDA in October 2015 as a complementary but not required diagnostic test for nivolumab

in lung cancer, and subsequently approved in January 2016 as a complementary test for nivolumab in melanoma.[109] As compared to the pembrolizumab assay, this assay uses a threshold of more than 1% for a "positive" PD-L1 result for both melanoma and nonsquamous NSCLC. Moreover, there are a number of pitfalls associated with PD-L1 biomarker assays, including the age of the tumor specimen, the timing of biopsy in relation to treatment course, and the means of sampling (i.e., core biopsy vs. fine-needle aspiration) highlighting the need for a standardized approach.[138,139] A cross-industry initiative, termed the Blueprint Working Group, has been established to provide an analytical comparison of several PD-L1 IHC tests currently in use or in development that use different antibodies and different scoring criteria for PD-L1 positivity.

"Immunoscoring" of cancers is emerging as a useful tool to assess the proximity and infiltration of T cells into the TME. In a study of human colorectal carcinoma specimens detailing the relationship among T cell densities at the invasive tumor margin and those in the center of the tumor, high densities of CD3+CD8+CD45+ T cells (antigen-experienced Teff cells) was associated with a lower likelihood of tumor relapse and improved OS.[140] The colorectal cancer "immunoscore" also outperformed internationally accepted clinical staging criteria (Union for International Cancer Control [UICC]-tumor, node, metastasis [TNM]) in predicting disease-free survival (DFS) and OS in a multivariate analysis. In the context of anti-PD-1 therapy for melanoma, CD8+ T cell density at the invasive tumor edge has also been correlated with favorable response to anti-PD-1 treatment.[141]

Mutational burden has also been correlated with higher likelihood of response to checkpoint inhibition, and is particularly relevant for carcinogen-induced tumors, such as melanoma (UV radiation) and smoking-associated lung cancers. However, to date no specific oncogenic driver or tumor suppressor gene has been associated with response to anti-PD-1 therapy as an independent variable. In melanoma, the response to anti-PD-1 therapy seems to be similar in BRAF[V600E] and BRAF wild-type tumors,[109,142] and in lung cancer, the anti-PD-1 response is lower in EGFR-mutant adenocarcinomas.[143] However, this might reflect the association of mutant EGFR with never-smoker status, which correlates with a considerably lower RR to anti-PD-1 than smoking-associated lung cancer, independent of driver oncogene mutations.

As a corollary, it has been suggested that mutation-inducing cancer therapies, such as certain chemotherapies or radiation therapy, may predispose to subsequent successful therapy with immune checkpoint blockade,[71] although this mechanism is not entirely elucidated and may also be related to neoantigen release. As described earlier, the synergistic effects of chemotherapy and radiation therapy with immune checkpoint blockade are at least partly explained by immune priming with neoantigen release after cancer cell death. Neoantigen exposure and priming may also account for the high RRs seen in mismatch-repair deficient tumors, as in the case of MSI in colorectal cancer. The MSI phenotype as it relates to response to anti-PD-1 was formally tested in a three-arm clinical trial of pembrolizumab.[144] An ORR of 60% was seen in MSI-high colorectal carcinoma (CRC), whereas patients with microsatellite stable (MSS) tumors did not respond. The responsiveness of PD-1 blockade was also seen in patients with non-CRC MSI-high tumors (chemotherapy-refractory endometrial, duodenal, and ampullary cancers), who also demonstrated an RR of approximately 60%. Additionally, based on data from multiple trials (KEYNOTE-016, -164, -012, -028, -158) that included patients with MSI-H or mismatch repair deficient (dMMR) solid tumors, pembrolizumab was granted accelerated approval for all tumors carrying MSI-H/dMMR aberrancies. In 149 patients evaluated from these trials, an ORR of 39.6% (CR of 7.4% and PR of 32.2%) was observed, and median duration of response was not reached.

Patient Profiling

In addition to extensive tissue biomarker studies, a number of assays are being evaluated to track patient responsiveness to checkpoint inhibition. As an example, biomarker studies of anti-CTLA-4 therapies (ipilimumab and tremelimumab) have focused on the diversity, phenotype, and function of peripheral blood lymphocytes (PBLs) before and after therapy. Increased diversity and expression of activation markers on PBLs have been reported, including a rise in the absolute lymphocyte count (ALC) correlating with a higher rate of response to ipilimumab.[145–147]

Baseline assessments of patients before receiving immunotherapy may also be clinically useful: Peripheral blood biomarkers associated with clinical outcome were studied in 209 advanced melanoma patients before treatment with ipilimumab.[148] Low baseline lactate dehydrogenase (LDH), low absolute monocyte counts (AMCs), and low MDSC frequencies, coupled with high absolute eosinophil counts (AECs), relative lymphocyte counts (RLCs), and $CD4^+CD25^+Foxp3^+$ T_{reg} cell frequencies, were significantly associated with better survival. In a multivariate analysis, patients presenting with the best biomarker signature had a 30% ORR and median OS of 16 months, compared with 3% ORR and median OS of 4 months in patients with the poorest biomarker signature. AEs correlated with neither baseline biomarker signatures nor the clinical benefit of ipilimumab. In another model, limited to the routine parameters LDH, AMC, AEC, and RLC, the number of favorable factors (4 vs. 3 vs. 2–0) was also associated with OS ($p < 0.001$ for all pairwise comparisons) in the main study and additionally in an independent validation cohort. In another peripheral blood analysis, patients with ipilimumab-responsive melanoma who developed $CD4^+$ and $CD8^+$ PBLs with specificity against NY-ESO-1 had superior survival outcomes.[149] Flow cytometry has also identified clonal expansion of T cells following RT and PD-1 inhibition and may serve as a dynamic (and early) marker of clinical response.[150]

In contrast, other factors in peripheral blood, such as high levels of soluble CD25 (also known as interleukin-2 receptor-alpha [IL-2Rα]), have been correlated with resistance to anti-CTLA-4 therapy.[151] Expression of the co-stimulatory molecule inducible T cell co-stimulator (ICOS) on PBLs and TILs has been observed following anti-CTLA-4 therapy as a positive predictor of response;[152,153] however, its expression on $Foxp3^+$ T_{reg} cells has been associated with immune escape and thus poorer survival outcomes.[153,154] Despite these correlations, no predictive biomarker for selection of patients to receive ipilimumab, nor any on-treatment pharmacodynamic marker, has yet proved sufficiently robust to be used clinically. Studies to identify biomarkers from circulating PBLs in patients treated with anti-PD-1 therapy have been similarly unrevealing.[132,145]

Another means of patient immunoprofiling is the gut microbiome, as one study in mice suggested that hosts with high levels of commensal *Bifidobacteria* species had enhanced tumor response to anti-CTLA-4 therapy.[155] In addition, another study in humans suggested that *Bacteroides* species (*Bacteroides fragilis* and *Bacteroides thetaiotaomicron*) present among the microbiome might enhance the response of patients with melanoma to anti-CTLA-4 therapy.[154,155] Even though the mechanisms by which these species may enhance systemic antitumor immunity are unknown at this time, these data suggest that microbiome-derived biomarkers may be developed to guide immunotherapy and are currently being investigated in patients with advanced colorectal cancer undergoing chemo- and immunotherapy (NCT02960282). Furthermore, the gut microbiome has shown to be a potentially valuable biomarker to differentiate nonresponders and responders to immunotherapies in clinical settings. A number of studies have established that gut microbiota can help modulate the response to immunotherapy.[156] Gopalakrishnan et al. showed metastatic melanoma patients treated with anti PD-1 antibodies had significant differences in diversity and composition of gut microbiomes of responders versus nonresponders. These data show that responders had relative abundance of bacteria of the *Ruminococcaceae* family and enrichment of anabolic pathways. This study also revealed that responding patients had improved systemic and antitumor immunity due to favorable gut microbiomes that was transferrable via fecal transplant (carried out in mouse models). Similar data were reported by Zheng et al. in hepatocellular carcinoma showing an interaction between gut microbiome and response to anti-PD-1 mAb.[157] Based on this work, a clinical trial is underway to evaluate fecal material transplant in combination with anti-PD-1 therapy (NCT03817125). Another Phase 1 study has evaluated fecal microbiota transplant with anti-PD-1 in refractory advanced melanoma and preliminary results show that this strategy is feasible and possibly leads to alteration in intratumoral immune responses.[158] However, this study is very early in its accrual and data on only four patients have been presented.

An emerging and dynamic biomarker may be gene signatures of innate PD-1 resistance (IPRES). Investigators analyzed whole-exome sequences of pretreatment biopsies obtained from 38 melanoma patients treated with either pembrolizumab or nivolumab (responders, n = 21; nonresponders, n = 17) and patient-matched normal tissues.[159] Responders were defined as patients who had CR, PR, or stable disease (SD), and nonresponders defined as patients who had progressive disease. Genes expressed higher in nonresponding pretreatment tumors included mesenchymal transition genes (WNT5A, familial adenomatous polyposis [FAP]), immunosuppressive genes (interleukin 10 [IL-10], vascular endothelial growth factor [VEGFA], VEGFC), and monocyte and macrophage chemotactic genes (chemokine [C–C motif] ligand 2 [CCL2], CCL7, CCL8, and CCL13). Moreover, genes associated with wound healing and angiogenesis, which are considered T cell suppressive, were expressed at higher levels among nonresponding relative to responding pretreatment tumors. IPRES has yet to be validated in other tumors and models but may serve as a future useful tool for pretreatment, and on-treatment, surveillance with anti-PD-1 therapies.

Another biomarker that has become more readily available is multispectral imaging of fixed tissue. In a small study reported by Feng et al., select tumors that can generate TILs were analyzed using multispectral imaging, which allows for a maximum of eight markers to be evaluated using a specialized camera.[160] Five markers (CD3, CD8, Foxp3, CD13, and PD-L1) were found to predict successful TIL generation in patients undergoing adoptive TIL transfer. The data indicated that CD8+ to Foxp3+ ratio carried a positive predictive value of 91% and negative predictive value of 86% for TIL generation. Methods such as these will allow clinicians to select patients who will have successful TIl generation or should be selected for other therapeutic approaches.

The most successful biomarker strategy will likely be a combination of different approaches to assess tumors. For example, Higgs et al. analyzed pretreatment biopsy specimen for PD-L1 by immunohistochemistry and mRNA analysis for immune gene expression.[161] In patients who were dual positive (PD-L1 and mRNA analysis for

immune gene expression), objective response rate was 46%; for those who were dual negative, the response rate was 3%. Such biomarkers will perhaps help with deselecting patients who are unlikely to respond and can be spared adverse events. Similarly, Ott et al. evaluated GEP, PD-L1, and TMB as predictive markers for pembrolizumab in patients treated in KEYNOTE-028 study.[162] The retrospective biomarker analysis of prospective study showed that patients with each of the biomarkers (GEP, PD-L1, and TMB) were associated with antitumor activity of pembrolizumab. Furthermore, combination of PD-L1 and TMB or T cell inflamed GEP and TMB was also able to predict response to pembrolizumab. This observation can potentially help in patient selection. In a similar report by Cristescu et al., GEP and TMB when high predicted clinical benefit. They also demonstrated that GEP was interchangeable with PD-L1 when combining with TMB for biomarker assessment.[163] These approaches remain to be validated prospectively.

CONCLUSION

Within the next 5–10 years, the hundreds of ongoing immunotherapy combination trials will undoubtedly produce novel combinations with enhanced clinical activity, thus necessitating unique trial designs, nuanced patient selection, and expansion of predictive and prognostic biomarkers. The list of targets and agents employed in combination trials continues to grow at a rapid pace. Oncologists are currently practicing in a fortunate time, as such scientific advances are quickly changing the treatment landscape and our understanding of the immune response to cancer.

Because many novel therapies are being studied in conjunction with PD-1 pathway inhibition, and a majority of these clinical trials are in their early stages, there are as yet no validated biomarkers to predict which patients will benefit most, and which dual or higher order combination therapy is most beneficial. Ultimately, validation of any immunotherapy strategy will rely heavily on clinical outcomes and must be weighed carefully against expected (and unexpected) toxicity risks. Future combination trials—even early exploratory ones—should be biomarker driven in order to derive the most information as efficiently as possible.

KEY REFERENCES

Only key references appear in the print edition. The full reference list appears in the digital product on Springer Publishing Connect: connect.springerpub.com/content/book/978-0-8261-3743-2/part/part02/chapter/ch32

1. Topalian SL, Hodi FS, Brahmer JR, et al. Safety, activity, and immune correlates of anti-PD-1 antibody in cancer. N Engl J Med. 2012;366(26):2443–2454. doi:10.1056/NEJMoa1200690
4. Larkin J, Chiarion-Sileni V, Gonzalez R, et al. Combined nivolumab and ipilimumab or monotherapy in untreated

melanoma. *N Engl J Med*. 2015;373(1):23–34. doi:10.1056/NEJMoa1504030

83. Sullivan RJ, Hamid O, Gonzalez R, et al. Atezolizumab plus cobimetinib and vemurafenib in BRAF-mutated melanoma patients. *Nat Med*. 2019;25(6):929–935. doi:10.1038/s41591-019-0474-7

85. Andtbacka RH, Kaufman HL, Collichio F, et al. Talimogene laherparepvec improves durable response rate in patients with advanced melanoma. *J Clin Oncol*. 2015;33(25):2780–2788. doi:10.1200/JCO.2014.58.3377

136. Brahmer J, Reckamp KL, Baas P, et al. Nivolumab versus docetaxel in advanced squamous-cell non-small-cell lung cancer. *N Engl J Med*. 2015;373(2):123–135. doi:10.1056/NEJMoa1504627

156. Gopalakrishnan V, Spencer CN, Nezi L, et al. Gut microbiome modulates response to anti-PD-1 immunotherapy in melanoma patients. *Science*. 2018;359(6371):97–103. doi:10.1126/science.aan4236

161. Higgs B, Morehouse C, Streicher K, et al. Interferon gamma mRNA signature in tumor biopsies predicts outcomes in patients with non-small cell lung carcinoma or urothelial cancer treated with durvalumab. *Clin Can Res*. 2018;24(16):3857–386. doi:10.1158/1078-0432.ccr-17-3451

Immune Function in Cancer Patients

Lisa H. Butterfield

33

Introduction to Immune Function in Cancer Patients

Lisa H. Butterfield

For immune surveillance to be successful in preventing cancer development, the immune system has to function robustly. For immunotherapy vaccines, effector cells, and antibodies to be successful at eradication of existing tumors, again, the immune system must function well. Section I of this textbook presented the basic principles of immunity and its intersection with cancer biology. Section II presented the wide array of approaches to clinical immunotherapy. In Section III, a series of more translational chapters are presented which describe the many ways in which the presence of cancer can impact and deregulate immune function in patients. These chapters present our current understanding of immune function at the tumor site, and immune function throughout the human system as generally measured in the blood. This section also focuses on specific cell types and molecules that have important protumor and antitumor effects including key aspects of the tumor cell biology.

The section begins with an examination of tumor infiltrates and focuses on the function and characterization of myeloid cells and their immune suppressive capabilities (Chapter 34). These diverse and multifunctional cells can have a major impact on antitumor immunity. In Chapter 35, the transcriptional signatures of an effective response across disease states are presented. This analysis approach provides mechanistic insights to further improve antitumor responses. Next (Chapter 36), the somatic mutations that can impact the development of an immune response are presented, which identify critical pathways of tumor resistance. The chapter also discusses the way in which such tumor-specific mutations can be harnessed to promote more effective antitumor effects. The subsequent chapter, Chapter 37, presents the topic of tumor antigen profiling, including another perspective on neoantigens, T cell responses to such antigens, and ways to identify them.

The next several chapters examine systemic immune function in cancer patients. Cancers, even those localized to a single organ site, can have a significant and often negative impact on immunity, and can also skew the activity of many immune cells. One of the areas of enormous impact in immunotherapy involves biomarkers: those

that can predict outcomes and toxicities, as well as those that are prognostic for outcome to a given therapeutic. In Chapter 38, measures of immune function, particularly those made from blood samples, are discussed and an overview of critical investigated immune measures is presented. Next, Chapter 39 presents a mechanistic view of regulatory T cell biology and its impact in cancer. These cells have an important regulatory function across multiple tumor types and can suppress needed antitumor immunity. The subsequent chapter, Chapter 40, gives a broader view of multiple types of suppressive cells and cells skewed to a more suppressive function in the setting of cancer, including myeloid-derived suppressor cells (MDSCs), neutrophils, and cancer-associated fibroblasts. In Chapter 41, a newer area of cancer immunobiology is presented, focused on circulating mediators of immune suppression, including exosomes, which can be derived from both tumor cells and immune cells with opposing immune impact.

In the next part of this section, there are chapters that give fresh perspectives on other systemic measures of immune function, as well as newer areas of cancer biology that are now understood to have potent effects on immune function. First, in Chapter 42, there is a thorough presentation of B cells and humoral immunity in cancer, which have important pro- and antitumor effects and are an important component of tertiary lymphoid structures. In Chapter 43, systems biology approaches for dealing with the complexity of immune–cancer interactions are presented. Such profiling approaches can deconvolute highly multiplexed data and identify overarching regulatory networks. Subsequently, in Chapter 44, new advances in immune biomarker analysis are presented, with an emphasis on highly multiplexed analysis of nucleic acid and protein level measures. That is followed by Chapter 45, which presents areas of already validated biomarkers such as PD-L1 expression, tumor mutation burden, and genomic instability, which impact checkpoint blockade response.

In the final part of this section, starting with Chapter 46, the substantial effects of cancer on cellular metabolism are presented, as well as how cancer metabolism and immune metabolism intersect in the tumor microenvironment. This active area of investigation is identifying new areas for therapeutic intervention. In Chapter 47, the impact of aging is discussed. Most cancers develop in aged individuals, and the role of aging on the immune function is understudied. Aging impacts antitumor immune memory development, treatment toxicity, and other areas addressed in this chapter. Finally, Chapter 48 describes how imaging approaches, long used to detect and measure tumor size, can be used to better understand antitumor immunity, tumor metabolism, and pseudoprogression.

As a whole, this section presents a thorough discussion of many aspects of immune activity at the tumor site and throughout the patient. It presents critical molecular mechanisms and cellular networks of antitumor activity and discusses how complex immune activity is affected by the basic biology of metabolism and aging.

34

Tumor-Infiltrating Myeloid Cells in Cancer Progression and Therapy Response

Sushil Kumar, Amanda Poissonnier, Courtney B. Betts, Dhaarini Murugan, Eivind Valen Egeland, Femke Ehlers, Jacklyn Woods, Nicky Beelen, and Lisa M. Coussens

KEY POINTS

- Inflammation is a dynamic tissue response that accompanies neoplastic progression in tissues.

- Myeloid cells, composed of multiple subtypes, functionally contribute to cancer-associated inflammation by producing numerous mediators impacting pro- as well as antitumor pathways within tumor microenvironments.

- Multiparametric analytical methods are used to analyze cellular phenotypes and molecular changes while studying myeloid cells in cancer.

- Myeloid cell activities can suppress T cell activation, proliferation, cytoxicity, and infiltration in neoplastic microenvironments.

- Cytotoxic chemo- and radiotherapy influences cancer inflammation in an immunosuppressive as well as, in rare instances, an immunostimulatory manner.

- The inhibitory immune checkpoint function of tumor-infiltrating T cells is critically dependent upon myeloid cell activities in tumor microenvironments.

- Targeting myeloid cell activities in cancer can improve response to cytotoxic chemo- and radiotherapy, as well as other immunotherapies.

INTRODUCTION

As early as the 19th century, Rudolf Virchow observed that inflammation was closely associated with cancer development;[1] two centuries later, cancer-related inflammation within tumor microenvironments (TME) represents one of the most actively studied areas of modern cancer research.[2] Tumor-associated inflammation is now acknowledged as a significant factor impacting not only clinical outcome of patients but also how patients respond to cytotoxic, targeted, and immune-based therapies.[3] As we understand today, tumor-associated inflammation reflects a diversity of leukocyte lineages, each including a range of differentiation and bioeffector states impacting a myriad of cancer hallmark functions,[3] chief among them being subsets of myeloid lineage cells, the focus of this chapter. Although differentiating from hematopoietic stem cells in bone marrow during development and in response to damage sustained within peripheral tissues where they further differentiate into heterogeneous subpopulations comprising various aspects of the innate immune response, myeloid cells also represent resident sentinel cells within select organs/tissues, including spleen, lung, gut, skin, brain, and liver, where their bonafide "role" involves safeguarding the organ as first responders. Myeloid cells that infiltrate tissues from bone marrow and blood precursors orchestrate initial innate immune responses to "damage," in addition to their indispensable role in shaping adaptive immune responses. In cancer, the functional heterogeneity of myeloid subsets bestows both pro- and antitumor functionality, largely dependent on the context of the TME, including would-be tumor cells (Figure 34.1). In this chapter, we provide characteristics of myeloid subtypes, their bonafide homeostatic functions in healthy tissue, their skewed functions in tumors, and their impact on "standard-of-care" therapies and newly developed immunotherapies for cancer.

MONOCYTES AND IMMATURE MYELOID CELLS

Monocytes are the precursors of tissue-resident macrophages (Mφ) and monocyte-derived dendritic cells (mo-DCs). Under steady-state conditions, they are generated from granulocyte/macrophage progenitors (GMPs) in the bone marrow and are predominantly found in the blood and spleen.[4,5] Upon tissue recruitment, and under the influence of local environmental cues consisting of

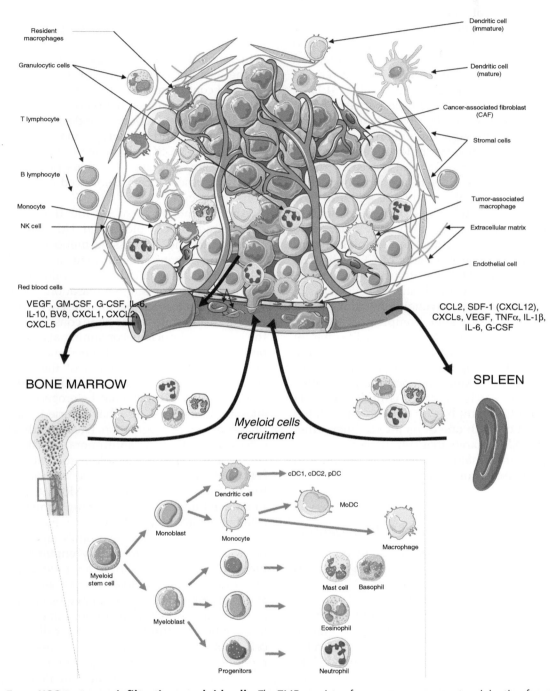

Figure 34.1 From HSC to tumor-infiltrating myeloid cells. The TME consists of numerous components originating from mesenchymal, epithelial, and hematopoietic origins. Within established tumors, both innate and adaptive immune subsets are present where the balance between pro- and antitumorigenic actors is key to malignancy. Various immune cell subsets (such as tumor-associated macrophages, DCs, mast cells, eosinophils, neutrophils with immunosuppressive functions) contribute to fuel tumor progression. These cells are generated during induced myelopoiesis in bone marrow in response to secreted factors by TMEs where a spectrum of myeloid subsets reside. In tumor-bearing context, splenic myelopoiesis is mediated through a distinct hematopoiesis progenitor response where generated cells migrate to TMEs and maintain immunosuppressive environments by producing protumoral factors in a complex regulatory network.

BV8, Bombina variegate; CCL, CC chemokine ligand; cDC, conventional dendritic cell; CSF, colony-stimulating factor; CXCL, chemokine (C-X-C motif) ligand; G-CSF, granulocyte colony-stimulating factor; GM-VEGF, granulocyte-macrophage vascular endothelial growth factor; HSC, hematopoietic stem cells; IL, interleukin; TME, tumor microenvironment; TNF, tumor necrosis factor.

chemotactic gradients of chemokines, cytokines, and bioreactive mediators, monocytes can differentiate into Mφ and/or mo-DCs.[6,7] Monocytes are categorized into classical or inflammatory, nonclassical or patrolling, and intermediate subsets, classified in part based on relative expression of cell surface markers (see Table 34.1).[8–11] Inflammatory monocytes (iMo) shuttle between blood and bone marrow and eventually give rise to patrolling monocytes (pMo), although an alternative model wherein iMo and pMo develop independently from a common progenitor in bone marrow also exists.[116,117] The aforementioned monocyte subsets are phenotypically and functionally distinct.[7] iMo comprise ~80% to 95% of circulating monocytes and have a half-life in blood of less than 1 day in humans and mice at steady state.[118] iMo emigrate from bone marrow using the chemokine receptor CCR2 and traffic along gradients of CCR2 ligands (CCL2, CCL7, and CCL12) to enter tissues.[119] Once there, iMos differentiate into Mφ or dendritic cells (DCs).[12] Monocytes can also perform scavenging functions to aid resident Mφ. pMo, at steady state, comprise ~2% to 11% of circulating monocytes, but have a longer life span of 7 days in humans, and at least 2 days in mice.[118] These utilize CX$_3$CR1 and sphingosine-1 phosphate receptor 5 (S1PR5) axis for trafficking and patrolling endothelium,[120] where their search for injury is undertaken via the ß2 integrin LFA (lymphocyte function-associated antigen 1) interaction with one of its intercellular adhesion molecule (ICAM) ligands that stimulates migration. pMo have a pro-inflammatory function in response to infection and are also involved in antigen presentation leading to T cell stimulation.[121]

Monocytes and Immature Myeloid Cells in Cancer

While monocyte expansion at steady state occurs in bone marrow, injury or neoplastic progression instigates monocyte reservoirs in the spleen to expand.[4,122] Splenic monocytes in turn produce new monocytic and granulocytic cells, which continually "feed" growing tumors.[122] Monocytes are recruited to primary tumor sites mainly through cytokines initially produced by tumor cells, of which CCL2 and colony-stimulating factor-1 (CSF-1) are key chemotactic factors.[123–125] Significant recruitment of iMos have been reported in breast, pancreatic, and colorectal carcinomas regulated by the CCR2/CCL2 axis,[126,127] while CX$_3$CL1 has also been reported to facilitate recruitment of CX$_3$CR1+ iMo and pMo to tumors.[13,128]

One predominant population of heterogeneous immature myeloid cellsiMCs) generated under "emergency" hematopoiesis scenarios (i.e., peripheral tissue injury, cancer) commonly found in TMEs is Gr-1 (a GPI-linked myeloid differentiation marker, also known as Ly-6G) expressing iMCs, frequently described as myeloid-derived suppressor cells (MDSCs).[129] MDSCs,

comprised of both granulocytic (G-MDSCs) and monocytic (M-MDSCs) subpopulations, possess T cell suppressive functions, as well as pro-angiogenic properties.[130] While the MDSC terminology has been widely accepted by the scientific community, it is prone to misinterpretation and controversy due to widespread use of Gr-1 as a sole biomarker in combination with CD11b (an integrin), thus bypassing functional validation. Further, overlapping functions and phenotypic markers between monocytes and M-MDSCs challenge the notion that they are a distinct myeloid subset. Others postulate that MDSC merely represent a cancer-induced cell state of a transitional monocyte.[131]

Another monocyte subset identified in humans and mice found in both blood and TMEs are the angiopoietin receptor Tie2-expressing monocytes (TEMs). TEMs are protumorigenic due to their angiogenic-promoting role in TMEs, as well as by their ability to aid metastasis by fostering tumor cell extravasation.[132,133] Other known subsets of monocytes that are present at lower frequency during steady state but become conspicuous in TMEs are the segregated nucleus-containing atypical pMo (SatM), neutrophil-like iMo, and trained-monocytes; however, origin and thorough function of these rare monocyte subsets in cancer have yet to be elucidated.

In addition to functional heterogeneity of monocyte subsets, monocytes also have varied roles in discrete phases of cancer progression. During early phases, monocytes can exert several antitumoral functions to limit cancer growth. Through cytokine-mediated induction of cell death and phagocytosis, monocytes can directly kill tumor cells.[134] Moreover, both iMo and pMo are known to induce tumor cell death through antibody-dependent cellular cytotoxicity (ADCC).[135,136] Furthermore, tumor-derived factors such as exosomes and other microparticles in circulation are readily engulfed by monocyte-mediated phagocytosis. pMo are particularly implicated in tumor-cell-phagocytosis given their longer life span and patrolling activities and have been reported to play an essential role in limiting tumor cell seeding and metastasis, where natural killer (NK) cell-mediated tumor cell cytotoxicity also aides this process[137,138] as has been reported during the early stages of lung cancer.[139]

To establish within a tissue, initiated neoplastic cells must successfully evade initial (antitumor) host immune responses; once established, emergent data from the past two decades has revealed that subsets of immune cells within TMEs shift their functionality toward favoring tumor progression.[3] For instance, tumor-recruited iMos release vascular endothelial growth factor (VEGF) and thereby stimulate angiogenesis (formation of new blood vessels), thus facilitating both primary tumor expansion and cancer metastasis.[140,141] Heightened levels of bioavailable VEGF in tumors in turn upregulates monocyte-derived arginase 1 (ARG1) and inducible nitric

Table 34.1 Main Biomarkers for Cell Type Identification in Human and Mouse, and the Cells' Molecules Involved in Pro- and Antitumor Functionality, Including Therapeutic Targets

CELL TYPE	MAIN MOUSE MARKERS FOR IDENTIFICATION	MAIN HUMAN MARKERS FOR IDENTIFICATION	PROTUMOR ACTIVITY MOLECULES	ANTITUMOR ACTIVITY MOLECULES	THERAPEUTIC TARGETS
Monocytes[8-23]	CD11b, CCR2, CD16/CD32, CD31, CD43, CD44, CD45, CD62L, CD115, CX3CR1, F4/80, Gr1, Ly-6C, VEGF	CD11b, CD2, CD14, CD16, CD31, CD56, CD62L, CD115, CD192, CX3CR1, CXCR3, CXCR4			CSF1R- blockade
iMo	$Ly6C^{hi}$, $CD43^{lo}$, $CX3CR1^{hi}$	$CD14^{hi}$, $CD16^{-}$	Arg1, iNOS, F13a1		CCR2
pMo	$Ly6C^{lo}$, $CD43^{hi}$, $CX3CR1^{hi}$	$CD14^{lo}$, $CD16^{hi}$	IL-10, CXCL5, CXCR4		CX3CR1, CXCR4
iMCs	$CD11b^{+}$, $Gr-1^{+}$, $Ly6C^{+}$, $Ly6G^{-}$, CCR5	$CD14^{+}$, $CD33^{+}$, $HLA-DR^{lo}$	VEGF-A, MMPs, IL-1β, Arg1, iNOS, CD40, TGF-β		TRAIL-R2, Entinostat, ATRA
Tumor-associated macrophages[24-34]	$CD11b^{+}$, Ly6CLo, $Ly6G^{-}$, $F4/80^{+}$, $MHCII^{Lo/Hi}$	$CD11b^{+}$, $CD14^{+}$, $CD163^{+/-}$, $CD206^{+/-}$, $HLA-DR^{Lo/Hi}$	IL-10, MMP9, EGF, TGF-β, Arginase, VEGF, Cathepsins, PD-L1	CXCL10, CXCL9, CCL5, TNF-α	CSF1R, PI3Kγ, BTK, HDAC
DCs[35-54]					
cDC1	CD11c, MHC-class II, CD8a (resident), CD103 (migratory), Flt3, Clec9a, CD205	CD11c, HLA-class II, CD141, XCR1, Clec9a, CD205	IL-10, IL-6, TIM3, SIRPα, PD-L1	IL-12, CD40, Flt3L-R, TLRs, Type I IFN, TNF-α, CXCL9, CXCL10	Anti-CD47 (SIRPα ligand), CD40 agonist, anti-PD-L1, TLR agonists (Imiquimod, BCG), cancer vaccines
cDC2	CD11c, MHC-class II, CD11b, Flt3, SIRPα	CD11c, HLA-class II, CD11b, SIRPα, CD1c, BDCA1			
pDC	CD11clo, MHC-class IIlo, B220, Flt3, Clec9a, Siglec-H, SIRPα	$CD11c^{lo-}$, HLA-class II^{lo}, CD123, CD303, CD304			
Neutrophils[34,55-73]	$Ly6G^{+}$ $Ly6C^{-}$ $CD11b^{+}$	$CD10^{+}$, $CD33^{+}$, $CD13^{high}$, $CD14^{-}$, CD15/$CD65^{+}$, $CD16^{high}$, $CD123^{+}$, $HLA-DR^{lo/int}$			
TAN-N1		$CD66b^{+}$, $CD33^{+}$, $CD15^{+}$ $CD16^{+}$ $CD11b^{+}$ $CD62L^{low}$ $HLA-DR^{-}$ $Arg-1^{+}$		IL-2, CCR5, CCR7, CXCR3, CXCR4, CXCL12, TNF-α	

(continued)

Table 34.1 Main Biomarkers for Cell Type Identification in Human and Mouse, and the Cells' Molecules Involved in Pro- and Antitumor Functionality, Including Therapeutic Targets (continued)

CELL TYPE	MAIN MOUSE MARKERS FOR IDENTIFICATION	MAIN HUMAN MARKERS FOR IDENTIFICATION	PROTUMOR ACTIVITY MOLECULES	ANTITUMOR ACTIVITY MOLECULES	THERAPEUTIC TARGETS
TAN-N2		CD66b+, CD33+, CD15+ CD16+ CD11b+ HLA-DR- Arg-1+	VEGF, MMP9, CCL2, CCL5, Arginase-1, Cathepsin G, Oncostatin M, ROS, CCL4, CXCL8, IL-17		Blockade of TGF-β, type I interferon treatments
G-MDSCs or PMN-MDSCs		CD14- CD11b+ CD15+ CD66b+ HLA-DR-CD33+ LOX-1+	CXCL6, CXCL8, CCL15, Arginase-1, Cathepsin G, ROS, iNOS, MMPs, TGF-β, IL-10, PD-L1		Low doses of Gemcitabine, 5-fluorouracil, TRAIL-R, S100A9-derived peptides conjugated to Fc fragments, COX-2 inhibition
PMN-II		CD49d^{Lo} CD11b^{Hi} TLR2^{Hi} TLR4^{Hi} TLR7^{Hi} TLR9^{Hi}	IL-10		
Circulating	CXCR4^{Hi} CXCR2^{Hi} CD62L^{Lo} CD11b+ Ly6G+	CXCR4^{Hi} CXCR2^{Hi} CD62L^{Lo} CD11b+			
Mast cells[74–80]	FcεRI+, cKit+, mMCP-1, MMCP-2, mMCP-6, mMCP-7, mMCP-4, mMCP-5	FcεRI+, cKit+, Tryptase, Chymase	VEGF, FGF2, MMP9, TGF-β, Tryptase, IL-6, IL-10, IL-13,	IL-4, TGF-β	Angiogenic potential
Eosinophils[81–105]	F4/80, CD11b, CD193, GR1^{Lo}, MBP-1, SIGLEC-F, IL-5Rα	CD11b, CD193, MBP-1, IL-5Rα, SIGLEC-8, EMR1	VEGF-A, FGF-2, CXCL8/ IL-8, SPP1	TNF-α, Grzα, Grzβ, IL-18	IL-5
Basophils[106–115]	FcεRI, CD49b, CD123, MCP-8	FcεRI, CD123, CD203c, BB1, 2D7	IL-4, VEGF, HGF		

CX3CR1, CX3C motif containing receptor 1; CXCR3, CXC motif containing receptor 3; CXCR4, CXC motif containing receptor 4; VEGF, Vascular endothelial growth factor; CSF1R, colony stimulating factor 1 receptor; iMO, inflammatory monocytes; Arg1, Arginase; iNOS, Inducible nitric oxide synthase; F13a1, Coagulation factor XIII a; CCR2, CC motif chemokine receptor type 2; pMO, Patrolling monocytes; IL-10, Interleukin 10; CXCL5, CXC motif chemokine receptor type 5; HLA-DR, human leukocyte antigen DR; MMPs, Matrix metalloproteases; IL-1b, Interleukin 1 beta; TGF-β, Transforming growth factor beta; TRAIL-R2, TNF related apoptosis inducing lignad-receptor 2; MHC, Major histocompatibility complex; EGF, epidermal growth factor; CXCL10, CXC motif chemokine 10; CXCL9, CXC motif chemokine 9; PI3K, phosphatidylinositol 3 kinase; BTK, Brutton tyrosine kinase; HDAC, histone deacetylase; DCs, Dendritic cells; cDC1, conventional dendritic cell type 1; Flt3, FMS related tyrosine kinase 3; CLEC9a, C type lectin domain family 9 a; IL-6, Interleukin 6; TIM3, T cell immunoglobulin and mucin domain containing 3; SIRPa, Signal regulatory protein alpha; IL-12, Interleukin 12; TLR, Toll-like receptor; IFN, Interferon; TNF, Tumor necrosis factor; PD1, Programmed cell death protein 1; PD-L1, Programmed cell death ligand 1; cDC2, Conventional DC 2; BDCA, Blood dendritic cell antigen; pDC-Plasmacytoid dendritic cells; TAN-N1, Tumor associated neutrophil type N1; IL-2, Interleukin 2; CCR7, CC motif containing receptor 7; TAN-N2, Tumor associated neutrophil type N2; CCL4, CC motif containing chemokine 4; CXCL8, CXC motif containing chemokine 8; G-MDSC, granulocytic myeloid derived suppressor cells; PMN-MDSC, Polymorphonuclear myeloid derived suppressor cells; LOX1, Lysil oxidase 1; CXCL6, CXC motif containing chemokine 6; CCL15, CC motif containing chemokine 15; ROS, Reactive oxygen species; PMN-II, polymorphonuclear cell type II; COX2, Cycloxygenase 2; FcεR1, Fc epsilon receptor 1; MCP, Monocyte chemoattaractant protein; FGF2, Fibroblast growth factor 2; IL-6, Interleukin 6; IL-13, Interleukin 13; HGF, Hepatocyte growth factor; Grz, Granzyme; IL-4, Interleukin 4; IL-5, Interleukin 5; IL-4, Interleukin 13

oxide synthase (iNOS) leading to T cell inactivation.[142,143] Notably, CCR5-expressing iMCs possess enhanced angiogenic properties as compared to their CCR5-negative counterparts.[144,145]

Monocytes also play a key role in promoting tumor metastasis. iMOs, recruited through the CCR2/CCL2 axis from bone marrow, are abundant in premetastatic niches where they promote tumor colonization by secreting VEGF-A, as well as promoting cross-linking of extracellular matrix (ECM) to increase stiffness,[146,147] and accelerate metastatic colonization.[148,149] In the B16F10 murine model of metastatic melanoma, accumulation of CXCR3+ monocytes in lung is a prerequisite for establishment of lung metastases.[150] iMOs also facilitate formation of an immunosuppressive premetastatic niche;[151,152] tumor-derived exosomes enter lung premetastatic niches by extravasating alveolar capillaries, where they are taken up by alveolar and interstitial Mϕs, that in turn signal iMO recruitment.[153–155] Recruited iMOs differentiate into tumor-associated macrophages (TAMs) that promote tumor growth by secretion of interleukin (IL)-6, IL-10, and VEGF, and induce fibrin deposition.[3] Altogether, monocytes and their subtypes play rate-limiting roles in promoting tumor-permissive microenvironments.

MACROPHAGES (Mϕ)

Macrophages are housekeepers of healthy tissue where they maintain tissue homeostasis by performing scavenging functions to remove cellular debris and aid in wound healing. While Mϕ intrinsic ability to phagocytose debris is necessary for scavenging functions, their ability to support tissue regeneration during wound healing requires coordinated activities with other stromal cells (e.g., endothelial cells and fibroblasts) to modulate cell proliferation/death, vascularization, and tissue regeneration). Due to these virtues, Mϕs are regarded as central regulators of inflammation; however, like other myeloid cells, there exists a diversity of Mϕ phenotypes and functions, each characterized by expression of distinct effector proteins.

Mϕs activate their phagocytic action and inflammatory activities by sensing tissue changes using unique cell surface receptors, called pattern recognition receptors (PRRs).[156] These recognize pathogen-associated molecular patterns (PAMPS) and damage-associated molecular patterns (DAMPS) that originate from microbial cell fragments or autologous cellular constituents released from dead or necrotic cells.[157–159] In addition to activating Mϕ phagocytic ability, PRRs also endow Mϕ with the ability to orchestrate adaptive immune responses by increased secretion of chemokines/cytokines that then mobilize T cells in tissues for cytotoxic activities to remove infected or damaged cells.[160,161] Mϕ

functions are further enhanced by feed-forward signaling from interferons (IFNs) released by recruited T cells in tissues.[162] Altogether, these activities are an important aspect of innate defense where dysregulation of any process can lead to progression of chronic diseases, including cancer.[1,163,164]

Macrophages in Cancer

Mϕs residing in TMEs are distinct in molecular and functional characteristics as compared to their healthy tissue counterparts and are therefore commonly referred as tumor associated macrophages (TAMs). TAMs are derived from progenitors recruited to tumors from blood, spleen, or bone marrow, whereas tissue-resident homeostatic Mϕ are instead derived from yolk sac or other tissue-specific progenitors at an embryonic stage.[122,165–167] Across cancer indications, it is appreciated that recruited TAMs are rate-limiting for malignant conversion of otherwise benign tumors;[123,168] TAMs induce or aggravate a wide range of hallmark cancer characteristics that include, but are not limited to, tissue remodeling, angiogenesis, invasion and metastasis, and immune (T cell) evasion, as well as imparting resistance to several cytotoxic drugs.[3,24,25,169–171] One of the bonafide Mϕ activities underlying their tumor-promoting function is secretion of matrix metalloproteases (MMPs), cysteine proteases, and growth factors that together support tumor growth and disease progression to advanced stage cancer.[24,172–175] Release of these molecules within TMEs impacts cell proliferation, cell survival, and migration of endothelial, immune, and tumor cells, and together regulates development of angiogenic vasculature, tumor growth, and eventually metastasis. Among these tumor-promoting hallmarks, their ability to modulate T cell functionality is also significant due to implications for not only tumor progression but also response to therapy;[26,176,177] thus, definitive biomarkers indicative of a pro- versus an antitumorigenic, or T cell activating/suppressing, TAM are highly sought-after. Mϕ ablation strategies in preclinical murine tumor models have confirmed that Mϕ are indeed rate-limiting for angiogenesis, as well as cancer dissemination for some tumor types.[27,123,178]

One predominant simplistic paradigm describing TAM phenotype in cancer is termed the "M1-like" and "M2-like" nomenclature describing antitumor or pro-tumor functionality, respectively. Accordingly, Mϕ that metabolize arginine through nitric oxide synthase (NOS) pathway are generally found to be immunostimulatory and thus loosely referred to as M1-like, whereas Mϕ that utilize arginine preferentially by arginase pathway are found to be (T cell) immunosuppressive and are termed M2-like.[179,180] These metabolic states are now characterized in greater detail where there are in excess of 50 molecules expressed or suppressed in these opposing activation states[181,182] While these phenotypes can reproducibly be generated under defined culture conditions using cytokine/Toll-like receptor (TLR) ligand cocktails, in vivo, TAMs exhibit a spectrum of these phenotypes where TMEs are more dynamic and complex.[183]

Since TAMs often exist within a spectrum of phenotypes, it is imperative to understand the molecular basis of TAM phenotype in vivo.[184] Colony-stimulating factor-1 receptor (CSF-1R) represents a key molecular mechanism regulating a diversity of Mϕ tumor-associated phenotypes.[185] Many TMEs are rich in CSF-1 derived largely from epithelial cells and fibroblasts that aid accumulation of myelomonocytic cells.[123,186,187] However, there are a plethora of other cytokines and growth factors that also impact the abundance of TAMs as well as influence their phenotypes (e.g., GM-CSF, IL-1α and β, and CCL2).[188–192] Cellular cross-talk due to paracrine signaling also alters TAMs. Notably, B cells and their products have well-described roles in regulating TAM phenotype. Autoantibodies produced during neoplastic progression in premalignant skin can induce Mϕs to acquire protumorigenic activities, which in turn can be attenuated by therapies neutralizing or depleting B cells.[193] Interestingly, immune complexes (IC), adducts formed by antigens and their respective immunoglobulins (Igs), modulate Mϕ phenotype to upregulate expression of IL-10,[194] which induces immunosuppression by direct and indirect mechanisms in part due to activation by IC.[25,193,195,196] Another important cellular nexus in breast cancer is between Th2 CD4+ T cells that produce high levels of IL-4 and IL-13 to activate protumorigenic properties of M2-like TAMs.[170] In addition, IL-33 also induces M2-like TAM properties leading to invasive progression of otherwise benign tumors.[197] TAMs are also instructed by immune-stimulating cytokines such as IFNs produced by various cell types in TMEs that lead to M1-like TAM properties.[198–200] Such synchronous or opposing signals in addition to PRR signaling (e.g., TLRs) are transcribed in TAMs to give rise to a complex phenotype that TAMs display in a variety of tumor types.[201]

The role of intracellular signaling in exerting transcriptome changes in TAM phenotype has gained considerable traction based on implications for both biomarker development, as well as potential for identification of novel targets for cancer therapy. Depending upon the cell surface receptors, TAMs are used for sensing TME cues, and specific intracellular signals are generated, for example, phosphoinositide 3-kinase (PI3K) or mitogen-activated protein kinase (MAPK) induced by either receptor tyrosine kinases such as CSF-1R, or instead Janus kinase-signal transducer and activator of transcription (JAK-STAT) signaling, which is primarily induced upon engagement of interleukins and interferons (IFNs). Overt PI3K, MAPK, STAT3, or STAT6 signaling is generally identified in protumorigenic M2-like

TAMs, whereas STAT-1 and stress-related MAPK (e.g., JNK or p38) is more associated with immune-stimulatory or antitumorigenic M1-like TAMs.[28,202,203]

Taken together, TAM gene expression or surface marker expression can be analyzed for functional characterization of TMEs and serve as surrogates indicating a tumor's propensity to mount an antitumorigenic response. In summary, while TAMs display complex traits, these phenotypes are dependent upon molecular mechanisms highly regulated in these cells by signals present in the tumor milieu, with divergent outcomes on tumor progression. Further, their role as master orchestrator of the TME has placed great emphasis on therapeutically "depleting" or reprogramming TAMs for the purpose of tumor therapy.

DENDRITIC CELLS

Dendritic cells (DCs) comprise a group of specialized antigen-presenting cells (APCs) that bridge innate and adaptive immune responses in tissues. DCs are capable of orchestrating T cell activation or tolerance based upon integration of diverse tissue environmental inputs (cytokines and cell-cell contacts) and constant antigen sampling.[35,204,205] One of the main attributes of DCs that make them unique among other myeloid cells is their propensity to emigrate to T cell-rich secondary lymphoid organs once loaded with antigenic peptides on their major histocompatibility complexes (MHCs).[206] Apart from the existence of various subtypes of DCs, DCs are also categorized as mature and immature; immature DCs reside in peripheral tissues where they constantly patrol and sample TMEs,[206] and upon encountering a foreign antigen (e.g., bacterial component), immature DCs transition to mature DCs.[206] Similar to macrophage activation, PRRs play an essential role in DC maturation, which enables increased functionality for both processing and presenting antigens to T cells, as well as increased mobility to transition into the lymph nodes and spleen where they can interact with and prime naïve T cells to orchestrate adaptive immune responses. Therefore, it is essential to understand the DC maturation process as it can unleash antigenic T cell responses against an infected or transformed cell.

Dendritic Cells in Cancer

Although DCs are capable of activating antitumor adaptive immune responses, DCs are often dysfunctional and/or hypofunctional in TMEs and exist, like other myeloid cells, in a diversity of functional states within TMEs. Understanding what regulates the balance of pro- versus antitumor DC function has led to development of therapeutic strategies aimed at harnessing potent DC-mediated antitumor immunity.

Conventional Dendritic Cells

"Classical" or "conventional" DCs (cDCs) arise from myeloid-lineage common DC precursors (CDPs) in bone marrow under the influence of FMS-like tyrosine kinase 3 ligand (Flt3L), macrophage-colony stimulating factor (M-CSF or CSF1), and granulocyte-macrophage colony-stimulating factor (GM-CSF).[36] Two major subsets of cDCs have been described in both human and mouse, termed cDC1 and cDC2. cDC1, are specialized to elicit immunity against intracellular pathogens and tumors owing to their efficient presentation of exogenous antigens on MHC class I (MHCI) to CD8+ T cells, resulting in activation (cross-presentation) and subsequent activation of Th1 CD4+ T cells.[36,37,207–210] cDC2 are instead largely skewed toward inducing CD4+ T cell responses.[211,212]

Within the context of cancer, there is plentiful evidence that DCs prime (or re-prime) robust antitumor T cell responses. The main mechanism of DC-mediated antitumor activity is cross presentation of tumor neoantigens to CD8+ effector T cells. cDC1 are most credited with eliciting antitumor T cell immunity via their superior priming ability of CD8+ effector T cells and Th1 CD4+ T cells.[25,38,39,213,214,215] Consistent with these observations, BATF3 (basic leucine zipper transcriptional factor ATF-like 3)-derived cDC1 are necessary for tumor rejection, where vaccination with tumor-antigen loaded cDC1 is sufficient for reducing tumor growth in murine tumor models, supporting the conclusion that cDC1 are both necessary and sufficient for eliciting antitumor T cell-mediated immunity.[25,38,39,213,214,215] However, cDC2 and MoDCs may also be capable of cross-presenting antigen to effector CD8+ T cells, and cDC2 are necessary for priming of antitumor CD4+ T cell responses.[216] That said, while cDCs may be capable of activating antitumor T cell responses, many TMEs exhibit reduced DC recruitment, development, survival, and APC functionality, all of which contribute to dampening DC-mediated T cell antitumor immunity.[215]

In TMEs, there are relatively few cDC1 at steady state, thus indicating likely defects in DC differentiation, recruitment, retention, and/or survival. Tumors with relatively reduced TME abundance of cDC1 correlate with decreased survival and diminished response to newer immunotherapies (discussed in the text that follows) as compared to tumors with relatively higher abundance of cDC1.[217–219] Reduced DC recruitment to TMEs may be due to reduced chemokines attracting DCs from blood or peripheral tissues; examples include reduced secretion of CCL4 by tumor cells with active-β-catenin and loss of NK-derived CCL5 and XCL1.[218, 220, 221]

Another hurdle that DCs must face in TMEs is maturation; pre-DCs are known to exit bone marrow and enter peripheral tissues, where they complete their final steps of differentiation;[36,215] however, DC differentiation in situ is reduced in tumor settings. NK cells are notable producers of Flt3L, a cytokine that is essential for DC differentiation.[36,222] Reduced NK cells in TMEs, regulated by diverse mechanisms, have been reported to correlate with reduced DC abundance.[219] Further, VEGF, an abundant cytokine in many TMEs, functionally opposes Flt3L-mediated DC differentiation in vivo.[40]

DC maturation and antigen presentation can also be dampened by factors within TMEs. Dying cells can release high-mobility-group box 1 (HMGB1), an alarmin protein that binds to TLR4 on DCs, resulting in DC maturation and cross presentation of antigen to T cells. This effect has been observed to result in antitumor immunity following chemo- and/or radiation therapy.[223] However, DC expression of TIM3 (T cell immunoglobulin mucin-3), which is commonly upregulated in cancer settings, sequesters HMGB1 and thwarts this effective avenue of antitumor immunity.[224] Another mechanism by which tumors reduce DC APC activity is through the CD47-SIRPα (signal-regulatory protein alpha) axis. Tumor cells commonly upregulate expression of CD47, also known as the "don't eat me" signal, that interacts with SIRPα on DC surfaces, resulting in reduced phagocytosis and reduced DC antigen uptake and presentation to effector T cells.[41]

In addition to TME suppressing DC-mediated T cell activation, TMEs can actively enforce DC-mediated immune tolerance. Immune tolerance, the functional opposite of immune activation, is a common occurrence in TMEs. Tumor-derived versican binds TLR2 on DCs resulting in IL-10 and IL-6 production and cognate receptor expression to induce autocrine signaling.[225] IL-10- and IL-6-dependent STAT3 (signal transducer and activator of transcription 3) activation reprograms DCs into immunosuppressive cells that are poor T cell activators.[25,226] In addition, prostanoids, a subclass of eicosanoids, that are common in TMEs also reduce DC abundance, maturation, and ability to mount antitumor T cell responses[220] as do some metabolic byproducts, such as tumor-associated lipid peroxidation and lipid byproducts that reduce APC capacity[227–229] and directly influence APC functions.

Plasmacytoid Dendritic Cells

Plasmacytoid DCs (pDCs) are a rare subset, representing only 0.3% to 0.5% of total immune cells in blood and lymphoid organs.[230] pDCs differ in development and function from other cDC subsets: pDCs develop from both myeloid and lymphoid precursors in bone marrow under the action of Flt3L.[231] pDCs are highly specialized to produce high levels of type I IFNs in response to viral infections, and thus play important roles in antiviral immunity.[230,232,233] However, pDC are also involved in allergy and asthma, response to nonviral pathogens, and antitumor immunity.[230] Similar to cDCs, pDCs regulate antitumor T cell responses in vivo; in a murine melanoma model, TLR9-activated pDC delivered locally to TMEs resulted in tumor regression via activation of NK cells, cDCs, and CD8[+] T cells.[234] In another study, vaccination with activated and tumor-antigen loaded pDC in a small cohort of patients with melanoma resulted in T cell priming, IFN-γ production, and a modest survival benefit.[235] However, also similar to cDCs, pDCs are often dysfunctional and/or hypofunctional in TMEs. Notably, pDCs in breast and ovarian tumors produce little type I IFN and preferentially induce regulatory CD4[+] T cells (T$_{reg}$ cells).[236–239] In fact, pDC abundance in tumors can be a poor prognostic indicator in part due to pDC support of T$_{reg}$ cell populations in an ICOSL (inducible T cell co-stimulator ligand)-dependent manner.[240] Tumor-derived transforming growth factor (TGF)β and prostaglandin E2 (PGE2) are implicated in pDC support of T$_{reg}$ cells in tumors.[241–243] It is important to consider the variability of cancer therapy effects on the ability of DCs to mediate potent and long-lasting antitumor T cell immunity. Further, there is great promise for designing cancer immunotherapies with the direct intent of restoring antitumor DC mediated T cell activity.

GRANULOCYTES

Granulocytes are a group of specialized myeloid cells involved in allergic disease and protecting tissues against viral infections. Common for all three types of granulocytes, namely basophils, eosinophils, and neutrophils, are the abundance of cytoplasmic protein-filled granules often released into extracellular spaces upon cell activation. Emerging in the bone marrow from a common precursor, they differentiate and mature before entering blood. Granulocytes act as first responders to infections.

NEUTROPHILS

Neutrophils represent the most abundant population of white blood cells in the human circulatory system. Granulocyte colony-stimulating factor (G-CSF) is an essential regulator of neutrophil generation and differentiation.[244,245] Like other myeloid cells, neutrophils are a population of complex cells with great plasticity endowing them with wide-ranging activities, challenging the old view associating neutrophils merely with tissue damage and early phases of infection.[246,247] Due to their high motility, neutrophils also act as early responders during infection or tissue injury, where activated neutrophils are known to generate reactive oxygen species (ROS), release granular constituents, and create neutrophil extracellular traps (NETs), to target microbial infection in tissues and prevent their dissemination.[248–251] While these pathways are beneficial in the context of trauma and infection, such

activities in the context of a tumor can either potentiate or slow tumor progression depending on context.[252]

During the last decade, a variety of subtypes among tissue-resident neutrophils have emerged, differing in their phenotype, function, package of cytokines produced, degree of maturation, and site of action.[253,254] Their various polarization states add to the complexity of their role in cancer, beyond implications for promoting or slowing tumor initiation, progression, and metastasis. Apart from constituting a significant fraction of peripheral blood and splenic cells, neutrophils are also abundant constituents in lungs. At steady state, neutrophils protect lungs from infections due to tissue exposure to outer environments from oro- and nasopharyngeal cavities.

Neutrophils in Cancer

In many advanced stage cancer patients, elevated counts of neutrophils are found in peripheral blood and tumors, where when correlated with survival, neutrophils are associated with the worst outcomes.[255,256] However, TME complexity is involved in generation of stimulatory or suppressive neutrophil subsets, thus highlighting the importance of carefully evaluating neutrophil regulatory networks and functions. In fact, the complex interplay between immune cells, tumor cells, and stromal cells dictates neutrophil behavior.[257] Neoplastic cell secretions stimulate granulopoiesis in the bone marrow and actively induce release and recruitment of both mature neutrophils and their progenitors.[257–259] Newly emerging data from single cell RNA sequencing indicates that early progenitors of neutrophils could be programmed to give rise to a heterogenous neutrophil pool comprised of immature and mature subtypes.[260] Depending on the spectrum and quantity of soluble mediators produced by cancer cells, and cancer-associated cells, neutrophils can be polarized into different activation states by which they elicit various pro- or anti-tumor functions.

Interactions between neutrophils and other immune cells are key in exerting their function(s). Genetically engineered mouse models for cancer have been crucial for identifying underlying mechanisms by which neutrophils influence tumor initiation, growth, and metastasis as they exert multifaceted, and sometimes opposing, roles during cancer development.[261,262] Together, studies from patients with cancer and mouse models point to cancers reprogramming the myeloid compartment resulting in an expansion of myeloid cells, including neutrophils. These granulocytic cells infiltrate tumors and can promote tumor progression, in a manner similar to many other myeloid subtypes, by inducing tumor cell proliferation,[56] stimulating angiogenesis and matrix remodeling, and disabling T cell-dependent antitumor immunity.[56,143,263–266] Tumor cells are subjected to high

ROS levels in TMEs where ROS exerts protumor roles during progression.[267] For instance, in breast cancer, multinucleated cells produce ROS to stabilize hypoxia inducible factor (HIF)-1α, which in turn promotes increased VEGF production and macrophage migration inhibition factor (MIF), facilitating cancer progression and chemotherapy resistance.[264] In addition, neutrophils release Oncostatin M, a member of the IL-6 superfamily, that supports tumor progression by increasing angiogenesis and metastasis through induction of VEGF.[56] Another crucial player is TGF-ß secreted by tumor-associated myeloid cells including neutrophils, and known to be involved in cancer metastasis. Another inflammatory mediator produced by neutrophils is IL-17, which can act as a pro-inflammatory cytokine by upregulating CXCR2 ligand expression and elicit neutrophil mobilization as part of a feedforward loop to fuel cancer development.[268]

There is evidence that activated neutrophils can interact with T cells in paradoxical ways. Several studies have reported that neutrophils can present antigens and provide accessory signals for T cell activation.[269–272] However, a multitude of studies have reported that, similar to iMCs, peripheral blood neutrophils can migrate to tumors and suppress T cell proliferation through release of arginase-1 and the production of ROS.[273–274] Due to the divergent impacts that neutrophils can have on tumor progression, several complex subtypes of regulatory neutrophils have been recently described.[275] The most prominent regulatory neutrophil subtypes are tumor-associated neutrophils (TAN) G-MDSCs, also called polymorphonuclear myeloid-derived suppressor cells (PMN-MDSCs), polymorphonuclear type II (PMN-II), and circulating neutrophils (NCs).[55,57,276,277,278] These subtypes are defined based on their functional attributes and specific molecular expression.[254,279] Their phenotypic heterogeneity is mainly modulated according to individual conditions and capacity to induce an anti-inflammatory response, either by interacting directly or indirectly with other immune cells in TMEs.[280–282] In addition to these categorizations, TANs are further subdivided into antitumor "N1 neutrophils" versus protumoral "N2 neutrophils" similar to TAMs.[55] Phenotypically, the N1 type presents a hypersegmentated nuclei with high expression of FAS (a type-II transmembrane protein belonging to the tumor necrosis factor family), ICAM, and tumor necrosis factor (TNF)α production, enabling them to activate CD8+ T cells, thereby aiding in tumor cell elimination.[283–285] Polarization of TANs depends on many factors including cytokines, chemokines, and adhesion molecules secreted by other immune cells or by tumor cells. The immune profile of N1 TANs is characterized by high levels of a TNF-α, CCL3, ICAM-1, and low levels of arginase axis, whereas N2 neutrophils are characterized by upregulation of the chemokines CCL2, CCL3, CCL4, CCL8, CCL12, and CCL17, as well as CXCL1, CXCL2,

IL-8/CXCL8, and CXCL16.[286] The anti-inflammatory cytokine TGF-β has an important role in this scenario: in its presence, TANs can be directed to a protumor N2 phenotype, and in its absence (using blocking antibodies), TANs are driven to an antitumor N1 phenotype.[58,287,288] On the other hand, neutrophils can also interfere with the TME through release of cytokines (TNF-α, IL-1β, IL-12), chemokines (CCL2, CCL3, and CCL5), ROS, and growth factors, creating a diverse niche amplifying or downregulating inflammatory responses.[289]

Translation of these phenotypic paradigms from murine tumor models to human cancer is now beginning.[59,254,279,290] In humans, neutrophil to lymphocytes ratios have been used to assess the prognostic value of circulating neutrophils. However, with acknowledgment that neutrophils constitute a substantial proportion of immune infiltrates in a wide variety of cancer types, an increasing number of studies have examined the prognostic value of tumor-infiltrating neutrophils. Correlative studies using immunohistochemistry (IHC) have demonstrated that TAN infiltrates are associated with a poor prognosis for patients with head and neck cancer, renal cell carcinoma, melanoma, and gastric cancer with the only exception being colorectal cancer where high neutrophil counts have been associated with favorable outcomes.[268,291–302] Therefore, it would be interesting to analyze TAN polarization to N1 or N2 states in these cancers to determine if different outcomes are due to differences in such polarization states. Further, as with the other myeloid cells discussed in this chapter, therapeutic intervention to alter neutrophil abundance or polarization is a promising approach in cancer therapy.

MAST CELLS

Mast cells are derived from CD34+ CD117+ pluripotent hematopoietic stem cells that migrate from the bone marrow and circulate in the blood before their recruitment to peripheral tissues by chemokine/cytokine interactions, where differentiation and maturation are finalized.[303,304] Like other granulocytes, mast cells were initially characterized for their function as first-line responders against pathogens and their role in allergic reactions. Crosslinking of antigen-IgE complex to the high-affinity IgE receptors, FcεRI, leads to mast cell activation and release of granules containing inflammatory, vasoactive, and/or chemo-attractive mediators.[305] In addition, mast cells contribute to innate defense against bacteria and helminths in skin, airways, and the digestive tract where they are commonly found.[306] Further, mast cells are also categorized into different subtypes based on the repertoire of proteolytic enzymes expressed in their granules (chymases, tryptases, MMPs), or due to the tissues where they reside. During inflammation, migration and frequency of mast cell progenitors rapidly increase.

Mast Cells in Cancer

Mast cells have been described in a variety of malignancies, including cancers of the breast, lung, pancreatic ductal adenocarcinoma, glioblastoma, and melanoma.[307-313] Mast cell recruitment and infiltration in tumors is mainly mediated by tumor-derived stem cell factor (SCF) and c-kit receptor (CD117). In addition to its role in transmigration of mast cells to the tumor tissue, SCF/c-kit signaling is critical for survival and activation. Mast cell activation leads to release of granule contents into TMEs where MMP-9 is significant.[24,314,315] MMP-9 is known for inducing angiogenesis, and is thereby an early instigator of tumor development and metastasis.[316,317] Furthermore, mast cells secrete other classical pro-angiogenic factors such as VEGF, fibroblast growth factor (FGF)-2, platelet-derived growth factor (PDGF), and IL-6, in addition to nonclassical factors such as chymase and tryptase.[74]

Mast cells are critical in early stage tumors; however, in advanced stages, mast cells are dispensable for tumor growth.[24,193] For example, as compared to normal prostatic epithelial cells cultured in vitro, benign prostatic hyperplasia proliferation is stimulated by presence of mast cells.[318] Consistent with this, mast cell infiltration has been observed in adenomatous polyps, the precursors of invasive colon cancer, where depletion of mast cells leads to remission of existing polyps.[319] In addition to their important role in angiogenesis based on production of MMP-9 and VEGF, mast cells are also critical in immunomodulation. Mast cells release adenosine and IL-4 which increases T_{reg} cells and TAMs in TMEs.[315,320] Due to their role as early responders, intrinsic mast cell functions can induce divergent phenotypes in tumors with both anti- and protumorigenic activities. Growth factor secretion can also activate the Ras-MAPK pathway in mast cells, which is essential for their protumorigenic function.[321,322] Altogether, mast cells reside at the crossroads of benign tumors developing into a bona fide malignancy; thus, mast cells may serve as candidate biomarkers for early cancer detection, as well as a means to limit tumor development beyond benign stages.

EOSINOPHILS

Under normal conditions, eosinophils are recruited to tissues through Th2-derived cell signals,[323] in particular, eotaxins and IL-5 mediate eosinophil development, survival, and recruitment.[324-326] Like other granulocytes, eosinophils circulate in the blood before recruitment to peripheral tissues in response to inflammatory stimuli. At destination sites, eosinophils release cytotoxic granule proteins and major basic protein, along with a wide range of cytokines and lipid mediators upon encountering helminths, viral or microbial pathogens.[327] Eosinophil degranulation contributes to parasite destruction, in addition to often resulting in extensive inflammation and tissue damage. Eosinophils store, synthesize, and release excessive amounts of cytokines, chemokines, growth factors, enzymes, and lipid mediators; thus, they are able to arbitrate pathogen demolition. Their destruction of other cells in the TME, however, can cause pathologies, such as asthma. When these tissue-damaging properties are directed toward tumors, eosinophils can be beneficial and even protective against cancer, however at a cost. In gastrointestinal tissue, eosinophil presence can lead to eosinophilia, an overt reaction against helminths or allergic reactions, which can be life-threatening.[327,328]

Eosinophils in Cancer

In cancer, eosinophils have been given little attention as compared to other myeloid cells, even though they are present in both solid tumors and hematologic malignancies.[329,330] Tumor-associated eosinophilia is frequently observed in patients with cancer, as eosinophils can be recruited by factors secreted from necrotic cancer cells.[329] Both peripheral eosinophils and tumor-infiltrating eosinophils have been associated with beneficial prognoses in several cancer types, including gastrointestinal, head and neck, and colorectal cancer.[331,332] In triple negative and HER2-positive breast cancer, a low peripheral eosinophil count could be a good prognostic indicator.[333] In contrast, eosinophils in Hodgkin lymphoma and cervical carcinoma are associated with a poor prognosis,[334,335] thus indicating that eosinophil presence in TMEs may reflect either pro- or antitumorigenic conditions depending on context. Nevertheless, the majority of these studies focus solely on the association between eosinophils and clinical outcomes, without considering functional differences and infiltration of other leukocytes in respective tumors. In addition, existence of subpopulations of eosinophils with distinct phenotypes has also begun to emerge[336] where it has been proposed that eosinophils can be distinguished into E1 or E2 polarization states akin to macrophages and neutrophils, based on expression patterns of Th1/Th2 cytokines, that likely play a role in determining pro- versus antitumorigenic activities.[81,337,338]

Tumor-infiltrating eosinophils are limited by activities of T_{reg} cells. T_{reg} cell depletion leads to not only enrichment of eosinophils but also TME changes with increased presence of cytotoxic T cells[338] owing to secreted chemokines associated with T cell chemotaxis, and vascular normalization that may aid T cell transmigration into tumors. These changes could also be linked to eosinophil-derived IL-18, a cytokine that upregulates endothelial adhesion molecules (LFA-1 and ICAM-1) and supports leukocyte adhesion and trafficking.[82] One therapeutic approach to increase eosinophils in tumors being investigated is recombinant IL-33; increased IL-33 is accompanied by increased CD8+ T cell recruitment along with tumor rejection and reduced lung metastasis.[81] Similarly, increased

CCL11 concentration, based on its diminished degradation, enhances eosinophil tumor infiltration, degranulation, and eosinophil-mediated tumor cell cytotoxicity.[339] Eosinophils have the ability to counteract tumor growth; however, the TME is critical for determining these outcomes. For instance, lung metastasis is accelerated by IL-5 and eosinophil recruitment with heightened T_{reg} cell activity that otherwise is known to control metastatic colonization.[340,341] The importance of the TME is emphasized, however, by the fact that distinct models of lung metastasis demonstrate how eosinophil can suppress metastasis.[342] In conclusion, eosinophils can contribute to both tumor regression and progression based upon distinct tissue context leading to unique polarization and functional states.

BASOPHILS

Basophils are another type of granulocyte, with similar fundamentals to neutrophils and eosinophils. Namely, the presence of cellular granules released upon cell activation that result in immune modulation. Basophil activation occurs either by antigen crosslinking of IgE molecules bound to the FcƐR on basophils or by IgE-independent manners utilizing allergen components, TLRs, or cytokines such as IL-3, IL-18, and IL-33. Activated basophils are recruited to inflamed tissue (from the circulation) and rapidly release a variety of factors stored in their preformed granules including histamine, several growth factors, and cytokines such as IL-4 and IL-13 and thereby impact monocyte, macrophage, DC, and T cell functionality.[343,344]

Basophils in Cancer

Basophils have long been considered passive bystander cells, even though in cancer, high numbers of basophils have been described in several cancer types including hematological tumors (basophilia is considered a negative prognostic factor for chronic myeloid leukemia),[345] such as myelodysplastic syndromes, and in solid tumors, including lung and pancreatic.[106,346-348] To evaluate their functional relevance, recently basophil-depleting antibodies (anti-FceRI) and basophil-deficient murine models have become available, resulting in improved ability to focus on this relatively understudied myeloid cell type in cancer.

Basophils can exert protumor characteristics by secreting factors that promote tumor growth and suppress anticancer immune cells. For example, tumor growth can be supported through basophil secretion of VEGF and hepatocyte growth factor (HGF) released upon basophil activation that in turn induces angiogenesis and migration of endothelial cells.[349] Similar to mast cells, basophils also release histamine, a factor known to act on endothelial cells and stimulate angiogenesis.[350] Basophils can support tumor progression also by their production of large amounts of IL-4, which is required for induction of Th2 CD4+ T cell responses and involved in alternative activation of monocytes and macrophages.[351,352] IL-4 expressing basophils have been identified in tumor-draining lymph nodes of pancreas cancer patients and correlated with protumoral Th2 inflammation that predicts reduced survival.[106] In murine pancreatic tumor models, basophil recruitment to lymph nodes was required for full tumor development and was partly mediated by chemokines released by alternatively activated protumor monocytes demonstrating a mechanistically defined protumor function for basophils.[106] However, basophils also contribute to antitumor immunity when they secrete high levels of CCL3 and CCL4, thereby leading to CD8+ T cell infiltration and tumor rejection,[107] thus supporting the notion that in some contexts, basophils contribute to tumor regression, highlighting cellular plasticity as has been noted in all myeloid cells discussed thus far.

METHODS FOR PROFILING MYELOMONOCYTIC CELLS IN CANCER

There is a need to better understand tumor immunity in order to design immunotherapeutic strategies to improve clinical outcomes as well as to reveal prognostic signatures based on biomarker expression characteristics. To achieve this, several well-established methods for profiling immune contexture of either the TME or peripheral blood to uncover mechanisms and biomarkers have been employed with the goal to improve precision immunotherapeutics/diagnostics. Immune cell profiling, including myeloid cells, in healthy tissues and tumors has been conventionally performed by either multi-parametric flow cytometry or IHC detection in tumor sections. However, gene and soluble molecule expression analysis using molecular methods as well as immune assays are also critical for understanding the diverse and dynamic role myeloid cells play in different tissues. Finally, while IHC approaches have been instrumental historically, the advent of advanced multiplexed IHC approaches are now illuminating the TME cellular nexus and provide high content information on a per cell basis similar to flow cytometry. Altogether these multifaceted approaches singly and in combination provide robust and detailed information on myeloid cells in the TME.

Multiparametric Flow Cytometry

Flow cytometry allows quantitative analysis of single cells based on size and granularity, and when combined with fluorochrome-conjugated antibodies to bind protein antigens for further characterization. Such flow cytometry-based analyses have been invaluable for defining myeloid cell subsets in different cancer contexts, as well as in identifying cell types correlating with patient prognosis.[29,30,353] Further, the continual advancement of flow cytometric technology allows for utilization of ever-increasing numbers of antibodies to distinguish immune subsets, not only in terms of presence and abundance within a tissue compartment (spleen, thymus, draining lymph nodes, bone-marrow, circulating blood, or within the TME), but also assessing functional, differentiation, and maturation states of leukocytes. We can indeed now analyze millions of cells at once (when the sample size allows it) with 18 to 50 antibodies (or more). Not to mention that flow cytometry is one of the fastest techniques to study heterogeneous populations of cells, with both quantitative and qualitative endpoints. New cytometers are being constantly developed in conjunction with associated antibody conjugates to break the boundaries of numbers of parameters analyzed per cell for quantitative readouts. Spectral cytometry is one such new development where the emission spectrum of every fluorescent molecule is captured by a set of detectors or an array of channels, across a defined wavelength range. Every molecule's fluorescent spectrum can be recognized and recorded as a spectral signature, only limited by the number of fluorophores currently available. This power to distinctly record unique spectra will aid in expanding the number of markers multifold than current state-of-the-art that can be analyzed in a single reaction. Mass cytometry using CyTOF technology is another new development in conventional flow cytometry where mass of different metals conjugated to protein antibodies are analyzed using an in-built mass spectrometer. Due to the uniqueness of metal particles that can be identified, a significantly greater number of parameters (i.e., bound antibodies) can be studied per cell.

Imaging

Consistent with the old adage "a picture is worth a thousand words," the TME has long been imaged. Starting with the advent of microscopy and special histological stains in the 1800s, most notably hematoxylin and eosin, pathologists have long appreciated the value in seeing biology with their own eyes. Imaging the TME, of which myeloid cells are a large component, has advanced tremendously over the years. Advent of standard chromogenic-based IHC in 1942 allowed for visualization of a single bound antibody in a tissue specimen with relative low cost and broad accessibility. However, albeit powerful, single antibodies do not allow for confident identification of leukocyte subsets, usually requiring several antibodies, and even more antibodies for delineation of cell phenotypes/states. In recent years, highly multiplexed imaging platforms, whereby between 8 and 50+

antibodies can be applied and quantitated in a single tumor specimen, have rapidly accelerated understanding of immune contexture (immune cell abundance and localization) of tumors.[354,355] There are at least 15 distinct categories for multiplexed imaging, all of which rely upon distinct chemistries. One such class is the adaptation of standard IHC, where alcohol-soluble chromogens are removed after every immunodetection and imaging step, followed by iterative addition of additional primary antibodies on formalin-fixed tissue specimens.[356] There are many fluorescence-based multiplexed imaging platforms including those based on signal amplification and bleaching, oligo-barcode-based antibody detection, and mass-spec detection of antibodies, to name a few.[354] While multiplexed imaging platforms are highly unique and diverse, most platforms afford single cell proteomics in situ. These powerful approaches can provide data on both the abundance and composition of the immune contexture of a tumor, while maintaining tumor architecture. Thus, a deep understanding of spatial relations between tumor and immune cells is unveiled, unlike any other approach to date. Data generated from multiplexed IHC platforms increases exponentially due to the number of biomarkers that can be analyzed by new modalities that not only promise to discover unique immune cell subtypes but also help generate intricate spatial relationships that can be meaningful in cancer patient stratifications for diagnostic and prognostic purposes. Therefore, imaging modalities provide an unprecedented understanding of tumor immune contexture that is sure to rapidly advance both our understanding of, and our ability to treat, tumors well into the future.

Gene Expression Analysis

Methods of analyzing gene expression have been instrumental in our understanding of the biological phenomenon across the whole spectrum of life forms. Such analysis not only aids in uniquely identifying different cell forms but also in understanding the molecular basis of cellular behavior. To this point, gene expression analysis in cancer can be analyzed in great detail, either at a global level or within the context of specific leukocyte populations, to provide understanding of the molecular machinery of cancer inflammation. There are now several methods available that can be utilized to analyze gene expression that differ in extent of the number of genes or gene length, biased or unbiased (targeted arrays or whole genome/transcriptome sequencing), nucleotide or histone modifications analysis, as well as whether these analyses can be generated from single cells versus bulk tissue/tumor.[357–359] Utility of these methods is highly dependent upon the downstream data analysis; for example, knowledge-based databases can be used to determine cell state (e.g., M1 or M2 state of macrophages), signaling pathways can be studied using gene set enrichment analysis, or cell function inferred using gene ontology.[360] Gene expression analysis can also provide information as to myeloid cell enrichment in different tumor types and changes in population due to application of therapeutics that may directly target them or may have indirect impact on frequency or functionality.[357] Such gene expression analyses can provide mechanistic insight into cancer inflammation that amplifies precision medicine and biomarker discovery efforts.

Analysis of Soluble Mediators of Inflammation

One of the main effector functions of a cell is release of soluble mediators that facilitate cell-to-cell communications and/or influence cell behaviors. Soluble mediators include a broad variety of molecules, such as proteins and miRNAs, sometimes loaded into extracellular vesicles, and therefore represent a diverse and complex biological communication network. The enzyme-linked immunosorbent assay (ELISA) and bead-based multiplexed immunoassays allow for routine measurement of a multiplex of antigens or analytes in small volumes of (patient) samples. Such analysis is helpful for detection of inflammatory diseases as well as assessment of the nature/quality of inflammation to identify cytokine(s) potentially driving inflammatory disorders. A limitation is that these techniques rely upon measurement of predefined antigens/analytes (biased); thus, unbiased high-throughput strategies to analyze inflammatory mediators or proteomes using mass spectrometry provides functional information on cellular states at a global level, and is particularly useful in explorative studies without the need for a priori knowledge of analytes.[361,362] These technologies for secreted protein analysis have allowed in-depth analysis of factors regulating TMEs, and pose a relevant source for biomarkers to predict cancer development and progression, response rate to treatments, novel targets for therapeutics, and stratification of patients.[363]

MYELOID CELLS AND RESPONSE TO CANCER CHEMOTHERAPY

Cytotoxic chemotherapy is the most common therapy used in cancer for tumor debulking, but it has provided limited benefit for improving overall survival for most cancer types. Therefore, understanding mechanisms underlying chemorefractoriness in tumors is a significant area of investigation. Cancer inflammation is now acknowledged as an important determinant of response to chemo- and radiotherapy in various tumor types where activities of different myelomonocytic cell populations are found to be indispensable contributors to chemotherapy outcome (Figure 34.2).[3,364] It has also become evident that

anticancer therapy, whether genotoxic chemicals or small molecule inhibitors of oncogenic signals, require cytotoxic activity of T cells against tumor cells.[365–370]

Chemotherapy modulates myelomonocytic cell activity in tumors by at least two mechanisms resulting in different outcomes: (a) by activating/maturing DCs resulting in antitumor T cell priming for enhanced tumor debulking and (b) by increasing recruitment of immature monocytes, granulocytes, or macrophages in tumors, leading to dampening of cytotoxic T cell responses to incur a subverted response to chemotherapy. The effect of chemotherapy into these two main outcomes is dependent upon the cellular complexity of the tumor and tumor stage.[27,371]

In early stage cancer or low volume tumors, chemotherapy results in enhanced priming of T cell response by increasing DC activities in a process defined as immunogenic cell death (ICD) where cell death activates immune responses.[372] ICD in turn fuels widespread tumor cell death due to heightened activity of cytotoxic T cells. ICD is activated by select classes of chemotherapies (e.g., anthracyclines, certain platinum analogues, and antifolates in chemoresponsive tumors).[371,373–376] In chemotherapy-induced ICD, release of "alarmins" and other cellular content from dying cells enhances DC maturation, cross presentation of tumor antigens to effector T cells, and secretion of inflammatory cytokines.[371] These processes are critical for activation of T cell immunity against tumor cells and therefore critically determine the extent of immunogenic response of a chemotherapy.[371,377] Another known impact of chemotherapy in eliciting immunogenic responses is observed in the metronomic regimen where a low dose of cyclophosphamide produces a favorable outcome[378,379] by suppressing T_{reg} cells in tumors; that, in turn, leads to improved antitumor T cell immunity.[368,380,381] In addition, other classes of chemotherapy can negatively impact immature monocytes in tumors and thereby improve antitumor immunity where chemotherapy can elicit CD8+ T cell response in tumors by engaging eosinophils.[81] Unfortunately, eosinophilia is a known side effect for many immunotherapies or vaccination approaches that hamper patient survival.[382] Although we have a relatively poor understanding of eosinophil biology in cancer, these myeloid cells appear to be potent in engaging antitumor T cell activities and therefore hold promise for future cancer therapy development.

Heightened inflammation in advanced stages or in bulky tumors, on the other hand, is known to suppress antitumor T cell responses associated with abnormal vessel remodeling (angiogenesis), as well as increased proliferation of tumor cells;[383–387] thus, inflammation in tumors is now also regarded as an underlying regulator of resistance to chemotherapy. Indeed, tumors that poorly respond to chemotherapy exhibit enhanced recruitment

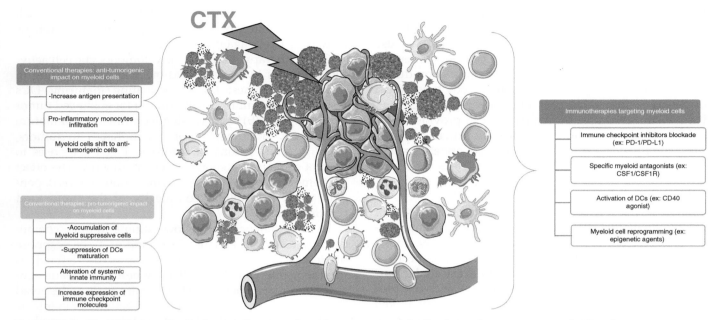

Figure 34.2 Chemotherapy/radiotherapy/immunotherapy outcome critically depends upon tumor microenvironment. Conventional therapies have demonstrated efficacy to limit tumor growth by eliciting antitumorigenic functions in some myeloid subsets. As depicted, in many cases, these therapies are also able to increase antigen presentation, infiltration of pro-inflammatory subsets, and induce a shift within TMEs to favor tumor destruction. These therapies, however, trigger protumorigenic activities as well, such as accumulation of emerging granulocytic and/or monocytic suppressive cells within TMEs, further suppression of DCs leading to accumulation of more immature phenotypes, and less cross-talk with other immune components to leverage ongoing antitumor processes. With extensive antitumor action, and to regulate their fate, myeloid cells also tend to express a broader repertoire and higher levels of immune checkpoint molecules that in turn promote immune evasion. Immunotherapies targeting myeloid cells (or their activities) are being developed to mainly target these critical points: inhibit tolerogenic cells, reprogram suppressive cells toward a more protumorigenic phenotype, enhance efficacy and quantity of APCs, and enhance cytotoxic functionality. Therapies are often combined for an optimal result to counteract possible compensating mechanisms from the remaining protumorigenic actors.

of myeloid cells with lower frequencies of cytotoxic T cells.[27,196,388] In turn, targeting of discrete myeloid cells or their effector programs using various signaling inhibitors or select toxins can result in improved response to chemotherapy.[27,28,195,389,390] Paradoxically, chemotherapy can also aggravate inflammatory processes in tumors due to increased recruitment of myeloid cells, for example, immature monocytes and granulocytes that subsequently can also give rise to immunosuppressive macrophages.[27,195,391] Therefore, chemotherapy can induce changes that oppose generation of potent antitumor responses. These chemotherapy-dependent inflammatory changes are likely due to stress signaling in tumor cells leading to secretion of myeloid cell recruiting cytokines in TMEs.[392,393] Stress responses are also observed independent of exposure to cytotoxic chemicals, for example, during tissue injury due to bacterial infection or physiological stress;[4,394,395] therefore, stress responses instigating myeloid cell-dependent inflammation is likely an intrinsic program evolved in multicellular organisms to aid tissue repair and for maintaining homeostasis, but is co-opted by tumors for fueling growth, and is exacerbated during chemotherapy exposure.

Since a major percentage of cancer patients present with advanced disease, it must also be considered that chemotherapy can exacerbate inflammation and thereby negatively impact cytotoxic T cell responses and in turn diminish therapeutic outcome. Researchers have tested this supposition by targeting tumor-associated (protumoral) inflammation to improve efficiency of chemotherapy using small molecule inhibitors of essential signaling pathways in myeloid cells and macrophage-specific toxins where improved efficacy of chemotherapeutics has been observed dependent on cytotoxic T cells.[27,28,396–398] Other changes associated with myeloid cell ablation in murine tumor models involves normalization of tumor vasculature and stromal remodeling that demonstrate increased penetrance of chemotherapeutics and intensifying cell death signaling in cancer cells.[399,400] It is possible that myeloid cell targeting by one of these modalities may also be engaging ICD programs to activate T cell responses by alleviating suppressive signals hindering DC maturation. To this point, it has been reported that targeting macrophage-derived IL-10 results in enhanced DC maturation and expression of IL-12 with subsequent activation of CD8+ T cells for enhanced tumor cell killing in a murine breast cancer model.[25] Therefore, one can anticipate many more inflammation-based targeting strategies to evolve as combination therapies to pair with standard of care chemotherapeutics for cancer patients arise.

An important side effect of chemotherapy is unselective killing of highly proliferative cells throughout the body in addition to proliferating tumor cells. Myelomonocytic cells, especially neutrophils, are highly proliferative with a short half-life; thus, neutrophils are significantly impacted by chemotherapy, and prolonged exposure without intervention can lead to febrile neutropenia in cancer patients.[401,402] An effective treatment to overcome this debilitating condition is administration of GM-CSF to rejuvenate bone marrow cells to supply neutrophils, thereby allowing continuation of chemotherapy cycles.[403] However, recent studies demonstrate that use of such bone marrow supplements can also harm durability of chemotherapy as increased neutrophils in blood transit to ectopic tissues where they can enable metastatic colonization to critically limit overall survival.[404,405] Continuation of such studies to understand how inflammation impacts chemotherapy response and vice versa is necessary for achieving optimal therapy response to significantly improve outcomes for cancer patients.

MYELOID CELLS AS TARGETS FOR CANCER IMMUNOTHERAPY

Streptococcus inoculum, introduced by William Coley in the last century for therapy to treat sarcoma, represents the earliest documented use of an immunostimulating agent to treat cancer.[406] Subsequent development of various classes of biologic-based immunotherapies for cancer management have followed (e.g., immune-stimulating cytokines, inactive whole microbe vaccines, and oncolytic viruses).[407] The advent of more recent immunotherapeutics has been developed with recognition that T cell proliferation, activation, and recruitment can be regulated by a large family of "checkpoint" molecules, inhibition or activation of which, dependent on mechanism(s) of action, can result in robust enhancement of T cell functionality.[408–410] These therapeutics, also referred to as immune checkpoint blockers (ICBs), have been highly successful for generating meaningful clinical responses in some of the most difficult to treat cancer types, where they collectively activate or sustain cytotoxic T cell responses to elicit tumor cell killing.[411–413]

T cell checkpoint molecules act as "brakes" to control T cell activation in response to antigen where co-stimulatory molecules potentiate antigenic T cell activation.[414] Interestingly, while checkpoints and co-stimulatory molecules are primarily expressed on T cells, ligands of many of these are expressed on myeloid cells, especially APCs.[415] Two

key checkpoint molecules therapeutically targeted by U.S. Food and Drug Administration (FDA)-approved biologics are PD-1 and CTLA-4 (program cell death molecule-1 and cytotoxic T-lymphocyte-associated protein-4, respectively). Both molecules critically impact CD28 signaling to attenuate T cell receptor (TCR)-dependent T cell activation by interaction with CD80 on APCs.[416] CTLA-4 competes with CD28 to impact CD80 expression on APCs, whereas PD-1, upon engagement with its ligand PD-L1 (programmed death ligand 1) largely expressed by myeloid cells in tumors, negatively regulates CD28 activation by phosphatase-dependent activity.[408,416] Recent findings have further elucidated a rate-limiting role for APCs in T cell checkpoint signaling where cis interaction of CD80 with PD-L1 regulates CD80 expression by APCs and in turn regulates T cell activation,[417] in addition to APC-expressed PD-L1 directly regulating PD-1-dependent T cell activation.[418] Together, recognition of the diverse role of myeloid cells in regulating T cell functionality via impacting "checkpoint" responses is now also shaping efforts toward biomarker discovery for predicting immunotherapy response, as well as novel therapy development for combination with ICBs.[407]

While efficacy of ICBs has improved overall survival for some cancer types, not all cancers respond and, within cancers, not all patients respond; thus, understanding resistance mechanisms for these immunotherapies is of paramount importance.[419] Since myeloid cells are major components of TMEs and can suppress T cell functionality by a multitude of mechanisms including T cell checkpoint regulation, therapeutic targeting of myeloid-expressed checkpoint molecules, in addition to or in combination with T cell-expressed checkpoints, is being examined (Figure 34.2). For example, myeloid cells express high levels of CD39 leading to accumulation of adenosine that lowers the frequency of cytotoxic T cells while simultaneously enhancing frequency of T_{reg} cells; thus, therapeutically neutralizing CD39 activity could theoretically reverse this effect.[420] TIM3, a coinhibitory receptor expressed by DCs, affects their ability to cross-prime or activate CD8+ T cells.[421,422] On the other hand, *LAG-3* (lymphocyte activation gene-3) is expressed on T_{reg} cells and interacts with major histocompatibility complex (MHC)-II on DCs and macrophages, thereby inhibiting their maturation, cytokine production, and T cell activation;[419,423,424] thus, targeting TIM-3 and/or *LAG-3* could greatly improve efficacy of anti-PD-1/PD-L1 therapies.[419,425,426] As previously discussed, DC maturation is downstream of TLR signaling; thus, agonistic TLR ligands are also being evaluated in combination with ICBs for cancer therapy. Intracellular TLRs as well as cGAS-STING antagonists are in clinical trials to enhance antitumor T cell response and improve ICB efficacy. CD40 activation has also been reported to activate DCs and newly recruited TAMs to enhance T cell priming as well as direct tumoricidal activity.[427–429]

Table 34.2 Select Drugs Targeting Myeloid Cells in Preclinical or Clinical Stages of Immunotherapy Development

TARGET MOLECULE	COMPOUND	TARGETED MYELOID CELL TYPE	CANCER TYPE	COMBINATION WITH CHEMO +/- ICB	CLINICAL TRIAL	PHASE
CSF-1/CSF-1R axis	PLX3397 (pexidartinib)	Monocytes, macrophages	Advanced solid tumors	Pembrolizumab	NCT02452424	1/2
	MCS-100			PDR001	NCT02807844	1/2
	RG7155 (emactuzumab)			Atezolizumab	NCT02323191	1
	BLZ945			PDR001	NCT02829723	1/2
CCR2/CCR5	BMS-813160 (CCR2, CCR5 antagonist)	Monocytes, macrophages	Colorectal, pancreatic	Chemotherapy or nivolumab	NCT03184870	1/2
All transretinoic acid	ATRA	iMCs	Neuroblastoma	IFN-α2a	NCT00001509	2
BTK	Ibrutinib	B cells, myeloid cell migration, iMCs	Lymphocytic leukemia and lymphoma	Nivolumab	NCT02420912	2
			NSCLC, breast, pancreatic	Durvalumab	NCT02403271	1/2
PI3Kδ	Idelalisib	Macrophages	CLL	Rituximab	NCT02044822	2
	INCMGA00012		Advanced solid tumors	Retifanlimab, epacadostat	NCT03589651	1
PI3Kγ	IPI-549	Macrophages	HNSCC	Monotherapy	NCT03795610	2
CX3CL1	JMS-17-2; KAND567	pMOs	Pancreatic		Preclinical	
C5aR1	PMX-53	Macrophages	SCC	Paclitaxel	Preclinical	
Trabectedin	Chemotherapy	Preferential toxicity for monocytes and macrophages	Metastatic sarcoma	Trabectedin monotherapy	NCT04076579	2
CD47/SIRPα axis (SIRPα-Fc fusion proteins)	TTI-621	Macrophages	Hematological, select solid tumors	Rituximab, nivolumab	NCT02663518	1
	ALX148	Macrophages	Advanced solid tumors	Pembrolizumab	NCT03013218	1
TLR9	MGN1703 (lefitolimod)	DC activation	Melanoma Solid tumors	Ipilimumab	NCT02668770	1
	SD101	DC activation	B-cell non-Hodgkin lymphoma	Anti-OX40 and radiation therapy	NCT03410901	1
	CMP-001	DC activation	Melanoma	Pembrolizumab	NCT02680184	1

(continued)

Table 34.2 Select Drugs Targeting Myeloid Cells in Preclinical or Clinical Stages of Immunotherapy Development (*continued*)

TARGET MOLECULE	COMPOUND	TARGETED MYELOID CELL TYPE	CANCER TYPE	COMBINATION WITH CHEMO +/- ICB	CLINICAL TRIAL	PHASE
STING ligands	MK-1454	DC activation	Solid tumors, lymphoma	Pembrolizumab	NCT03010176	1
DC vaccines	Autologous mature DCs	DC/therapeutic vaccination	Metastatic melanoma	Monotherapy	NCT01042366	2
CD40	APX005M	DC, APCs	NSCLC	Nivolumab	NCT03123783	2

APCs, antigen-presenting cells; BTK, Bruton tyrosine kinase; CCR, CC chemokine receptor; C5aR, complement 5a receptor; CLL, chronic lymphocytic leukemia; CSF, colony-stimulating factor; CX3CL, C-X3-C-motif chemokine ligand; DC, dendritic cells; HNSCC, head and neck squamous cell carcinoma; ;iMCs, immature myeloid cells; NSCLC, non-small cell lung cancer; PI3K, phosphoinositide 3-kinase; pMO, patrolling monocyte; SCC, squamous cell carcinoma; SIRPα signal-regulatory protein α; STING, stimulator of interferon genes; TLR, Toll-like receptor.

This approach is now also being evaluated in pancreatic cancer as a single agent, as well as in combination with ICBs (Table 34.2).

The immunosuppressive capacity of TAMs, as well as monocytic and granulocytic cells, thus reveals their potential as candidate therapeutic targets for improving ICB responses. It has been reported that tumor-associated myelomonocytic cells represent a major determinant of ICB resistance in nonresponding murine tumor models;[430,431] thus, targeting these cells by abrogating growth factor signaling, such as the CSF-1/CSF1R axis or its downstream intracellular signaling molecules (e.g., PI3Kγ), improves ICB response in preclinical tumor models, resulting in enhanced T cell activation accompanied by tumor regression.[430,431] Such responses could result from heightened recruitment of T cells due to increased expression of chemokines, increased co-stimulatory ligand expression, or a combination of both. Future research will improve our understanding of underlying mechanisms of improved mechanisms of these combination therapy approaches. TEK kinases, especially Bruton tyrosine kinase (BTK), while important for B cell activity, also relays immunosuppressive signals in myeloid cells.[407,432] BTK inhibitors have been transformative in B cell malignances and are also undergoing clinical testing for their utility in solid tumors for relieving T cell suppression by tumor-associated myeloid cells.[28] Chemokine and cytokine targeting agents are also being evaluated to block infiltration of myelomonocytic cells in tumors and reduce inflammation in order to relieve immunosuppressive signals for improved efficacy of immunotherapies.[407] CXCR2 and CXCR4 inhibitors have shown efficacy in reducing neutrophils that accumulate in tumors in a Th1 TME to enhance the benefits of Th1 reprogramming.[433]

CONCLUSION

Our understanding of the complexity of TMEs is ever-evolving with new revelations where we now appreciate the diversity of activities bestowed on evolving tumors by myeloid cells reflecting a multitude of functional states. Going forward, aided by new emerging technologies, we will be better able to associate distinct myeloid subtypes to specific functional roles within cancers, as well as stratify patients for improved therapeutic outcomes based on nuances of myeloid functionality.

KEY REFERENCES

Only key references appear in the print edition. The full reference list appears in the digital product on Springer Publishing Connect: connect.springerpub.com/content/book/978-0-8261-3743-2/part/part03/chapter/ch34

3. Hanahan D, Coussens LM. Accessories to the crime: functions of cells recruited to the tumor microenvironment. *Cancer Cell.* 2012;21(3):309–322. doi:10.1016/j.ccr.2012.02.022
12. Geissmann F, Manz MG, Jung S, et al. Development of monocytes, macrophages, and dendritic cells. *Science.* 2010;327(5966):656–661. doi:10.1126/science.1178331
27. Denardo DG, Brennan DJ, Rexhepaj E, et al. Leukocyte complexity predicts breast cancer survival and functionally regulates response to chemotherapy. *Cancer Discov.* 2011;1(1):54–67. doi:10.1158/2159-8274.CD-10-0028
35. Wculek SK, Cueto FJ, Mujal AM, et al. Dendritic cells in cancer immunology and immunotherapy. *Nat Rev Immunol.* 2020;20(1):7–24. doi:10.1038/s41577-019-0210-z
59. Coffelt SB, Wellenstein MD, de Visser KE. Neutrophils in cancer: neutral no more. *Nat Rev Cancer.* 2016;16(7):431–446. doi:10.1038/nrc.2016.52
365. Ruffell B, Coussens LM. Macrophages and therapeutic resistance in cancer. *Cancer Cell.* 2015;27(4):462–472. doi:10.1016/j.ccell.2015.02.015
407. Gotwals P, Cameron S, Cipolletta D, et al. Prospects for combining targeted and conventional cancer therapy with immunotherapy. *Nat Rev Cancer.* 2017;17(5):286–301. doi:10.1038/nrc.2017.17

Intratumoral Gene Signatures and Host Genetic Variations Associated With Immune Responsiveness

Davide Bedognetti, Eiman I. Ahmed, Jessica Roelands, Zohreh Tatari-Calderone, Francesco M. Marincola, and Ena Wang

KEY POINTS

- Gene expression profiling studies in humans have enhanced our understanding of mechanisms associated with immune responsiveness.

- Transcriptomic studies have defined common themes associated with immune-mediated tumor rejection. Overlapping signatures have been observed in tumors with favorable prognostic connotation, in pretreatment lesions more likely to respond to immune manipulation, and in tumors about to regress following immunotherapy administration.

- These signatures summarize a phenomenon characterized by the activation of the signal transducer and activator of transcription 1 (*STAT1*)/interferon regulatory factor 1 (*IRF1*)/*IFNG* signaling, the expression of genes encoding for C-C motif chemokine receptor 5 (CCR5) and C-X-C motif chemokine receptor 3 (CXCR3) ligands (e.g., *CCL5*, *CXCL9*, and *CXCL10*), and induction of immune effector function genes (e.g., perforin [*PRF1*], granulysin [*GNLY*], and granzymes [*GZMs*]) by cytotoxic cells with consequent development of a T helper 1 (Th1) immune response.

- The favorable Th1 cancer phenotype is also typified by the activation of adaptive counterregulatory mechanisms, as signified by the overexpression of indoleamine-pyrrole 2,3-dioxygenase 1 (*IDO1*), programmed death ligand 1 (PD-L1), and Forkhead Box P3 (*FOXP3*).

- The prognostic and predictive connotations of this immune active disposition are enhanced in high-proliferative/high-mutational load tumors and impaired in presence of high TGF-β signaling.

- Correlative and functional studies have demonstrated that tumor genetic programs can influence the

development of an effective immune response, including MAPK, PI3K, and Wnt- β catenin-activating mutations.

- Associations between responsiveness to immunotherapy and polymorphism of human leukocyte antigen (HLA), *CCR5*, *IL-2* to *IL-21*, *IRF5*, *HLA*, Fc-receptor, and cytotoxic T lymphocyte–associated protein 4 (*CTLA-4*) have been reported, particularly in melanoma patients.

- Emerging data from germline pan-cancer analyses indicates that the functional orientation of the tumor immune microenvironment is partially heritable, and identified germline variants associated with poor immune disposition, including missense polymorphisms in key interferon-signaling genes such as *IFIH1* and *TMEM173* (STING).

- HLA polymorphisms have been consistently associated with susceptibility to leukemia and virally induced tumors such as head and neck, cervical, and nasopharyngeal cancer.

- Associations between killer cell immunoglobulin–like receptor (*KIR*) polymorphisms and cancer susceptibility have been reported with some conflicting results, particularly in leukemia and lymphoma.

- Associations between killer cell immunoglobulin–like receptor (*KIR*) polymorphisms and cancer susceptibility have been reported with some conflicting results, particularly in leukemia and lymphoma.

INTRODUCTION

The efficacy of a given immunological treatment is related to its ability to induce, directly or indirectly, a cytotoxic response against tumor cells.

Going beyond the use of proinflammatory cytokines or vaccines, scientists and clinicians have tested the possibility of enhancing antitumor immune reaction by targeting immune regulatory pathways,[1,2] now broadly known as "immune checkpoints."[3,4] The dramatic results of such approaches have revolutionized the field of tumor immunology. In early studies on metastatic melanoma patients, blockade of the T cell inhibitory receptor cytotoxic T lymphocyte–associated protein 4 (CTLA-4) was shown to induce prolonged immune responses and increased overall survival in Phase 3 trials.[5,6] Subsequently, the inactivation of the programmed cell death protein 1 (PD-1)–programmed death-ligand 1 (PD-L1) pathway was found to induce long-lasting tumor regression in several tumor types.[7–14] The remarkable achievements of other refined immunotherapies, such as adoptive transfer therapy with autologous tumor-infiltrating lymphocytes (TILs) or with engineered T cells, which entered the clinical practice in hematological malignancies and demonstrated signs of activity in solid tumors, have amplified the enthusiasm in the field.[15–19]

At the same time, the strong prognostic impact of pre-existing immunity in several tumors, and in particular in breast and colon cancer, has triggered vigorous research in the field.

Nevertheless, in solid tumors, objective responses to immune checkpoint blockade (ICB) occur in only a minority of patients, ranging from 10% (e.g., glioblastoma and ovarian cancer) to 40% (e.g., melanoma, and microsatellite instable (MSI-H) tumors).[20] Complete remission is still, and unfortunately, a rare phenomenon.[14,21] Globally, less than 15% of patients with cancer is estimated to respond to such as a treatment.[22]

The precise definition of molecular features associated with treatment response is a critical step for the development of a more efficient, personalized immunotherapy.[4,23]

In humans, ex vivo transcriptomic approaches in the context of cancer immunology have defined molecular mechanisms associated with immune-mediated tumor rejection. Such studies have observed that common signatures are shared by tumors bearing favorable prognostic connotations and those that will respond to immune manipulations.[19,24–27] Moreover, following immunotherapy administration, the induction of such signatures, or immune modules, is observed in neoplastic lesions before clinical response is detectable. In the first part of this chapter, we discuss how gene expression studies in humans have enhanced our understanding of mechanisms associated with immune responsiveness.

The intrinsic genetics of the tumor cells, the genetic makeup of the host bearing the disease, and environmental factors such as the microbiome likely act in concert to modulate spontaneous or treatment-induced antitumor immune response (Figure 35.1). Strong data from mice and humans suggest that the composition of commensal microbiota can influence the efficacy of immunotherapeutic approaches.[28] Comprehensive studies assessing

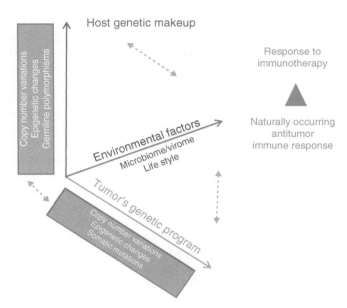

Figure 35.1 Putative variables influencing tumor immune responsiveness. Putative interdependent variables influencing the development of naturally occurring or treatment-induced antitumor immunity are represented.

the contributions of the genetic makeup of the host on antitumor immunity are emerging in the last couple of years, and polymorphisms of specific genes have been correlated with neoplastic development, polarization of the tumor immune microenvironment, and responsiveness to immunotherapy as discussed in the second part of this chapter.

PART 1: INTRATUMORAL SIGNATURES ASSOCIATED WITH IMMUNE RESPONSIVENESS

It is difficult to overstate the contribution of transcriptomic studies on our understanding of tumor-host interactions and on identifying features associated with spontaneous and treatment-induced immune response. In this part of the chapter, we summarize main findings derived from bulk transcriptomic studies on tumor tissues in humans. We try to follow, when possible, a chronologic order to better elucidate the progressive gains of knowledge.

Intratumoral Transcriptomic Changes Induced By Immunotherapy: Mechanistic Signatures

Early Studies: Cytokine-Based Therapies, Imiquimod, and Vaccines

Because of the challenges in accessing the tumor microenvironment (TME) in humans, immune monitoring has been limited for decades to the analysis of circulating immune cells.

In early 2000, in parallel with the implementation of reliable high-throughput gene expression profiling approaches (i.e., microarrays), an emphasis was placed on complementing the analysis of immune response in peripheral blood with the study of the tumor–host interactions by directly analyzing tumor samples. This approach offered the opportunity to capture in real time the physiology of the disease by simultaneously assessing the expression of thousands of analytes. In those years, in parallel with the optimization of microarray technology, the development of refined assays for linear amplification of messenger RNA[29] allowed the profiling of minimal starting materials, such as those from fine needle aspiration biopsies. It was therefore possible to study intratumoral transcriptomic modifications by profiling the same lesion before and after treatment. In the first study of this kind, lesions from metastatic melanoma were studied before and 3 hours after the first and the fourth dose of interleukin (IL)-2 (i.e., 24 hours after the first dose).[30] This approach revealed that the immediate effect of systemic IL-2 administration on the TME predominantly consists of the induction of genes associated with monocytic cell activation. Contrary to what was expected, there was no effect on lymphocytic migration, as demonstrated by the absence of changes in the expression of transcripts encoding proteins constitutively expressed by immune cells such as CD4 and CD8. Rather, the early effects induced by IL-2 were represented by the induction of cytotoxic mechanisms in monocytes and natural killer (NK) cells (e.g., calgranulin, grancalcin, NKG5, and NK4), activation of the antigen-presenting machinery (e.g., human leukocyte antigen [HLA] class II molecules), and production of chemoattractants (especially C-X-C motif chemokine receptor 3 [CXCR3] and C-C motif chemokine receptor 5 [CCR5] ligands such as CXCL9, CCL3, and CCL4) that may recruit activated CXCR3/CCR5 expressing T helper 1 (Th1), T cytotoxic, and natural killer (NK) cells. Central to this signature was the presence of the interferon regulatory factor 1 (IRF1) and other interferon γ (IFN-γ)-inducible transcripts. Such monocytic/macrophagic activation appeared shifted toward a M1-type response, which is thought to exert important antitumoral functions by sustaining Th1 inflammation[31] (see Chapter 11).

The following step was to characterize molecular variations associated with immune-mediated rejection through the comparison of treatment-induced transcriptomic changes between responding and nonresponding lesions. By studying melanoma patients treated with IL-2 and various vaccination schedules, it was evident that nonresponding lesions lacked post-treatment transcriptional modifications.[32] Conversely, tumors that would subsequently undergo complete remission displayed signs of an early switch from chronic to acute inflammation substantiated by the activation of IRF1. Despite the fact that observations were in part hampered by the use of prototype platforms querying only a proportion of the transcriptome, they were confirmed by subsequent investigations employing genome-wide arrays. The following genome-wide transcriptomic analysis of a cohort of patients homogeneously treated with high-dose IL-2 showed that the majority of molecular pathways induced by such agents reflect a positive modulation of immunological processes, including induction of the CCR5 chemokine pathway.[33] Transcriptomic differences between post-treatment responding and nonresponding lesions (collected 3 hours after the sixth dose of IL-2) were centered on the induction of the IFN-γ/IRF1 signaling, such as the upregulation of HLA class II transcripts. However, signatures qualitatively similar, but quantitatively lower, were already detectable in baseline samples from responding patients, suggesting that tumor lesions are preconditioned to respond by an immunologically active TME.[33]

Another seminal study investigated the transcriptional changes induced by the Toll-like receptor-7 (TLR-7) agonist imiquimod, a local immunotherapeutic agent approved for the treatment of basal cell carcinoma. The high clinical activity of imiquimod (80%–90% of complete remission rate) and the easy accessibility of basal cell carcinoma lesions make this therapeutic agent an outstanding model for the study of treatment-induced microenvironmental changes. The perturbations induced by imiquimod qualitatively overlapped with those induced by IL-2, although they were more pronounced with an enhanced activation of IFN-stimulated genes (e.g., signal transducers and activator of transcription 1 [STAT1], and IFN-γ-inducible HLA class I and II molecules), and transcripts associated with immune effector functions (IEF; e.g., perforin [PRF1], granulysin [GNLY], and granzymes [GZMs]) and Th1 chemotaxis (e.g., the CCR5 and CXCR3 ligands CCL3, CCL4, CXCL9, and CXCL10), in line with the higher activity of such an agent. However, the magnitude of the treatment-induced changes was maximal in lesions treated with a highly effective dose-intense schedule, indirectly implying a relationship between the intensity of local inflammation and clinical response.[34] A validation of these findings has been recently obtained by analyzing breast cancer skin metastases, in which a coordinated activation of these sets of genes following imiquimod treatment was strongly associated with durable clinical response.[35]

In another study, investigators compared melanoma metastases undergoing tumor regression after immunotherapy (vaccination or IFN-α) to synchronous lesions that continued to progress from two patients who experienced mixed responses.[36] The analysis of opposite evolution of tumor lesions treated simultaneously allowed the elimination of variables related to genetic background of the host and environmental factors. Again, regressing lesions displayed activation of the STAT1/IRF1 signaling pathway associated with the induction of CCR5 ligands and immune effector (cytotoxic) function (IEF) transcripts.[36] Furthermore, in a recent longitudinal study of 31 metastases from two colorectal cancer patients experiencing exceptionally long survival, the activation of pathways reflecting adaptive immunity was associated with genetic immunoediting, which characterized clones less likely to generate other metastases.[37]

Molecular pathways captured by early studies greatly overlap with those observed in other forms of immune-mediated rejection such as graft-versus-host disease (GvHD), allograft rejection, and flares of autoimmunity.[23,31–33] It has been proposed that although the trigger leading to tissue destruction varies in distinct pathologic states, the immune effector response converges into similar molecular pathways.[16] These pathways reflect a process typified by the coordinated modular activation of IFN-stimulated genes orchestrated by the transcription factors IRF1 and STAT1, the recruitment of cytotoxic cells through the production of specific chemokine ligands with subsequent Th1/cytotoxic polarization of the intratumoral immune response and activation of IEF/cytotoxic genes. Activation of these pathways coexist with the counteractivation of adaptive immune-modulatory pathways,[15–18] which follows, rather than precedes, CD8 T cell infiltration.[38] These modules, which overall include more than 500 genes,[27,34] have been defined as the "immunologic constant of rejection (ICR)."[19,27,39,40] The ICR has been optimized into a 20-gene signature which include: IFN-γ/Th1 signaling (*IFNG, CD8A, CD8B, TBX21, IRF1, STAT1, IL-12B*), CXCR3/CCR5 chemokine signaling (*CXCL9, CXCL10, CCL5*), IEF/cytotoxic function (*GNLY, PRF1, GZMA GZMB, GZMH*), and adaptive counterregulatory transcripts (*CD274, PD-L1, CTLA-4, Foxp3, IDO1, PD-1*).[35,41–43]

Studies in the Context of Immune Checkpoint Blockade: Melanoma

These early findings have been confirmed and expanded in the context of ICB, with the first observation being reported in 2012 by Ji et al.[44] In excised melanoma metastases profiled before and after the second ipilimumab (CTLA-4 blockade) administration (i.e., 3 weeks after the first dose), the induction of HLA class II genes, IFNG, CXCR3/CCR5 ligand genes, and IEF/cytotoxic transcripts such as GZMs was greater in lesions from patients who subsequently experienced clinical benefit as compared with those who did not.[44] A comprehensive list of transcriptomic studies in the context of ICB is presented in Table 35.1.

Furthermore, in patients treated by anti-PD-1 monoclonal antibody (mAb) within early trials across different tumors, Herbst et al. showed that on-treatment responding lesions display a Th1-dominant immune infiltrate, while nonresponding tumors lack tumor CD8+ T cell infiltration and T cell activation/cytotoxic markers and CXCR3 chemokines (e.g., GZMA, PRF1, CXCL9, CXCL10, and inducible T cell co-stimulatory [ICOS]).[45] Similarly, Chen et al. reported that posttreatment melanoma metastases collected at early time points following PD-1 blockade treatment in responding patients showed a greater upregulation of HLA molecules, Th1/IFN-γ-related transcripts (including PD-L1), and chemokines, as compared to the ones from the nonresponding patients.[69] In fact, pre- versus on-treatment fold changes of those genes perfectly segregated responding and nonresponding lesions.[69]

In another study in melanoma patients, while PD-1 blockade overall induced upregulation of several immune-related genes, such changes were broader in samples from patients achieving a clinical response, and include upregulation of ICR modules such as Th1/cytotoxic polarization (*IFNG, CD8A, CD8B*), IEF genes (*GZMA, GZMB, GZMH, GNLY, PRF1*), CXCR3/CCR5 ligands (*CXCL9, CXCL10, CCL5*), and immune regulation (*CTLA-4, IDO1, PD-1*),[52] confirming and expanding early observation in the context of CTLA-4 blockade.[44] These changes were accompanied by upregulation of additional immune checkpoint genes such as *TNFRSF4* (OX40), *TIGIT, HAVCR2* (TIM-3), *C10orf54* (VISTA), and *LAG-3*.[52] Upregulation of similar transcripts were observed after a single dose of PD-1 blockade neoadjuvant treatment in another independent study in melanoma.[63]

Studies in the Context of Immune Checkpoint Blockade: Glioblastoma and Head and Neck Cancers

Beyond the melanoma setting, a higher activation of IFN-γ genes and IEF/cytotoxic transcripts were observed in glioblastoma tumors treated with neoadjuvant PD-1 blockade (posttreatment lesions) as compared to the ones treated with adjuvant PD-1 blockade (pretreatment lesions), and were associated with increased survival.[65] In another glioblastoma study, increase of CD8 T cells after neoadjuvant treatment was only evident in patients with PTEN wild type and not in the ones with PTEN mutations, which were resistant to treatment.[61]

Different results were observed in HPV-unrelated head and neck cancers treated with PD-1 blockade.[68] While at baseline several immune-related genes encompassing ICR modules were significantly higher in responding versus nonresponding lesions, the investigators observed that, in nonresponding lesions only,

Table 35.1 Transcriptomic Studies in the Context of Immune Checkpoint Blockade

AUTHOR ACCESSION #	TUMOR	SAMPLES N (PATIENTS N)	IMMUNE CHECKPOINT BLOCKADE	BIOPSY TIME	PREDICTIVE VALUE OF T CELL/CYTOTOXIC/IFN-Γ SIGNATURES (ICR-RELATED PATHWAYS)	PLATFORM
Ji et al. (CA184004)[44]	Melanoma	90 (45)	CTLA-4	Pre/Post	+/+	Affymetrix microarrays
Herbst et al. (NCT01375842)[45]	Solid tumors and hematological malignancies	76*	PD-1	Pre/On	+/+	Real-time PCR-based platform (Fluidighm)
Van Allen et al. (phs000452.v2.p1)[46]	Melanoma	42 (42)	CTLA-4	Pre	+	RNA-Seq
Ascierto et al. (GSE67501)[47]	Renal cell carcinoma	11 (11)	PD-1	Pre	−	Microarrays
Chen et al.[48]	Melanoma	102 (53)	PD-1 CTLA-4	Pre/On	− (CTLA-4) + (PD-1)	NanoString
Hugo et al. (GSE78220)[49]	Melanoma	28 (27)	PD-1	Pre	−	RNA-Seq
Ayers et al.[50]	Pan-cancer (9 tumors)	220 (220)	PD-1	Pre	+	NanoString
Prat et al. (2017) (GSE93157)[51]	NSCLC Head and neck squamous cell Melanoma	65 (65)	PD-1	Pre	+	NanoString
Riaz et al. GSE91061[52]	Melanoma	109 (65)	PD-1 (CTLA-4-treated, and CTLA-4-naïve)	Pre/On	+/+ (in CTLA-4-treated group only)	RNA-Seq
Tarhini et al.[53]	Melanoma	54 (27)	CTLA-4	Pre/Post (Neoadjuvant)	+/+	Microarrays
Auslander et al. GSE11582142[54]	Melanoma	37 (11)	PD-1 CTLA-4	Pre/On	Unclear	RNA-Seq
Cristescu et al.[55]	Pan-cancer† (22 tumor)	304 (304)	PD-1	Pre	+	NanoString
Mariathasan et al. EGAS00001002556[56]	Urothelial cancer	297 (297)	PD-1	Pre	+	RNA-Seq
McDermott et al. (EGAD00001004183)[57]	Renal cell carcinoma	263 (263)	PD-1/ /VEGF PD-1+VEGF	Pre	−/−/+	RNA-Seq
Miao et al. (phs001493.v1.p1)[58]	Renal cell carcinoma	32 (32)	PD-1 CTLA-4	Pre	−/−	RNA-Seq
Kim et al. (2018) (PRJEB25780)[59]	Gastric cancer	45 (45)	PD-1	Pre	+	RNA-Seq

(continued)

Table 35.1 Transcriptomic Studies in the Context of Immune Checkpoint Blockade (*continued*)

AUTHOR ACCESSION #	TUMOR	SAMPLES N (PATIENTS M)	IMMUNE CHECKPOINT BLOCKADE	BIOPSY TIME	PREDICTIVE VALUE OF T CELL/CYTOTOXIC/IFN-Γ SIGNATURES (ICR-RELATED PATHWAYS)	PLATFORM
Rodig et al.[60]	Melanoma	90 (90)‡	PD-1 → CTLA-4 CTLA-4 → PD-1	Pre	+/−	RNA-Seq
Cloughesy et al. (GSE121810)[61]	Glioblastoma	29 (29)	PD-1	Pre/Post (Neoadjuvant)	−/+	RNA-Seq
Gide et al. (PRJEB23709)[62]	Melanoma	158 (120)	PD-1 PD-1 + CTLA-4	Pre/On	+/+	RNA-Seq
Huang et al. (GSE123728)[63]	Melanoma	24 (14)	PD-1	Pre/Post	+	NanoString
Liu et al. (phs000452.v3.p1) [64]	Melanoma	103 (103)	PD-1 (CTLA-4-treated, CTLA-4-naïve)	PD-1	+	RNA-Seq
Zhao et al. (PRJNA482620)[65]	Glioblastoma	38 (17)	PD-1	Pre/Post	+/+	RNA-Seq
Braun et al.[66]	Renal cell carcinoma	297 (297)	PD-1	Pre	−	RNA-Seq
Hwang et al. (GSE136961)[67]	NSCLC	21 (21)	PD-1	Pre	+	RNA-Seq
Uppaluri et al. (NCT02296684)[68]	Head and heck	34 (19)	PD-1	Pre/Post	+/−	RNA-Seq

*Baseline numbers derived from figures, number of "on treatment" samples unspecified.

†Include samples previously described in Ayers et al.

‡Data extracted from figures plots.

"-", no predictive value.

"+", positive predictive value.

CTLA-4, cytotoxic T lymphocyte associated protein 4; NSCLC, non-small cell lung cancer; PD-1, programmed cell death 1; On, on treatment; Post, posttreatment; pre, pretreatment.

the increase of lymphocyte infiltration (estimated by gene expression) was associated with upregulation of immune-regulatory genes such as *PD-1*, *CTLA-4*, *ICOS*, *TIGIT*, *IDO1*, and *TNFSF4*.[68] The inability of this study to detect significant upregulation of immune-related genes in responding lesions might be due to the limited sample size, and/or time point selections. However, it might also suggest the existence of tissue-dependent regulatory mechanisms.

Qualitatively similar signatures are observed in pretreatment tumor lesions that are more likely to respond to immunotherapy (as discussed in the following paragraph) as well as in excised tumors from patients experiencing prolonged survival, as discussed in detail in the following paragraph. Therefore, a certain degree of activation of the ICR pathways is observed in the presence of growing tumors in the absence of tumor rejection. In these settings, it is possible that the ICR signatures underline a subacute inflammatory process in which tumor growth is either partially counteracted or not suppressed at all until its magnitude is amplified by the treatment.

Pretreatment Transcriptomic Features Associated With Responsiveness to Immunotherapy: Predictive Signatures

Early Studies: Cytokine-Based Therapies and Vaccines

The therapeutic index of immunotherapeutic approaches is limited by the inability to select patients more likely to benefit to such therapies before treatment.[70] In this respect, gene expression profiling studies have contributed to define dominant and shared themes linked to the effectiveness of distinct approaches.

The early study by Wang et al. on melanoma patients[32] introduced the notion that tumors displaying a functional active immune phenotype are more likely to undergo tumor regression. Such study revealed that pretreatment lesions undergoing complete remission following IL-2 and various vaccination schedules bear an inflammatory status characterized by the preactivation of cytotoxic mechanisms and the upregulation of IFN signaling. The expression of lymphocytic cell phenotypic markers was similar in pretreatment responding versus nonresponding lesions, suggesting that the functional orientation is a critical determinant of reactivity to IL-2 administration.[32] This observation was corroborated by a second study on melanoma patients homogeneously treated with the same high-dose IL-2 regimen. In that investigation, Weiss et al. showed that baseline responding lesions displayed a signature of immune activation centered on IFN-γ signaling.[33] As anticipated, such differences were magnified by comparing posttreatment lesions according to their clinical response, suggesting that treatment-induced inflammation represents a magnification of a preexistent inflammatory condition. Similarly, a gene signature centered on immune-related genes has been reported to be predictive of IL-2 efficacy by Sullivan et al.[71] Furthermore, in melanoma patients treated with IL-12 and vaccination, Gajewski et al. reported that the pretreatment upregulation of CXCR3 and CCR5 ligands (i.e., CXCL9, CXCL10, CCL4, and CCL5, respectively) correlated with clinical response.[72,73] In line with these findings, an inflammatory signature characterized by T cell markers, inflammatory chemokines, and IFN-related genes was associated with clinical benefit in metastatic melanoma patients treated with a dendritic cell-based vaccine.[74,75] Similarly, Bedognetti et al. showed that a coordinated overexpression of CCR5 and CXCR3 ligand transcripts (i.e., *CCL5* and *CXCL9-11*) could segregate pretreatment metastatic melanoma lesions according to the responsiveness to adoptive transfer therapy and IL-2.[76]

These observations have been reinforced by the results of correlative studies within two randomized Phase 2 trials employing MAGE-A3 vaccination for the treatment of early non-small cell lung cancer and metastatic melanoma patients.[26,77] Genes included in the predictive classifier, developed by global transcriptomic analysis of pretreatment metastatic melanoma biopsies, were centered on immune-related functions. IRF1 and STAT1 represented the master regulators of the genes included in the signature. The signature included transcripts encoding Th1 chemokines (e.g., *CXCL9*, *CXCL10*, and *CCL5*), cytotoxic granules (*GZMs*), HLA class I and II molecules, T cell activation markers, T cell surface markers, NK cell-associated genes, and other classical IFN-stimulated genes.[26,77] Unfortunately, the final validation is lacking due to the premature interruption of the subsequent Phase 3 trial.[78]

Studies in the Context of Immune Checkpoint Blockade: Melanoma

Remarkably, while these findings have been generated from trials testing agents with direct proinflammatory properties, overlapping signatures have been described in the context of ICB studies,[44] and especially, in metastatic melanoma patients.

By comparing baseline biopsies from patients treated with CTLA-4 blockade according to treatment responsiveness, Ji et al. observed molecular perturbations that closely resemble those that predict responsiveness to proinflammatory cytokines.[44] Genes overexpressed in responding lesions recapitulated the ICR pathways. Such transcripts include *CD8A*, *NKG7*, *GZMB*, and *PRF1* (IEF/cytotoxic genes), *HLADQA1*, *CCL4-5* (CCR5 ligands), and *CXCL9-11* (CXCR3 ligands).[44] Van Allen and coworkers reported that the baseline expression of immune effector transcripts reflecting ongoing cytolytic activity of local immune infiltrates (i.e., *GZMA* and *PRF1*) was associated with clinical benefit and prolonged survival in the same clinical setting (i.e., CTLA-4 blockade in metastatic melanoma).[46] Superimposable signatures have been recently observed in responding lesions from melanoma patients treated with neoadjuvant ipilimumab.[53] Despite these positive associations other small cohort studies did not detect pretreatment immunological differences in patients receiving CTLA-4 blockade.[60,69]

The association between preexisting immunity and therapeutic response is, however, much stronger in the context of PD-1 blockade. Herbst et al., by analyzing pretreatment biopsies of metastatic patients (including melanoma and other tumor types) treated with PD-1 blockade, showed that biopsies from responding patients had a higher expression of *IFNG*, *IDO1*, and *CXCL9*.[45] A 10-gene IFN-γ signature developed within Merck Keynote Trials from a panel of more than 700 genes assessed with NanoString technology[50,79] has been associated with responsiveness to anti-PD-1 therapy in melanoma (*IFNG*, *STAT1*, *CCR5*, *CXCL9*, *CXCL10*, *CXCL11*, *IDO1*, *PRF1*, *GZMA*, and *HLA-DRA*). The 10-gene Merck IFN-γ signature was tested independently in metastatic melanoma patients enrolled in the BMS PD-1 blockade Checkmate064 and confirmed its predictive role in baseline tumors.[60] In addition, authors extracted from RNA-Seq the top 25 genes associated with response to PD-1 blockade, and among them eight were ICR genes (*IDO1*, *STAT1*, *IRF1*, *CXCL9*, *CXCL10* [and *CXCL11*], *IFNG*, *TBX21*, and *CD8A*), together with other related genes including *CXCL13*,[60] a chemokine secreted by T follicular helper cells involved in the formation of tertiary lymphoid structures, often associated with favorable prognosis and response to immunotherapy.[80–83] Exactly 50% (11/22) of responding patients and only around 5% (1/17) of the nonresponding patients exhibited a coordinated expression of those genes.[60] Enrichment of IFN-γ, JAK-STAT, and allograft rejection pathways were also associated with PD-1 blockade response in a relatively large melanoma study, and genes such as CXCR3 and CXCL9-10 together with IFN-γ signatures were predictive to response.[64] Superimposable results have been observed in two additional independent melanoma studies within PD-1 blockade[52,62] or PD-1 and CTLA-4 combinatorial treatment.[62]

Two studies that stratified the analyses according to previous treatment (i.e., CTLA-4 blockade naïve or CTLA-4-blockade pretreated) observed that the association between intratumoral adaptive immunity (T cell/IFN signatures) and response to PD-1 blockade was largely driven by the group of patients pretreated with CTLA-4 blockade.[52,64] Tumors with scant immune response at progression following ipilimumab treatment were completely resistant to PD-1 blockade, while the disposition of an immune silent phenotype did not prevent PD-1 responsiveness.[52,64] Therefore, predictive variables might be significantly altered by previous immunotherapeutic exposure. Overall, the large majority of studies in melanoma in patients detected an association between preexisting adaptive antitumor immunity and response to PD-1 blockade, with few exceptions in small case series.[49,69]

Studies in the Context of Immune Checkpoint Blockade: Pan-Cancer Predictors

Optimization of gene signatures using NanoString technology occurred within the Merck Keynote PD-1 blockade trials. The 10-gene IFN-γ signature was initially downsized to a six-gene signature (CXCL9, CXCL10, IDO1, IFNG, HLA-DRA, and STAT1), and subsequently validated in head and neck cancer patients.[84] A further stepwise marker selection process in 220 patients and nine cancer types culminated into a pan-cancer 18-gene signature, further validated into a clinical-grade assay (tumor inflammation signature [TIS],[50] and expanded in additional Keynote participants for a total of more than 300 patients and 22 tumor types.[55] The TIS contains genes related to antigen presentation (HLA-DQA1, HLA-DRB1, PSMB10), IFN response (such as CD27, STAT1, IDO1, and CXCR3/CCR5), chemokine genes (CCL5, CXCL9), other chemokine receptors (CXCR6, CMKLR1), cytotoxic cells (CD8A, NKG7, HLA-E), and adaptive immune resistance (TIGIT, LAG-3, CD274, CD276, PDCD1LG2). Notably, the TIS correlates tightly ($R = 0.97$) with the 20-gene ICR signature across the TCGA data sets and shared core genes.[43]

Similar signatures in baseline lesions were strongly associated with responsiveness to PD-1 blockade in head and neck HPV-unrelated tumors in independent studies.[68] Among all transcriptome, the list of 41 genes discriminating responders and nonresponders reflect activation of ICR modules and included CD8A, CXCL9-11, STAT1, and IFNG, which were coherently upregulated in all the six responder tumors and in two out of 13 nonresponding lesions.[68] Once again, in a study assessing archival and baseline biopsies from 63 patients with melanoma, NSCLC, and head and neck cancers treated with PD-1 blockade, the cluster of genes associated with objective response and survival overlap with ICR genes.[51] A 12-chemokine signature including CCL3-5, CXCL9-11, and CXCL13[85,86] also has been associated with PD-1 blockade response in gastric cancer,[59] and T cell signatures were associated with PD-1 blockade response in NSCLC[67] and in a large study in urothelial cancer.[56]

It is remarkable that across the large majority of the studies, the only chemokines that are consistently represented are the CXCR3 chemokine CXCL9-11 and the CCR5 chemokine CCL5.

Among all the chemokines, these (and in particular CXCL9 and CCL5) are the only ones that consistently correlate with CD8 T cell infiltration across tumor types.[87] It has been recently observed that CXCL9 is specifically upregulated by IFN-γ and not by type I interferon in tumor-associated macrophages and dendritic cells (DCs) and cooperate with tumor-derived CCL5 for the engraftment of tumor-reactive TILs.[87]

The Enigmatic Case of Kidney Cancer

As for tumor types, an outlier is represented by clear cell renal cell carcinoma (ccRCC), the most frequent, and most studied, kidney cancer histology (>75% of the cases). This remains an enigmatic tumor as (a) it displays, across tumor types, a relatively low mutational burden but is among the tumors with the highest T cell infiltration,[88] cytolytic score,[89] ICR score,[43] or TIS score;[90] and (b) the degree of T cell infiltration is inversely correlated with prognosis.[43,88,90–93] Despite this, renal cell carcinoma has been known for many years to be responsive to immunotherapy; in fact, together with melanoma, it is the only tumor type in which IL-2 and interferon have been broadly employed in clinical practice before the advent of ICB.[94]

The negative correlation between immune signatures and survival has been observed by multiple independent studies in the TCGA and other cohorts,[43,88,90–93] overall encompassing >1,000 patients, and across other renal cell carcinoma histological subtypes such as papillary and chromophobe renal cell carcinoma.[93] While studies differ in the metrics used to quantify immune response, in general and consistently, the T cell-enriched group that expresses high level of IFNG and GZMB was strongly associated with worse survival.[88,93] A potential explanation is that the worse prognosis is driven by a group of tumors with abnormally high immune-regulatory signals (M2 macrophages and regulatory T [T_{reg}] cells), in which T cells are passenger rather than reactive, as suggested by subgroup analyses.[91] Supporting this hypothesis is the observation that the ratio between CD8 T cells and T_{reg} cell estimates might be associated with better survival.[88] Additionally, ccRCC are characterized by high levels of TGF-β, hypoxia, and vascular endothelial growth factor (VEGF) angiogenic signaling, all known immune-suppressive factors.[43] However, in ccRCC, T cell infiltration is associated with a more advanced stage,[43] and systemic manifestations of inflammation such as thrombocytosis and anemia,[93] which are strong predictors of poor prognosis. In fact, when analysis is stratified by stage, the negative prognostic value of T cell infiltration disappears, and T cell infiltration/ICR become a neutral prognostic factor.[43] It is therefore possible that, in this particular tumor type, the signal captured by bulk transcriptome does not reflect an active ongoing antitumor immunity.[43] This can explain the complete lack of an association between immune signatures and response to PD-1 blockade observed in independent cohorts Immotion[57,58,66] and Checkmate Trials[58,66] and at the same time the strong association with response of T cell signature when PD-1 blockade atezolizumab is associated with the anti-angiogenic agent bevacizumab.[57] In fact, the objective response rate (ORR) in T effector (cytotoxic) high tumors treated with atezolizumab and bevacizumab was three times higher as compared to the one observed in the T effector low group (49% vs. 16%, respectively).[57] Moreover, the combination of atezolizumab and bevacizumab outperformed in term of progression-free survival (PFS) both anti-angiogenic treatment alone (sunitinib) or PD-1 blockade alone (atezolizumab) in the T effector high group[57] only. As a note, mutations of PBRM1 have been associated with responsiveness to PD-1 blockade although with conflicting results.[57,58,66] Balances between metabolic and immunologic signaling also have been posed in relationship with PD-1 blockade's outcome.[47]

Increasing the Predictive Value of Immune Signatures

The association between the presence of an active TME and treatment responsiveness, and especially in the context of PD-1 blockade, has been shown by multiple studies across different cancer types. However, a T cell inflamed phenotype has been observed in similar proportions in pretreatment lesions from responder and nonresponder patients in some (small) cohorts.[49,69] Besides the fact that response to immunotherapy is a complex trait, and several factors can contribute to its development (as previously discussed), an important confounding variable is represented by tumor heterogeneity. A recent study compared the response to anti-PD-1 treatment of multiple lesions in a single extensively metastasized melanoma patient.[95] Intriguingly, while the metastases were highly similar with respect to their genomic and immunologic characteristics, response to treatment displayed notable variability. Gene expression analysis[95] revealed that progressing metastases showed an upregulation of genes involved in cellular adhesion and extracellular matrix formation (LAMA3, CCM2L, CST2, and DACT1), neutrophil function (FAM183B, PTPRC, and CXCR2), and Wnt signaling (Wnt3 and WN5A) and genes encoding for protein with mechanical barrier functions such as filaggrin (FLG2), and desmocolin (DSC1 and DSC3), which have been previously observed to be associated with lack of T cell infiltrate and ICR transcripts in melanoma and ovarian cancer.[96] The relevance of intratumor immunologic heterogeneity is further exemplified by a recent comprehensive study of melanoma patients treated with targeted therapy or immunotherapy encompassing phenotypic, genotypic, and transcriptional analysis.[97] A high degree of immunologic heterogeneity was observed among synchronous metastases, which was much greater than genomic heterogeneity.[97] A unique transcriptomic profile in synchronous metastases was observed in all patients studied, with differences in the expression of cytokines and chemokines, HLA molecules, adhesion molecules, and IFN-related genes.[97] Dramatic differences were also observed in T cell frequency and T cell clonality, with less than 8% shared T cell clones across the cohort. Importantly, divergent immune profiles were associated with differential responsiveness to treatment, suggesting that the analyses of more than one lesions (in patients with multiple metastases) might better guide therapeutic choice.[97] Other studies in ovarian[98] and colorectal[37] cancers indicates that regressing metastases are characterized by a dense oligoclonal T cell infiltration while the progressing or recurrent ones are immune-excluded[37,98] and lack immune-editing (i.e., depletion of neoantigens due to T cell-mediated killing).[37] It is noteworthy that despite this heterogeneity, in colorectal cancer metastases at least, the predictive accuracy of the T cell infiltrates from a single biopsy was superior to the one of PD-L1.[99] Overall, going forward, it will be critical to study in depth multiple lesions longitudinally, which will also allow people to better understand mechanisms of secondary resistance (i.e., a resistance that is acquired weeks or months after initial clinical benefit).[100]

Assessing multiple lesions might not be practical in a clinical context for the purpose of selecting patients that might benefit from treatment. A partial mitigation of this problem might be to consider long-term PFS as an endpoint for correlative studies.[23] It is, however, unlikely that immune signatures alone will be used to select patients for immunotherapy treatment, also considering that other metrics, such as the neoantigen load, have strong prediction values.[101]

Integration of immune signatures capturing a "bona fide" active immune response with other analytes might increase their predictive power. For instance, the prognostic and predictive role of T cell/IFN-related signatures (i.e., ICR, TIS, and others) might be decreased or even absent in the presence of certain immune-suppressive signaling such as TGF-β and other inhibitory pathways activated in cancer or stromal cells,[56] as demonstrated in urothelial cancers,[56] in three meta-analyses across different tumor types.[43,102,103] Complex predictive models might, however, suffer from the problem of data overfitting[104] and need to be carefully addressed and validated prospectively. For instance, a predictive model based on pairwise interactions of genes involved in the immune checkpoint pathways has been shown to outperform existing methods for predicting ICB response in 11 independent melanoma data sets,[54] but failed to reproducibly predict response when the algorithm was run on the same cohorts by an independent group,[104] triggering a rampant discussion in the field.[104,105]

T cell-related signatures might be integrated with other analytes strongly associated with immunotherapeutic responses such as the mutational load.[55,101,106] It is, in fact, possible that in tumors with higher mutational load the T cell infiltration might capture a "true" tumor-reactive, rather than a "bystander," immune infiltration.[55,101,106]

Critical pathways associated with immune responsiveness, such as the IFN signaling, are activated not only in immune cells but also in tumors and stromal cells and might lead to T cell exhaustion through chronic PD-L1 to PD-1 signaling activation,[107] therefore exerting opposite functions. Transcriptomic analyses of different compartments such as stroma, immune cells, and cancer cells might better elucidate the tumor-host dynamic interplay.[23]

Single-cell sequencing approaches have contributed to broaden our understanding of the complexity of intertumoral T cell states associated with cancer development and immune escapes, and proposed novel parameters/transcripts related to T cell dysfunction or exhaustion differentially associated with treatment outcomes.[108,109,110] Undoubtedly, upcoming single-cell sequencing investigations will increase even further our understanding of tumor-host interactions and might unveil novel therapeutic targets. At the moment, because of costs and technical complexity, this method is not scalable for clinical application, but it might be in the future. For reliable measurement, it requires either single-cell dissociation from fresh tissue or single-nuclei isolation from frozen material, while bulk transcriptomic analysis has been shown to generate robust data from formalin-fixed-paraffin-embedded (FFPE) samples,[50,55] which are usually available in clinical practice.

Whether single-cell sequencing approaches or emerging TCR single-cell sequencing,[108] might be superior in predicting responsiveness to treatment as compared to bulk transcriptomic analysis likely will be addressed in the future years. In addition, single-cell sequencing might propose novel markers that can be extracted by bulk transcriptomic analyses to improve treatment outcome prediction. Single-cell sequencing approaches, however, disrupt the geographical relationship among cells in different tumoral areas. Other methods that retain the spatial information such as quantitative spatial profiling[111] might increase the interpretation and digestion of data derived from single-cell analysis.[23]

Immune Signatures Associated With Favorable Outcome Following Surgical Resection: Prognostic Signatures

For years, cancer prognostication has been based on tumor-centered parameters, such as the extent of the tumor burden (T), the presence of tumor cells in lymph nodes (N), and the detection of distant metastases (M). While the prognostic role of the TNM classification is well documented, a wide margin of error exists. As clinical outcome varies greatly among patients with the same stage of cancer, a significant effort has been placed into finding prognostic biomarkers. In specific tumors, the analysis of molecular markers (e.g., tyrosine-protein kinase kit [c-KIT] and V-Ki-ras2 Kirsten rat sarcoma viral oncogene homolog [KRAS] mutations, Ki-67, epidermal growth factor receptor [EGFR], estrogen receptor [ER], and human epidermal growth factor receptor 2 [HER2] expression) has increased survival prognostication. In addition to such tumor cell–centric features, biomarkers based on the host immune response are emerging as powerful prognostic tools.

It is now accepted that the evolution of the tumor is modulated by the microenvironment in which it develops. Epidemiological studies in humans have substantiated the experimental hypothesis that chronic inflammation supports tumor growth.[112] However, when a temporal dimension is added to the analysis of the intratumoral immune response and patients are prospectively followed, intriguing hypotheses on the role of TME in counteracting tumor growth emerge.[19,37]

Immunohistochemistry studies, and more recently, deconvolution algorithms applied to transcriptomic data to infer subset leucocyte abundance or proportion,[113,114] have shown a considerable interpatient variation in the frequency of leukocyte subpopulations such as B, T, NK cells, macrophages, DCs, and granulocytes.[113,115–119] While a differential role of such populations in modulating cancer development has been described, most of the studies have highlighted a positive correlation between the intratumoral frequencies of lymphocytic infiltration and prolonged disease-free or overall survival.

The density of TILs has been positively correlated with better prognosis in most tumors such as melanoma,[120] breast (in particular triple-negative breast cancers),[121,122] ovarian,[123] head and neck, gastric, urothelial, and colorectal cancer.[124-126] In particular, the most consistent association with favorable prognosis has been observed for CD3+ and CD8+ T cells.[124-126]

Colon Cancer

The SITC Immunoscore worldwide consortium has recently validated the prognostic role of TILs by analyzing more than 2,500 individuals affected by stage I to III colon cancer, and has been included in the group of "essential and desirable diagnostic criteria for colorectal cancers" in the current edition of the WHO classification of tumors. Notably, the Immunoscore outperforms, as a prognostic variable, all clinical-pathological criteria including the microsatellite instability status.[124]

In mammary carcinoma, the prognostic role of TILs has been conclusively demonstrated in patients with triple-negative breast tumors.[127-130] Guidelines for the implementation of TIL scoring in breast cancer have been proposed.[122]

The analysis of the tumor transcriptional program has added molecular precision to these observations. In the context of colon cancer, phenotypic characteristics associated with favorable prognosis have been associated with specific transcriptomic features.[131,132] Such signatures reflect the activation of Th1-related transcripts such as *IFNG*, *STAT1*, *IL-12*, and *IRF1*, and the transcription factor T-bet (*TBX21*), the induction of cytotoxic mechanisms (*GZMs*, *PRF1*, and *GNLY*), and the production of Th1 chemoattractants such as CXCR3 and CCR5 ligands (e.g., *CXCL9*, *CXCL10*, and *CCL5*) and other chemokines (e.g., *CX3CL1* and *CXCL13*).[19,83,131] These specific chemokine transcripts were associated with differing densities and spatial organization of T cell subpopulations within tumor regions and were associated with prolonged patient survival.[83,132] Such signatures overlap significantly with those being predictive of responsiveness to immunotherapy or observed in lesions about to undergo clinical regression after immunotherapeutic administration (see preceding discussion). By mining more than 4,000 gene expression profiles, a robust transcriptomic classification of colorectal cancer has been proposed.[133] Immune infiltration is present in two subtypes.[133,134] These are the CMS1/immune, mostly consisting of hypermutated microsatellite-instable tumors, and CMS4/mesenchymal, displaying stromal cell invasion and angiogenesis. Although the lymphocytic count, as predicted by transcriptomic data, was similar between the two subtypes, only the CMS1 tumors exhibited a Th1 polarization, as substantiated by the overexpression of *IFNG*, *IL-15*, and the Th1 chemokine transcript

CXCL9-10, which was invariably accompanied by the counteractivation of the PD-1/PD-L1 pathway.[133,134] In contrast, CMS4 tumors, which exhibited the worse prognosis, displayed a high expression of myeloid chemokines (i.e., CCL2), angiogenic factors (e.g., vascular endothelial growth factor B [VEGFB]), and transforming growth factor-β (TGF-β) signaling–related immunosuppressive molecules.[133,134]

Breast Cancer

Significant progress has been made in the characterization of gene signatures in the context of early breast cancer. In view of the robustness of the intrinsic molecular subtype classification and other classifiers mainly capturing tumor-intrinsic features, a flurry of gene expression studies have been performed in this setting since early 2000.[135,136] However, only in the last decade have such repositories been queried to investigate the prognostic role of tumor–host interactions.

Because of the known prognostic role of ER and HER2 status, analyses have often been stratified according to these parameters. A seminal study conducted a decade ago by Teschendorff et al. (in approximately 200 ER⁻ primary breast cancers from different microarray data sets) reported that tumors enriched in immune-related transcripts were characterized by good prognosis.[137] Markers included in the predictive module consist of B cell transcripts and other genes linked to immune response. A few years later, Desmedt et al., in a large meta-analysis of almost a thousand samples, showed that the intensity of a metagene centered on STAT1 was strongly associated with decreased risk of relapse in ER⁻/HER2⁻ and HER2⁺ patients, even when corrected for other prognostic variables through multivariate analysis.[138] In 2009 to 2011, several investigations assessing additional internal cohorts of samples or employing meta-analytic approaches have demonstrated the association between immune-related metagenes (or "immunological subtypes") and decreased risk of recurrence, especially in the ER⁻HER⁻/triple-negative or HER2⁺ subsets. Examples include a T cell metagene centered on lymphocytic kinase (LCK);[139] a HER2-derived prognostic signature enriched in immune-related genes, such as *CD69*, *CD3D*, and *CD247*;[140] a kinase metagene consisting of several immune kinases;[141] a medullary breast cancer (MBC)-derived signature enriched in immune genes including CD8⁺ T and B cell transcripts;[142] and a triple-negative breast cancer (TNBC)-derived prognostic signature enriched in immune genes (i.e., IFN signaling, B cell, and T cell transcripts),[143] as well as a B/plasma cell gene signature.[144] In 2012, Curtis et al. analyzed a new cohort consisting of 2,000 early breast cancers (i.e., the METABRIC data set).[145] By using joined copy number and gene expression clustering analysis, the authors defined discrete different breast cancer subtypes, of which one, enriched in immune-related genes including ICR genes, showed a favorable prognosis.[145] Critical genes include *CD8A, CXCL9, CXCL10, CCL5, CXCR3, STAT1*, and several other IFN-related transcripts. A few years later, Burstein et al. defined specific subclusters of TNBC including a basal-like immunosuppressed and a basal-like immunoactivated phenotype, characterized by a poor and good prognosis, respectively.[146]

Rather than profiling entire tumors and dissecting the signal according to biological functions, other approaches have been represented by separate analysis of the stromal compartment. By profiling microdissected tumor stroma from primary breast cancer, Finak et al. observed that tumors from patients experiencing prolonged relapse-free survival were enriched in transcripts indicative of a Th1 immune response, such as *CD8A, GZMA, CD52*, and *CD247*.[147] Additionally, by sorting CD4 T cells from tumor specimens, Gu-Trantien et al. observed that polarization of CD4 T cells differed among extensively and minimally infiltrated tumors.[82] Although all the Th subsets were present in the analyzed tumors, the highly infiltrated ones were enriched in Th1 and follicular helper T cells (T-fh), as demonstrated by the expression of *CCL4, CXCL9-11*, and *TBX21* (Th1 transcripts) and *ICOS, CXCL13, IL-21*, and PD-1 (T-fh markers). Furthermore, by mining publicly available data sets, the authors observed that Th1 and T-fh signatures correlated with decreased risk of relapse in HER2[+] tumors, while the T-fh signature was also associated with prolonged relapse-free survival in patients bearing ER[+]/HER2[-] cancers. Bonsang-Kitzis et al.[148] assessed the performance of the 10 previously published immune gene signatures (described earlier) upfront in TNBC from the METABRIC data set.[145] Remarkably, eight of them[82,137–139,142,146] predicted clinical outcome, including the STAT1-centered signatures described by Desmedt (STAT1 module)[138] and Gu-Trantien (Th1 signature).[82] In addition, the authors defined an additional immune-related signature that was able to outperform the other ones when tested in a multivariate analysis.[148]

Although the breast cancer prognostic immune signatures mentioned earlier differ in terms of specific genes, it is interesting to note that the large majority of them include ICR genes, as reviewed in detail elsewhere.[149] A large meta-analysis on more than 7,000 transcriptome profiles from patients affected by early breast cancer has systematically assessed the prognostic role of leukocyte subpopulations and previously described immune signatures.[150] Strikingly, the previously published metagene tested (i.e., the Teschendorff signature, the Gu-Trantien T-fh signature, and the STAT1 signature by Desmedt)[137,138,147] was associated with decreased risk of relapse or death in all but the ER[+]/HER2[+] tumors. As

for lymphocytic subpopulations, a higher proportion of plasma cells and M1 macrophages and a lower frequency of M0 macrophages and activated mast cells displayed the most consistent positive correlation with outcome across the subgroups.[150]

Because the adjuvant treatment (e.g., endocrine therapy, chemotherapy, anti-HER2 therapy, combined chemohormone therapy, or no treatment) of patients included in these meta-cohorts was not randomized, it is difficult to determine whether immune signatures can bear a predictive role. To overcome this limitation, Perez et al. profiled tumors from HER2 patients randomly treated with chemotherapy alone or chemotherapy plus the anti-HER2 mAb trastuzumab.[151] Among patients receiving chemotherapy and adjuvant trastuzumab, but not in those treated with chemotherapy alone, the most significant pathways associated with prolonged relapse-free survival were centered on immune response such as IFN-γ, cytokine-receptor activation, T cell receptor (TCR) signaling in CD8[+] T cells, and TNF signaling. Again, ICR transcripts such as *CXCL9, CCL5, CXCR3, PRF1*, and *GZMB* were central in the nodes identified by the pathway analysis,[151] suggesting perhaps that an active immune microenvironment could potentiate the elimination of residual disease via antibody-dependent cell-mediated cytotoxicity induced by trastuzumab. It is interesting to note that the density of TILs and the levels of ICR/Th1 and immune regulatory transcripts (e.g., IDO1, Foxp3, and PD-L1) have been strongly associated with responsiveness to neoadjuvant chemotherapy.[81,149,150,152–158] It is presently unclear how an immunologically active microenvironment can enhance the efficacy of antineoplastic drugs. It has been proposed that certain chemotherapeutic agents, such as doxorubicin, cyclophosphamide, and oxaliplatin, act as immune adjuvants by inducing an immunogenic cell death through the stimulation of dendritic cell-mediated uptake of apoptotic corpses and consequent induction of antigen-specific T cell response (see Chapter 13).[159] Moreover, anthracyclines might directly stimulate the production of type I IFN by cancer cells with subsequent release of the CXCR3 ligand CXCL10 through the activation of autocrine and paracrine loops.[160] It could be speculated that a chemotherapy-mediated enhancement of antitumor immunity, facilitated by a permissive microenvironment, could facilitate a more effective immune-mediated clearance of residual cancer cells.

Pan-Cancer

Besides breast and colon cancer, large meta-analyses using deconvolution approaches to estimate the absolute or relative abundance of leukocyte subpopulations have confirmed the positive prognostic role of metagenes related to T cell/CD8 T cells and/or B cells in most of the solid tumors (including melanoma and lung cancer), with the exception of kidney cancer and glioblastoma, although the reasons for these paradoxical discrepancies are elusive (see previous paragraph).[43,102,113,116,119,161–163] In particular, a comprehensive meta-analysis of the TCGA cohort has proposed that solid tumors can be classified in six immune subtypes, with the inflamed subtype characterized by a high Th1 infiltration being associated with the best survival, while the TGF-β dominant subtype had the worst prognosis.[116]

Interaction Between Host-Derived and Tumor-Centric Factors: Prognostic and Predictive Implications

Several commercially prognostic gene-expression classifiers have been approved by the U.S. Food and Drug Administration for clinical use or endorsed by American Society of Clinical Oncology (ASCO), National Comprehensive Cancer Network (NCCN), and Saint-Gallen guidelines to guide clinicians in making decisions about treatment, in particular, to omit chemotherapy or prolong hormone therapy for patients with HR+/HER2− tumor. Those classifiers, such as Mammaprint, Onco-type DX, and Prosigna, are centered on cell-cycle/proliferation-related genes.[164] A reasonable question to ask is why, if a correlation between immune-related genes and survival has been established, immune-related genes reflecting adaptive immunity activation are not included in commercially available, robust, clinical-grade gene-expression classifiers.

There are two main reasons. First, as a single variable, the main prognostic factor in early breast cancer is not the immunological composition but rather the proliferation capacity, and this is the signal that is captured by the proposed classifiers.[41,165,166] Second, the prognostic connotation of immune signatures is limited to proliferation and/or mutational load[41,43,106,165,166] high tumors, in which they might capture a tumor reactive rather than bystander immune infiltration. This is on par with the observation that TIL infiltration is prognostic only in triple-negative breast cancer and not in HR+ tumors, which have overall lower proliferative capacity.[129,167]

Importantly, in HR+ breast cancer, for instance, a recent meta-analysis showed that all the main prognostic classifiers (Mammaprint-, Oncotype-DX, or Prosigna-like signatures) identify well high and low risk group.[41] However, among the high-risk group (highly proliferative tumors), the presence of a T cell/cytotoxic response (ICR high tumors) identifies a group of patients with an extremely low risk or relapse, which would have been otherwise classified at high risk.[41] This observation is critical as it suggests that a subgroup of patients classified at high risks by main clinical, cancer-cell centered, assays, and therefore candidate to chemo-hormone therapy, might be actually treated with hormone therapy alone. Notably, tumors with high ICR/T cell infiltration and low proliferation are also characterized by high TGF-β signaling.[43,166] This notion might not be restricted to breast cancer. A recent pan-cancer analysis showed that, across different tumor types, the prognostic connotation of ICR score is abolished in tumors with low proliferation/low mutational load and/or high TGF-β signaling. Similarly, as mentioned in the previous paragraph, the predictive value of ICR and other immune signatures is impaired in the presence of high TGF-β signaling.[43,56,103] In conclusion, integration of immune cell and cancer or stromal cell-driven signatures might increase both prognostic and predictive values of gene expression signatures.

Mining Transcriptomic Studies to Disentangle the Relationship Between the Tumor Genetic Program and Immune Responsiveness

Copy Number Alterations

Strong associations have been demonstrated by TCGA pan-cancer analyses between a high copy number alteration (aneuploidy), the absence of a cytotoxic T cell infiltration[43,168–170] (as estimated by gene expression), and resistance to CTLA-4 and PD-1 blockade.[52,169–171] This might be due to the loss of genes required for immune activity such as antigen-presentation and HLA genes.[169]

Moreover, copy number loss of the IFN gene cluster was associated with reduced expression of IFN and T cell-related transcripts in melanoma.[172] However, amplifications of immune-related genes, such as CXCL chemokines (including CXCL9-11 and CXCL13), have been found more frequently in tumors displaying an immune active microenvironment in breast and colon cancer.[42,83,173] Additionally, overexpression of nitric oxide synthase (NOS), driven by genomic amplification of NOS1 locus within segment 12q22-24, impairs IFN-α responsiveness of peripheral blood mononuclear cells.[174] Interestingly, baseline expression of NOS1 in tumor metastases was negatively associated with response to adoptive therapy in metastatic melanoma patients, therefore linking genetic tumors with specific immune dysfunctions, leading to impaired response to immunomodulatory approaches.[174]

Somatic Mutations

Exome sequencing studies have consistently shown that a high mutational load, which in turn equates to an elevated number of predicted neoantigens, correlates with the response to checkpoint blockade.[46,55,101,175,176] Additionally, mutations or deletions of genes of IFN-γ signaling and antigen presentation genes have been reported in patients with primary or acquired resistance

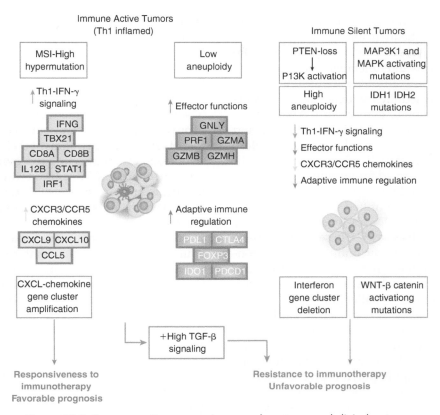

Figure 35.2 Tumor genetic program, immune phenotypes, and clinical outcome.

to ICB (also called deletion signatures).[177–180] However, those mutations are rare and the number of patients analyzed in such studies is small. In additional studies, such mutations have also been found in responding patients,[52,181,182] questioning the clinical implications of such deletion mutational signatures.[183]

Although the degree of the intratumoral inflammation and number of somatic mutations (or the number of predicted neoantigens) are significantly correlated in some tumors,[89] such association is in general weak or even absent in some histotypes,[42,184] with the exception of tumor with extremely high heterogeneity of mutational load such as colorectal cancer.[133] In fact, a considerable proportion of tumors display the Th1 phenotype despite a low number of mutations, and vice versa; a fraction of tumors with high number of mutations lack T cell infiltration. Therefore, it is likely that other modulators contribute to the development of the favorable immune phenotype.[42]

Transcriptomic data have often been queried to investigate hierarchically relevant relationships between the tumor genetic program and immune response in humans (Figure 35.2). The contribution of specific mutations on cancer immune responsiveness is discussed in detail in Chapter 14. Overall, strong evidence exists regarding

a relationship between MAPK mutations resulting in MAPK activation,[42,49,116,127,185–187] Wnt/β-catenin activating mutations,[188,189] and PTEN-loss mediated PI3K activation[190–193] and immune exclusion and/or ICB therapeutic resistance. Other emerging genes associated with immune-exclusion include *IDH1* and *IDH2*, in both solid[43,116] and hypermethylation status characterizing *IDH1/2* mutant tumors.[117,118]

In conclusion, correlative studies in humans have unveiled meaningful relationships between tumor-specific genomic alterations of tumor cells and immune responsiveness (see also Chapter 28). Targeting oncogenic pathways prohibiting the development of an efficient antitumor immune response offers a promising approach to potentiate the efficacy of agents with direct immuno-modulatory properties.[23,40,187]

PART 2: HOST GENETIC VARIATIONS ASSOCIATED WITH IMMUNE RESPONSIVENESS

The study of families affected by inherited immune-related diseases through next-generation exome sequencing led to the identification of critical genes involved in controlling immune homeostasis.[194–198] Moreover, genome-wide association studies (GWASs) have identified more than 300 loci associated with the development of autoimmune diseases.[199,200] Sequencing and genotyping approaches have recently been used to assess the heritability of immune cell levels and functions[201] in steady-state conditions. In a large study enrolling thousands of individuals, Orru et al. assessed the frequency of 95 immune cell populations corresponding to almost 300 immune traits. The authors estimated that trait-heritability could account for about 40% of the observed variance, therefore indicating a large genetic effect size.[201] The greatest estimated heritability was observed for immune populations implicated in fine immunological tuning such as in T_{reg} cells. Importantly, variants identified in some loci (e.g., HLA and IL-2RA) overlapped with those identified by GWASs of autoimmune diseases.[201] These findings have important implications for cancer immunotherapy, considering that stable baseline differences of immune cell traits across healthy individuals are associated with differential response to immune challenging, such as with influenza vaccination.[202] As for cancer development, GWAS case–control studies have frequently reported genes related with immune function, but the causal relationship is largely lacking. More targeted investigations have assessed the role of highly polymorphic genes critical for immune functions such as the HLA and the killer cell immunoglobulin-like receptor (KIR) genes. Some of these studies are reviewed later in this chapter.

Regarding immunotherapy, large GWASs in patients affected by chronic hepatitis C virus (HCV) infection have identified a strong association between the λ3/IL-28B gene and response to IFN-α treatment.[203–205] Such comprehensive investigations have been facilitated by the fact that IFN-α has for decades represented the gold standard for the treatment of HCV infection. Conversely, cancer immunotherapy has only recently been implemented in clinical practice.

Before the advent of checkpoint inhibitors, immunotherapy was accessible, through enrollment in early phase clinical trials, by only a small proportion of metastatic cancer patients. Early phase trials, which assessed drug toxicity and activity, are frequently monocentric and enroll a limited number of patients. Such trials are in general not suitable for GWASs. Instead, associative studies have been focusing on specific genes. The genes tested by such approaches include HLA, CTLA-4, IRF5, and CCR5.

In melanoma patients treated with the anti-CTLA-4 mAb ipilimumab, a single study has assessed multiple single-nucleotide polymorphisms (SNPs) and deletions in immune-related genes (i.e., CCR5, CD86, butyrophilin like [2BTNL2], IFN-α and -β receptor subunit 1 [IFNAR1] and 2 [IFNAR2], CTLA-4, IFNG, nucleotide-binding oligomerization domain–containing protein 2 [NOD2], IL-23R, and protein tyrosine phosphatase, nonreceptor type [22PTPN22]) as well as HLA-A and HLA-B genotypes. No correlations between the tested genetic variants and

clinical outcome[206] were observed, although the small sample size might have prevented the detection of statistically significant associations. Interestingly, a recent investigation has reported an association between two PD-L1 polymorphisms (i.e., rs2297136 and rs4143815) and responsiveness to first-line chemotherapy in metastatic NSCLC patients.[207] Moreover, a number of investigations in breast cancer and lymphoma patients have assessed the role of crystallizable fragment (Fc)-γ receptor and responsiveness to mAbs targeting receptors expressed by tumor cells, such as anti-HER2 and anti-CD20 mAbs, with conflicting results.[208] Polymorphisms of P2RX7, TLR4, and FPR1 have been found to be associated with differential outcome in early breast and colon cancer patients treated with adjuvant chemotherapy, likely through modulation of immune-mediated cell death mechanisms.[209,210]

Recently, polymorphisms of Fc-γ receptor were associated with treatment outcome in a small cohort of patients treated with CTLA-4 blockade displaying an immunologically active tumor phenotype.[211] Studies that have evaluated CTLA-4, IRF5, and CCR5 polymorphisms are presented in more detail as follows.

Cytotoxic T Lymphocyte-Associated Protein 4 Polymorphisms and Responsiveness to Immunotherapy

CTLA-4 is an inhibitory receptor expressed on CD4[+] and CD8[+] cells, which is crucial for maintaining T cell homeostasis and tolerance to self. CTLA-4 signaling pathways play critical roles in T cell activation and regulation. Its key role consists of the regulation of T CD4[+] populations through downmodulation of helper T cell function and induction of regulatory T cell immunosuppressive activity.[212,213] CTLA-4 germline mutations have been associated with susceptibility to organ-specific autoimmune diseases.[198,214]

Three studies assessed the association of a total of 12 SNPs of CTLA-4 with metastatic melanoma patients treated with anti-CTLA-4 mAbs.[206,215–217] In addition, Gogas et al. investigated the association of six SNPs in high-risk melanoma patients treated with adjuvant IFN-α therapy (Table 35.1).[218] Although some significant associations were detected by such studies, the overall results are inconclusive. Comparison of such reports is challenging, as the SNPs tested only partially overlap among the studies. Moreover, different statistical models have been used to test association with either allele or genotype frequency. Three polymorphisms (rs4553808, rs11571317, and rs231775) were significantly associated with response to treatment with ipilimumab in the study by Breunis et al.[216] Among the five SNPs assessed by Hamid et al., including those described by Breunis et al., no significant associations were reported. Only a trend was observed for rs4553808, rs11571317, and rs231775. In a third study from the Italian Melanoma Intergroup on metastatic patients treated with ipilimumab, Queirolo et al. reported a significant association with clinical benefit for rs11571316 and rs3087243 polymorphisms. Both polymorphisms were significantly associated with overall response.[217] For both variants, the GG genotype had the best 4-year overall survival, GA the worst, and AA the intermediate survival. Furthermore, in a separate report from the same group, rs4553808 was reported to be associated with immune-related endocrine adverse events.[219]

Polymorphism rs3087243 was not associated with any clinical response in Breunis's study, while Hamid's study showed only a trend toward significance, but in the opposite direction. Moreover, Gogas et al. studied six CTLA-4 polymorphisms that partially overlapped with the three previously discussed studies. In this study, patients were treated with adjuvant IFN-α. At first glance, no association between CTLA-4 polymorphisms and risk of relapse or death was observed.[218] Subsequently, using a multivariate approach and combining rs3087243CT polymorphism with HLA variants (i.e., HLA-B38, -C15,

-C3, -DRB1*15), Wang et al. demonstrated that rs3087243 significantly contributed to the predictive survival models.[1] Indeed, rs3087243 GG genotype was correlated with shorter overall survival, similar to what was observed by Queirolo et al. in patients receiving ipilimumab.[217]

IRF5 Polymorphisms and Responsiveness to Immunotherapy

IRF5 is a member of the IRF family, and plays an important role in the induction of antiviral and inflammatory response and, therefore, is implicated in host defense (Table 35.2).[220] IRF5 is involved in the induction of IFN-α and inflammatory cytokines.[221,222] IRF5 polymorphisms have been associated with susceptibility to several autoimmune diseases such as systemic lupus erythematosus,[223] multiple sclerosis,[224] rheumatoid arthritis,[225] and inflammatory bowel diseases.[226]

Treatment-induced symptoms suggestive of autoimmunity (e.g., vitiligo, thyroiditis, enterocolitis) are observed in patients with metastatic melanoma treated successfully with immunotherapeutic approaches.[227–230]

Table 35.2   Polymorphisms and Responsiveness to Immunotherapy

TESTED POLYMORPHISMS	SETTING	MAIN FINDINGS	REFERENCE
rs3087243* rs231775 rs5742909 rs7565213 rs11571297 rs11571302	Resected melanoma treated with adjuvant interferon (N = 286)	No significant association with clinical outcome was found.	218
rs4553808 **rs11571317** **rs231775** rs5742909 rs3087243 rs7565213 rs733618	Metastatic melanoma treated with ipilimumab (N = 152)	rs4553808 (−1660 G vs. A allele); rs11571317 (−657 T vs. G allele), and rs231775 (49 A vs. G allele) were associated with increases in overall response rate.	216
rs11571317 rs3087243 rs4553808 rs1863800 rs231775	Metastatic melanoma treated with ipilimumab (N = 55–57)†	No significant associations with clinical benefit were found; a trend was observed for rs1863800, rs231775, rs3087243, and rs4553808.	206
rs5742909 rs231775 **rs3087243** rs4553808 rs11571317 **rs11571316**	Metastatic melanoma treated with ipilimumab (N = 173)	rs11571316 (−1577 G allele) and rs3087243 (CT60 G allele) were associated with overall response (p <.01) and prolonged survival. For rs11571316 overall survival was 27%, 11%, and 9% for GG, GA, and AA, respectively. For rs r087243 overall survival was 27%, 13%, and 17% for GG, GA, and AA, respectively.	217

*In a subsequent analysis, rs3087243 (CT60) was correlated with overall survival in a multivariable Cox regression model including HLA-B38, HLA-C15, HLA-C3, DRB1*15, and CT60*G/G. G/G genotype was associated with shorter overall survival.

†Genotype data not available in some patients; SNPs significantly associated with clinical outcome are in bold.

Source: Adapted from Wang E, Zhao Y, Monaco A, et al. A multi-factorial genetic model for prognostic assessment of high risk melanoma patients receiving adjuvant interferon. *PLos One.* 2012;7(7):e40805. doi:10.1371/journal.pone.0040805

However, the Hellenic IFN trial reported a direct correlation between clinical and/or molecular manifestation of autoimmunity after high-dose IFN-α treatment,[231] although such findings were not validated by the pooled analysis of the EORTC and the Nordic IFN clinical trials.[232,233]

In the context of cancer immunotherapy, Uccellini et al. studied five IRF5 polymorphisms in metastatic melanoma patients treated with adoptive therapy and high-dose IL-2.[234] These variants include rs10954213, rs11770589, rs6953165, rs200464, and rs2004640. All but rs2004640 were in linkage disequilibrium and associated with response to therapy. For example, lack of the A allele in rs10954213, which confers protection to lupus erythematosus, was predominant in nonresponders ($P = .005$). Therefore, the IRF5 polymorphisms associated with the development of autoimmune diseases can influence the degree of antitumor response, emphasizing the genetic analogies between distinct tissue destruction processes.[234]

CCR5 and CXCR3 Polymorphisms and Responsiveness to Immunotherapy

The CCR5 and CXCR3 chemokine receptors are coexpressed by activated Th1, cytotoxic T, and NK cells. Recruitment of activated T cells by CXCR3 and CCR5 chemokine ligands plays a key role in immune-mediated tissue destruction, including tumor rejection.[19,24,26,34,235] However, the systemic administration of IL-2 and checkpoint inhibitors induces, directly or indirectly, the production of chemoattractants such as CXCR3 and CCR5 ligands, leading to migration of lymphocytes to the site of inflammation.[27,30,33,236] Therefore, polymorphisms and/or expression levels of CXCR3 and CCR5 may influence the migration of TILs to a tumor site and, possibly, the tumor rejection. The CCR5Δ32 polymorphism consists of a 32-base deletion encoding for a truncated protein that is not transported to the cell surface. CCR5Δ32 heterozygosity results in decreased, and homozygosity in the absence of, receptor expression.[58] As CCR5 is used as a coreceptor by the human immunodeficiency virus (HIV) to infect the target cells, subjects carrying the CCR5Δ32 homozygous mutations are resistant to HIV infection, while heterozygous patients show a considerable delay in disease progression.[237]

The polymorphism seems to be protective against the development of some autoimmune diseases (i.e., rheumatoid arthritis), but is associated with increased risk of others, such as systemic lupus erythematosus and sclerosing cholangitis.[238-241] Conflicting reports exist on the role of CCR5Δ32 in response to immunotherapy in metastatic melanoma. A retrospective study on patients treated with immunotherapy or immunochemotherapy observed a decreased survival in patients carrying this polymorphism.[242] Conversely, Hamid et al., by studying

responsiveness to ipilimumab, did not report any significant association with CCR5Δ32 or CCR5 rs1799987 polymorphisms.[206] A polymorphism in the CXCR3 gene (*rs2280964*) has been associated with a risk of developing asthma, impaired lymphocyte chemotactic activity, and altered receptor expression.[243] The role of both CCR5Δ32 and CXCR3 rs2280964 polymorphisms has been assessed in patients with metastatic melanoma who were treated with adoptive therapy and high-dose IL-2.[76] In a univariate analysis, the CCR5Δ32 was slightly associated with an increased overall response rate, but no significant association was found for rs2280964 (CXCR3). However, a lower expression of CXCR3 and CCR5 as a consequence of the downregulation of the corresponding genes and/or the presence of CCR5Δ32 mutation was strongly correlated with both the frequency and the degree of response ($p < .001$).[76] These counterintuitive results could be explained in relation to concomitant IL-2 administration and TIL migration to the tumor, which follow multiphasic kinetics.[244] In fact, a few hours after IL-2 infusion, TILs mainly localize in the lung, spleen, and liver, but not in neoplastic sites. TILs at the tumor sites can be detected between 1 and 2 days after infusion, with a partial clearance of the TILs from the lung.[244] However, the concentration of CCR5 and CXCR3 ligands in peripheral blood increases shortly after IL-2 administration, while the variations within tumor are less intense.[236] It can be speculated that the administration of IL-2 leads to a release of specific chemokines (primarily CXCR3 and CCR5 ligands) by resident immune cells and/or stromal cells from peripheral organs (e.g., spleen, lung, and liver), leading to the early compartmentalization. It is possible that TILs with low expression of CXCR3 and CCR5 are not sequestrated by extratumoral tissue and can subsequently migrate into the tumor after the cytokine storm has receded and when the tumor becomes the predominant source of such chemokines.[76] This explanation matches with the observation that high levels of CXCR3 and CCR5 ligand transcripts in pretreatment tumors are associated with an increased response to adoptive therapy and IL-2.[76] It is possible that during the administration of other types of treatments (e.g., combination of immunochemotherapy,[242] or vaccine therapy), the induction of the CXCR3 and CCR5 ligands is less unbalanced than it is during administration of high-dose IL-2, leading to a different kinetic modulation of T cell activities, and therefore reconciling different results. More recently, a preliminary analysis of an exome-wide scan assessing rare and common variants on 250 metastatic melanoma patients treated with CTLA-4 identified associations between the 3p21 CCR5 locus (which also include CCR2 and CCRL2) and treatment resistance, suggesting the relevance of CCR5 variants in the therapeutic setting, according to preliminary analyses (T Kirchhoff, Melanoma Bridge, Naples 2019).

HLA Polymorphisms

Early studies have investigated HLA variants in relation to treatment responsiveness. Marincola et al. reported a lack of association between HLA genotype (HLA-A, HLA-B, and HLA class II) and response to IL-2 in a large cohort of metastatic melanoma patients,[245] while Gogas et al. observed a modest, although statistically significant, association between HLA-DRB1*15, Cw6, Cw7, and B44 and survival in melanoma patients treated with adjuvant IFN-α.[220,246]

But with the availability of more advanced technology for HLA typing and the development of a refined analytic pipeline, the predictive role of HLA polymorphisms has been revived.

A large study on more than 1,500 patients (two cohorts) on melanoma and lung cancer patients treated with CTLA-4 or PD-1 blockade observed that loss of HLA-I heterozygosity was associated with poor outcome, an effect that was enhanced by tumor mutational burden.[247] It is possible that patients with HLA homozygosity would present a reduced and less diverse repertoire of neoantigens to T cells. This was substantiated by an increased on-treatment coloniality of TCR from infiltrating lymphocyte in patients with heterozygous versus homozygous HLA-I. Mechanistically, molecular dynamics simulations of HLA super-types associated with poor outcome identified the presence of specific elements that might alter cytotoxic T cell recognition. Somatic loss of HLA heterozygosity was also associated with poor outcome.[248] Further validations in independent cohort will determine whether the proposed effect conferred by germline HLA loss of heterozygosity can be implemented as clinical predictive biomarkers.

Genome-Wide Scans Assessing the Germline Genetic Contribution to the Functional Orientation of the Tumor Microenvironment: Emerging Data

Expression quantitative trait loci (eQTL) in immune-related genes (i.e., the associations between gene polymorphisms and expression) can be found in different tissue types,[249] including immune cells[250] and tumors,[251] which are a mixture of cancer and stromal/immune cells. But a critical and unexplored question in cancer immunology is whether and how the functional orientation of the TME is influenced by the genetic background of the host.[252]

A recent pan-cancer analytic effort analyzing the entire TCGA solid tumor cohort (>9,500 subjects with either array genotyping or whole-exome sequencing data available), supported by the Society for Immunotherapy of Cancer (SITC),[253] sought to fill this knowledge gap. Sayaman et al.[253] performed heritability and GWAS analyses for common variants, and pathway burden analysis for rare pathogenic cancer variants,[253] using 139 immune phenotypes (Immune traits) compiled by the TCGA Pan-Immune working group.[116]

The first question addressed by the group was whether, and to what degree, genotypic differences can explain microenvironmental variations, as calculated by heritability analysis. From a quantitative point of view, one-fourth of the traits had significant heritability. The abundance or gene-expression estimates of CD8 T cells, Th1 cells, and the activation of IFN signaling have been consistently associated with favorable prognosis and responsiveness to immunotherapy. Notably, they were among the traits displaying the highest heritability (15%–20%).[253] This magnitude is similar with what was observed for some other complex traits such as body mass index, hemoglobin, and fasting glucose levels.[254]

In addition to obvious associations driven by known eQTL of *HLA* and *IL-17RA* genes that were included for the estimation of HLA traits and Th17 abundance, respectively, the GWAS analysis identified 21 loci significantly associated with 17 immune traits likely modulating the immune microenvironment.[253] This observation expands the number of loci identified by another recent GWAS study in the TCGA ($n = 2$, of which one being the result of the *IL-17RA* eQTL) which, however, included only patients with European ancestry ($N = 5,800$) and was restricted to a limited number of immune traits.[255]

Extensive and stringent colocalization analysis using orthogonal data sets mapped variants associated with differences in abundancy of T cells with genes involved with immune functions or oncogenic processes.[253] Additionally, rare variant analyses identified a link between Wnt-β catenin pathway germline mutations and regulatory mechanism (PD-L1 and T_{reg} cell), corroborating the immune-modulatory role of genetically sustained alteration of this pathway observed by somatic analysis in melanoma and other cancers.[188,189] The effect on leukocyte infiltration and mutational load of germline mutations of mismatch-repair genes was dependent upon the acquisition of the microsatellite unstable/hypermutated phenotype at the somatic level, suggesting that germline mismatch-repair gene deficiency might not be sufficient to predict response to immunotherapy.[253] Furthermore, rare pathogenic variants in telomere stabilizing genes and in BRCA1 were associated with decreased and increased expression of immune-related signatures.

What was remarkable is that the top loci associated with differential IFN signaling in the GWAS analysis includes genes that are critical for the IFN signaling such as the Interferon Induced With Helicase C Domain 1 (*IFIH1*) and *TMEM173* (STING). *IFIH1* polymorphisms overlapped with those described by GWAS in the context of autoimmune diseases and include a functionally characterized missense variant.[256] The top IFIH1 hit (rs2111485) was recently associated with response to ICB in metastatic melanoma patients.[201]

Furthermore, another top hit was represented by a missense variant of TMEM173 (STING) rs1131769,[253] which results in a defective protein.[257] The allele encoding for the defective protein was associated with lower IFN signaling in the tumor, strongly indicating a causal relationship.[257] This variant has been recently found associated with decreased production of type I IFN in a large GWAS study in patients vaccinated with smallpox virus, according to a preliminary report.[258]

STING is a critical modulator of the immune-mediated tumor rejection.[259,260] The STING pathway is activated by cyclic GMP-AMP (cGAMP), which is synthesized by the corresponding synthase (cGAS) following binding of cytosolic DNA.[260] STING induces IFN-I production via IRF3 and NFKB, which results in the secretion of CXCL9-11 and recruitment of activated CD8 T cells.[260]

As experimental studies in mice suggest that STING activation is necessary for the optimal activity of checkpoint inhibition[261] and radiation therapy,[262] and

considering that STING agonists are in clinical trials,[260] this observation might have clinical implications.

Those data, which have been all generated in the last couple of years, support the important role of the host's genetic background in shaping antitumor immunity. Studies focusing on specific cancer types and using whole-genome approaches for a comprehensive assessment of common and rare variants in both coding and noncoding regions could further expand our understanding of antitumor immunity.

Furthermore, these observations corroborate the existence of molecular mechanisms shared between autoimmunity, response to pathogens, and antitumor immunity, as predicted early by the immunologic constant of rejection hypothesis.[39]

Genome-Wide Scans Assessing the Germline Genetic Contribution to Outcome and Toxicity of Immunotherapeutic Agents: Work in Progress

Because of the multitude of possible ways in which germline variants can control antitumor immunity (Figure 35.3), it is imperative to use a comprehensive approach to

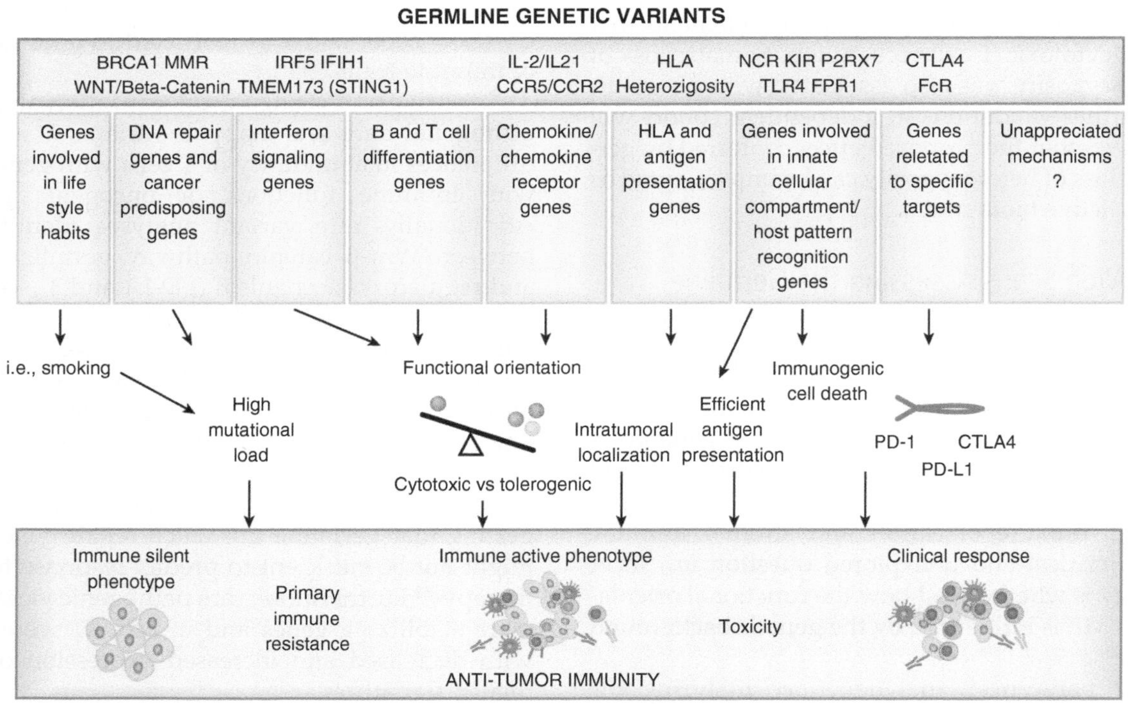

Figure 35.3 Germline genetic contribution to antitumor immunity. Genetic germline variants can influence cancer immune responsiveness in different ways, which are tightly interconnected. Genes or gene categories whose polymorphisms have been associated with either treatment outcome or differential immune microenvironmental features are highlighted in the top panel.

Source: Modified from Ref. (253). Bedognetti D, Ceccarelli M, Galluzzi L, et al. Correction to: toward a comprehensive view of cancer immune responsiveness: a synopsis from the SITC workshop. *J Immunother Cancer.* 2019;7(1):167. doi:10.1186/s40425-019-0640-y

identify variants associated with either clinical outcome or the development of immune-related adverse events. While this approach is necessary at this early stage of the research in the field as no genome-wide analyses have been published and made available to the scientific community, it is expected that variants identified by wide-genome scans could be condensed in variant panels for clinical use. These panels might be used to compute a polygenic risk score predictive to either adverse events or outcome.

It has been estimated that a sample size of 5,000 subjects (50% cases and 50% controls) will be needed to achieve a power of 80% for detection of low-penetrance loci (effect size between 1.1 and 1.5) by GWAS.[263] Large collaborative consortia are therefore needed, as recommended by the SITC Cancer Immune Responsiveness Taskforce.[23] Consortia have been created by different investigators, and it is expected that data will be available in the near future.[23,263]

In the absence of a large cohort, a reasonable approach is to test variants selected based on a predefined hypothesis, either extracted from genotyping arrays or from next-generation sequencing assays. Kirchhoff's group has selected 25 variants, each associated with multiple autoimmune diseases and profiled germline DNA from 465 melanoma patients treated either with CTLA-4 or PD-L1 blockades.[264] The rs7388568 SNP, a risk variant in the *IL-2-IL-21* locus, was associated with response to PD-1 blockade (OR 0.26; 95% CI 0.12–0.53), which was statistically significant after multiple test correction ($p = .0002$). Additionally, in the combined cohort (CTLA-4 and PD-1), the *IFIH1* rs2111485 variant was the second top SNP associated with outcome (OR 0.21, 95% CI 0.04–0.98), with a nominally significant p value. Remarkably, rs2111485 was also the most significant variant associated with IFN signaling across the entire genome in the TCGA study.[253]

Implementation of germline genetics represents an emerging challenge in the immuno-oncology biomarker field. Importantly, variants associated with immune-related adverse events can increase the therapeutic index of immunotherapeutic modalities, especially in patients with comorbidities, and might favor patient selection. This might be particularly relevant in the adjuvant setting, in which predicting toxicity in patients unlikely to benefit from treatment is particularly important for clinical decision-making.

As germline DNA is easily accessible (i.e., through blood or saliva), and considering that sequencing costs are decreasing rapidly, it is reasonable that data on the germline genetic contribution to an immunotherapeutic agent efficacy will exponentially increase in the next few years. Correlative data from immune-germline studies paired with functional validations of the results could lead to the implementation of more effective immunotherapeutic approaches.

KIR Polymorphisms and Tumor Development

NK cells are at the front line of early innate immune response. In contrast to T cells, which recognize foreign antigens through TCR in the context of the major histocompatibility complex (MHC), NK cells are modulated by the expression of self-MHC molecules, which allows them to eliminate virally infected or transformed cells (see Chapter 22). The impact of missing MHC class I expression on NK cell activation is known as the "missing-self" model. Later, the "missing self" model was completed with the "induced-self" model in which NK receptors, in particular NKG2D, are activated by stress-induced molecules. It is now accepted that NK cell lytic activity depends on a fine-tuning between activating and inhibitory signals.[265–267]

The KIR genes represent a key component of NK activity. They are located on chromosome 19q13.4 in the leukocyte receptor complex region and are highly polymorphic.[268,269] Fifteen distinct KIR genes (*KIR2DL1-5A,5B, KIR2DS1-5, KIR3DL1-3, KIR3DS1*) and two pseudogenes (*KR2DP1* and *KIR3DP1*) have been characterized (www.ebi.ac.uk/ipd/kir). KIR genes encode for either two (2D) or three (3D) extracellular immunoglobulin-like domains that might be associated with short (S) or long (L) cytoplasmic domains. KIRs can exert either activating or inhibitory activities. Two types of haplotypes have been described. The presence or absence of different KIR genes gives rise to haplotype diversity. Two haplotypes (A and B) are described based on KIR gene content (Figure 35.4). The haplotype A mainly encodes inhibitory KIRs, with the exception of *KIR2DS4*, which is an activating receptor. Although genes in the A haplotype do not generally vary in content, they show large allelic variations. In contrast, B haplotype exhibits lower allelic polymorphism, but higher variation in gene content. In view of the role of NK cells in host immunity against tumor, the role of KIR polymorphisms in cancer control, and in particular in the context of hematological malignancies, has been extensively studied.

Recently, germline mutations in NK cell-related genes (including NCRs and KIRs) have been correlated with an immune-excluded subtype in cancers from the TCGA cohorts and were enriched in patients with tumor versus healthy controls.[270] These data suggest that germline variants of NK-related gene influence not only tumorigenesis but also the development of a protective antitumor immunity.

KIR Polymorphisms in Hematological Malignancies

In 2004, Verheyden et al. reported an association between inhibitory KIR2DL2 and the disease in Belgian White patients affected by leukemia.[271] Haplotype analysis of the same cohort detected an increased frequency of the inhibitory KIRs in patients as compared to controls, suggesting that a large proportion of leukemic patients expressed a

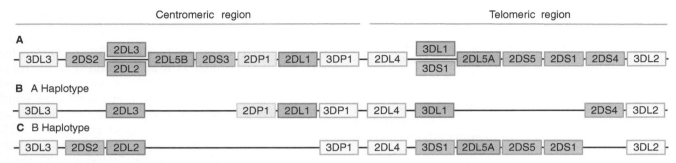

Figure 35.4 KIR haplotypes. (A) The four conserved framework genes are represented in blue. Inhibitory KIRs are in red and the activating ones in green. Pseudogenes are represented in yellow. **(B)** The group A haplotype is generally nonvariable. **(C)** The group B haplotype is more variable, and one example is shown in the panel. There is some evidence that the *3DL1* and *3DS1* genes are two alleles belonging to the same gene. Similarly, *2DL2* and *2DL3* are sometime considered alleles.

KIR phenotype that favors innate immunity escape. One major limitation of this study was the lack of stratification for different subtypes of the diseases. Indeed, all four types of leukemia (i.e., T acute lymphocytic leukemia [ALL], B-ALL, acute myeloid leukemia [AML], and chronic myeloid leukemia [CML]) were included in the study. In 2009, Middleton et al. described, in a cohort of patients from Turkey, that the frequency of *KIR2DL2* and *KIR2DS2* was decreased in CML and AML, but not with ALL, as compared to controls.[272] Although such a study emphasizes the importance of differentiating patients by the type of leukemia, the reason for the discrepancy with the previous study by Verhyden et al. remains unclear. Later, Zhang et al.,[273] in a relatively large cohort of Chinese leukemic patients, found that the rate of activating *KIR2DS4* was higher in patients with CML, while *KIR2DS3* was lower in patients with ALL. Interestingly, by studying a small number of adult T cell leukemia (ATL) patients, Obama et al. suggested that the expression of the inhibitory *KIR3DL2* might confer a survival advantage to ATL cells.[274]

Some additional studies reported discrepant results, therefore underscoring the complexity of NK modulation in cancer progression. In particular, in a pediatric cohort of Canadian-French patients, Almalte et al. showed that harboring activating KIRs (i.e., *KIR2DS1*, *KIR2DS2*, *KIR2DS3*, *KIR2DS4*, *KIR2DS5*, and *KIR3DS1*) was associated with decreased risk for developing B-ALL, with a very strong association between *KIR2DS1* and *KIR2DS2* with B-ALL.[275] Unfortunately, inhibitory KIRs were not assessed. To overcome the lack of data on inhibitory KIRs, Babor et al. examined a similar cohort of pediatric white patients with B-ALL and T-ALL. No association between KIR gene frequencies and disease susceptibility was detected.[276,277] Additionally, de Smith et al. studied the KIR haplotypes in Hispanic and non-Hispanic North American patients with ALL. The authors showed a significant increased frequency of individuals with KIR A/A haplotype among Hispanic patients only, suggesting

that the role of the KIR genes in pediatric ALL might be dependent on the ethnic origin of the patients.[278]

In multiple myeloma, Hoteit et al. demonstrated that *KIR2DS5* and some alleles of *KIR2DS4* were associated with an increased risk of the disease.[279] In non-Hodgkin lymphoma (NHL) patients, Vejbaesya et al. showed that the frequency of *KIR3DL1* with HLA-Bw4 was significantly lower in patients with diffuse large B cell lymphoma than in controls.[280] However, Pamuk et al. did not observe any significant association between KIRs and their ligands in NHL, while *KIR2DS1*, *KIR2DL5A*, and *KIR3DS1* were associated with a poor prognosis in this context.[281] In contrast, in a study of French families with first-degree siblings, Besson et al.[282] observed a dominant protective effect of *KIR3DS1* and/or *KIR2DS1* against Hodgkin lymphoma (HL).[282] Considering the role of NK cells in virus elimination, the authors also addressed the effect of the Epstein–Barr virus, as it represents a major environmental factor associated with HL. They found that the protective effect of *KIR3DS1* and *KR2DS1* was even stronger in patients with a detectable viral load. Nevertheless, the authors failed to validate the results in an additional smaller cohort of patients.

KIR Polymorphisms in Bone Marrow Transplantation

The interplay between HLA and KIRs is crucial for the positive outcome of hematopoietic stem cell transplantation (HSCT). Seminal investigations by Velardi's group examined the role of KIR-HLA mismatch by studying ALL, AML, and CML patients who had received haplotype-mismatched transplants.[283,284] The authors observed that absence of HLA ligands against the inhibitory KIRs present in the donor favors the development of graft-versus-leukemia and showed for the first time that the residual leukemic cells can be lysed by allogeneic NK cells. The results of such reports led many laboratories to implement KIR typing for the selection of HSCT donors. Elegant models explaining the consequences of mismatch between HLA and activating or inhibitory KIRs have been proposed.[285]

To investigate the influence of KIRs on the outcome of unrelated HSCT, Wu et al. retrospectively analyzed the HLA and KIR genotypes of donor recipients with leukemia in Chinese patients. Missing KIR ligands in recipients with myeloid diseases were significantly associated with a decreased risk of relapse or death. In addition, the presence of donor-activating KIR2DS3 gene was associated with decreased overall and disease-free survival. No effect was seen in patients with lymphoid disease.[286] More recently, in a comprehensive analysis of 1,277 AML patients, Venstrom et al.[287] described that activating KIR genes from donors were associated with differential outcomes of allogeneic HSCT. However, donor KIR2DS1 was associated with a reduced risk of relapse in an HLA-C-dependent manner.

KIR Polymorphisms in Solid Tumors

There are only a few studies focusing on the association between KIR polymorphisms and solid tumors. A study of 33 patients from Turkey demonstrated a negative correlation between KIR2DS1 and breast cancer. In addition, the authors performed allelic genotyping for KIR2DS4 and found a higher expression of KIR2DS4*003/4/6/7 in the control group, suggesting that KIR polymorphisms can influence the risk of disease development.[288] However, the results should be considered with caution because of the small sample size. Another study of interest was performed on a relatively large cohort of Brazilian breast cancer patients from predominantly European descendants, in which a strong association between KIR2DL2 and the disease was detected.[289]

Campillo et al. analyzed the influence of both KIR genes and KIR/HLA combinations on melanoma susceptibility and/or prognosis in a Spanish Caucasian population.[290] The frequency of the KIR2DL3/HLA-C1 combination was decreased in the overall melanoma population, while KIR2DL3 behaved as a protective condition in nodular and ulcerated melanoma patients.

A study of KIRs in patients with ovarian cancer showed that the frequency of KIR2DS4 full length was higher in patients with endometrioid than in other histological subtypes and controls.[291] In Korean colorectal cancer patients, Kim et al. observed a higher frequency of KIR2DS5 compared with controls.[292] They also showed a lower frequency of KIR3D1, KIR2DS2, and KIR2DS4 in the rectal cancer subgroup.

Among pediatric cancers, neuroblastoma is one of the most common extracranial solid tumors. The early onset of the disease suggests the potential role of genetic factors. By studying KIRs and HLA genotypes in this

setting, Keating et al. found a significant increase in the frequency of KIR2DL2 and KIR2DS2 independent of the presence of their ligand HLA-C.[293]

Kaposi's sarcoma (KS) is a severe complication of KS-associated herpes virus (KSHV), and is frequent in HIV-infected patients. Goedert et al. studied KIRs and their ligand HLA class I gene frequencies in a total of more than 1,000 KS patients, including classic KS (AIDS unrelated), KSHV-seropositive, and KSHV-seronegative patients. The authors detected a consistent association across the three cohorts with activating KIR3DS1 plus HLA-B Bw4-80I and homozygosity for HLA-C group. Interestingly, in patients with KIR3DS1 plus HLA-B Bw4-80I, the risk of KS was doubled despite KSHV seroprevalence being 40% lower. This observation led to the hypothesis that KIR-mediated NK cell activation may decrease the risk of KSHV infection but at the same time enhance KSHV dissemination and progression to KS if infection occurs.[294]

Although some positive associations between KIR polymorphisms and cancer susceptibility have been reported, the results are overall inconclusive due to the small number of large and homogeneous studies. These results highlight the importance of studying the influence of KIR variations in a specific clinical setting and advocates for considering the overall balance between activating and inhibitory KIR genes and their interaction with the respective HLA class I ligands and with environmental factors. Other factors such as the epigenetic regulations should also be considered.

HLA Polymorphisms and Tumor Development

The HLAs are part of the MHC located in a region of approximately 4,000 kilobases of the short arm of chromosome 6.[295] The (classical) HLAs are designated as class I (HLA-A, -B, and -C) and class II (HLA-DR, -DP, and -DQ). Class I molecules are composed of a heavy chain (45 kD) with $\alpha 1$ and $\alpha 2$ domains that are noncovalently associated with a β_2 microglobulin (12 kD) light chain encoded by a gene on chromosome 15. In contrast, class II molecules are heterodimers formed by α (32 kD) and β (28 kD) chains. The main function of HLA class I and II molecules is the recognition of self and nonself by presenting antigenic peptides to $CD8^+$ and $CD4^+$ T cells. Both class I and II molecules are highly polymorphic, and currently more than 12,000 distinct alleles of these genes have been identified (IMGT/HLA database, www.ebi.ac.uk/ipd/imgt/hla).

In contrast to highly polymorphic classical HLAs, nonclassical HLA molecules are characterized by a lower genetic diversity and by a particular expression pattern, structural organization, and functional profile.[296] Here, we focus on the association between polymorphisms of classical HLA molecules and tumor development.

HLA variants have been associated with more than 100 diseases. One of the most studied diseases is ankylosing spondylitis, which is associated with HLA-B*27 in 90% of Caucasian patients.[297,298] HLA polymorphisms have been described as a critical genetic determinant of susceptibility to several other autoimmune and infectious diseases, such as type 1 diabetes mellitus and HIV.[299–302]

HLA Polymorphisms in Bone Marrow Transplantation

With the clinical implementation of tissue and organ transplantation, the analysis of HLA variations has been the subject of intensive investigation. Following bone marrow transplantation (BMT), HLA mismatch between the donor and host can have life-threatening consequences. The outcome of BMT between the donor and an unrelated recipient is inversely correlated with the degree of HLA matching. All HLA loci have been reported to influence the BMT outcome, with some ethnic specificities.[303–305]

GvHD constitutes a significant cause of morbidity and mortality in transplanted patients. Several factors can trigger GvHD, with the most critical being the disparity in HLA alleles between the donor and recipient.[306] It is well established that the severity of GvHD is strongly correlated with the degree of HLA mismatch between donor and recipient. Because of the high morbidity and mortality related to GvHD grade II or higher, the favorable clinical outcome of BMT is directly associated with the degree of HLA match between donor and recipient.[307–311] Unfortunately, due to the high diversity of HLA molecules, only a minority of patients find an HLA-compatible donor. Extensive research has been focused on the identification of permissible HLA mismatches. The National Marrow Donor Program (NMDP) guidelines recommend HLA-A, -B, -C, and -DRB1 high-resolution matching to maximize survival.[312] However, the level of HLA disparity between the host and the donor can affect the success of the BMT with different degrees.[313,314] This fluctuation might be dependent upon other factors such as the intensity of conditioning protocol[315] and variations of other critical loci such as those of KIR genes. Further functional and correlative studies are needed to better understand the role of HLA/KIR interaction on the outcome of BMT.

HLA Polymorphisms in Hematological Malignancies

Polymorphisms of HLA class I and II genes may also influence the risk of developing different types of cancers. Several alleles of HLA class I have been associated with the onset of leukemia.[316,317] It is now well established that HLA allele frequency varies noticeably among different ethnicities. To evaluate the role of the HLA polymorphisms in a population-specific manner, Gragert

et al.[318] studied the HLA frequencies in a large cohort of patients with chronic lymphocytic leukemia (CLL), consisting of 3,616 U.S. Caucasians, 413 African Americans, and 97 Hispanics and compared it with 50,000 controls from the NMDP. Their finding confirms the association of a severe form of CLL with HLA-A*02:01 only in Caucasian patients. In patients with an African American background, a predisposing effect for HLA-DRB4*01:01, -DRB1*09:01 haplotype was detected. Interestingly, the authors described a universal association for HLA-DRB4*01:01, DRB1*07:01, DQB1*03:03 haplotype across the three populations, suggesting a similar disease etiology. A large study on 3,700 multiple myeloma patients based on NMDP and the Center for International Blood and Marrow Transplant Research (CIBMTR) HLA genotyping data conclusively demonstrated the role of HLA variations in susceptibility to B cell malignancies.[319]

Other smaller studies have confirmed the existence of an association between HLA variants and NHL susceptibility.[320,321] Moreover, large GWASs enrolling globally more than 3,500 follicular lymphoma[322–324] and 4,500 multiple myeloma patients have detected loci in the HLA region strongly associated with disease development.[325]

HLA Polymorphisms in Solid Tumors

Cervical cancer (CC), the second most frequent cancer in women worldwide, is almost invariably associated with human papillomavirus (HPV) infection. However, despite HPV infection being relatively common in women, only a small proportion develop the neoplasia. For this reason, the genetic variability of the host has been proposed as one of the key factors influencing disease development and progression. In this context, polymorphisms of classical and nonclassical HLA class I and II antigens have been widely investigated. Studies conducted in different ethnicities have found significant associations of CC with different HLA-A or B alleles in Chinese, Japanese, Swedish, and Costa Rican women and with HLA C alleles in Chinese, Korean, and American women.[236,326] In a North American study employing high-resolution genotyping, Madeleine et al. showed that co-occurring HLA alleles can increase the risk of CC. Combinations of HLA-B*4402-DRB1*1101 and -DQB1*0301 conferred a strong risk of developing CC, whereas HLA-Cw*0701 and -DQB1*02 were associated with a decreased risk of developing CC.[327] HLA-DQ and HLA-DR polymorphisms have been associated with CC in one of the first complete studies of HLA regions (conducted in Dutch patients).[328] Subsequent studies have confirmed the correlation between HLA-DQ/DR and CC in Argentine, Tunisian, and Chinese women.[326] Associations between nonclassical HLA class I (HLA-G) and CC have also been reported in different ethnicities by several reports.[326] Recently, two GWASs on more than 2,000 Swedish[329] and Chinese[330] CC patients reported an association with loci in the HLA region. In addition, HLA variants have been found to be associated with advanced cervical intraepithelial neoplasia by a large pooled analysis of GWASs in the Swedish population.[48]

Associations between HLA-B and HLA-DR variants with head and neck squamous cell carcinomas, which are also associated with HPV infection, have been reported in the Dutch population.[331] Several studies have reported associations between HLA variants and predisposition to nasopharyngeal carcinoma (NPC), which is another virally induced tumor, in different ethnic groups.[332–334] A meta-analysis of 13 studies on a Southern Chinese population found a positive association between NPC and HLA-A2, -B14, and B-46, and a negative association for HLA-A11, -B13, and -B22.[335] A large GWAS in 1,538 Chinese patients[336] and two smaller GWASs in Taiwanese[337] and Malaysian Chinese[338] patients have corroborated the role of HLA variants in NPC susceptibility.

In Caucasian breast cancer patients, Chaudhuri et al. showed a protective role of HLA-DQB*03032 and -DRB1*11.[339] In another study on breast cancer patients from a Mexican mestizo background, HLA-DQ0301 had a protective effect. In contrast, HLA-DQ0302 was associated with an increased risk of the disease.[340] Moreover, in Indian women, the frequency of HLA-B*40:06 was higher in breast cancer patients as compared to controls. The authors also observed a low frequency of HLA-B*08 and increased homozygosity at the HLA-Cw locus in these patients.[341] A number of studies with limited sample size focused on the association of HLA class II and melanoma, but no consensus could be reached.[246,342–347]

In conclusion, strong evidence supports the existence of a relationship between HLA variants and tumor development, particularly in leukemia and virally induced tumors. The clinical relevance of such association in different clinical settings and the interaction between HLA variants, environmental factors, and cancer-specific alterations must be further elucidated.

CONCLUSION

Bulk transcriptome studies have corroborated the existence of a continuum between prognostic, predictive, and mechanistic signatures. Such studies have defined representative genes consistently associated with better prognosis and responsiveness to immunotherapy. These genes reflect the activation of a cytotoxic/Th1 response, the induction of IFN signaling, and the secretion of specific chemokines. From a mechanistic point of view, analyses of multiple biopsies during treatment (e.g., at relapse), single cell sequencing, and spatial transcriptomic, integrated with somatic analyses (e.g., whole exome or whole genome sequencing), will be needed to better understand the complex interaction between cancer cells and the immune system to implement more effective immunotherapeutic approaches. To be translated into clinical practice, prospective trials will be needed. It is likely that, rather than being used as isolated biomarkers, gene signatures could be used together with other metrics (e.g., tumor mutational burden) to identify patients in which immunotherapy could be more beneficial than standard therapy in that specific context (e.g., targeted therapy or chemotherapy). In addition, transcriptomic analyses have identified a relationship between antitumor immunity and specific oncogenic pathways leading to the conceptualization of several combinatorial approaches currently in clinical trial.

Studies in large data sets annotating germline data have demonstrated that the host's genetic background contributes to the functional orientation of the tumor immune microenvironments and proposed genetic variants and genes responsible for this phenomenon. Large genome or exome scans in the context of cancer immunotherapy are expected to define the clinical impact of germline variants in the near future. Such information could be integrated with other predictive biomarkers (including gene signatures) to increase the therapeutic index of immunotherapeutic approaches.

Strong evidence supports the existence of a relationship between HLA variants and tumor development, particularly in leukemia and virally induced tumors. The clinical relevance of such association in different clinical settings and the interaction between HLA variants, environmental factors, and cancer-specific alterations must be further elucidated.

KEY REFERENCES

Only key references appear in the print edition. The full reference list appears in the digital product on Springer Publishing Connect: connect.springerpub.com/content/book/978-0-8261-3743-2/part/part03/chapter/ch35

37. Angelova M, Mlecnik B, Vasaturo A, et al. Evolution of metastases in space and time under immune selection. *Cell.* 2018;175(3):751–765. doi:10.1016/j.cell.2018.09.018
43. Roelands J, Hendrickx W, Zoppoli G, et al. Oncogenic states dictate the prognostic and predictive connotations of intratumoral immune response. *J Immunother Cancer.* 2020;8(1):e000617. doi:10.1136/jitc-2020-000617
55. Cristescu R, Mogg R, Ayers M, et al. Pan-tumor genomic biomarkers for PD-1 checkpoint blockade-based immunotherapy. *Science.* 2018;362(6411):eaar3593. doi:10.1126/science.aar3593
60. Rodig SJ, Gusenleitner D, Jackson DG, et al. MHC proteins confer differential sensitivity to CTLA-4 and PD-1 blockade in untreated metastatic melanoma. *Sci Transl Med.* 2018;10(450):eaar3342. doi:10.1126/scitranslmed.aar3342
62. Gide TN. Distinct immune cell populations define response to anti-PD-1 monotherapy and anti-PD-1/anti-CTLA-4 combined therapy. *Cancer Cell.* 2019;35:238–255. doi:10.1016/j.ccell.2019.01.003
116. Thorsson V, Gibbs DL, Brown SD, et al. The immune landscape of cancer. *Immunity.* 2018;48(4):812–830. doi:10.1016/j.immuni.2018.03.023
253. Sayaman RW, Saad M, Thorsson V, et al. Germline genetic contribution to the immune landscape of cancer. *bioRxiv.* 2020;54(2):367–386. doi:10.1101/2020.01.30.926527

Impact of Somatic Mutations on the Local and Systemic Antitumor Immune Response

Paul F. Robbins

KEY POINTS

- T cell infiltration into the tumor microenvironment (TME) is correlated with increased response to immunotherapeutic interventions, including checkpoint blockade and adoptive T cell transfer.

- Tumor cell-intrinsic signaling pathways—for example, activation of the Wnt/β-catenin pathway or phosphatase and tensin homolog (PTEN) deletion—are associated with the lack of T cell infiltration.

- Alterations of oncogenic pathways are often mediated by mutational events associated with or causal for tumor progression.

- Tumor-infiltrating, tumor-reactive T cells often recognize tumor-specific antigens generated by mutations (neoantigens). Neoantigens resemble foreign antigens for which the T cell repertoire has not been negatively selected against.

- Clinical benefit from immunotherapy may be more tightly correlated with the number of potential neoepitopes predicted to bind to a patient's major histocompatibility complex (MHC) than to overall mutational burden.

INTRODUCTION

Tumors represent complex mixtures of malignant cells with normal or stromal components that include immune cells, fibroblasts, vasculature, and extracellular matrix. Within the context of immunotherapeutic interventions, this aggregation of cells has been termed the "tumor microenvironment" (TME), as these cells appear to interact in a complex manner with each other and with metabolic factors such as oxygen and energy supplies. This chapter discusses to what extent tumor cell-intrinsic changes in gene expression, protein function, and/or metabolic turnover affect the composition of the TME and the implications of those changes for immunotherapy.

IMPACT OF SOMATIC MUTATIONS ON GENE EXPRESSION AND PROTEIN FUNCTION

For decades, cancer biologists have focused on somatic mutations, gain of function of oncogenes, or loss of function of tumor-suppressor genes, as tumor cell-intrinsic events impact tumor cell proliferation, tumor cell senescence, tumor cell migration, and formation for metastasis. Results from those studies have provided us with a deep understanding of how somatic mutations affect cell-intrinsic signaling and thereby drive tumor progression. The majority of nucleotide changes can be grouped into three general categories: (1) single nucleotide changes (often referred to as single nucleotide variants; SNVs), which are limited to substitutions at one position or two adjacent genomic positions, (2) insertions or deletions (indels), in which relatively short sequences are removed or inserted into genes or chromosomal segments, and (3) large scale changes such as the amplification or deletion of individual or multiple genes, loss or amplification of chromosomal arms, and whole chromosomes and chromosomal fusion events. Although indels and chromosomal fusions occur at higher frequencies in tumors with deficiencies or mutations in mismatch repair genes, designated dMMR, SNVs can be generated by multiple endogenous and exogenous mutagens that result in different mutational profiles. For example, substitutions representing interchanges of two-ring purine residues or one-ring pyrimidine bases frequently occur in response to ultraviolet (UV) exposure or alkylating chemotherapy and predominate in cutaneous cancers, whereas interchanges of purine for pyrimidine bases or transversions are primarily caused by tobacco smoke, intracellular reactive oxygen species (ROS), or deamination in CpG-rich DNA segments. In addition, SNVs can either lead to no change in the amino acid sequence of the protein, termed synonymous SNVs, or result in protein sequence changes, termed nonsynonymous SNVs.

Different mutations have the potential to have different effects on protein function or protein expression. Gene or gene segment amplifications or deletions, referred to as copy-number changes, generally result in overexpression or lack of expression of the encoded protein, respectively. For example, overexpression of *c-myc* as a result of gene amplification leads to enhanced cellular proliferation whereas bi-allelic deletion of the gene encoding for phosphatase and tensin homolog (PTEN) results in lack of PTEN protein function.[1,2] The majority of nonsynonymous SNVs have no impact on protein function and are termed "passenger mutations," but can nevertheless potentially give rise to "foreign" antigens or neoantigens that are recognized by the adaptive immune system (T and B lymphocytes). Single amino acid substitutions at certain positions in a protein, such as the substitution of glutamic acid for valine at position 600 of the *BRAF* gene ($BRAF^{V600E}$) or substitutions at position 12 in the *KRAS* gene such as $KRAS^{G12D}$, $KRAS^{G12V}$, or $KRAS^{G12R}$ result in constitutive activation of the Ras/Raf/MAPK/ERK kinase (MEK)/mitogen-activating protein kinase (MAPK) signaling pathway.[3] These mutations have been shown to exert a dominant effect on the protein functionality and thereby are only required to occur as a mono-allelic event. Indels can have a relatively small or large effect that depends upon their size, location, and whether they represent in-frame or out-of-frame indels but can all potentially be recognized by the immune system as they result in altered protein sequences.

Protein function can also be dramatically altered by the modification of specific phosphorylation sites. Protein phosphorylation, mainly of the amino acids serine, threonine, and tyrosine, acts as a major regulator for protein activation but also for protein degradation. For instance, loss of PTEN function results in increased activity of phosphatidylinositol-4,5-bisphosphate 3-kinase (PI3K), which in turn activates protein kinase B (AKT) through phosphorylation of specific amino acids. Another example of phospho-site–specific regulation are the serine and threonine residues located between amino acids 37 to 42 of the CTNNB1(β-catenin) protein, which, if phosphorylated, marks β-catenin for degradation. Upstream signaling cues resulting from Wnt–Frizzled interactions can lead to de-phosphorylation of those sites, leading to downstream signaling resulting from translocation of β-catenin into the nucleus. Substitutions of serine or threonine amino acids within this region resulting from somatic mutations can stabilize β-catenin, resulting in constitutive activation of downstream signaling pathways. Although these examples are primarily focused on constitutive activation of oncogenes, which comprise pro-survival/pro-proliferation tumor cell-intrinsic properties, SNV can also affect tumor-suppressor genes. Tumor-suppressor genes encode proteins that can either inhibit uncontrolled proliferation or enhance cellular senescence, and their loss is generally thought to be required for tumor development. The most common and most detrimental SNVs are the generation of a stop codon, which leads to early termination of protein translation, and frameshift mutations, which can generate a nonfunctional protein, depending on the location of the frameshift. Mutations abolishing kinase/phosphatase activity or protein–protein interactions can also cause loss of protein function (see Weinberg et al.[4] for an additional discussion of this topic).

Although some somatic mutations that result in alterations of the amino acid sequence of a protein may have an impact on tumor cell-intrinsic signaling, alterations in signaling pathways can also have detrimental effects on the TME, particularly the immune infiltrate into the tumor. This chapter focuses on the impact of somatic mutations on an antitumor immunity through alterations of tumor cell-intrinsic signaling.

ESTABLISHING A LOCAL AND PRODUCTIVE ANTITUMOR IMMUNE RESPONSE

In order to understand the effects of somatic alterations on the local immune response, it is crucial to understand the critical components of potent and productive antitumor immune responses. From seminal work, our current understanding is that innate immune cells, predominantly dendritic cells (DCs) driven by the transcription factor Batf3, are activated and produce high amounts of type 1 interferons (IFN).[5,6] Activation of Batf3-DC depends on antigen-presenting cells (APCs) that are usually activated through the pattern recognition receptor pathway cyclic GAM-AMP synthesis (cGAS)/stimulator of IFN genes (STING), which has been shown to sense tumor-derived DNA.[7] Additional work suggests that Batf3-driven DCs migrate to the tumor-draining lymph node (TdLN), where they contribute to the antigen presentation and activation of tumor-specific T cells.[8,9] Successful T cell priming presumes the existence of T cells specific for tumor-associated or mutant tumor-specific antigens, termed neoantigens. Following effector T cell activation, tumor-specific T cells are recruited back into the TME through a chemokine gradient, predominantly CXCL9 and CXCL10, and a local adaptive antitumor immune response is initiated.[10] Additional immune inhibitory mechanisms within the TME dampen this local response, as discussed further in Chapters 39 and 40. Several studies illustrated the importance of CD8+ T cells in the response to immunotherapies, including checkpoint blockade therapy, and therefore, it is important to understand why some tumors fail to recruit a potent antitumor immunity into the TME.[11]

Antigens Recognized by Tumor-Reactive T Cells Associated with Responses to Cancer Immunotherapy

Extensive studies carried out in murine tumor model systems demonstrated that T cells could not only recognize nonmutated antigens, primarily consisting of tissue-specific antigens and cancer germline antigens whose expression is limited to germ cells, but also could frequently recognize mutated gene products or neoantigens. Additional studies showed that T cells from either of these classes can mediate both tumor protection and the rejection of established tumors, and indicated that immune surveillance may play a significant role in mediating the regression of tumors that express highly immunogenic tumor antigens, which appear to predominantly consist of mutated gene products.[12]

In vitro cultured human tumor-infiltrating lymphocytes (TILs) and T cells derived from peripheral blood mononuclear cells (PBMCs) have also been shown to recognize both tissue-specific nonmutated gene products and mutated gene products. Objective clinical responses were observed in human trials involving transduction of autologous PBMCs with T cell receptors (TCRs) that target the shared melanocyte differentiation antigens MART-1 and gp100,[13] but a durable complete response was only observed in one of the 36 patients treated in these trials. Long-term complete tumor regressions were observed in approximately 20% of patients receiving autologous PBMCs transduced with a TCR that recognizes the cancer germline antigen NY-ESO-1,[14] but attempts to target other members of the CG gene family, such as MAGEA3, have led to severe neurological[15] and cardiac[16] toxicities. Regression of bulky metastatic tumor lesions has been observed after adoptive immunotherapy with bulk populations of autologous neoantigen-reactive TILs from patients with metastatic melanoma[17-20] and with metastatic colorectal cancer,[21] cholangiocarcinoma,[22] and breast cancer;[23] however, it is difficult to discern the role of T cells with particular specificities in mediating these responses because of the polyclonal nature of these cell products.

Gene products that are not encoded in the normal human genome represent attractive targets for therapy, as they obviate issues resulting from expression in normal tissues. These include both neoantigens and antigens expressed by viruses such as HPV, a virus associated with the etiology of many cervical and head and neck cancers. Neoantigens can potentially arise from random mutations that occur in any expressed gene product, including those that play a functional role in promoting tumorigenicity, termed "driver mutations," and those that have no functional significance, termed "passenger mutations." There is a wide range in the mutation frequencies seen in different cancer types,

varying from fewer than 10 nonsynonymous somatic mutations in some hematological malignancies to several thousand in dMMR tumors and some melanomas.[24] The likelihood that tumor cells elicit neoantigen reactivity is thus at least in part dependent on the tumor type being evaluated; at the same time, however, the mutation frequency rather than tissue of origin is likely to be an important factor influencing the generation of neoantigen reactivity as there is a two log or more variation in the mutation rates of individual tumors of a given histology. Significantly, recent studies indicate that tumor regressions seen in response to a variety of immunotherapies may be predominantly mediated by neoantigen-reactive T cells. Evidence supporting this hypothesis, along with potential strategies for addressing challenges arising from attempts to target neoantigens, is discussed in the following section.

Immune Checkpoint Blockade Therapies: Association Between Mutational Load and Predicted Neoantigen Reactivity

Immune checkpoint blockade therapies or treatments that involve administration of antibodies directed against inhibitory molecules, such as cytotoxic T-lymphocyte associated protein 4 (CTLA-4) and programmed death 1 (PD-1), have provided long-term clinical benefits to patients with a variety of tumor types that include melanoma,[25] non-small cell lung cancer (NSCLC),[26] renal cancer,[27] and Hodgkin lymphoma.[28] Results of a study carried out to identify factors associated with the response of metastatic melanoma patients to treatment with antibodies directed against the inhibitory ligand CTLA-4 indicated that long-term benefit in response to treatment with these reagents was associated with tumor mutational load and the number of candidate human leukocyte antigen (HLA) class I–restricted mutant peptides MHC identified using MHC binding prediction algorithms.[29,30] A study was also carried out to evaluate antitumor immunity in a melanoma patient who exhibited a partial response to ipilimumab, which was carried out by screening a library of major histocompatibility complex (MHC)–peptide tetramers consisting of mutated candidate epitopes identified by combining whole exome sequencing (WES) and whole transcriptome (RNA-Seq) analysis of autologous tumor cells with the use of an MHC class I peptide-binding algorithm.[31] A TIL population generated from a lesion resected before ipilimumab treatment of this patient reacted with two neoepitopes present in the screening panel, one of which corresponded to approximately 3%, and a second corresponded to 0.003%, of the TIL population. Cells with the same specificity as the dominant TIL clonotype appeared to undergo a fivefold increase in the patient's peripheral blood 1 month following treatment, at which time they had expanded to 0.3% of total peripheral CD8[+] T cells, indicating that they may have played some role in the tumor regression observed in this patient.

The potential association between mutational load and response to immune checkpoint blockade was further evaluated in clinical trials evaluating responses to pembrolizumab. In a study evaluating responses of metastatic melanoma patients to treatment with antibodies directed against the immune checkpoint inhibitor PD-1, response to therapy was not associated with total mutational load, and was not associated with the number of predicted HLA class I or class II neoepitopes.[32] Nevertheless, in this study, extended survival was seen in patients whose tumors were within the top third of the distribution of total nonsynonymous somatic mutations relative to patients whose tumors were within the bottom third of the distribution of nonsynonymous mutation. A positive association of neoantigen burden with both clinical benefit and progression-free survival (PFS) has been noted in patients with metastatic NSCLC receiving pembrolizumab.[33] Evaluation of the impact of intratumor heterogeneity and predicted neoantigen burden on response to immune checkpoint blockade in patients with metastatic melanoma or NSCLC indicated that high neoantigen burden was associated with longer overall survival (OS) in a predominantly early stage cohort of patients with lung adenocarcinoma but not in early stage patients with squamous cell carcinoma.[34] An inflamed tumor signature, as determined by expression of genes associated with effector function such as CD8 and genes involved with antigen processing and presentation, was associated with the load of candidate neoepitopes identified using an HLA-binding algorithm that were also predicted to be clonally represented in the tumor population. In this study, the intratumoral heterogeneity of predicted neoepitopes expressed by patient tumors also appeared to have a relatively small but significant negative influence on PFS in patients with advanced NSCLC treated with pembrolizumab and on OS in metastatic melanoma patients treated with ipilimumab or tremelimumab.

In an initial study, patients with dMMR carcinomas derived from either colon or additional tumor types that possessed relatively high mutational burdens exhibited objective clinical response rates of 40% and 71%, respectively, whereas none of the 18 patients with colorectal cancers that did not contain MMR defects, termed "mismatch-repair proficient" or pMMR, responded to therapy.[35] These observations have been confirmed in further studies demonstrating clinical responses in patients bearing colorectal,[36,37] endometrial, gastroesophageal, and pancreatic cancers[37] that possess relatively high mutational burdens resulting from defective MMR. As a result of these and other studies, in June 2020 the U.S. Food and Drug Administration (FDA) granted approval for the use of pembrolizumab as a treatment for adult and pediatric patients with unresectable or metastatic solid tumors with a high tumor mutational burden (TMB) of greater than 10 mutations per megabase who have progressed following prior therapy and who have no satisfactory alternative treatment options.

Targeting Nonself Antigens in Adoptive Immunotherapy and Tumor Vaccine Clinical Trials

Vaccination of patients against viral proteins such as the human papillomavirus (HPV) E6 and E7 oncogenes, gene products highly expressed in HPV-driven cancers, has been shown to have clinical benefit in patients with premalignant disease,[38] whereas vaccination with HPV peptides alone did not appear to be effective in patients with invasive cervical cancer.[39] Reports from a recent clinical trial indicate that there was a positive association between the frequency of peripheral HPV-reactive T cells administered during multiple cycles of chemotherapy and prolonged patient survival.[40] Objective clinical responses were also observed in five of 28 metastatic cervical cancer patients, two of which have ongoing complete regression lasting more than 7 years, and two of 11 noncervical cancer patients with HPV positive cancers who received autologous TIL cultures that were selected on the basis of multiple characteristics, including responsiveness to the HPV E6 and E7 oncoproteins and in vitro proliferation.[41] The indication that clinical response to therapy may be associated with the frequency of E6- and E7-reactive T cells has led to additional studies to evaluate the clinical efficacy of autologous PBMC transduced with TCRs that target E6 or E7.[42]

The availability of relatively inexpensive high-throughput sequencing methods, including whole genome sequencing and WES analysis of tumor and matched normal DNA and RNA-Seq analysis, has led to the development of methods that facilitate the rapid and efficient identification of candidate neoepitopes targeted by patient tumor-reactive T cells. Using this approach, a mutated spectrin-a2 neoepitope was found to represent a dominant tumor rejection antigen for d42m1 murine methylcholanthrene-induced sarcoma cells, which were derived from an immune-deficient Rag2 knockout mouse, when injected into normal Rag2-proficient mice.[43] Eleven of 50 mutated 27-mer peptides identified by WES of the B16F10 murine melanoma induced T cells specific to mutated epitopes but with little or no cross-reactivity to the corresponding wild-type peptides. Immunization of tumor-bearing mice with an immunodominant mutated peptide significantly slowed tumor growth and enhanced survival.[44] Tumor rejection antigens have also been identified using novel approaches in tumor model systems that are potentially relevant to patient treatment trials. In one study, mass spectrometric analysis carried out on peptides eluted from MHC class I molecules isolated from the surface of MC-38 and TRAMP-C1 murine tumor cells was combined with WES and RNA-Seq analysis to identify naturally processed candidate neoepitopes.[45] Vaccination with candidate tumor neoepitopes identified using this approach was effective in preventing MC-38 tumor growth and appeared to treat mice with established subcutaneous tumors. Using a similar peptide elution approach, an MHC class-I restricted epitope was identified as a target of human TIL.[46] In another study, RNA constructs encoding tandem arrays of candidate neoepitopes identified by WES and RNA-Seq analysis of murine B16F10 and CT26 colon carcinoma cells were complexed with cationic lipids and injected into tumor-bearing mice.[47] The results indicated that vaccination predominantly elicited HLA class II and not class I-restricted responses, and that immunization with constructs encoding individual CD4 epitopes that induced robust immune responses, or with constructs encoding multiple HLA class I- and class II–restricted epitopes, was capable of treating mice with established B16F10 and CT26 tumors.

Analysis of the specificity of human tumor-reactive T cells derived from TILs or PBMCs has also provided correlative evidence of an association between tumor regression and neoepitope recognition. A total of seven neoepitopes recognized by three populations of human melanoma TILs were identified by screening TILs for their ability to respond to candidate neoepitopes that were also identified using WES and RNA-Seq analysis in combination with a similar MHC class peptide binding peptide algorithm.[48] Two of the three patients analyzed in this study exhibited durable complete regressions of multiple metastases in response to the transfer of autologous TILs that appeared to predominantly or uniquely recognize neoantigen targets.

Neoepitopes recognized by two bulk populations of melanoma TILs that were associated with durable complete responses to adoptive immunotherapy were identified using a screening approach using transient transfection of COS-7 or HEK293 cell lines with tandem minigene constructs (TMGs) encoding mutated residues plus the 12 flanking normal amino acids and autologous HLA constructs.[49] In addition, a patient who received bulk TILs that did not appear to recognize shared nonmutated gene products, but that contained a dominant clone (representing approximately 50% of the TIL population) which recognized a mutated HLA class I-restricted PPP1R3B epitope, exhibited a complete regression of all metastatic melanoma lesions lasting more than 10 years following adoptive transfer.[19]

Studies have also been carried out to evaluate the use of WES and RNA-Seq analysis to identify neoantigen-reactive T cells from patients with cancer types other than melanoma. Use of a screening method that involved transfection of autologous DCs with a panel of TMGs identified by WES of tumor samples, combined with the pulsing of autologous DCs with 25 amino acid peptides encompassing the mutations, led to the identification of between one and three neoepitopes targeted by nine of the 10 gastrointestinal TILs that were evaluated using this approach.[50] All of the T cells evaluated in this study recognized unique neoepitopes that were restricted to an individual tumor, with the exception of T cells from two patients that recognized an identical peptide containing a substitution of aspartic acid for glycine at position 12 of the KRAS oncogene (KRAS^{G12D}) in the context of HLA-C*08:02. Mutated KRAS gene products containing substitutions of aspartic acid as well as substitutions of valine or cysteine at this position, termed "driver mutations," stimulate cell growth through constitutive activation of the RAS/MAPK signaling pathway and are commonly expressed in multiple tumor types that include pancreatic, colon, and lung cancers. The KRAS^{G12D} and KRAS^{G12V} mutations are expressed by 60% to 70% of pancreatic adenocarcinomas[51,52] and 20% to 30% of colorectal adenocarcinomas.[53,54] Multiple TCRs that mediate recognition of KRAS^{G12V} and KRAS^{G12D} epitopes in the context of HLA-A*11:01,[55] an HLA class I allele expressed by approximately 14% of the patient population, and TCRs that mediate recognition of the KRAS^{G12D} HLA-C*08:02, expressed by approximately 10% of patients, are currently being evaluated in adoptive immunotherapy trials. Gene products encoded by common driver mutations in TP53 have also been found to be frequently targeted by HLA class I and class II restricted T cells identified by screening patient TIL[56,57] and peripheral blood[58] populations, and TCRs mediating recognition of these products are being evaluated in ongoing trials, including TCRs that mediate recognition of a TP53 p.R175H mutant peptide, encoded by a mutation that is found in between 5% and 10% of gastrointestinal cancers, in the context of HLA-A*02:01, an HLA class I allele expressed by approximately 50% of the patient population.

Although driver mutations represent the most attractive targets for immunotherapy, additional therapies will be needed for the treatment of patients whose tumors do not express any of the common driver mutations or patients whose T cell repertoire does not contain T cells reactive with these neoantigens. In a recent study, 62 of 85, or over 80% of, patients bearing gastrointestinal tumors that are MMS and consequently have relatively low TMBs possess T cells reactive with one or more autologous neoantigen targets,[59] and ongoing clinical trials are being carried out to evaluate the ability of T cells targeting these neoantigens to mediate tumor regression.

Evidence for the importance of neoantigen reactivity in clinical responses to immunotherapy was provided by a case study of a metastatic cholangiocarcinoma patient who received an autologous TIL culture, approximately 95% of which consisted of a CD4⁺ T cell clone that recognized a single HLA class II-restricted neoepitope derived from the ERBB2IP protein.[22] A dramatic, nearly complete regression of all metastatic lesions, which has been ongoing for nearly 7 years following treatment, was observed following adoptive transfer of this TIL population.

Neoantigen-reactive CD4[+] T cells have also been identified within populations of tumor-reactive T cells from four of five metastatic melanoma patients who were screened for their ability to recognize panels of 31 amino acid synthetic peptides encompassing individual, patient-specific mutations.[60] Approximately 4% of the CD4[+] T cells present within autologous TILs that were administered to a patient in this study who was a partial responder to autologous TIL therapy recognized a single neoepitope, and a total of 13% of the CD4[+] T cells that were administered to a patient who exhibited a complete response to autologous T cells recognized three unique mutated epitopes.

Taken together, these results indicate that T cells recognizing neoepitopes expressed by patients' tumors may play a significant role in mediating responses to immune checkpoint inhibitors and may play a similarly important role in mediating responses to adoptive immunotherapy.[61]

Vaccine trials evaluating responses against candidate neoantigens have been carried out using a variety of delivery platforms that include synthetic peptides, messenger RNA, viral and bacterial vectors, and ex vivo antigen-loaded DCs (reviewed in Vormehr et al.[62]). Currently, there is little evidence that vaccination can lead to objective clinical responses in patients with metastatic disease, but some evidence for disease stabilization has been observed in patients receiving a vaccine based upon injection of synthetic mRNAs encoding candidate mutant antigens encapsulated by cationic liposomes[63] or admixed with the adjuvant polyinosinic–polycytidylic acid (poly-ICLC).[64]

Influence of Somatic Mutations on the Tumor Microenvironment

Somatic Mutations in the Wnt/β-Catenin Pathway Result in Lack of T Cell Infiltration

The Wnt/β-catenin signaling pathway is upregulated in numerous cancer types, and its activation is generally associated with increased invasiveness of cancers.[65] Studies carried out in BRAF-mutant (BRAF[V600E]) genetically engineered mouse models has shown that activation of β-catenin signaling does not accelerate tumor development or growth but results in an increased frequency of metastasis at distant sites.[66] Activation of β-catenin signaling through somatic mutations can occur either by ablation of the phosphorylation sites that normally mark

β-catenin for degradation, or through loss-of-function mutations in regulatory genes (APC, APC2, axin1, axin2, GSK3β).[65]

Activation of the Wnt/β-catenin pathway was correlated with a reduction in the levels of T cell infiltration into the TME of patients with a variety of tumor types.[67] Lack of T cell infiltration was further observed in a genetically engineered melanoma mouse model based on constitutive BRAF (BrAF[V600E]) activation as well as PTEN inactivation combined with a stabilized β-catenin variant. In contrast, tumors lacking the stabilized β-catenin variant showed evidence of a productive T cell infiltrate into the TME.[68] Consistent with the observation that the presence of CD8[+] T cells correlates with response to anti-PD-1 checkpoint blockade made in human melanoma patients,[11] murine tumors with activated β-catenin signaling and lack of T cell infiltration were insensitive to checkpoint blockade therapy.

Mechanistically, mice bearing tumors with activated β-catenin signaling showed reduction in tumor-specific T cell activation in the tumor-draining lymph node (TdLN), which was associated with a failure to recruit CD103[+] DCs, a DC subset driven by expression of the Batf3 transcription factor, into the TME.[68] Studies carried out in additional mouse model systems have shown that CD103[+] DCs are required for effective T cell priming in the TdLN through production of type-I IFN and antigen presentation.[5,8,9] Lack of CD103[+] DC recruitment into the TME of β-catenin-positive tumors was associated with a reduction in proinflammatory chemokines, in particular CCL4.[68] Tumor cell-intrinsic, β-catenin signaling was found to result in the expression of a transcriptional repressor, ATF3, which represses the expression of CCL4 by tumor cells (see Figure 36.1A).[69] In agreement with these findings, resistance to PD-1 blockade immunotherapy in patients with melanoma arising following treatment was associated with defects in IFN-receptor signaling and antigen presentation pathways.[70] In addition, clinical responses of melanoma patients to anti-PD-1 therapy were associated with both T cell infiltration and IFN-γ signaling signatures that were manifested as a reciprocal decrease in cell-cycle and Wnt signaling pathways in responding biopsies.[71]

The lack of T cell infiltration into tumors with activated β-catenin signaling has been shown to be reversible through local injection of FLT3-ligand-derived DCs, a therapeutic intervention that also renders β-catenin-positive tumors sensitive to checkpoint blockade therapy.[68] Similar results were also obtained when FLT3-ligand, the growth factor for the Batf3-linage of DC, was administered systemically, further strengthening the importance of this subtype of DC for the local antitumor response.[72] The mechanism by which tumor cell-intrinsic Wnt/β-catenin signaling mediates T cell exclusion seems not to be limited to melanoma, because similar observations

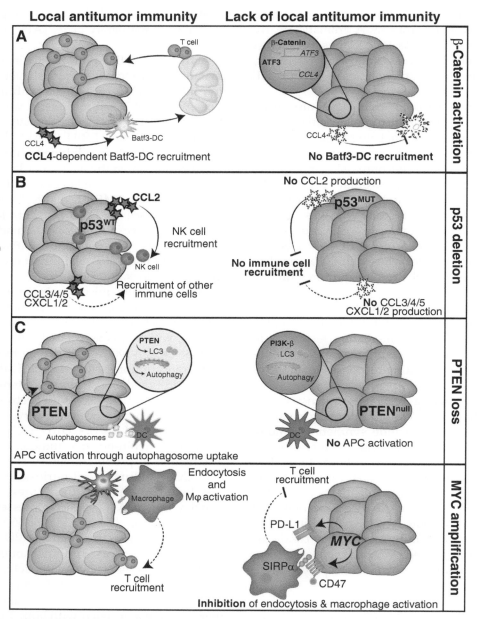

Figure 36.1 Tumor cell-intrinsic oncogene activation or tumor-suppressor gene loss affecting the local antitumor immune infiltration. From top to bottom: illustrations of the effects of β-catenin activation (**A**), p53 deletion (**B**), PTEN loss (**C**), and *MYC* activation (**D**) on the local antitumor immune response. The left side (gray tumors) depicts the generation of a local antitumor immune response with an unperturbed signaling pathway, whereas the right side (red tumors) depicts the impact of altered tumor cell-intrinsic signaling on the local immune response. Zoom-ins illustrate tumor cell-intrinsic changes resulting or contributing to the lack of immune infiltration. Solid arrows indicate a direct effect, whereas dashed arrows indicate a distal effect in which multiple steps could be involved.

APC, antigen-presenting cell; DC, dendritic cell; NK, natural killer; PD-L1, programmed death-ligand 1; PTEN, phosphatase and tensin homolog; SIRPα, signal regulatory protein α.

have been made in bladder and in head and neck cancer patients.[73,74] Taken together, these results demonstrate that the strength of antitumor T cell responses and corresponding downstream activation of the IFN-γ signaling pathway influenced clinical responses to immune checkpoint blockade therapy in multiple cancer types.

P53-Mediated Senescence of Tumor Cells Induces a Proinflammatory Tumor Microenvironment

The tumor-suppressor protein p53 is a critical mediator of the DNA damage response and mediates cell cycle arrest; it can drive cells into a senescent state.[75,76] One of the initial studies providing a link between TP53 protein function and immune infiltration involved the use of an orthotopically transplanted Hras mutant hepatoblastoma cell line that had been engineered to express a microRNA silencing p53 in a doxycycline-dependent manner.[77] Reactivation of wild type TP53 protein expression resulted in rapid and complete regression of the tumor which was associated with a significant increase in the number of senescent cells without an apparent increase in the number of apoptotic or necrotic cells. Subsequent gene expression profiling indicated that the senescent tumor cell state observed after up-regulation of TP53 gene expression was associated with increased expression of molecules involved with immune invasion that included chemokines CSF-1, CCL2, and CXCL1, along with the cytokine IL-15 and adhesion molecules, intercellular adhesion molecule 1 (ICAM-1), and vascular cell adhesion protein 1 (VCAM-1).[77] Results presented in a subsequent study indicated that while a T cell response was dispensable for the acute rejection of the hepatocellular carcinoma cell line, natural killer (NK) cells and NKG2D-mediated recognition of tumor cells were required.[78] Furthermore, tumor cells appeared to produce significant levels of multiple chemokines that included CCL2, CCL3, CCL4, CCL5, CXCL1, and CXCL2 and multiple cytokines that included IL-1β, IL-12β, and IL-15. Additional studies are needed to address the molecular link between tumor cell senescence and expression of proinflammatory signals. Enhanced expression of CCL2 appeared to play a predominant role in the NK-mediated acute rejection observed in this murine tumor model system[78] (see Figure 36.1B).

The hypothesis that a loss of p53-mediated senescence may play a causal role in limiting cytotoxic lymphocyte infiltration was further supported by a study carried out in patients with basal-like breast cancer, a tumor type that is highly associated with a loss of p53 protein function.[79] Loss of p53 was associated with the absence of a T cell infiltration gene signature in basal-like breast cancers, and the lack of immune cell infiltration was even more profound in tumors containing a mutation in the TP53 gene combined with loss of heterozygosity of the TP53 gene locus. Similar results were also observed in ER-negative but not ER-positive breast cancer patients.[79]

The results presented in these studies indicate that loss of p53 protein function and the consequent loss of p53-mediated tumor cell senescence is associated with a reduction the recruitment of innate and adaptive immune cells into the TME. Although tumor cell-intrinsic molecular mechanisms involved with this process have not been elucidated, mutations in p53 may play an important role in immune evasion due to the reduced levels of cytokines and chemokines by effector cell exclusion.

Activation of PI3K Pathway Through Phosphatase and Tensin Homolog Loss Is Correlated With Reduced Responses to Immunotherapy

The PI3K/PTEN pathway is one of the most commonly affected oncogenic pathways in human cancers (reviewed in Alvarez-Garcia et al.).[80] Although loss-of-function mutations within the PTEN are observed in some cancers, deletion or downregulation of protein expression is more commonly seen in most tumor types.[80] Loss of PTEN expression in melanomas has been found to synergize with BRAF-MEK activation to drive tumorigenesis, and loss-of-function mutations have been reported in roughly 30% of all melanomas.[81,82] Loss of PTEN, which is a lipid phosphatase that inhibits PI3K activity, resulting in the loss of AKT phosphorylation, has been associated with increased survival of tumor cells and a reduced rate of apoptosis.[83] The loss of PTEN function has also been associated with a lack of response to anti-PD-1 checkpoint blockade therapy in patients with metastatic melanoma.[84] In addition, the ability to culture TILs in vitro for subsequent adoptive transfer therapy was significantly reduced in patients lacking PTEN protein expression. These data, together with data from preclinical models, indicate that T cell activation and recruitment to the TME may be compromised in tumors that lack functional PTEN protein. Use of a PI3K-beta-isoform-specific inhibitor resulted in increased T cell infiltration and restored sensitivity to checkpoint blockade. A global decrease in the expression of autophagy-related genes was also observed.[84] Results presented in this study also indicated that PTEN loss resulted in reduced activation of autophagy in tumor cells, which may lead to further activation of APCs through the STING pathway, enhanced priming, or recognition of tumor cells (Figure 36.1C).[84] Enhanced T cell activation and accumulation within the tumor may be mediated by a T cell/IFN-γ-driven positive feedback loop resulting in enhanced effector T cell chemokine production following activation of APCs by innate immune mechanisms,[85] but additional studies are needed to further clarify the factors that influence these responses and to determine their relevance for additional cancer types. The potential role of the STING pathway in mediating antitumor immune responses is being evaluated in ongoing clinical trials evaluating systemic and local administration of STING agonists (reviewed in Gajewski & Higgs[86]). Although evidence for their effectiveness in mediating tumor regression has not been obtained to date, these studies are focusing on evaluating the effects of systemic versus intratumoral administration of agonist agents and identifying agonists with enhanced in vivo stability profiles.

Overexpression of the *MYC* Proto-Oncogene Induces Expression of Immunosuppressive Molecules on Tumor Cells

The normal product of the *MYC* proto-oncogene represents a transcription factor that plays a critical role in regulating cell proliferation, differentiation, and survival, and is overexpressed in many cancers.[87,88] *MYC* gene expression is often increased through gene duplication, whereas point mutations are relatively rare in tumor cells.[1] Tumor cells generally require stable and consistent expression of *MYC*,[89] and loss of *MYC* expression leads to an arrest in cell proliferation and tumor cell death.[90] Furthermore, the enhanced tumor infiltration and activation of T cells observed following *MYC* downregulation appeared to play an important role in the tumor control observed in these model systems.[90,91] Decreased expression of PD-L1 and CD47 was observed in multiple tumor types that included lymphoma, melanoma, lung cancer, and hepatocellular carcinoma following *MYC* downregulation.[91] While T cell activation is suppressed following the interaction of PD-L1 with PD-1 molecules expressed on activated T cells,[92] CD47 limits APC activation and tumor antigen presentation by inhibiting antigen uptake through endocytosis.[92,93] Expression of both PD-L1 and CD47 on the tumor cells was directly dependent on the transcriptional activity of *MYC*, and stabilization of either of those two molecules was sufficient to prevent an increased immune infiltrate from occurring (see Figure 36.1D). The expression of the immune inhibitory molecules was further linked to stabilization of CD31+ microvessels as well as expression of proangiogenic molecules (Tie2 and Ang1). Consistent with previous reports, inactivation of *MYC* was also associated with an increase in senescent tumor cells, indicating *MYC* inactivation might lead to transcriptional changes that influence multiple cellular pathways.[91] While these studies indicate that multiple oncogenic pathways may influence local antitumor immune responses, the tumor-derived factors responsible for enhanced T cell infiltration following *MYC* inactivation have not been identified.

Additional Somatic Alterations That Appear to Influence the Local Antitumor Immune Response

Activation of the NFκB (nuclear factor kappa-light-chain-enhancer of activated B cells) signaling pathway has often been associated with increased tumor incidence and appears to play an important role in tumor formation,[94,95] but in addition represents another oncogenic pathway that can potentially impact on host immune responses. The activation signal for tumor cell-intrinsic NFκB activation has been shown to be derived from immune cells in some inflammation-mediated cancer models.[96] Increased immune-derived tumor necrosis

factor (TNF) signaling has been shown to augment NFκB signaling in liver cells and promoted tumor progression in a hepatocellular carcinoma model[97] and constitutive activation of NFκB was found to increase expression of tumor cell-derived chemokines that could enhance immune cell infiltration and activation.[96,98] Increased chemokine levels were observed following inhibition of NFκB signaling in lung adenocarcinoma,[99] indicating that the impact of tumor-intrinsic NFκB activation on local antitumor immune response also depends on the cellular context and balance between tumor-promoting inflammatory cells and antitumor adaptive immunity. Furthermore, the mechanisms involved with the activation of NFκB signaling may also influence the genes activated and repressed transcriptional profile.

Similarly, activation of the signal transducer and activator of the transcription 3 (STAT3) signaling pathway might impact infiltration into the TME. Although expression of a dominant negative STAT3 variant resulted in augmented expression of proinflammatory molecules, constitutively active STAT3 signaling has been reported to lead to decreased expression of proinflammatory mediators, including CCL5 and CXCL10.[100,101] Similar results have also been obtained using a genetically induced prostate cancer model, providing further evidence that intrinsic tumor cell signaling through the STAT3 pathway can have a significant impact on the local immune response.[102,103] Somatic mutations affecting the NFκB and STAT3 pathways have also been described, but to date a direct linkage between specific alterations in these gene products and immune infiltration has not been established.

Somatic alterations in CpG-rich domains might result in differential epigenetic upregulation or downregulation of gene expression in tumor cells. Reduced production of the CXCL9 and CXCL10 chemokines by human ovarian cancer, which was linked with epigenetic silencing of the gene loci controlling expression of these proteins, was associated with decreased effector T cell recruitment to these tumors,[104] and similar mechanisms might apply to other genetic loci that influence the TME.

Influence of Metabolic Factors on the Local Tumor Microenvironment

One of the most profound metabolic changes within the TME is the generation of a hypoxic environment associated with deprivation of nutrients such as glucose[105] that may have less of an impact on tumor cell growth than on antitumor immune infiltrate (see also Chapter 46 on immune metabolism). Although local immune responses can be influenced by multiple metabolic changes in the TME, reduced angiogenesis associated with hypoxia, established through rapid proliferation combined with delayed vascularization,[105] appears to play an important role in the immune exclusion seen in some tumors. The master regulator hypoxia-inducible factor 1-alpha (HIF1-α) activates multiple factors including vascular endothelial growth factor (VEGF) and cyclooxygenase (Cox) gene transcription in tumor cells or stroma cells, including endothelial cells.[106] This response mediates the formation of new blood vessels, supplying the tumor with oxygen and nutrients.[107] Besides this natural response, the expression of VEGF and Cox genes has been shown to prevent a productive antitumor immune response from being established within the TME.[108,109] These studies were prompted by the initial observation that tumor vasculature appeared to be less adhesive for immune cells than vasculature from normal tissue. This notion is supported by the observation that VEGF mediates downregulation of the adhesive molecules VCAM-1 and ICAM-1 on the tumor vasculature (see Figure 36.2).[110] Lack of these adhesive molecules on endothelial cells results in a reduction of lymphocyte rolling and lymphocyte extravasation. In addition to the reduction in adhesion molecules, a subsequent study provided evidence that hypoxia induced Cox1-dependent prostaglandin E_2 (PGE_2) expression, and VEGF expression resulted in upregulation of Fas-ligand

expression on endothelial cells where it led to apoptotic cell death.[108] Expression of Fas-ligand was found on endothelial cells present in multiple human cancer types, including ovarian, breast, and bladder cancer, and was associated with a reduction of CD8+ T cell infiltration. In a preclinical mouse model and in vitro cell culture assays, overexpression of Fas-ligand was found to lead to the death of effector T cells (CD4 and CD8) but not appear to have a significant impact on regulatory T cells (see Figure 36.2). The reduction of CD8 T cell infiltration mediated by Fas-ligand-expressing stromal cells could also be reversed using Cox inhibitors such as acetylsalicylic acid and anti-VEGF-blocking antibodies, establishing a direct link between hypoxia, Fas-ligand expression, and lack of effector T cell entry into the TME.[108]

The effects of tumor cell–derived PGE_2 on immune evasion were explored in a model system involving the use of a BRAF-mutant melanoma cell line in which PGE_2 expression was driven by Cox2, which could either be induced through Ras/Raf signaling or in response to a hypoxic microenvironment.[109] Under steady state, high levels of PGE_2 are generated, leading to an IL-6-driven immune response, that has been associated with an

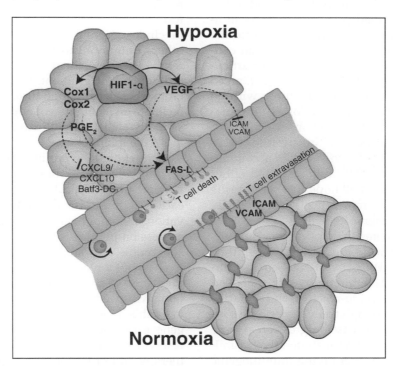

Figure 36.2 Impact of hypoxic conditions on the local antitumor immune infiltrate. The figure depicts a tumor growing in hypoxic conditions (upper half, hypoxia, red) or normal oxygen levels (lower half, normoxia, gray) separated by a blood vessel. Although ICAM/VCAM-mediated T cell (purple cells) extravasation is uneffaced in the nonhypoxic tumor, no T cells are able to migrate into the hypoxic tumor. Effector T cells adhering to vessels in a hypoxic tumor undergo Fas/Fas-ligand-mediated apoptosis. Solid arrows among signaling molecules imply proven effects on the signaling cascade occurring within a tumor cell under hypoxic conditions, whereas dotted arrows imply effects on protein expression in other cell types within the TME.

HIF1-α, hypoxia-inducible factor 1-α; ICAM, intercellular adhesion molecule; PGE_2, prostaglandin E_2; TME, tumor microenvironment; VCAM, vascular cell adhesion protein; VEGF, vascular endothelial growth factor.

unproductive antitumor immune response.[109] By contrast, productive type-I IFN immune responses were observed when PGE$_2$ was knocked-out or when Cox2 was inhibited following administration of acetylsalicylic acid. This immune response was primarily altered through an increased recruitment of Batf3-driven DCs associated with increased effector T cell recruitment, which enhanced the sensitivity to checkpoint blockade therapy.[109] Taken together, these examples provide strong evidence that metabolic changes within the TME can have substantial impact on local antitumor immune responses.

CONCLUSION

Further progress in developing novel approaches to the treatment of patients for whom current immunotherapies are of limited or no clinical benefit may depend on gaining a better understanding of the biological basis of these responses. The observation that renal cell carcinomas that possess relatively low mutational loads respond to immune checkpoint blockade[111] indicates the difficulties in modeling the complex cellular interactions that take place in the TME. A recent summary and meta-analysis of 35 randomly controlled clinical studies carried out in over 21,000 patients confirmed previous analyses indicating that OS and PFS was more advantageous for the treatment of advanced and metastatic cancer than conventional therapies, and indicated that this was particularly beneficial for male patients, those younger than 65 years of age, current or former smokers, those with no CNS or liver metastasis, those negative for *EGFR* mutations, and those with PD-L1 expression on >1% of tumor cells.[112] The results of clinically evaluating the role of activating molecules such as CD40[113] and OX40[114] and inhibitory molecules such as TIGIT[115] and LAG-3,[116] either alone or used in combination, will hopefully provide the basis for the development of more effective and widely applicable cancer immunotherapies.

Vaccination of three metastatic melanoma patients with autologous DCs that were pulsed with neoepitope peptides identified using WES and RNA-Seq in combination with peptide–MHC binding algorithms led to in vivo expansion of peptide-reactive and putative tumor-reactive T cells.[117] Although no evidence for a clinical impact of vaccination on disease progression in these patients was found, this study demonstrated the feasibility of using this approach for identifying immunogenic neoepitope targets.

The development of more effective therapies will be dependent on gaining a better understanding of the factors that limit antitumor immune responses. Although tumor immune editing has been found in murine tumor model systems to lead to the elimination of tumors that express potent neoepitopes,[12] adoptive immunotherapy and immune checkpoint inhibitor–based therapies are effective

in mediating regression of multiple cancer types. For these patients, failure of the immune system to control tumor growth may primarily result from inhibitory factors within the TME, rather than a lack of potent target antigens.

Nevertheless, the characteristics of target antigens expressed by patients' tumors are likely to have a significant impact on their effectiveness. Attractive therapeutic targets include neoantigens derived from trunk (shared between all cancer cells) mutations that have arisen before clonal diversification[118] or driver mutations, which are essential for carcinogenesis or metastasis, such as common KRAS and TP53 mutations, as previously discussed. Future studies are likely to result in the identification of T cells that recognize neoepitopes encompassing hotspot driver mutations in TP53 and KRAS as well as in additional driver genes such as IDH1 and PIK3CA, potentially leading to the development of personalized adoptive immunotherapies for a relatively broad patient population.

In addition to generating de novo antigens, mutations affect protein function and signaling within tumor cells, which affects the local TME. Identifying which somatic mutations impact the local antitumor immune response in what way could be an extremely powerful tool, because SNVs and indels can be readily assessed in clinical testing. Furthermore, in contrast to many other immunohistochemistry-based biomarkers currently discussed, the result is binary rather than a threshold-dependent gradient. Similarly, the development of biomarkers based upon tumor sequence analysis would facilitate an evaluation of additional therapeutic options, as many signaling pathways are targetable using small molecule inhibitors.

Gene expression profiling and somatic mutation analyses now being carried out in many clinical trials are providing data that is critical for testing hypotheses based upon earlier trials and tumor model systems. In one trial, activation of an epithelial-to-mesenchymal transition (EMT) expression profile, as well as a hypoxia-response expression profile, appeared to be associated with poor response to checkpoint blockade, while mutations in BRCA2 were predictive of an enhanced response,[32] but these observations will need to be evaluated in larger patient cohorts to establish the validity of these findings. Mutational and gene expression profiles of tumors from patients who respond to immune checkpoint and adoptive immunotherapy and of tumors from refractory patients enrolled in sequential trials involving multiple immunotherapies are also currently being carried out and should provide valuable data that will help to guide future trials.

Many challenges remain for the field of cancer immunotherapy, particularly the development of effective treatments for cancers such as pancreatic and prostate cancer that do not appear to be responsive to current treatments. Continued efforts to identify true tumor rejection antigens will hopefully facilitate the development of enhanced responses in patients with a variety of cancer types. Responses to multiple immune checkpoint inhibitors and combinations of immune checkpoint inhibitors with antitumor vaccines and adoptive immunotherapies directed against the appropriate target antigens, when coupled with thoughtful studies evaluating the optimal timing and dosage of treatment regimens, represent the best strategy for the development of more effective cancer immunotherapies.

ACKNOWLEDGMENTS

I would like to thank Dr. Stephanie Spranger for her assistance in the preparation of this manuscript.

KEY REFERENCES

Only key references appear in the print edition. The full reference list appears in the digital product on Springer Publishing Connect: connect.springerpub.com/content/book/978-0-8261-3743-2/part/part03/chapter/ch36

7. Woo SR, Fuertes MB, Corrales L, et al. STING-dependent cytosolic DNA sensing mediates innate immune recognition of immunogenic tumors. *Immunity*. 2014;41(5):830–842. doi:10.1016/j.immuni.2014.10.017

12. Vesely MD, Schreiber RD. Cancer immunoediting: antigens, mechanisms, and implications to cancer immunotherapy. *Ann N Y Acad Sci*. 2013;1284:1–5. doi:10.1111/nyas.12105

32. Hugo W, Zaretsky JM, Sun L, et al. Genomic and transcriptomic features of response to anti-PD-1 therapy in metastatic melanoma. *Cell*. 2016;165(1):35–44. doi:10.1016/j.cell.2016.02.065

33. Rizvi NA, Hellmann MD, Snyder A, et al. Cancer immunology. Mutational landscape determines sensitivity to PD-1 blockade in non-small cell lung cancer. *Science*. 2015;348(6230):124–128. doi:10.1126/science.aaa1348

48. Robbins PF, Lu YC, El-Gamil M, et al. Mining exomic sequencing data to identify mutated antigens recognized by adoptively transferred tumor-reactive T cells. *Nat Med*. 2013;19(6):747–752. doi:10.1038/nm.3161

68. Spranger S, Bao R, Gajewski TF. Melanoma-intrinsic β-catenin signalling prevents anti-tumour immunity. *Nature*. 2015;523(7559):231–235. doi:10.1038/nature14404

92. Topalian SL, Taube JM, Anders RA, et al. Mechanism-driven biomarkers to guide immune checkpoint blockade in cancer therapy. *Nat Rev Cancer*. 2016;16(5):275–287. doi:10.1038/nrc.2016.36

37

Tumor Antigen Profiling

Robert Saddawi-Konefka, Bryan S. Yung, and Jack D. Bui

KEY POINTS

- Tumor neoantigens offer tremendous potential as targets for immune-based cancer therapies by virtue of their restricted expression in tumors and their freedom from mechanisms of central immune tolerance.

- Most mutated tumor neoantigens result from nonsynonymous single-nucleotide variants (SNVs), which imbue immunogenicity onto the neoantigen in one of three ways: increasing the neoantigen affinity for the major histocompatibility complex (MHC; anchor amino acid), increasing the neoantigen-MHC affinity for the T cell receptors (TCR), and activating novel mechanisms of antigen processing and presentation.

- The majority of neoantigen-specific T cell antitumor responses are directed toward passenger mutations, implying that successful cancer immunotherapies will most likely need to be personalized.

- Only a fraction of nonsynonymous mutations in tumors beget immunogenic neoantigens to which CD4 or CD8 T cells can respond, highlighting the importance of robust methods for neoantigen detection.

- The advent of next-generation sequencing (NGS) among other innovations makes it possible to profile the tumor mutanome and identify neoantigens on an individual patient basis, enabling researchers and clinicians to develop personalized immunotherapies.

- Two stipulations define the current set of parameters within which we may develop immunotherapies: one, mutational load must be large enough to allow for the expression of one or more neoantigens to which the host immune system can respond; two, there should be an endogenous neoantigen-specific T cell response that presumably is suboptimal but can be boosted to achieve complete antitumor immunity.

INTRODUCTION

This chapter discusses novel tumor antigens commonly referred to as tumor "neoantigens." We review the genesis and biology of these unique antigens, the preclinical and clinical evidence supporting the importance of tumor neoantigens, the methodologies employed to identify them, and the current state of neoantigen-based therapies.

BIOLOGY OF NEOANTIGENS

Tumor Neoantigens

In the 1950s, various groups hypothesized and, subsequently, demonstrated that cancer cells, by virtue of their genomic anomalies, could be recognized as foreign by the immune system.[1-3] For example, mice, immunized with cancer cell lysate, displayed antitumor immunity such that when challenged with the same live tumor cells, mice mounted immune responses against the tumor. Early on, tumor antigens were postulated to be self-antigens that were immunogenic secondary to the inflammatory nature of cancer itself. It was not until almost 40 years later, in 1995, that Hans Schreiber's group demonstrated that tumor antigens are, in fact, gene products arising from mutations in cancer cells and, consequently, intrinsically immunogenic by virtue of representing "non-self" as recognized by host immunity.[4]

These distinctive tumor antigens have come to be known as neoantigens and are central to the revolution we have witnessed in anticancer immunotherapies. Figure 37.1 illustrates the landmark studies and discoveries that shape our current understanding of tumor neoantigens and how tumor neoantigen-based anticancer strategies have evolved over time.

Most mutated tumor neoantigens result from nonsynonymous single-nucleotide variants (SNVs),[5] which code for single amino acid changes in translated peptides. As we currently understand, these SNVs can imbue immunogenicity onto the neoantigen in one of three ways (Figure 37.2).[6] First, the neoantigen can acquire a higher affinity for major histocompatibility complex (MHC), known as an anchor amino acid.[7] Second, the neoantigen-MHC can

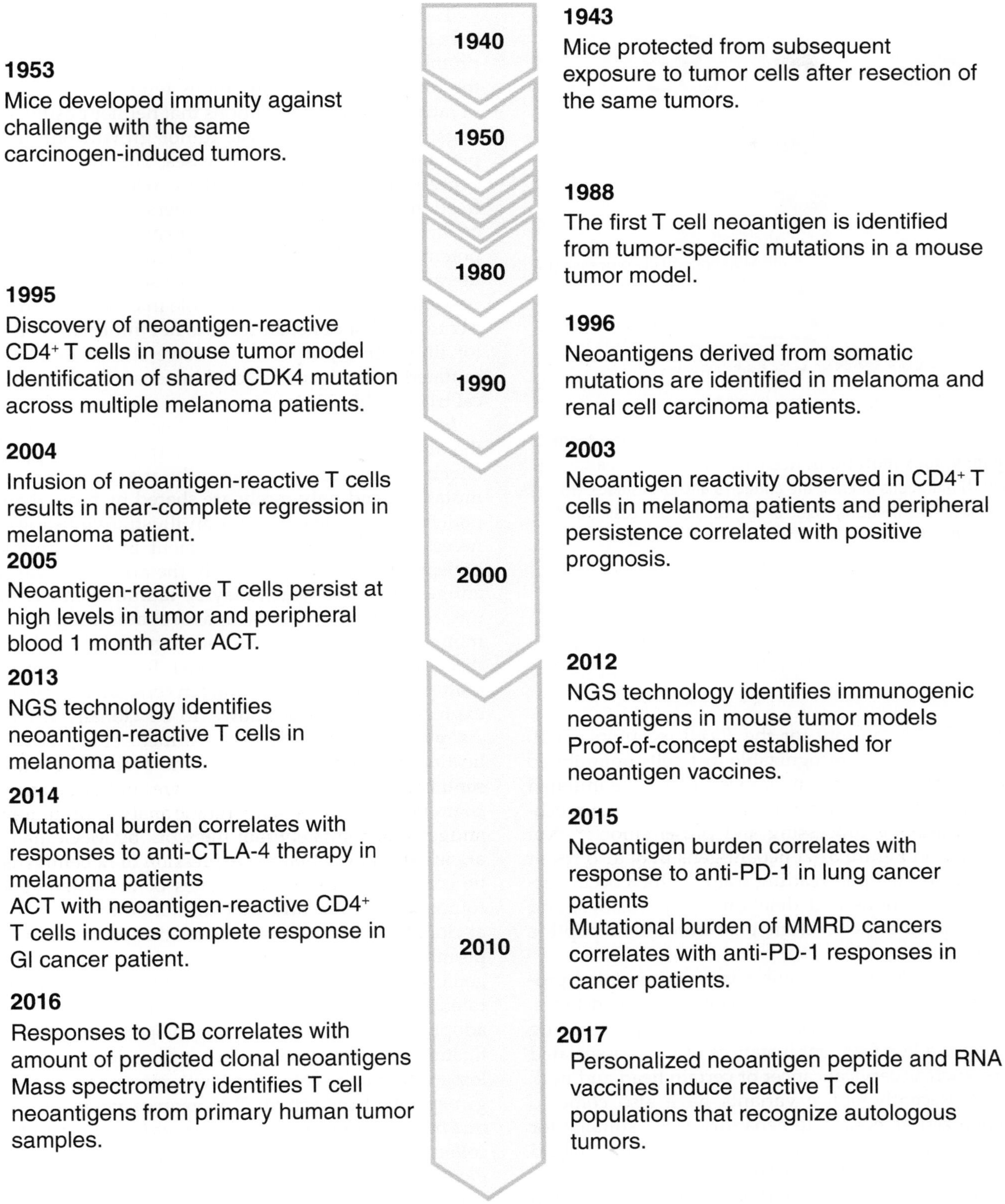

1953

Mice developed immunity against challenge with the same carcinogen-induced tumors.

1995

Discovery of neoantigen-reactive CD4+ T cells in mouse tumor model Identification of shared CDK4 mutation across multiple melanoma patients.

2004

Infusion of neoantigen-reactive T cells results in near-complete regression in melanoma patient.

2005

Neoantigen-reactive T cells persist at high levels in tumor and peripheral blood 1 month after ACT.

2013

NGS technology identifies neoantigen-reactive T cells in melanoma patients.

2014

Mutational burden correlates with responses to anti-CTLA-4 therapy in melanoma patients ACT with neoantigen-reactive CD4+ T cells induces complete response in GI cancer patient.

2016

Responses to ICB correlates with amount of predicted clonal neoantigens Mass spectrometry identifies T cell neoantigens from primary human tumor samples.

1940

1950

1980

1990

2000

2010

1943

Mice protected from subsequent exposure to tumor cells after resection of the same tumors.

1988

The first T cell neoantigen is identified from tumor-specific mutations in a mouse tumor model.

1996

Neoantigens derived from somatic mutations are identified in melanoma and renal cell carcinoma patients.

2003

Neoantigen reactivity observed in CD4+ T cells in melanoma patients and peripheral persistence correlated with positive prognosis.

2012

NGS technology identifies immunogenic neoantigens in mouse tumor models Proof-of-concept established for neoantigen vaccines.

2015

Neoantigen burden correlates with response to anti-PD-1 in lung cancer patients Mutational burden of MMRD cancers correlates with anti-PD-1 responses in cancer patients.

2017

Personalized neoantigen peptide and RNA vaccines induce reactive T cell populations that recognize autologous tumors.

Figure 37.1 Landmark neoantigen discoveries.

ACT, adoptive cell transfer; CTLA-4, cytotoxic T-lymphocyte-associated protein 4; ICB, immune checkpoint blockade; MMRD, microsatellite instability and mismatch repair deficiency; NGS, next generation sequencing; PD-1, programed cell death protein 1.

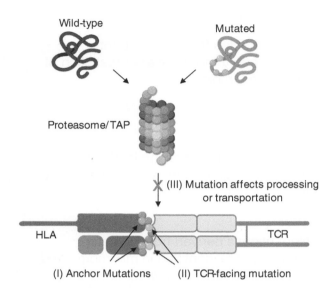

Figure 37.2 Mechanisms of neoantigen generation from nonsynonymous mutations. Neoantigens can arise as a result of (**I**) mutations altering the antigen's anchor residues, (**II**) T cell receptor (TCR)–facing motif, or (**III**) cellular processing and presentation machinery.

HLA, human leukocyte antigen; TAP, transporter associated with antigen processing; TCR, T cell receptor.

Source: Adapted with permission from Vormehr M, Diken M, Boegel S, et al. Mutanome directed cancer immunotherapy. *Curr Opin Immunol.* 2016;39:14–22. doi:10.1016/j.coi.2015.12.001

acquire a higher affinity for the T cell receptors (TCR) or otherwise become recognizable to T cells uninhibited by mechanisms of central tolerance.[8] Third, the mutated residue can cause the peptide to undergo novel mechanisms of antigen processing and presentation.[9,10] Not represented in Figure 37.2, neoantigens may also result from shifts in the open-reading frame, which occur secondary to insertions and deletions, gene fusions, and mutated splice sites or from post-translation peptide splicing.

Although most neoantigens arise from mutated proteins, there are other sources of neoantigens. For instance, neoantigens can also arise from viral open-reading frames in the less frequent instances of virus-associated tumors, such as cervical cancer or certain head and neck cancers.[11] Recently, splice variants have also come to be recognized as bona fide neoantigens,[12,13] suitable for targeted vaccine development.[14] In addition, "hybrid peptides"[15] were identified as "neoantigens" within pancreatic beta islet cells that could be recognized as foreign and lead to autoimmune diabetes. These hybrid peptides could also be found in cancer cells,[16] and so could represent a source of neoantigens. The relative contribution of hybrid peptides versus mutated peptides to the neoantigen repertoire of any cancer cell is not known.

Tumor neoantigens can be broadly categorized as either "driver" or "passenger."[17] While driver antigens promote growth by affording a selective advantage to the tumor, passenger mutations represent the products of random, somatic mutations that neither positively nor negatively impact intrinsic tumor growth but are perpetuated as the tumor progresses. The tumor-restricted expression of neoantigens along with their presumed freedom from central immune tolerance—a consequence of their aberrant expression[18]—explain the tremendous potential they harbor as targets for immune-based cancer therapies. As most neoantigens arise from mutations in passenger genes without any role in cancer progression, a complete list of neoantigens is not informative. Rather, for illustrative purposes, we have shown examples of mutated neoantigens targeted in neoantigen-based clinical trials (Table 37.1).

Immunotherapies based on neoantigens can take the form of a vaccine or cellular therapy approach. Given that neoantigens typically arise from passenger mutations and only rarely are shared by more than one patient[5,17] (see Table 37.1 for an illustrative listing), it is necessary to personalize treatment in each individual patient by identifying not only the array of tumor neoantigens but also which may be immunogenic antigens (i.e., recognized by T cells capable of mounting an antitumor immune response; methodology and clinical use are discussed in subsequent sections). To further complicate matters, tumor neoantigens are in constant flux, and their expression pattern is known to be clonally restricted. As reviewed in the study by Vormehr et al.,[6] DNA replication and repair, as well as the processing and presentation machinery in tumors, are imprecise and ever changing, thereby making a static analysis of tumor neoantigens inadequate. From the work by McGranahan et al., we also know that the expression of neoantigens can be confined to certain subclones of the heterogeneous tumor population and that immunotherapies directed at clonally restricted neoantigens can counterintuitively promote tumor growth by negatively selecting immunogenic subclones.[19] This paradoxical finding was corroborated in a clinical study of melanoma patients receiving adoptive therapy with neoantigen-specific T cells; investigators found that neoantigen expression is selectively lost in the tumor coincident with intratumoral neoantigen-specific T cell activity.[20] As exome sequencing of cancers becomes routine, and sequences from longitudinally collected samples become available for study, a clearer picture will emerge regarding the stability of a neoantigen repertoire during cancer progression.

There are several outstanding questions regarding the functional value of the neoantigen repertoire in cancer: What are the dynamics of neoantigen presentation and/or recognition that determines the efficacy of immunotherapies directed toward those neoantigens? Are there

Table 37.1 Illustrative of Neoantigen-Based Clinical Trials

THERAPEUTIC STRATEGY	PHASE	TARGETED CANCER POPULATION	INVESTIGATION THERAPY	CLINICAL TRIAL IDENTIFIER
Neoantigen-agnostic vaccine	Phase 1/2	Colorectal	PolyPEPI1018 Vaccine	NCT03391232
Neoantigen-agnostic vaccine + checkpoint blockade inhibitor	Phase 1	Glioma	IDH1R132H Vaccine +/− avelumab	NCT03893903
	Phase 1	Colorectal, gastric, gastroesophageal, endometrial	Nous-209 + pembrolizumab	NCT04041310
	Phase 1/2	Colorectal, pancreatic, NSCLC (select other solid tumor)	GRT-C903/GRT-R904 +/− nivolumab or ipilimumab	NCT03953235
Neoantigen-personalized vaccine	Phase 1	Pancreatic	Personalized vaccine	NCT03558945
	Phase 1	Solid tumor	Personalized vaccine	NCT04087252
	Phase 1	Melanoma, NSCLC, renal	EVAX-01-CAF09b	NCT03715985
Neoantigen-personalized vaccine + checkpoint blockade inhibitor	Phase 1	Renal	NeoVax + ipilimumab	NCT02950766
	Phase 1	Urothelial	PGV001 + atezolizumab	NCT03359239
	Phase 1	Glioblastoma	Personalized vaccine + radiation + pembrolizumab	NCT02287428
	Phase 1	Melanoma, NSCLC, urothelial, breast, renal, head and neck, (select other solid tumors)	RO7198457/mRNA + atezolizumab	NCT03289962
	Phase 1	Prostate	Personalized vaccine + PROSTVAC-V + PROSTVAC-F + nivolumab/ipilimumab	NCT03532217
	Phase 1b	Melanoma, NSCLC, urothelial	NEO-PV-01 + nivolumab	NCT02897765
	Phase 1/2	NSCLC, colorectal, gastroesophageal, urothelial	GRT-C901/GRT-R902 + nivolumab/ipilimumab	NCT03639714
	Phase 2	Breast (triple-negative)	Personalized vaccine + conventional therapy + durvalumab	NCT03606967

NSCLC, non-small cell lung cancer.

quantitative and qualitative aspects of the repertoire that determine responsiveness to immunotherapy? How stable is the neoantigen repertoire throughout cancer progression? And finally, how does the immune system interact and sculpt the neoantigen repertoire?

Tumor Antigens and Immunity

Cancer immunoediting describes the process by which tumor cells interact with the host immune system resulting in measurable changes in the immunogenicity of the cancer cells.[21–23] It occurs in three phases: elimination, where subclinical tumors are recognized and rejected by innate and adaptive immunity; equilibrium, where elimination is incomplete but tumor progression is held in check by immune activity; and escape, where tumor cells have survived and are capable of progression in an immunocompetent environment.[24] There is also evidence demonstrating that innate immunity drives the editing process in the absence of the adaptive immune system, which implies a greater role for innate immunity in the design of future antitumor immunotherapies.[25]

We now know that the process of cancer immunoediting can shape the neoantigen repertoire. The strongest evidence to support this claim comes from a recent study in which human tumors, analyzed from the extensive Cancer Genome Atlas (TCGA) database, were found to have fewer than expected expressed antigens, implying that an active editing process influences the expression of tumor neoantigens.[26] This elegant study provided important correlative data but did not establish causality—did tumor progression cause loss of neoantigens because of immune cell editing? Using a mouse model of neoantigen editing, Schreiber et al. identified a dominant neoantigen by exome sequencing of highly immunogenic "regressor" methylcholanthrene (MCA)-sarcoma cells.[27] This neoantigen was created by a mutation in the *LAMA4* gene. Although the regressor underwent rejection in most cases, 20% of animals challenged with the regressor cells failed to completely reject cancer, leading to escape variants. These escape variants had "edited" their neoantigen repertoire, leading to loss of the *LAMA4* gene. Notably, exome sequencing had identified dozens of mutations that could have produced neoantigens, but the loss of a single neoantigen allowed the cancer cells to escape immune rejection. Interestingly, secondary subdominant neoantigens in progressively growing tumors can be revealed and targeted by endogenous T cells after checkpoint blockade.[28] Together, these studies show that endogenous or induced antitumor T cells can actively shape the neoantigen repertoire.

There are multiple ways to alter the neoantigen repertoire. Cancers are known to be genetically heterogeneous, and this can translate into immunologic heterogeneity.[25,29] This immunologic heterogeneity forms the substrate for cancer immunoediting, resulting in a more homogeneous repertoire. Therefore, it is possible that the nascent cancer cell repertoire contains clones that have different neoantigens, and over time, a single clone can emerge that lacks the major immunogenic neoantigens. Indeed, the negative immunoselection of tumor cells expressing strongly immunogenic neoantigens was shown to underly the development of cancer escape variants.[27] Functional expression of the neoantigen repertoire can also be diminished through mutations in genes involved in antigen processing and presentation.[26] Finally, the genes coding for neoantigens could be epigenetically silenced under the pressure of prolonged exposure to T cell recognition.[30] Of interest, this last study made use of a murine, oncogene-driven sarcoma model that was engineered to express known antigens. The intention of this model system was to address the phenomenon of immunoediting in the presence or absence of tumor antigens. Strikingly, it was observed that, absent antigens, tumors did not necessarily undergo immunoediting by the adaptive immune system, demonstrating that immunoediting not only shapes the tumor neoantigen repertoire but that neoantigens may, in fact, drive the adaptive immune component of the process.

EVIDENCE FOR CLINICAL RELEVANCE OF NEOANTIGENS

Tumor Mutational Burden as a Biomarker for Response to Immunotherapy

Presuming that the recognition and response to tumor neoantigens is a key initial step in mounting effective antitumor immunity, we would expect the tumor mutanome—responsible, in part, for neoantigen expression—to operate as a biomarker to gauge the eventuality of successful immunotherapeutic interventions. Accordingly, we should expect a correlation to exist between mutational burden and antitumor immunity and that the efficacy of the immune checkpoint inhibitors (ICI) is linked with the presence and generation of neoantigen-specific T cells. These presumptions have been borne out in the clinical and preclinical literature. A host of recent clinical studies seeking to identify the biomarkers of responsiveness to ICI in advanced cancers reveal that the overall mutational load and neoantigen load predict clinical benefit with therapy.[31] Specifically, several recent clinical studies find that both the mutanome and neoantigenome significantly associate with cytolytic markers in the immune microenvironment and clinically benefit from cytotoxic T-lymphocyte–associated protein 4 (CTLA-4) ICI.[32] In addition, a recent cohort study on patients with non-small cell lung cancers (NSCLCs) documents a correlation between neoantigen-specific CD8 T cell reactivity and tumor regression after treatment with pembrolizumab. This study also demonstrated the association of tumor mutational burden after checkpoint blockade therapy with neoantigen burden and DNA repair pathway mutations as well as overall clinical response and progression-free survival (PFS).[27] Later, a Phase 2 clinical study of patients with metastatic carcinoma revealed that the efficacy of checkpoint blockade therapy relies on the integrity of the DNA repair pathways in tumors. In this study, 41 patients whose tumors had either proficient or deficient DNA mismatch-repair received programmed cell death protein 1 (PD-1) blockade with pembrolizumab. Those with mismatch repair deficiency had 40% to 78% survival compared with those who did not (survival: 0%–11%), suggesting that the number of mutations in colorectal cancer directly affected responsiveness to immunotherapy.[33] In addition, hypermutator tumors with large mutational burden respond better to anti-PD-1/programmed cell death ligand 1 (PD-L1) therapy than tumors that have intact repair mechanisms. Several investigators found a correlation between the tumor mutational load and the cytolytic activity of T cells and NK cells across a variety of human tumors.[26,34,35] And, tumor mutational and neoantigen burden correlate with survival—both progression-free and overall—in addition to responsiveness to adoptive T cell therapy.[31]

Although it is tempting to rely on mutational tumor burden as a stand-alone surrogate for predicting the success of immunotherapeutic interventions, it would necessarily fall short as it encompasses only one part of effective tumor immunosurveillance. In their comprehensive review, Chen and Mellman espouse the cancer-immunity cycle—the process by which immunity to cancer is initiated and effected. The cycle is multistep: beginning with the processing and presentation of neoantigens by antigen-presenting cells (APCs), involving the subversion of central and peripheral tolerance mechanisms and priming of T cell responses, and ending with activated neoantigen-specific effector cells infiltrating the tumor to initiate cytolytic rejection.[36,37] The tumor mutanome and antigenome represent only one aspect of this complex cycle, precluding its use as a sole biomarker for immunotherapy. This particular claim is substantiated by recent evidence from Subudhi et al. in their clinical study examining antigen-specific T cell responses in tumors with low tumor mutational burden (TMB). Specifically, they find a heterogeneity of responsiveness to ICI in advanced prostate cancers with low TMB that can be parsed out by measuring immune-correlated biomarkers—namely, the CD8 response and IFN-γ gene expression signature.[38] In addition, it is now appreciated that "cold" tumors that lack T cell infiltration could have a limited response to immunotherapy despite having a high mutational burden, thus providing additional nuance to the prognostic value of total tumor mutational burden.[39]

Moreover, for reasons related to the genesis of neoantigens, only a fraction of the total number of somatic mutations within a tumor will beget an immunogenic neoantigen. And, even those mutations that do code for a bona fide tumor neoantigen are heterogeneously expressed within tumors, as a consequence of heterogeneity in tumor clonality, as elegantly demonstrated in a recent publication from Wolf et al.[40] In their work, they employ syngeneic murine melanoma models and human data to explore intratumoral neoantigen heterogeneity, finding that within-tumor clonal heterogeneity in neoantigen expression artifactually increases total mutational burden without increasing the overall immunogenicity of the tumor. In other words, tumor clonal-neoantigen heterogeneity is more important than the total mutational burden in predicting immunogenicity and response to ICI; and, an otherwise immunogenic neoantigen may fail to engender a clinically appreciable neoantigen-specific T cell response by virtue of its relatively low, clonally restricted expression.[19,41-45] Interestingly, a previously mentioned clinical study examining biomarkers of responsiveness to CTLA-4 ICI in advanced melanoma failed to identify a patterned neoantigen sequence predictive of responder patient populations.[32] Likewise, a meta-analysis from Brown et al., culling data from 515 patients across six tumor sites, revealed that mutational

epitopes not only correlated with survival and infiltration of cytotoxic lymphocytes but also the expression of PD-1 and CTLA-4 on those lymphocytes, suggesting that tumors deploy mechanisms to circumvent T cell-neoantigen recognition and tumor killing.[46]

Exceptions notwithstanding, a central dogma emerges as follows: a greater mutational burden begets a greater neoantigen load and portends a greater potential for tumor-immune infiltrate and immune-mediated rejection.[19,31,32] The actual observed level of neoantigen-directed immune responses could be restricted by active immune suppression or a lack of immune activation/infiltration due to inadequate activation of innate immunity.

Evidence of Neoantigen-Specific T Cell Activity

Investigating the mechanistic underpinnings of immune checkpoint blockade reveals that its success hinges on the activity of tumor-specific T cells. Supporting this claim, a preclinical study interrogating the downstream targets of checkpoint blockade in mice demonstrated an enhanced neoantigen-specific T cell antitumor response after therapy.[27] In this study, orthotopic tumor transplantation and treatment with anti-PD-1 and anti-CTLA-4 therapy, followed by exome sequencing, led to the identification of two neoantigens. These neoantigens were confirmed to induce anti-specific CD8+ T cell responses. Moreover, vaccination to these two immunogenic epitopes was sufficient to mediate tumor rejection comparable to checkpoint blockade alone. This preclinical observation has since been convincingly corroborated in several human studies (see Table 37.1 for an illustrative listing). In a case report of a patient with metastatic melanoma, investigators identified that tumor-infiltrating T cells following ipilimumab treatment were neoantigen-specific with reactivity against mutant epitopes of ATR and Rad3 gene products, which were highly expressed after checkpoint blockade therapy.[47] Likewise, another study on 64 patients with melanoma showed that CTLA-4 blockade with either ipilimumab or tremelimumab induced neoantigen-specific T cells that could be harvested from tumors. In addition, in this study, the investigators characterized a signature common among treatment-responsive tumors, which was validated in the second set of 39 melanoma patients.[48] New technology now allows for the detection of neoantigen-specific T cells in the blood and tumor of patients, demonstrating that these T cells could mediate tumor regression.[49] In contrast, other studies have found that only a minority of T cells infiltrating tumors have specificity for tumor antigens, while the vast majority have undefined specificity or even recognize viral antigens.[50] In fact, using viral peptides to activate tumor-specific T cells was shown to synergize with checkpoint blockade in a mouse model.[51]

NEOANTIGEN DISCOVERY

Methodologies to Identify Neoantigens

The identification of single mutated antigens in UV-induced murine cancers in 1995 was a tedious process involving the isolation of UV-induced tumor antigens from nuclear extracts by reversed-phase high-performance liquid chromatography (RP-HPLC) and sodium dodecyl sulfate–polyacrylamide gel electrophoresis (SDS–PAGE) immunoblot assays, using T cell hybridomas. Now, more than 20 years later, exciting, recent advances in technology make it possible to interrogate complete tumor genomes. The advent of next-generation sequencing (NGS) among other innovations makes it possible to profile the tumor mutanome and to identify neoantigens (antigenome) on an individual patient basis. With access to the mutanome and antigenome for the first time, researchers and clinicians can begin to develop personalized tumor immunotherapies.

What can we learn from sequencing entire tumor genomes? A landmark paper published in *Nature* in 2013 cataloged the number of mutations that are present in different individuals with different types of cancer.[5] This manuscript shows that melanoma, lung, and bladder cancers, as groups, have the most mutations among more than 7,000 tumors sequenced. Notably, even within a single cancer type, the number of mutations varied greatly. For example, some patients with melanoma had ~1,000 mutations in their tumors, whereas others had ~10 mutations. This type of study has been reproduced and expanded, and it is now appreciated that almost all tumors have detectable mutations in expressed proteins.[6,52]

The methods used to define the tumor "mutanome" have also proliferated. It is important to review these methods because the definition of mutanome can be directly related to the methods used. For example, the conceptual definition of mutanome is the collection of mutations that are present in a tumor. This can be identified by sequencing the DNA of the tumor and comparing it to a reference genome obtained from normal lymphocytes of the same individual. Figure 37.3 provides a bird's eye view of the methodologies in current use to profile the tumor mutanome and to identify immunogenic neoantigens.[52] All methodologies begin similarly: harvested tissues are screened for nonsynonymous SNV.[53] These SNVs are "called" as bona fide mutations based on the depth of sequencing and the number of reads. Typically, once the mutations are called, the mutanome can be defined, and the total number of SNVs can be quantitated.

The complete mutatome will have mutations in coding and noncoding genes. The "expressed mutanome" is more relevant for immunologists. This can be defined by exome sequencing or high-depth RNA sequencing. Although the expressed mutanome is considered as the driving force of cancer immunogenicity, it is not clear whether every single expressed mutation is immunogenic. The "antigenome or neoantigenome" is the subset of expressed mutated genes that could be recognized by the immune system. This is a theoretical definition, as there are currently no exact ways to definitively elucidate and quantify the antigenome.

The analyses employed to identify neoantigens from an expressed mutatome are diverse and without uniformity in the literature (see comprehensive review in the study by Fritsch et al.[54]). In the beginning, most groups made use of prediction algorithms that identify neoantigens with higher binding affinity for MHC molecules, which narrows the pool of candidate neoantigens to those more likely to be recognized by T cells.[27,48,55–58] Specifically, these predictive MHC-binding analyses filter neoantigens by identifying novel MHC anchor residues on the neoantigen—most of the cases—or assessing the conformational stability of the MHC–peptide interaction.[7] Likewise, a few reports document the identification of immunogenic neoantigens by measuring the antigen-specific T cell responses in the combinatorial encoding of MHC multimers.[47,59] Making use of a flow cytometry–based system to screen several reactive T cell populations simultaneously, the MHC multimer method significantly reduces the biological material necessary to identify candidate neoantigens.[60] Building on MHC prediction methods, some groups have succeeded in narrowing the neoantigen candidate pool even further by employing mass spectrometry to model structural binding to MHC molecules.[8,27] Although the silico approach can define potentially immunogenic mutations, further testing is required to prove that T cells can react to the predicted neoantigen repertoire.

The methods used to define T cell reactivity are numerous and evolving. These include tandem minigene library analysis[61] or in vitro functional screens with immortalized APCs to present candidate neoantigens.[34] Direct functional assays can also be done, including reactivity of neoantigens to CD8 T cells[29,47,48,58,62] and to CD4 T cells.[34,57,63] Methods to identify tumor neoantigens have been and continue to be an active area of research. As we learn more about which neoantigens most effectively engender immunosurveillance of tumors, methods employed to filter candidate neoantigens will likely become uniform and streamlined.

It should be noted that the final steps in defining whether a putative expressed SNV is recognized by T cells are highly dependent on host factors. For example, "T cell editing," where the T cell repertoire is actively tolerized to tumor antigens,[64] could impact whether a neoantigen elicits immunity. Indeed, a recent study found that melanoma neoantigen peptides could elicit broader T cell reactivity when using responder T cells from normal human leukocyte antigen (HLA)-matched donors compared with autologous T cells.[65] This study suggests

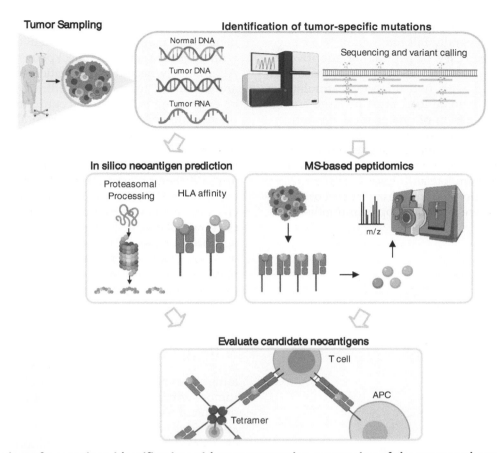

Figure 37.3 **Overview of neoantigen identification with next-generation sequencing of the expressed tumor genome.** Tumor tissue is harvested and mutations within the expressed genes are identified. Mutations in expressed genes are then expressed as peptides—most often, modeled in silico—for further analysis with MHC-binding algorithms or mass spectrometry. Finally, candidate neoantigens can be validated for immunogenicity with MHC multimer-based screening or functional assays.

APC, antigen-presenting cell; HLA, human leukocyte antigen; MHC, major histocompatibility complex.

Source: Adapted from Schumacher TN, Schreiber RD. Neoantigens in cancer immunotherapy. *Science.* 2015;348(6230):69–74. doi:10.1126/science.aaa4971

that cancer patients may develop antineoantigen T cell responses early during cancer development, but once the cancer progresses, these neoantigen-specific T cells become unreactive or are deleted from the repertoire. Therefore, current methods in defining T cell reactivity to neoantigens using autologous T cells from cancer patients may actually underestimate the number of neoantigens in any one cancer cell. To circumvent this issue, neoantigen-reactive T cells can be found and generated from allogeneic normal donors.[65]

Standardization for Neoantigen Identification

The variables inherent in pipelines for neoantigen prediction are a testament to innovation in the field, but ultimately preclude standardization and, therefore, the clinical potential of neoantigen-based therapies. In response, there has been a call for a consensus in the reporting of neoantigen prediction algorithms and

protocols. Harkening back to an analogous circumstance involving the standardization of T cell protocols (minimal information about T cell assays [MIATA]),[66] there has been a push toward developing a consensus "minimal information about neoantigen assays" (MIANA). Conceptually, the MIANA framework should include information regarding (a) sequencing, (b) genomic aberration nomenclature, (c) prediction algorithms, and (d) techniques for validation. This emerging discipline within the field of tumor neoantigen research is comprehensively addressed in a recent review.[67]

TRANSLATION APPLICATION FOR NEOANTIGENS

Vaccine-Based Therapies

Using the wealth of data gleaned from the tumor mutanome, researchers and clinicians can implement personalized anticancer immunotherapies. To date, these immunotherapies generally fall into one of two categories: vaccines (DNA, RNA, or peptide) or adoptive cell transfer (ACT; Figure 37.4).[52] In both cases, these therapies are developed with two important stipulations. First, the tumor mutational load must be large enough to allow for the expression of one or more neoantigens to which the host immune system can respond. Second, there should be an endogenous neoantigen-specific T cell response that presumably is suboptimal but can be boosted to achieve complete antitumor immunity.

These two stipulations define the current set of parameters within which we may develop immunotherapies.

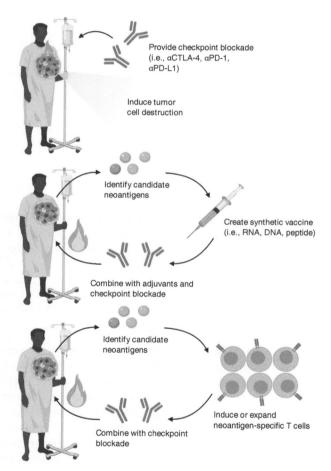

Figure 37.4 Overview of contemporary, personalized, neoantigen-based anticancer immunotherapies. Synthetic vaccines—DNA, RNA, peptide—can be designed against patient-specific tumor neoantigen targets and combined with checkpoint blockade inhibitors. Alternatively, neoantigen-specific T cells can be expanded ex vivo and adoptively transferred along with checkpoint blockade infusions.

Source: Adapted from Schumacher TN, Schreiber RD. Neoantigens in cancer immunotherapy. *Science.* 2015;348(6230):69–74. doi:10.1126/science.aaa4971

As shown in Figure 37.4, vaccines, engineered after neoantigen mapping, may be delivered in conjunction with adjuvant and/or checkpoint blockade therapy. Alternatively, neoantigen-specific T cells—either isolated and expanded from tumor-infiltrating leukocytes (TILs) or engineered in vitro to recognize and react to neoantigens—are adoptively transferred along with adjuvant and/or checkpoint blockade therapy. It is also standard of care (SOC) in various cancers to induce tumor cell destruction with adjuvant therapies, such as radiotherapy and chemotherapy. Adjuvant therapies promote the expression of tumor neoantigens, rendering subsequent checkpoint blockade more effective.[68–70] These SOC practices may, of course, be combined with the vaccine-based approach or the ACT-based approach. As of yet, however, an analysis of the impact that adjuvant therapies may have on the tumor antigenome has not been performed. In moving forward, it will be important to determine the particular combination of therapies that allows for optimal neoantigen-driven immunosurveillance and immunotherapy.

The overarching goal of these personalized vaccines targeting neoantigens is to prime and amplify neoantigen-reactive T cells in vivo to boost adoptive antitumor immunity in patients. Several recent studies document the efficacy of vaccine-based antitumor therapies. The earliest tumor vaccines in preclinical models were designed to target common driver mutations, such as Ras and p53.[71–73] These reports were promising but ultimately limited to a small pool of common, identifiable tumor antigens, a barrier that, when overcome with NGS technology, re-invigorated the interest in personalized tumor vaccines. A proof-of-principle experiment was published in 2012 by Castle et al. wherein the commonly used cell line B16F10 was sequenced using next-generation exome sequencing to detect expressed mutations. Interestingly, this group found that B16F10 had 962 mutations, and when these mutations were formulated into peptides for vaccination, 60% of the peptides induced immune responses. These studies show that mutated proteins identified by exome sequencing could be used to stimulate immune responses.[55] In the same year, Matsushita et al. found that T cells infiltrating highly immunogenic "regressor" MCA-sarcoma cell lines were specific for a mutated peptide presented on K[b]. This study combined exome sequencing with T cell antigen cloning and elegantly showed that endogenous immune responses to immunogenic cancer cells could target mutations. Moreover, when the cancer cell line was "edited" to become poorly immunogenic, it lost the mutation, proving that tumor cell immunogenicity could be affected by a single mutated peptide.[29]

Later preclinical work revealed that an array of unique neoantigens—both MHC class I and class II restricted—were adequate targets in designing immunogenic tumor vaccines.[7,8,27,57] These preclinical studies afford important insights regarding the design of personalized antitumor vaccines. In particular, they demonstrate the importance of precision in neoantigen prediction and of identifying immunogenic antigens. With respect to neoantigen prediction in antitumor vaccine design, Duan et al. observed that predicting the degree to which mutated antigen will bind to MHC-I determines the efficacy of the resulting antitumoral vaccine.[7] Work from Yadav et al. combined mass spectrometry along with exome sequencing and analyses of MHC-binding to narrow the pool of candidate neoantigens from more than 150 after exome sequencing and MHC-binding analyses alone to just three candidate CD8 T cell-specific epitopes after mass spectrometry. Vaccines designed from these three predicted epitopes were all sufficient to effectively control tumors in vivo.[8] Duperret et al. reported immune activation, expansion of neoantigen-specific T cells, and antitumor immunity using a synthetic DNA vaccine with electroporation-mediated delivery.[74] This study revealed that their multineoantigen targeting vaccine induced a predominantly MHC class I restricted CD8+ T cell response. Regarding the identification of immunogenic antigens, Gubin et al. showed that tumor vaccines designed against antigens determined to be targets for neoantigen-specific T cells were commensurate in clinical response to checkpoint blockade alone.[27] Kreiter et al. made use of three independent murine tumor models to identify several nonsynonymous mutations against which tumor vaccines were designed; antigens encoded from these mutations were found to largely be MHC class II-restricted. They found that a majority of these vaccines were immunogenic and elicited protective antitumor immunity by recruiting neoantigen-specific CD4 cells.[57] A separate study conducted by Schumacher et al. reported the effective vaccination against glioma in a mouse model using synthesized neopeptides of mutant IDH1 (R132H), which bound to transgenic human MHC class II.[75]

These exciting preclinical findings quickly gave way to clinical studies, which have documented the efficacy of dendritic cell vaccines[76] and have recently yielded promising results for the development of personalized neoantigen vaccines. In 2015, the first reported Phase 1 clinical trial using neoantigen-based vaccines came from Carreno et al. In their study, they used a dendritic cell vaccine to boost preexisting neoantigen-specific immunity in three patients with advanced melanoma. Using a multimodal approach for neoantigen identification, including whole-exon sequencing, a neoantigen prediction pipeline, and mass spectrometry, they were able to identify neoantigens that could be presented on HLA-A*02:01 and design patient-specific vaccines that can redirect T cell immunity toward naturally occurring neoantigens. More recently in 2019, Keskin et al. reported a Phase 1 study in which a multiepitope peptide vaccine promoted the expansion of neoantigen-specific CD4+ and CD8+ responses in patients with methylguanine methyltransferase-unmethylated glioblastoma.[77] They report an induction of Th1 response, enrichment of memory-like phenotypes, and enhancement of tumor infiltration in a highly immunosuppressive tumor with the low mutational burden. Further advancements in the field have included the design and implementation of nucleic acid vaccines, which are appealing because they allow for the delivery of multiple antigens with one immunization, are not restricted to HLA type, have great safety profiles, and are easily manufactured at a bulk scale. Sahin et al.[78] developed an RNA-based vaccine against multiple neoantigens in patients with melanoma. In their trial, 13 patients received the RNA vaccine and developed no related serious adverse events, and eight had no tumor development during follow-ups. This study demonstrated that these vaccines can enhance preexisting neoantigen-reactive T cell responses as well as generate de novo responses.

In summary, personalized dendritic cell, peptide, DNA, and RNA vaccines against neoantigens have demonstrated the ability to induce potent CD8+ and CD4+ responses in preclinical and clinical studies, highlighting the potential of this immunotherapy. Although neoantigen vaccines can stimulate and augment preexisting antitumor immunity in patients, tumor cells possess various escape mechanisms, including subverting immune recognition and recruiting suppressive immune subtypes to the tumor microenvironment (TME), resulting in many failures in clinical development. These vaccines alone may not be enough to overcome the suppressive barriers, such as the upregulation of immune checkpoints, and must be combined with ICI, adjuvants, or other therapies to modify the TME. Indeed, multiple preclinical models have demonstrated the synergistic potential of combining antitumor vaccines and immune checkpoints,[79–81] and as such clinical trials combining neoantigen vaccines with ICI are now ongoing. Notably, the presence of immunogenic neoantigens seems to also permit responses to immunotherapies that do not directly target neoantigens, such as checkpoint blockade.[27,48]

Cell-Based Therapies

In patients with suboptimal preexisting immunity or otherwise vaccine-unresponsive endogenous T cells, ACT of antigen-specific T cells represents a solution to engender protective antitumor immunity.[82] ACT imparts antitumor activity by introducing large numbers (up to 10^{11}) of in vitro selected T cells with both high specificity and effector function—a consequence of developing in an environment free of the endogenous inhibitory mechanisms that curtail T cell activation—into patients. Typically, ACT is done in an autologous setting, but research is underway to provide ACT from "off-the-shelf" products or alloge-neic donors.[83,84] In the autologous setting, the persistence of adoptively transferred cells in the host was once a limiting factor in the efficacy of this therapy.[85] Interestingly, it was determined that lymphodepletion of the host, namely with cyclophosphamide and fludarabine, prior to ACT combined with IL-2 treatment after ACT enhances the longevity of transferred cells as well as the duration of clinical responses.[86] Lymphodepletion enhances ACT by removing suppressor cells—both CD4+ Foxp3 and myeloid-derived suppressor cells (MDSCs)—from the TME,[87–89] increasing the levels of T cell-activating cytokines[90,91] and mobilizing commensal microflora, which activates APCs by signaling through TLRs.[92]

Initial commonly used ACT protocols did not specifically target antigens. In these protocols, tumor biopsies are harvested, and the T cells that infiltrate the biopsies (TILs) are expanded under the assumption that a certain percentage of these T cells would be tumor-specific. In most cases, the antigen is not even known. Thus, it cannot be proven that current TIL-based ACT protocols expand mutanome-specific T cells. Nevertheless, this "antigen agnostic" approach has shown efficacy. Several recent reports demonstrate durable responses after TIL-based ACT in several cancers, primarily melanoma as well as some epithelial cancers and leukemia/lymphomas.[86,93] In order to target a specific neoantigen, TIL-based ACT must overcome several obstacles: first, the mutated peptide must be identified; second, T cells specific for the peptide must be isolated from the tumor; and third, the expansion of the T cells to specific peptide must be performed in a validated facility, ideally with "clean room" specifications and following current good manufacturing practice (cGMP). A few pioneering studies have overcome these obstacles and indeed have generated neoantigen-specific T cells for ACT. Figure 37.5[82] shows the basic idea behind this process.

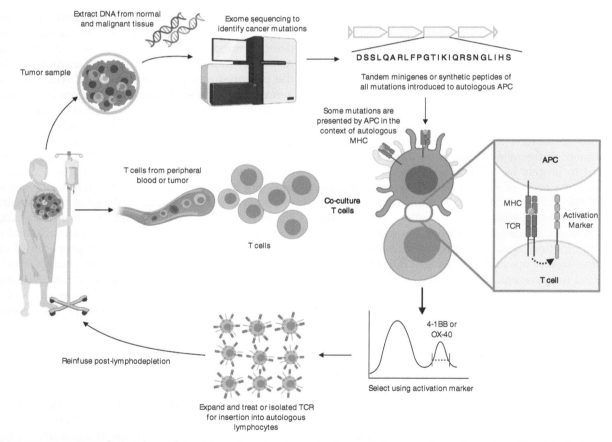

Figure 37.5 Preparation of peripheral blood lymphocytes for adoptive cell therapy. Neoantigens, identified by whole-exome sequencing, are loaded onto antigen-presenting cells (APCs). Neoantigen-loaded APCs activate host T cells, which have been isolated from peripheral blood. Neoantigen-specific T cells are expanded in vitro and sorted based on their activation profiles by flow cytometry—41BB on CD8+ cells, OX40 on CD4+ cells.

APC, antigen-presenting cell; MHC, major histocompatibility complex; TCR, T cell receptor.

Source: Adapted from Rosenberg SA, Restifo NP. Adoptive cell transfer as personalized immunotherapy for human cancer. *Science.* 2015;348(6230):62–68. doi:10.1126/science.aaa4967

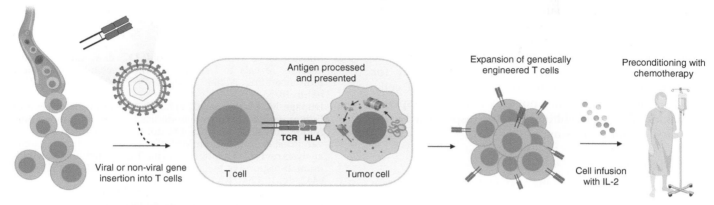

Figure 37.6 **Illustrative methodology for T cell receptor (TCR)–specific T cell adoptive therapy.** T cells isolated from patient peripheral blood are engineered to express an antigen-specific TCR, expanded ex vivo and adoptively transferred back into the host who has been lymphodepleted in advance of adoptive therapy.

HLA, human leukocyte antigen.

Source: Adapted from Rosenberg SA, Restifo NP. Adoptive cell transfer as personalized immunotherapy for human cancer. *Science.* 2015;348(6230):62–68. doi:10.1126/science.aaa4967

Of particular clinical interest, durable clinical responses were noted in several studies involving ACT to treat patients with metastatic melanoma.[58,94,95] In an attempt to define an effective strategy to isolate neoantigen-specific T cells from peripheral blood before ACT, Cohen et al. studied eight patients with metastatic melanoma. They characterized nine candidate neoantigens and then used an MHC tetramer screen to identify T cells in peripheral blood that were specific to those particular antigens; they found neoantigen-specific T cells at frequencies ranging between 0.4% and 0.002% in peripheral blood.[96] In addition to reports of ACT in patients with melanoma, one report documents a significant clinical response in one patient with metastatic cholangiocarcinoma following ACT with a pure neoantigen-specific CD4 population. In this work, an analysis of TILs from a patient with metastatic cholangiocarcinoma revealed CD4+ T cells specific for the mutated tumor antigen in Erbb2-interacting protein (ERBB2IP). ACT of CD4+ T cells, of which 25% were ERBB2IP-specific, led to tumor control and PFS; in addition, treatment of disease recurrence with a more than 95% ERRB2IP-specific CD4 transfer again led to durable tumor control.[63]

The interest in genetically engineering T cells with non-native receptors for use in ACT developed first in the preclinical model[97] and then in the clinical setting when a T cell isolated from peripheral circulation was engineered with a TCR to recognize the melanoma-specific antigens MART-1 and gp100[98–100] as well as NY-ESO-1.[95,101] The advancement of TCR engineering allowed for the identification of antigen-specific TCR sequences and the ex vivo generation of antigen-specific T cells, which overcame previous barriers such as isolating tumor-specific T cells from patients and producing a therapeutic number of cells needed for infusion.

Clinical applications of TCR-based cell therapies generated considerable enthusiasm as studies demonstrated positive objective responses in patients with synovial cell sarcoma, melanoma, myeloma, and esophageal cancers.[95,98,102–104] Figure 37.6 provides an illustrative overview of engineered TCR-specific T cell therapy.

However, most of these clinical trials were tested in a small number of cancer patients and unexpected toxicities have occurred. In a study using a TCR-engineered T cell therapy targeting metastatic colorectal cancer, three patients developed severe inflammatory colitis due to cross-reacting to normal colon epithelium.[105] In another study, TCRs that were engineered to recognize melanoma-associated antigen 3 (MAGE-A3) also recognized a MAGE-A12-derived epitope, which resulted in two patients lapsing into comas and subsequently dying.[106] While TCR-engineered T cell therapies are promising therapeutics in the treatment of a variety of cancers, identifying cross-reactivity and appropriate antigens is required for its safe and efficacious application in the clinical setting.

CONCLUSION

In summary, it is clear that cancer cells possess antigens that can be recognized by the immune system. In 1909, Ehrlich posited that the immune system should restrict the growth of cancers, but it was not until 1957 that Burnet offered that tumor cells, "because of their possession of new antigenic potentialities, provoke an effective immunological reaction...." Indeed, we now know that mutation can not only drive cancer but also consequently drive its immunogenicity. These "new antigenic potentialities" have a molecular basis as neoantigens, and our current understanding of this forms the foundation for future therapies, personalized or otherwise. Although Burnet and Ehrlich proposed a qualitative aspect to tumor recognition, our modern tools have provided more nuance to this model, defining certain quantitative parameters, including mutational burden, affinity for MHC molecules, and number of cancer-specific T cells, which ultimately determine not only whether a response occurs but also the likelihood that the response achieves complete tumor regression.

KEY REFERENCES

Only key references appear in the print edition. The full reference list appears in the digital product on Springer Publishing Connect: connect.springerpub.com/content/book/978-0-8261-3743-2/part/part03/chapter/ch37

5. Alexandrov LB, Nik-Zainal S, Wedge DC, et al. Signatures of mutational processes in human cancer. *Nature.* 2013;500(7463):415–421. doi:10.1038/nature12477

19. McGranahan N, Furness AJ, Rosenthal R, et al. Clonal neoantigens elicit T cell immunoreactivity and sensitivity to immune checkpoint blockade. *Science.* 2016;351(6280):1463–1469. doi:10.1126/science.aaf1490

27. Matsushita H, Vesely MD, Koboldt DC, et al. Cancer exome analysis reveals a T-cell-dependent mechanism of cancer immunoediting. *Nature.* 2012;482(7385):400–404. doi:10.1038/nature10755

30. Dupage M, Mazumdar C, Schmidt LM, et al. Expression of tumour-specific antigens underlies cancer immunoediting. *Nature.* 2012;482(7385):405–409. doi:10.1038/nature10803

47. van Rooij N, van Buuren MM, Philips D, et al. Tumor exome analysis reveals neoantigen-specific T-cell reactivity in an ipilimumab-responsive melanoma. *J Clin Oncol.* 2013;31(32):e439–e442. doi:10.1200/JCO.2012.47.7521

76. Carreno BM, Magrini V, Becker-Hapak M, et al. Cancer immunotherapy. A dendritic cell vaccine increases the breadth and diversity of melanoma neoantigen-specific T cells. *Science.* 2015;348(6236):803–808. doi:10.1126/science.aaa3828

82. Rosenberg SA, Restifo NP. Adoptive cell transfer as personalized immunotherapy for human cancer. *Science.* 2015;348(6230):62–68. doi:10.1126/science.aaa4967

38

Assessment of Antitumor Immunity in Blood and Lymph Nodes

Priyanka B. Subrahmanyam, Lei Wang, Lisa H. Butterfield, Peter P. Lee, and Holden T. Maecker

KEY POINTS

- Testing immune function in the blood yields information about the systemic immune competence of the patient.

- Tumor-associated antigen (TAA)-specific immune responses may indicate increased antitumor immunity and immune responses to intervention but may not indicate improved clinical outcomes.

- It is important to assess both antitumor effect-promoting (T helper 1 [Th1], CD8+) T cells and dampening (regulatory T cell [T_{reg} cell], myeloid-derived suppressor cells [MDSC]) immune cell populations and soluble factors.

- The tumor microenvironment (TME) is complex and involves many cell types and interactions; therefore, measuring numerical and spatial changes in immune cell populations can be informative.

- Tumor-draining lymph nodes (TdLNs) are important sites of immunecancer interactions and should be analyzed.

- More comprehensive and multifactorial measures of immune function will be most likely to yield predictors of immunotherapy success.

ASSESSMENT OF ANTITUMOR IMMUNITY IN BLOOD AND LYMPH NODES

Predictive Biomarkers for Cancer Immunotherapy in Peripheral Blood

The recent advancements in cancer immunotherapy are promising in terms of long-term progression-free survival (PFS) and easier management of toxicities. However, the rapid and widespread implementation of these strategies is greatly hampered by the fact that effective antitumor responses are observed only in a subset of patients. This has necessitated an urgent search for predictive biomarkers, which can be used to identify likely responders for a specific type of immunotherapy, as well as biomarkers of the mechanisms of effective immunotherapy. These two classes of biomarkers are worth differentiating; those that are clinically useful for patient stratification need to be distinct and largely nonoverlapping in responders versus nonresponders. In other words, patient selection can be guided by such biomarkers if the probability of predicting response correctly is very high. However, many biomarkers show significantly different levels in responders and nonresponders but have high overlap between the two groups. These markers can still give us insight into the biology that underlies an effective antitumor response but may not be useful on their own for patient decision-making.

Immunotherapy targets a patient's immune system, and understanding the immune "landscape" or status before the administration of such therapy is vital. Different types of immunotherapy target different immune cell types or signaling pathways, making it important to understand the baseline frequency, phenotype, and function of these cell subsets in patients. In other words, it is important to understand the underlying differences in the immune system of patients who respond to certain therapies, compared to those who do not. These differences, once identified and validated, will allow us to develop relevant clinical tests to identify the right therapy for a particular patient. Tailoring cancer immunotherapy to specific patient immune profiles is instrumental in maximizing the probability and magnitude of an effective antitumor immune response. The identification of specific immune biomarkers can aid in appropriate patient selection, which is even more important as the range of available immunotherapies expands rapidly. The discovery, standardization, validation, and clinical implementation of biomarker testing will be instrumental in the appropriate and effective use of cancer immunotherapy. Understanding the mechanisms of antitumor immunity is critical to optimize therapeutics and combinations.

Arguably, the most direct site at which to measure cellular biomarkers of immunotherapy response is the tumor itself. However, there are advantages to looking for biomarkers in peripheral blood.[1,2] Most notably, blood is much more universally and repeatably accessible than tumor tissue, and it is also more homogeneous. Robust biomarkers in tumor tissue will be harder to identify, simply because of heterogeneity between tumor sites and metastatic sites, and even between repeated biopsies from the same site.[3] Sampling tumor tissue through biopsies is invasive and also increases healthcare costs associated with cancer treatment. In addition, biomarkers identified in the tumor microenvironment (TME), once specified, could be sought in blood, where they might be rare but detectable. Moreover, it could be hypothesized that certain systemic immune factors might be necessary if not sufficient for local tumor responses. For these reasons, blood biomarkers should be considered as important as biomarkers derived from tumors and/or the TME.

One of the most general parameters of the immune system, absolute lymphocyte count (ALC), is routinely measured in clinical blood tests and can serve as an indicator of immune competence. ALC has been reported to be a potential biomarker predictive of clinical response to ipilimumab, an anticytotoxic T-lymphocyte-associated protein 4 (CTLA-4) monoclonal antibody.[4,5] However, ALC correlated significantly with clinical outcome only after the first or second ipilimumab treatment cycle. Although some reports have shown that patients with higher baseline ALC are more likely to respond to therapy, the difference between responders and nonresponders reached statistical significance only after ipilimumab treatment. This implies that the inhibition of a negative signaling pathway through CTLA-4 blockade leads to immune activation and expansion of lymphocyte populations, resulting in elevated ALC levels. Martens et al. have reported that early increases in ALC, and delayed increases in CD4$^+$ and CD8$^+$ T cell count, predicted favorable clinical outcome, while decreases in these parameters portended poor prognosis. ALC greater than 1,000/mm^3 (normal range: 800–2,600/mm^3) and an increase in absolute eosinophil count greater than 100/mm^3 (normal range: 0–400/mm^3) at the second ipilimumab dose have been associated with improved overall survival (OS) in metastatic melanoma.[6] Also, ALC has recently been shown to be significantly lower in non-small cell lung cancer (NSCLC) and renal cell carcinoma patients who had progressive disease on anti-PD-1 therapy.[7] Baseline neutrophil count and derived neutrophil-to-lymphocyte ratio have also been found to have prognostic value in response to ipilimumab, warranting further investigation and validation.[8] The neutrophil-to-lymphocyte ratio has been reported to have potential as a predictive biomarker in NSCLC patients treated with anti-PD-1 (nivolumab), as well as urothelial cancer patients treated with various immune checkpoint inhibitors.[9,10] In cutaneous melanoma patients

treated with ipilimumab, responders were found to have a higher baseline frequency of nonclassical CD16$^+$ monocytes in peripheral blood.[11] Ex vivo, these CD16$^+$ monocytes could be engaged by ipilimumab and lyse regulatory T cells (T$_{reg}$ cells) through antibody-dependent cellular cytotoxicity (ADCC), which could potentially be the basis for the association of this subset with improved outcome. In a recent study by Krieg et al., the frequency of monocytes, specifically CD14$^+$CD16$^-$HLA-DR^{hi}, was found to be predictive of response to anti-PD-1 immunotherapy in metastatic melanoma.[12]

Besides CBC parameters, soluble factors have also been studied for correlation with response to cancer immunotherapy. Baseline C-reactive protein (CRP) has been significantly correlated with OS but will need further evaluation as a prognostic biomarker for anti-CTLA-4.[13] Delyon et al. have reported that patients with normal lactate dehydrogenase (LDH) levels before the first ipilimumab infusion were more likely to respond to therapy.[6] In general, low LDH levels are associated with better clinical outcome in melanoma after treatment with ipilimumab, as compared to patients with high LDH at baseline.[14,15] General measures of the immune system such as ALC, total CD4$^+$ and CD8$^+$ T cell counts, eosinophils, neutrophils, CRP, and LDH have all shown promise as potential biomarkers, awaiting further investigation and validation. However, compared to CTLA-4 blockade, there is limited knowledge on the potential use of these parameters as prognostic biomarkers in programmed death 1 (PD-1)/programmed death-ligand 1 (PD-L1) blockade[16] and other immune-modulatory interventions.

The PD-1/PD-L1 axis is an important regulatory target for cancer immunotherapy with potent clinical results. PD-L1 expression on tumor and tumor-infiltrating lymphocytes (TILs) has been approved as a companion diagnostic for PD-1 immunotherapy, using immunohistochemistry on tumor biopsies. Free soluble PD-L1 in serum has also been evaluated as a pharmacodynamic biomarker. Suppression of free PD-L1 in serum was indicative of target engagement by anti-PD-1 antibody.[17] PD-L1 expression on peripheral T cells and myeloid cells has shown promise in predicting response to anti-PD-1/PD-L1, as well as anti-CTLA-4 immunotherapy.[18–20] PD-1 on immune cells may also be a predictive biomarker, with early increases in proliferating PD-1$^+$ CD8$^+$ T cells being associated with clinical benefit in NSCLC patients treated with anti-PD-1.[21] PD-1 may also have predictive value in combination with other T cell exhaustion markers and tumor characteristics. Huang et al. have reported that the ratio of exhausted T cells to tumor burden was predictive of response to PD-1 blockade in melanoma.[22] Aside from expression of the direct target of an immunotherapy, there are substantial data on the activation of T cells following immune checkpoint blockade. Expansion of inducible co-stimulator (ICOS)⁺CD4⁺ T cells has been reported following CTLA-4 blockade, in peripheral blood as well as in the tumor.[23] This ICOS⁺ interferon gamma (IFN-γ)-producing CD4⁺ T cell subset correlates with improved clinical outcome, including OS, and may be a potential biomarker for ipilimumab response.[24,25] Di Giacomo et al. have reported that patients who showed an increase in ICOS⁺CD4⁺ and ICOS⁺CD8⁺ T cells in peripheral blood have significantly better overall survival after ipilimumab treatment.[26] Ki67 and EOMES have also shown promise as activation markers. Low levels of Ki67⁺EOMES⁺CD8⁺ T cells at baseline were found to correlate with the likelihood of relapse.[27] On the other hand, low numbers of Ki67⁺EOMES⁺CD4⁺ T cells were found to correlate with immune-related adverse events (irAEs) in metastatic melanoma patients treated with ipilimumab. The frequency of Ki67⁺EOMES⁺ peripheral blood T cells shows promise in predicting not only clinical response to treatment but also the occurrence of irAEs. Another study reported expansion of the activated human leukocyte antigen—antigen D related (HLA-DR)⁺Ki67⁺CD8⁺ T cell subset (where HLA-DR serves as an activation marker)—following treatment with anti-PD-L1 antibody MPDL3280A, but there was no correlation with clinical outcome.[28] Increased HLA-DR⁺CD4,⁺ along with concomitant decreases in naïve CD4⁺ and CD8⁺ T cells, have been reported at 4 weeks after ipilimumab treatment.[29] Comparison of pretreatment and posttreatment samples from patients treated with ipilimumab also showed increases in HLA-DR⁺ T cells in the periphery, which is in line with T cell activation by CTLA-4 blockade.[30–32] These studies also reported increases in CD45RO, a memory marker on both CD4⁺ and CD8⁺ T cells, following treatment, implying that ipilimumab treatment can trigger not only activation but also long-term memory responses. Memory CD4⁺ and CD8⁺ T cells in peripheral blood have now emerged as predictive biomarkers of response. Several studies have reported that in melanoma patients treated with anti-CTLA-4, responders had higher central/effector memory T cells compared to nonresponders at baseline and during treatment.[33–36] So far, these memory subsets have not correlated with response to anti-PD-1 treatment in melanoma. However, higher central memory CD4⁺ T cells and CD62L^lo CD4⁺ T cells have been reported in responders to anti-PD-1 therapy in NSCLC or renal cell carcinoma.[7,37] Sander et al. studied the dynamics of CD8⁺ T cell subsets in patients treated with histamine dihydrochloride and low-dose interleukin-2 (IL-2) in patients with acute myeloid leukemia (AML).[38] They compared memory CD8⁺ T cells before and after the first treatment cycle and found that some patients showed a reduction in effector memory cells, with a concomitant induction of the effector subset. These patients, who showed an early shift from effector memory to effector CD8⁺ T cells,

were less likely to relapse, and had better leukemia-free survival and overall survival. Thus, it should be noted that in addition to baseline predictive biomarkers, there is also potential for early changes in cell subsets to be predictive of outcome, underscoring the importance of immune monitoring, especially during initial treatment cycles. Aside from general immune cell subsets, CD8⁺ T cells in the peripheral blood that are specifically reactive to melanoma-associated peptide antigens may also be investigated for use as biomarkers.[39] Other subsets like T helper 17 (Th17) cells in the peripheral blood of patients treated with anti-CTLA-4 have shown more promise in the prediction of irAEs than in predicting response to therapy.[40,41]

Activated cell subsets can be important indicators of patient immune competence. However, it is equally important to evaluate the regulatory cell subsets like T_{reg} cells[42] and myeloid-derived suppressor cells (MDSCs) that can suppress the antitumor response (for greater detail, see Chapters 39–41). Effective antitumor immunity can be triggered only when the balance between immune activation and immune suppression is tipped. T_{reg} cells are known to express CTLA-4, which can play an important role in their suppressive function.[43] It then follows that CTLA-4 blockade will alter T_{reg} cell frequency and/or function in a patient. However, correlations between T_{reg} cells and clinical outcome following immunotherapy have been controversial.[44] Normal ranges for T_{reg} cells are between 4% and 9% of circulating CD4⁺ T cells, varying with the specific markers chosen for identification. Some groups have reported a decrease in circulating Foxp3⁺ T_{reg} cells as treatment progressed and found that it correlated with improved clinical outcome.[45] However, many studies have reported no changes in circulating T_{reg} cells, and some have even reported increases in circulating T_{reg} cells following ipilimumab or nivolumab treatment.[25,29,41,46,47] One study even reported that higher baseline circulating T_{reg} cells were prognostic of better clinical outcome in response to ipilimumab treatment.[15] A major issue that needs to be considered is T_{reg} cell migration between the periphery and tumor sites. Apparent increases or decreases in circulating T_{reg} cell numbers must be interpreted with caution as they may indicate migration to/from tumor sites. Also, combinations with other T_{reg} cell modulating factors like IL-2 can confound results by exerting their own effects independent of immune checkpoint blockade.

MDSCs are another suppressive cell type that has been found to play a major role in inhibiting antitumor responses. Meyer et al. reported that melanoma patients have a higher frequency of circulating MDSC compared to healthy donors.[48] In patients with advanced melanoma treated with neoadjuvant ipilimumab, circulating MDSCs were decreased from baseline to 6 weeks posttreatment.[46] Low baseline MDSCs have been reported to be predictive of response to ipilimumab and improved clinical outcome.[15,49] Other studies have also associated lower MDSC frequency with response to ipilimumab treatment and prolonged OS.[48,50,51] An inverse correlation between baseline MDSC and peripheral blood CD8[+] T cell expansion following treatment has also been reported.[50] To date, normal ranges of MDSC have not been delineated due to the differences in blood or tissue handling and the phenotypic markers used. This supports the idea that MDSC can suppress antitumor immunity triggered by immune checkpoint blockade, and therefore a lower MDSC frequency can be prognostic of response to ipilimumab, and potentially other immunotherapies. Besides T cells and regulatory subsets, it is interesting to note that natural killer (NK) cells have also correlated with response to anti-PD-1 immunotherapy. Recent studies have reported that higher frequencies of functionally active NK cells, such as IFN-γ producing, or CD69[+]MIP1β[+] NK cells correlate with response to anti-PD-1, while higher PD-L1[+] NK cells correlate with progressive disease.[7,52,53]

Various CD4[+] and CD8[+] T cell populations, such as naïve, central memory, effector memory, and terminal effector cells, as well as functional markers like cytokines and cytotoxicity molecules, hold high potential to become biomarkers for various immunotherapies targeting T cells. However, the limitation in the number of channels that can be included in conventional flow cytometry poses a major obstacle to their discovery and validation. Emerging technologies like mass cytometry have been instrumental in overcoming this hurdle.[54,55] Mass cytometry (CyTOF) is a single-cell proteomic technique that uses the principles of mass spectrometry using antibodies tagged with metal isotopes. This currently allows the simultaneous detection of 40 different markers with potential for expansion up to 100. Since CyTOF eliminates the use of fluorochromes, there is less need for compensation to correct for spectral overlap. Indeed, the use of mass cytometry for comprehensive immune monitoring in cancer patients has led to rapid advancement in the identification of predictive biomarker candidates.[12,53]

Cancer immunotherapy-mediated activation of the immune system certainly involves the induction of various cytokines. However, serum cytokine levels have generally not proven reproducible as biomarkers to date. Interestingly, two studies on PD-L1 blockade using the MPDL3280A antibody have reported increases in serum cytokines like type 1 immunity-promoting IFN-γ and IL-18 during the second cycle of treatment.[28,56] However, neither study found any correlation between these parameters and the clinical outcome of the patients. IL-8 has been identified as a baseline negative prognostic serum cytokine in multiple checkpoint trial studies.[57] Another interesting prognostic biomarker for ipilimumab is soluble CD25 (sCD25; an activation marker and part of the IL-2 receptor complex when membrane bound) in the serum.[58] CTLA-4 blockade helps in releasing negative regulation of T cell responses, and consequently relies heavily on IL-2 signaling, which is required for T cell function. sCD25 acts as a decoy IL-2 receptor, making IL-2 unavailable for T cells. Hannani et al. found that serum sCD25 was a predictor of OS, with high sCD25 prognostic of resistance to anti-CTLA-4 therapy in melanoma. Vascular endothelial growth factor (VEGF), which is an angiogenesis promoting factor, has also been associated with response to ipilimumab, although the exact mechanism remains elusive. Yuan et al. have reported that pretreatment serum VEGF levels correlated with clinical benefit of ipilimumab treatment.[59] High VEGF levels (greater than or equal to 43 pg/mL) correlated with decreased OS, as assessed at week 24. Antibodies against melanoma antigens in the serum have also been studied by several groups. Yuan et al. have reported that patients with baseline seropositivity to NY-ESO-1 had a higher likelihood of clinical benefit from ipilimumab treatment.[60] Peripheral blood transcriptome analysis has revealed the development of distinct gene expression signatures, which may also serve as a "fingerprint" for prediction of clinical outcomes in patients treated with immunotherapy, or even for the prediction of irAEs.[61,62] Genes related to the immune response, such as *ICOS*, *IFN-γ*, and *Granzyme B*, as well as cell cycle-related genes like *Ki67*, showed transcriptional upregulation after treatment with anti-CTLA-4 and anti-PD-1. Shahabi et al. reported that increases in genes belonging to three functional categories (immune system, cell cycle, and intracellular trafficking) correlated with gastrointestinal irAEs after the first cycle of ipilimumab therapy.[62,63]

Tumor Antigen-Specific T Cells

An extremely important development in the early 1990s was the initial identification of the tumor-associated antigens (TAAs), the tumor-expressed antigens that were recognized by TIL. This work was initially performed in melanoma due to accessibility of tumors, as well as the frequency with which melanomas are infiltrated with T cells. The first antigens identified came to be known as cancer testes antigens (melanoma antigen A [MAGE-A] family)[64] and melanoma lineage antigens (MART-1/Melan-A,[65] gp100, tyrosinase) based on their patterns of expression. Tumor antigens are described in detail in Chapter 4.

Two other key developments led to the ability to measure tumor-specific T cell responses: first, the identification of major histocompatibility complex (MHC)-restricted peptides that are presented by commonly expressed tissue types like HLA-A2. Determination of the biophysical "rules" of binding of these 8–11aa peptides allowed prediction and testing of candidate peptide epitopes for processing and presentation in MHC class I molecules. Second, the development of tetrameric

MHC molecules that are fluorescently labeled,[66] which, when loaded with these peptide epitopes, bind to the surface of T cells expressing T cell receptors (TCRs) that recognize the peptide–MHC complex, was another key. Since that time, many modifications of MHC tetramers have been created around this technology. These developments allowed the easier isolation and testing of antigen-specific T cell responses.

The most commonly used techniques for measuring tumor antigen-specific immunity in cancer patients are MHC multimers (4–10 MHC molecules loaded with peptide bound together), proliferation, cytokine production, and cytotoxicity assays (Table 38.1). Most of these assessments over many years have been focused on the cells that are most feasible to measure, shared (or commonly overexpressed) tumor antigen-specific CD8+ T cells. Because of the substantial murine model data supporting IFN-γ-producing, cytotoxic CD8+ T cells as being the critical denominator for successful antitumor effect, these cells have been a major focus.

Table 38.1 Approaches for Measuring Immune Status

ASSAY	WHAT IS MEASURED
CBC and differential	ALC, AEC, and neutrophil-to-lymphocyte ratio
Serum and plasma testing	CRP, LDH, inflammatory cytokines, and antibody responses
Multiparameter flow cytometry or CyTOF	Naïve/memory T cells, T_{reg} cells, MDSC, NK cells, and detailed phenotype of cell subsets
Multiplex/multispectral IHC or IF	Lymph node and tumor architecture, cellularity, and tumor infiltrate
MHC multimer (flow cytometry)	Frequency of antigen-specific T cells
ELISPOT (cytokine capture)	Frequency of antigen-reactive cytokine-producing cells
Proliferation	^{3}H-thymidine uptake (population measure) CFSE dye dilution (flow cytometry)
Cytotoxicity (^{51}Cr release, granzyme B ELISPOT, CD107a release flow cytometry)	Ability of cells to degranulate or lyse target (tumor) cells
Single-cell sequence analysis	Detailed molecular profile at the level of individual cells

ALC, absolute lymphocyte count; AEC, absolute eosinophil count; CBC, complete blood count; CFSE, carboxyfluorescein succinimidyl ester; CRP, C-reactive protein; CyTOF, cytometry-time of flight; ELISPOT, enzyme-linked immunospot; IF, immunofluorescence; IHC, immunohistochemical; LDH, lactate dehydrogenase; MDSC, myeloid-derived suppressor cell; MHC, major histocompatibility complex; NK, natural killer; T_{reg}, regulatory T.

What Has Been Learned From Measuring Shared Tumor Antigen-Specific T Cells?

Over the years of measuring T cell responses to shared TAA, it is clear that most patients have T cells reactive to these self-antigens in their repertoire. Interestingly, while the frequency of most self-antigen-specific T cells is approximately $1/10^5$ to $1/10^6$, the frequency of CD8+ T cells specific to MART-1 is unusually high,[67] allowing easier evaluation of these particular T cell populations. These self-antigen-specific T cells can be activated by vaccination, and derepressed by checkpoint blockade. They can also be boosted by a variety of therapeutic interventions that reduce tumor burden (see Sections II and IV of this book).

Indication of Successful T Cell Expansion From Immunotherapy

An important role for measuring TAA-specific T cells in patients is to determine whether or not tumor-specific immunity exists or has been enhanced by an intervention. As the technology available and assay sensitivity have improved, the ability to detect low-frequency immune responses has improved. Initially, TAA-specific responses were difficult to detect at baseline before a vaccine, adoptive T cell transfer, or other immune stimulatory intervention. Subsequently, limited dilution cell cloning, multimers, cytokine production, flow cytometric sorting, and TCR cloning have allowed the measure of frequency, function, and phenotype of TAA-specific T cells with greater sensitivity.[68] Such assessments have shown evidence of successful expansion of tumor-specific T cells after vaccination (with peptides, DC vaccines, or other vaccine platforms). These important assays also permit tracking of labeled or clonal populations of adoptively transferred effector cells. Proliferation and longevity of adoptively transferred T cells is an important correlate of their clinical impact.[69,70]

Limitations to Correlation With Clinical Outcome

While many cancer vaccine trials have shown a positive impact on T cell expansion by measuring activation, expansion, and effector function of targeted antigen-specific T cells, the correlation of these systemic measures with clinical outcome has been limited. There are examples of positive correlations,[71] as well as lack of any significant correlation.[72] There are many reasons why blood effector cell measures of activation and expansion may be insufficient to confer tumor eradication in cancer patients. First, the cells in blood circulation may not traffic to tumor deposits. Indeed, expression of chemokine receptors like CXCR3 on antigen-specific T cells is an important correlate for improved clinical outcome.[73] Second, the specificity of the measured T cells may not match the specificity of true tumor rejection antigens (see subsequently). Third, the TAA-specific T cells available after positive and negative thymic selection during T cell development may be of insufficient affinity to be potent tumor-eradicating T cells. Lastly, the state of immune skewing and immune suppression in the TME may be such that potent effectors are functionally neutralized when they successfully traffic to the tumor.

Determinant or Epitope Spreading and In Vivo Cross-Presentation

A number of investigators have observed that in the setting of a multiple peptide or multiple antigen vaccination, the broader the immune response promoted (the greater the number of antigens or peptides responded to), the better the clinical outcome.[74] Taking another approach, several groups have examined T cell and antibody responses to not only the antigens patients were immunized with but also additional commonly expressed tumor antigens. This could be considered a measure of cross-presentation of antigens released from dying tumor cells by endogenous antigen-presenting cells (APCs) to subsequently activate T cells with specificities to a broader array of tumor antigens.[75] This phenomenon, which is a known mechanism of autoimmune disease, is known as determinant spreading[76] or epitope spreading. It can occur between different antigens, as well as between regions of a single antigen.[77] In many clinical trials, detection of spreading from immunizing antigens to other tumor-expressed antigens has correlated with improved clinical outcomes.[78] More recently, the measure of TCR clonality in peripheral blood mononuclear cell (PBMC) has suggested that an increase in TCR diversity correlates with improved clinical outcome.[79] This is the opposite from the correlation with measures of TCR clonality in tumor deposits, where greater clonality (reduced diversity) correlates with improved clinical outcome.[80] It is possible that the improvement of greater diversity of TCR detected in the blood represents a broadening of the epitopes and antigens responded to by circulating T cells, and a more intact host immune system.

Measuring Tumor Rejection and Mutated Neoantigens

Tumors are well known to accumulate genetic mutations over time. It is also understood that the development of a potent and robust T cell response to foreign pathogens and their proteins that are unrelated to human proteins is much easier and stronger than anti-self-immunity. Therefore, it is expected that as tumors grow and evolve, they express mutated forms of proteins. There are common driver mutations (like those in ras, p53, and BRAF) and a vast array of unique, patient-specific (private)

mutations in most tumors. Tumors whose etiologies involve environmental mutagenesis (melanoma from UV exposure, lung cancer from cigarette smoking) can be particularly high in tumor mutation load.[81]

Until the technological advance of high-throughput and reduced-cost DNA sequencing, the analysis of patient-specific mutations was a technically challenging, time-consuming, and very expensive endeavor. At that time, there were very few reports in which identification of patient-specific mutated antigens was accomplished, and their immunogenicity confirmed.[82,83] These important advances demonstrated that such antigens were recognized by high-affinity TCR and highly avid T cells that could kill tumors. Since then, exome sequencing and full DNA sequencing of tumors have been more efficient and cost-effective, and the ability to identify patient-specific mutations that are recognized by T cells is feasible. Isolating and characterizing T cells specific for private mutated antigens is now feasible. In addition, the diversity of the TCR in peripheral blood has also been studied for the discovery of potential biomarkers. Metastatic melanoma patients with higher TCR diversity were more likely to receive clinical benefit from ipilimumab treatment, although the TCR diversity did not significantly correlate with OS.[84] Another study has reported that patients who had better clonal stability and maintained high-frequency TCR clonotypes from baseline were significantly more likely to benefit clinically and had higher OS.[85]

IMPORTANCE OF T CELL AVIDITY

T cell recognition is not Boolean but driven by TCR affinity for specific peptide–MHC (pMHC) complexes on target cells. It has been demonstrated that cancer vaccine-elicited T cells are heterogeneous with respect to tumor-killing capacity, and only a small subset of vaccine-elicited T cells are efficient at tumor cell lysis.[86,87] This is largely due to differences in functional avidity (also known as recognition efficiency): Peptide-specific T cells that are indistinguishable by tetramer staining may still differ by up to 1,000-fold in peptide requirement for target lysis.[87] Only high-avidity cytotoxic T lymphocytes (CTLs), which may represent 10% or less of a vaccine-elicited response, could lyse tumor targets.[86,87] Low-avidity T cells, which are nontumor cytolytic, represent the predominant cell population elicited via vaccine conditions that involve high, supraphysiological antigen doses. Importantly, low-avidity CTLs do not kill tumor cells but can inhibit tumor lysis by high-avidity CTLs in an antigen-specific manner.[88] This phenomenon operates in vivo, and the mechanism involves stripping of specific pMHC complexes via trogocytosis by low-avidity TAA-specific CTLs without degranulation, leading to insufficient levels of specific pMHC complexes on the target cell surface to trigger lysis by high-avidity CTLs.[88] As such, it is critical to include avidity in immune monitoring. This can be incorporated via a flow cytometric method for rapid assessment of recognition efficiency and functional capacity of antigen-specific T cell responses.[89] In this method, antigen-specific T cells that otherwise appear homogeneous on tetramer staining are stimulated with graded amounts of cognate peptides. Individual T cells downmodulate surface TCRs and thus lose tetramer reactivity with variable dynamics within the T cell population. The dynamics of TCR downregulation represent an accurate assessment of an individual cell's antigen sensitivity, avidity, and relative functional state within an antigen-specific population and have direct correlation to killing capacity by chromium release, as well as degranulation by CD107 mobilization.

The development of antigen-specific T cell immunity has been critical in many models for tumor rejection. There are tumor-intrinsic reasons why effective T cell responses may not translate to antitumor effector function, including tumor heterogeneity, antigen loss variants, antigen processing, and presentation mutants. CD8+ CTL requires MHC class I expression, in addition to target antigen presentation. Antigen presentation requires that the antigen protein be expressed, processed through the many antigen-processing machinery proteins (TAP1, TAP2, etc.) and that the peptides be presented in MHC class I/β_2 microglobulin complexes. This topic is presented thoroughly in Chapter 5. There are many examples of human tumors (or subsets of tumor cells) that have downregulated or entirely lost expression of these key molecules, making those tumor cells invisible to CTL.[90] Some of these defects may make the tumor cells more visible to and targetable by NK cells (where loss of "self" or MHC class I is a key NK cell cytotoxicity response trigger). In later stage tumors, NK cell defects may already be present, reducing the positive compensatory impact of innate immune responses. With the advent of single cell-sequencing approaches, the ability to determine the extent of the heterogeneity of tumor cells and how that impacts antitumor immunity is poised to dramatically expand.[91]

Analysis of Tumor-Infiltrating Lymphocytes

The clinical significance of TILs came into focus over the past decade, with large studies of sufficient size to detect statistically significant correlations with survival. The strongest evidence for tumor infiltration by T cells and favorable clinical outcomes has been established in colorectal carcinoma.[92,93] Similar correlations have now been observed in essentially all tumor types,[94] including melanoma,[95] head and neck cancer,[96] lung cancer,[97] and others. Several large studies have also firmly established the clinical significance of TILs in breast cancer. The largest study followed clinical outcomes of 12,339 newly diagnosed breast cancer patients in the UK and Canada over 10 years.[98] Cytotoxic (CD8+) and regulatory (CD4+ Foxp3+) T cells within tumors were quantified via immunohistochemical (IHC) staining. The study showed a survival benefit of CD8+ T cells within breast tumors (within tumor—iTIL, within stroma—sTIL) in triple-negative and estrogen receptor (ER)-negative/HER2-positive patients: Presence of iTIL was associated with 28%, and sTIL with 21%, reduction in breast cancer-specific mortality. For ER-positive/HER2-positive patients, there was also a 27% reduction in hazard when iTIL was present but not for ER-positive/HER2-negative patients. In this study, the presence of Foxp3+ T_{reg} cells within tumors was not associated with breast cancer-specific survival after adjustment for known prognostic factors. A survival benefit from CD8+ T cells within triple-negative breast tumors was also shown in two additional studies: the ECOG (75)[99] and FinHER (76)[100] studies representing an additional 1,491 patients analyzed. Together, these studies firmly establish the prognostic significance of tumor-infiltrating CD8+ T cells in triple-negative and HER2+ breast cancer. Furthermore, these studies also found that tumor-infiltrating CD8+ T cells were predictive of clinical benefit from trastuzumab (76)[100] and anthracyclines (74).[98] Thus, the presence of intratumoral CD8+ T cells can help guide breast cancer patient management and should be included in routine pathologic examinations—a concept being put forth called "Immunoscore" (see also Chapter 56).[101,102]

Importantly, T cells are often exhausted and dysfunctional within the TME (79).[103] Their metabolism may be inhibited due to oxygen and nutrient depletion. Tumor-infiltrating T cells often express a number of immune checkpoint molecules—CTLA-4, PD-1, T cell immunoglobulin and mucin domain-containing 3 (TIM-3), lymphocyte activation gene 3 protein (LAG-3), and others—which, when engaged with their counter ligands (B7, PDL-1, etc.), lead to inhibition of T cell function. Antibodies that block immune checkpoint molecules have demonstrated exciting clinical efficacy and have been U.S. Food and Drug Administration (FDA) approved for metastatic melanoma, NSCLC, renal cell carcinoma (RCC), and lymphoma. These results definitively demonstrate that the host immune system can respond to cancer, the success of the endogenous antitumor immune response determines clinical outcome and response to even conventional therapies, and that this immune response can be further enhanced for clinical benefit.

Checkpoint blockade works only in a subset of patients. There is still no definitive test to select patients who will respond clinically. For anti-PD-1/PD-L1 antibodies, IHC staining for PD-L1 expression in the tumor is currently the only predictive test. This correlation is not present in all cancer types, and patients with PD-L1-negative tumors may still respond. Other immune cell types also infiltrate human tumors, including B cells, NK cells, and myeloid cells. The balance of these different immune cell populations within tumors drives the clinical outcome. Further studies need to account for this additional complexity, which is possible using novel image analysis approaches.[104,105] A deeper understanding of the interplay between different immune cell populations within tumors and tumor-draining lymph nodes (TdLNs) will uncover ways to enhance the total effect of cancer immunotherapies, including checkpoint inhibitors and adoptive T cell therapy.

Immune Profiles in Tumor Draining Lymph Nodes and Spatial Patterns

In breast cancer, melanoma, and other cancers, tumor invasion of draining lymph nodes is an important prognostic parameter.[106] This has led to the sentinel lymph node (SLN) biopsy technique in which the first TdLN(s) is/are identified via injection of a blue dye and/or a radioactive tracer into the tumor prior to surgical resection. An often overlooked site of immune–cancer interactions is the TdLN. It is the site where tumor antigens are typically first presented to the immune system and a critical initial decision between immune activation and tolerance is made. It has been shown that significant changes in immune cell populations arise within TdLNs in breast cancer,[107] specifically in CD4+ T cells and CD1a+ DCs—reduction in these cells is strongly correlated with a worse clinical outcome.[108]

In one study, IHC analysis of sentinel and axillary (nonsentinel) nodes was performed in 77 breast cancer patients with 5 years of follow-up to determine if alterations in CD4, CD8, and CD1a cell populations predict nodal metastasis or disease-free survival. Sentinel and axillary node CD4 and CD8 T cells were decreased compared to control nodes. CD1a dendritic cells (DCs) were similarly diminished in sentinel but increased in axillary nodes. Importantly, axillary node CD4 T cell and DC populations were highly correlated with disease-free survival and were independent of axillary metastasis. Immune profiling of a test set of axillary lymph nodes (ALNs), applying CD4 T cell and CD1a DC population thresholds of CD4 greater than or equal to 7.0% and CD1a greater than or equal to 0.6% determined from learning set analysis, provided significant risk stratification into favorable and unfavorable prognostic groups superior to clinicopathologic characteristics, including tumor size, extent, or size of nodal metastasis (CD4, p <.001 and CD1a, p <.001). Moreover, axillary node CD4 T cell and CD1a DC populations allowed more significant stratification of disease-free survival of patients with T1 and T2 tumors than all other patient characteristics. Lastly, SLN immune profile correlated primarily with the presence of infiltrating tumor cells, while ALN immune profile appeared largely independent of nodal metastases, raising the possibility that, within ALNs, immune profile changes and nodal metastases represent independent processes. These findings demonstrated that the immune profile of TdLNs is of novel biologic and clinical importance for patients with early stage breast cancer (Figure 38.1).

Beyond numerical changes, spatial distributions of immune cells are also altered within TdLNs as compared to healthy lymph nodes (HLNs).[105] DCs are key mediators of the antitumor immune responses. Many DC-based vaccination approaches have been and are in clinical testing. Further studies showed that the degree of clustering of DCs may be reduced in some TdLNs compared to HLNs, and such changes correlate with clinical outcome in breast cancer.[104] Collectively, these findings point to the importance of examining TdLNs, including spatial distribution/patterns of immune cells.

Dendritic Cell Clustering

DCs are important mediators of the antitumor immune responses. An in-depth analysis of DCs and their spatial relationships to each other, as well as to other immune cells within TdLNs, provides a better understanding of immune function and dysregulation in cancer. In another study, immune cells within TdLNs from 59 breast cancer patients with at least 5 years of clinical follow-up were analyzed using IHC staining with a novel quantitative image analysis system. Algorithms to analyze spatial distribution patterns of immune cells in cancer versus HLNs were developed to derive information about possible mechanisms underlying immune dysregulation in breast cancer. Maturation and clustering of DC was reduced in TdLNs compared to HLNs. Importantly, clinical outcome analysis revealed that DC clustering in tumor-positive TdLNs was correlated with the duration of disease-free survival in breast cancer patients.

The important technological advance of multiplexing of immunohistochemistry and immunofluorescence staining[109] of lymph node and tumor samples has enabled more detailed phenotyping of tumor and immune cells. For example, the results of single stains for Foxp3 may identify a T_{reg} cell; the simultaneous identification of CD3, CD4, and Foxp3 on the same cell gives much greater confidence that the cell in question is a T_{reg} cell. Similarly, the determination of DC and other myeloid lineage cells necessitates multiple phenotypic markers. It is now possible to multiplex up to 40 markers using metal ion–labeled antibodies and multiplexed ion beam imaging (MIBI).[110]

As discussed earlier, the special relationships between cells can also yield novel and important insights. The ability to quantify the interactions and locations of

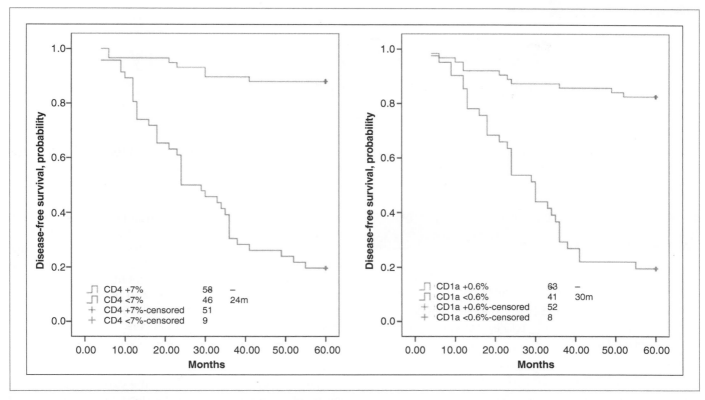

Figure 38.1 Axillary node CD4 T cell and CD1a DC populations allowed more significant stratification of disease-free survival of patients with T1 and T2 tumors than all other patient characteristics.

Source: From Kohrt HE, Nouri N, Nowels K, et al. Profile of immune cells in axillary lymph nodes predicts disease-free survival in breast cancer. *PLOS Med*. 2005;2:e284. doi:10.1371/journal.pmed.0020284

immune and tumor cells will help to convey the critical parameters of tumor and immune cell cross-talk.

CONCLUSION

In summary, many different approaches are currently being used to find relevant biomarkers for immunotherapy. These efforts utilize a wide range of technologies including sequencing, proteomic technologies to detect soluble factors in serum, and single-cell technologies like flow and mass cytometry or single-cell RNA-Seq and Ab-Seq. The results of these studies, once validated and standardized for implementation in the clinic, could give rise to routine pretreatment immune-profiling practices, to maximize clinical benefit and minimize irAEs.

KEY REFERENCES

Only key references appear in the print edition. The full reference list appears in the digital product on Springer Publishing Connect: connect.springerpub.com/content/book/978-0-8261-3743-2/part/part03/chapter/ch38

12. Krieg C, Nowicka M, Guglietta S, et al. High-dimensional single-cell analysis predicts response to anti-PD-1 immunotherapy. *Nat Med*. 2018;24:144–153. doi:10.1038/nm.4466
15. Martens A, Wistuba-Hamprecht K, Geukes Foppen M, et al. Baseline peripheral blood biomarkers associated with clinical outcome of advanced melanoma patients treated with ipilimumab. *Clin Cancer Res*. 2016;22:2908–2918. doi:10.1158/1078-0432.CCR-15-2412
22. Huang AC, Postow MA, Orlowski RJ, et al. T-cell invigoration to tumour burden ratio associated with anti-PD-1 response. *Nature* 2017;545:60–65. doi:10.1038/nature22079
62. Shahabi V, Berman D, Chasalow SD, et al. Gene expression profiling of whole blood in ipilimumab-treated patients for identification of potential biomarkers of immune-related gastrointestinal adverse events. *J Transl Med*. 2013;11:75. doi:10.1186/1479-5876-11-75
81. Alexandrov LB, Nik-Zainal S, Wedge DC, et al; Australian Pancreatic Cancer Genome Initiative; ICGC Breast Cancer Consortium; ICGC MMML-Seq Consortium; ICGC PedBrain. Signatures of mutational processes in human cancer. *Nature*. 2013;500:415–421. doi:10.1038/nature12477
91. Tirosh I, Izar B, Prakadan SM, et al. Dissecting the multicellular ecosystem of metastatic melanoma by single-cell RNA-Seq. *Science*. 2016;352:189–196. doi:10.1126/science.aad0501
93. Pagès F, Galon J, Dieu-Nosjean MC, et al. Immune infiltration in human tumors: a prognostic factor that should not be ignored. *Oncogene*. 2010;29:1093–1102. doi:10.1038/onc.2009.416

Regulatory T Cell Biology and Its Applications in Cancer Immunotherapy

Michael R. Pitter and Weiping Zou

KEY POINTS

- Regulatory T cells (T_{reg} cells) infiltrate various types of tumors and mediate immunosuppression.

- Forkhead box protein 3 (Foxp3) is an indispensable transcription factor for T_{reg} cell development, homeostasis, and function.

- Foxp3 is genetically, epigenetically, and metabolically regulated in the tumor microenvironment.

- T_{reg} cells are phenotypically and functionally plastic.

- Targeting T_{reg} cells may improve tumor immunity.

- Several dispensable components on T_{reg} cells can be targeted to disrupt T_{reg}-mediated immunosuppression and promote antitumor immunity.

INTRODUCTION

Regulatory T cells (T_{reg} cells) are the essential mediators of immune tolerance to self, preventing autoimmunity.[1,2] Meanwhile, T_{reg} cells demonstrate significant functional heterogeneity.[2] The means by which T_{reg} cells maintain self-tolerance are diverse. Therefore, the capacity with which T_{reg} cells mediate tolerance and immune suppression is determined by a wide range of distinct components. Genetic, epigenetic, and metabolic regulatory factors direct T_{reg} cell phenotypes and thereby serve to distinguish T_{reg} cells into separate functional subsets. Comprehensive study of the components unique to the various T_{reg} cell subsets is needed so as to identify novel approaches to control T_{reg}-mediated tumor progression. Infiltration of T_{reg} cells into tumor tissues is often associated with poor prognosis.[1,3] T_{reg} cell immunosuppression continues to pose major challenges in tumor immunity and cancer immunotherapy. While, across the spectrum of T_{reg} cell subsets, there are conserved, shared characteristics—according to which T_{reg} cells as a whole are classified—specific T_{reg} cell subsets exhibit particular dispensable features sufficient to disrupt tumor immunity and cancer immunotherapy. To inhibit T_{reg} cell function without triggering autoimmune disorder constitutes a major goal in clinical oncology. A comprehensive survey of the current literature reveals the significant T_{reg} cell heterogeneity and how understanding this heterogeneity is critical to effectively and safely targeting T_{reg} cells in a variety of cancers.

T_{reg} CELL IDENTITY

T_{reg} cell subtypes are unified by the exhibition of a classical set of features. Foxp3[+] CD25[+] CD4[+] T_{reg} cells exist apart from conventional T cells (T_{conv}) by the expression of Foxp3 and CD25, interleukin 2 receptor (IL-2R).[4–7] During thymic development, the T cells that recognize self-antigens presented by the epithelial tissue of the thymus are deleted through the process of negative selection while a small amount of these cells develop into T_{reg} cells.[2] Thymic T_{reg} cells (tT_{regs}), therefore, maintain a T cell receptor (TCR) repertoire that tends to recognize self-antigens while still overlapping with T_{conv} in phenotype.[8–10] Nevertheless, Foxp3 expression constitutes a central determining factor identifying T_{reg} cells.

Genetic and Epigenetic Stabilization of Foxp3 Expression

Foxp3 expression is controlled by three conserved noncoding sequence (CNS) elements within the first intron of the mouse *Foxp3* gene.[11,12] The human *Foxp3* gene contains several CNSs, including two in intron 2 and in the promoter, as well as many others in downstream areas.[13] Both mouse and human CNSs contain binding sites for several transcription factors crucial for the stabilization of *Foxp3* expression.[12] TCR signaling regulates the genetic stabilization of Foxp3 expression.[14] T_{reg} cell TCR activation initiates calcium and calmodulin-dependent calcineurin activity, drives the transcription factor NFAT to bind to CNS1 (Figure 39.1).[13,15] The complex formed by NFAT and *Foxp3* is required for T_{reg} cell suppressive activity demonstrated

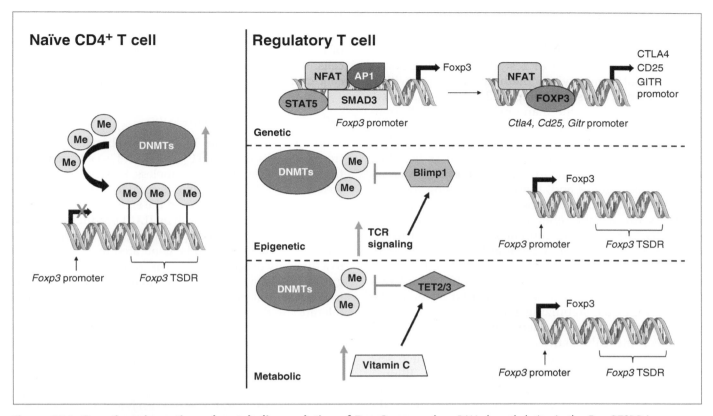

Figure 39.1 Genetic, epigenetic, and metabolic regulation of Foxp3 expression. DNA demethylation in the *Foxp3* TSDR is required for Foxp3 expression, stability, and immunosuppression. By contrast, nonsuppressive naïve CD4+ T cells and T$_{conv}$ cells contain a highly methylated TSDR. In T$_{reg}$ cells, NFAT binds and joins a complex of transcription factors on the *Foxp3* gene, resulting in upregulation of immunosuppressive phenotype. Blimp1 and TET proteins inhibit methyltransferase activity, stabilizing Foxp3. Vitamin C, for example, potentiates TET-mediated demethylation.

AP1, activator protein 1; CD25, IL-2 receptor; CTLA4, cytotoxic T lymphocyte-associated protein 4; DNMTs, DNA methyltransferases; GITR, glucocorticoid-induced tumor necrosis factor-related receptor; Me, methyl; NFAT, nuclear factor of activated T cells; SMAD3, mothers against decapentaplegic homolog 3; STAT5, signal transducer and activator of transcription 5; TCR, T cell receptor; TET, ten-eleven translocation; T$_{reg}$, regulatory T; TSDR, T$_{reg}$-specific demethylated region.

Source: From Huehn J, Polansky JK, Hamann A. Epigenetic control of Foxp3 expression: the key to a stable regulatory T-cell lineage? *Nat Rev Immunol.* 9:83–89. doi:10.1038/nri2474; Iyer LM, Tahiliani M, Rao A, Aravind L, et al. Prediction of novel families of enzymes involved in oxidative and other complex modification of bases in nucleic acids. *Cell Cycle.* 2009;8(11):1698–1710. doi:10.4161/cc.8.11.8580; Lozano T, Villanueva L, Durántez M, et al. Inhibition of Foxp3/NFAT interaction enhances T cell function after TCR stimulation. *J Immunol.* 2015;195(7):3180–3189. doi:10.4049/jimmunol.1402997; Tahiliani M, Koh KP, Shen Y, et al. Conversion of 5-methylcytosine to 5-hydroxymethylcytosine in mammalian DNA by MLL partner TET1. *Science.* 2009;324(5929):930–935. doi:10.1126/science.1170116; Wu Y, Borde M, Heissmeyer V, et al. FOXP3 controls regulatory T cell function through cooperation with NFAT. *Cell.* 2006;126(2):375–387. doi:10.1016/j.cell.2006.05.042

by the upregulation of the suppressive markers and the suppression of IL-2 expression.[16,17] Also downstream of TCR signaling, transcription factor activator protein 1 (AP-1) can bind to CNS2 and trigger TGF-β secretion, a central hallmark of T$_{reg}$-mediated immunosuppressive activity.[18] Additionally, IL-2 signaling via signal transducer and activator of transcription 5 (STAT5) leads to Foxp3 expression and subsequently endows the T$_{reg}$ cell with its immunosuppressive functions.[19] Other transcription factors downstream of TCR signaling include cAMP

response element-binding (CREB) and NF-kB, which further tune and modulate T$_{reg}$ cell suppressive activity.[16,17,20–24]

Crucial epigenetic events occur downstream of TCR ligation preceding the expression of Foxp3. Key transcriptional factors binding to the *Foxp3* promotor are under epigenetic control at both the DNA and the histone modification level. Since the CNS1 lacks CpG motifs, it is regulated only through histone modifications. TGF-β induces histone acetylation permitting NFAT and SMAD3 to bind to the CNS1 region activating

Foxp3, all as a consequence of TCR engagements.[25] In activated T_{reg} cells, Foxp3 binds to multiple DNA sites, recruits and forms complexes with a number of proteins including enhancer of zeste homolog 2 (Ezh2)—the chromatin-modifying methyltransferase within the polycomb repressive complex 2 (PRC2)—as a necessary condition for the maintenance of T_{reg} cell identity and function.[26-28] At the Foxp3-bound sites, Ezh2 tri-methylates lysine 27 on the exposed N-terminal tail of histone H3 (H3K27me3); these markings facilitate the formation of heterochromatin, decreasing accessibility at select genes and, thereby, repressing the non-T_{reg} transcriptional programs. This prevents T_{reg} cell plasticity toward the other T helper subsets and consequently supports the cellular commitment toward functioning as a T_{reg} cell. Unlike in the CNS1 element, DNA demethylation occurs at the CNS2, also known as the T_{reg}-specific demethylation region (TSDR), a CpG-rich, noncoding sequence within the first intron of the *Foxp3* gene locus, stabilizing Foxp3 expression in T_{reg} cells.[22] A fundamental distinction between T_{reg} cells and T_{conv} cells is the fully methylated DNA in the T_{conv} TSDR. In T_{reg} cells, Blimp1 prevents methylation in the CNS2 (Figure 39.1).[29] In response to TCR signaling, Blimp1 negatively regulates IL-6 and STAT3-dependent methyltransferase DNMT3a expression, restraining methylation events at the TSDR and, therefore, serving to stabilize Foxp3 expression. Although Blimp1 alone is not responsible for Foxp3 expression, ablation of Blimp1 regulation disrupts stable Foxp3.

TCR ligation density and affinity serve as a fundamental factor in Foxp3 induction and therefore T_{reg} cell suppressive activity.[30,31] Naïve tT_{regs} enter the circulation and emigrate to peripheral tissues, where TCR signals promote their conversion from $CD44^{lo}CD62L^{hi}$ central T_{reg} cells (cT_{regs}) into the more suppressive $CD44^{hi}CD62L^{lo}$ effector T_{reg} cells (eT_{regs}).[32-35] Suboptimal TCR stimulation is associated with partial calcineurin activity which abrogates T_{reg} cell expansion.[36-38] However, excessive TCR stimulation could also disrupt eT_{reg} fitness.[39] Healthy T_{reg} cell homeostasis requires a balance between cT_{reg} and eT_{reg} populations, as well as between the peripherally induced T_{reg} cells (pT_{regs}). Downstream of TCR signals, transcriptional regulator Bach2 maintains the balance eT_{regs} and pT_{regs} by limiting the effector differentiation and responsiveness of mature T_{reg} cells so as to maintain a longer term expansion and systemic maintenance of T_{regs}.[40] pT_{regs} in the gut—$CD4^+$ T_{conv} cells that acquire T_{reg} cell suppressive phenotype through the de novo upregulation Foxp3—must tolerate a variety of innocuous antigens, such as from food or commensal microbes. Bach2 is required for the development and maintenance of pT_{reg} cells in the gut contributing to local immunological homeostasis.[41,42] Collectively, T_{reg} cell stability and, therefore, Foxp3 expression is stabilized by genetic and epigenetic mechanisms.

In the following sections, we will provide details as to the means by which Foxp3 is induced, the consequences of Foxp3 induction, and the heterogeneity of $Foxp3^+$ T_{reg} cells. These insights can be applied in the development of cancer immunotherapeutic strategies.

Induction of Foxp3 Expression

While pT_{regs} refer to the T_{reg} cells peripherally generated from T_{conv} cells in vivo, iT_{regs} refer to T_{reg} cells generated from T_{conv} cells in vitro; nevertheless, these subsets generated from $CD4^+$ T_{conv} assume natural T_{reg} cell identity via the upregulation of Foxp3 and the exhibition of immunosuppressive properties, such as IL-10 production. While T_{reg} cells commonly develop their regulatory functions in the thymus, pT_{regs} tend to be generated in areas exposed to a diversity of antigens, such as from food, allergens, or gut microbes in the gastrointestinal tract or to the fetus in the maternal placenta, so as to extend immunological tolerance to those areas.[43,44]

In the gastrointestinal tract, TGF-β and the dietary metabolite, retinoic acid (RA), induce Foxp3 expression in activated naïve T cells.[45] A population of $CD103^+$ mesenteric lymph node dendritic cells (DCs) produces these factors, promoting naïve $CD4^+$ T_{conv} cells to acquire Foxp3 expression and immunosuppressive functions. pT_{regs} serve a crucial homeostatic role in the gut, where a myriad of antigens need to be interpreted and processed by host immunity. The maintenance and stability of T_{reg}-like features in pT_{regs} and iT_{regs} depends principally, as previously mentioned, on the DNA demethylation status in the CpG-rich TSDR. While natural tT_{regs} indeed have fully demethylated TSDRs, i- and pT_{regs} display a transiently and sometimes a fully methylated TSDR, which compromises the stable expression of Foxp3.[9,41,46]

In addition to this molecular distinction in TSDR methylation status, tT_{regs} and pT_{regs} differ cellularly in the expression of receptor neuropilin-1 (Nrp1) such that tT_{regs} are $CD4^+$ $CD25^+$ $Foxp3^+$ $Nrp1^{hi}$ and pT_{regs} are $CD4^+$ $CD25^+$ $Foxp3^+$ $Nrp1^{lo}$.[2,41,47-51] Nrp1 expression initially served as a marker to distinguish tT_{regs} from pT_{regs}; however, Delgoffe et al. later designated that Nrp1 was required by T_{reg} cells to limit antitumor immunity.[47] Importantly, tumor-infiltrating T_{reg} cells were largely observed to be $Nrp1^{hi}$ and Nrp1 was found to be dispensable for disruption without causing autoimmune events. Immune-cell-expressed ligand semaphorin-4a binds to T_{reg}-expressed Nrp1, enforcing T_{reg} cell stability and survival by restraining Akt phosphorylation, which consequently increased the nuclear localization of transcription factor Foxo3a. This activity enhances quiescence and survival programs, inhibiting further T_{reg} cell differentiation and exhaustive expenditure of effector functions.

TGF-β is enriched in the tumor microenvironment (TME). Many cells, including tumor, macrophages,

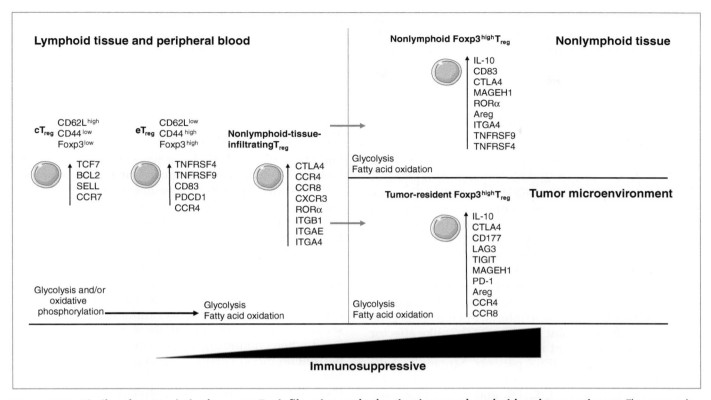

Figure 39.2 Similar characteristics between T_{reg} infiltration and adaption into nonlymphoid and tumor tissues. The process by which mouse and human naïve T_{regs} in circulation become activated and then are recruited into nonlymphoid tissues involves key phenotypic and metabolic changes that facilitate adaptation, survival, and suppressive functioning as seen when T_{regs} adapt to the TME. T_{reg} naïvety and T_{reg}-mediated immunosuppression is governed by the expression of signature cytokines, surface markers, integrins, and other factors.

Source: From Green JA, Arpaia N, Schizas M, Dobrin A. A nonimmune function of T cells in promoting lung tumor progression. *J Exp Med.* 2017;214:3565–3575. doi:10.1084/jem.20170356; Lee GS, Pan Y, Scanlon MJ, et al. Fatty acid-binding protein 5 mediates the uptake of fatty acids, but not drugs, into human brain endothelial cells. *J Pharm Sci.* 2018;107:1185–1193. doi:10.1016/j.xphs.2017.11.024; Miragaia RJ, Gomes T, Chomka A, et al. Single-cell transcriptomics of regulatory T cells reveals trajectories of tissue adaptation. *Immunity.* 2019;50:493–504. doi:10.1016/j.immuni.2019.01.001; Plitas G, Konopacki C, Wu K, et al. Regulatory T cells exhibit distinct features in human breast cancer. *Immunity.* 2016;45:1122–1134. doi:10.1016/j.immuni.2016.10.032.

myeloid cells, and fibroblasts, produce sufficient TGF-β to induce T_{reg} cell identity in naïve CD4+ T cells generating pT_{regs}, a de novo subset of nonlymphoid and/or tumor-infiltrating T_{reg} cells capable of promoting tumor growth. Thus, T_{reg} cell accumulation in the TME constitutes a major hurdle in the deliverance of antitumor treatment. Our understanding of the phenotypic consequences of Foxp3 upregulation has served to explain the impact of T_{reg} cells on tumor growth in the TME.

Immunosuppressive Mechanisms of Foxp3+ T_{reg} cells in the Tumor Microenvironment

In the TME, activated T_{reg} cells dominate in maintaining immune tolerance, outcompeting antitumor effector T_{conv} cells.[1] Ectopic Foxp3 expression confers immunosuppressive activity in T_{reg} cells and can induce T_{reg}-like qualities in T_{conv}. The latter will be discussed in a later section. Through several mechanisms—including the expression of cytotoxic T lymphocyte-associated protein 4 (CTLA4), glucocorticoid-induced TNF receptor (GITR), lymphocyte-activation gene 3 (LAG-3) expression, and/or IL-10, IL-35, TGF-β, adenosine production, and/or IL-2 absorption—T_{reg} cells can control the immune balance in a microenvironment among many cell types (Figure 39.2). For example, CTLA4 on T_{reg} cells downmodulates expression of co-stimulatory CD80 and CD86 on DCs, preventing the activation of antitumor T_{conv}.[52–54] CD25 or IL-2R on T_{reg} cells absorbs IL-2 from the environment, which limits the amount of IL-2 available to promote the activation and proliferation of

T_{conv}.[55] While Foxp3 expression supports the means by which T_{reg} cells maintain immune tolerance in the TME leading to tumor growth, disruption of Foxp3 expression impairs T_{reg} cell development and promotes spontaneous autoimmune disease.

Fundamental Consequence of Foxp3 Mutation on T_{reg} Cell Phenotype

Mutations of the gene encoding the T_{reg}-specific transcription factor Foxp3 impair T_{reg} cell development and cause a fatal autoimmune disease called immune dysregulation, polyendocrinopathy, enteropathy, and X-linked (IPEX) syndrome, affecting multiple organs.[56] In mice, the depletion of Foxp3+CD25+CD4+ T_{reg} cells by a variety of methods is sufficient to cause similar autoimmune diseases.[57] In human IPEX patients and in the rodent M370I (substitution of methionine for isoleucine at amino acid 370) mutant counterparts, there is a point mutation in the domain-swap interface of the *Foxp3* gene driving T_{reg} cells to exhibit T helper 2 (Th2)-like effector function.[58] M370I mutant mice recapitulate the T_{reg} cell phenotype observed in IPEX patients. Mutant T_{reg} cells from M370I mice do exhibit suppressive activity, still expressing Nrp1, CTLA4, GITR, and IL-10. However, they are aberrantly proliferative, highly expressing Ki67 and CD44 with downregulated CCR7. In addition, surface IL-2R was decreased in M370I mutant T_{reg} cells. Above all, the M370I mutation in the *Foxp3* gene disrupts the ability of T_{reg} cells to regulate and maintain immune homeostasis.

Foxp3 endows T_{reg} cells with their identity as immunosuppressive, self-tolerant immune cells. Foxp3 stability relies on a network of genetic and transcriptional programs, which support the production of cytokines and other factors sufficient to tip the immune balance in a TME. While Foxp3 regulates the development, homeostasis, and activity of T_{reg} cells in a TME, the T_{reg} cell population is composed of a diverse range of subsets. In the next section, we will survey the heterogeneity among Foxp3+CD25+CD4+ T_{reg} cells, explore the components that distinguish T_{reg} cell subsets, and show how certain components contribute to T_{reg}-mediated immunosuppression.

HETEROGENEITY AND PLASTICITY AMONG FOXP3+ T_{reg} CELL SUBSETS

Although Foxp3 expression gives T_{reg} cells their immunomodulatory functions, many other cellular components determine the phenotype of T_{reg} cells and form distinctions between T_{reg} cell subsets. Moreover, single-cell transcriptomic analysis provides unprecedented amounts of information as to the heterogeneity T_{reg} cell in circulation and diverse tissues, including TMEs. This calibration in our knowledge of T_{reg} cell heterogeneity of Foxp3+ endows researchers and clinicians with insights on novel molecular targets for specific control of distinct T_{reg} cell populations in order to achieve tumor immunity without disrupting the vital self-tolerance mediated by T_{reg} cells.

Three Major T_{reg} Cell Subsets

Dr. Sakaguchi and his team have demonstrated that human T_{reg} cells were composed of three phenotypically distinct subpopulations determined by the differential expression of CD25 and CD45RA, a marker for naïve T cells (Figure 39.3). So-called Fraction I (Fr. I) consists of CD25loCD45RA+ resting T_{reg} cells (rT$_{regs}$), Fr. II consists of CD25hiCD45RA- effector T_{reg} cells (eT$_{regs}$), and Fr. III consists of CD25loCD45RA (Figure 39.3).[49,50,59–61] Unlike Fr. I and Fr. II, Fr. III cells were nonsuppressive and more proinflammatory. We will discuss this particular subset more deeply in a later section. The proportion of these three subsets differed when comparing T_{reg} cell composition in cord or peripheral blood versus in aged individuals versus in patients with immunological diseases. Furthermore, these three subgroups also differ in terms of differentiation dynamics. Fr. II or eT$_{regs}$ express the highest Foxp3, IL-2R, Ki67, and CTLA4 demonstrating a highly proliferative, potent effector T_{reg} cell phenotype. Comparatively, Fr. I or resting T_{reg} cells (rT$_{regs}$) express lower Foxp3 and IL-2R and are less proliferative and immunosuppressive than the Fr. II aT$_{regs}$. In vivo, Fr. I rT$_{regs}$ localize predominantly in the peripheral and cord blood and can proliferate upon TCR stimulation. rT$_{reg}$ homeostasis persists throughout life but this cell number drops with age.[2,59,62,63] When stimulated, rT$_{regs}$ differentiate into eT$_{regs}$ and acquire Fr. II phenotype. eT$_{regs}$ demonstrate strong suppressive phenotype, but these cells are terminally differentiated and this activity is short-lived. The Fr. II eT$_{regs}$ compose a major proportion of the tumor-infiltrating T_{reg} cells that contribute to poor prognoses.

The TSDR methylation status varies from Fr. I to III, which results in differences in the maintenance of Foxp3 and immunosuppressive phenotypes across groups. The separation of T_{reg} cells into these three functional subpopulations continues to serve as a foundation in our understanding of T_{reg} cell heterogeneity. With this knowledge, a specific subset of Foxp3+ cells could be targeted and manipulated to modulate immune responses in a TME without destabilizing self-tolerance and promoting systemic autoimmune disorder. These three T_{reg} cell subdivisions could be further dissected according to more granular/modular components expressed by the T_{reg} cells, which further regulate the phenotype and function.

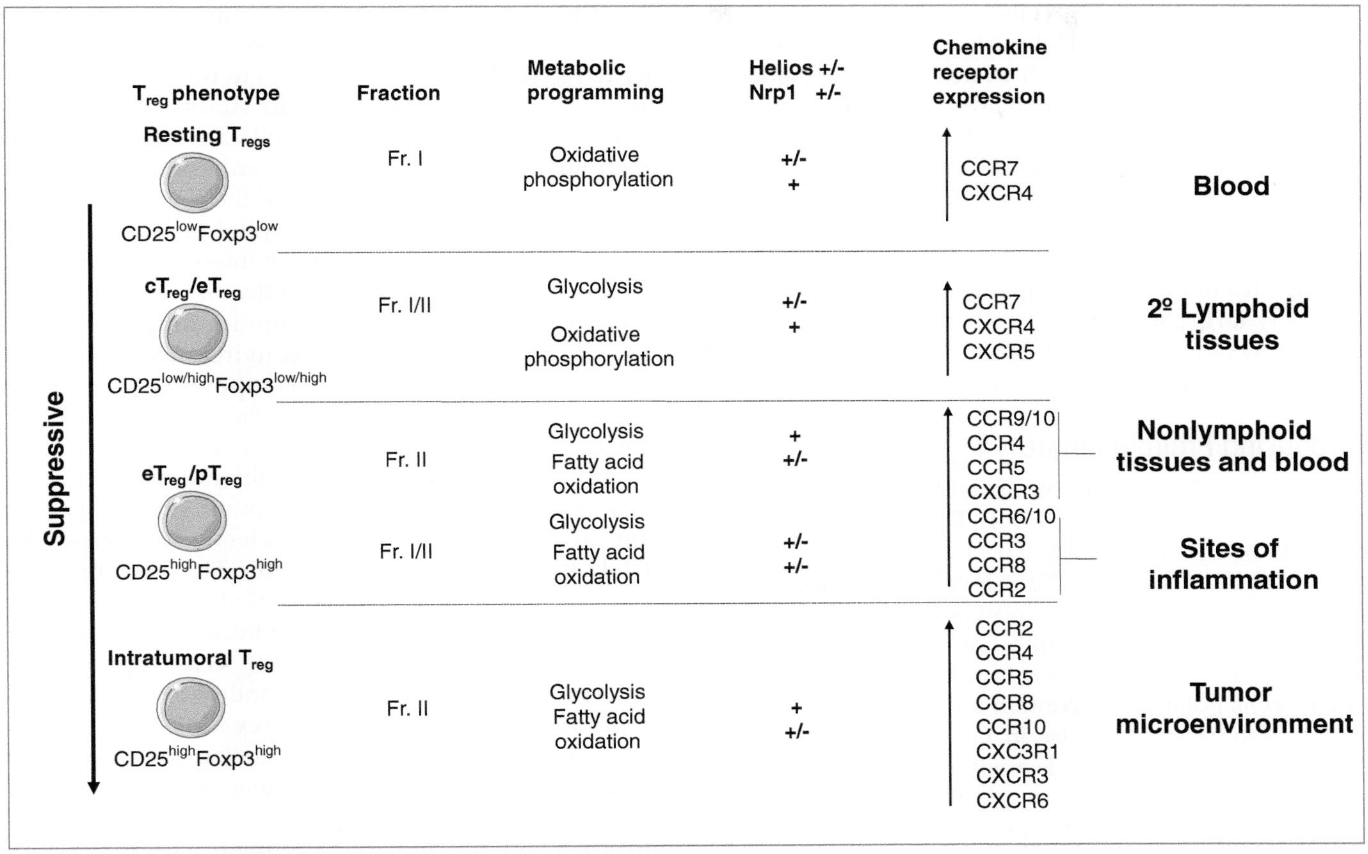

Figure 39.3 **Stratification and classification of T$_{reg}$ cell subsets across microenvironments.** Major human T$_{reg}$ subsets are distinguished according to metabolic programming, surface expression of Helios and neuropilin-1 molecules, chemotactic profile, and immunosuppressive phenotype.

Source: From Delgoffe GM, Woo SR, Turnis ME, et al. Stability and function of regulatory T cells is maintained by a neuropilin-1-semaphorin-4a axis. *Nature.* 2013;501:252–256. doi:10.1038/nature12428; Miragaia RJ, Gomes T, Chomka A, et al. Single-cell transcriptomics of regulatory T cells reveals trajectories of tissue adaptation. *Immunity.* 2019;50:493–504. doi:10.1016/j.immuni.2019.01.001; Plitas G, Konopacki C, Wu K, et al. Regulatory T cells exhibit distinct features in human breast cancer. *Immunity.* 2016;45:1122–1134. doi:10.1016/j.immuni.2016.10.032; Saxton RA, Sabatini DM. mTOR signaling in growth, metabolism, and disease. *Cell.* 2017;169:361–371. doi:10.1016/j.cell.2017.03.035; Thornton AM, Korty PE, Tran DQ, et al. Expression of Helios, an Ikaros transcription factor family member, differentiates thymic-derived from peripherally induced Foxp3+ T regulatory cells. *J Immunol.* 2010;184:3433–3441. doi:10.4049/jimmunol.0904028; Wing JB, Tanaka A, Sakaguchi S. Human FOXP3+ regulatory T cell heterogeneity and function in autoimmunity and cancer. *Immunity.* 2019;50:302–316. doi:10.1016/j.immuni.2019.01.020.

Helios Expression Delineates T$_{reg}$ Cell Origin and Phenotype

Phenotypic and functional differences among circulating and intratumoral T$_{reg}$ cells could also be defined by the expression of Helios, an Ikaros family transcription factor (Figure 39.3).[48] Developmentally, Helios expression differentiates tT$_{regs}$ from pT$_{regs}$. Across the three main T$_{reg}$ cell subgroups, Fr. II T$_{reg}$ cells in human blood uniformly express Helios, whereas Fr. I and III T$_{reg}$ cells contain both Helios-positive and -negative cells. Helios expression regulates Foxp3 stability such that Helios+Foxp3^{lo} and Helios+Foxp3^{hi} demonstrate similar levels of TSDR demethylation.[64,65] Since Helios

expression impacts TSDR demethylation, whether a T$_{reg}$ cell is Helios-positive or -negative determines the suppressive phenotype. Despite Foxp3 expression levels, Helios-deficient T$_{reg}$ cells exhibit effector phenotypes, producing proinflammatory cytokines.[66] Helios expression is positively correlated with immunosuppressive cell-surface receptor TIGIT, whereas Helios-deficient T$_{reg}$ cells are CD226-positive, which antagonizes the suppressive impact of TIGIT+ T$_{reg}$ cells in a microenvironment.[67] Helios-deficient T$_{reg}$ cells are not immunosuppressive; therefore, in the TME, Helios expression has functional and prognostic consequences. While Helios-Foxp3+ T$_{reg}$ cells show instability characterized by higher levels of TSDR methylation compared to Helios+ T$_{reg}$ cells, greater infiltration of Helios⁻ T_{reg} cells in a TME is associated with a better prognosis. Helios$^{fl/fl}$ Foxp3^{cre} mice demonstrate reduced tumor growth in multiple subcutaneous tumor models compared to wild-type counterparts. In addition, the majority of tumor-infiltrating Foxp3$^+$CD4$^+$ T_{reg} cells in these mice produced significant quantities of IFNg and TNF-α, while the tumors of wild-type mice had been infiltrated largely by immunosuppressive and anergic Foxp3$^+$CD4$^+$ T_{reg} cells. In a later section, we will discuss current immunotherapeutic interventions, which especially target strategic T_{reg} cell components, and will revisit how manipulating Helios expression can serve as a novel treatment option for a variety of cancers.

Introducing Proinflammatory T_{reg} Cells

Fr. III T_{reg} cells largely exhibit unstable Foxp3 expression and, unlike rT$_{regs}$ and eT$_{regs}$, Fr. III T_{reg} cells produce high amounts of IL-2 and IFNg. The Fr. III subset contains effector Th1 and Th17-like Foxp3$^+$ cells that demonstrate a more proinflammatory phenotype as opposed to Fr. I and II subsets. During autoimmune diseases such as systemic lupus erythematosus (SLE), the proportion of Fr. I-III T_{reg} cells polarizes to contain a significant increase in the Fr. III subset, a decrease in Fr. II, and no change to the Fr. I subset. In colorectal carcinoma (CRC), the tumor infiltration and accumulation of Fr. II cells results in poor prognosis, whereas Fr. III tumor infiltration shows a better prognosis, given the production of proinflammatory cytokines. Within the pT$_{reg}$ subset in the gut, Fr. III T_{reg} cells in CRC could be generated by the presence of particular gut microbes, such as Fusobacteria.[68] The proinflammatory T_{reg} cell population can be further fractioned into subsets that vary in suppressive activity.

Th-Like T_{reg} Cells

T_{reg} cell heterogeneity is further demonstrated by subsets of Th-like T_{reg} cells. Previously, we discussed how point-mutated Foxp3 drives T_{reg} cells to exhibit Th2 phenotypes, which is the source of the dysregulation to T_{reg} cell homeostasis, consequently causing autoimmune disorders such as IPEX in humans.[58] However, T_{reg} cells can demonstrate Th-like qualities in both healthy and pathologic conditions. Within the past decade, Duhen et al. characterized a novel subpopulation of so-called memory T_{reg} cells, also known as Th-like T_{reg} cells.[69] In addition to Foxp3 expression, these cells also express CXCR3, CCR6, CCR4, chemokines, typically expressed by T-bet$^+$-Th1, RORgt$^+$-Th17, and GATA3$^+$-Th2 subsets, respectively.[70] Importantly, these IFNg$^+$Th1 and IL-17$^+$Th17-like T_{reg} cells express higher amounts of Foxp3 than the IL-4$^+$IL-5$^+$IL-13$^+$ Th2-like T_{reg} cells. Indeed, Foxp3 expression among these Th-like T_{reg} cell subsets serves as a proapoptotic metric.[71] Since the Th2-like T_{reg} cells express a low amount of Foxp3, this subset exhibits an enhanced survival and viability.[58,70] In addition, the

Th2-like T_{reg} cell subset produces autocrine IL-2, propagating its own activation and proliferation. This quality to resist cell death contributes to the Th2-like T_{reg} cell ability to promote tumor growth. Across the Th-like T_{reg} cell subsets, the Th2-like T_{reg} cells are most associated with supporting a tumorigenic environment. Th2-like T_{reg} cells compose the majority of the T_{reg} cells that infiltrate and accumulate in nonlymphoid tissues as well as melanoma and colorectal cancer. Interestingly, Halim et al. showed how Th2-polarized effectors and T_{reg} cells can "collaborate" in promoting immunosuppression over the other subsets in a microenvironment. Following TCR activation, Th-like T_{reg} cells suppress the proinflammatory cytokines produced by the Th effectors except the IL-10 produced by the Th2 effectors. The Th2-like T_{reg} cells do not suppress the proliferation of Th2 effectors as much as they do to the other subsets, perhaps due to differences in how the Th effectors respond to TIGIT$^+$T$_{regs}$. Co-inhibitory molecule TIGIT expressed by Th2-like T_{reg} cells selectively inhibits proinflammatory Th1 and Th17 cells but not Th2 effector cells. Therefore, the process by which Th2-like T_{reg} cells suppress only Th1 and Th17 effectors and the ability for Th2 effectors to produce IL-10 unabated and to evade TIGIT-mediated immunosuppression constitute major contributions to maintaining a TME. Taken together, while Th-like phenotypes can occur naturally in T_{reg} cells, Th2-like T_{reg} cells are especially capable of promoting tumor growth.

While both Th1- and Th17-like T_{reg} cells can exhibit more proinflammatory phenotypes, each subset has distinct qualities. Moreover, the Th17-like RORgt$^+$ T_{reg} cells demonstrate superior suppressive activity during inflammation and cancer. Th1-like Foxp3$^+$CXCR3$^+$T-bet$^+$ T_{reg} cells accumulate at sites of inflammation and are essential for the homeostasis and regulation during type 1 inflammation.[72] Importantly, activated Th1-like T_{reg} cells produce IFN-g and are, therefore, capable of promoting antitumor responses in the TME[70,73,74] The Th17-like Foxp3$^+$CCR6$^+$RORgt$^+$ T_{reg} cells exhibit a strong suppressive phenotype during colitis.[75] Whether the Th17-like T_{reg} cells exhibit a pro- or anti-inflammatory phenotype depends on the balance between concentrations of cytokines such as IL-6, IL-21, and IL-23 or TGF-β, respectively.[76–79] Th17-like T_{reg} cells localize mainly in the gastrointestinal tract and therefore adapt to local cues including the composition of the gut microbiota.[74,76] RORgt$^+$ T_{reg} cells constitute a stable T_{reg} cell lineage demonstrated by fully demethylated TSDR and *CTLA4* regions. Notably, they exhibit superior suppressive capacity during T cell–mediated intestinal inflammation.[75] Furthermore, substantial numbers of IL-17$^+$Foxp3$^+$ T_{reg} cells accumulate in the mucosa of colitis-associated colon cancer carcinoma.[80] The RORgt$^+$ Foxp3$^+$ T_{reg} cells exhibit higher expression of IL-10, CTLA4, CCR4, and CCR6 than the RORgt⁻Foxp3$^+$ T_{reg} cells indicating that RORgt expression endows T_{reg} cells with a higher suppressive potency.[75]

T$_{reg}$ Cell Plasticity

T$_{reg}$ cells exhibit significant developmental and functional plasticity within and across tissues, in health, and in disease. The means by which activated T$_{reg}$ cells adapt to nonlymphoid tissues informs us on the transcriptional programs established as T$_{reg}$ cells infiltrate and accumulate within tumors (Figure 39.3). As we endeavor to characterize the range of variation across T$_{reg}$ cell subsets, we rely on the power of modern computational tools, such as single-cell sequencing, processing, and analysis, in order to observe T$_{reg}$ cell subset-specific differences in gene expression. For example, Azizi et al. profiled over 45,000 immune cells from eight breast carcinomas, as well as from various matched tissues, and they were able to selectively observe that the terminally differentiated immune cells found in the tumor included GITR$^+$OX40$^+$CTLA4$^+$TIGIT$^+$IL-2RA$^+$CD39$^+$Foxp3$^+$ T$_{reg}$ cells, among other subsets.[81,82] These T$_{reg}$ cell clusters featured similar patterns for distinct anti-inflammatory, exhaustion, hypoxia, and metabolism gene sets. Knowledge of the distinct transcriptional profiles, which lead to specific T$_{reg}$ cell phenotypes, provides insight into how to modulate T$_{reg}$ cell activity. Comprehensive understanding of the plasticity of T$_{reg}$ cell phenotypes prepares our understanding for the ways in which T$_{reg}$ cells can acquire defective functions suitable to promote tumor growth. Genetic, epigenetic, and metabolic events control T$_{reg}$ cell phenotype and function both in health and in disease. Knowledge of the modular components of these events sufficient to drive T$_{reg}$ cell phenotypes is used in the development of treatment strategies and therapeutics.

Single-cell transcriptomics permits a calibrated view and characterization of a wide variety of T$_{reg}$ cell subsets. Modern sequencing technologies and analytic methods enhance the resolution of our scope of T$_{reg}$ cell heterogeneity. Tissue-specific conditions govern T$_{reg}$ cell phenotype and plasticity, as well as disease states. During development and steady-state conditions, T$_{reg}$ cells traffic into nonlymphoid tissues (Figure 39.3).[83,84] Migrating T$_{reg}$ cells acquire tissue-specific integrins, chemokines, and receptors sufficient to promote distinct phenotypes across a diversity of T$_{reg}$ cell subsets.[85,86] Importantly, single-cell RNA sequencing data reveals phenotypically and functionally distinct properties of the subsets localized in specific tissue types. Transcriptional profiles form distinct clusters between T$_{reg}$ cell subsets from lymphoid tissues versus those from nonlymphoid tissues. As T$_{reg}$ cells adapt from lymphoid tissues to nonlymphoid tissues, such as barrier regions like the skin or the colon, they exhibit more activated and suppressive gene expression signatures. Compared to lymphoid tissue T$_{reg}$ cells, nonlymphoid tissue T$_{reg}$ cells upregulate IL-10, CD83, CCR4, CCR8, CTLA4, and granzyme B, as well as multiple TNF receptors and transducers and other components along the TNF receptor superfamily-NF-kB axis.[49] Importantly,

these cells upregulate several chemokines and integrins as they migrate and infiltrate nonlymphoid tissues (Figure 39.3). Functionally, the lymphoid tissue T$_{reg}$ cells are associated with the naïve or Fr. I (CD45RA$^+$Foxp3^{lo}) T$_{reg}$ cell phenotype distinguished by the expression of Tcf7, Bcl2, Sell, and Nrp1, among, other factors. Among the lymphoid tissues, central T$_{regs}$ (cT$_{regs}$) have been identified to express these naïve-like markers whereas the eT$_{regs}$ exhibit a transcriptional program closely associated with the more activated nonlymphoid tissue T$_{reg}$ cells. eT$_{regs}$ may demonstrate this phenotype as a means to prepare to migrate and to adapt to nonlymphoid tissues and to exhibit strong immunosuppression amid the diversity of antigens found in the barrier tissues.[40] For example, along the trajectory from the mesenteric lymph node to the lamina propria of the colon, cT$_{regs}$ differentiate into eT$_{regs}$ acquiring a Fr. II T$_{reg}$ cell transcriptional program, followed by a nonlymphoid tissue-like and then back to a lymphoid tissue-like phenotype before gaining the full suppressive T$_{reg}$ cell phenotype characteristic of the nonlymphoid tissue T$_{reg}$ cells.[49] T$_{reg}$ cell migration and phenotype heterogeneity across tissue types involve common mechanisms with the process by which tumor tissues recruit T$_{reg}$ cells into a TME.

The Resemblance Between Nonlymphoid T$_{reg}$ Cells and Tumor T$_{reg}$ Cells

The means by which T$_{reg}$ cells can migrate from lymphoid tissues, polarize, and adapt to nonlymphoid tissues are consistent with the processes by which T$_{reg}$ cells are recruited by tumor tissues (Figure 39.3). Tumor T$_{reg}$ cells are likely recruited de novo from lymphoid tissues and not from adjacent nonlymphoid tissues despite tumor T$_{reg}$ cells exhibiting a phenotype similar to that of nonlymphoid T$_{reg}$ cells.[50,87] Tumor T$_{reg}$ cells upregulate exhaustion marker LAG-3, as well as CXCR3, CCL5, CCR8, and TIGIT.[49,88] Importantly, the transcriptional signatures that T$_{reg}$ cells acquire along the trajectory toward tumor infiltration, which include genes in the TNF receptor superfamily -NF-kB axis, are shared by normal cT$_{regs}$ adapting to nonlymphoid tissues at steady-state.[49] Therefore, some of the characteristic phenotypes found in nonlymphoid tissue T$_{reg}$ cells may also be present in tumor-infiltrating T$_{reg}$ cells.

In addition to the immune phenotype of "emigré" T$_{reg}$ cells in nonlymphoid tissues, this subset can participate in "nonimmune" functions that also take place during tumorigenesis. Nonlymphoid tissue T$_{reg}$ cells engage in tissue repair.[89] Beyond suppressing proinflammatory chemokine and cytokine production and endothelial cell activation, T$_{reg}$ cells can mediate tissue repair and remodeling through the production of amphiregulin, a ligand to epidermal growth factor receptor (EGF-R).[90,91] T$_{reg}$ cells isolated from visceral adipose tissue, muscle, and in the gut lamina propria during inflammation express amphiregulin. Importantly, amphiregulin was upregulated in lung tumor-resident T_{reg} cells, including other genes involved in wound healing, such as *Mmp12, Plau, Hpse, and Fn1*.[60] While both Foxp3[+] and Foxp3[-] CD4[+] T cells produce high amounts of amphiregulin in the lung TME compared to CD4[+] T cells from normal lung tissue, CD4[+] Foxp3[+] T_{reg} cells produced notably more amphiregulin promoting lung tumor growth.[92] Ablation of T_{reg} cells in Foxp3[DTR] mice-harboring Lewis lung carcinoma tumors caused a reduction in tumor size, along with an upsurge in activated CD4[+] and CD8[+] T cell infiltration into the tumor. This tumor growth-promoting role of T_{reg} cells is independent of tumor cell signaling and alterations in vasculature across a variety of cancers. Therefore, we see here the nonimmune means by which T_{reg} cells can adapt to functioning in non-lymphoid tissues and how these adaptive features in the scenario of cancer contribute to tumor growth.

Distinct Features of Tumor-Resident T_{reg} Cells

Within the diversity of immune phenotypes in a TME, T_{reg} cells exhibit a distinct range of features. The capacity with which T_{reg} cells adapt within a TME is originally required for the processes by which T_{reg} cells migrate and adapt into nonlymphoid tissues, as previously mentioned. For example, in breast cancer, tumor-resident T_{reg} cells showed very similar gene expression patterns as normal breast parenchyma-resident T_{reg} cells.[50] Both normal nonlymphoid tissue and tumor-resident T_{reg} cell populations contain mostly highly expanded clones, proliferating similarly to the CD45RO[+] T_{reg} cells as found in the Fr. II of peripheral T_{reg} cells. The transcriptional profile exhibited by T_{reg} cells resident in nonlymphoid tissues can inform us as to the gene change characteristics that occur in tumor-infiltrating T_{reg} cells. Nevertheless, while the tumor-resident T_{reg} cells share phenotypic and functional qualities with nonlymphoid tissue T_{reg} cells, the tumor-resident T_{reg} cells show increased expression of genes involved in cell activation and inflammatory response, as well as cytokine and chemokine signaling. Importantly, a range of effector-like chemokine receptors, including CCR5, CCR8, CCR10, CXC3CR1, CXCR3, and CXCR6, are especially upregulated in tumor-resident T_{reg} cells. Notably, CD177—a receptor known to be implicated in neutrophil extravasation and survival—was highly expressed in tumor-resident T_{reg} cells in melanoma, lung, breast, and colorectal cancers and associated with the most suppressive T_{reg} cell subsets.[93,94] In addition, tumor-resident T_{reg} cells specifically express higher proinflammatory IL-1R2, IL-27, and OX40 in comparison to nonlymphoid tissues, such as normal breast parenchyma. These highly activated tumor-resident T_{reg} cells are also strongly suppressive characteristics of the Foxp3[hi] Fr. II T_{reg} cell subset. As tumor-resident T_{reg} cells transcriptionally and functionally

resemble T_{reg} cells that have migrated into nonlymphoid tissues, the tumor-resident T_{reg} cells are demonstrating an adaptive phenotype in response to the local factors in the TME. Among the various chemokine receptors selectively upregulated in tumor-resident T_{reg} cells, CCR8 has been identified to be robustly expressed in breast cancers and, therefore, can serve as a prognostic metric.[50]

T_{reg} Cell Tumor Trafficking Into Tumor Microenvironment

T_{reg} cells traffic to different environments via distinct chemokine receptor and chemokine pathways.[95] Bone marrow CD4[+] T_{reg} cells express functional CXCR4, the receptor for CXCL12. In patients with tumor bone marrow metastasis, CXCR4/CXCL12 signals are crucial for CD4[+] T_{reg} cell bone marrow trafficking and retention. Bone marrow T_{reg} cells contribute to tumor bone marrow pathology.[96] Using human ovarian cancer as an example, early study has defined that human tumor CD4[+] T_{reg} cells express functional CCR4, the receptor for CCL22, and migrate toward tumor microenvironmental CCL22 in vitro and in vivo. The source of tumor CCL22 appears to be cancer cells and tumor-associated macrophages.[97] Subsequent studies have confirmed this observation and extended to many other solid epithelial carcinomas.[98] In addition to CCR4, CCR8 facilitates the migration of T_{reg} cells into sites of inflammation as well as into the tumor tissue.[99–101] Intratumoral myeloid CCL1, one of the cognate ligands of CCR8, serves as a chemoattractant for the highly activated and suppressive T_{reg} cells to infiltrate the tumor tissue.[102–104] In studying the distinct trafficking features of tumor T_{reg} cells, we can devise strategies to therapeutically target specific components on T_{reg} cells so as to disrupt their protumor activity without disrupting homeostatic global T_{reg} cell self-tolerance.

METABOLIC REGULATION OF T_{reg} CELL PHENOTYPE

Metabolism also contributes to the stabilization of Foxp3 expression and, therefore, to T_{reg} cells suppressive activity. As previously mentioned, the TSDR methylation status determines the Foxp3 stability. Mammalian ten-eleven translocation (TET) enzymes maintain the demethylated status of several regulatory regions in the mouse *Foxp3* gene.[23,24,105,106] TET family members oxidize methylated cytosine to the intermediate stages in DNA methylation. Vitamin C induces TET family demethylase activity in the *Foxp3* TSDR (Figure 39.1). Importantly, vitamin C has been shown to stabilize Foxp3 expression in iT$_{regs}$ in vitro by modulating the TSDR demethylation.[74,107] Various other metabolic components, such as nutrients and metabolites, contribute to the induction and stability of Foxp3. As previously mentioned, in the gastrointestinal (GI) tract, retinoic acid RA and TGF-β produced by CD103[+] DCs can induce Foxp3 expression and consequently suppressive activity in naïve CD4$^+$ T cells producing pT$_{reg}$ cells.[45] Also in the gut, other dietary metabolites, such as short-chain fatty acids (SCFAs) produced by commensal microbes, can promote the development and function of colonic T$_{reg}$ cells through the induction of Foxp3 in a histone deacetylase-dependent manner.[108–111] While the fundamental stabilization of Foxp3 expression is regulated by metabolic factors, other aspects of T$_{reg}$ cell phenotype and activity are determined by specific metabolic programs and nutrient signals.

T$_{reg}$ Cell Versus T$_{conv}$ Metabolism

T cell differentiation states differ by phenotype and therefore also by metabolic programming. T$_{conv}$ cells use aerobic glycolysis and not oxidative phosphorylation (OXPHOS), while T$_{reg}$ cells primarily use fatty acid oxidation (FAO).[112–115] mTOR serves as a sensor of the metabolic environment and regulates glucose metabolism in activated T cells.[116,117] Downstream of TCR signaling, mTOR kinase signaling cascades regulate T$_{reg}$ cell homeostasis and proliferation.[118,119] mTOR-deficient T cells are converted into Foxp3$^+$ T$_{reg}$ cells.[120,121] Fundamentally, inhibition of glycolysis and mTOR signaling may favor FAO and facilitate the generation of T$_{reg}$ cells.[122,123] Further, inhibition of mTOR leads to TSDR region demethylation and increase in Foxp3 expression and therefore the suppressive phenotype of T$_{reg}$ cells.[124,125] Nevertheless, T$_{reg}$ cells implement alternating metabolic programs—glycolysis, OXPHOS, or FAO—depending on the differentiation state and the microenvironment.

Metabolism and T$_{reg}$ Cell Phenotype

T$_{reg}$ cell metabolism is governed by the level of Foxp3 expression and by microenvironment conditions, which, in turn, shape the T$_{reg}$ cell suppressive activity. As previously mentioned, T$_{conv}$ cells undergo aerobic glycolysis; similarly, Foxp3-deficient T$_{reg}$ cells implement heightened aerobic glycolysis, which is associated with low suppressive capacity. Contrarily, in homeostatic conditions, Foxp3 controls T$_{reg}$ cell metabolism by promoting FAO and by limiting glycolysis through the inhibition of c-myc and mTORC2 pathways, resulting in more potent suppressive activity.[126] During inflammatory conditions, signals as from Toll-like receptors promote glycolysis by inducing Glut1 expression via mTORC1 and simultaneously modulate Foxp3 expression exhibiting less FAO but more glycolysis and OXPHOS than in the homeostatic conditions. The highest suppressive ability achieved by T$_{reg}$ cells occurs when they implement FAO. Still, T$_{reg}$ cells activated through mTOR signaling can demonstrate immunosuppressive properties depending on the differentiation state and microenvironment.

Introducing mTOR Signaling in Suppressive Effector T$_{reg}$ Cells

As previously mentioned, once T$_{reg}$ cells from the thymus emigrate to the peripheral tissues, the TCR signals along the way promote the conversion of the CD44^{lo}CD62L^{hi} cT$_{regs}$ into the more suppressive CD44^{hi}CD62L^{lo} eT$_{regs}$. eT$_{regs}$, or effector T$_{reg}$ cells, belong to the Fr. II subset and, accordingly, produce potent immunosuppressive factors, notably in nonlymphoid tissues or site of inflammation.[1,49,126] At these capacities, eT$_{regs}$ use both glycolysis and OXPHOS to fuel their suppressive activity. mTORC1 signaling in T$_{reg}$ cells promotes cholesterol and lipid metabolism, including the mevalonate pathway critical for coordinating T$_{reg}$ cell proliferation, differentiation, and upregulation of suppressive molecules, such as CTLA4 and ICOS.[119] Effector T$_{reg}$ cells depend on mTOR signaling, balancing between OXPHOS to exhibit immunosuppressive phenotypes and to maintain cellular fitness; and glucose uptake and glycolysis to facilitate migration.[127,128]

Nutrient Signaling Permits mTOR Activity in Effector T$_{reg}$ Cells

The mTOR kinase activity responsible for the T$_{reg}$ cell demonstration of immunosuppressive phenotypes requires amino acid triggers. Amino acids stimulate mTORC1 activity through the coordinated signaling of small G proteins Rag and Rheb. Fundamentally, mammalian cells express amino acid sensors that activate Rag GTPases.[51,129] Amino acid-dependent activation of mTORC1 requires RagA; also, amino acids can activate mTORC1 by inactivating the Tsc complex, a negative regulator of the small G protein Rhe127.[1,130–132] In T$_{reg}$ cells, amino acid signals are integrated by the Rag and Rheb proteins to permit TCR-induced mTORC1 activation and to maintain mTORC1 signaling in eT$_{reg}$ cells. Compared to naïve CD4$^+$ T cells, T$_{reg}$ cells show higher expression of Sestrin 1 (a leucine sensor) and CASTOR1/2 (an arginine sensor), suggesting that their critical functions depend on amino acid signals. Deficiency in the RagA/B proteins and/or depriving T$_{reg}$ cells of amino acids impairs TCR-induced mTOR activity and therefore mTOR localization to the lysosome in T$_{reg}$ cells.[133] Importantly, genetic deletion of Rag and Rheb proteins results in the development of fatal autoimmunity, revealing the necessity of mTOR signaling in T$_{reg}$ cell survival and function. Both RagA/B- and Rheb1/2-deficient T$_{reg}$ cells show significantly downregulated OXPHOS pathway and Myc targets that induce glycolytic programs. RagA/B deficiency, however, more significantly impacts the expression of mitochondrial genes and therefore OXPHOS.[76] RagA/B promotes eT$_{reg}$ differentiation, accumulation, and function. The generation of eT$_{regs}$, not cT$_{regs}$, requires mTOR functioning.[134] Compared to cT$_{regs}$, eT$_{regs}$ exhibit increased expression of

CD98 and SLC7A1, leucine, and arginine transporters, respectively. Metabolomics analysis of T_{reg} cells reveals increased intracellular concentrations of multiple amino acids upon activation, which initiates and maintains mTORC1 activation in eT_{regs}.[128] Arginine and leucine have been identified to significantly induce mTOR activation in eT_{regs} consistent with the observations of upregulated arginine and leucine sensors and transporters in effector T_{reg} cells (in vivo) and activated T_{reg} cells (in vitro). Taken together, the transcriptional programs maintaining T_{reg}-mediated immunosuppression depends on mTOR activity, which is fueled by amino acid signaling through small G proteins.

Foxp3 Expression Can Occur Independently of mTOR Signaling

mTORC1 plays a central role in maintaining the balance between anabolic and catabolic processes.[51] While mTOR signaling regulates T_{reg} cell homeostasis and function, the networks linking mTOR activity to the specific metabolic programs responsible for T_{reg} cell immunosuppressive phenotype remain complex. $CTLA4^+KLRG1^+CD98^+Ki67^+$ eT_{regs} have higher mTOR activity than the $CD62L^+CD25^+Bcl2^+$ cT_{regs} with no difference in Foxp3 expression.[132] Nevertheless, inappropriate mTORC1 activation and dysregulated glycolysis in T_{reg} cells lead to decreased Foxp3 expression and consequently reduced suppressive activity.[135] Still, Foxp3 stability does not always depend directly on metabolic programming. T_{reg}-specific deletion of mitochondrial transcription factor A (Tfam), an essential component in mitochondrial respiration and mitochondrial DNA replication, impairs T_{reg} cell maintenance specifically in nonlymphoid and tumor tissues under inflammatory contexts. In this situation, Tfam deficiency in T_{reg} cells switches OXPHOS toward glycolysis, simultaneously destabilizing Foxp3 associated with the enhancement of TSDR methylation in the Foxp3 locus.[136] Tissue-resident T_{reg} cells require Tfam for Foxp3 stability and OXPHOS-dependent suppressive functions only in low-glucose, inflammatory environments, whereas in the absence of inflammation, Tfam is dispensable for Foxp3 stability.[136] In addition, Weinberg et al. showed that specific deletion of mitochondrial complex III in T_{reg} cells impairs suppressive function without altering Foxp3 expression.[137] Taken together, while metabolic programs do impact T_{reg} cell phenotypes, they do not necessarily directly impact Foxp3 stability. Metabolic factors can modulate Foxp3 stability and, as we will see, Foxp3 can impact metabolism. Importantly, T_{reg} cell suppressive functions depend on specific metabolic programs and metabolism does play a major role in shaping T_{reg} cell phenotypes in both homeostasis and cancer.

T_{reg} cells rely less on glycolysis for energy production compared to the other $CD4^+$ subsets: Th1, Th2, Th17.[76,114] Again, Foxp3 expression is actually sufficient to reprogram T cell metabolism by suppressing glycolysis and enhancing OXPHOS.[138,139] In certain scenarios, elevated glycolysis may impede T_{reg} cell suppressive activity as inhibition of glycolysis promotes the induction of Foxp3 expression upon stimulation with IL-2 and TGF-β.[112,140] While c-Myc promotes glycolysis, the autophagy that occurs to maintain suppressive T_{reg} cell phenotypes inhibits c-Myc expression.[39,141] Still, T_{reg} cells rely on glycolysis during migration.[142] Reasonably, T_{reg} cells balance metabolic programs depending on the situation. Nevertheless, both at a steady state and in the TME, mitochondrial metabolism, OXPHOS, and FAO support T_{reg} cell suppressive activity.[75,137, 143,144]

Metabolism and T_{reg} Cell-Mediated Tumorigenesis

T_{reg} cell metabolism shapes the phenotypes necessary to adapt to different immune scenarios and environments. Understanding how metabolic programs permit T_{reg} cells to acquire different functions and activities provides insight into certain metabolic events implicated in T_{reg}-mediated tumor growth. Tumor-resident T_{reg} cells have been shown to rely on a combination of glycolysis and fatty acid synthesis and oxidation permitting survival and proliferation in the hostile TME.[145] As previously mentioned, T_{reg}-cell proliferation, survival, and upregulation of suppressive molecules rely on lipid metabolism-fueled OXPHOS promoted by mTORC1 signaling.[30] To meet metabolic needs, tumor-resident T_{reg} cells resort to acquiring and using extracellular free fatty acids.[146]

Fatty acid-binding proteins (FABPs) are lipid chaperones responsible for fatty acid uptake from the microenvironment, trafficking lipids to select organelles, such as nucleus, peroxisomes, endoplasmic reticulum (ER), and mitochondria.[61,147,148] FABP5 is particularly highly expressed in T_{conv} and T_{reg} cells; but more so in T_{reg} cells.[149,150] Inhibiting or knocking down FABP5 in T_{reg} cells disrupts T_{reg} cell proliferation, mitochondrial respiratory functioning, and lipid metabolism. Unexpectedly, FABP5 inhibition increases T_{reg} cell suppressive activity despite the compromised OXPHOS.[100] FABP5 disruption impairs mitochondrial Tfam, damaging mitochondrial integrity and respiratory functions. Under these metabolic stress conditions, the mitochondria release their mtDNA molecules into the cytosol, which ultimately serves as agonists on the cGAS-STING pathway. The cGAS-STING system senses the mtDNA, which consequently drives type I IFN signaling in the T_{reg} cells.[151] Importantly, the type IFNs can promote IL-10 production by T_{reg} cells in vitro, ex vivo, and in vivo in the TME.[152,153] Indeed, the nutrient-sparse TME prevents T_{reg} cell OXPHOS simulating the FABP5-deficient conditions, and promotes type I IFN signaling and subsequently IL-10 production by T_{reg} cells.[61] This IL-10 enhances T_{reg} cell suppression despite the disruption of OXPHOS by the low nutrient TME and, with the enhanced immunosuppression, effector T cell function is disrupted and the tumor can continue to grow.

Given the metabolically abnormal TME, how tumor-resident T_{reg} cells behave in the TME continues to be an area of intense research study. The protumor immunosuppressive phenotype exhibited by T_{reg} cells does not always depend on the expression of factors such as PD-L1, CTLA4, TGF-β, IL-35, and IL-10. T_{reg}-derived adenosine mediates immunosuppression sufficient to abolish the antitumor efficacy of PD-L1-blockade therapy.[154] The highly proliferative T_{reg} cells in the TME become highly apoptotic, and those apoptotic T_{reg} cells release ATP and metabolize it into adenosine. The hypoxic TME favors glycolytic metabolism, which strongly impacts and disrupts the activity of effector T cells.[155–157] Glucose restriction in the TME does not disrupt T_{reg} cells as it typically does T_{conv} but the oxidative stress from the TME induces apoptosis in the T_{reg} cells.[150] Apoptotic T_{reg} cells release high levels of ATP via pannexin-1-dependent channels and convert it to adenosine through the CD39 and CD73 enzymatic activity.[158] Effector T cells interact with adenosine through their A2A receptors, which specifically mediate IL-2 suppression; thus, antitumor immunity is disrupted.[104,159,160]

T_{reg} cell adaptation to the lactic acid-enriched TME serves as a driving factor in tumor progression. The previously described single-cell transcriptomic studies on T_{reg} cells migrating and then adapting into nonlymphoid tissues underscores the plasticity of T_{reg} cell phenotypes and the vast set of transcriptional changes necessary to achieve adaptation.[49] Many of the phenotypic changes that occur within T_{reg} cell infiltrating nonlymphoid and/or tumor tissues drive an increase in T_{reg} cell suppressive activity.[49,50] As previously mentioned, the TME imposes metabolic stressors on infiltrating cells, including acidosis, hypoxia, and nutrient deprivation.[104,161] Consequently, intratumoral T_{reg} cells must adjust their metabolic preferences to support their survival and functions in response to this environment. Contrary to circulating T_{reg} cells, intratumoral T_{reg} cells upregulate CD36 to support mitochondrial fitness and biogenesis in the TME.[162] CD36 serves as a "scavenger receptor" tasked with long-chain fatty acid and oxidized low-density lipoprotein uptake.[163] Heightened CD36 expression in tumor-resident T_{reg} cells positively correlates with increased lipid metabolism, proliferation, immunosuppression, and T_{reg} cell survival. CD36 lipid uptake in tumor-resident T_{reg} cells activates peroxisome proliferator-activated receptor (PPAR) b/g signaling known to enhance mitochondrial oxidation, supporting metabolic fitness and endurance.[164–166] Importantly, CD36 is dispensable; genetic ablation does not elicit T_{reg} cell autoimmunity, and therefore CD36 constitutes a practical target in cancer immunotherapy. Indeed, blocking CD36 activity in the TME with an anti-CD36 monoclonal antibody results in reduced tumor infiltration by T_{reg} cells and consequently reduced tumor growth, while maintaining the integrity of T_{reg} cell function in regions outside of the tumor. In addition, PD-1 blockade therapy spontaneously potentiates the antitumor effects of CD36 blockade.[158]

TARGETING T_{reg} CELLS IN CANCER PATIENTS

In recent years, there have been close to 20 million new cancer diagnoses and close to 10 million deaths due to cancer annually.[167] Tumors enriched with T_{reg} cells are associated with aggressive cancers and therefore poor prognoses.[1,50] Therefore, targeting T_{reg} cells constitutes a reasonable treatment strategy, given the involvement of T_{reg} cells in tumor progression (Figure 39.3). The essential homeostatic role of T_{reg} cells in maintaining self-tolerance continues to pose significant obstacles in achieving tumor immunity. Tumor antigens resemble self- and quasi-self-antigens, thereby protecting tumors from tumor immunity.[1] Therefore, identifying dispensable components of T_{reg} cell structure and function that can be manipulated as a treatment strategy without triggering an autoimmune response remains as one of the utmost priorities in cancer immunotherapy.[168] Foxp3 expression, in particular, is indispensable for balanced T_{reg} cell functioning and cannot be safely modified.[1] Nevertheless, many alternative strategies have been devised to target T_{reg} cell components so as to modulate T_{reg} cell suppressive activity without impairing Foxp3 expression and self-tolerance. Continued progress in this endeavor requires the study of T_{reg} cell heterogeneity so as to identify the parts and functions of T_{reg} cells that can be targeted.

Throughout the chapter, we surveyed the T_{reg} cell properties according to which T_{reg} cells are delineated into distinguished functional subsets. In pointing out the differences among T_{reg} cell subsets, we aim to clarify which parts of T_{reg} cells can be targeted in therapies. The following studies demonstrate the range of strategies taken to target T_{reg} cell components beyond CTLA4, PD-1, PD-L1, and TGF-β production so as to either thwart or redirect T_{reg} cell function for the purpose of favoring antitumor immunity.

Targeting CD25

As previously mentioned, IL-2R or CD25 plays a central role in T_{reg} cell development, homeostasis, and suppressive activity.[210–213] Through CD25, T_{reg} cells mediate immunosuppression by "starving" the environment of immunostimulatory IL-2, partially depriving effector T cells of the means to carry out antitumor responses.[214] Targeting CD25 so as to induce antitumor immunity without disrupting vital T_{reg} cell Foxp3 expression constitutes an important and reasonable therapeutic strategy. Daclizumab, a U.S. Food and Drug Administration (FDA)-approved CD25-blocking monoclonal antibody (mAb), downregulates the intratumoral CD25^{hi} CD45RA^{-} or the Fr. II eT_{reg} subset associated

Table 39.1 Current and Emerging Clinical Targeting of T$_{regs}$ Cells

	TARGET	TARGET CATEGORY	FUNCTION	INTERVENTION METHOD	NAME	COMPANY STUDIES REFERENCES
EXISTING	CCR4	Chemokine receptor	Blocks trafficking	Monoclonal antibody	Mogamulizumab	Kyowa Hakka Kirin Co., Ltd[169–171]
	CD21	Cytokine receptor	T$_{reg}$ cell depletion	Monoclonal antibody	Daclizumab	Biogen and Abbvie[172–175]
	Neuropilin-1 (NRP1)	Inhibitory surface molecule	Neutralizes T$_{reg}$ cell surface inhibition	Monoclonal antibody	Anti-NRP (MNRP1685A)	Genentech[176–178]
	TGF-β2	Cytokine	Neutralizes suppression	Monoclonal antibody	Fresolimumab	Cambridge Antibody Technology[179,180]
	TGF-β2	Cytokine	Neutralizes suppression	Antisense molecule	Trabedersen	Antisense Pharma[181,182]
	TGF-β receptor	Cytokine receptor	Neutralizes suppression	Monoclonal antibody	Anti-TGF-βR1 (PF-03446962)	Pfizer[183–186]
	TGF-β receptor	Cytokine receptor	Neutralizes suppression	Monoclonal antibody	Galunisertib	Eli Lilly[187–191]
	TGF-β receptor	Cytokine receptor	Neutralizes suppression	Kinase inhibitor	ALK5 inhibitor (TEW-7197)	MedPacto[192]
	CTLA4	Inhibitory surface molecule	Neutralizes T$_{reg}$ cell surface inhibition	Monoclonal antibody	Ipilimumab	Bristol-Meyers Squibb/Medarex[193,194]
	PD-1	Inhibitory surface molecule	Neutralizes T$_{reg}$ cell surface inhibition	Checkpoint inhibitor	Nivolumab	Bristol-Meyers Squibb/Medarex[195,196]
	PD-L1	Inhibitory surface molecule	Neutralizes T$_{reg}$ cell surface inhibition	Checkpoint inhibitor	Atezolizumab	Genentech/Roche[197,198]
ONGOING TRIALS	Adenosine receptor (A2A)	Adenosine metabolism	Blocks adenosine binding	Antagonist	Ciforadenant	NCT02655822[199]
	Adenosine receptor (A2A)	Adenosine metabolism	Blocks adenosine binding	Antagonist	PBF-509	NCT02403193[200]
	CD73	Adenosine metabolism	Inhibits CD73 enzymatic activity	Monoclonal antibody	Oleclumab	NCT02503774[201]
	CBM complex	TCR signaling	Neutralizes suppression	Inhibitor	MALT1 inhibitor (JNJ-67856633)	NCT03900598[202]
	OX40	Inhibitory surface molecule	Neutralizes T$_{reg}$ cell surface inhibition	Monoclonal antibody	Anti-OX40 antibody (MEDI0562)	NCT03336606[203]
	LAG3	Inhibitory surface molecule	Neutralizes T$_{reg}$ cell surface inhibition	Monoclonal antibody	Anti-LAG-3 antibody (LAG525)	NCT02460224[204]

(continued)

Table 39.1 Current and Emerging Clinical Targeting of T_{regs} Cells (*continued*)

	TARGET	TARGET CATEGORY	FUNCTION	INTERVENTION METHOD	NAME	COMPANY STUDIES REFERENCES
NOVEL INTER VENTIONS	CD36	Metabolic	T_{reg} cell depletion, neutralizes suppression	Monoclonal antibody	Anti-CD36 monoclonal antibody	Wang et al. (2020)[162]
	CMB complex	TCR signaling	Neutralizes suppression	Inhibitor	CARMA1 inhibitor	Di Pilato et al. (2019)[205]
	CTLA4	Inhibitor surface molecule	Neutralizes T_{reg} cell surface inhibition	Monoclonal antibody	"Fc-engineered" anti-CTLA4	Ha et al. (2019)[206]
	CD25	Cytokine receptor	T_{reg} cell depletion	Monoclonal antibody	"Fc-optimized" anti-CD25	Vargas et al. (2017)[207]
	CD25	Cytokine receptor	T_{reg} cell depletion	Photoimmunotherapy	Near-infrared photoimmunotherapy	Sato et al. (2016)[208]
	Small G patients: Rag/Rheb	mTOR signaling	Block amino acid-mediated suppression	Inhibitor	N/A	Shi et al. (2019)[133]
	CD39	Adenosine metabolism	Blocks CD39 enzymatic activity	Monoclonal antibody	OREG-103/BY40	Nikolova et al. (2011)[209]
	Amphiregulin	Epidermal growth factor	Blocks T_{reg}-mediated tumor growth	Inhibitor	N/A	Green et al. (2017)[60]
	cGAS-STING signalling	Type 1 IFNs	Neutralizes suppression	Antagonist	N/A	Field et al. (2020)[150]
	CCR8	Chemokine receptor	Blocks trafficking	Monoclonal antibody	Anti-CCR8 antibody	Plitas et al. (2016)[50]; Villarreal et al. (2018)[101]

CTLA4, cytotoxic T-lymphocyte-associated protein 4; IFN, interferon; PD-1, programmed cell death 1; PD-L1, programmed cell death ligand 1; TCR, T cell receptor; T_{reg}, regulatory T.

with strong suppressive activity and poor prognosis.[2,215] Mechanistically, the drug reduces Foxp3 and CD25 expression in T_{reg} cells, weakening T_{reg} cell suppression and survival, which is required for persistent antitumor CD8$^+$ T cell effector activity. Still, there remain some critical issues in targeting CD25 with blocking agents. Several CD4 and CD8 T_{conv} cells also express CD25, and treatment with daclizumab has shown to decrease the bystander Foxp3$^-$ CD4$^+$CD8$^+$ populations in circulation. Moreover, therapeutic use of anti-CD25 against established versus recent tumors fails to thwart tumor growth for a variety of reasons, including the depletion of activated effector CD8$^+$ and CD4$^+$ T cells that upregulate CD25.[216] In addition, certain isotypes of the anti-CD25 antibody may fail to deplete intratumoral T_{reg} cells because of upregulation of Fc-g receptor IIb (FcgRIIb) within tumors. FcgRIIb is expressed on a range of immune cells as well as on tumors and is known to be particularly inhibitory when binding to a range of antibodies.[217] Daclizumab is a humanized IgG1 antibody, and

both human and murine studies have shown that the IgG1 isotypes of anti-CD25 mAbs often fail to deplete tumor-infiltrating T_{reg} cells.[121,172] Therefore, in murine studies, Vargas et al. optimized the anti-CD25 mAb by replacing the constant regions of the original IgG1 isotype with IgG2a and k constant regions, making it capable of overcoming this FcgRIIb-mediated inhibition of antitumor immunity.[207] While this optimized anti-CD25 isotype does more effectively deplete the tumor-infiltrating T_{reg} cells and synergizes with PD-1 blockade to eradicate established tumors, it still reduces CD25 expression on T_{conv} and reduces the number of T_{reg} cells in circulation and in the lymph nodes.

Another innovative strategy has been implemented to selectively deplete tumor-infiltrating T_{reg} cells through the use of targeted phototherapy. Near-infrared photoimmunotherapy (NIR-PIT) is a method of treating cancers that uses activation of an antibody-photoabsorber conjugate activated by NIR light to kill specific cells.[218] The antibody binds to the specific cell-surface antigen and the photoactivatable silicon phthalocyanine dye (IRDye 700DX) causes irreversible damage to the cell membrane after exposure to the NIR light irradiation. The 690 nanometer wavelength of the NIR light selectively induces necrotic cell death to cancer cells without damaging adjoining cells. There are ongoing clinical trials using this technology to target tumor epidermal growth factor receptor (NCT02422979). This method has been primarily tested in antibodies directed at cancer antigens; however, it can also be employed to kill any cell type as long as appropriate antibody is available.[219-221] Sato et al. pioneered the use of NIR-PIT to selectively target and control the accumulation of CD4$^+$CD25$^+$Foxp3$^+$ T$_{reg}$ cells without disturbing the nontumor CD25$^+$Foxp3$^-$ T$_{conv}$ cells. They generated the anti-CD25-F(ab')$_2$ fragments and conjugated them with the IR700 dye. In vivo, the NIR-PIT targeting CD4$^+$CD25$^+$Foxp3$^+$ T$_{reg}$ cells induced tumor regression, due to depleting these T$_{reg}$ cells and therefore facilitating the activation and infiltration of natural killer and CD8$^+$ T cells.[208]

Anti-CD25 NIR-PIT treatment also induced upregulation of MHC I complex and co-stimulatory molecules, such as CD86 and CD40, on dendritic cells. Other antigen-presenting cells, such as B cells, monocytes, and macrophages, upregulated co-stimulatory CD69, showing an activated phenotype in response to treatment. Still, the NIR-PIT-mediated induction of the antitumor effector T cell response requires that these effector T$_{conv}$ cells exhibit a CD25^{lo} phenotype before treatment or else the CD25-expressing antitumor effector T$_{conv}$ cells may also be depleted, defeating the purpose of treatment altogether. In addition, this therapy may initially promote a systemic as well as an intratumoral "cytokine storm" whereby cytokine and chemokine production is elevated to near clinically harmful levels.[222,223] Importantly, the therapeutic benefit of the NIR-PIT treatment requires optimally that the antibody-photoabsorber conjugate is bound to the cells and that it is exposed to the NIR light; both conditions must be met for an antitumor effect. Given the complexities that can arise here as well as the remaining potential problems with therapeutically blocking T$_{reg}$ cell CD25, other T$_{reg}$ cell targets have been reasonably proposed to more seamlessly deplete the tumor-infiltrating T$_{reg}$ cells.

Targeting CCR4 and CCR8

Other dispensable components on T$_{reg}$ cells that can be therapeutically targeted to mediate antitumor immunity include chemokine receptors CCR4 and the previously mentioned CCR8. Indeed, some clinical studies have shown that depleting CD25-expressing can augment antitumor immune responses, whereas other similar studies have failed to support this effect of anti-CD25 mAbs.[20,59,121,224,225] CCR4 was specifically highly expressed in the suppressive and terminally differentiated CD45RA$^-$Foxp3^{hi}

eT$_{reg}$ cells, which compose most of the tumor-infiltrating T$_{reg}$ cells. Nontumor T$_{reg}$ cells do not upregulate CCR4 as the tumor-resident T$_{reg}$ cells, and therefore CCR4-blocking antibodies do not negatively impact the T$_{reg}$ cells in circulation or in lymphoid tissues.[226] Importantly, while in vivo administration of anti-CCR4 mAb reduced the number of tumor-infiltrating T$_{reg}$ cells, it also evoked the augmentation of tumor antigen-specific CD4$^+$ and CD8$^+$ T cell responses. Targeting CCR4 allows for selective inhibition of specifically tumor-resident T$_{reg}$ cells and does not hinder nontumor T$_{reg}$ cells.

High CCR8 expression in tumor-resident T$_{reg}$ cells is associated with a highly activated and proliferative T$_{reg}$ cell phenotype and consequently a poor prognosis.[99] CCR8 binding to its respective ligand CCL1 in the tumor tissue plays a role in enhancing T$_{reg}$ cell suppressive activity and survival.[50,227] Since CCR8 serves as a unique marker for the highly suppressive T$_{reg}$ cells, strategies to specifically manipulate CCR8$^+$Foxp3$^+$ T$_{reg}$ cells are reasonable. Distinguishing that CCR8^{hi} Foxp3$^+$ T$_{reg}$ cell accumulation correlates with a poor prognosis provides rationale for the therapeutic targeting of T$_{reg}$ cells through a CCR8-depleting antibody. This would be particularly critical for breast cancers since common checkpoint blockade therapies have had limited success.[50] An anti-CCR8 mAb has shown promise in inducing antitumor immunity and even enhancing vaccine-induced responses.[101] CCR8 mAb reduces the accumulation of suppressive T$_{reg}$ cells in the TME and thereby helps to facilitate the robust antigen-specific tumor-infiltrating CD8$^+$ T cells. Therapeutically targeting CCR8$^+$ allows for the specific blocking of suppressive T$_{reg}$ cells and not effector T$_{conv}$ without disrupting T$_{reg}$ cell homeostasis.

Targeting Components of the CARMA1-BCL10-MALT1 Complex

Indeed, TCR signaling constitutes a central component in the activated T$_{reg}$ cell contribution to tumor growth. The interaction between the tumor-infiltrating T$_{reg}$ cells and the cognate TAAs spurs T$_{reg}$ cell activation and therefore propagates the immunosuppressive activity of T$_{reg}$ cells in the TME.[228] In this sense, aspects of TCR signaling could be targeted in T$_{reg}$-based therapeutic intervention. Through the CARMA1-BCL10-MALT1 (CBM) signalosome, antigens stimulate the TCR triggering PKCθ activity, promoting various functions such as canonical NF-kB signaling, AP-1, and mTOR pathways.[229] Mempel and colleagues showed that strategic disruption of the CBM signalosome rewires tumor-infiltrating T$_{reg}$ cells from exhibiting immunosuppressive activity to secreting IFNγ and enhancing local antitumor immunity.[205] Genetic deletion of CARM1, BCL10, or MALT1 abrogates thymic development of T$_{reg}$ cells.[230-234] The CBM complex is essential for T$_{reg}$ cell homeostasis; however, partial reduction in CARMA1 expression of up to 50% is permissible while maintaining Foxp3 expression, without causing systemic autoimmunity.[205] Partially CARMA1-deficient T_{reg} cells in the TME produce IFNg and also potentiates PD-1 blockade therapy. Pharmacological inhibition of MALT1 reproduces these effects.[205] Partial disruption of the CBM complex constitutes a reasonable strategy to target dispensable components on T_{reg} cells without compromising T_{reg} cell development and homeostasis.

CONCLUSION

T_{reg} cells play a role in tumor growth and, therefore, constitute a reasonable and an important target in cancer immunotherapy. Several novel T_{reg} cell components have been identified as both contributors to tumor growth and as targetable entities in immunotherapeutic strategies. The distinct homeostatic mechanisms that allow T_{reg} cells to tolerate self-antigens and adapt to non-lymphoid tissues are responsible for the T_{reg}-mediated malignancy in tumors. Identification of T_{reg} cell subsets and ways in which T_{reg} cells exhibit plasticity provides insight into the number of ways T_{reg} cells can promote tumor growth. With this insight, targeted treatments can be developed to thwart and control T_{reg} cell activity to achieve antitumor immunity.

ACKNOWLEDGMENTS

This work was supported in part by the research grants from the U.S. NIH/NCI R01 grants (W.Z) (CA217648, CA123088, CA099985, CA193136, and CA152470), and the NIH through the University of Michigan Rogel Cancer Center Grant (CA46592).

KEY REFERENCES

Only key references appear in the print edition. The full reference list appears in the digital product on Springer Publishing Connect: connect.springerpub.com/content/book/978-0-8261-3743-2/part/part03/chapter/ch39

1. Tanaka A, Sakaguchi S. Regulatory T cells in cancer immunotherapy. *Nat Cell Res.* 2017;27:109–118. doi:10.1038/cr.2016.151
2. Wing JB, Tanaka A, Sakaguchi S. Human FOXP3+ regulatory T cell heterogeneity and function in autoimmunity and cancer. *Immunity.* 2019;50:302–316. doi:10.1016/j.immuni.2019.01.020
49. Miragaia RJ, Gomes T, Chomka A, et al. Single-cell transcriptomics of regulatory T cells reveals trajectories of tissue adaptation. *Immunity.* 2019;50:493–504. doi:10.1016/j.immuni.2019.01.001
50. Plitas G, Konopacki C, Wu K, et al. Regulatory T cells exhibit distinct features in human breast cancer. *Immunity.* 2016;45:1122–1134. doi:10.1016/j.immuni.2016.10.032
70. Halim L, Romano M, McGregor R, et al. An atlas of human regulatory T helper-like cells reveals features of T_h2-like T_{reg} cells that support a tumorigenic environment. *Cell Rep.* 2017;20:757–770. doi:10.1016/j.celrep.2017.06.079
107. Nair VS, Song MH, Oh KI. Vitamin C facilitates demethylation of the Foxp3 enhancer in a Tet-dependent manner. *J Immunol.* 2016;196:2119–2131. doi:10.4049/jimmunol.1502352
128. Chapman NM, Zeng H, Nguyen TLM, et al. mTOR coordinates transcriptional programs and mitochondrial metabolism of activated T_{reg} cell subsets to protect tissue homeostasis. *Nature Communications.* 2018;9:2095. doi:10.1038/s41467-018-04392-5
133. Shi H, Chapman NM, Wen J, et al. Amino acids license kinase mTORC1 activity and T_{reg} cell function via small G proteins Rag and Rheb. *Immunity.* 2019;51:1012–1027. doi:10.1016/j.immuni.2019.10.001
136. Fu Z, Ye J, Dean JW, et al. Requirement of mitochondrial transcription factor A in tissue-resident regulatory T cell maintenance and function. *Cell Reports.* 2019;28:159–171. doi:10.1016/j.celrep.2019.06.024
137. Weinberg SE, Singer BD, Steinert EM, et al. Mitochondrial complex III is essential for suppressive function of regulatory T cells. *Nature.* 2019;565:495–499. doi:10.1038/s41586-018-0846-z

Systemic Measures of Immune Function in Cancer Patients: Other Suppressive Cellular Mechanisms

Thomas A. Mace, Raju R. Raval, and William E. Carson III

KEY POINTS

- Most precancerous lesions likely undergo immune surveillance and elimination through a variety of immunological pathways.

- Clinical tumors may develop, proliferate, and metastasize in part through mechanisms that evade the normal immune response.

- Immunosuppressive tumor microenvironments (TMEs) are now well characterized, and contribute to tumor progression even in the setting of modern immunotherapies.

- A deeper understanding of the variety of immunosuppressive cell subtypes and the functional mechanisms these cells use is of significant importance in overcoming immune-based therapeutic resistance in cancer patients.

- Numerous cell subtypes, in addition to the well-characterized roles of regulatory T cells (T_{reg} cells) and myeloid-derived suppressor cells (MDSCs), can have important roles in tumors evading elimination through the normal immune system or in the setting of modern immunotherapy.

- Significant research is taking place to better characterize these immunosuppressive cell populations and to target their effects in clinical trials. Depleting or inhibiting these cellular populations could lead to improved efficacy of immunotherapy approaches in the clinic.

INTRODUCTION

The immune system is known to have multiple roles in relation to the development of cancer. Tumor cells undergo immune surveillance as they contain mutations that can be translated into potential neoantigens and have increased cellular stress with release of inflammatory cytokines that recruit immune cells. Thus, it is believed that the majority of early precancerous lesions are eliminated from the body through such mechanisms. However, clinically detectable tumors necessarily evolve mechanisms to evade or suppress the normal immune response. In addition, tumors can use a variety of mechanisms to increase growth and metastasize through modifying the tumor microenvironment (TME).

Advancements in immunotherapy, specifically immune checkpoint blockade and adoptive cell therapies, have led to remarkable gains for patients with a variety of malignancies, with U.S. Food and Drug Administration (FDA) approval of numerous treatments for patients with melanoma, non-small cell lung cancer (NSCLC), kidney cancer, and head and neck cancer.[1-5] However, the immunosuppressive TME can limit effective immunotherapy through a variety of mechanisms. These mechanisms leading to tumor immune escape and metastasis may be central to why many patients have not derived benefit from these remarkable new therapies, in both the approved indications and in many other solid and hematologic malignancies. There is mounting evidence that a variety of immunosuppressive cell subtypes play a central role in allowing tumor cells to escape immune surveillance and elimination.

Tumor cells also undergo constant modification of epigenetic markers, metabolic pathways, and cell surface expression of antigens, receptors, and ligands to decrease apoptosis and avoid immune recognition. In addition, these signals, along with the release of cytokines, help to recruit a variety of suppressive immune cell subtypes to the TME as well. Significant focus has been placed on the role of regulatory T cells (T_{reg} cells) and myeloid-derived suppressor cells (MDSCs) in contributing to these immunosuppressive and tumor-promoting mechanisms. However, there are a number of other interactions and mechanisms that may play a role in creating an immunosuppressive TME.

Tumor progression may require cooperation among cancer cells, immune cells, and other stromal and inflammatory components of the TME.[6] There is a growing body of literature suggesting that, in addition to MDSCs and T_{reg} cells, other immune cell subtypes, such as tumor-associated macrophages (TAMs), T helper cells (Th17), regulatory B (B_{reg}) cells, tumor-associated neutrophils (TAN), cancer-associated fibroblasts (CAFs), and bone marrow-derived cells (BMDCs), play crucial roles in tumor cell immune evasion and tumor progression.[7–10] Although much has been elucidated, there are numerous questions to be answered as to the mechanisms and functions of immunosuppressive cell types in both tumor development and metastasis (Table 40.1). Indeed, the stimulation and expansion of many of these immunosuppressive cells may lead to tumor progression and spread in patients.[11,12]

Table 40.1 Immunosuppressive Cell Types

CELL TYPE	MECHANISMS
Regulatory T cells (T_{reg} cells)	Maintains limits on normal autoimmune responses, and can suppress effector T cell function in tumors through expression of negative co-stimulatory molecules
Myeloid-derived suppressor cells (MDSCs)	Heterogeneous group of immature myeloid cells that can create an immunosuppressive TME through suppression of NK cells, DCs, and effector T cells
Tumor-associated macrophages (TAMs)	Can form dense tumor stromal infiltrates in many cancer types leading to immune evasion
T helper cells (Th17)	Through cytokine release may recruit CAFs, attract MDSCs, and promote tumor cell metastasis
regulatory B (B_{reg}) cells	Promote conversion of effector T cells to T_{reg} cells and enhance tumor metastatic potential
Tumor-associated neutrophils (TANs)	Directly inhibit the function of cytotoxic T cells, which can thus promote tumor growth
Cancer-associated fibroblasts (CAFs)	Stimulate an immunosuppressive TME through secretion of proinflammatory cytokines

CAFs, cancer-associated fibroblasts; DCs, dendritic cells; MDSCs, myeloid-derived suppressor cells; NK, natural killer; TME, tumor microenvironment; T_{reg}, regulatory T.

CAFs can secrete proinflammatory cytokines and may help to promote an immunosuppressive TME. Though normal mesenchymal stem cells (MSCs) are immune stimulatory, MSCs recruited to the TME may become immunosuppressive by secreting transforming growth factor-β (TGF-β) and hepatocyte growth factor (HGF; suppressing T cell proliferation), and inducing indoleamine 2,3-dioxygenase (IDO; promoting apoptosis of activated T cells).[13] Elimination of CAFs in a 4T1 model of breast cancer metastases has been shown to promote antitumor activity by shifting the immune phenotype from Th2 to Th1.[14]

Recent ongoing research has improved our knowledge of the mechanisms by which immunosuppressive cells can contribute to tumor immune evasion.[15] Immunosuppressive cells can be recruited during tumor progression through the release of a variety of cytokines and chemokines such as CXCL5-CXCR2 and TGF-β, among many others.[16–18] Overall, these immunosuppressive cells invading the TME maintain their own function and allow continued tumor immune evasion by a variety of mechanisms, including disruption of dendritic cell (DC) antigen presentation,[19] further secretion of immunosuppressive cytokines (IL-10),[20] inhibition of effector cell (natural killer [NK] cells or cytotoxic T lymphocytes) cytotoxicity,[21,22] and regulation of B and T cell proliferation or activation through expression of molecules such as IDO,[23] arginase, or inducible nitric oxide synthase (iNOS).[24]

REGULATORY T CELLS

T_{reg} cells (CD4+CD25+Foxp3+) are an immunosuppressive cell type that maintains limits on autoimmune responses and thus has been shown to have a role in tumor immune evasion. T_{reg} cells can inhibit the function of effector T lymphocytes through expression of negative co-stimulator molecules, such as cytotoxic T lymphocyte antigen-4 (CTLA-4), programmed death 1 (PD-1), or its ligand PD-L1, or by releasing immunosuppressive cytokines (TGF-β or IL-10).[25] Hypoxic conditions within a tumor can lead to the recruitment of T_{reg} cells through expression of CCL28, leading to angiogenesis (vascular endothelial growth factor A [VEGF-A] release) and continued suppression of effector T cells.[26] TGF-β secreted by T_{reg} cells can directly inhibit cytotoxic T cells, decreasing antitumor activity in the melanoma microenvironment.[27] Further, expression of PDL1 in the TME may expand and sustain T_{reg} cells, leading to greater immunosuppression.[28]

MYELOID-DERIVED SUPPRESSOR CELLS

MDSCs are a heterogeneous group of immature myeloid cells able to foster an immunosuppressive TME. Elevated levels of MDSCs circulating in the blood can directly correlate to worse overall survival in many gastrointestinal cancers such as pancreatic cancer.[29,30] Many growth factors and cytokines secreted by the TME like IL-6, granulocyte-macrophage colony-stimulating factor (GM-CSF), granulocyte colony-stimulating factor (G-CSF), and vascular endothelial growth factor (VEGF) can drive the expansion of these MDSC in patients.[31,32] In humans, MDSC are phenotypically characterized as CD11b$^+$CD33$^+$HL-DR$^-$ and separated into either CD14$^+$ monocytic or CD15$^+$ granulocytic populations.

MDSCs can suppress the function of other immune cells such as NK cells, DCs, and effector T cells through release of IL-6 and through the CCAAT/enhancer-binding protein (C/EBP) homologous protein (Chop) cellular stress sensor pathway.[33,34] Indeed, it has been shown that some of the immunosuppressive function of MDSCs can be abrogated in a mouse model of lung carcinoma with this pathway (Chop) deleted.[35] In general, it has also been shown that the immunosuppressive activity of MDSCs can limit the success of using checkpoint blockade.[36] Recently, it was discovered that PD-1 expression by MDSC was just as effective at limiting antitumor growth and that expression can dampen antitumor T cell responses.[37] Inhibition of glutamine metabolism reduced MDSC accumulation, inhibited IDO expression, and rendered checkpoint blockade-resistant glioma tumors susceptible to immunotherapy.[38] Additionally, inhibition of CCR2 expressed by MDSC decreased numbers in the tumor and enhanced the efficacy of checkpoint blockade.[39] Recent studies have reported that expression of CD200 in the TME (brain and pancreatic cancer) can enhance the suppressive activity of MDSC.[40,41] Also, MDSCs that release IL-10 have been shown to decrease L-selectin expression on circulating naïve T cells and to limit the antigen-mediated activation of CD4$^+$ and CD8$^+$ T cells.[42] MDSCs may also decrease available amino acids required for T cell function, among other mechanisms of immune suppression.[43] In addition, MDSC production of nitric oxide (NO), reactive nitrogen species (ROS), arginase, IDO, peroxynitrite, and cytokines, such as TGF-β and IL-10, are also classical mechanisms by which these cells may suppress immune effector cell function.

TUMOR-ASSOCIATED MACROPHAGES

TAMs are derived from circulating monocytes or resident tissue macrophages and can form the major leukocytic infiltrate found within the stroma of many tumor types. Cytokines such as IL-4, IL-10, and M-CSF expressed by the TME can drive the expansion of TAMs.[44] TAMs can function to be protumorigenic, though they may also have some tumor-suppressing properties. Specifically, TAMs can inhibit CD8$^+$ T cell–mediated antitumor immune responses, thus allowing increased tumor immune evasion.[45] Breast cancer TAMs have been shown to release high levels of the immunosuppressive cytokine IL-10, suppress intratumoral DC production of IL-12, and thus block CD8$^+$ T cell-dependent antitumor immune responses.[46] Specifically, these TAMs are derived from CCR2$^+$ inflammatory monocytes, depend on Notch signaling via the transcription factor RBPJ, and lead to tumor promotion.[47] TAMs can inhibit the function of cytotoxic CD8$^+$ T cells through expression of PD-L1 and B7-H4/VTCN1 or can indirectly affect them through recruitment of T$_{reg}$ cells.[48] TAM-infiltration levels have been shown to be of significant prognostic value, and in certain tumor types, such as breast cancer, ovarian cancer, certain types of glioma, and lymphoma, have been associated with a poor prognosis. In a study of classic Hodgkin lymphoma patients, an increased number of CD68$^+$ macrophages in biopsies correlated with increased relapse and decreased survival.[49]

Tumors can promote progression and metastasis by reprogramming and switching the functional status of recruited immune cells within the TME. Macrophages are known to be a cell type with a high level of plasticity, and can have a variety of functions depending on environmental stimuli. The first subgroup, M1-type macrophages, play a classical role in the innate immune response to external pathogens. On the other hand, M2-type macrophages can be activated by a variety of cytokines and can lead to tumor progression through expression of low levels of IL-12 and high levels of IL-10. The interconversion of M1 to M2 macrophages depends on the TME. For example, the expression of retinoic acid-related orphan receptor (RORC1/RORγ) in animal models and cancer patients has been shown to lead to M2 polarization and TAM differentiation. Experimentally, it was shown that deletion of RORC1 in the hematopoietic compartment led to decreased tumor growth and metastasis.[50] M2-type macrophages in many tumor types make up the bulk of TAMs and have been shown to promote tumor progression and metastasis expression of cytokines and other factors such as VEGF, matrix metallopeptidase 9 (MMP9), and TGF-β.[51] In addition, the release of cytokines from the TME, such as GM-CSF, IL-1, IL-4, IL-6, IL-10, and tumor necrosis factor (TNF)α, can lead to the polarization of TAMs through activation of STAT signaling. Also, a hypoxic TME can lead to expression of the angiopoietin receptor TIE2, which can polarize M1 into M2 macrophages, and has shown to promote TAM-associated metastasis.[52]

The process of epithelial to mesenchymal transition (EMT), which is thought to be central to the process of metastatic tumor development, can be induced by immunosuppressive cells such as T$_{reg}$ cells, MDSCs, and TAMs. For example, TAMs can promote tumor metastasis by releasing TGF-β, and the JAK/STAT3 pathway is necessary for TGF-β-induced EMT and tumor cell migration and invasion. Thus, both JAK/STAT3 and TGF-β/

SMAD signaling can enhance EMT in lung carcinomas, leading to further metastatic disease progression.[53]

A variety of immunosuppressive cells can promote tumor cell invasion during the process of metastatic development through the release of a variety of cytokines including TNF-α, IL-1, and IL-6 that can activate matrix metalloproteinase (MMP) expression through nuclear factor kappa β (NF-κB)/STAT3 signal transduction pathways. Macrophages, including TAMs, can induce tumor cell migration through release of migration-stimulating factor (MSF). In addition, TAMs can secrete epidermal growth factor (EGF), leading to potentiation of tumor cell invasion and motility through EGF receptor signaling and downstream effects.[54] This TAM-mediated tumor invasion mechanism may be regulated by a HRGβ1 and CXCL12 dependent EGF/CSF-1 paracrine loop between TAMs and tumor cells.[55] Thus, TAMs in tumors can promote movement away from the primary tumor site, invasion into surrounding tissue, and intravasation into systemic circulation, whereas another class of TAMs termed "metastasis-associated macrophages" (MAMs) within secondary sites facilitates tumor cell extravasation and metastatic growth.[56] This less-described population of TAMs promotes extravasation and survival of metastasizing cancer cells.[57] These cells differentiate from classical macrophages into MAMs at the metastasis site, have similar function in their ability to suppress T cells, and do not require CSF1R signaling for their accumulation.[58]

OTHER IMMUNOSUPPRESSIVE CELL TYPES

There are also other immunosuppressive cells that are not as well characterized, though mounting evidence has begun to elucidate their roles as well. Subsets of DCs, such as tolerogenic DC (Tol-DC), which are alternatively activated or maturation resistant DCs (low major histocompatibility complex [MHC] and low co-stimulatory molecule expression levels), play a role in the induction of immune tolerance.[59-61] Thus, regulatory DCs (DCregs) can be induced by tumors and subsequently suppress antitumor immune responses.[19] A subset of human CD14+ CTLA-4+ DCreg in hepatocellular carcinoma has been shown to suppress T cell responses through CTLA-4-dependent IL-10 and IDO production.[35] Thus, this piece of evidence shows that CTLA-4 expressed on DCs also plays a potential role in tumor cell immune evasion. A hypoxic TME or apoptotic cells can induce the presence of Tol-DCs through TGF-β and IL-10 signaling, and these cells can promote the expansion of T_{reg} cells through cell surface PD-L1 expression.[62] Aberrant DC function and differentiation are commonly seen during cancer progression.[19] Research has shown that human lung carcinoma cells can cause DCs to secrete TGF-β, and mouse models have revealed increased levels of VEGF, arginase 1 (ARG1), NO, and IL-10.[63] In addition

to TAMs and MDSCs suppressing CD8+ T cells through ARG1 production, tumor-infiltrating DCs have also been shown to use this immunosuppressive mechanism.[64] It is important to note that cytokines released from tumor cells can directly affect myeloid differentiation toward more immunosuppressive cell types, such that tumor-derived IL-6 and TGF-β have been shown to increase the expression of inhibitor of differentiation 1 (Id1) and can skew bone marrow-derived DC differentiation toward MDSCs expressing high levels of Id1.[65] This also leads to a decrease in functional DC numbers, and this increased Id1 expression was shown to promote an immunosuppressive phenotype leading to inhibition of CD8+ T cell proliferation and both tumor growth and metastatic progression. Clinically, it has been observed that melanoma patients have increased plasma TGF-β levels and higher levels of Id1 expression in myeloid peripheral blood cells.[65]

The immunosuppressive TME can promote a shift from a Th1 CD4+ (helper) T cell, which can assist cytotoxic CD8+ T cells in rejecting tumor cells, to a Th2 tumor-promoting (regulatory) phenotype, which can abrogate CD8+ T cell activity.[52,66] In addition, other subsets of regulatory NK cells and B cells can inhibit immune effector cell responses to tumors as well. Neutrophils have been found to transition from an N1 phenotype to a protumoral N2 phenotype within an immunosuppressive TME.[67] Protumoral neutrophils (N2) can degrade extracellular arginine (needed for effective T cell function) through release of ARG1 and thus inhibit CD8+ T cell function.[68] Within animal lung tumor models, it was shown that TGF-β induced the development of N2 neutrophils (high ARG1 and low TNF), and thus these cells could play an immunosuppressive role.[69] B_{reg}s have also been shown to express IL-10 to reduce Th1 cells, leading to lower tumor-infiltrating CD8+ T cells in the melanoma microenvironment.[70]

Tumor cells can also secrete a variety of cytokines and attract other immunosuppressive cells such as TANs and B_{reg}s to primary tumor and metastatic sites. These cells, among many others, can decrease the function of cytotoxic CD8+ T cells and NK cells, which can indeed allow for both tumor growth and potential movement of cells from the primary tumor to the circulation.[71] It has been shown that IL-1β expression can lead to IL-17 release from gamma delta (γδ) T cells, leading to G-CSF-dependent systemic expansion and polarization of neutrophils in animal models. The TANs can subsequently inhibit the function of cytotoxic T lymphocytes, and thus promote tumor growth and potential metastases.[72] Th17 cells may also play a role in decreasing antitumor immune activity, as an EL4 lymphoma model showed that IL-17 produced from Th17 cells promoted CAFs to express G-CSF, attracting MDSCs to the tumor, and promotion of tumor cell metastasis.[73] B_{reg}s have been shown to potentially enhance metastatic disease progression in a 4T1 model of breast cancer metastasis in which there were increases in the baseline number of circulating CD25[+] B cells, and the targeted depletion of these cells using a B20-specific antibody significantly decreased lung metastases.[74] In addition, it was observed that B$_{regs}$ within lung metastases also induced the conversion, through TGF-β release, of CD4[+] T cells into T$_{reg}$ cells.[74]

THERAPIES FOR TARGETING IMMUNOSUPPRESSIVE POPULATIONS

Many groups are researching methods for targeting immunosuppressive populations. Leading therapeutic efforts are examining treatment options for depleting circulating and tumor-infiltrating immunosuppressive cells, preventing the recruitment and trafficking of these cells, inhibition of their suppressive functions, and abrogating the differentiation of cells into a nonresponsive immune state.

Utilization of chemotherapeutic, targeted therapies, or antibody therapy, has provided promising evidence that suppressive immune populations can be depleted. A study in patients with pancreatic cancer found that treatment with gemcitabine reduced myeloid and T-regulatory populations sparing the T cell prolific capacity.[75] Preclinical data using either paclitaxel or 5-fluorouracil resulted in the inhibition and reduction of MDSC in select tumor-bearing animal models.[76,77] Cyclophosphamide in combination with GVAXs can inhibit T-regulatory cell populations.[78] MDSC in humans are characterized by their expression of CD33; recent data elucidates a mechanism for utilizing an antibody against CD33 (gemtuzmab ozogamicin) in vitro resulting in an increase in human MDSC cell death with a restoration of T cell proliferation.[79] A study by Stiff et al. provides additional evidence that depletion of MDSC using ibrutinib (Bruton's tyrosine kinase inhibitor) can enhance anti-PD-L1 checkpoint inhibitor therapy in preclinical animal models.[80]

Therapeutic approaches that target the trafficking of these suppressive immune populations is another strategy for reducing immunosuppression. One promising approach is targeting chemokine receptors (CXCR1 and CXCR2) expressed by MDSC and TAMS to reduce their trafficking to the TME. Using a head and neck squamous cell carcinoma (HNSCC) murine model, investigators observed that inhibition of MDSC trafficking with a small molecule inhibitor of CXCR1 and CXCR2 (SX682) significantly abrogated tumor MDSC accumulation and enhanced the tumor infiltration, activation, and therapeutic efficacy of adoptively transferred murine NK cells.[81] Another study genetically ablated CXCR2 expression, which prevented the accumulation of tumor-associated neutrophils and led to a T cell dependent suppression of

tumor growth.[82] Current clinical trials are testing the efficacy of AZD5069 (CXCR2 inhibitor) in combination with durvalumab (anti-PD-L1) in patients with metastatic pancreatic cancer (NCT02583477). Tumors that produce colony-stimulating factor 1 (CSF-1) can recruit myeloid populations such as TAMs and MDSC. Inhibition of CSF-1R has been another promising approach for reducing the trafficking of these cell populations. Preclinical work provides evidence that inhibition of CSF-1R using PLX3397 or pexidartinib in mice with melanoma significantly reduced tumor-infiltrating myeloid cells and increased CD8[+] T cell responses.[83] Several trials are currently testing the efficacy of CSF-1R inhibitors (pexidartinib, caliralizumab, IMC-CS4) in combination with checkpoint inhibitors (nivolumab, pembrolizumab) to determine whether reducing suppressive cells in patients can improve antibody responses.

Inhibiting suppressive factors secreted by MDSC such as arginase and iNOS can improve T cell activity and the success of immunotherapy. Inhibition of iNOS by MDSC improves Fc-receptor-mediated NK cell function.[84] MDSCs from patients with cancer were found to significantly inhibit NK-cell FcR-mediated functions, including antibody-dependent cellular cytotoxicity, cytokine production, and signal transduction in a contact-independent manner. Inhibition of iNOS in vivo significantly improved the efficacy of mAb therapy in a mouse model of breast cancer. TAMs can secrete the proinflammatory cytokine IL-1β. A recent study provides evidence that BTK physically associates with the NLRP3 inflammasome and that inhibition of BTK with ibrutinib can impair the production of in vitro-generated TAM.[85] Suppressor cells secrete IDO which can deplete tryptophan, rendering T cells inactive. Inhibition of IDO is one approach to targeting a secreted factor that limits T cell responses in the TME. IDO inhibition has progressed to clinical trials in combination with checkpoint immunotherapies. A large Phase 3 randomized double-blinded study in patients with metastatic melanoma was conducted treating patients with epacadostat (IDO1 inhibitor) plus pembrolizumab (anti-PD-1).[86] Epacadostat plus pembrolizumab did not improve progression-free survival or overall survival compared with placebo plus pembrolizumab in patients with unresectable or metastatic melanoma. Another recent Phase 1 study treated NSCLC patients with epacadostat in combination with atezolizumab (anti-PD-L1); it was well tolerated but provided limited efficacy.[87] The current landscape of IDO inhibition to enhance checkpoint immunotherapy in cancer patients remains unclear.

Another approach to target these suppressive populations is to utilize treatments that reprogram or affect differentiation pathways of these cells. Targeting a bromodomain using the inhibitor i-BET762 suppresses HCC patient-derived M-MDSCs and enhances tumor-infiltrating lymphocytes and ICB efficacy in a fibrosis-associated hepatocellular carcinoma (HCC) model.[88] One group pharmacologically inhibited fatty acid transport 2 (FATP2), leading to the inhibition of the activity of PMN-MDSCs and substantially delayed tumor progression. The authors suggest the main mechanism of FATP2-mediated suppressive activity involved the uptake of arachidonic acid and the synthesis of prostaglandin E$_2$.[89] Another example of a targeted approach is the blockade of leukocyte immunoglobulin-like receptor LILRB2, which effectively suppressed granulocytic MDSC and T$_{reg}$ cell infiltration and significantly promoted in vivo antitumor effects of T cell immune checkpoint inhibitors.[90] Furthermore, LILRB2 blockade polarized tumor-infiltrating myeloid cells from NSCLC tumor tissues toward an inflammatory phenotype. All-trans retinoic acid (ATRA) has been previously described to effect myeloid populations, and recent clinical results suggest treatment may improve immunotherapeutic approaches.

Recent reports suggest ATRA in combination with ipilimumab in patients with melanoma observed a reduction in MDSC and increased T cell activity compared to the single agent ipilimumab group.[91] Cytokines such as IL-6 are highly elevated in cancer patients and promote the differentiation of suppressive immune cells in patients through signaling of the JAK/STAT3 pathway. Many research groups have examined ways to target this pathway to target differentiation of MDSC and TAMs to reduce immunosuppression.[53,92,93] These preclinical results suggest targeting STAT3 is a reasonable approach to inhibit the differentiation of these suppressive populations; however, few efficacious studies have been observed in the clinic.

CONCLUSION

A variety of immunosuppressive cell subtypes have important roles in promoting tumor immune evasion and

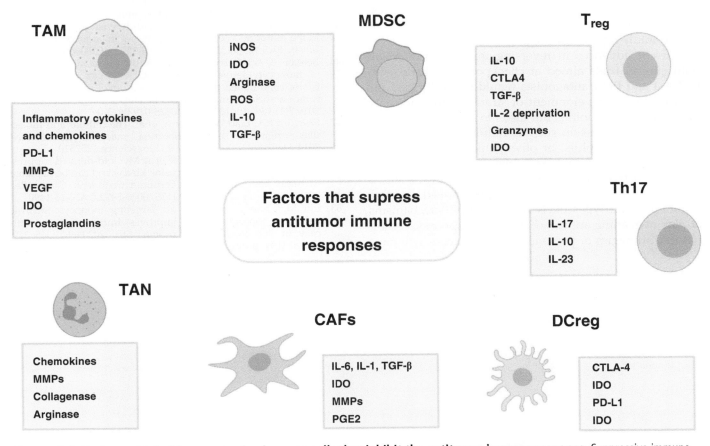

Figure 40.1 **Factors secreted by suppressive immune cells that inhibit the antitumor immune response.** Suppressive immune populations in the TME can secrete soluble factors, cytokines, chemokines, and express checkpoint ligands that lead to inhibition of antitumor immune responses.

CAFs, cancer-associated fibroblasts; DCreg, regulatory dendritic cells; IDO, indoleamine 2,3-dioxygenase; INOS, inducible nitric oxide synthase; MDSC, myeloid-derived suppressor cells; MMP, matrix metallopeptidase; PD-L1, programmed cell death ligand 1; TAM, tumor-associated macrophages; Th17 cells, T helper 17 cells; TAN, tumor-associated neutrophils; TME, tumor microenvironment; T$_{reg}$, regulatory T cell; VEGF, vascular endothelial growth factor.

in the development of metastases through a variety of mechanisms. These immunosuppressive cells can secrete a host of factors that can directly affect the ability of anti-tumor immune cells to traffic to the TME and kill tumor cells (Figure 40.1). Multiple new treatment approaches are leading to significant clinical advancements such as adoptive cellular immunotherapy (modified T cells or NK cells) or through immune checkpoint blockade and other forms of immune modulation. The future of the field of immunotherapy will definitely focus on targeting these peripheral, though critically important, immunosuppressive immune cell subsets. It is important that combinatorial strategies incorporating other modalities, such as chemotherapy and radiation, in addition to immune-directed therapies will be required to achieve greater clinical success for patients. A variety of physical and temporal targets will need to be considered; in addition, an assessment of opportunities to prevent differentiation of myeloid cells into mature immunosuppressive cells, and specific techniques of directly preventing the recruitment—and later depleting—of immunosuppressive cells within the TME, will need to be considered as important therapeutic strategies.

Current advances in reversing immunosuppression with clinical trials aimed at checkpoint blockade with CTLA-4 and PD-1 antagonists would naturally lead the field to further development of strategies that not only block other checkpoints, but also block other mediators of immunosuppression such as cellular processes (B_{regs}, TAMs, N2 neutrophils) or other inhibitory soluble targets such as TGF-β and IDO. Many of these pathways are being actively explored in multiple clinical trials in patients with a variety of tumor types. Indeed, because different tumor types likely have multiple mechanisms at play in evading antitumor immune responses, combinatorial strategies or personalized approaches will have

to be—and are being—used in clinical trials to overcome the current limitations of immunotherapy response rates in patients. Future research further detailing the cellular and molecular characteristics of the mechanisms of the immunosuppressive TME, tumor–host immune relationships, and the methods used by tumors for progression and metastasis in the setting of current immunotherapy approaches will help develop new and combinatorial strategies for cancer immunotherapy.

KEY REFERENCES

Only key references appear in the print edition. The full reference list appears in the digital product on Springer Publishing Connect: connect.springerpub.com/content/book/978-0-8261-3743-2/part/part03/chapter/ch40

7. Gajewski TF, Schreiber H, Fu YX. Innate and adaptive immune cells in the tumor microenvironment. *Nat Immunol.* 2013;14(10):1014–1022. doi:10.1038/ni.2703
31. Lechner MG, Liebertz DJ, Epstein AL. Characterization of cytokine-induced myeloid-derived suppressor cells from normal human peripheral blood mononuclear cells. *J Immunol.* 2010;185(4):2273–2284. doi:10.4049/jimmunol.1000901
43. Marvel D, Gabrilovich DI. Myeloid-derived suppressor cells in the tumor microenvironment: expect the unexpected. *J Clin Invest.* 2015;125(9):3356–3364. doi:10.1172/JCI80005
44. Benner B, Scarberry L, Suarez-Kelly LP, et al. Generation of monocyte-derived tumor-associated macrophages using tumor-conditioned media provides a novel method to study tumor-associated macrophages in vitro. *J Immunother Cancer.* 2019;7(1):140. doi:10.1186/s40425-019-0622-0
47. Franklin RA, Liao W, Sarkar A, et al. The cellular and molecular origin of tumor-associated macrophages. *Science.* 2014;344(6186):921–925. doi:10.1126/science.1252510
80. Stiff A, Trikha P, Wesolowski R, et al. Myeloid-derived suppressor cells express Bruton's tyrosine kinase and can be depleted in tumor-bearing hosts by ibrutinib treatment. *Cancer Res.* 2016;76(8):2125–2136. doi:10.1158/0008-5472.CAN-15-1490
88. Liu M, Zhou J, Liu X, et al. Targeting monocyte-intrinsic enhancer reprogramming improves immunotherapy efficacy in hepatocellular carcinoma. *Gut.* 2020;69(2):365–379. doi:10.1136/gutjnl-2018-317257

41

Circulating Mediators of Tumor-Induced Immune Suppression

Theresa L. Whiteside

KEY POINTS

- Human tumors produce and use cellular or soluble mediators to induce immune suppression and escape from the host immune system.

- Regulatory T cells (T$_{reg}$ cells) suppress functions of various types of immune cells using mechanisms ranging from contact-dependent signaling to secretion of inhibitory cytokines or soluble factors mediating juxtacrine or paracrine interactions.

- Tumor-derived exosomes (TEX) emerge as a major mechanism for carrying messages from the tumor to immune cells.

- TEX promote functions of T$_{reg}$ cells and myeloid-derived suppressor cells but suppress activity of antitumor effector cells.

- TEX carry proteins, miRNA, mRNA, and DNA from the tumor to immune cells and utilizing this cargo reprogram recipient cell functions.

- TEX-mediated reprogramming of antitumor immune cells represent a major and underestimated mechanism of tumor immune escape.

- TEX reprogram immunoregulatory mechanisms including maturation, differentiation, proliferation, and survival of immune effector cells.

- Mechanisms that TEX employ for reprogramming immune cells involve receptor/ligand signaling at the surface of receptor cells and/or genetic alterations in the transcriptome and proteome of the cells after exosome uptake.

- The TEX cargo and their ability to reprogram immune cells are of great interest as potential biomarkers of cancer progression and immune competence in patients with cancer.

INTRODUCTION

Tumor-derived immune suppression has been recognized as one of the main reasons for the ability of tumors to escape immune surveillance and to progress.[1] Tumor cells are known to produce a variety of factors that exert inhibitory effects on the development, differentiation, progression, or recruitment of immune cells to tumor sites, including those mediating innate immune responses as well as tumor-antigen-specific T cells.[2] At the same time, tumor cells are characterized by genetic and molecular heterogeneity, which has been implicated in differential sensitivity of human tumors to various therapies. Tumor heterogeneity is driven by genetic and epigenetic changes in the tumor and the tumor microenvironment (TME), respectively. Further, these changes benefit the tumor, and select for tumor cells that are resistant to immune intervention by the host or to administered therapies. The key question of how the developing tumor manages to overcome the natural host defense mechanisms against malignant invasion remains largely unanswered. It is clear that the disarming of host antitumor immune responses may be mediated by many different molecular mechanisms, which operate not only in the TME but also in the periphery.[3] How many or which of these mechanisms play a key role in tumor escape is critically important, yet it remains debatable. If we are to overcome tumor immune escape, it seems essential to identify the responsible mechanisms and therapeutically inhibit their effects. In this chapter, we discuss several types of circulating mediators of immune suppression in cancer, stressing the relatively novel mechanism that appears to involve vesicular-mediated interactions between the tumor and immune cells in the TME. This mechanism does not dispense with previously emphasized concepts of intercellular immune regulation involving suppressor and effector immune cell cooperation. It only introduces an additional component (i.e., small extracellular vesicles [EVs]), to the process of intercellular communication that underscores and probably determines the effects tumors impose on the host immune system.

REGULATORY T CELLS IN CANCER

CD4[+] regulatory T cells (T_{reg} cells) play a crucial role in the maintenance of peripheral tolerance and represent 4% to 8% of CD4[+] T cells in the periphery.[3] The essential function of T_{reg} cells is to suppress activation, clonal expansion, and effector functions of various immune cells, including CD4[+] and CD8[+] T cells, NK cells, and antigen-presenting cells (APCs), comprising B cells, monocytes, and dendritic cells (DCs). T_{reg} cells can utilize a variety of different mechanisms to do so.[4] While recent studies of T_{reg} cells have identified many of these mechanisms, expression of Foxp3, a transcription factor, appears to be required for the development of T_{reg} cells.[4] T_{reg} cells can be broadly divided into two subsets: thymus-derived T_{reg} cells (tT_{regs}) and peripherally induced T_{reg} cells (p-T_{regs}), which are also called inducible T_{reg} cells (iT_{regs}). While the former regulated reactivity against self, the latter are induced in the periphery from naïve or T effector cells under inflammatory or non-inflammatory conditions and regulate responses to self or foreign antigens, including tumor-associated antigens. In cancer, iT_{regs} accumulate both in the TME and in the periphery.[4] They are a heterogeneous population of CD4[+] T cells, only some of which are Foxp3[+] and which may or may not produce IL-10, TGF-β, IL-35, or adenosine.[4] The production of immunosuppressive cytokines is only one of various mechanisms used by iT_{regs} to suppress antitumor immunity. These mechanisms operate by direct cell-to-cell contact or indirectly, often at considerable distances, and result in suppression of antitumor immune responses. They seem to involve signaling pathways common to most tumors such as programmed cell death 1/programmed cell death ligand 1 (PD1/PD-L1), TGF-β1, or adenosine. Importantly, accumulations and suppressor activities of iT_{regs} in cancer have been correlated to poor prognosis in some human malignancies.[5] However, in other cancers (e.g., colorectal carcinomas), the presence of iT_{regs} is associated with a better outcome.[6] This suggests that iT_{regs} are themselves under a regulatory oversight that may be different in various cancers. The question of how iT_{regs} are regulated and how this regulation impacts on tumor progression is critical for our understanding of how tumors execute immune escape.

MYELOID-DERIVED SUPPRESSOR CELLS IN CANCER

Much has been written about the critical role of myeloid cells in cancer progression.[7] There is no doubt that the development, differentiation, and frequency of myeloid-derived suppressor cells (MDSCs) have a major impact on cancer development and on tumor escape from immune surveillance.[8] The M1 to M2 transition in the TME has been extensively investigated and shown to be the major pathway for promotion of tumor escape in murine models of tumor growth and in humans with cancer.[9] Here also numerous mechanisms for the promotion of M1 to M2 transition have been proposed.[9] Cellular interactions as well as various tumor-derived soluble factors have been described that promote the development and differentiation of MDSC.[10] Nevertheless, no consistent mechanism for MDSC accumulation and activity in cancer has been available so far. While the elegant studies by Mantovani's group go a long way to explain the importance of cytokines/chemokines in the process, there remains a question of what regulates M1 to M2 transition in the TME.[11]

TUMOR-DERIVED EXOSOMES

Emerging evidence indicates that tumors communicate with nonmalignant cells in their microenvironment by various means, including soluble factors such as cytokines and chemokines or small membranous vesicles. Tumors release vesicles of different sizes either by "blebbing" or active extrusion. Virus-size exosomes (currently called small extracellular vesicles or sEVs) are the smallest of these vesicles (30–150 nm).[12] They originate in the endocytic compartment of the parent cell by invagination of the endosome membrane and are released when multivesicular bodies (MVB) containing numerous exosomes fuse with the cell surface membrane.[13] All cells produce exosomes, but tumor cells produce large numbers of tumor-derived exosomes (TEX), which freely distribute throughout the body. Plasma and other body fluids of patients with cancer contain many more exosomes than those of healthy individuals.[14] TEX are a subset of sEVs found in the plasma of all cancer patients.[14,15] TEX differ from other sEVs in their molecular and genetic cargos, because the TEX surface membrane (containing proteins, lipids, and glycans) and TEX lumen (containing DNA, mRNA, and microRNA) in part resemble contents of the parent tumor cells.[13] TEX may carry oncogenes, and those vesicles that do are referred to as "oncomirs."[16] Because they mimic parent tumor cells, TEX in body fluids of cancer patients have been of great interest as potential cancer biomarkers.[15,17] Importantly, TEX carry and deliver to recipient cells molecular signals and nucleic acids, which alter functions of these cells.[18,19] This phenotypic and functional alteration is referred to as TEX-mediated reprogramming. It is tumor driven; it can involve nonmalignant or malignant cells; and it results in changes of cellular behavior benefitting the tumor.[18,19] It is responsible for converting antitumor functions of nonmalignant normal cells, such as immune cells, to functions that promote tumor growth and immune escape.

INTERACTIONS OF TUMOR-DERIVED EXOMES AND IMMUNE CELLS

Local and systemic distribution and transfer of TEX to other circulating or tissue cells represents a newly recognized mechanism responsible for exchange of genetic and molecular materials between cells residing at close or distant locations. TEX contribute to cancer development by interference with immune surveillance mechanisms, thus promoting tumor cell proliferation and differentiation, angiogenesis, drug resistance, invasion, and metastasis as well as maintenance of cancer stem cells.[17] In the TME, TEX carrying various immunoinhibitory molecules and factors are highly effective mediators of immune suppression.[20,21] TEX can alter functions of immune cells directly or indirectly. Direct interactions of TEX and immune cells involve a receptor-ligand type signaling or an uptake by endocytosis or phagocytosis of TEX and release of their content in the recipient cell.[22] In either case, TEX are highly efficient in delivering inhibitory signals to immune cells, as well as reducing or abolishing antitumor activities of the recipient immune cells. Indirect TEX-mediated suppression is executed by T_{reg} cells or MDSC, which upon interaction with TEX are induced to expand and/or increase their suppressive activities.[23,24] This, in turn, results in TEX-orchestrated increase in local as well as systemic immunosuppression.[25] In this context, TEX emerge as a tumor-driven mechanism regulating activities of T_{reg} cells and MDSC.

TUMOR-DERIVED EXOME AND REGULATORY T CELL COLLABORATION

The frequency of circulating $CD4^+CD25^{high}Foxp3^+$ T_{reg} cells is often elevated in patients with cancer.[25] TEX appear to be responsible, at least in part, for elevated T_{reg} cell numbers in the blood of cancer patients. Ex vivo coincubation experiments showed that TEX induced the conversion of human conventional $CD4^+CD25^-$ T cells to $CD4^+CD25^{high}Foxp3^+$ T_{reg} cells, which was dependent on the presence of TGF-β1; this led to increased levels of phosphorylated SMAD2/3 and phosphorylated STAT3 in T_{reg} cells and promoted their proliferation.[26] TEX coincubated with neutralizing antibodies against TGF-β1 or IL-10 lost the ability to induce T_{reg} cell expansion. Further, T_{reg} cells coincubated with TEX upregulated expression levels of various inhibitory molecules, including Fas-L, TGF-β1/LAP/ GARP, IL-10, CTLA-4, PD-1, granzyme B (GrB), and perforin.[27] After coincubation with TEX, T_{reg} cells mediated enhanced suppression of proliferation in autologous $CD4^+$ T cells and acquired enhanced apoptotic activity in cultures with activated $CD8^+$ T cells.[27,28] T_{reg} cells that proliferated in response to TEX were completely resistant to TEX-mediated apoptosis.[27] These data indicate that TEX influence not only the frequency of T_{reg} cells but also their suppressor functions.

EFFECTS OF TUMOR-DERIVED EXOMES ON FUNCTIONS OF CD8+ EFFECTOR CELLS AND NATURAL KILLER CELLS

TEX carrying PD-L1, TGF-β, CTLA-4, CD39/CD73, and other inhibitory proteins interact not only with regulatory cells but also with effector immune cells, including $CD8^+$ T cells and natural killer (NK) cells. Recent studies documented that these interactions are mediated by TEX isolated from plasma of cancer patients by size exclusion chromatography and immune capture of TEX to separate them from non-TEX present in plasma.[29] The proteins present on the TEX surface of the separated subsets were evaluated by on-bead flow cytometry,[30] and the acquired data were presented as relative fluorescence intensity (RFI) values. Stimulatory/inhibitory functions were measured in coincubation assays of primary activated human T cells or NK cells +/− TEX, and the stim/ supp ratios were determined.[31] The analysis of molecular content of TEX was showed enrichment in immunosuppressive proteins and paucity of immunostimulatory proteins, such as OX40L or OX40, in agreement with data previously reported by us for TEX from tumor cell supernatants.[26] TEX had significant immunosuppressive activity (i.e., induced downregulation of CD69 expression on $CD8^+$ T cells, inhibition of $CD8^+$ T cell proliferation, apoptosis of activated $CD8^+$ T and NK cells).[31] The separated non-TEX, consisting largely of $CD3^+$ sEVs, were also tested in coincubation assays with primary human immune responder cells and, surprisingly, were found to mediate immune suppression, albeit to a lesser extent than the paired TEX.[31] Also, non-TEX of cancer patients were phenotypically and functionally different from sEV in the plasma of healthy donors (HDs) tested in parallel assays. They were more similar to TEX. These results suggested that in patients with cancer, non-TEX subpopulations were reprogrammed and acquired immunosuppressive properties.[31] Thus, both TEX and non-TEX in cancer plasma were capable of inhibiting functions of immune effector cells, and this suppression was dependent on the ratios of suppressive/stimulatory proteins present in their respective cargos.

EVALUATION OF REPROGRAMMED NON-TUMOR-DERIVED EXOMES IN CANCER PATIENTS' PLASMA

The possibility that reprogrammed nonmalignant sEVs (i.e., non-TEX) contributed to tumor-induced immune suppression and immune escape was directly tested by using the immunocapture strategy with anti-CD3 monoclonal antibodies (mAbs) to separate $CD3^+$ sEV from CD3(-) sEV in cancer plasma.[32] Since only T cells express CD3, this strategy separates sEV that are produced by T cells from all other sEV in plasma. It can be separated from CD3(-) sEV and recovered on beads. Surprisingly, CD3(+) sEV represented >50% of total plasma sEV in patients with head and neck squamous cell carcinoma (HNSCC).[32] Also, both CD3(+) and CD3(-) sEV fractions were enriched in the immunosuppressive proteins (PD-L1, CTLA-4, COX2, CD39/CD73) and patients with high levels (i.e., above the mean level for the entire patient cohort) of immunosuppressive proteins in CD3(+) sEV had stage III/IV tumors and positive lymph nodes, while patients with low levels of the suppressive cargo in CD3(+) sEV had less advanced (stage I/II, N0) disease.[32,33] In HNSCC patients with early stage I/II disease, CD3(+) sEV carried high levels of immunostimulatory cargo (i.e., had high expression of OX40 or OX40L), while in patients with advanced disease and positive lymph nodes, CD3(+) sEV had low levels of OX40 or OX40L, and in coincubation assays induced apoptosis of CD8$^+$ effector T cells and promoted expansion of T$_{reg}$ cells.[32,33] These data provided preliminary evidence that the molecular content of CD3(+)(T cell derived) sEV fractions correlated with disease activity and disease progression in patients with HNSCC. It appears that in patients with cancer, plasma sEV produced by reprogrammed CD3$^+$ T cells acquire the ability to suppress immune responses and thus contribute to tumor immune escape.

MECHANISMS INVOLVED IN SMALL EXTRACELLULAR VESICLE-MEDIATED IMMUNE SUPPRESSION IN CANCER

As previously described, coincubation of TEX with subsets of immune cells isolated from human peripheral blood was shown to result in phenotypic and functional reprogramming of these cells. Mechanisms that TEX utilize for altering the molecular profile and functions of regulatory as well as effector immune cells are not yet entirely clear. Mechanistically, TEX were shown to induce massive changes in expression levels of mRNA coding for numerous genes in recipient cells, consistent with miRNA-mediated effects.[34] Because TEX carry miRNAs, it has been suggested that the uptake of TEX by recipient cells results in the delivery of miRNAs followed by miRNA-driven changes in gene expression.[35] Following TEX-induced changes in expression levels of 24 randomly selected immunoregulatory genes by qRT-PCR analyses in CD4$^+$ T cells, CD8$^+$ T cells, and T$_{reg}$ cells, it was possible to demonstrate either down- or upregulation of all of these genes.[35] Thus, TEX induced changes in the transcriptional profile of T cells. Further, these transcriptional changes had functional consequences, as shown by simultaneous measurements by flow cytometry of expression levels of selected proteins in activated T cells coincubated with TEX. For example, CD69 (an activation marker) expression level (MFI) on the surface of these T cells was found to be significantly reduced ($p < 0.0005$) after interaction with TEX, suggesting that TEX interfered with T cell activation.[35] TEX were also shown to increase expression levels of genes encoding proteins involved in suppression of immune responses, such as COX2, Fas-L, Fas, CTLA-4, or TGF-β1 in activated CD4$^+$ or CD8$^+$ T cells. This

suggested that TEX promoted the synthesis and translation of mRNA encoding these inhibitory proteins, resulting in a molecular profile consistent with a loss of activation and a gain in immune suppression.[35] The results are in agreement with previous reports of TEX inducing immune suppression in activated T cells,[21] including a loss or downregulation of the zeta chain associated with the T cell receptor (TCR) and of activation markers such as CD69 on the T cell surface.[26] TEX profoundly inhibited T cell proliferation and induced rapid apoptosis of effector T cells.[26,27] In NK cells, TEX inhibited (in a dose-dependent manner) surface expression of NKG2D and blocked NK cell lytic activity against tumor cell targets.[36] Coincubation of DCs with TEX led to downregulation of CD80 and CD86 on the DC surface and inhibited DC maturation.[37] Another report demonstrated inhibition of the antigen-processing machinery (APM) components such as TAP1 upon coincubation of matured DC with TEX.[37] These direct suppressive effects of TEX on functions of various immune effector cells suggested that TEX interactions with immune cells involved the complementary receptors/ligands (e.g., Fas/Fas-L or PD-1/PDL-1) on the surface of recipient cells, ultimately resulting in the observed immunosuppression.

To further investigate cellular consequences of TEX interactions with T cells, TEX were labeled with the PKH26 dye and their uptake by T cells, B cells, and monocytes isolated from human peripheral blood was monitored. Image analyses using an Amnis Image Stream cytometer showed that CD14$^+$ monocytes and CD19$^+$ B cells readily internalized PKH26$^+$ TEX during 24-hour coincubation.[38] However, resting or activated T$_{reg}$ cells or conventional CD4$^+$ and CD8$^+$ T cells did not internalize TEX even after prolonged incubation. This suggested that uptake, internalization of TEX by T cells, and TEX-mediated miRNA transfer were not required for delivery of a message responsible for the observed reprograming of T cell functions. Instead, signals delivered by TEX to receptors on the surface of activated T cells appear to be sufficient for inducing TEX-mediated genetic and molecular changes.

Almost all of the previously described effects of TEX in recipient immune cells involved activation of common suppressive pathways by signals carried on the vesicle surface. We showed that suppression of T cell or NK cell functions by TEX was concentration dependent, was absent when TEX were pretreated with proteinase K or heat denatured, and was significantly reversed by: (a) neutralizing Abs to inhibitory ligands (Fas-L, TRAIL, PD-L1, CTLA-4, MICA/B); (b) blocking of TEX uptake by recipient cells; and (c) pharmacologic inhibitors of TGF-β, adenosine, AKT/PI-3K, or NF-KB pathways.[31] The amelioration in vitro of TEX-mediated immune cell suppression simultaneously by several different inhibitors suggests that not one but many molecular pathways may be engaged when TEX are interacting with T cells.[39] Such a simultaneous engagement of several inhibitory receptors on the surface of a T cell would result in a rapid T cell exhaustion and/or demise.

One of the major mechanisms of suppression utilized by T_{reg} cells is production of immunosuppressive adenosine.[40] Adenosine signaling via A2a receptors on T effector cells inhibits their proliferation and cytokine production by the cAMP-dependent mechanism.[41] Interestingly, TEX carry enzymatically active CD39 and CD73, the two ecto-nucleotidases catalyzing adenosine production from exogenous ATP, and to deliver CD73 to CD4+CD39+ human T_{reg} cells, thus facilitating adenosine synthesis and enhancing T_{reg} cell suppressor functions.[42] Coincubation of T_{reg} cells with TEX significantly increased expression levels of CD39, leading to a burst of enzymatic activity, upregulated adenosine production, and enhanced suppression by T_{reg} cells.[23,42] While TEX-mediated signaling promoted suppressor functions of T_{reg} cells in CD4+ T cells via the adenosine pathway, TEX-induced signals in CD8+effector T cells promoted translation of the genes encoding various inhibitory proteins, as previously described. Thus, TEX-mediated effects in CD4+T_{reg} cells were distinct from those observed in CD4+ or CD8+ effector T cells, suggesting that the nature of recipient cells might determine the outcome of TEX-immune cell cross talk.

BIOLOGICAL SIGNIFICANCE OF TUMOR-DERIVED EXOMES IN CANCER

Functional responses of immune cells interacting with TEX are likely to have an impact on cancer progression and outcome. The presence of numerous inhibitory ligands or soluble factors such as PGE_2 or adenosine in the cargo of TEX isolated from body fluids of cancer patients has been well documented.[41] It appears that common inhibitory pathways are activated in various immune cells by TEX decorated with the immunosuppressive ligands and/or carrying immunosuppressive soluble factors. Activation by TEX of the Fas/Fas-L pathway in CD8+ T cells is well known;[26,43] suppression of NK cell activity by TEX via TGF-β/TGF-βR or MICA and MICB/NKG2D pathways has been reported;[37,44] T_{reg} cell suppressor functions are upregulated by TEX promoting activation of the adenosine or PGE_2 pathways;[40] and T effector cells can be suppressed by TEX via PD-1/PD-L1 pathway.[45]

The TEX-mediated blockade of immune cell functions via these various inhibitory pathways results in compromised antitumor immunity and predicts poor outcome in cancer.[46] A large deal of attention is currently directed at TEX, because of its potential importance as a biomarker of disease presence, progression, and outcome, as well as a biomarker of immune dysfunction and response to immune therapies. Despite this attention, there is a lack of understanding of the vicious pathway of immune suppression that TEX perpetrate in cancer patients with advanced malignancies. The pervasive nature of TEX-mediated immune suppression and reprogramming of immune cells underlie the tumor immune escape and a lack of response to immune therapies by many patients with cancer.

CONCLUSION

This chapter introduces a novel and perhaps the most efficient mechanism yet discovered of tumor-induced immune suppression. The mechanism involves EVs otherwise known as exosomes and focuses on EVs produced by tumor cells or TEX. Among the many and various mechanisms responsible for tumor escape from the host immune system, TEX, which are present in all body fluids, are currently emerging as highly effective facilitators of tumor escape through protein-based negative signaling or microRNA-mediated functional reprogramming of immune cells. By interfering with antitumor functions of immune effector cells, TEX actively impair immune competence of cancer patients, promote cancer progression, and reduce responses to therapy. Recent progress in our understanding of the mechanisms and role TEX play in tumor immune escape provides hope that TEX-mediated immune suppression is amenable to immunotherapy. While TEX represent another barrier to cancer treatment that we need to cross, there is preliminary evidence that TEX might be useful as cancer biomarkers and that their removal or blockade might reverse tumor escape.

KEY REFERENCES

Only key references appear in the print edition. The full reference list appears in the digital product on Springer Publishing Connect: connect.springerpub.com/content/book/978-0-8261-3743-2/part/part03/chapter/ch41

12. Zijlstra A, di Vizio D. Size matters in nanoscale communication. *Nat Cell Biol.* 2018;20(3):228–230. doi:10.1038/s41556-018-0049-8
15. Whiteside TL. The potential of tumor-derived exosomes for noninvasive cancer monitoring. *Expert Rev Mol Diagn.* 2015;15(10):1293–1310. doi:10.1586/14737159.2015.1071666
17. Melo SA, Luecke LB, Kahlert C, et al. Glypican-1 identifies cancer exosomes and detects early pancreatic cancer. *Nature.* 2015;523(7559):177–182. doi:10.1038/nature14581
18. Peinado H, Alečković M, Lavotshkin S, et al. Melanoma exosomes educate bone marrow progenitor cells toward a pro-metastatic phenotype through MET. *Nat Med.* 2012;18(6):883–891. doi:10.1038/nm.2753
21. Whiteside TL. Exosomes and tumor-mediated immune suppression. *J Clin Invest.* 2016;126(4):1216–1223. doi:10.1172/JCI81136
38. Muller L, Simms P, Hong CS, et al. Human tumor-derived exosomes (TEX) regulate T_{reg} cell functions via cell surface signaling rather than uptake mechanisms. *Oncoimmunology.* 2017;6(8):e1261243. doi:10.1080/2162402X.2016.1261243

42

Harnessing B Cells and Tertiary Lymphoid Structures for Antitumor Immunity

Ayana T. Ruffin and Tullia C. Bruno

KEY POINTS

- Intratumoral B cells and tertiary lymphoid structures (TLSs) are key components of the immune response to cancer but have been severely understudied in the context of immunotherapy.

- Intratumoral B cells and TLS correlate with better survival in multiple cancer indices and can predict response to current immune-based therapies.

- Intratumoral B cells and TLS are heterogeneous in the tumor microenvironment (TME) with distinct phenotypes that have been associated with better prognosis and reduced risk of recurrence.

- Intratumoral B cells may promote antitumor immunity by presenting antigen to intratumoral T cells, producing cytokines and chemokines that drive TLS formation, and generating tumor-reactive antibodies that can activate NK and macrophage-mediated killing of tumor cells.

- The B cell/TLS axis provides exciting, new opportunities for immunotherapy, such as adoptive cell transfer (ACT), therapeutic induction of TLS, B cell vaccines, and targeting of novel B cell specific pathways with new therapeutic antibodies.

INTRODUCTION

Harnessing the immune system to detect and destroy tumors has revolutionized the treatment of cancer patients. U.S. Food and Drug Administration (FDA)-approved immunotherapies have focused on blocking immune checkpoints such as programmed cell death 1 (PD-1) and cytotoxic T lymphocyte-associated protein 4 (CTLA-4) (immune checkpoint blockade; ICB), which are cell-intrinsic inhibitors of T cell function. There has been remarkable clinical success with ICB in some patients, but only 20% to 30% of patients treated with ICB have durable therapeutic benefit.

Therefore, understanding the role of other immune cells in the tumor microenvironment (TME) will be paramount for generating new and effective therapies. Intratumoral B cells are the second most abundant tumor-infiltrating immune cell and correlate with increased survival in a variety of cancers. In human solid tumors, intratumoral B cells can be found in ectopic, lymph node-like structures termed "tertiary lymphoid structures" (TLSs), which have been implicated in driving antitumor immune responses. Recent advances indicate that B cells and TLS can predict whether patients will respond to current immunotherapies. Strong and effective immune responses require cooperation of B and T cells; thus, further investigation of the function of B cells in the TME is warranted. This chapter reviews our current understanding of B cells and TLS in cancer with a focus on patient-based studies. We discuss both antibody-dependent and antibody-independent functions of B cells within different TMEs and compare B cell and TLS composition within TMEs. Finally, we discuss potential ways to therapeutically enhance antitumor B cell responses and induce TLS formation to complement current T cell-focused immunotherapies with the ultimate goal of improving patient survival.

BRIEF PRIMER ON B CELL DIFFERENTIATION AND MATURATION

Early B cell differentiation and maturation steps begin in the bone marrow (BM), resulting in naïve CD19+ CD20+ B cells characterized by expression of unmutated immunoglobulin (Ig) isotypes, IgM and IgD.[1] Upon activation by cognate antigen, circulating naïve B cells expressing chemokine receptor CXCR5 migrate into primary follicles within secondary lymphoid organs (SLOs) such as lymph nodes.[2] Antigen-activated B cells then receive growth and differentiation signals from T follicular helper (TFH) cells, which results in either short-lived plasmablast differentiation (extrafollicular pathway) or formation of germinal centers (GCs).[3,4] During a GC reaction, antigen-activated B cells migrate into the two polarized zones of the GCs, which include a dark zone (DZ) and a light zone (LZ).[3] Within these specialized sites, high-affinity B cell clones are created through rapid proliferation, mutation of Ig genes (somatic hypermutation [SHM]), and class switching to the IgG, IgA, or IgE isotypes. They are selected based on their ability to capture and present antigen to TFH cells (affinity maturation).[5] These events are regulated by a host of genes including transcription factor B cell lymphoma 6 protein (BCL6), which is essential for GC formation and controls gene expression in GC B cells.[5] Successful B cell clones differentiate into memory B cells (MBC) or long-lived plasma cells (PC). MBC can be distinguished by CD27 and CD21 expression and are responsible for differentiation into antibody-secreting cells upon re-encountering antigen (recall response).[6] Several studies have demonstrated that MBC are also capable of re-entering GCs during recall responses in mice and that is likely the case in humans.[7-11] PCs, distinguished by CD138 and CD38 expression, produce the majority of antibodies found in serum and can migrate to sites of inflammation to produce high concentrations of local antibodies.[12] These maturation steps for B cells are paramount for mounting effective immune responses against invading pathogens. We will discuss how these processes can shape B cell responses against tumors in later sections of this chapter.

CLINICAL SIGNIFICANCE OF B CELLS AND TERTIARY LYMPHOID STRUCTURES IN HUMAN TUMORS

Mouse Versus Human Cancer Studies: Are B Cells Friend or Foe?

Within the last decade, several studies have highlighted that increased infiltration of B cells in human solid tumors is associated with favorable outcomes in a variety of cancers.[13-18] However, B cells have been overlooked as a potential target for immunotherapy. In fact, mechanistic studies interrogating how B cells contribute to anti- or protumor immune response in humans are very limited despite their abundance within the TME. Perhaps this neglect of B cells as an immunotherapeutic target can be attributed to the contradictory evidence regarding B cell function in the TME in preclinical mouse models.[19,20] Most mouse models demonstrate that B cells promote tumor progression or play no role in the antitumor immune response. For example, in melanoma and sarcoma murine models, depletion of B cells enhanced CD8[+] T cell antitumor reponses.[21] However, a different study demonstrated that depletion of B cells in a B16 melanoma model significantly accelerated melanoma growth and metastasis and reduced the antitumor response of CD4[+] and CD8[+] T cells.[20] Depletion of B cells, either genetically (RAG[−/−], μMT mice) or via therapeutic antibodies (anti-CD20; rituximab), overlooks the fact that B cells are a heterogeneous population and it may be more physiologically relevant to enhance some B cell subsets while inhibiting others. Preclinical mouse models will be needed to perform critical mechanistic studies to assess B cell function in the TME. Thus, developing physiologically relevant mouse models with immunogenic TLS to study B cells in cancer should be prioritized.

B cell infiltration in human solid tumors is associated with favorable outcomes in hepatocellular carcinoma (HCC), colorectal carcinoma (CRC), melanoma, pancreatic ductal adenocarcinoma (PDAC), breast cancer (BRCA), non-small cell lung cancer (NSCLC), esophageal cancer (ESCA), stomach adenocarcinoma (STAD), ovarian cancer (OV), and head and neck squamous cell carcinoma (HNSC) patients.[15,22-28] TLS are also associated with better survival in at least 10 different types of cancers including HCC, OV, HNSC, melanoma, BRCA, and NSCLC.[14,16,27,29,30] Thus, immunotherapies targeting B cells and TLS could potentially benefit multiple cancer indices and perhaps enhance responses to current T cell-focused therapies. Recently, B cells and their presence in TLS were shown to predict whether patients would respond to ICB.[13,17,31] Patients with high-risk resectable melanoma and metastatic renal cell carcinoma (RCC) that responded to ICB had more B cells and TLS prior to and after treatment.[17] Additional studies corroborated these findings in melanoma, demonstrating that TLS in melanoma patients contained high densities of B cells and patients without TLS had worse outcomes while on ICB.[31] B cell-rich TLS are also predictive of response to ICB therapy in soft tissue sarcomas (STSs) and B cells were shown to be the strongest prognostic factor in comparison to CD8[+] T cells in STS patients.[13] These complementary studies highlight the prognostic importance of B cells and TLS. More importantly, they emphasize the potential of B cells and TLS to inform whether patients should be treated with current immunotherapies.

HETEROGENEITY OF B CELLS AND TERTIARY LYMPHOID STRUCTURES IN THE TUMOR MICROENVIRONMENT

Primer on Tertiary Lymphoid Structure Formation

TLS are ectopic lymphoid aggregates that form at the sites of chronic inflammation in nonlymphoid tissues, including tumors.[32] TLS have been implicated as critical mediators of antitumor immunity in cancer patients as the absence of TLS is associated with worse outcomes.[31,33] TLS share many structural characteristics with SLOs including T cell-rich immune clusters, B cell follicles consisting of naïve B cells surrounding an active GC, specialized blood vessels called high endothelial venules (HEVs), mature dendritic cells (DCs), and follicular dendritic cells (FDCs).[33,34] Murine studies suggest that TLS formation in nonlymphoid tissues occurs by similar mechanisms of SLO neogenesis.[32,35] In SLO neogenesis, CD4[+]CD3[-]RANK[+]IL-7Rα[hi] lymphoid tissue inducer (LTi) cells are recruited to sites of inflammation by local production of CXCL13 and IL-7 by immune or tissue-resident stromal cells.[32,36,37] LTi cells also express lymphotoxin LTα$_1$β$_2$ which binds LTβR (lymphotoxin beta receptor) on stromal cells.[33,37,38] This interaction leads to the production of chemokines CCL19, CCL21, CXCL12, and CXCL13, as well as vascular endothelial growth factor C (VEGFC), which recruits B cells, T cells, and DCs and supports the development of HEVs.[32,36–38] While LTi cells are required for SLO development in the LN, spleen, and Peyer's patches, CD4[+] T helper 17 cells (Th17), M1-polarized macrophages, and B cells can induce TLS formation in the absence of LTi cells.[39,40] Although TLS formation has largely been studied in chronic infection and autoimmunity, studies in human cancer (i.e., NSCLC, BRCA, and melanoma) suggest that similar chemokine and cytokine gene signatures may also regulate TLS formation in human tumors.[41–43]

Tertiary Lymphoid Structure Heterogeneity Within the Tumor Microenvironment

TLS have been detected within the tumor bed but are more abundant in the invasive margin and stroma of the TME.[33,37] Significant variability in TLS organization and immune cell composition can be observed from patient to patient within a given cancer type and between different cancer types, suggesting that some TMEs are more conducive to TLS formation and maintenance.[27,41,44,45] For example, in treatment-naïve lung squamous cell carcinoma (LUSC) and nonmetastatic colorectal carcinoma (nmCRC) patients, three distinct phenotypes of TLS were identified using multispectral immunofluorescence (mIF): (a) early TLS (E-TLS): dense immune cell aggregates without FDCs; (b) primary follicle-like TLS (PFL-TLS): B cell clusters with FDCs but without GCs; and (c) secondary follicle-like TLS (SFL-TLS): TLS with GCs (Figure 42.1).[41,46] In nmCRC, high numbers of E-TLS and low numbers of SFL-TLS were associated with increased risk of recurrence.[46] Further, in LUSC, patients with high densities of TLS also had increased expression of genes involved in TLS formation such as CXCL13, CXCL12, LTB, CCL19, CCL21, IL-7, and genes associated with the adaptive immune response including B cell (CD20, CD40) and T cell (CD3, CD8, IL-21, PD-1) gene signatures.[41] In high-grade serous ovarian cancer (HGSOC), similar TLS phenotypes were described: (a) *Type I:* small aggregate of CD20[+] B cells, CD4[+] and CD8[+] T cells, and some DCs; (b) *Type II:* larger aggregate of CD20[+] B cells and CD4[+] and CD8[+] T cells without clear zones or follicles; (c) *Type III:* defined B cell follicle with GC and a network of CD21[+] FDCs, discrete CD4[+] and CD8[+] T cell zones, and HEV.[27] Active immune responses within TLS

were observed in HGSOC patients by immunohisto-chemistry (IHC) staining of transcription factor BCL6, which regulates GC reactions and activation-induced cytidine deaminase (AID), which regulates SHM of Ig genes and class switch recombination (CSR).[5,27] Notably, patients with tumors containing CD8[+] and CD4[+] T cells and CD20[+] B cells and plasma cells had increased dis-ease-specific free survival.[27]

Oncogenic drivers such as environmental exposure to carcinogens or viral infection may influence the type of TLS present within a given TME. For example, TLS phenotypes are distinct within the TME of HNSC patients, which is caused by both carcinogen exposure (alcohol and tobacco use) and infection with human papillomavirus (HPV).[47,48] TLS-containing GCs were significantly increased in HPV[+] HNSC patients compared to HPV[-] HNSC.[47,49] Viral and carcinogen stimuli can activate the lymphotoxin/CXCL13 pathway which is key for TLS formation; however, chemical carcinogens present in tobacco can also suppress immune responses, which could perhaps explain poor TLS formation in HPV[-] HNSC.[50–52] Additionally, it is possible that poor TLS formation in HPV[-] HNSC could be attributed to extrafollicular differentiation of intratumoral B cells and lack of GC formation.[4,53] While TLS and the key TLS-associated inflammatory gene signatures are increased in virally associated cancers such as HNSC and HCC, whether viral infection in tumors plays a direct role in maturation of B cells and TLS remains unclear.[54] Further, there is a growing interest in understanding how organisms (microbiome) that live on barrier surfaces where tumors occur such as skin and colon affect tumor immunity.[55] While direct effects of the microbiome on intratumoral B cells and TLS in human solid tumors are largely unknown, early studies in murine models of CRC reveal that modifying the microbiome of CRC with colonization of *Helicobacter hepaticus* (Hhep) can drive microbiome-specific TFH differentiation and TLS formation in CRC tumors.[56]

Cancers caused by exposure to carcinogens such as UV exposure or tobacco and alcohol use often have an increased mutational burden, which has been associated with increased TLS and TLS-associated gene signatures.[43,46,54] It is clear from mouse and human studies that at least three key events are needed for TLS formation: (a) inflammatory cytokine expression, (b) lymphoid chemokine production by stromal cells, and (c) HEV development.[35] Future studies should investigate how oncogenic drivers play a role in initiation of these events as this may provide insight into why TLS formation is absent in some TMEs. Additionally, it will be important to understand the stimuli and factors necessary for mature TLS (SFL-TLS) development and maintenance as this TLS phenotype is associated with better survival and reduced risk of recurrence.

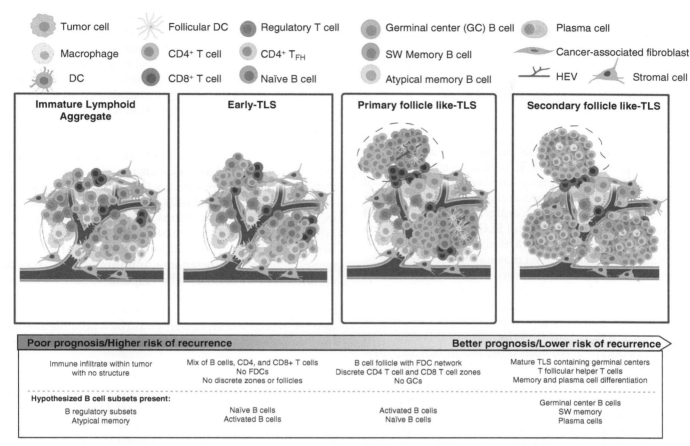

Figure 42.1 **B cells and TLS are heterogeneous within the tumor microenvironment.** The schematic depicts the different stages of tertiary lymphoid structures (TLS) maturation within the TME as well as the immune cell composition within each. Four distinct phenotypes of TLS have been identified in human tumors: (**A**) **Immature lymphoid aggregates:** small collections of B and T cells, with immature DCs scattered throughout the tumor with no organized structure formation. (**B**) **Early-TLS:** B cells and T cells begin to form larger aggregates but DCs remain undifferentiated. (**C**) **Primary-follicle like:** TLS begins to resemble primary B cell follicle in lymph node with defined naïve B cell cluster with a network of FDC within the follicle, defined T cell zone, and HEV formation. (**D**) **Secondary-follicle-like:** mature TLS with active germinal centers (GC); GC B cells can be found interacting with CD4+ T follicular helper cells. Class-switched memory B cells and plasma cells have been detected *in situ* in patients with mature TLS. Patients can have one or more of these TLS phenotypes, with mature TLS correlating with better survival and reduced risk of recurrence. Intratumoral B cells within TLS are often identified using only CD20 staining; thus, its not yet clear which B cell subsets are present in each type of TLS. Here, we hypothesize which B cell subsets could be present in each TLS based on what is known about their function and impact on overall patient survival.

DC, dendritic cell; FDC, follicular dendritic cell; HEV, high endothelial venule; SW, class-switched; TLS, tertiary lymphoid structures.

Source: Figure created with Biorender.com.

How Many Subtypes of Tumor-Infiltrating Lymphocyte-Bs Exist Within the Tumor Microenvironment?

B cells continue to be quantified within tumors and TLS using only surface expression of CD20. However, it is known that multiple B cell phenotypes exist in normal tissues and peripheral blood (PBL) and these different subsets of B cells have unique gene and protein expression profiles as well as distinct function.[57–59] Deeper phenotypic characterization of B cell phenotypes within different TMEs will be necessary to determine which B cell subsets carry out anti- or protumor functions in vitro and in vivo. These types of analyses are paramount for identifying B cell-specific proteins and pathways that may be of therapeutic value. Advances in gene sequencing technologies such as single-cell RNA sequencing (scRNAseq) and high dimensional flow cytometry platforms including mass cytometry (CyTOF) and spectral cytometry (Cytek Aurora), as well as traditional flow cytometry, have allowed for deeper characterization of immune cells within tumors, including B cells.[60,61] Studies using these technologies have revealed that multiple B cell phenotypes with unique gene expression profiles are present in cancers such as NSCLC, BRCA, melanoma, HCC, CRC, and HNSC.[17,47,62–65] Here, we will discuss the different B cell subsets that have been described in different TMEs and highlight key surface markers that define them. For the remainder of this chapter, we will refer to B cells within tumors as intratumoral B cells.

Naïve B Cells

In normal SLOs, naïve B cells become activated by capturing antigen via their BCR which results in downstream BCR signaling, processing, and presentation of antigen on MHC class II molecules (HLA-DR,DP,DQ).[66] Expression of CCR7 allows antigen-activated naïve B cells to migrate to T cell zones of SLOs to present antigen to TFH.[2,66] Following this interaction, naïve B cells can differentiate into: (a) short-lived plasma cells, (b) GC B cells, and (c) GC-independent memory B cells.[66] Canonically, naïve B cells can be distinguished by expression of IgM and IgD as well as CD21 and CD23.[57,58] CD23 can be used to mark naïve B cells within B cell follicles (also marks FDCs) using IHC or mIF.[24,37,67] Intratumoral B cells with a naïve phenotype have been observed in NSCLC, metastatic melanoma, HNSC, BRCA, and CRC. In NSCLC, naïve intratumoral B cells were associated with favorable outcomes.[61] However, patients with metastatic melanoma who did not respond to ICB had increased naïve intratumoral B cells in their tumors compared to patients who responded.[17] It is not yet abundantly clear what role naïve intratumoral B cells play in tumor immune responses. Deeper characterization of transcriptomes and protein expression of naïve intratumoral B cells may give insight into whether effector functions (BCR signaling, TFH interaction, differentiation into GC B cells) of naïve intratumoral B cells are intact or impaired.

Germinal Center B Cells

GCs are paramount for producing high affinity and durable B cell responses.[68] Detecting intratumoral B cells with a GC phenotype within TLS suggests that active, antitumor B cell immune responses are occurring within different TME.[32] GC B cells can be distinguished by staining for transcription factor BCL6, which regulates the GC reaction.[5] Active GC reactions can also be detected in TLS by staining for AID, which regulates SHM and CSR.[69] GC B cells also express glycoprotein CD38 and co-stimulatory molecules CD40 and CD27.[70] Chemokine receptor CXCR4 and co-stimulatory molecule CD86 can be used to distinguish GC B cells in the dark zone (CXCR4[+]; centroblasts) and light zone (CD86[+]; centrocytes) in the GC reaction.[70] Intratumoral B cells with a GC phenotype have been described in melanoma, NSCLC, HNSC, HCC, and BRCA.[16,17,24,41,41–49,71] In HNSC, intratumoral GC B cells with both centroblast and centrocyte phenotypes are increased in patients with HPV+ disease.[47] Intratumoral

GC B cells in HNSC and GC B cells within SLOs also express semaphorin-4A (SEMA4A).[47] SEMA4A is a membrane-bound and secreted glycoprotein that plays a role in CD4[+] and CD8[+] T cell, DC, and macrophage function and regulatory T cell (T_{reg} cell) stability.[72,73] SEMA4A has been implicated as a potent co-stimulatory molecule for T cell activation through interaction with ILT4 receptor.[74] In HNSC and SLO tissue, SEMA4A expression increases as naïve B cells differentiate into GC B cells.[47] The precise role of SEMA4A in GC reactions has not been determined, but given that SEMA4A can also bind to neuropilin-1 (NRP1), which is expressed on T_{reg} cells and TFH, plexins on DCs and endothelial cells suggest it may play a role in T cell-GC B cell interactions in normal SLO tissue and HNSC tumors and TLS formation.[47,75–77] Intratumoral GC B cells in HNSC correlate with better survival in treatment-naïve patients.[47] In melanoma, intratumoral GC B cells are increased in patients who respond to ICB.[17,71] Given the importance of GCs in developing antigen-specific B cell responses, increasing differentiation of naïve B cells into GC B cells within tumors could be a possible avenue for B cell-specific therapeutic intervention.

Memory B Cells

Memory B cells (MBCs) are an important B cell subset for establishing life-long protection against foreign invaders. Several key characteristics distinguish MBCs from other B cell subsets including: (a) increased life span, (b) faster proliferation and/or differentiation following antigen or polyclonal stimulation, and (c) expression of somatically mutated and affinity matured Ig genes.[78–82] Upon re-activation, MBCs upregulate co-stimulatory molecules (CD40, CD86, CD27), anti-apoptotic proteins (bcl-2, bcl-xL), and signal transducer molecules (SLAM family, STAT3, TACI, TLR-9, IL-21R), which allow them to persist and perform effector functions such as differentiation into PCs, re-entering GCs, cytokine production, and antigen presentation.[59,79,80,83–85] MBCs are localized in normal tissues and SLOs where they are able to encounter antigen more readily; however, phenotypic and functional characterization of MBCs in humans thus far mostly comes from nondiseased PBL and tonsils.[57,86,87] MBCs, classically defined as CD27[+] CD38[-], in normal tissues are quite heterogeneous with several phenotypically distinct subsets including the following: (a) Class-switched: IgD[-] express either IgA or IgG; can be activated (CD21[-] CD95[+]) or resting (CD21[+]CD95[-]); (b) Non class-switched: IgD[+]IgM[+]; and (c) IgM only: IgM[+] IgD[-].[6,58,88] Recently, a deeper characterization of MBCs using high level flow cytometry and RNA-sequencing across healthy tissues including gut and spleen has revealed novel tissue-resident MBC populations defined by CD45RB and CD69.[89] Chronic infections such as HIV-AIDS, malaria, and tuberculosis (TB) are characterized by a large expansion of functionally "exhausted" MBCs within PBL, referred to as tissue-like memory (TLM) or atypical memory B cells (aMBC).[90–94] aMBCs, which are defined by significantly low expression of the canonical MBC markers, CD27 and CD21, have increased expression of a variety of inhibitory receptors (IRs) including members of the FcRL family: FcRL4 and FcRL5.[92,94,95] aMBC also have abnormal expression of transcription factor Tbet and altered homing receptors (CD11c and CXCR3) but appear to have undergone class-switching as they express a predominant IgG isotype. Chronic antigen exposure is hypothesized to drive upregulation of IRs, which inhibit MBC effector functions including BCR signaling, differentiation, cytokine production, and antibody production.[91,96,97] Of note, this aberrant accumulation of aMBC in infections like HIV and malaria is thought to contribute to poor immunity against these diseases.[90] Further understanding the mechanisms that drive this expansion and loss of function in vivo may aid in vaccine development as these infections have eluded vaccine efforts thus far.

Intratumoral B cells with a memory (MBC) phenotype are the predominant intratumoral B cell subset in NSCLC, metastatic melanoma, HNSC, BRCA, CRC, and HCC, making up >60% of all intratumoral B cells.[16,17,24,47,64,65] Of note, intratumoral MBCs are also heterogeneous within these tumor types with multiple subsets being observed, non-class switched, class-switched MBC, and aMBCs.[26,47,48,64] While there is some shared heterogeneity within the intratumoral MBC population across these tumor types, different surface markers are being used to describe these populations, which makes cross-tumor comparisons challenging. For example, both resting (CD21+) and activated (CD21-) CD27+ class-switched MBC are increased in HNSC and NSCLC.[47,98,99] However, in HCC, class-switched intratumoral MBCs are distinguished solely using CD27 and IgD, revealing both CD27+ and CD27- class-switched MBCs in these patients.[64] Further, in metastatic melanoma, class-switched MBCs are distinguished by CXCR4, CXCR3, or CD11c expression, with CXCR3+ and CXCR4+ being increased in the tumors of patients who responded to ICB.[17] The intratumoral aMBC phenotype has been largely uncharacterized in the TME beyond low CD27 and CD21 expression.[16,26,99–101] However, in HCC, intratumoral aMBCs do express IgG and functional tumor necrosis factor (TNF)-related apoptosis-inducing ligand (TRAIL).[26] More detailed characterization is needed of intratumoral aMBC to determine if they are analogous to those in chronic infections, which could present unique targeting avenues in regards to IR pathways and potentially reversing the dysfunction of aMBCs.[97] Despite these differences in characterization, intratumoral MBCs correlate with improved patient survival and can predict response to ICB therapy.[17,26,47,101] Class-switched cells and aMBCs have also been shown to independently correlate with survival in HNSC, OV, and HCC, suggesting that

they may be functionally distinct from those in chronic infection.[26,47,101] Pan-tumor analysis using high level sequencing and flow cytometry of intratumoral MBCs may provide more consistency in characterization and reveal unique pathways for targeting. Additionally, consensus on surface markers used to distinguish intratumoral MBCs will also allow for uniform functional analysis across tumor types.

Intratumoral Plasma Cells

Antigen-activated mature B cells can differentiate into: (a) short-lived PCs (SLPCs)/plasmablasts (PB) or (b) long-lived PCs (LLPCs).[12,102,103] SLPCs primarily form in extrafollicular sites of SLOs and secrete low-affinity IgM antibodies.[12,102,103] LLPCs form in secondary follicles during GC reactions and secrete high affinity antibodies.[12,102,103] Both LLPCs and SLPCs express CD138, CXCR4, IL-6R, and B cell maturation antigen (BCMA).[12,104] BCMA is the receptor for APRIL and BAFF, which promote B cell survival.[105,106] Additionally, LLPCs and SLPCs express high levels of CD27 and CD38 and downregulate CD19 and CD20.[12] PC populations also express the transcription factors Blimp-1, XBP1, and IRF4. The major difference between SLPCs and LLPCs is life span and proliferative capacity. SLPCs are actively proliferating and only last for 3 to 5 days unless they migrate to a survival niche for PCs, which is primarily the BM. Here, they can become a LLPC.[12,103] LLPCs can persist for months or a lifetime and can secrete antibodies without T cell help.[102,103,107] Intratumoral PCs are present in NSCLC, triple-negative breast cancer (TNBC), HCC, HNSC, OV, CRC, esophageal cancer, and STAD.[18,27,48,64,98,108,109] Within these tumor types, intratumoral PCs are distinguished by CD138, CD38, and multiple myeloma oncogene 1 (MUM1).[18,98,108,110] Intratumoral B cells correlate with better survival in some indices such as OV, esophageal, gastric, TNBC, NSCLC, and HCC[27,28,64,108,111]. However, in HNSC, CRC, and lung adenocarcinoma (LUAD), intratumoral PCs correlate with worse prognosis.[47,48,109,110] Additionally, one study in BRCA demonstrated that tumors predominantly infiltrated with intratumoral PC were associated with worse prognosis, which contradicts previous studies in TNBC.[112] It is not clear why intratumoral PCs could correlate with worse prognosis in some cancers and not others. Perhaps the location of intratumoral PCs within the TME play a role as these cells in TNBC and OV can be found in TLS, which correlates with better prognosis in these indices.[27,113] In mice, PC can have an immunosuppressive phenotype (IgA+ IL-10+, PD-L1+, LAG-3+), which can impede T cell responses in the TME; however, this phenotype has not been well defined in humans.[114,115] Thus, deeper characterization of intratumoral PCs within different TMEs is needed.

Intratumoral Regulatory B Cells

Regulatory B (B_{reg}) cells are a subset of B cells that can suppress immune responses via cytokine production (IL-10, IL-35, TGF-β) and cell-to-cell contact. The phenotype of human B_{reg} is not well defined as a master transcription factor like Foxp3 for T_{reg} cells has not been identified. Additionally, the surface markers used to define human B_{reg} subsets are not the same as murine B_{regs}, which makes comparisons between mouse and human systems challenging. Nevertheless, several human B_{reg} subsets have been identified and characterized in peripheral blood: (a) B10: CD24[hi] CD27[+]; (b) transitional B: CD19[+] CD24[hi]CD38[hi]; (c) IgM-only memory: CD19[+] CD27[+]IgM[+]; (d) plasmablasts: CD19[+]CD38[hi] CD24[hi] CD27[int]; (e) GrB[+] B cells: CD19[+]CD38[+]CD1d[hi] IgM[+]CD147[+]; and (f) Br1 cells: CD19[+]CD25[hi]CD71[hi] CD73[lo].[116] With the exception of GrB[+] B cells, which secrete granzyme B, all other peripheral B_{reg} subsets suppress CD4[+] T cell and DC effector functions through IL-10 production.[116–118] Intratumoral B_{regs} are associated with worse prognosis in HCC, STAD, and tongue squamous cell carcinoma (TSCC).[119–122] HCC, cervical cancer (CESC), and melanoma patients with late-stage disease (III and IV) and/or metastases also have higher levels of intratumoral B_{regs}.[119,123] Of note, the phenotype of intratumoral B_{regs} is distinct across many tumor types. For example, in STAD and HNSC, intratumoral B_{regs} are CD19[+]CD24[hi]CD38[hi] while intratumoral B_{regs} in CESC are CD19[+]CD5[+]CD1d[+].[98,122,124] CD1d[+]CD5[+] intratumoral B_{regs} are also present in PDAC.[125] Additionally, CD39[+]CD73[+] intratumoral B_{regs} are present in HNSC patients and produce immunosuppressive adenosine (ADO).[126] Program death receptor ligand 1 (PD-L1) has also been used to describe intratumoral B_{regs} in BRCA and melanoma.[123,127] Further, a subset of intratumoral B_{regs} in HCC also express PD-1 and are increased in late-stage disease.[119] The heterogeneity in intratumoral B_{reg} populations across tumor types is intriguing. Understanding what factors (i.e., environment, transcriptional regulators) regulate the intratumoral B_{reg} phenotype and function may provide further insight into how to target this population as a form of immunotherapy as it is associated with disease progression and poor outcomes.

HOW DO INTRATUMORAL B CELLS CONTRIBUTE TO TUMOR IMMUNITY?

While intratumoral B cells and TLS correlate with better prognosis in many cancers, it is not yet clear why and how intratumoral B cells provide a survival advantage to patients. Further, patients on ICB therapy have better outcomes when their tumors have high levels of intratumoral B cells; however, the mechanisms by which intratumoral B cells are supporting improved outcomes to ICB remain unclear. Nevertheless, insights into potential functions of intratumoral B cells can be gained from other disease models such as autoimmunity, transplantation, and infectious disease.[128] Additionally, some cancer studies have revealed that intratumoral B cells can support antitumor immunity in a number of ways including: (a) producing tumor-reactive antibodies, (b) presenting tumor-antigen to CD4[+] T cells, (c) providing co-stimulation to CD4[+] or CD8[+] T cells, (d) directly killing tumor cells via Fas/FasL or TRAIL pathways, (e) generating pro-inflammatory cytokines, and (f) inducing TLS formation. Alternatively, in some cancer indices, intratumoral B cells can promote tumor progression by producing immunosuppressive cytokines (IL-10, IL-35, TGF-β) and adenosine. It is not yet clear whether the same intratumoral B cell subset can perform multiple functions or if there is a "division of labor" whereby multiple intratumoral B cell subsets carry out distinct functions. Linking intratumoral B cell phenotypes to distinct function will aid in the development of B cell-based immune therapies.

Tumor-Reactive Antibodies

Targets of Tumor-Reactive Antibodies

Intratumoral B cells and PCs and circulating B cells and PCs can be a potent source of tumor-reactive antibodies, which recognize a variety of aberrantly expressed or mutated self-antigens and tumor-specific antigens.[129–131] Mucin 1 (MUC1) is a self-antigen that is overexpressed in its unglycosylated form in several tumor types including OV, PDAC, gastric, BRCA, and NSCLC.[132–136] Serum IgG antibodies directed at MUC1 are associated with favorable prognosis in patients with early stage PDAC and BRCA.[134–136] Circulating antibodies to cancer/testis (CT) antigens such as melanoma-associated antigen1 (MAGE1) and New York esophageal squamous cell carcinoma-1 (NY-ESO-1) are found in serum of HNSC, OV, NSCLC, and esophageal adenocarcinoma (EAC).[98,137–139] In NSCLC, intratumoral PCs also produce antibodies to MAGE proteins and NY-ESO-1.[24] Interestingly, serum antibodies to NY-ESO-1 and X antigen family member 1A (XAGE1) in NSCLC also correlate with better survival and response to anti-PD-1 therapy.[137] In medullary BRCA, serum and intratumoral antibodies were also directed at intracellular self-antigens aberrantly exposed on the surface of apoptotic tumor such as β-actin.[140,141] Mutations to tumor suppressor gene *p53* is a common feature of most human cancers and antibodies directed to mutated p53 can be detected in the sera of patients.[142–146] In some NSCLC patients, anti-p53 antibodies are associated with favorable outcomes.[145,147]

Circulating antibodies to growth factor receptors that are overexpressed in tumors including human epidermal growth factor receptor 2 (HER2) and epidermal growth factor receptor (EGFR) have also been detected.[131,148–151] Treatment-naïve patients with BRCA have naturally occurring serum antibodies directed to the intracellular domain of HER2 and this is associated with favorable outcomes.[148] The level of circulating anti-HER2 IgG is increased in patients treated with chemotherapy and trastuzumab, a HER2 monoclonal antibody.[149] While increased circulating antibodies to self-antigens (autoantibodies) are a sign of disease progression in autoimmune disorders, it is thought that they can be used as biomarkers for detection of early stage cancer and a positive prognostic indicator in some indices including OV, CRC, HCC, BRCA, and NSCLC.[132,136,152–154] However, there is some contradictory evidence demonstrating higher levels of circulating, and intratumoral antibodies to tumor-associated self-antigens are associated with poor prognosis in BRCA.[155] Additionally, antibodies can be directed at novel tumor-specific antigens known as "neoantigens" as well as new epitopes of known antigens (cryptic epitopes), both of which are associated with improved survival.[156,157] Further, circulating antibodies from plasmablasts in metastatic melanoma, LUAD, and RCC were shown to be reactive to autologous and heterologous tumor tissue and tumor cell lines, suggesting that shared tumor antigens are present in these cancer types.[144,158]

Intratumoral and circulating antibodies can also be directed at viral proteins present in cancers caused by oncogenic viruses including HPV, hepatitis B (HBV), hepatitis C (HCV), and Merkel cell polyomavirus (MCPyV).[49,98,159–162] In HPV+ HNSC, intratumoral B cells and PCs produce IgG antibodies directed at E6, E7, and E2 HPV viral proteins.[49] Additionally, circulating antibodies to early (E2, E4, L1) and late (E6 and E7) HPV antigens are detected in HNSC and oropharyngeal squamous cell carcinoma (OPSCC).[98,163] Serum antibodies to HBV surface antigen (HBVsAg) and HCV core protein are prevalent in HCC patients.[160–162] HBV-specific intratumoral B cells are present in HBV-driven HCC; however, they have an atypical memory phenotype and poor antibody production.[93,162,164] Several technologies are available to study antigen-specific B cells including: (a) *ELISPOT*; (b) *flow cytometry*: using fluorescently labeled antigen probes; and (c) *reversed B-cell FluoroSpot assay*: uses recombinant tagged antigens and fluorescently labeled detection systems (streptavidin or IgG antibodies) to detect antigen-specific IgG secreted by B cells. Given the role of antibodies in immune memory, more studies should assess antigen specificity of intratumoral B cells and PCs and ways to increase tumor-specific antibody production.[165–167]

Antibody-Mediated Effector Mechanisms

Antibody effector functions are an important part of the humoral immune response against invading pathogens.[129,168,169] These effector functions are mediated by the Fc portion of antibodies, which interact with complement proteins or Fc-receptors expressed on innate immune cells such as NK, neutrophils, macrophages, and DCs.[168,169] There is very limited evidence regarding the effector function of tumor-reactive antibodies within the TME of human solid tumors. However, we can hypothesize how tumor-specific antibodies can contribute to tumor immunity by taking cues from humoral responses to viral infection.[168,169] The major Fc-mediated effector functions include: (a) antibody-dependent cellular cytotoxicity (ADCC), (b) antibody-dependent cellular phagocytosis (ADCP), and (c) complement-dependent cytotoxicity (CDC; Figure 42.2).[168,169] ADCC in vivo is thought to mostly be carried out by NK cells, although in vitro other innate immune cells such as monocytes and macrophages are also capable of ADCC.[168] ADCC is mostly mediated by IgG1 isotype which interacts with Fc gamma receptor III a (FcγRIIIa) or CD16a on NK cells, causing release of granzyme b and perforin that lyse infected or tumor cells.[168,169] In melanoma, melanoma-reactive antibodies derived from patients have been shown to be capable of ADCC in vitro.[170] Although not well studied in the context of intratumoral antibodies from B cells or PCs, ADCC is a key mechanism of action for therapeutic monoclonal antibodies.[171–174] ADCC is carried out by phagocytic cells such as macrophages, which express a number of FcγR that interact with IgG1 antibodies bound to infected or tumor cells.[168,169,175] Additionally, antigen:antibody complexes can also bind FcγRs on macrophages which can allow them to uptake these complexes and present antigen to T cells.[168,169] It appears that the complement system plays a complex role in the TME in murine models, but is severely understudied in human tumors.[176,177] During immune responses to infection, CDC is mediated by IgG and IgM antibodies which activate the complement pathway.[168,169] Classical complement protein C1q binds to antibodies on infected or tumor cells, which activates the complement cascade, ultimately leading to formation of membrane attack complex (MAC), which directly causes cell lysis.[168,169,176] Whether intratumoral IgG and IgM antibodies can mediate complement pathway activation in tumors and what effect this has on tumor immunity remains unknown. However, expression of classical and alternative complement genes can be found in a variety of tumors.[176] In addition to Fc-mediated effector functions, antibodies can form immune complexes which can: (a) activate degranulation of neutrophils and eosinophils (cytokine/chemokine release; reactive oxygen species [ROS]), (b) induce DC maturation which can skew T cell responses, (c) activate macrophages, and (d) regulate B cell antibody responses.[168,169] Future studies should focus on isolating intratumoral B cells and PCs from patients, stimulating them to make antibodies and subsequently testing the effector function capabilities (ADCC, ADCP, CDC, immunomodulation) in vitro.[171,174,178,179] This may provide insight to the potential in vivo roles of tumor-specific antibodies.

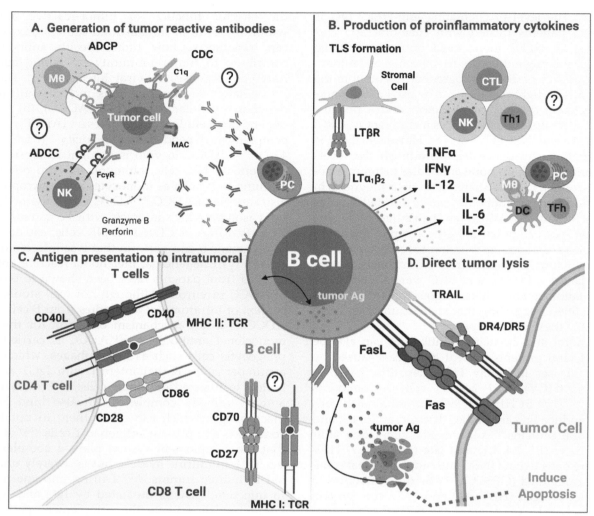

Figure 42.2 **B cells and TLS are heterogeneous within the tumor microenvironment.** B cells can potentially promote antitumor immunity in several ways: (**A**) **Generation of tumor-reactive antibodies:** Intratumoral B cells and PCs can produce antibodies that are specific to surface proteins expressed on tumor cells. These antibodies are then recognized by the Fc-receptors on NK cells, which can induce ADCC via the release of granzyme B and perforin or monocytes/macrophages, which induce ADCP. Tumor-specific antibodies can also opsonize tumor cells, making them targets for CDC by complement cascade proteins such as C1q. (**B**) **Production of pro-inflammatory cytokines:** Intratumoral B cell can produce lymphotoxin (LT$\alpha_2\beta_1$) which interacts with LTβR on stromal cells. LTβR signaling leads to chemokine production by stromal cells, initiating TLS formation. Th1 effector cytokines (TNF-α, IFN-γ, IL-12) produced by intratumoral B cells can support immune cells associated with antitumor function such as CTLs, NK cells, and Th1 cells. However, in some patients intratumoral B cells may produce more Th2 effector cytokines, which typically support more suppressive populations but can also support DCs, PCs, and TFH. (**C**) **Antigen presentation to intratumoral T cells:** Intratumoral B cells are found in close proximity to CD4 T cells and CD8 T cells within TLS, suggesting that they may be interacting. Intratumoral B cells have been shown to present tumor antigen via MHC II to CD4+ T cells, and co-stimulatory molecules associated with antigen presentation such as CD86 and CD40 are present on activated intratumoral B cells. Cross presentation of tumor antigen on MHC I by intratumoral B cells has not been investigated in humans but has been shown in mice models. In humans, intratumoral B cells can support intratumoral CD8 T cell function via CD27/CD70 interactions. (**D**) **Direct tumor lysis:** Intratumoral B cells can induce apoptosis in tumor cells through expression of TRAIL, which only induces apoptosis in tumor cells, leaving healthy cells intact, or expression of FasL, which binds Fas and induces apoptosis; however, it is not necessarily restricted to tumors. Apoptosis of tumor cells can lead to exposure of intracellular tumor antigens that can be presented to T cells.

ADCC, antibody-dependent cellular cytotoxicity; ADCP, antibody-dependent cellular phagocytosis; CDC, complement-dependent cytotoxicity; CTL, cytotoxic T lymphocyte; DC, dendritic cell; LTβR, lymphotoxin beta receptor; MHC I, major histocompatibility complex I; MHC II, major histocompatibility complex II; NK cell, natural killer cell; PC, plasma cell; TFH, T follicular helper; Th1, T helper 1; Th2, T helper 2; TRAIL, TNF-related apoptosis-inducing ligand.

Source: Figure created with Biorender.com.

Antigen Presentation

Although DCs are regarded as the main antigen-presenting cell (APC) in immune responses to infection and tumors, DC function is often rendered dysfunctional by the immunosuppressive TME.[180–182] B cells are also a professional APC; however, their role as APCs in human solid tumors remains understudied. There are several key features of B cells that make them an effective APC: (a) BCR-mediated endocytosis: high-affinity BCRs produced after GC reactions allow B cells to concentrate small amounts of antigen and internalize them faster than DCs, which allows for efficient antigen presentation; (b) HLA-DO expression: inhibits HLA-DM, allowing loading of MHC II peptides to occur in the MHC class II-enriched compartment (MIIC) where BCR:antigen complexes can be degraded and processed; (c) BCR signaling: antigen binding to BCR sends internal signals to the B cell for activation, directs antigen-processing machinery, and upregulates expression of co-stimulatory molecules CD40, CD86, and MHC II.[183–186] It has been shown that activated B cells CD21⁻CD86⁺ are potent APCs while resting B cells (CD21⁺CD86⁻/lo) are more tolerogenic.[187–189] Indeed, in NSCLC patients, activated intratumoral B cells were shown to be capable of presenting tumor antigen to CD4⁺ T cells.[99] Additionally, activated intratumoral B cells in NSCLC were shown to influence CD4⁺ T cell phenotypes.[99] CD40-stimulated B cells were able to generate tumor-specific CD4⁺ T cells after being pulsed with tumor-associated antigens gp100 and NY-ESO-1.[190] Cross presentation by B cells to CD8⁺ T cells in humans has not been well investigated. However, activated B cells can promote CD8⁺ T cell proliferation and survival independent of antigen via CD27/CD70 interactions.[191] In OPSCC, activated intratumoral B cells and CD8⁺ T cells are found in close proximity within TLS, and depletion of B cells from tumor-derived cell suspensions resulted in decreased survival and functionality of CD8⁺ T cells.[192] Activated, antigen-experienced (CD27⁺CD21⁻ CD86⁺CD95⁺) intratumoral B cells have been described in HNSC, TNBC, NSCLC, and gastric cancer.[16,24,98,99,138] Thus, further investigation of the antigen-presentation capabilities of different intratumoral B cell subsets is warranted.

Cytokine Production

Intratumoral B cells also have the potential to shape tumor immunity via cytokine and chemokine production, although this has not been well investigated in human solid tumors.[59,193–195] B cells primed by CD4⁺ T helper (Th1) cells or CD4⁺ T helper 2 (Th2) cells can polarize B cells to produce IFN-γ, TNF-α, and IL-12 (Th1 effector) or IL-2, IL-13, IL-6, and IL-4 (Th2 effector) cytokines, respectively.[59,195] Th1 effector cytokines promote Th1 T cells, NK cells, and M1 macrophage responses. Th2 effector cytokines promote Th2 T cells, M2-macrophages, and T_{reg} cells. However, IL-6 is also important for TFH responses. In TNBC, intratumoral B cells had higher mRNA expression of Th1 effector cytokines IFN-γ and TNF-α as compared with B cells from nondiseased lymph nodes and tonsils. Th2 effector cytokines IL-4 and IL-5 mRNA were also detected.[16] However, this study did not directly assess soluble protein production of cytokines by intratumoral B cells. In HCC, intratumoral aMBC, located in the margin of the tumor, produced IFN-γ, IL-12-p40, and granzyme B by flow cytometry and confocal microscopy.[26] Granzyme B production by B cells has been reported in the context of viral infection. In fact, B cells from patients recently vaccinated against tickborne encephalitis virus (TBEV) produce granzyme B when rechallenged with TBEV antigens.[196] Granzyme B production by B cells is driven by IL-21 and BCR stimulation in the absence of help from T cells through CD40 ligation.[197] Depending on the context, IL-21-induced granzyme B production by B cells could be an important mechanism of killing tumor cells within the TME.[196–198] There is more evidence regarding the production of immunosuppressive cytokines (IL-10, IL-35, TGF-β) by intratumoral B_{reg} subsets. IL-10 production is induced by intratumoral B cells when co-cultured with tongue squamous cell carcinoma (TSCC). Tumor cell lines can induce differentiation of resting CD4⁺ T cells into T_{reg} cells.[121] IL-10 production by intratumoral B cells has been detected in OV, CESC, HNSC, and HCC, and can suppress CD4⁺ T cell and DC effector responses.[21,98,122,199] In HCC, IL-10 production by PD-1ʰⁱ intratumoral B_{regs} inhibit cytokine production by CD8⁺ T cells.[119] IL-35 production by intratumoral B cells has been detected in STAD patients and is associated with disease progression of STAD.[200] Future studies should further assess soluble cytokine production by intratumoral B cells and cytokine production across intratumoral B cell subsets. Using different stimuli (tumor-specific vs. polyclonal) may provide insight into how B cell cytokine production is influenced by different TMEs.

Direct Tumor Lysis

There is evidence that intratumoral B cells are capable of killing tumor cells directly in the absence of antibodies through expression of death ligands: Fas Ligand (FasL) and TRAIL.[26,201,202] Expression of FasL has not been well characterized on intratumoral B cells in humans but increased expression of FasL on B cells is observed in infection models, particularly on CD5⁺ B cells. IL-10 and IL-4 can also regulate FasL expression. Human B cells express TRAIL following stimulation with CpG-A (ODN2007) and IFN-α and can directly kill tumor cells via TRAIL.[203] In HCC, intratumoral aMBC express TRAIL and granzyme B and were shown to kill HCC tumor cells in an *in vitro* co-culture.[26] Further studies are needed to solidify the cytotoxic function of intratumoral B cells.

HARNESSING B CELLS AND TERTIARY LYMPHOID STRUCTURES FOR CANCER IMMUNOTHERAPY

Given the strong correlation between intratumoral B cells and TLS with patient survival in many cancers and response to current immunotherapies, it is important to consider the B cell compartment in the design of new cancer immunotherapies. Therapeutically enhancing antitumor functions of B cells or blocking or depleting immunosuppressive B cell populations could be beneficial for patients. Further, rescuing B cell populations whose function may be impaired by the TME may also be a viable therapeutic option. Lastly, inducing TLS formation in patients with immunologically "cold" tumors could enhance responses to current immunotherapies. To this end, we will review how current immunotherapies affect intratumoral B cells and how to enhance B cell function and TLS formation with novel immunotherapies.

Effects of Standard of Care Therapies

Standard of care treatments for cancer patients including radiation, chemotherapy, and hormone therapies have all been shown to impact antitumor immunity.[204–206] These studies have been largely focused on T cells, but B cells and TLS can also be affected. For example, corticosteroids are often given to LUSC patients treated with chemotherapy to manage side effects; however, TLS density is greatly impaired in chemotherapy-naïve LUSC patients treated with corticosteroids before surgery.[41] Notably, in chemotherapy-treated LUSC patients, TLS density was similar to untreated patients, but GC formation was significantly impaired.[41] In patients with HGSOC metastases, chemotherapy enhanced MBC cell responses.[207] Radiotherapy enhanced activation of B cells, GC formation, and increased tumor-specific B cell and PC differentiation in a murine model of HNSC.[14] More studies should assess the changes that B cells and TLS can undergo following standard therapies as these could be leveraged in combinatorial treatments with immunotherapies directed at B cells.

Effects of Checkpoint Blockade

Therapeutic monoclonal antibodies (mAbs) targeting the PD-1/PD-L1 pathway have had remarkable success in cancer patients. While blocking this pathway on T cells enhances antitumor responses in patients, the effects of anti-PD-1 and anti-PD-L1 mAbs have been severely understudied in the context of B cell responses in tumors. Both human and murine B cells express PD-1 and PD-L1.[119,208–210] There is a basal level of PD-1 on resting B cell populations (naïve and MBC) within nondiseased PBL and lymph nodes and is significantly upregulated after stimulation.[208] In HCC, PD-1 marks an immunosuppressive B cell population that suppresses CD8+ T cell responses.[119] Recently, we learned that B cell and TLS promote responses to anti-PD-1 therapy in melanoma, RCC, and STS patients, although it is not clear if anti-PD-1 is acting directly on B cells.[13,17,31] PD-1 is also expressed on TFH cells and is important for GC B cell survival and differentiation into PC.[128,211,212] PD-L1 is also used to mark B_{reg} subsets in many tumors and nondiseased tissues.[116,118,123] In HNSC, anti-PD-L1 enhanced B cell antibody responses, GC formation, and B cell clonality in mice and antibody responses in patients who responded to ICB.[14] Thus, more studies should assess direct effects of ICB, especially anti-PD-1 and anti-PD-L1 on intratumoral B cells in patients.

Therapeutically Inducing Tertiary Lymphoid Structure Formation

There is overwhelming evidence that TLS drive antitumor responses and patients without TLS have overall poor prognosis and are nonresponsive to ICB.[17,31–33,213] However, it is not yet clear why TLS form in some patients and not others. Extensive studies in mice and human models of infection and autoimmune disease reveal the key events needed for TLS formation, including: (a) inflammatory cytokine expression, (b) lymphoid chemokine production by stromal cells, and (c) HEV development.[32–34,214] Developing therapies that can initiate one or more of these events in patients without TLS could be a promising new avenue for therapeutic intervention. Inducing inflammatory cytokine expression could be accomplished using Stimulator of Interferon Genes response cGAMP interactor 1 (STING1) agonists (Figure 42.3).[215–217] STING1 is an endoplasmic reticulum (ER) resident protein important for sensing cytoplasmic double-stranded DNA (dsDNA) during viral and bacterial infection and promoting type 1 interferon gene expression (IFN-α/β, IL-6, TNF-α) through canonical and noncanonical NF-κB signaling pathways.[215–217] There are at least 15 STING agonists being investigated in clinical trials as single agents and in combination with ICB for treating cancer patients due to the success of STING agonists to promote antitumor activity in preclinical models.[215–217] Type 1 IFNs regulate chemokines such as CXCL13 which are important for TLS formations, which suggests that STING agonists could be used for TLS induction.[218,219] Indeed, in vivo models using STING agonists to induce TLS are being developed.[220]

Tumor necrosis factor superfamily member 14 (TNSF14) or LIGHT is an activation-inducible inflammatory cytokine homologous to lymphotoxins that binds to herpesvirus entry mediator (HVEM) and LTβR. LIGHT provides co-stimulation to T cells via HVEM and can induce SLO formation through LTβR signaling.[221,222] Further, activated CD4+ and CD8+ T cells, NK cells, and monocytes can also express membrane-bound LIGHT, suggesting it also has immunomodulatory functions.[221] Additionally, LIGHT

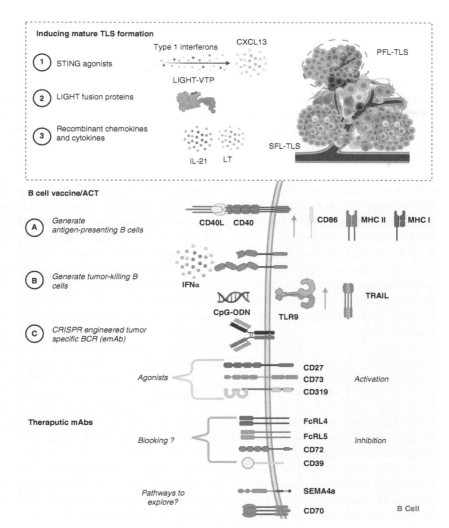

Figure 42.3 Targeting TLS and B cells for cancer immunotherapy. B cell/TLS axis may provide new and exciting avenues for developing B cell-based immunotherapies. This schematic lists potential mechanisms that could be leveraged for future therapeutics. **Inducing TLS: (1) STING agonists:** Compounds that can induce activation of the STING pathway (Stimulator of Interferon Genes) are being investigated as a potential immunotherapy as this pathway leads to induction of type 1 interferons and promotes antitumor immunity through T cells in preclinical models. Type 1 interferons also regulate chemokines and cytokines important for TLS formation, suggesting this pathway could be leveraged to induce TLS. Using STING agonists for inducing TLS is an active area of research. **(2) LIGHT fusion protein:** Tumor necrosis factor superfamily member 14 (TNFSF14) or LIGHT is a secreted protein important for TLS formation. Fusing LIGHT to vascular targeting peptide (VTP) allowed for de novo TLS formation in solid tumors in mice. **(3) Recombinant cytokines/chemokines:** Delivering recombinant cytokines that are important for TLS formation and maintenance such as lymphotoxin , IL-21, and IL-7 to tumors without TLS could induce TLS in these patients. IL-21 is important in regulating GC reactions and B cell differentiation and thus could be used to mature TLS in patients. Recombinant IL-21 as an immunotherapy is actively being investigated in clinical trials. **B cell vaccines/ adoptive cell therapy: (A) Generating antigen-presenting cells:** This process involves activating B cells from patient tumors or blood via CD40, pulsing these CD40-activated B cells with tumor Ag, and then transferring them back to the patient as an ACT. **(B) Generating tumor-killing B cells:** This process involves activating B cells isolated from patient tumors or blood via CpG-ODN (TLR-9 agonist) and IFN-α, which induce TRAIL expression on B cells, and then transferring them back to the patient as ACT. **(C) CRISPR engineering tumor-specific BCRs:** This process involves using CRISPR/Cas9 technology to engineer B cells and plasma cells to target specific tumor Ag to use as a B cell vaccine. **Therapeutic mAbs:** This process involves leveraging current immunotherapies that target activation pathways in B cells. mAb against CD27, CD73, and CD319 are actively being investigated in clinical trials to target other immune cell types but are also important for B cell function. SEMA4a and CD70 have not been well investigated in the TME for B cells but are also important for B cells in normal tissues. This involves developing new mAbs to targeting pathways that inhibit B cell function or are immunosuppressive.

ACT, adoptive cell transfer; Ag, antigen; CpG-ODN, CpG oligodeoxynucleotides; CXCL13, chemokine ligand 13; FcRL4, Fc receptor like 4; FcRL5, Fc receptor like 5; IFNα, interferon alpha; IL-21, interleukin 21; IL-7, interleukin 7; LT, lymphotoxin; mAb, monoclonal antibody; MHC I, major histocompatibility complex class I; MHC II, major histocompatibility complex class II; PFL-TLS, primary follicle like TLS; SEMA4a, semaphorin 4a; SFL-TLS, secondary follicle like TLS; TLR-9, Toll like receptor 9; TME, tumor microenvironment; TRAIL, TNF-related apoptosis-inducing ligand.

Source: Figure created with Biorender.com.

can enhance CD40L co-stimulation of B cells whereby it increases IgM and IgG production and proliferation of naïve cells and MBCs, which express HVEM.[223] In a murine model of spontaneous pancreatic neuroendocrine tumors, LIGHT fused to a vascular targeting peptide (VTP) was used to study de novo TLS formation.[224] VTP aided in targeting delivery of LIGHT to angiogenic tumor blood vessels. LIGHT-VTP fusion protein was able to normalize blood vessels, enhance immune cell infiltration, and induce TLS formation.[224] Thus, LIGHT could be a potential pathway for TLS induction in patients (Figure 42.3).

Recombinant cytokines, IFN-α (rIFN-α), and IL-2 (rIL-2) were some of the first FDA-approved immunotherapies to treat several malignancies.[225] Given the potent antitumor activity of these pro-inflammatory cytokines and their role in TLS formation and maintenance, delivering specific TLS-associated cytokines to the TME could be used to induce TLS in patients. rLT-α and rTNF-α can induce chemokine expression (CXCL13, CCL19, CCL21) in stromal cells and macrophages, which is important for recruiting immune cells.[32,40,51,218] rIL-21 and rIL-7 could potentially play an important role in GC formation, B cell differentiation, and TFH development within the TME and TLS.[82,226,227] Several clinical trials are ongoing to assess rIL-21 and rTNF-α in combination with other cancer therapies and ICB.[225] One key consideration for TLS-inducing therapies will be also developing delivery vehicles that can deliver therapies to the TME and minimize off target effects and toxicities that can be associated with cytokine-mediated inflammation. Additionally, future therapies will need to consider how to induce GC formation within TLS as this remains understudied. New spatial transcriptomic platforms 10X Visium and NanoString DSP may allow researchers to identify genes and pathways that are important for GCs and TLS within tumors.[228,229]

Adoptive Cell Therapy/B Cell Vaccine

Adoptive cell transfer (ACT) is a form of cellular immunotherapy that harnesses the natural ability of T cells to kill tumors by isolating and reinfusing T cells to patients after (a) expanding naturally occurring tumor-specific T cells, (b) engineering T cells to have a TCR directed at specific tumor antigens, or (c) creating a chimeric antigen receptor (CAR) that can bypass the need for tumor antigens to be presented on MHC.[230] There is evidence suggesting that ACT mechanisms could be employed with B cells to harness their ability to present tumor antigens, potentially directly kill tumor cells, and generate long-lasting protective tumor-specific antibodies.[231] The CD40L/CD40 signaling pathway is a key stimulator of the antigen presentation capacity in B cells.[99,185,190,232] Ligation of CD40 increases B cell proliferation and expression of co-stimulatory molecules (CD86, CD27, MHC molecules).[190,231,233,234] There are several studies that show that antigen-presenting

B cells can be generated from PBL using CD40 agonistic antibodies, soluble CD40 ligand, and CD40L-expressing cell lines.[231] In fact, a few early stage clinical trials have shown that CD40-activated B cells could be used in ACT in RCC and metastatic melanoma.[235,236] B cells are isolated from PBL, activated and expanded in a CD40L culture, pulsed with tumor antigen, and reinfused into the patient.[231] In addition to CD40 activation, TLR-9 agonists (CpG ODN) can induce antibody production and B cell differentiation when coupled with cytokines (IL-2, IL-10, IL-15), which could be used to enhance tumor-specific antibody production by B cells.[79,237] When coupled with IFN-α, TLR-9 agonist can induce expression of functional TRAIL on B cells, which could license B cells with cytotoxic capabilities as an ACT.[203] Lastly, CRISPR/Cas9 technology could potentially be used to engineer B cells from patients to express BCRs to different tumor-specific antigens and subsequently be used as an B cell-based vaccine (Figure 42.3). This technique has already been developed and employed to generate pathogen-specific antibodies to respiratory syncytial virus (RSV) that protect against re-infection in mouse models and can be used on human primary B cells from blood to produce RSV-specific antibodies.[238] In this technique, CRISPR/Cas9 technology replaces endogenous membrane antibody, with an engineered monoclonal antibody (emAb) that recognizes RSV antigens.[238] These emAb engineered B cells can also be expanded using traditional methods, and PC differentiation can also be induced.[238]

Therapeutic mAb

With anti-CTLA-4 and anti-PD-1 mAbs only being successful in a subset of patients in some cancer types, development of new mAbs targeting other immune checkpoints as well as co-stimulatory molecules has been prioritized. While most of these are still T cell- and tumor cell-focused, markers of interest such as CD27, PD-L1, and CD73 are also expressed on B cells and could be leveraged in B cell-based immunotherapies. CD27 is expressed on MBC subsets and is important for B cell differentiation and antibody production. Two CD27 therapeutic agonistic antibodies have been developed and are in current clinical trials: Varlilumab (anti-CD27) and CDX-527 (anti-CD27 and anti-PD-L1-bispecific) have shown efficacy in boosting T cell responses in solid tumors; however, effects on B cells with these therapies has not yet been reported.[239,240] Additionally, other molecules that are in clinical trials that are also important for B cell activation, antibody production, and proliferation and could affect B cells include CD73 (CPI-006), CD319, or SLAMF7 (elotuzumab).[241-246] Further, pathways that inhibit B cell function could be considered for the development of new B cell therapeutics such as inhibitory receptors unique to B cells including FcRL4, FcRL5, and CD22, which could rescue dysfunctional B cell populations.[95,247,248] Further, SEMA4a and CD70 are expressed on B cells during activation but their role on intratumoral B cells has yet to be explored. CD70 is the receptor for CD27 and plays an important role in IgG production in B cells.[249] Targeting the CD70 signaling pathway in intratumoral B cells could be combined with other therapies to enhance tumor-specific antibody production. SEMA4a/NRP1 axis is currently being investigated in the clinic context of intratumoral T_{reg} cells.[76] It is not clear whether SEMA4a on GC intratumoral B cells is playing a role in interactions with TFH or T_{reg} cells or both in the TME of HNSC or if SEMA4a is a feature of GC intratumoral B cells in other human cancers. Additionally, T_{reg} cells are not a prominent feature in TLS in human tumors, but they are present in a mouse model of LUAD.[250] There are still many major questions that exist regarding the phenotype of intratumoral B cells; thus, there may be many underappreciated targets that will be revealed as we further define the phenotype intratumoral B cell subsets across tumor types.

CONCLUSION

Early murine models led researchers to believe that intratumoral B cells only promoted tumor progression with no role in the antitumor response. However, as reviewed here, intratumoral B cells are a key feature of TLS and antitumor responses in humans correlating with better overall survival and therapeutic response. The increased heterogeneity of B cells within tumors should be further explored across tumor types to determine which B cell subsets can carry out antitumor function.

Antigen specificity of intratumoral B cells remains largely unknown but several methods exist to explore this further. Whether antibodies from intratumoral B cells have antitumor capabilities is a major knowledge gap for the field. Linking intratumoral B cell phenotypes to antigen-presentation function, tumor-specific antibody production, and cytokine production will aid in the development of B cell-based therapies. It will be paramount to prioritize B cells and TLS in the next generation of immunotherapies to coordinate B and T cell immune responses to ensure more patients can benefit from cancer immunotherapy.

KEY REFERENCES

Only key references appear in the print edition. The full reference list appears in the digital product on Springer Publishing Connect: connect.springerpub.com/content/book/978-0-8261-3743-2/part/part03/chapter/ch42

17. Helmink BA, Reddy SM, Gao J, et al. B cells and tertiary lymphoid structures promote immunotherapy response. *Nature.* 2020;577(7791):549–555. doi:10.1038/s41586-019-1922-8

27. Kroeger DR, Milne K, Nelson BH. Tumor-infiltrating plasma cells are associated with tertiary lymphoid structures, cytolytic T-cell responses, and superior prognosis in ovarian cancer. *Clin Cancer Res.* 2016;22(12):3005–3015. doi:10.1158/1078-0432.CCR-15-2762

41. Siliņa K, Soltermann A, Attar FM, et al. Germinal centers determine the prognostic relevance of tertiary lymphoid structures and are impaired by corticosteroids in lung squamous cell carcinoma. *Cancer Res.* 2018;78(5):1308–1320. doi:10.1158/0008-5472.CAN-17-1987

238. Moffett HF, Harms CK, Fitzpatrick KS, et al. B cells engineered to express pathogen-specific antibodies protect against infection. *Sci Immunol.* 2019;4(35):eaax0644. doi:10.1126/sciimmunol.aax0644

Blood Transcriptomic Approaches to Cancer Immunotherapy

Darawan Rinchai, Davide Bedognetti, and Damien Chaussabel

KEY POINTS

- Blood transcriptomics encompasses profiling of leukocyte RNA abundance *ex vivo* in whole blood, fractionated cell populations or single cells, as well as *in vitro* following stimulation.

- The field is technology-driven and evolving rapidly with development of new data acquisition platforms and new approaches for data analysis and interpretation.

- Analysis of blood transcriptional profiles served to elucidate disease signatures for a wide range of diseases and is also used to monitor responses to therapy or disease progression.

- Over 50 studies have been undertaken to profile transcript abundance in the blood of cancer patients on a genome-wide scale.

- Much is left to be done, notably with regards to monitoring of changes in transcript abundance or immune function through different stages of the disease and especially in response to therapy.

- The development of fixed module repertoires supported by extensive resources for analysis, visualization. and interpretation may provide a means to streamline and democratize the use of blood transcriptomics in cancer immunotherapy trials.

BACKGROUND: IMMUNOMONITORING AND CANCER IMMUNOTHERAPY

Studies of tumor immunity have commonly relied on the use of tissue samples for the quantitative and qualitative characterization of immune-cell infiltration at the tumor site. However, tumor lesions are not always accessible and cannot be repeatedly biopsied for longitudinal immunomonitoring. Given these limitations, blood-based analyses, which are usually not as constrained in terms of sampling frequency or accessibility, have been proposed as alternative methods. Given the systemic nature of tumor immunity,[1] blood assessments allow changes in circulating immune cells to be identified and, hence, provide a more global view of drug-mediated immunoconditioning. Furthermore, with the recent breakthroughs in cancer immunotherapies, the development of immunomonitoring platforms that can be implemented in the clinical setting is a priority. This is, partly, to facilitate the characterization of variations among individuals prior to and during therapy and the possible associations these variations have with treatment outcomes (e.g., response, survival, and adverse immune reactions). Additionally, immunomonitoring could also prove to be indispensable for extending the traditional pharmacokinetic and pharmacodynamic studies into the selection of drug doses and administration schedules.[2]

Immunological monitoring is not new to clinical science, even in the context of cancer treatment. In 1979, DiSaia and Rich discussed the merits of measuring immune parameters following an "immunopotentiation" regimen consisting of the intravenous (IV) administration of *Corynebacterium parvum* to patients being treated for ovarian or cervical cancer.[3] As a result, the measurement of immune parameters has been integral to the development of currently approved checkpoint inhibitors.[4] In the context of cancer immunotherapy, immune phenotyping can be applied to both tumor immune infiltrates and peripheral blood leukocytes. We will focus on the latter in this review, as they have the advantage of being suitable for the longitudinal monitoring of immune responses.

When employed in large clinical studies, immunomonitoring typically involves the combined characterization of leukocyte cellular composition/activation, the measurement of cytokines/chemokines in serum or plasma, or the use of functional antigen-stimulation assays of cell cultures, with proliferation and cytokine production as the typical determinants. Such approaches have been widely implemented as part of immunotherapy trials and studies, with a tendency toward an emphasis on T cell phenotyping panels and functional assays because of the importance attributed to this cell population in mediating therapeutic responses.[4-7]

Technological advances over the past two decades have motivated the development of more advanced immunomonitoring approaches that have added depth to the analyses, with the introduction of mass spectrometers being a good example. Newly engineered instruments combine flow cytometry and mass spectrometry to vastly increase the number of markers that can be detected at the individual cell level, and they have been used to enhance cancer immunotherapy studies.[8-10] Moreover, the introduction of breakthrough technologies—such as microarrays and, more recently, next-generation sequencing (NGS)—has given rise to new immunomonitoring methods. Of particular relevance to cancer immunotherapy is the development of T cell receptor (TCR) repertoire sequencing, which, again, has already been employed for cancer immunotherapy monitoring.[11-13]

Another method enabled by the introduction of NGS platforms is RNA sequencing (RNA-Seq); this, and microarray platforms that have been employed earlier, permit the measurement of transcript abundances on a genome-wide scale. It can, therefore, be referred to as a "systems approach," as all the quantifiable transcript species present in a given sample are profiled using this technique. Blood transcriptome profiles have been generated from whole blood, leukocyte cell populations, and, more recently, from single cells. Short RNAs, which are also present in serum, can be quantified using similar approaches. For the remainder of this review, we will focus on "bulk" whole blood transcriptome profiling, as it is probably the most relevant approach to modern large-scale immune monitoring, which may entail hundreds of subjects, thousands of samples, and multiple collection time points.

An important caveat is that changes in transcript abundance in whole blood, as in all tissues, cannot be attributed solely to gene regulation. Indeed, the relative changes in cell abundance or the appearance of new populations may also be due to differential expression. This consideration somewhat limits the interpretation of the results; however, as with bulk tumor transcriptome profiling, the derived information remains highly valuable, both clinically and mechanistically.

BLOOD TRANSCRIPTOMICS TECHNOLOGY PRIMER

Sample Collection

A wealth of information can be gathered about the immune status of an individual through profiling of abundance of cellular leukocyte RNA on a genome-wide scale.

Bulk, whole-blood transcriptome assays have become the preferred approach for generating such profiles on large scales. Initially, the use of peripheral blood mononuclear cells (PBMCs) to extract high-quality RNA from blood proved rather challenging, and the fractionation procedure was found to be a significant source of technical variability. Collection systems have since been introduced that allow blood to be drawn into a vacutainer tube containing an RNA-stabilizing solution. Homogenization by vigorously shaking the tube after sampling disrupts blood cells and releases the RNA, which is immediately precipitated. This protects the RNA from degradation, even when kept for a few hours at room temperature or a few days at 4°C, and it can be preserved for years when the lysates are stored at −20°C. Two of the most common vacutainer tubes used are the PaxGene and Tempus tubes manufactured by Qiagen and Thermo-Fisher, respectively. Lastly, it should be noted that, while the volume of blood sampled using vacutainer tubes can be relatively small (3 mL), it is possible to employ fingerstick sampling to obtain volumes as low as 15 µl, which have been used successfully for the in-home collection of blood.[14] Solutions are also commercially available whereby study participants are mailed sampling packs that are returned to the laboratory by courier.[15]

Data Generation

As technology has progressed, microarrays have been largely replaced by RNA-Seq. This methodology relies on the same high-throughput sequencing platforms that are used for whole-genome sequencing. In simple terms, it consists, starting from RNA in (1) generating and sequencing tens of millions of cDNA fragments per sample, (2) aligning the sequence of each fragment against a reference human genome, (3) measuring expression by counting the number of fragments aligned to a given gene, and (4) applying further normalization steps to account for the length of each gene (e.g., the count value is expressed per thousand bases). A description of the various downstream analysis methodologies, the choice of which is largely dependent on the design of a particular study, is beyond the scope of this review and has been covered in detail elsewhere.[16]

Limitations

Some inherent limitations to whole blood transcriptional profiling approaches should be noted. First, it may not always detect immunological changes, especially if they are subtle or involve rare cell populations (e.g., T_{reg} cells, dendritic cell subsets). Thus, the suitability of the method should be considered based on, for instance, the study hypotheses, research field, or clinical settings. Often, pathologies or physiological states, such as pregnancy, have a robust and systemic immune component. When immune involvement is less pronounced or localized, the signals detected in whole blood may be more muted or transient. As mentioned earlier, it is also important to account for the fact that transcriptome profiles of tissues may reflect both gene regulation and relative changes in cellular composition. In cancer, as would be expected, blood transcriptional profiling appears to be relatively subtle, but robust signatures would be expected in the context of immunotherapy, especially prior to and during the development of adverse immune-mediated events.

Although cost can be another limiting factor, transcriptome profiling is relatively economical compared with the resolutions achieved. The cost of running microarrays, while initially high (USD 1,000/sample range in the early days), eventually decreased to USD 100/sample range or less for Illumina Beadarrays (now discontinued). Over time, microarrays have been replaced by the more expensive RNA-Seq, which may have prevented the wider adoption of blood transcriptomics for large-scale immune monitoring. However, costs have again steadily reduced to around the current price of ±USD 100/sample (reagents only) using 3' biased library preparation protocols.[17,18]

Access to bioinformatic resources may be another limitation, as the costs, whether they be direct (to the project) or indirect (to the institution), are substantial. Furthermore, large volumes of data are generated, which must be stored, processed, and interpreted, although there have also been improvements made over the years on that front. While, nowadays, data storage and processing may be quite manageable on a small to medium scale, the problems involved may limit the employment of the technique on a larger scale. This is especially true for organizations with fewer resources in terms of IT infrastructure and bioinformatics staff.

THE USE OF BLOOD TRANSCRIPTOMICS

Blood Transcriptome Monitoring in Cancer Studies

The transcriptomic analysis of peripheral blood[19,20] has been extensively used to dissect the mechanisms of action involved in vaccinations against infectious diseases;[21] to elucidate the pathogenic mechanisms behind immunological disorders;[22,23] and to identify the perturbations associated with parasitic,[24] bacterial,[22,25] and various viral infections,[26,27] including COVID-19.[28,29] However, the approach remains relatively underexploited in the field of cancer therapy, including immunotherapy, research.[30] Pioneering blood transcriptomic studies conducted on cancer patients treated with interleukin 2 (IL-2) have contributed to the characterization of the systemic changes induced by this cytokine. More recently, peripheral blood transcriptomic analyses have been used to identify the signatures associated with responsiveness of melanoma to anti-cytotoxic T lymphocyte-associated protein

4 (CTLA-4)[31] and to describe the changes differentially associated with CTLA-4 and a combined CTLA-4/programmed cell death protein-1 (PD-1) blockade.[30,32]

While preparing this chapter, we identified 55 studies in which blood transcriptomic approaches were employed to investigate solid tumor cancers. The topics of the studies are listed in Table 43.1,[25,33,34] and the cancer types investigated were: breast (13 studies), colorectal (11), prostate (seven), pancreatic (four), lung (five), liver (three), melanoma (four), and a single study each of cervical, renal, ovarian, head and neck, gastric, nasopharyngeal, and bladder cancers. MicroRNA profiling studies are not included in this table and neither are hematological malignancies. The studies listed were manually curated out of thousands retrieved from a PubMed query that employed broad search criteria to minimize false negatives. However, despite these precautions and careful curation of the results, it is possible that relevant studies have been inadvertently omitted. Many of the studies listed in this table were interested in the identification of biomarkers for the early detection of disease, while other studies aimed to identify prognostic markers to aid therapeutic decision-making or to assess the effects of therapy. Of the 55 studies, 42 were cross-sectional (76%), with only a small minority measuring changes in blood transcript abundance before and after treatment (eight studies) or longitudinally with multiple time points (four studies). Of the latter, only two examined responses to immunotherapies: one following the administration of IL-2 to melanoma patients,[35] and another after a gene-modified allogeneic tumor cell vaccine was administered to renal cancer patients.[36] The cohort sizes included in the studies listed in Table 43.1 ranged from a few to hundreds of patients.

It is evident from this literature survey that much more could be done to bring blood transcriptomics approaches to bear in the investigation of cancer immunobiology and responses to immune-modifying agents, in particular. Collecting samples prospectively can account for inter-individual variations and allow the identification of changes associated with pathogenesis or therapeutic responses that cannot be measured in a cross-sectional study. The measurement of transcriptional changes in whole blood following the initiation of immunotherapy could identify molecular changes predictive of therapeutic responses or, conversely, life-threatening adverse events. More generally, the research field would benefit from an increase in the frequency of sampling, testing, and monitoring of large patient cohorts. This may be possible through the adoption of the methods mentioned earlier that allow the at-home self-collection of small volumes of blood via fingerstick sampling. Changes in isolated leukocyte populations or even variations at the single-cell level could also be measured, although feasibly, the latter would be

Table 43.1 Blood Transcriptome Studies on Cancer

CANCER TYPE	AIM	STUDY DESIGN/*N*=	PMID	NOTES
Breast cancer	Early detection	Cross-sectional/121	20078854	
	Early detection	Cross-sectional/130; re-analysis	24371830	
	Early detection	Cross-sectional/130	23369435	Early detection of breast cancer
	Classification/Prognosis	Case control/36	26884644	Subtyping HER2- breast cancer patients
	Diagnosis	Cross-sectional/594	24931809	
	Response to therapy	Longitudinal/4	25000515	
	Effect of radiation therapy	Pre- and postintervention/12	22687815	
	Other	Cross-sectional/254	21129856	Signature of breast cancer survivors experiencing fibrosis
	Diagnosis	Cross-sectional/178	20930549	Signature to distinguish breast cancer and benign breast disease in nonconclusive mammography patients
	Other	Cross-sectional/21	20854893	Signature of breast cancer survivors with persistent fatigue
	Other	Cross-sectional/403	19546881	Signature of breast cancer survivors with persistent fatigue
	Other	Cross-sectional/30	19352458	Signature of BRCA1 mutation carriers
	Characterize molecular phenotypes	Unsupervised/33	31632916	Identified two distinct subtypes
Colorectal cancer	Early detection	Meta-analysis of public data	18949363	Detection of circulating tumor cells
	Early detection	Cross-sectional/31	18203981	Validation by PCR in an independent cohort of 115 subjects
	Early detection	Cross-sectional/85	24428642	
	Diagnosis	Cross-sectional/40	23650534	
	Diagnosis	Cross-sectional/403	23536436	18 gene signature
	Diagnosis	Cross-sectional/642	19795455	Assess performance of select panel of 196 genes
	Diagnosis	Case-control/338	25339833	
	Diagnosis	Cross-sectional/6	17054783	
	Response to therapy	Pre- and postintervention/23	12657164	VEGF receptor tyrosine kinase RTK inhibitor
	Response to therapy	Cross-sectional/27	24040155	Compare chemoradiation responders and nonresponders
	Methods development	Pre- and postintervention Healthy and CRC patients/20	25306939	Assess effect of colonoscopy on blood transcriptome
Prostate cancer	Classification/Prognosis		26297150	
	Classification/Prognosis		26261420	Candidate predictive biomarker signature of response to docetaxel
	Classification/Prognosis	Cross-sectional/255	23071848	Markers for aggressive prostate cancer

(*continued*)

Table 43.1 Blood Transcriptome Studies on Cancer (*continued*)

CANCER TYPE	AIM	STUDY DESIGN/*N*=	PMID	NOTES
	Classification/Prognosis	Cross-sectional/202	23059047	Signature to classify patients in low- and high-risk groups
	Classification/Prognosis	Cross-sectional/94	23059046	Identify prognosis biomarker
	Classification/Prognosis	Cross-sectional/40	22071976	Long-term vs. short-term survivors after peptide vaccination
	Effect of radiation	Longitudinal: pre- and 24 hours posttreatment	27552618	
Pancreatic cancer	Diagnosis	Cross-sectional	23732782	
	Diagnosis	Cross-sectional/177	22820136	Also includes 35 patients with chronic pancreatitis
	Diagnosis	Cross-sectional/59	21347333	
	Other	Cross-sectional/102	20571492	Signature in pancreatic cancer-induced diabetes mellitus
Lung cancer	Diagnosis	Cross-sectional/50	23451142	Non-small cell lung cancer patients
	Diagnosis	Cross-sectional/233	21558400	Early detection
	Diagnosis	Cross-sectional/228	19951989	Signature of patients with lung cancer vs. nonmalignant lung disease
	Classification/Prognosis	Cross-sectional/108	22479623	Prediction of survival
	Early detection	Cross-sectional/248	30425263	Compare cases and controls using samples collected before diagnosis
Liver cancer	Early detection	Cross-sectional/20	27461685	PBMCs, Affymetrix, case-control
	Early detection	Cross-sectional/166	24332572	
	Methods development		27600246	Investigate collection tube bias
Melanoma	Diagnosis	Cross-sectional/10	21698244	Signatures for detection and monitoring
	Response to immunotherapy	Pre- and postintervention	12184809	Response to systemic IL-2 administration
	Predict response to checkpoint inhibitor	Pretreatment samples	28807052	Pretreatment samples before receiving chemotherapy and anti-CTLA-4
	Response to DC vaccine	Pre- and postvaccination	doi:10.1038/s43018-020-00143-y	Response to Fl3t ligand before receiving DC vaccine
Cervical cancer	Early diagnosis	Cross-sectional/42	20497704	
Renal cancer	Response to immunotherapy		25242680	Measure effects of a gene-modified allogeneic tumor cell vaccine; longitudinal
	Response to immunomodulator drug (TKI)	Longitudinal (three timepoints); pre and posttreatment	doi:10.1101/2020.05.01.071613v2	Monitoring immune response to Pazopanib
Ovarian cancer	Diagnosis	Cross-sectional/63	23551967	
	Response to checkpoint inhibitors	Longitudinal (seven timepoints); pre and posttreatment	31694725	Predict response to treatment and AE

(*continued*)

Table 43.1 Blood Transcriptome Studies on Cancer (*continued*)

CANCER TYPE	AIM	STUDY DESIGN/*N*=	PMID	NOTES
Head and neck cancer	Effects of radiation therapy	Cross-sectional/87	23009663	
Gastric cancer	Diagnosis	Cross-sectional/14	22977563	
Nasopharyngeal carcinoma	Response to treatment	Cross-sectional; pre- and posttreatment	22986368	
Bladder cancer	Diagnosis	Cross-sectional/45	16740760	
"Various malignancies"	Effect of treatment	Pre- and posttreatment/4	17390994	Effect of hyperthermia and chemotherapy

AE, adverse events; CRC, colorectal carcinoma; CTLA-4, cytotoxic T-lymphocyte-associated protein 4; DC, dendritic cell; FlT3, FMS-like tyrosine kinase 3; HER2, human epidermal growth factor receptor 2; IL-2, interleukin 2; PBMCs, peripheral blood mononuclear cells; PCR, polymerase chain reaction; RTK, receptor tyrosine kinase; TKI, tyrosine kinase inhibitor; VEGF, vascular endothelial growth factor.

conducted using a smaller subset of patients given the greater technical complexity and cost. Research at the single-cell level presents challenges associated with the high costs and the need to amplify the starting material, but by employing microfluidic technology, the amount of sample manipulation required during isolation and preparation can be minimized. Therefore, single-cell genomics may, in time, become amenable to implementation in multicenter clinical studies. Finally, blood-based in vitro assays employing transcriptomic readouts could be employed to assess the immune function of patients at various disease stages, with uses ranging from early detection to the selection and monitoring of immunotherapy regimens.

Implementation of Blood Transcriptome Monitoring on Large Scales

To provide context to the potential uses of the technique, illustrative examples of studies that have implemented blood transcriptome monitoring on a large scale outside of the cancer research field are provided in Table 43.2.[37–43] These studies involved longitudinal sample collection, used systems-scale profiling approaches (RNA-Seq or arrays), and had sample sizes greater than 500 patients (our arbitrary definition for "large scale").

The research setting and the questions addressed in these studies were remarkably diverse. Those that investigated responses to treatment form the first category, as is the case in the work by Fourati et al., who sought to identify the key determinants of the immunogenicity of an experimental HIV vaccine.[37] In another study, Thompson et al. generated blood transcriptome profiles for blood samples from patients with active tuberculosis during the course of antimicrobial therapy,[38] and they were successful in identifying a signature predictive of tuberculosis treatment outcomes. The same signature

was found to correlate with the pulmonary inflammatory state measured by PET-CT.

The second category includes observational studies. A good example is the work by Banchereau et al.,[39] who collected study samples from 158 children with systemic lupus erythematosus (SLE) during clinical visits over a duration of almost 4 years, with data representing 996 time points. The main achievement of this study was the molecular classification of patients according to their "correlation patterns." It appeared that patients with SLE could be broadly categorized according to which signatures correlated with changes in the activity of their disease over time. As this case demonstrated, immunomonitoring permits us to follow the "natural" evolution of the disease; however, it is also possible to observe changes that occur under "perturbed" physiological states. Hong et al., for instance, followed the immunological trajectories of women during pregnancy, both in control subjects and those with prior SLE diagnosis, with the latter being more prone to adverse pregnancy outcomes.[40] In another observational study, Altman et al. endeavored, instead, to identify the signatures associated with episodes of asthma exacerbation caused by viral respiratory illnesses.[41]

As illustrated by these examples, valuable knowledge has already been gained from the use of blood transcriptomics for immune monitoring, but the implementation of more intensive sampling regimens could, potentially, pave the way for even more applications. For instance, being able to capture the changes in transcript abundance that precede adverse clinical events may lead to the development of novel preventive therapies.[44] In the context of cancer immunotherapy, this notion could apply, for example, to the study of adverse immune-related events, making it possible to make individual adjustments to dosage or regimens to interrupt immunopathogenesis and prevent the onset of clinical symptoms.

Table 43.2 Large-Scale Blood Transcriptome Monitoring Studies (Illustrative Examples)

DISEASE/SETTING	AIM	STUDY DESIGN/*N*=	PMID (REFERENCE)	FINDINGS
Asthma	Identify mechanisms of asthma exacerbation in children	1,034 samples from 208 subjects monitored over a 6-month period (number of time points variable) and profiled via RNA-Seq	20078854 (Altman et al.[41])	Distinct pathways are associated with virus-associated and nonvirus associated exacerbations.
Systemic lupus erythematosus (SLE)	To assess molecular heterogeneity among pediatric SLE cases	996 samples from 158 subjects monitored for up to 1,412 days (number of time points variable) and profiled via microarrays	27040498 (Banchereau et al.[39])	SLE patients can be classified based on which transcriptome signatures correlate with their disease severity.
HIV vaccine	To identify correlates of immunogenicity	598 samples from 263 subjects monitored for 2 weeks (2 time points) and profiled via microarrays	30787294 (Fourati et al.[37])	Identified IRF7 as mediator of protection.
Tuberculosis	Prediction of tuberculosis treatment outcome	914 samples from subjects monitored for 24 weeks (three time points) and profiled via RNA-Seq	29050771 (Thompson et al.[38])	A five-gene panel can be used for stratification of patients according to risk of treatment failure.
Intensive care	Discrimination of infectious and noninfectious sources of critical illness	802 samples obtained from subjects at admission in the ICU and throughout length of stay	26121490, 28864056 (Scicluna et al.[42,43])	A 140-gene signature used for the classification of sepsis
Systemic lupus erythematosus and pregnancy	Identify mechanisms responsible for increased complications in pregnant women with SLE	512 samples obtained from 189 subjects monitored for 44 weeks (five time points) using microarrays.	30962246 (Hong et al.[40])	Neutrophil, interferon, and plasma cell signatures were associated with complicated pregnancies.

BLOOD TRANSCRIPTOME MODULE REPERTOIRES

To this day, data analysis and interpretation remain significant rate-limiting steps when considering the routine adoption of systems-scale profiling approaches for immunomonitoring applications. These may be even more relevant now that the cost has decreased and represents less of a barrier to mainstream implementation. We have worked for well over a decade on the development of transcriptional module repertoires that can be employed to streamline the analysis and interpretation of blood transcriptome profiling data (Figure 43.1).[20,45,46] A starting point for this is the identification of coexpression patterns among the transcripts in which abundance is being measured. The sets (or repertoires) of transcriptional modules that can be identified as a result are employed as a fixed framework for data analysis and interpretation. This means that, once formed, the module repertoire can be reused in the analysis of any new data set. This is in contrast to the more common practice of forming a new set of modules every time a new data set is analyzed. The method employed for the construction of such reusable module repertoires is described in the text that follows as well as in Figure 43.1. Since these repertoires are meant to be stable over time, the main imperative is to factor in the coexpression observed across a wide range of immune states. The major benefit of reusing such module

repertoires is that it allows researchers to dedicate significant amounts of time toward the development of ad-hoc data analysis visualization and interpretation resources, such as the ones that are described in the text that follows. Finally, we also outline how such fixed module repertoires can be employed in the development of targeted assays.

The Construction of Module Repertoires

Blood transcriptional module repertoires were constructed based on coexpression patterns observed across several immune "states" (Figure 43.1), which correspond to patient pathologies (e.g., infections, autoimmune diseases, or cancer) as well as physiological "variants" (e.g., pregnancy, maintained pharmacological immunosuppression). Each framework is developed independently of the data set it serves to analyze. In other words, each framework is based on the coexpression observed in the multiple data sets or immune states used for its construction and does not account for any coexpression present in the data set(s) being analyzed. Since 2008, we have established two such repertoires,[45,47] and a third is being finalized[46] ("BloodGen3" repertoire, which serves as an illustrative use case for Figure 43.1). Each repertoire differs by only two parameters: the first is the platform

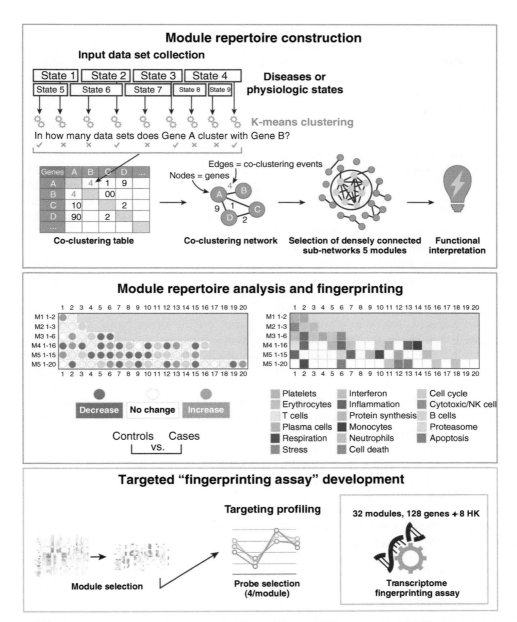

Figure 43.1 **Overview of module repertoire construction, downstream analyses, and targeted assay development.** *Top panel:* The approach described here has been previously reported in detail in earlier publications.[20,45,46] Briefly, blood transcriptional module repertoire construction involves the collection of transcriptome data sets for use as input. Each data set corresponds to a different "state" of the system—primarily pathological (disease) or physiological variants (e.g., pregnancy). The clustering behavior of gene pairs is recorded for each independent data set, and the information is compiled in a co-clustering table. Subsequently, the co-clustering table serves as input for the generation of a graph, in which the nodes are the genes and the edges represent co-clustering events. Next, the largest, most densely connected subnetworks are parsed mathematically (graph theory) and assigned a module ID. The genes constituting the module are removed from the selection pool and the process is repeated. *Middle panel:* Changes in transcript abundance can be visualized using a fingerprint grid. A red spot on the grid denotes an increase in abundance for a set of coexpressed genes constituting a given module, while a blue spot denotes a decrease in abundance. The position of each module on the grid is fixed, so they can be related to the functional annotations shown on the adjacent grid. For instance, the first two modules on the first row are functionally associated with platelets and interferon, respectively. *Bottom panel:* The module repertoire framework can serve as the basis for the development of targeted assays, which involves two major steps. First, representative modules are selected from among the modules constituting the framework. Second, representative probes are selected from among those modules. The process can be adjusted according to practical constraints, such as assay throughput and cost. For instance, the selection of 32 modules, and four representative genes from each, would yield a 128-gene fingerprinting assay.

HK, housekeeping.

employed for transcriptome profiling (e.g., Affymetrix or Illumina arrays), and the second is the number of data sets and breadth of immune states used as input. For our second modular repertoire, coexpression was determined across nine data sets and seven immune states, including autoimmune/inflammatory diseases such as systemic lupus erythematosus and juvenile arthritis, infections such as HIV and tuberculosis, and melanomas. The third and latest iteration encompasses 16 immune and physiological states.[46]

Module Repertoire Analyses

The analysis workflow is relatively simple. In the first step, the expression matrix (samples × genes) is annotated to indicate which genes included in the matrix belong to which module for a given preexisting module repertoire (e.g., one of the 382 modules comprising the BloodGen3 repertoire we have recently finalized). Typically, 70% to 80% of genes expressed in whole blood samples can be assigned to a given module. The next step consists of identifying the differentially expressed genes, and the methods and parameters used at this stage can be adapted to the study design and hypotheses. Generally, either a group comparison (e.g., cases vs. controls; responders vs. nonresponders) or a comparison with baseline samples (e.g., pretreatment) is performed. The differences are then expressed as the proportion (percentage) of transcripts constituting a given module that are either increased or decreased in comparison to a control group or baseline sample analyzed earlier. By design, the genes constituting the modules tend to be coexpressed; therefore, changes are coordinated in most instances, with the majority of genes being either increased or decreased. When divergences occur, the overall trend is retained for further interpretation and visualization. Indeed, for the next and final steps, the changes are visually represented by a grid, often referred to as a "module repertoire fingerprint" (Figure 43.1). For this type of representation, each module is assigned a fixed position on the grid. The changes in each module, observed through the comparisons performed in the previous step, are shown as either a red or blue spot, representing an increase or decrease in abundance, respectively. No spots are shown when percent changes are below a given threshold (it is adjustable but typically set to 15%—this is to avoid representing changes that may be deemed marginal and may not be reproducible). When spots are present, their color and position on the grid are used to represent the functional changes, and the interpretations assigned to various modules are mapped on the grid with the aid of a color key (Figure 43.1). A collection of fingerprints generated for well-characterized patient populations can also be employed as a reference to assist with interpretation of the results, allowing for

instance, the use of viral infection responses or systemic inflammation as benchmarks (Figure 43.1).

The previously described analysis is performed to determine overall differences at the "group level," for instance, between a group of cases and controls. But importantly, differences can also be mapped for individual samples (e.g., subjects) within a group in comparison to a baseline (e.g., pretreatment sample for the same individual, or a group of healthy controls that serves as a reference). This type of representation is simple to interpret when presented as a report card: when the grid is clear of any spots, the analyst can immediately see that no immune perturbations or deviations from normal or baseline were detected.

It is apparent that employing a fixed modular repertoire can facilitate the analysis and interpretation of transcriptome profiling data. This is due to, on one hand, a reduction in the scale of the analysis (dealing with "only" hundreds of parameters rather than thousands), and, on the other hand, the development of a framework for data visualization and interpretation, which initially allows in-depth functional profiling of the data, and then, access to collections of reference fingerprints. We next describe a recently published illustrative case in which the previously described analysis workflow was employed to evaluate the immune response in melanoma patients receiving DC vaccines (Figure 43.2).[33,47] Specifically, the study aimed to evaluate the immunogenicity of FMS-like tyrosine kinase 3 (Flt3L: CDX-301) combined with poly-ICLC (a TLR3 agonist that activates DCs) and a DC vaccine comprising anti-DEC-205-NY-ESO-1, a fusion antibody targeting CD205, linked to the NY-ESO-1 antigen. Melanoma patients were randomized into two groups that received the vaccine with and without CDX-301 (cohorts 1 and 2, respectively). Blood samples were collected from 23 subjects on at least 10 time points for transcript profiling, and the abundance of a targeted set of transcripts was measured on a Nanostring nCounter instrument (using the NanoString PanCancer Immunology Panel that can measure an abundance of 770 transcripts). Compared with the prevaccination baseline, the immunological changes were dramatic in cohort 1 but absent in cohort 2 (Figure 43.2A). Changes in transcript abundance mediated by CDX-301 peaked on day 8, were sustained on day 15, and had returned to almost baseline by day 22. Mapping changes at the module level against the fingerprint grid identified the cell types/pathways that were perturbed following treatment at the peak of the response (Figure 43.2B). Increases in transcript abundance compared with the pretreatment baseline were observed for 18 modules associated with a wide range of biological/immunological processes, such as inflammation, cell death, interferon, and proliferation immune suppression, as well as with cell types such as monocytes and neutrophils. The abundance of 10 modules, including

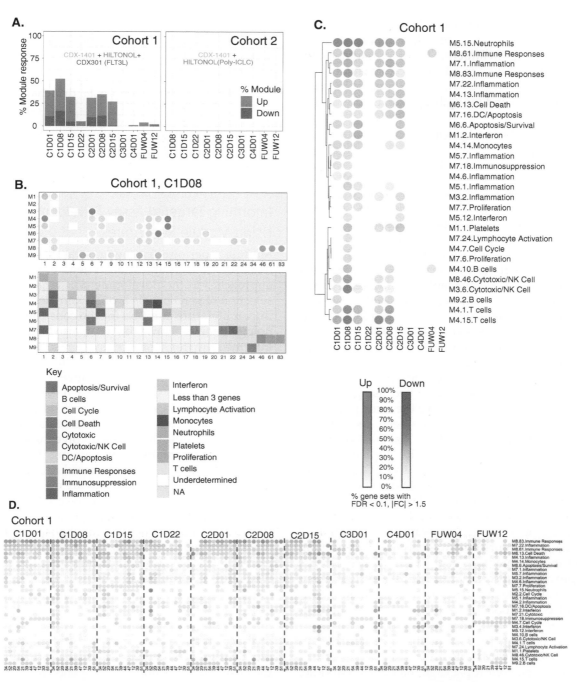

Figure 43.2 Measuring responses to immune-modifying treatments in cancer patients using blood transcriptional profiling.
Changes in transcript abundances in peripheral blood mononuclear cells (PBMCs), measured using NanoString, were mapped against a preconstructed, second-generation modular analysis framework.[47] (**A**) The proportion of modules found to be responsive to treatment are represented by a bar graph for both study cohorts. The naming convention for the time points is as follows: C indicates the cycle number (C1 = cycle 1, C2 = cycle), D indicates the number of days posttreatment, FUW indicates the follow-up week number. (**B**) Changes observed at C1D08 in the first treatment cohort (with CDX301/FLT3L) are mapped against a module fingerprint grid plot (see Figure 43.1). Red spots indicate increased and blue spots indicate decreased abundance compared with prevaccination baseline. Functional associations are shown on the color grid on the right. (**C**) Changes in transcript abundance for the modules found to be responsive are shown across all time points on the heatmap, with columns representing posttreatment time points. (**D**) Changes in transcript abundance for responsive modules are shown on the heatmap, with columns representing increases or decreases for individual subjects across different time points.

Source: Reproduced with permission from Bhardwaj N, Friedlander PA, Pavlick AC, et al. FLT3 ligand augments immune responses to anti-DEC-205-NY-ESO-1 vaccine through expansion of dendritic cell subsets. *Nat Cancer.* 2020;1(12):1204–1217. doi:10.1038/s43018-020-00143-y

those for T cells, B cells, platelets, leukocyte activation, cell cycle, proliferation, and cytotoxic and NK cells, was decreased following treatment. The representation of the "responsive modules" in a heatmap format gave the authors the ability to map changes over time, at both the group (Figure 43.2C) and individual level (Figure 43.2D).

Resources Available to Support Module Repertoire Analyses

Over the years, our research team has developed and made available three successive fixed blood transcriptional module repertoires. The first, published in 2008, was based on PBMC profiles generated using Affymetrix GeneChips across eight data sets.[45] The second, which we published in 2013, was based on whole-blood profiles generated using Illumina Beadarrays across nine data sets.[47] We have now made available a "third-generation" repertoire (BloodGen3) that, again, is based on whole-blood profiles generated using Illumina Beadarrays, but this time, across 16 data sets and nearly 1,000 individual profiles.[46] Finally, another collection of blood transcriptional modules (BTMs) has also been made available via our collaborators; these are based on larger collections of publicly available data and generated using different methodologies, but essentially serve the same purpose.[48]

A significant amount of effort has been dedicated to the functional interpretation of the established blood module repertoires, including via the implementation of literature profiling approaches (BloodGen1[45]) and the development of an annotation wiki (BloodGen2[47]). For our third generation of modules (BloodGen3), the functional profiling work was expanded to comprise the outputs from gene ontology, pathway, and transcription factor binding site enrichment analyses. In addition, for each of the 382 modules comprising this repertoire, we now provide transcriptional profiles derived from several reference data sets (fractionated circulating leukocytes and cord blood progenitors). This plethora of information is made available to end users via interactive "circle packing plots" (for instance: prezi.com/view/GqtUO22JJlSf16zMJKbB/).

In addition, a custom R package, BloodGen3Module, was developed to support data analysis and visualization using this latest generation of modules[49] (github.com/Drinchai/BloodGen3Module and bioconductor.org/packages/release/bioc/html/BloodGen3Module.html), and the package has functions that allow the generation of fingerprint grid plots representing changes in transcript abundance for a group of subjects. Heatmaps can also be generated that permit the visualization of changes in individuals at the module level.

Finally, to complete the interpretation framework for this BloodGen3 repertoire, several R shiny web applications were developed that provide access to the fingerprints of the reference cohorts used for the construction of this repertoire (16 data sets), as well as disease-specific collections:

1. Sixteen reference cohorts,[46] drinchai.shinyapps.io/BloodGen3Module
2. Six respiratory syncytial virus studies,[26] drinchai.shinyapps.io/RSV_Meta_Module_analysis
3. Two COVID-19 studies,[28] drinchai.shinyapps.io/COVID_19_project

Informing Targeted Assay Development Using Module Repertoires

Module repertoire frameworks can also help fulfill the demand for more streamlined immunomonitoring approaches in the development of targeted assays. The selection of gene panels is often knowledge-driven, relying on literature curation for the constitution of "immunology panels." However, it can also be data-driven and informed by, for instance, system-scale-profiling data, such as transcriptomic data. Modular repertoires happen to be well-suited for the development of targeted gene panels. One simple approach consists of selecting a subset of modules, based on gene functional relevance or on the patterns of change observed across studies, for example. The next steps then involve the selection of one or a few representative genes among those constituting the chosen modules. This is based on the premise that the genes forming the modules are coexpressed and can serve as surrogates to represent the changes observed for the entire gene set. Gene selection at this stage can also be data-driven, for instance, for choosing genes that are the most representative (e.g., those that show patterns closest to the mean for the entire module) or deciding which levels of expression are optimal (i.e., neither too low nor too high). Additionally, gene selection can be based on function, such as known cell markers, and may take into account assay design limitations, such as probe/primer design for PCR-based assays. For example, the BloodGen3 repertoire was used as the basis for the design of a 44-module/184-gene "transcriptome fingerprinting assay" (TFA) panel. A manuscript describing the selection process and examples of studies that have used this TFA has been deposited in BioRxiv.[50] More recently, we also employed the BloodGen3 repertoire to design targeted blood transcript panels specifically for the monitoring of immune trajectories in patients infected with SARS-CoV-2.[28] The initial data-driven approach, which utilized the module repertoire, was accompanied by a knowledge-driven approach supported by the BloodGen3 interpretation framework; this permitted the development of three different panels with distinct functional connotations (immunobiology, therapy, and viral biology).

CONCLUSION

In conclusion, understanding immune variation in cancer patients both prior to and during therapy may prove critical for guiding therapy choices, such as when balancing efficacy with the risk of adverse events and achieving optimal outcomes. For this, leveraging the available deep immune phenotyping and multi-omics platforms may prove especially useful, and blood transcriptomics may have a role to play with that regard. Although with recent technological advances it has been necessary to implement increasingly more sophisticated analytical approaches, efforts must now also be made toward streamlining and democratization in order to permit more routine use and on larger scales. The development of well-annotated and reusable module repertoires along with supporting resources may partly address this need. The development of targeted profiling assays based on such repertoires is another potential avenue for enabling routine implementation of blood transcriptome-based immune monitoring in cancer immunotherapy trials.

KEY REFERENCES

Only key references appear in the print edition. The full reference list appears in the digital product on Springer Publishing Connect: connect.springerpub.com/content/book/978-0-8261-3743-2/part/part03/chapter/ch43

26. Rinchai D, Altman MC, Konza O, et al. Definition of erythroid cell-positive blood transcriptome phenotypes associated with severe respiratory syncytial virus infection. *Clin Transl Med.* 2020;10(8):e244. doi:10.1101/527812

33. Bhardwaj N, Friedlander PA, Pavlick AC, et al. FLT3 ligand augments immune responses to anti-DEC-205-NY-ESO-1 vaccine through expansion of dendritic cell subsets. *Nat Cancer.* 2020;1(12):1204–1217. doi:10.1038/s43018-020-00143-y

35. Panelli MC, Wang E, Phan G, et al. Gene-expression profiling of the response of peripheral blood mononuclear cells and melanoma metastases to systemic IL-2 administration. *Genome Biol.* 2002;3(7):research0035.1–research0035.17. doi:10.1186/gb-2002-3-7-research0035

39. Banchereau R, Hong S, Cantarel B, et al. Personalized immunomonitoring uncovers molecular networks that stratify lupus patients. *Cell.* 2016;165(3):551–565. doi:10.1016/j.cell.2016.03.008

41. Altman MC, Gill MA, Whalen E, et al. Transcriptome networks identify mechanisms of viral and nonviral asthma exacerbations in children. *Nat Immunol.* 2019;20(5):637–651. doi:10.1038/s41590-019-0347-8

45. Chaussabel D, Quinn C, Shen J, et al. A modular analysis framework for blood genomics studies: application to systemic lupus erythematosus. *Immunity.* 2008;29(1):150–164. doi:10.1016/j.immuni.2008.05.012

Advances in Techniques for Immunotherapy Biomarker Analysis

Theresa M. LaVallee, Pier Federico Gherardini, and Cheryl Selinsky

KEY POINTS

- Immuno-oncology therapies have transformed the cancer treatment landscape and afforded long-term survival to some cancer patients. The mechanisms of response and resistance involve a complex multicomponent system associated with host characteristics and tumor and immune interactions.

- Precision medicine for targeted therapy has advanced cancer treatments using single-omic approaches but precision immunotherapy requires advancement in technology to derive a multi-omic, multiparameter algorithm.

- Precision immunotherapy will require predicative assays to inform patient selection, stratification, and rational combinations to define who to treat with single-agent immunotherapy, such as programmed cell death protein 1 (PD-1) therapy or chimeric antigen receptor T cell (CAR T cell) therapy, or who to treat with combination immunotherapy therapies.

- Biomarker discovery to derive precision immunotherapy tests requires generating baseline and on-treatment biomarker data utilizing methods that broadly assess the genome, epigenome, transcriptome, proteome, microbiome, and metabolome in tumor, blood, and stool.

INTRODUCTION

Immune checkpoint inhibitors (ICI), such as anti-programmed cell death protein 1 (anti-PD-1), anti-programmed cell death protein-ligand 1 (anti-PD-L1), and anti-cytotoxic T lymphocyte associated protein 4 (anti-CTLA-4) monoclonal antibodies, and cell and gene therapies, such as chimeric antigen receptor (CAR) T cells, are successful classes of immunotherapy drugs and have resulted in remarkable clinical benefits for cancer patients, including durable clinical responses and improved survival.[1,2] Despite important advancements with immunotherapy and broad use across a range of tumor indications and lines of treatment, the benefits of these drugs are limited to a minority of patients.[3] There is an urgent need to identify biomarkers to select cancer patients who are likely to benefit or not from immunotherapy treatments. These predictive biomarkers will define who to treat with single-agent immunotherapy but, importantly, may also inform biology-directed immuno-oncology combinations to expand the number of cancer patients who derive clinical benefit.

Historically, precision medicine has focused on single-omic approaches to identify oncogenic "driver" mutations that cause uncontrolled tumor growth and matching the biomarker directly to targeted therapies that inhibit the specific oncogenic pathway. Examples include evaluating the tumor by immunohistochemistry (IHC) for hormone receptor expression[4] or human epidermal growth factor receptor 2 (HER2) amplification in breast cancer,[5] and by genomic sequencing to detect genetic alterations either by a gene-specific polymerase chain reaction (PCR) assay or, more recently, by next-generation sequencing (NGS) with a targeted panel of genes to detect lung cancer somatic mutations.[6]

Certain tumors are primed and ready to respond to immunotherapy treatment such as ICI therapy, and others are not. Cancer patients who benefit from ICI treatment are characterized as having immunologically responsive tumors, whereas those who do not respond to ICI treatment are characterized as having immune nonresponsive tumors. Several biomarkers have been proposed to classify a tumor as immune responsive versus immune nonresponsive, including PD-L1 expression, tumor mutation burden (TMB) as a measure of the number of somatic mutations acquired in the tumor genome that the immune system may recognize,[7,8] a tumor-immune gene signature that is indicative of the immune responsiveness of the tumor microenvironment (TME),[9,10] fecal microbiome profile that is thought to influence immune tone,[11–14] and the extent of the CD8 T cell infiltrate[15] as an indicator that T cells are present and available for anti-tumor immunity.[3] PD-L1 expression using IHC assays[16] has demonstrated clinical utility, and while it has been shown in some tumor types to enrich for cancer patients who are likely to benefit, it does not have robust positive and negative predictive values.[17]

The mechanism of action of immunotherapy is to induce antitumor immunity by activating the patient's own immune system. The immune system is composed of a multitude of cell types and can be divided into lymphocytes: B cells, T cells, and natural killer (NK) cells and myeloid cells: macrophages, dendritic cells, and monocytes.[18] Improvements in immunotherapy biomarker technologies that increase the ability to multiplex have enabled sensitive methods for subtyping the phenotype of the immune cells involved. Much focus is on the CD8 T cell given it is the effector cell (Teff) for antitumor immunity in response to ICI treatment and the drug for CAR T and TCR-based therapies. Recent work has further subtyped Teff cells into terminal differentiation (PD-1, TIM3, CD39) and states of exhaustion (T_{EX}) characterized by transcription factors TOX and TCF7.[19,20] The complex interplay between the multitude of immune cells to initiate and maintain an effective immune response, evaluating other immune cells including B cells, CD4 T cells, dendritic cells, and immunosuppressive cells, such as myeloid-derived suppressor cells (MDSC) and macrophages,[21,22] may further inform immunotherapy treatment. Advances in immunotherapy biomarker technologies that can multiplex to enable characterization of multiple immune cell types including differentiation state and inform regional spatial relationships in the TME are critical to fully understanding how to design immunotherapy treatment and enable immunotherapy precision medicine.

Additionally, precision immune profiling to guide clinical management with immunotherapy treatment will need to assess host genetics, lifestyle behaviors, tumor characteristics, and a complex multicomponent immune system. The relationship between host and tumor genotypes, immune phenotypes, and tumor-immune escape mechanisms is complex. Thus, precision immunotherapy will require an "immunogram"[23]—a comprehensive, multi-omic portrait of host-tumor-immune interaction that leverages biological insight and computational analysis to predict cancer patient subsets and immunotherapy treatment regimens (Figure 44.1). Defining multifactorial biomarker algorithms for immunotherapy requires new approaches and methodologies that utilize deep molecular and cellular profiling of host factors, TME, and immune contexture with clinical metadata from clinical trials (Figure 44.2) to then develop reliable and reproducible biomarkers to distinguish patients whose tumors are immunotherapy responsive, from those with resistant tumors, with the goal of guiding treatment decisions for rational immunotherapy combinations or other treatments. Cristescu et al. have published an approach to use a multi-omic, multiparameter biomarker approach to select patients for PD1 therapy,[24] suggesting this may have utility in advancing precision immunotherapy. Given the complexities of the multifactorial components and diversity of cancer patients, biomarker discovery approaches beyond tumor DNA and RNA will be needed. Precision immunotherapy will include genomics but will need to bring together diverse data sets that go beyond the genome to characterize the epigenome, transcriptome, proteome, microbiome, and metabolome in tumor, blood, and stool (Figure 44.1). Developing reliable and robust predictive biomarker assays is out of scope for this review. For the purpose of the discussion in this chapter, we focus on recent advances in biomarker discovery technologies to generate high-dimensional data sets with a suite of assays to determine multiparameter, multi-omic factors from the host, tumor, and immune system (Table 44.1), with the aim of informing who and how to treat with immunotherapy and increase the number and types of cancer patients who benefit.

TUMOR-BASED BIOMARKERS

Tumor Genomics

Tumor Mutational Burden as a Predictive Biomarker of Immune Checkpoint Inhibitor Response

Tumor mutational burden (TMB), the total number of somatic mutations per sequenced area of a tumor genome, holds promise as a predictive biomarker of response to ICI therapy. The best responses to anti-PD-(L)1 monoclonal antibody therapies have been observed in cancers with the highest mutational loads (melanoma, NSCLC, SCCHN, gastric, and bladder cancer).[8,25–27] Tumors with low TMB, such as prostate, colorectal, pancreatic, and ovarian, have shown limited clinical benefit from PD-(L)1 therapy.[28] Further supporting the association between a high mutational burden and the response to ICI is the observation that mismatch repair (MMR)-deficient tumors, whose genomes contain high numbers of somatic mutations, are susceptible to PD-1 blockade.[29]

Comprehensive profiling of tumor genomes has become more routine in retrospective translational studies enabled by the availability of NGS technologies and computational methods to compare tumor and germline sequences and reliably call genetic variants. Advancements in the ability to identify genetic rearrangements, insertions, and deletions, paired with algorithms to predict the neoantigens they encode as immunogenic for both CD8 and CD4 T cells, provide a path forward for neoantigen vaccine development and discovery of targets for cell therapy.[30] Nevertheless, widespread adoption of TMB in the clinical setting is limited by the cost of whole-exome sequencing and the bioinformatics expertise necessary to interpret the results within a window amenable to inform treatment selection.

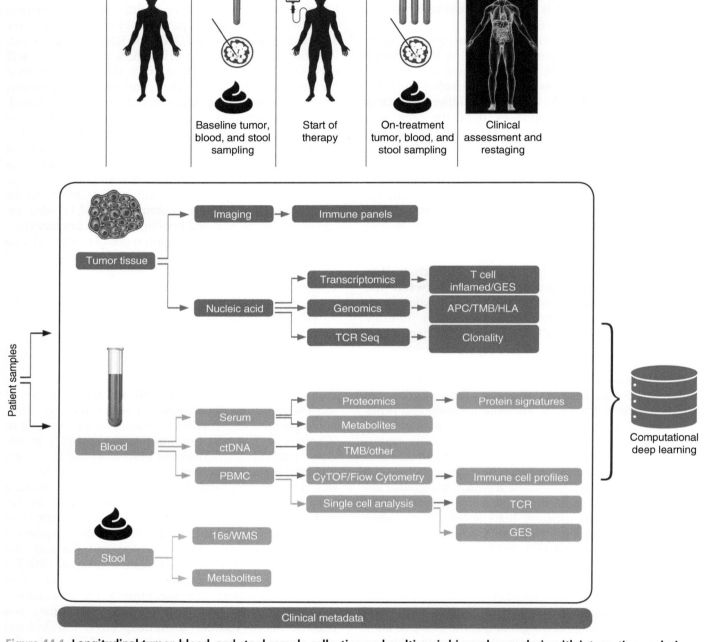

Figure 44.1 Longitudinal tumor, blood, and stool sample collection and multi-omic biomarker analysis with integrative analysis of clinical outcomes. Collection of patient samples for biomarker analysis including tumor, blood, and stool at baseline (before treatment) and over the course of immunotherapy treatment allows for multi-omic analysis. Biomarker discovery to inform immunotherapy precision medicine requires integrative multiparameter, multi-omic biomarker, and clinical data with state-of-the-art bioinformatic capabilities for computational deep learning.

APC, antigen-presenting cell; ctDNA, circulating tumor DNA; CyTOF, mass cytometry time of flight; GES, gene expression signature; HLA, human leukocyte antigen (major histocompatibility complex (MHC) in humans); PBMC, peripheral blood mononuclear cell; 16S, stands for 16S ribosomal ribonucleic acid (rRNA) sequencing; TCR, T cell receptor; TCR-Seq, T cell receptor high-throughput sequencing; TMB, tumor mutational burden; WMS, whole metagenomic sequencing.

Consequently, efforts are underway to estimate the total mutational load from next-generation gene panels and correlate the TMB with clinical benefit from ICI.

Mutational load of the whole genome has been extrapolated from sequencing smaller panels of a few hundred genes and comparing the results with whole-exome data

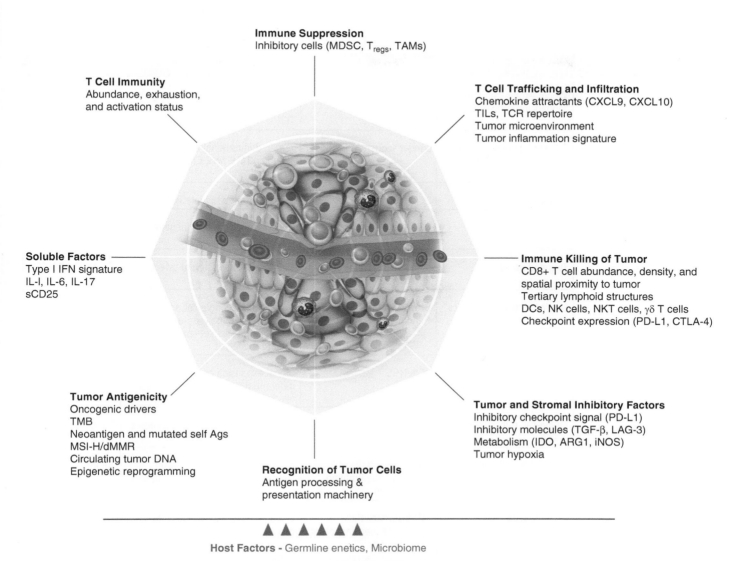

Immune Suppression
Inhibitory cells (MDSC, T_{regs}, TAMs)

T Cell Immunity
Abundance, exhaustion,
and activation status

T Cell Trafficking and Infiltration
Chemokine attractants (CXCL9, CXCL10)
TILs, TCR repertoire
Tumor microenvironment
Tumor inflammation signature

Soluble Factors
Type I IFN signature
IL-I, IL-6, IL-17
sCD25

Immune Killing of Tumor
CD8+ T cell abundance, density, and
spatial proximity to tumor
Tertiary lymphoid structures
DCs, NK cells, NKT cells, $\gamma\delta$ T cells
Checkpoint expression (PD-L1, CTLA-4)

Tumor Antigenicity
Oncogenic drivers
TMB
Neoantigen and mutated self Ags
MSI-H/dMMR
Circulating tumor DNA
Epigenetic reprogramming

Tumor and Stromal Inhibitory Factors
Inhibitory checkpoint signal (PD-L1)
Inhibitory molecules (TGF-β, LAG-3)
Metabolism (IDO, ARG1, iNOS)
Tumor hypoxia

Recognition of Tumor Cells
Antigen processing &
presentation machinery

Host Factors - Germline enetics, Microbiome

Figure 44.2 Precision immunotherapy will require an algorithm utilizing multiparameter, multi-omic biomarker data.
Integrated analysis can reveal relationships between host genetics, blood-based biomarkers (immune cells, circulating tumor DNA, proteins, and metabolites), tumor (mutations, gene expression signatures, soluble factors), tumor microenvironment variables (immune cell phenotypes, immunosuppressive cells, soluble factors), and stool microbiome (bacteria species and metabolites).

ARG1, arginase-1; DC, dendritic cell; dMMR, deficient mismatch repair; IDO, indoleamine 2,3-dioxygenase 1; iNOS, inducible nitric oxide synthase; IFN, interferon; MDSC, myeloid-derived suppressor cell; MSI-H, microsatellite instability high; NK, natural killer; NKT, natural killer T cell; sCD25, soluble CD25; TAM, tumor-associated macrophage; TCR, T cell receptor; TGF-β, tumor growth factor beta; TIL, tumor-infiltrating lymphocyte; T_{reg}, regulatory T cell.

sets that successfully predicted response to PD-1 therapy. Targeted gene sets were able to predict clinical benefit to PD-1 blockade in melanoma and non-small cell lung carcinoma (NSCLC) with accuracy similar to that reported using whole-exome sequencing.[31,32] Recently, the U.S. Food and Drug Administration (FDA) has granted accelerated approval to the anti-PD-1 monoclonal antibody (pembrolizumab) with a broad label for the treatment of adult and pediatric patients with unresectable or metastatic TMB-high; the information can be accessed at www.fda.gov/drugs/drug-approvals-and-databases. A consortium led by the Quality in Pathology (QiP) and Friends of Cancer Research is working to harmonize and standardize the use of gene panels for TMB assessment.[33] A composite predictive biomarker system that combines TMB with other parameters,[24] such as gene and protein expression signatures, neoantigens, MSI status, and immune status, is likely required to more accurately select patients who will benefit from immunotherapy.

Table 44.1 Biomarker Assays and Common Applications for Host, Tumor, and Immune Profiling

OMIC	TYPE	TECHNOLOGY	APPLICATION	MATRIX
Genomics: the analysis of genome using DNA sequencing technologies	Whole-exome/genome sequencing (WES/WGS)	NGS	Genome-wide mutational analysis including TMB, SNV, CNV, LOH, and TCR	Tumor and normal (tumor-adjacent tissue or blood)
	Targeted gene sequencing	Sanger sequencing; NGS	Targeted mutational analysis including TMB, SNV, CNV, LOH, and TCR	Tumor and normal (tumor-adjacent tissue or blood)
	ctDNA	PCR, NGS	Tumor mutational analysis	Plasma
Transcriptomics: the analysis of mRNA expression	RNA-Seq	NGS	Genome-wide differential gene expression	Tumor, PBMC
	Targeted panels	IO$_3$60 (Nanostring) Microarrays	Differential expression of select genes	Tumor, TIL, PBMC
	Single-cell transcriptomics	DropSeq, SMARTSeq, 10x Genomics	Droplet-based single-cell sequencing for cell-subset analysis; rare cell identification; subset-specific signature analysis	Tumor, TIL, PBMC
	TCR-Seq (bulk)	PCR, NGS	Clonal expansion analysis, differential clone analysis, repertoire overlap	Tumor, TIL, PBMC
	Single-cell transcriptomics + TCR	10x Genomics	Subset-specific clone tracing; subset-specific clonal expansion	Tumor, TIL, PBMC
	Spatial transcriptomics	10x Genomics, ReadCoor, Digital Spatial Profiling (Nanostring)	Spatially embedded cell-subset identification and signature analysis	Tumor
Epigenomics: the analysis of modifications on DNA or histones or accessible DNA that alters gene expression without changing the DNA sequence	DNA methylation	MS; Bisulfate whole genome sequencing; other NGS methods	Cytosine methylation across the genome or for a targeted panel within particular regulatory regions or genes	PBMC, cfDNA, tumor
	ChIP-Seq	NGS	Analysis of histone modifications and chromatin accessibility by chromatin immunoprecipitation (ChIP)	Tumor, TIL, PBMC
	ATAC-Seq	NGS	Chromatin accessibility across the genome, including in enhancer regions	Tumor, TIL
	Single-cell ATAC-Seq	10x Genomics	Chromatin accessibility of single cells; enable cell-subset identification and epigenomic regulation analysis	Tumor, TIL
Proteomics: the analysis of protein abundance	Unbiased deep profiling	MS	Genome-wide differential protein expression	Plasma, serum, tumor
	Glycoproteomics	MS	Post-translational modifications of glycans on proteins	Plasma, serum, tumor
	Immunoassays: ELISA type targeted panels (1-1000s)	ELISA, Luminex, PEA, aptamer-based	Differential protein abundance analysis	Plasma, serum, tumor

(continued)

Table 44.1 Biomarker Assays and Common Applications for Host, Tumor and Immune Profiling (*continued*)

OMIC	TYPE	TECHNOLOGY	APPLICATION	MATRIX
	Cellular immunoassays	CyTOF, flow cytometry	Differential protein abundance and immune cell phenotyping	Blood, TIL, tumor
	Immunohistochemistry Targeted panels (1-9 antibodies)	Chromogenic or fluorescence-based IHC	Differential protein abundance and tumor and immune cell phenotyping; spatial-regional characterization	Tumor
	High-dimensional spatial proteomics (10–100 antibodies)	MIBI, CODEX, IMC, DSP	High-dimensional imaging enabling spatial and regional tumor and immune cell phenotyping	Tumor
Bacteriomic: the analysis of types and amount of bacteria	Bacteria RNA or DNA sequencing	16S sequencing	Identifies bacteria at the taxonomic resolution and poor resolution at the species level	Stool, tumor
	Bacteria deep DNA sequencing	Whole metagenomic shotgun (WMS) sequencing	Identifies bacteria at the level of species and strain	Stool, tumor
Metabolomic: the analysis of small molecule substrates or intermediates that are products of cellular metabolism	Metabolite/small molecule	MS	Differential cellular metabolite abundance profiling	Stool, blood, tumor

ATAC-Seq, assay for transposase-accessible chromatin with high-throughput sequencing; ChiP-Seq, chromatin immunoprecipitation with high-throughput sequencing; CNV, copy number variant; CODEX, co-detection by indexing; ctDNA, circulating tumor DNA; CyTOF, mass cytometry time of flight; DSP, digital spatial profiling; ELISA, enzyme-linked immunosorbent assay; IHC, immunohistochemistry; IMC, imaging mass cytometry; LOH, loss of heterozygosity; MIBI, multiplex ion beam imaging; MS, mass spectrometry; PBMC, peripheral blood mononuclear cell; PEA, proximity extension assay; PCR, polymerase chain reaction; Seq, high-throughput sequencing; SMARTSeq, Switching Mechanism at s' End of RNA Template with high-throughput sequencing; SNV, single nucleotide variant; TCR, T cell receptor; TIL, tumor-infiltrating lymphocytes; TMB, tumor mutational burden; WES, whole-exome sequencing; WGS, whole-genome sequencing; WMS, whole metagenomic sequencing.

Tumor Transcriptomics

Gene Expression Signatures

Cancer patients who benefit from current ICI treatments are characterized as having "hot" or "inflamed" tumors with infiltrating CD8 T cells, while those who fail to respond have tumors characterized as immune-excluded or immune-deserts with few to none CD8 T cells within the TME rendering them "cold" or "non-inflamed." T cell-inflamed TMEs have signatures of activated T cell markers, chemokines, active antigen presentation, and a type I interferon (IFN) transcriptional profile suggesting a preexisting adaptive immune response; conversely, non-inflamed TMEs reflect expression profiles indicative of an adaptive immune response that is peripherally suppressed.[9,10] Currently, there are no approved assays to evaluate whether tumors are hot or cold and thus more or less likely to be immunologically poised to respond to immune-modulating agents. What is needed to predict response is a holistic view of the landscape within inflamed versus non-inflamed tumors—a signature of response versus resistance that comprehensively accounts for all the factors that drive the cancer-immunity cycle (Figure 44.2).

The complex and dynamic interplay between infiltrating T cells and the TME has made validation of robust predictive signatures of response and resistance for clinical utility challenging. Single analyte biomarkers such as PD-L1 expression or total TMB have limitations as surrogates of tumor permissiveness to immune attack.

Gene expression signatures (GES) are potentially the richest source of qualitative and quantitative data about the immune response within the tumor. A GES is a single or a combined gene expression pattern of a group of genes with validated specificity in terms of diagnosis, prognosis, or prediction of therapeutic response. Traditional methods of GES analysis used reverse transcription polymerase chain reaction (RT-PCR), which measures one gene at time, or microarray technology and RNA sequencing, which multiplex the expression profiling across many thousands of transcripts.[34] These technologies, while relatively high-throughput and easy to deploy, are somewhat intolerant to low-quality RNA samples such as those from FFPE, the typical matrix of clinical specimens. The nCounter platform from Nanostring Technologies (Seattle, WA) is an automated system that requires only small quantities (as little as 25 ng) of FFPE-derived RNA to generate a rich set of transcript information. Fluorescently labeled molecular barcodes hybridize directly to specific nucleic acid sequences, and each color-coded optical barcode is attached to a single target-specific hybridization probe corresponding to a gene of interest, allowing for the unamplified measurement of up to 800 targets within a single sample.[35] Merck, in collaboration with Nanostring Technologies, developed an nCounter assay to determine if quantifying the T cell-inflamed microenvironment pretreatment would be a useful pan-tumor signature of response to PD-1 therapy. The tumor inflammation signature (TIS) is an 18-gene signature that contains IFN-γ responsive genes related to antigen presentation, chemokine expression, cytotoxic activity, and adaptive immune resistance, features necessary but not always sufficient for clinical benefit from PD-1 blockade. The predictive value of the TIS was initially established in melanoma tumors and later independently confirmed in eight additional tumor types all treated with pembrolizumab.[36] Consistent with prior evidence, tumors with clinical response to PD-1 treatment had higher average TIS scores, a finding confirmed when the TIS algorithm was applied to more than 9,000 gene expression profiles from the TCGA database,[37] and when evaluated for its ability to predict response to immunotherapy in routine clinical settings. In a cohort consisting of melanoma, lung, RCC, urothelial carcinoma, and colon cancer, patients whose tumors had high TIS scores had better overall survival compared to patients whose tumor had lower TIS scores (hazard ratio = 0.37, 95% CI [0.18, 0.76], $p = 0.005$).[38]

The TIS is a gene expression signature derived from the larger Nanostring PanCancer IO360 gene CodeSet, which is a 770-plex panel designed for profiling tumor biopsies and characterizing gene expression patterns associated with the tumor, the immune response, and the microenvironment. The panel contains key driver genes, as well as genes, that contribute to tumor growth and invasiveness, angiogenesis, epithelial to mesenchymal transition, and extracellular matrix remodeling and metastasis. Assays such as the IO360 panel, which measures and integrates multiple transcripts across the biology of the tumor and of the host immune system, provide vast amounts of data for defining treatment approaches. Undoubtedly, more GES panels will be developed on the nCounter and other multiplex platforms as companies develop predictive biomarkers in conjunction with their checkpoint inhibitor programs.

Tumor Imaging

The ability to profile the tumor architecture, characterize immune cell infiltrates, and determine the cellular distribution and spatial relationships within the tissue microenvironment historically has been plagued by a lack of reagents and technologies that can detect, visualize,

and discriminate multiple features simultaneously. The choice of a tissue imaging platform for a given application is dictated by many factors, not the least of which is the quantity and quality of the tissue specimen under survey. Beyond potential limitations of the tissue itself, additional confounders include marker expression abundance, sensitivity, and specificity of the detecting reagent, and the hardware and software required to generate and segment the positive signals at a single cell or subcellular resolution. Recent advances in immunolabeling and multispectral imaging have enabled multiplexing of features within a single formalin-fixed paraffin-embedded tissue section with accurate cell discrimination and spatial information. Several platforms are commercially available or under development to visualize an ever-increasing number of cellular markers. As these are emerging technologies with limited applications published in the literature, we provide a brief description of the methods of each to highlight key technical differences and potential advantages and disadvantages. Common to most of the imaging technologies, segmentation to extract individual cellular features remains a challenge; while several groups work toward automated solutions for this process, manual curation and quality control of images remain a necessary part of the workflow.

Multiplex Immunohistochemistry

Multiplex IHC has been a mainstay of pathology facilities for immuno-oncology applications due to its ease of use, relatively inexpensive price point, and ability to visualize, analyze, and quantify phenotypes of immune cells in situ in solid tumors. Over the last decade, technologies like the Vectra automated multiplex IHC system (developed by Perkin-Elmer and acquired by Akoya Biosciences, Menlo Park, CA) have supplanted classical IHC, which relies on detecting one or two targets at a time, to enable multiple biomarkers to be detected simultaneously within complex tissues such as the TME. The first-generation Vectra system (the Vectra 3) can image up to seven protein markers and obtain per-cell and per-cell-compartment multiparameter data across multiple fields of views within FFPE tissue sections with 1 mm/pixel resolution at 10x magnification. The next generation Vectra system (the Polaris) advanced the platform to nine-color detection and whole slide imaging with comparable resolution to the Vectra 3. With both systems, biomarker panels can be constructed to detect individual markers for proliferation (Ki67), apoptosis (DAPI), and specific tumor proteins, immune cell populations (CD8 T cells, regulatory T cells (T_{reg} cells), B cells, NK cells, monocytes, dendritic cells, etc.), markers of immune suppression (PD-1, PDL-1, IDO, etc.), and markers indicative of cellular function (e.g., granzyme B). Typically, one channel is reserved for cytokeratin or vimentin staining, to distinguish epithelial from mesenchymal differentiation. Inevitably, the desired number of markers to address systems biology and tumor immunobiology questions exceeds the technical limitations of the Vectra system, and higher dimensional imaging platforms are required.

High-Dimensional Imaging

Multiparametric imaging of tissue must contend with the limitation imposed by the overlap in fluorophores emission spectra. In recent years, in parallel with advances in technologies for the analysis of cell suspensions (see the text that follows), multiple technologies have been developed that circumvent this limitation, thus enabling high-dimensional imaging of tissue section at the cell and subcellular resolution.

Co-Detection by indEXing (Codex, Akoya Biosciences, Menlo Park, CA) enables imaging of 40+ cellular markers on a single tissue section. The technology relies on antibodies conjugated to unique indexing oligonucleotide barcodes, and complementary fluorophore-labeled detection oligonucleotides. The workflow starts by staining the tissue section with the entire antibody panel in a single step. The tissue is then imaged in a cyclic process in which the bound antibodies are detected by adding three detection oligonucleotides at a time, which bind to their complementary barcodes on the antibodies. The tissue is then imaged using a conventional fluorescence microscope; the detection oligonucleotides are removed with a gentle wash; and the cycle is repeated with the next three markers until all markers are revealed and imaged. The integrity of the tissue is preserved throughout the process, which allows for region of interest analysis downstream. Once all the individual images are acquired, the software assembles them in a final composite.

Using CODEX and computational algorithms for single-cell antigen quantification, Goltsev et al. conducted deep molecular profiling of mouse splenic architecture in a model of lupus and were able to differentiate pathological changes associated with the disease process relative to normal splenic tissue.[39] The CODEX technology is early in its adoption but holds promise in moving tissue imaging forward from conventional multiplex IHC methods that are limited in the number of markers that can be interrogated.

Imaging technologies based on time-of-flight mass spectrometry include Imaging Mass Cytometry (IMC)[40] and Multiplexed Ion Beam Imaging (MIBI).[41] Both technologies dispense with fluorophores altogether by labeling antibodies directly with isotopically pure rare-earth metal. The tissue is then rastered pixel by pixel with either a laser (IMC) or an ion beam (MIBI) to ionize the reporters, which are then quantified by time-of-flight mass spectrometry. This approach enables simultaneous imaging of 40+ markers because mass spectrometry does not suffer from the same issues with channel interference, which limits fluorescence-based detection. While both technologies are based on similar concepts, there are important differences in the instrumentation. Contrary to IMC, MIBI is nondestructive, because only a very thin layer of the tissue is ablated during rastering. Also, because of the way that the ion beam rasters the tissue, and because of the fact that the sample stage does not move, MIBI has superior resolution compared to IMC.

The power of these approaches was demonstrated in two recent studies in breast cancer,[42,43] suggesting that the organization of the tumor-immune microenvironment, including the size and composition of the immune infiltrate, the spatial relationships at the tumor-immune border, and the temporal expression of inhibitory molecules, such as PD-1, PD-L1, and IDO, are linked to survival. These early findings support the broader use of high-dimensional imaging in immuno oncology studies to inform approaches to stratify patients to treatments, identify those more likely to benefit, and inform sequencing of therapies given the tumor-immune context in first line versus subsequent lines of treatment.

The imaging technologies discussed up to now achieve cellular and subcellular resolution, similar to conventional IHC. Additionally, other approaches have been developed that can image areas as small as a few cells but afford greater multiplexing. Nanostring's GeoMx Digital Spatial (DSP) is one such technology, and it couples cellular morphology and phenotyping with gene expression profiling. The DSP imager can detect up to 96 proteins or transcripts within a single tissue sample (individual tissue sections or tissue microarrays). GeoMx DSP relies on the nCounter barcoding technology, which includes photocleavable oligonucleotide tags coupled to antibodies or RNA via a light-sensitive linker. FFPE tissue sections are stained with fluorescently labeled antibodies to allow the GeoMx to capture the image for morphologic context, and regions of interest are selected based on tissue morphology, phenotype, on an individual cell basis, or by gridding or contouring. The imaged fluorophore-conjugate is used to create a binary mask, and after incubation with a cocktail of tagged antibodies or RNA, a selected area of the tissue (as small as 5 μm) is exposed to UV light to decouple the tags from the antibody or nucleic acid. The oligonucleotides are retrieved without disturbing the surface of the tissue, thus allowing it to be reused. The retrieved oligonucleotides are deposited into microtiter plates for quantification.

As a biomarker discovery tool, Toki et al. used GeoMx DSP to identify predictive biomarkers of ICI response in melanoma.[44] Their 44-plex assay characterized the macrophage, lymphocyte, and melanocyte compartments within the tissue, and identified 11 and 15 biomarkers that correlated with progression free survival (PFS) and overall survival (OS), respectively. The observed role of PD-L1 expression in macrophages in predicting relapse-free survival was consistent with two prior studies that used the GeoMx DSP. The first study investigated predictive biomarkers of melanoma response to adjuvant or neoadjuvant therapy with ipilimumab and nivolumab,[45] and the second study evaluated melanoma patients treated in the neoadjuvant setting with nivolumab alone or nivolumab in combination with ipilimumab.[46] The three studies found common roles for B2M, CD3, CD4, CD8A, PD-1, and PD-L1 in melanoma relapse-free survival following immunotherapy and pointed to several other potential biomarkers of response in the immune cell and tumor compartments that warrant further study.

Another powerful imaging technology with even greater multiplexing capability is spatial transcriptomics.[47] This approach is based on mounting the tissue on slides that are precoated with unique oligonucleotide barcodes, arrayed in a grid-like pattern. During library preparation, the RNA from the tissue is then tagged with the barcodes, which are unique for each grid point and encode the positional information. When the library is sequenced, it is possible to computationally create a synthetic image that encodes transcript abundance at each spot on the grid, and which can be overlaid on an optical image of the tissue if desired.

One important practical consideration, particularly for clinical studies, is that CODEX, MIBI, and spatial transcriptomics all require mounting the tissue on assay-specific slides. Therefore, access to the original FFPE blocks, as opposed to precut sections mounted on regular slides, is necessary to run these assays.

MINIMALLY INVASIVE BIOMARKERS

Tumor tissue biomarker analysis has resulted in several important insights and advances in precision medicine. However, there are several limitations with tumor tissue as a source for biomarker discovery for immunotherapy due to the invasive nature of tumor biopsies. The common adage "tissue is the issue" reflects a major constraint assessing a tumor at multiple time points; additionally, the quantity of tumor tissue available in a biopsy is often limiting: small core biopsies may not provide sufficient quantities for two, let alone more, multiplex platforms. Assays may require different tissue preparations, and biopsy of a single lesion may not capture tumor temporal and spatial heterogeneity as clonal differences often occur within and/or across metastatic sites.[48] Minimally invasive biomarkers, such as blood and stool have several advantages, including reduced risk and cost to the patient for sampling, the ability to assess longitudinal samples (before and at several time points on treatment including at the time of progression), and the ability to evaluate multiple analytes with a variety of different

collection tubes (Figure 44.3). Blood offers the ability to evaluate several important host, immune, and tumor factors for baseline characteristics, and, importantly, provides longitudinal assessment, which may enable discovery of biomarkers of response, as well as the ability to assess the development of treatment resistance as well.[49] Additionally, longitudinal sampling enables the normalization of measurements by baseline values, thus addressing the issue of patient heterogeneity.

Using peripheral blood mononuclear cells (PBMCs), serum, and/or plasma as a source for assessing host genetics and metabolomics may gather information regarding health and disease states. Additionally, PBMCs are readily available to characterize the circulating immune state, including the number, frequency, and activity of specific immune cell subsets at baseline and in response to treatment.[50] Liquid biopsy technologies are establishing blood as a source for tumor-derived information that can be analyzed at the cellular, genomic, and transcriptomic level.[49] The microbiome has emerged with increasing importance in influencing health, disease, and immune states and, moreover, favorable fecal microbiome signatures have association with increased T cell infiltration in the tumor.[11-13] This chapter will limit its discussion of minimally invasive multi-omic biomarker assays for blood and stool but acknowledges the fact that molecular and functional imaging with positron emission tomography (PET) and magnetic resonance imaging (MRI) allow repeated non-invasive whole-body measurement of molecular features of the TME, including novel PET tracers to detect PD-L1[51] or CD8 cells,[52,53] and clinical studies are being performed to evaluate if these may be informative in defining who to treat with or evaluating response to immunotherapy therapy (see Chapter 48 on metabolic imaging). Recent advances in biomarker technologies to evaluate multiple analytes with improved sensitivity are resulting in a plethora of research reports on new biomarkers for immunotherapy treatment. Integrating multiple tests may define algorithms for informing immunotherapy treatment. Minimally invasive approaches can rapidly collect and assess different biomarkers and may enable multi-omic tests not only for patient selection but also for guiding clinical management, which is particularly important for immunotherapy treatments since radiographic response assessments may be misleading due to delayed response, pseudo-progression, or prolonged stable disease.[54,55]

Immune Profiling Assays

Cellular Immune Assays

The function of the immune system depends on the complex interplay of a multitude of different cell types, and

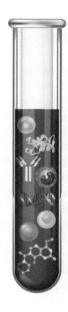

Biomarker assay	Matrix	Tube type
Immunophenotyping	PBMC	EDTA, CPT
Growth factors and other soluble mediators (e.g., antibodies)	Serum, plasma, and platelet poor plasma	Serum separator tube, EDTA, CPT
Cytokine and chemokines	Serum, plasma	Serum separator tube, EDTA, CPT
Circulating tumor cell	Whole blood	Cell save preservation tube[1]
MDSC	Whole blood	EDTA, CPT, Cyto-Chex BCT
Circulating tumor DNA	Plasma	Cell-free DNA BCP[1]
Cell metabolomics	Plasma, stool	Metabolite specific
Microbiome (16S/WMS)	Stool	OMNIGene GUT[2]

[1]Streck Laboratories, Omaha, NE
[2]DNA Genotek, Ottawa Ontario Canada

Figure 44.3 **Minimally invasive blood and stool biomarker sample collections**. Blood and stool samples are readily accessible for longitudinal biomarker assessment (baseline and on treatment) and have a wide variety of analytes that can be evaluated including PBMCs, protein factors (growth, angiogenic, and coagulation factors; cytokines; chemokines; and antibodies), circulating tumor cells, DNA (circulating tumor DNA or bacteria nucleic acids), and metabolites (e.g., short-chain fatty acids and butyrate). Preanalytical variables that can influence biomarker analysis include the matrix (e.g., serum versus plasma), type of tube used (e.g., EDTA chelates divalent metal cations that may affect certain proteins versus CPT tubes that often contain heparin), and sample processing methods. Each tube type has advantages and disadvantages depending on the biomarker of interest (e.g., while plasma can be used to evaluate proteins and circulating tumor DNA, it is preferred to use a nucleic acid stabilizing tube for circulating tumor DNA detection. Additionally, for microbiome analysis a DNA stabilizing tube is used for stool collection, but metabolite analysis generally requires stool samples in a different tube type). For biomarker discovery, baseline samples are essential; thus, it is recommended to maximize the amount of sample collected. It is advised to collect baseline samples at two different times not only to maximize the amount of sample available but also to mitigate from having any missing samples that would prevent evaluating before treatment (baseline) biomarker characteristics (e.g., collect at screening and before drug treatment on cycle 1 day 1).

BCT, blood collection tube; CPT, cell preparation tube; EDTA, ethane-1,2-diyldinitrilo tetraacetic acid; MDSC, myeloid-derived suppressor cell; PBMC, peripheral blood mononuclear cell; 16S, stands for 16S ribosomal ribonucleic acid (rRNA) sequencing; WMS, whole metagenomic sequencing.

as such single-cell analysis has long been the approach of choice in immunology. Accordingly, flow cytometry has been a mainstay of basic research in immunology for several decades. However, the number of parameters that can be simultaneously measured is limited by the breadth of available fluorophores and by the overlap in their emission spectra. In recent years, due to the development of new fluorophores that access a larger portion of the spectrum, as well as new instrumentation with increased number of lasers and filters that takes advantage of such fluorophores, the number of parameters that can be measured in a single experiment has increased to ~30.[56] Other advancements in the field include the development of spectral instruments that automatically deconvolve overlapping spectra, thus facilitating the

design of complex panels.[57] To circumvent the issues associated with fluorescence, mass cytometry employs isotopically pure rare earth metals for antibody labeling, which are then measured through time-of-flight mass spectrometry, thus enabling the routine measurement of more than 40 markers in individual cells with minimal interference.[58] The commercial Helios mass cytometry instrument (Fluidigm Inc, South San Francisco, CA, USA) can theoretically measure 135 channels, with the main limitation being the chemistry required for antibody labeling.

Panels for cytometry analysis can be designed for either "broad," that is, covering all major cell types, or "deep," that is focusing on specific subsets in cell types of interest, such as immunophenotyping. Even with the increased number of markers made possible by modern technologies, panel design still requires considerable care, as invariably the number of available slots limits the precision with which different cell subsets can be delineated.

One significant advantage of mass cytometry versus conventional flow cytometry is that the minimal interference between the measurement channels facilitates the design of modular panels, where a core set of markers can be complemented with specific drop-ins for individual studies.[50] Such a setup is more difficult to achieve with fluorescence-based flow cytometry because panel design needs to carefully take into account the overlap between fluorophores and how that relates to the co-expression of markers in individual cells.

Having a common core panel is necessary to integrate data across studies, a task that has traditionally been difficult because of the limited overlap between conventional flow cytometry panels, where fewer channels are available for measurement.[59] Another factor important to consider in panel design is whether the drug treatment interferes with antibody binding (e.g., nivolumab competing for binding with the antibody used to measure PD-1). Flow and mass cytometry have also been adapted for the simultaneous measurement of a panel of mRNA and proteins in single cells.[60,61]

Single-Cell Sequencing

Single-cell transcriptomics using RNA-Seq is an alternative profiling modality with complementary characteristics to cytometry. Initial approaches were based on physical separation of individual cells through either FACS sorting or microfluidic chips. While these methods are more sensitive, that is, they detect more genes per cell, they are limited to analyzing hundreds or thousands of cells per experiment and have been mostly supplanted by droplet-based cell barcoding approaches, such as those marketed by 10X Genomics, which can be used to measure tens of thousands of cells per experiment, albeit with a lower sensitivity due to limitations in RNA capture efficiency.[62,63]

Besides the advantages in cell throughput, droplet-based cell barcoding provides a powerful platform that can be leveraged for different types of analysis, including protein detection (through the use of oligo-tagged antibodies),[64] TCR and BCR repertoire sequencing, and measurement of accessible chromatin (ATAC-seq).[65]

It is important to note that the choice between cytometry versus sequencing-based assays involves a trade-off between the number of parameters and the number of cells that can be analyzed. While with flow or mass cytometry, millions of cells per sample can be analyzed in a single experiment (the only real limit being the amount of sample), the number of parameters is limited to 40+. Conversely, single-cell sequencing has the potential to measure thousands of parameters in individual cells, but the number of cells that can be analyzed per sample is limited to tens of thousands.

This is an important consideration when profiling PBMC to identify biomarkers in immunotherapy because of the fundamental question of how many cells is necessary to measure in order to reliably analyze the tumor-reactive cells, which are expected to represent only a small fraction of the total. While recent papers[66–68] have shed light on the role of the systemic versus peripheral response and highlighted the importance of taking the former into account, this remains an open question in the field. These limitations notwithstanding, single-cell TCR sequencing of both TIL and PBMC from the same patient[66,68] has demonstrated that tumor-reactive clones can be measured in the periphery with these approaches. Peripheral biomarkers of response to various immunotherapy-containing regimens that have been reported in the literature include reinvigoration of circulating CD8 T cells with an exhausted phenotype,[69] an increase in the proportion of CD27+FAS- central memory CD4+ T cells[70], the frequency of CD14+CD16-HLA-DRhi monocytes before the start of therapy,[71] higher levels of IL-2-producing CD8 T cells and central memory CD8 T cells,[72] a complex signature that includes the abundance of MDSC-derived suppressor cells and activated NK cells,[73] lower abundance of MDSC,[74,75] and the proportion of Th9 cells.[76] In a recent study that combined several high-dimensional assay technologies, peripheral T cell turnover, and the expansion of a specific subset of CD45RA-CD45ROhiCD27-CCR7- CD8 effector cells was found to be associated with response to checkpoint inhibition in melanoma.[77]

Critical questions remain around how these different signatures vary when CTLA-4 and PD-(L)1 targeting agents are used in combination with other therapeutic modalities and how they differ across indications.

Circulating Proteomics With Targeted Panels

Proteins regulate biological processes and enter the circulation in response to cell activation, damage, stress, or death, including angiogenic, coagulation, and growth factors, hormones, and cytokines. Clinical laboratory tests for blood proteins are commonly used as indicators of health status for liver, kidney, and cardiac function. Circulating tumor markers such as PSA, CA19-9, and CEA are used to monitor tumor burden and several markers have been validated as clinical biomarkers of disease response, including M protein for multiple myeloma[78] and CA-125 for ovarian cancer.[79] Cytokines play a critical role in regulating the immune system, as well as tumor and immune cells, and cells from the TME regulate cytokine production. These proteins may be biomarkers for understanding immune state and response to immunotherapy treatment. Cytokines are small proteins that generally act locally and are known by many different names including lymphokines, monokines, chemokines, interleukins (IL), interferons (IFN), and colony-stimulating factors.[80] Cytokines can cause activation or dampening of an immune response, and when overactivated can result in cytokine release syndrome that in the most severe cases results in death.[81]

Proteomics is the identification and quantification of the proteins in a biological sample. Blood-based proteomics have been hindered by the concern that blood as a surrogate tissue does not reflect the tumor state and due to technologic limitations compared to genomic methods to provide the sensitivity and dynamic range to robustly quantitate the proteome. Proteins consist of 20 amino acids in contrast to four nucleotides, have high complexity due in part to a variety of post-translational modifications, and lack the ability for amplification, so sensitivity of detection is more challenging than with genetic material. Proteomic analysis of serum or plasma often involves bead-based multiplex Luminex platform immunoassays, aptamer-based assays, or unbiased mass spectrometry. Protein arrays for auto- and tumor-reactive antibodies are also evaluated in serum for immunotherapy treatment but will not be discussed in this review.[82,83] Recent biomarker technology advances hold promise for this accessible biomarker that is a key regulator of health and disease.

Quantitative Multiplex Immunoassays for Serum or Plasma Proteins

Multiplex platforms used for quantitative protein evaluation are similar to ELISA immunoassays sandwiching analytes between a capture and a detection antibody. Luminex technology is commonly used by academic research centers and multiple technology companies (Myriad RBM, Millipore, Bio-Rad) and utilizes a magnetic or polystyrene bead-based technology that can detect dozens or hundreds of proteins[84] in a single sample using fluorophore-labeled antibodies and beads. These multiplex immunoassays can provide valuable data but have several limitations.[85] They utilize high-affinity reagents that are used to detect proteins within a range of concentrations in a complex matrix. Specificity and cross-reactivity issues can arise due to the reagents, as well as the level of abundance of the target protein and the complexity of the sample being analyzed. Additionally, secretion of factors from tumors into the blood may be expected to be at low levels and, thus, may not be detected. Given the wide array of modifications that can influence protein detection including protein–protein binding and post-translational modifications, the concordance between assays for a given target protein is low.[84,86] Additionally, the dynamic range and limits of detection of these assays can be limiting, and many

values are calculated based on extrapolation. Newer approaches including SOMAscan® using SOMAmer (Slow Off-rate Modified Aptamer)-based capture systems, which improve sensitivity in protein binding and increase the ability to multiplex, enable the capture of thousands of target proteins (www.somalogic.com). The single molecular array (SIMOA) technology improves detection sensitivity of the level of target proteins 1,000 times by trapping single molecules in femtoliter-sized wells and using digital readouts,[87] and the Proximity Extension Assay (PEA) technology improves sensitivity and ability to multiplex to the thousands of target proteins with a homogeneous assay that uses antibody pairs tagged with DNA reporter molecules that can be quantified by high-throughput real-time PCR.[88] While there are limitations with these immunoassays and knowing which assay is "the standard of truth" for a given protein is challenging, biomarker discoveries reporting circulating protein signatures that can classify health versus a range of diseases and also identify different lifestyle behaviors, such as smoking and amount of physical activity, have been reported.[89] Additionally, Lim et al. have reported the discovery of an 11-plex protein signature derived from a 65-plex Luminex panel that may predict immune-related adverse events in response to ICI treatment.[90]

Unbiased Proteomics in Serum or Plasma

Mass spectrometry (MS) is an unbiased and quantitative approach for proteomics that can overcome some of the limitations of immunoassays. MS can also be used for metabolomics in blood, but that application will be discussed in the text that follows with the biomarker assays for stool samples. MS typically analyzes a sample such as serum or plasma for proteins by protease digestion, usually trypsin, which can occur after an enrichment or fractionation step to rid the sample of high-abundance proteins. The digested peptides are then concentrated and separated on high-performance liquid chromatography, ionized, and assessed by MS. This gives quantitative information about the proteins present in the sample at the sequence level and may also provide information on post-translational modifications. However, there are several limitations that need to be appreciated including detection of only charged proteins, differential ionization, detection favoring high-abundance proteins, and the fact that the use of depletion steps to reduce abundant proteins may deplete lower abundance proteins, and variability exists in computational methods in reporting the target proteins.[91] Targeted proteomics such as multiple reaction monitoring (MRM), hyper-reaction monitoring (HRM) using label-free analysis, and machine learning-based approaches are improving MS sensitivity.[92,93] Improvements in deep learning tools improve reproducibility and the confidence in protein identifications, as well as automating generation of spectral libraries for data-independent acquisition (DIA).[91] Other novel approaches to MS proteomics are being reported, including an automated multinanoparticle platform, Proteograph, that is reported to identify low-abundance proteins and protein-protein interactions with improved sample processing time.[94] Post-translational modifications are another dimension of information on the proteome and the role of carbohydrate modifications by the addition of short sugar chains called glycans. Glycans play a major role in regulating protein folding, signaling, and numerous cellular functions. Aberrant patterns in protein glycosylation have been associated with immune function, inflammation, autoimmunity, and cancer.[95,96] Advances in machine learning and artificial intelligence algorithms with MS technology have improved the ability to assess patterns of glycans on proteins and may be referred to as the glycome.[97] Clinical trials evaluating the utility of this approach as a test for the diagnosis of ovarian cancer are currently ongoing (ClinicalTrials.gov NCT03837327).[98] As advances in these technologies and the computational methods to analyze the data improve, it warrants further exploration in precision immunotherapy biomarker discovery approaches.[99,100]

Liquid Biopsies

Diagnostic technological advances have enabled minimally invasive liquid biopsies as an exciting advancement in the field of precision medicine for oncology. In 2016 the FDA approved the first liquid biopsy test for the detection of EGFR gene mutations for lung cancer patients.[101] For ICI therapies, blood TMB (bTMB) is an area of active research to determine clinical utility for a progress in advancing precision immunotherapy.[7,102] The term "liquid biopsy" in oncology refers to the ability to analyze tumor-derived information at the cellular, genomic, and transcriptomic level and generally refers to the measurement of circulating tumor cells (CTC), circulating tumor DNA (ctDNA), and exosomes, from readily accessible samples such as blood, urine, and saliva. Liquid biopsy biomarker technologies hold an exciting potential in the diagnosis and treatment of cancer, including early screening and diagnosis, patient selection, and monitoring drug treatment for response and resistance.[49] For the purposes of this review, we will focus on the biomarker technologies to analyze ctDNA in blood and the relationship to immunotherapy treatment.

Circulating Tumor DNA (ctDNA)

Somatic genetic alterations in tumors such as mutations and amplifications are tumor-specific and can be detected in the blood of some cancer patients due to tumor cell shedding and death. Cell-free DNA (cfDNA), including tumor-derived ctDNA, is released into blood and other body fluids when cells die or through secretion. The overall abundance of ctDNA is generally low and reported to be less than 10% of the total cfDNA.[103] Disease characteristics affect the levels of ctDNA including tumor burden, histology, and treatment history. Thus, sensitive methods are required to detect the genetic alterations in ctDNA, and detection is influenced by the amount of total plasma cfDNA, the fraction of ctDNA in cfDNA, and the robustness of the assay.[104] Advances in the sequencing methods and the preanalytical plasma collection[105] are improving the ability to utilize this assay. Direct assessment of specific tumor mutations, such as EGFR or KRAS mutations, may have limited utility for predicting immunotherapy therapy treatment selection. However, longitudinal assessment of ctDNA for these disease-specific biomarkers may serve as a surrogate marker for antitumor activity and inform clinical benefit and the emergence of resistance and tumor progression.[104] TMB is under evaluation as a predictive biomarker for ICI treatment and has recently demonstrated clinical utility for pembrolizumab (ICI) monotherapy for the treatment of adult and pediatric patients with unresectable or metastatic solid tumors with TMB–high status (TMB-H; ≥ 10 mutations/mb; Keynote 158, NCT02628067).[106,107] A number of diagnostic companies (Grail, Foundation One, etc.) and academic centers have developed NGS-based bTMB assays. Gandara et al.[102] demonstrated using samples from two clinical studies of NSCLC that bTMB and tumor TMB positively correlated. An additional retrospective analysis bTMB has shown positive predictive value for ICI treatment of lung cancer patients.[108]

While the results are encouraging, TMB tests in blood and tissue are evolving and ctDNA test detection methods need further development in analytical and clinical validation and demonstration of clinical utility.[109] Continued advancement in the test methods and incorporating bTMB with other omic biomarkers may demonstrate improved clinical utility.[24]

Circulating Tumor DNA (ctDNA) With Other Omics

Evaluating ctDNA and other omic assays as a multiparameter liquid biopsy test with machine learning-based approaches is emerging with some early encouraging data. Others have utilized DNA sequencing of cfDNA coupled with analysis of DNA length and abundance to derive epigenetic information. If DNA is not actively transcribed, it is generally bound to nucleosomes and thus protected from degradation. The probability of gene activation and transcription factor activity can be inferred using machine learning approaches.[110] Vallania et al. recently reported the use of a composite assay evaluating cfDNA for the tumor fraction, estimated cell proportions, and transcriptional factor activity, by measuring both tumor- and non-tumor-derived biomarkers at baseline and on treatment. The study found associations with ICI treatment response (NCT02866149).[111] Using deconvolution methods of cfDNA fragmentation patterns, immune cell proportions were quantitated, and transcription factor activity was assessed by determining binding site accessibility across the genome and normalizing it to the ctDNA fraction. Baseline and on-treatment plasma samples from 30 NSCLC patients treated with ICI were evaluated and a decrease in immune-related transcription factor binding site accessibility at baseline and on treatment was associated with tumor response. Furthermore, a lower level of cfDNA compared to baseline and higher levels of the cellular proportion of monocytes in the plasma samples collected after ICI treatment were significantly associated with clinical benefit.[111] Additional approaches looking at cfDNA with other factors include the CancerSEEK blood test that is evaluating cfDNA and proteins as a diagnostic test.[112] Another approach to using cfDNA for predictive immunotherapy is using epigenomics and evaluating genome-wide DNA hydroxymethylation. Guler et al. analyzed longitudinal plasma samples from 19 NSCLC patients treated with ICI for hydroxymethylcytosine DNA signatures. Differential signatures in 5′ UTR and promoter regions of genes involved in tumorigenesis were observed in responders and nonresponders.[113] These reports support further evaluation of these minimally invasive longitudinal tests to guide clinical management of cancer patients with immunotherapy treatment.

STOOL-BASED BIOMARKER ASSAYS

Gut Microbiome Profiling

The microbiome is the collection of microbes—bacteria, viruses, and fungi—that live on and in the human body. The composition of the gut microbiome has received scientific attention due to its correlation with various disease processes. Our understanding of the bacterial component of the gut microbiome, in particular, has been advanced in the last decade due to the use of NGS to elucidate the complex and variable ecology of commensal species and pathobionts (commensal species that, under certain circumstances, can play a role in disease). The gut microbiome is thought to play a role in health in the following broad ways: promoting resistance to colonization and infection by pathogenic bacteria, educating and regulating the immune system, maintaining gut epithelial barrier integrity, modulating host metabolism, and potentially altering the function of the central nervous system.[114] The link between gut microbiota composition and immune state has prompted an evaluation in cancer, and particularly in regard to treatment with immunotherapy such as ICI (NCT03353402, NCT03341143, NCT03637803).[115–117]

Loss of microbial diversity (dysbiosis) is common in patients with cancer[118] and is also associated with poor prognosis. In animal models and studies in human cohorts, bacterial genera such as *Bacteroides*, *Clostridium*, and *Faecalibacterium* have been reported to modulate antitumor immunity via expansion of T_{reg} cells, activation of dendritic cells, or secretion of anti-inflammatory cytokines.[11–13] Furthermore, the relative abundance of *Akkermansia muciniphila* in patient stool samples prior to ICI initiation correlated with clinical response to PD-1 blockade.[11] Oral supplementation with this bacterium following fecal microbiota transplantation with feces from cancer patients who responded to ICI into germ-free or antibiotic-treated mice improved the PD-1 effect through IL-12 mediated immune mechanisms that promoted CD4T cell infiltration into the tumor bed.

The microbiome of metastatic melanoma patients prior to treatment with PD-1 therapy has been studied, and a recent publication demonstrated that the pre-treatment composition of the fecal microbiome in patients who respond to PD-1 therapy has a distinct bacterial signature compared to patients who do not respond to PD-1 therapy.[13] Specifically, higher alpha-diversity (i.e., a higher number of different species) and relative abundance of the bacterial genus *Faecalibacterium* (within the order *Clostridiales* and Family Ruminococcaceae) was associated with better treatment response and prolonged progression-free survival (PFS). Conversely, lower alpha-diversity and higher abundance of the bacterial order *Bacteriodales* were associated with lack of treatment response and shorter PFS. The bacterial signature in patients who achieved a response to PD-1 treatment was also associated with a more favorable tumor-immune profile in a subset of melanoma patients with available tumor samples. These data suggest that a gut microbiome signature may serve as a predictive biomarker of response to PD-1 therapy.

Microbiome analysis methods are rapidly advancing; considerations of experimental study design, data acquisition, incorporation of standards and controls, mapping sequencing data to reference genomes, and bioinformatic and statistical approaches have been extensively reviewed[119] and will not be discussed at length here. Several approaches for gut microbiome profiling are available, and the preferred application depends on, among other considerations, the desired taxonomic resolution (at the level of order, family, genus, species, or strain), whether functional diversity characterization of bacterial species is desired, and the cost per sample. Marker gene sequencing (such as 16S rRNA for bacteria and archaea) is the preferred method for high-level, but low-resolution analysis of microbial community composition at the genus level. The composition of the fecal microbiome is measured in terms of both the total number of unique types of bacteria (i.e., α-diversity) and the microbial composition (i.e., β-diversity). Genomic sequence read data sets are analyzed to assign a taxonomic identity at the resolution of an operational taxonomic unit (OTU) and, further, to define the proportion of each OTU relative to all other OTUs in a given sample. Differences between changes in the microbiome, for example, study intervention groups, pretreatment versus post-treatment, and normal versus disease state can be evaluated in terms of changes in α-diversity, β-diversity, and the prevalence and relative abundance of specific OTUs.

Marker gene sequencing is an inexpensive RT-PCR assay that works reasonably well for samples that are potentially contaminated with host DNA or are low-biomass; however, bias may be introduced in the latter due to preferential PCR amplification of DNA sequences with high-affinity primer binding sites, the amplicon size, and the number of PCR cycles, which can lead to an overrepresentation of contaminating organisms as the cycle number increases. For more detailed genomic information and taxonomic resolution, whole metagenomic sequencing (WMS) can be used to evaluate the total DNA in a sample. Depending on the sequencing depth (the number of sequencing reads per sample), taxonomic resolution at the species and strain level is possible,[120] and a profile of the functional diversity of the entire microbial community at the gene level is achievable, moving the depth of data far beyond the capacity of 16S marker gene sequencing.

Interpretation of WMS data must be performed within the broader context of the powerful influences of diet, antibiotic and probiotic usage, medications, physiology, lifestyle, and other factors that may transiently or temporally alter the gut microbiome composition and inadvertently ascribe observed changes as treatment effects. The ability to longitudinally capture these data points, along with relevant metadata, such as age, sex, ethnicity, disease state, treatment, viral status (e.g., EBV and CMV), and weight/BMI, impacts the quality of downstream microbiome data interpretation. Likewise, attention to stool sample collection and preservation techniques is important to prevent a skewing of the microbial populations due solely to sampling or handling pre-analytically.[121,122] Both marker gene sequencing and WMS can be performed from stool samples collected and preserved in tubes such as the OMNI-Gene Gut (DNA Genotek, now part of OraSure Technologies) with stability at room temperature for up to 60 days and longer-term stability for several months when stored frozen.[123]

Bacterial Metabolomics

Commensal bacteria have been shown to influence the generation of anti-inflammatory or pro-inflammatory responses within the intestine. Metabolic byproducts released through the fermentation of macromolecules influence the balance between T_{reg} cells, which express the transcription factor, Foxp3, and Th17 cells, which play a key role in host defense against extracellular pathogens by mediating the recruitment of neutrophils and macrophages to infected tissues and promoting B cell responses.[124,125] The molecular cues that shift the immune response from one of a pro-inflammatory state that can attack pathogenic invaders, to an anti-inflammatory state that dampens the response once the infection is cleared to prevent tissue damage, remain largely uncharacterized. Recent studies have shown that butyrate and propionate, short-chain fatty acids (SCFA) produced during the fermentation of partially and nondigestible polysaccharides, promote extrathymic generation of T_{reg} cells and de novo T_{reg} cell generation in the periphery, respectively.[126] As one of the major SCFA signaling mechanisms is the inhibition of histone deacetylases (HDACs), and HDACs regulate gene expression, propionate produced by commensal microorganisms could have far-reaching downstream effects and alter the way that the gut microbiome communicates with the immune system. The field of bacterial metabolomics and its role in response to immunotherapy is in its infancy, but methods to identify and quantify SCFA by HPLA and LC-MS are evolving quickly.[126]

METABOLOMICS

The TME is a harsh and inhospitable environment that immune cells must tolerate while they attempt to exert their antitumor effector functions. Cell migration and infiltration are metabolically demanding processes, and once immune cells successfully take up residence in the tumor bed, glucose and amino acids are critical substrates for effective activation and proliferation. Within the TME, competition for these resources favors tumor cells with their increased proliferative capacity and ability to commandeer the aerobic glycolysis pathway, the same metabolic pathway used to drive effector functions of immune cells. This nutrient deprivation is coupled with oxygen deprivation from insufficient blood perfusion, leading to a cascade of hypoxic effects that further set the tone for an immunosuppressive environment. We have only begun to dissect the role of the TME in antitumor-immune responses, but what is known suggests that a remodeling to reset the metabolic and hypoxic atmosphere within tumors may be required to unleash the immune system toward effective tumor cell killing.[127]

Over the last decade, several studies have provided insights into metabolism and lymphocyte function.[128,129] T cells use specific metabolic pathways during different phases of development that lead to their differentiation and functional capacity; therefore, metabolites may serve as important biomarkers of immune function and ability to respond to immunotherapy therapy. Naïve T cells exiting the thymus primarily use oxidative phosphorylation (OXPHOS) to drive their metabolism, while glycolytic metabolism is engaged once T cells are activated through ligation of the TCR and co-stimulatory receptors and stimulation with growth-inducing cytokines. Aerobic glycolysis, a process in which glucose is converted into lactate in the presence of oxygen, is less efficient than OXPHOS at yielding ATP per molecule of glucose, but it can generate metabolic intermediates important for cell growth and proliferation. However, while lactate is an effective substrate for tumor metabolism, elevated levels of lactate, like that found in the TME, suppress T cell and NK cell function, impair activation of their transcription factors and IFN-γ production, and decrease their cytolytic potential. Uptake of lactate by tumor-associated macrophages (TAMs) stimulates arginase-1 (Arg-1) production, which decreases the expression of the TCR CD3zeta chain and impairs T cell responses through hypoxia-inducible factor 1α, a metabolic checkpoint for the differentiation of Th17 and T_{reg} cells. Tumor-resident TAMs, MDSCs, and tolerizing DCs further suppress T cell expansion and antitumor activity by expressing enzymes that degrade essential amino acids such as indoleamine 2,3-dioxygenase (IDO), an enzyme involved in tryptophan metabolism. The net result is impairment of polyamine biosynthesis and reduced aerobic glycolysis by T cells, further shifting the balance toward cancer cell glucose utilization, more lactate release, and impaired T cell function.

As TILs acclimate in the TME, they lose their ability to respond to TCR stimuli, secrete cytokines, and proliferate in response to antigens, effectively entering a state of exhaustion or hyporesponsiveness. In this dysfunctional state, T cells fail to maintain bioenergetic requirements to sustain their effector functions and control tumor growth. Further, prolonged glucose and oxygen deprivation can upregulate expression of PD-1, CTLA-4, TIGIT, and LAG-3, checkpoints that inhibit T cell responsiveness to tumor antigen.[130]

Collectively, these findings support the development of cancer therapies directed at promoting a more favorable metabolic environment for immune cells to persist combined with immunotherapies to block inhibitory T cell receptors to potentiate their tumor cell killing activities. Indeed, clinical trials investigating inhibitors of IDO in combination with an anti-PD-1 antibody, for example, are underway (NCT03361228).[131] Methods to measure labile metabolites within the TME with techniques such as MS are evolving and adding to our understanding of the role of metabolism in directing antitumor-immune responses.

CONCLUSION

In the last decade, cancer immunotherapy, including the first FDA approval of an ICI in 2011 and cell and gene therapy in 2017,[3] has had a profound impact on some cancer patients. Given the complexities of tumor biology, the multitude of immune cells consisting of lymphocytes (B cells, T cells, and NK cells), myeloid cells (macrophages, dendritic cells, and monocytes), and host factors, including genotype and gut microbiome factors, defining who to treat with immunotherapy is going to require analysis of multiple cell types and assays beyond genomics. This is further complicated by the challenges associated with understanding temporal and spatial heterogeneity of tumors and the immune state. It is becoming apparent that understanding immunotherapy resistance by tumor intrinsic factors and immune and host-related defects will require a broad biomarker discovery approach using multi-omic technologies and patient samples that include tumor, blood, and stool (Figure 44.1). In this review, we summarize many of the current approaches using genomics, transcriptomics, epigenomics, proteomics, bacteriomics, and metabolomics (Table 44.1). There are several efforts by organizations to standardize immunotherapy biomarker methods, technologies, and data analysis including the Partnership for accelerating cancer therapies, accessible at https://fnih.org/what-we-do/programs/partnership-for-accelerating-cancer-therapies, which performs biomarker assays for NCI-funded trials, as has the Society for Immunotherapy of Cancer Immune Biomarkers Task Force[132] and the Parker Institute of Cancer Immunotherapy (PICI). These are important efforts to enable comparisons and learnings across clinical studies.

While there is enthusiasm for minimally invasive biomarkers from blood and stool, there are limitations to establish the biological association of peripheral markers and the tumor and immune tissue. There is still controversy regarding whether peripheral immune cells are informative for evaluating antitumor immunity as the TME plays a critical role, given that activated immune cells detected in the blood may be silenced at the disease site by tumor cells or by immunosuppressive cells such as MDSC, TAM, or T_{reg} cells.[3] Advances in multianalyte tests that use composite assays evaluating plasma for the tumor fraction, estimated cell proportions, epigenomics, and/or proteins by measuring both tumor- and nontumor-derived biomarkers[111,112] may hold promise. Kawaguchi et al. have recently reported using longitudinal PBMC, plasma, and serum samples from metastatic breast cancer patients treated with immunotherapy and analyzed with Cytof, RNA-Seq, and multiplex cytokine analysis, a systemic immune signature to identify patients who are likely to benefit from immunotherapy treatment (NCT03430479).[133]

Precision immunotherapy treatment may require some characterization of the tumor, given the influence of the TME on antitumor immunity. Several recent reports utilizing multiplatform biomarker analysis have reported important findings and are examples of multi-omic multiparameter biomarker discovery, shedding insights into immunotherapy treatment. Mitra et al. reported a remarkable study evaluating longitudinal genomic and immune analysis of tumor samples from a melanoma cancer patient who was treated with multiple therapies, including prolonged PD-1 therapy with progression.[48] This study featured deep longitudinal tumor and immune analyses of three metastatic lesions, including multiple subregions of one of the tumor samples, relationships between tumor genomics, copy number gain of chromosome 7, and unfavorable low T cell infiltrate, along with neutrophil activation. These biomarkers evaluating tumor genomics and T cell abundance and neutrophil activation in the TME should be further explored for the ability to predict treatment outcomes with immunotherapy therapy. Additionally, a long-term persistent T cell clonotype was identified that may inform new therapies such as tumor vaccines or TCR-based cell therapies.

Another example of the use of multi-omic multiparameter analysis of tumors that sheds insights into immunotherapy response was reported recently. Renal cell carcinoma (RCC) is characterized as an immunotherapy-responsive tumor despite having a low TMB. Braun et al. analyzed over 500 tumor samples from patients with RCC treated with PD-1 therapy with genomics, transcriptomics, and/or T cell (CD8) IHC analysis. Higher levels of CD8 T cells in tumors, which are usually associated with ICI response, were associated with chromosomal loss of 9p21.3 (associated with ICI resistance) and a low level of PBRM1 mutations (associated with ICI response). This integrated multi-omic biomarker analysis demonstrates the limitation of a single-omic approach, such as CD8 T cell infiltrate, to define tumors for ICI treatment, given the complex interaction between tumor, immune cells, and the TME. Biomarker discovery that can look at spatial-regional and spatial-temporal parameters will also be instructive given the dynamic nature of tumors and the immune system.[134]

Overall, recent and continued advances in biomarker technologies with broad profiling to enable deep molecular and cellular analysis of host tumor and immune states, paired with the ability to integrate tumor, blood, and stool biomarkers combining genomic, epigenomic, transcriptomic, proteomic, bacteriomic, and metabolomic multiplex approaches in clinical studies, should enable biomarker discovery and advance precision immunotherapy.

KEY REFERENCES

Only key references appear in the print edition. The full reference list appears in the digital product on Springer Publishing Connect: connect.springerpub.com/content/book/978-0-8261-3743-2/part/part03/chapter/ch44

24. Cristescu R, Mogg R, Ayers M, et al. Pan-tumor genomic biomarkers for PD-1 checkpoint blockade–based immunotherapy. *Science.* 2018;362(6411):eaar3593. doi:10.1126/science.aar3593

48. Mitra A, Andrews MC, Roh W, et al. Spatially resolved analyses link genomic and immune diversity and reveal unfavorable neutrophil activation in melanoma. *Nat Commun.* 2020;11(1):1839. doi:10.1038/s41467-020-15538-9

62. Papalexi E, Satija R. Single-cell RNA sequencing to explore immune cell heterogeneity. *Nat Rev Immunol.* 2018;18(1):35–45. doi:10.1038/nri.2017.76

77. Valpione S, Galvani E, Tweedy J, et al. Immune-awakening revealed by peripheral T cell dynamics after one cycle of immunotherapy. *Nat Cancer.* 2020;1(2):210–221. doi:10.1038/s43018-019-0022-x

111. Vallania F, Assayag K, Ulz P, et al. Plasma-derived cfDNA to reveal potential biomarkers of response prediction and monitoring in non-small cell lung cancer (NSCLC) patients on immunotherapy. *J Clin Oncol.* 2020;38(15 suppl):9588. doi:10.1200/JCO.2020.38.15_suppl.9588

132. Bedognetti D, Ceccarelli M, Galluzzi L, et al. Toward a comprehensive view of cancer immune responsiveness: a synopsis from the SITC workshop. *J Immunother Cancer.* 2019;7(1):131. doi:10.1186/s40425-019-0602-4

134. Braun DA, Hou Y, Bakouny Z, et al. Interplay of somatic alterations and immune infiltration modulates response to PD-1 blockade in advanced clear cell renal cell carcinoma. *Nat Med.* 2020;26:909–918. doi:10.1038/s41591-020-0839-y

45

Predictive Biomarkers (Programmed Death Ligand 1 Expression, Microsatellite Instability, and Tumor Mutational Burden) for Response to Immune Checkpoint Inhibitors

Kenneth Emancipator, Jianda Yuan, Razvan Cristescu, Deepti Aurora-Garg, and Priti S. Hegde

KEY POINTS

- The identification of biomarkers that can effectively predict response to immunotherapy is critical to guide treatment strategies and patient selection.

- The expression of programmed death ligand 1 (PD-L1) has become the most widely used biomarker for selecting patients for immunotherapy across a broad range of tumor types; four immunohistochemistry diagnostic assays have been approved in the clinic to guide use with a specific anti–PD-1/PD-L1 agent.

- Microsatellite instability status can be used to identify a unique patient population with highly immunogenic tumors that may respond to immunotherapy.

- Tumors with a higher mutational burden are more immunogenic and generally respond better to immunotherapy than nonimmunogenic tumors.

- The low but significant association between PD-L1 and tumor mutational burden highlights the complex biology and influence of tumor intrinsic and extrinsic signaling mechanisms that ultimately define these tumors and their response to immune checkpoint inhibitor therapy.

INTRODUCTION

Over the past decade, immune checkpoint inhibitor (ICI) therapy use has become increasingly important as improved understanding of the tumor microenvironment (TME) and pathways used by the tumor to evade immune system detection have led to the development and approval of agents targeting immune checkpoint pathways.[1,2] Programmed death ligand 1 (PD-L1) is primarily expressed on the surface of tumor cells (TCs) and immune cells (ICs) in solid tumors.[3–5] Binding of programmed cell death 1 (PD-1) on the surface of T cells to its ligand, PD-L1, on TCs or ICs led to the development of T cell tolerance, reduced T cell proliferation, decreased cytokine expression, and impaired antigen recognition.[6,7] Blocking the PD-1:PD-L1 interaction using anti–PD-1/PD-L1 antibodies restores T cell function and has been shown to increase antitumor immune activity, resulting in tumor regression and improved durable tumor control and survival outcomes across multiple types of solid tumors.[8–12] Despite the success of ICI therapies across numerous tumor types, only a subset of patients will respond to these agents. Therefore, the identification of biomarkers that can effectively predict response is critical to guide treatment strategies and patient selection with the intent to maximize clinical outcomes.

Malignancies arise due to the accumulation of DNA damage and genetic alterations, among other causes.[1]

Authors' Disclosures: Kenneth Emancipator is an employee and stockholder of Merck Sharp & Dohme Corp., a subsidiary of Merck & Co., Inc., Kenilworth, NJ, USA. He owns stock in Bayer AG, BMS, and Johnson & Johnson, and his spouse is an employee of BMS. He also has issued a patent for combined positive score. Jianda Yuan is an employee of Merck Sharp & Dohme Corp., a subsidiary of Merck & Co., Inc., Kenilworth, NJ, USA. Razvan Cristescu is an employee and stockholder of Merck Sharp & Dohme Corp., a subsidiary of Merck & Co., Inc., Kenilworth, NJ, USA. Deepti Aurora-Garg is an employee and stockholder of Merck Sharp & Dohme Corp., a subsidiary of Merck & Co., Inc., Kenilworth, NJ, USA. Priti S. Hegde is an employee of Foundation Medicine.

Highly mutated tumors are believed to be more likely to harbor immunogenic neoantigens, which are presented on the major histocompatibility complex (MHC) on the surface of TCs, thus rendering the TCs as foreign to the surveilling immune system.[13] For example, abnormalities in DNA mismatch repair (MMR) and replication pathways contribute to an increase in the rate of somatic tumor mutations, leading to a condition called microsatellite instability (MSI), which represents a hypermutated form of genetically unstable tumors.[1,14] Increased MSI has been shown to predict response to ICI therapy, and pembrolizumab is approved by the U.S. Food and Drug Administration (FDA) for patients with MSI-high (MSI-H) or mismatch repair deficient (dMMR) solid tumors that have progressed following prior treatment and have no satisfactory alternatives.[15] Retrospective data suggested that tumor mutational burden (TMB) might correlate with clinical response to anti–PD-1/PD-L1 and cytotoxic T lymphocyte–associated protein 4 (CTLA-4) inhibition.[1,8–10,16–20] This principle was subsequently investigated and confirmed, leading to the June 16, 2020, approval of pembrolizumab in patients with high TMB (TMB-H; ≥10 mutations/megabase) advanced solid tumors who have progressed following prior treatment and have no satisfactory alternative treatment options.[15]

This chapter reviews the role of PD-L1, MSI, and TMB as predictive biomarkers and their associated assays in the clinical development of cancer ICI therapies and the data demonstrating their clinical use across various solid tumor types.

PROGRAMMED DEATH LIGAND 1 EXPRESSION ANALYSIS

Biology of Programmed Death Ligand 1 Adaptive Resistance Mechanisms

The interaction of PD-1 with its ligand PD-L1, whose expression is induced by localized inflammatory stimuli, is a common mechanism by which normal cells avoid tissue damage and TCs evade immune responses.[2,21] PD-L1 expression suggestive of this adaptive immune resistance has been identified across numerous tumor types.[22] Within the TME, IC PD-L1 expression appears to be an important marker of both preexisting immunity and active immune suppression, and ICs play a key role in the regulation of T cell response independent of PD-L1 expression by TCs.[22–24] Inhibition of PD-L1 expression has been shown to overcome immune suppression, indicating that expression of PD-L1 on ICs provides a relevant biomarker for response to immune checkpoint inhibition.[22–24] Consequently, the expression of PD-L1 on TCs or tumor-infiltrating lymphocytes (TILs) determined via immunohistochemistry has become the most widely used biomarker for selecting patients for ICI therapy.

Programmed Death Ligand 1 Expression Assays

Four immunohistochemistry diagnostic assays have been approved for tumor PD-L1 protein assessment in the clinic, each individualized to guide use with a specific anti–PD-1/PD-L1 agent as summarized in Table 45.1.[15,25–31] The antibody clones used in each assay are raised against different epitopes on the PD-L1 molecule. VENTANA SP142 and SP263 antibodies (Roche Diagnostics, Tucson, AZ) target the intracellular domain on PD-L1, whereas Dako 22C3 and 28-8 antibodies (Dako North America, Inc., Carpinteria, CA) are raised against epitopes within the extracellular domain.[25,26] In addition, each assay has separate immunostaining protocols that depend on different antigen retrieval conditions and staining platforms.

Technical Aspects of Programmed Death Ligand 1 Testing

The Blueprint PD-L1 Assay Comparison Project was a novel industry-academic collaboration between the FDA, American Association for Cancer Research (AACR), and American Society of Clinical Oncology (ASCO), along with four pharmaceutical companies (AstraZeneca PLC, Bristol Myers Squibb, Genentech, Inc., and Merck & Co. Inc., Kenilworth, NJ, USA), and two diagnostic companies (Agilent Technologies, Inc./Dako Corp and Roche/VENTANA Medical Systems, Inc.) to evaluate the analytical comparability of currently available PD-L1 immunohistochemistry assays.[32,33]

Using real-world clinical lung cancer samples, the Blueprint Phase 1 and Phase 2 studies showed the interchangeability of three different PD-L1 expression assays: PD-L1 IHC 22C3 pharmDx, PD-L1 IHC 28-8 pharmDx, and VENTANA PD-L1 (SP263).[32] These assays showed high concordance with strong reliability among pathologists for the determination of PD-L1 expression on TCs; concordance of PD-L1 expression on ICs was also demonstrated, albeit with greater variability between assays.[32,33] Compared with the other immunohistochemistry assays, the VENTANA PD-L1 (SP142) assay demonstrated reduced sensitivity for the detection of PD-L1 expression on TCs.[32,33] Although the Blueprint PD-L1 Assay Comparison project concluded that the SP142 assay was equivalent to the other three assays for detecting PD-L1 on ICs, a similar project conducted by the National Comprehensive Cancer Network (NCCN) concluded that SP142 was less sensitive than 22C3 and 28-8 for IC detection of PD-L1 expression.[34]

The development and approval of multiple PD-L1 IHC assays designed to tailor therapy within one therapeutic class present a unique set of challenges, including the limited availability of tumor tissue for testing and the complexity of testing and interpretation with multiple tests.[28] The lack of standardization of PD-L1 assays may

Table 45.1 FDA-Approved IHC Methods of Assessing PD-L1 Expression

ASSAY	SCORE	CELLS	DESCRIPTION	APPROVED INDICATIONS
22C3[15,25]	TPS	Tumor	Percentage of TCs that exhibit membrane staining for PD-L1	Companion diagnostic for pembrolizumab: NSCLC, gastric or GEJ adenocarcinoma, ESCC, cervical cancer, urothelial cancer, HNSCC, TNBC
	CPS	Tumor and immune	Ratio (×100) of PD-L1-staining cells (membrane-staining TCs and any staining lymphocytes and macrophages) to all viable TCs	
SP263[26,27]	PD-L1 high	Tumor and immune	≥25% of TCs stain for PD-L1 *Or* >1% cross-sectional tumor area covered by ICs *and* ≥25% of those ICs stain for PD-L1 *Or* IC area ≤1% and 100% of ICs stain for PD-L1	Complementary diagnostic for durvalumab: Urothelial cancer
SP142[25,29,30]	IC	Immune	Cross-sectional tumor area occupied by PD-L1-staining ICs. Original classification defined IC0 as <1% occupied; IC1 as 1%–4%; IC2 as 5%–9%; and IC3 as ≥10%. Terminology is migrating to IC ≥X% where X is the percent area occupied.	Companion diagnostic for atezolizumab: NSCLC, urothelial cancer, TNBC
	TC	Tumor	Essentially equivalent to TPS. Original classification defined TC0 as <1% of cell staining; TC1 as 1%–4%; TC2 as 5%–49%; and TC3 as ≥50%. Terminology is migrating to TC ≥X%, where X is the percent of TCs stained.	
28-8[25,31]	% TC staining	Tumor	Essentially equivalent to TPS, although term is not used	Companion diagnostic for nivolumab-ipilimumab combination: NSCLC Complementary diagnostic for nivolumab: NSCLC, HNSCC, urothelial cancer

CPS, combined positive score; ESCC, esophageal squamous cell carcinoma; FDA, U.S. Food and Drug Administration; GEJ, gastroesophageal junction; HNSCC, head and neck squamous cell carcinoma; IC, immune cell; IHC, immunohistochemistry; NSCLC, non-small cell lung cancer; PD-L1, programmed death ligand 1; TC, tumor cells; TNBC, triple-negative breast cancer; TPS, tumor proportion score

have undermined the confidence of physicians in PD-L1 as a biomarker and limited its adoption into clinical practice. Ultimately, for an assay and scoring method to be approved in determining patient suitability to treatment (i.e., as a companion diagnostic), the proven association of clinical outcomes with PD-L1 levels and the reproducibility of this method is required. The extent to which an assay is able to document this association drives its adoption and uptake in clinical practice. Assays that have been adopted in clinical practice are those that clearly identified clinical benefit in appropriate patient subgroups in clinical trials.

Clinical assays intended for diagnostic use within the United States are required to adhere to FDA regulations. In contrast, research use only (RUO) or investigational use only (IUO) assays are defined by the FDA as products in the laboratory research phase or product testing phase of development, respectively, and, as such, are not considered for clinical use.[35] Therefore, in vitro companion diagnostic assays (which are FDA-approved medical devices) for PD-L1 have been developed for use with individual ICIs to determine populations that would have the highest clinical benefit from treatment, including PD-L1 IHC 22C3 pharmDx, which is approved for use with pembrolizumab.[25] Additional assays have since been developed for use with other ICIs, including VENTANA PD-L1

(SP142) approved for use with atezolizumab and PD-L1 IHC 28-8 pharmDx approved for use with nivolumab alone or in combination with ipilimumab.[25]

Scoring Programmed Death Ligand 1 Expression

Tumor proportion score (TPS) and combined positive score (CPS) are two methods used to score PD-L1 expression using PD-L1 IHC 22C3 pharmDx. Each method was developed to maximize the identification/enrichment of patients who are most likely to derive benefit from treatment with the ICI pembrolizumab.[36–38]

TPS is the percentage of TCs with partial or complete membrane staining, relative to all viable TCs present in the sample[39]:

$$TPS = \frac{\text{No. PD–L1 – stained tumor cells}}{\text{Total No. of viable tumor cells}} \times 100\%$$

CPS is the ratio of PD-L1–stained cells (TCs, lymphocytes, macrophages) divided by the total number of viable TCs, multiplied by 100[39]:

$$CPS = \frac{\substack{\text{No. PD–L1 – stained tumor cells}\\ \textit{(tumor cells, lymphocytes, macrophages)}}}{\textit{Total No. of viable tumor cells}} \times 100$$

Although the result of the calculation can exceed 100, the maximum score is defined as CPS 100. Although these scores are defined in terms of numbers of cells, pathologists typically score via visual estimation, rather than actual cell counting, except in very small biopsies.

The use of these different scoring methods in various solid tumor types is detailed in the text that follows. In short, PD-L1 expression on TCs assessed via TPS is a well-defined and validated biomarker in non-small cell lung cancer (NSCLC).[36,40–42] The CPS method was developed for use with PD-L1 IHC 22C3 pharmDx to aid in the selection/enrichment of patients with urothelial cancer (UC), gastric/gastroesophageal junction (GEJ) adenocarcinoma, triple-negative breast cancer (TNBC), and ovarian cancer who might benefit from pembrolizumab.[39,43] In gastric/GEJ cancer, CPS was better able to select patients for therapeutic benefit and capture more responders than TPS.[43]

By comparison, when the SP142 assay is used, PD-L1 IC expression is categorized according to the percentage of PD-L1–positive ICs: IC0 (<1%), IC1 (≥1% but <5%), and IC2/3 (≥5%).[9] In NSCLC and UC, the PD-L1 scoring algorithm includes both IC and TC expression to categorize as IC0TC0 (<1% for both IC and TC), IC1TC1 (≥1% but <5% for both IC and TC), IC2TC2 (≥5% but <10% for IC and ≥5% but <50% for TC), and IC3TC3 (≥10% for IC and ≥50% for TC).[44] Tumors are categorized as being PD-L1–high or PD-L1–low (do not meet criteria for high expression) by the SP263 assay, depending on PD-L1 expression levels in tumor and/or ICs as outlined in Table 45.1.[27]

Programmed Death Ligand 1 Expression and Companion Diagnostic Approvals

Non-Small Cell Lung Cancer

Recognizing the importance of PD-L1 as a biomarker has enabled the development of diagnostic assays that have the potential to identify patients most likely to benefit from ICI and to guide treatment decisions in patients with solid tumors. Landmark studies with pembrolizumab in NSCLC fully leveraged PD-L1 as a selective biomarker, defined a cutoff to identify a population with very high clinical benefit, and validated a companion diagnostic approach along with the drug.[36]

First, the KEYNOTE-001 study of single-agent pembrolizumab in patients with progressive locally advanced or metastatic NSCLC sought to define and validate the level of PD-L1 expression associated with clinical benefit.[36] Although a prototype assay[45] was initially used for enrollment, final scoring and selection of a cutoff value was determined using an investigational version of the eventual companion diagnostic.[36] PD-L1 expression in ≥50% of TCs correlated with improved efficacy (higher response rate; longer progression-free survival [PFS], and overall survival [OS]), demonstrating that

TPS ≥50% was a new predictive biomarker for pembrolizumab treatment in NSCLC.[36] Data from KEYNOTE-001 supported the FDA approval of pembrolizumab for the treatment of NSCLC, including approval of PD-L1 IHC 22C3 pharmDx as a companion diagnostic.[15,46]

The utility of PD-L1 as a biomarker was further evaluated in KEYNOTE-010, a Phase 2/3 randomized trial of pembrolizumab versus docetaxel for patients with previously treated PD-L1–positive NSCLC. This was the first randomized trial that prospectively enrolled patients based on tumor PD-L1 expression.[40] PD-L1 expression on ≥1% of TCs (TPS ≥1%) was a key criterion for eligibility in this trial, which enrolled 1,475 patients. The KEYNOTE-010 trial validated clinical benefit and the use of TPS ≥1% to determine PD-L1 expression in this population.[40]

Data from the Phase 3 KEYNOTE-024 study established in the first-line setting that pembrolizumab displays increased activity in PD-L1–positive tumors.[42] Pembrolizumab was compared with investigator's choice of platinum-based chemotherapy for previously untreated advanced NSCLC with no sensitizing *EGFR* mutations or *ALK* translocations. A key eligibility criterion was PD-L1 TPS ≥50%. PD-L1 expression was assessed at a central laboratory using the commercially available PD-L1 IHC 22C3 pharmDx. First-line pembrolizumab was associated with longer PFS and OS versus platinum-based chemotherapy in patients with advanced NSCLC and PD-L1 TPS ≥50% (5-year survival rate of 31.9% vs. 16.3%).[42,47]

In KEYNOTE-042, first-line pembrolizumab monotherapy significantly prolonged OS compared with investigators' choice of chemotherapy in patients with PD-L1–expressing NSCLC, regardless of the TPS cutoff used.[48] These results supported the approval of pembrolizumab as monotherapy for the first-line treatment of patients with NSCLC expressing PD-L1 TPS ≥1%, as determined by PD-L1 IHC 22C3 pharmDx, who have no *EGFR* or *ALK* genomic tumor aberrations, and patients with stage III disease who are not candidates for surgical resection or definitive chemoradiation or who do not have metastatic disease.[15] Consistent with the results of two randomized Phase 3 studies, KEYNOTE-189 and KEYNOTE-407, patients with NSCLC may be treated with combination pembrolizumab plus chemotherapy irrespective of PD-L1 status.[49,50]

Atezolizumab monotherapy is approved by the FDA for the first-line treatment for patients with metastatic PD-L1–positive NSCLC (≥50% of TC [TC3] or ≥10% of IC [IC3] per the SP142 PD-L1 IHC assay) with no *EGFR* or *ALK* genomic tumor aberrations.[30] The OS benefit of atezolizumab therapy was first demonstrated versus docetaxel in the OAK study of patients with previously treated advanced NSCLC (including at least one line of platinum therapy), particularly in patients with TC3/IC3 PD-L1–positive disease.[51] In the IMpower110 study, patients with TC3/IC3 (see SP142 scoring in Table 45.1) metastatic NSCLC also had significantly longer OS when administered atezolizumab rather than chemotherapy.[52] Atezolizumab, in combination with bevacizumab, carboplatin, and paclitaxel, is also approved for the treatment of NSCLC irrespective of PD-L1 status following the results of the Phase 3 Impower150 study.[28,30]

The FDA has also approved combination therapy with nivolumab plus ipilimumab as first-line treatment for patients with metastatic PD-L1–positive (≥1% TC staining per PD-L1 IHC 28-8 pharmDx assay) NSCLC with no *EGFR* or *ALK* genomic tumor aberrations after significantly longer OS was observed versus chemotherapy for this population in the CheckMate 227 study.[31,53]

Triple-Negative Breast Cancer

Patients with TNBC typically have a poor clinical prognosis and are generally treated with systemic chemotherapy, in accordance with guideline recommendations.[54] The results of the randomized Phase 3 IMpassion130 trial reinforce the usefulness of considering PD-L1 expression status on ICs to inform treatment choices for patients with metastatic TNBC.[55] In that trial, atezolizumab plus nab-paclitaxel prolonged PFS compared with placebo plus nab-paclitaxel in patients with previously untreated, PD-L1–positive metastatic TNBC.[55] PD-L1 expression was assessed using the VENTANA PD-L1 (SP142) IHC assay on tumor specimens (formalin-fixed paraffin-embedded [FFPE] archival, or fresh pretreatment relapsed-disease tumor tissue). PD-L1 positivity was defined as expression on "TILs ≥1%" (which means IC ≥1%; see Table 45.1). The FDA has approved atezolizumab, in combination with paclitaxel, for the treatment of patients with unresectable locally advanced or metastatic TNBC whose tumors express PD-L1 (PD-L1-stained ICs of any intensity covering ≥1% of the tumor area [IC ≥1%; see Table 45.1]).[49] Atezolizumab has also received EMA approval, in combination with nab-paclitaxel, for the treatment of adult patients with unresectable locally advanced or metastatic TNBC whose tumors have PD-L1 expression ≥1% and who have not previously received chemotherapy for metastatic disease.[56]

KEYNOTE-355 was a randomized Phase 3 study of pembrolizumab plus chemotherapy versus placebo plus chemotherapy in patients with untreated locally recurrent inoperable or metastatic TNBC.[57] Pembrolizumab plus chemotherapy significantly improved PFS versus chemotherapy alone in patients with PD-L1 CPS ≥10; this indication was recently approved by the FDA.[15]

Head and Neck Squamous Cell Carcinoma

In patients with HNSCC, higher PD-L1 expression on TCs and ICs has been associated with an improved response to pembrolizumab.[58] In the open-label Phase 3 KEYNOTE-048 trial, pembrolizumab monotherapy significantly prolonged OS compared with cetuximab plus chemotherapy in the PD-L1 CPS ≥20 and CPS ≥1 populations. PD-L1 was assessed at a central laboratory using PD-L1 IHC 22C3 pharmDx. In this same study, pembrolizumab, in combination with chemotherapy, significantly prolonged OS in the PD-L1 CPS ≥20, CPS ≥1, and total populations, compared with cetuximab plus chemotherapy.[58] Based on the positive findings of KEYNOTE-048, the FDA approved pembrolizumab as a single agent for the first-line treatment of patients with metastatic or unresectable, recurrent HNSCC whose tumors express CPS ≥1.[15]

In line with data from CheckMate 057 in patients with NSCLC,[59] evidence from an exploratory biomarker analysis in the CheckMate 141 trial indicated that PD-L1 expression was not a significant predictor of survival with nivolumab in patients with platinum-refractory HNSCC,[60] although it must be noted that the scoring method used in this study did not take into account IC PD-L1 expression. The randomized, open-label, Phase 3 CheckMate 141 trial compared nivolumab versus standard single-agent systemic therapy in patients with recurrent HNSCC whose disease had progressed within 6 months after platinum-based chemotherapy.[60] PD-L1 expression was evaluated using the PD-L1 IHC 28-8 pharmDx. Tumor PD-L1 expression was scored at ≥1%, ≥5%, and ≥10%. Patients treated with nivolumab had longer OS than those treated with standard therapy, regardless of tumor PD-L1 expression.

Urothelial Cancer

The IMvigor210 study was the first to suggest that PD-L1 is a potential biomarker for selection of patients with advanced UC who may benefit from ICI therapy. IMvigor210 was a single-arm, Phase 2 trial of atezolizumab in patients with locally advanced and metastatic UC who had progressed following treatment with platinum-based chemotherapy.[9] PD-L1 was prospectively and centrally assessed in tumor samples using the VENTANA PD-L1 (SP142) assay. Higher levels of PD-L1 expression on ICs were associated with higher response rates to atezolizumab, and longer OS although responses were observed across all PD-L1 expression levels.[9] These results supported the FDA approval of atezolizumab for the treatment of adult patients with locally advanced or metastatic UC who are not eligible for cisplatin-containing chemotherapy and whose tumors express PD-L1 (IC2/3).[30]

Two early phase studies in nivolumab and durvalumab further suggest that PD-L1 expression may not be a universal biomarker of response across the ICI classes. In the single-arm, Phase 2 CheckMate 275 trial of nivolumab in metastatic UC after platinum therapy, PD-L1 expression was assessed using the PD-L1 IHC 22-8 pharmDx on archived tissue from a previous biopsy of unresectable or metastatic disease or from previous surgical resection.[61] TC PD-L1 membrane expression, evaluated using cutoffs of ≥1% and ≥5%, demonstrated that nivolumab monotherapy provided meaningful clinical benefit in metastatic UC, irrespective of PD-L1 expression,[61] although, again, the study did not take into account PD-L1 expression by ICs. In the open-label, Phase 1/2 study (Study 1108) of durvalumab in locally advanced or metastatic UC, PD-L1 expression was evaluated by IHC analysis using the SP-263 anti–PD-L1 antibody assay on tumor tissue obtained prior to treatment. PD-L1 positivity was defined as ≥25% of either TCs or ICs.[63] Responses to durvalumab were early, durable, and observed regardless of PD-L1 expression.[62]

A single-arm Phase 2 study (KEYNOTE-052) investigated first-line pembrolizumab in cisplatin-ineligible patients with locally advanced and unresectable or metastatic UC.[63] PD-L1 expression was assessed using PD-L1 IHC 22C3 pharmDx. Two cutoffs were used: CPS 1 cutoff based on results from the UC cohort of KEYNOTE-012 and a strongly positive (high) PD-L1 expression cutoff identified in this study. CPS 10 was determined in the training set to be the optimum high cutoff; in the validation set, the highest response was seen in patients with CPS ≥10. However, responses with pembrolizumab monotherapy were observed across all PD-L1 expression categories.[63] In the KEYNOTE-045 study of patients with advanced UC that recurred or progressed after platinum-based chemotherapy, pembrolizumab was associated with significantly longer OS in all patients, as well as patients with PD-L1 CPS ≥10.[64] Pembrolizumab is approved by the FDA for the treatment of patients with locally advanced or metastatic UC who are ineligible for cisplatin-containing chemotherapy and whose tumors express PD-L1 with a CPS ≥10.[15,49]

Gastric/Gastroesophageal Junction Adenocarcinoma

Pembrolizumab is approved for the treatment of patients with recurrent locally advanced or metastatic gastric/GEJ adenocarcinoma whose tumors express PD-L1 CPS ≥1 with disease progression on or after two or more prior lines of therapy.[15] This approval is based on the results from KEYNOTE-059, in which pembrolizumab monotherapy demonstrated promising activity and durable responses in previously treated patients with PD-L1–positive (CPS ≥1 per PD-L1 IHC 22C3 pharmDx) gastric cancer.[65] Patients with PD-L1–positive versus PD-L1–negative tumors had a higher objective response rate (ORR; 15.5% vs. 6.4%, respectively) and more durable responses.[65] The findings of KEYNOTE-059 were expanded and confirmed in a post hoc exploratory subgroup analysis of the Phase 3 KEYNOTE-061 study in patients with gastric/GEJ adenocarcinoma.[66] Initially, patients were enrolled irrespective of PD-L1 status; enrollment was later restricted to patients with PD-L1 CPS ≥1 (assessed using PD-L1 IHC 22C3 pharmDx). Pembrolizumab did not significantly improve OS, compared with paclitaxel as second-line therapy

for advanced gastric/GEJ adenocarcinoma with PD-L1 CPS ≥1.[66] In the Phase 3 KEYNOTE-062 study, pembrolizumab monotherapy was noninferior to chemotherapy for OS in patients with untreated advanced gastric cancer in patients with CPS ≥1.[67] Pembrolizumab provided a clinically meaningful benefit in patients with CPS ≥10; however, this hypothesis was not tested per the statistical analysis plan.[67] These analyses indicate that the treatment effect of pembrolizumab may be enhanced in patients with higher levels of PD-L1 expression (CPS ≥10).

The global, randomized Phase 3 CheckMate 649 study enrolled patients with untreated, unresectable advanced or metastatic gastric/GEJ cancer or esophageal adenocarcinoma regardless of PD-L1 expression status.[68] Nivolumab plus chemotherapy showed a statistically significant improvement in OS and PFS versus chemotherapy in tumors expressing PD-L1 CPS ≥5. A significant improvement with nivolumab plus chemotherapy versus chemotherapy was also observed in PD-L1 CPS ≥1 and all-randomized populations.[68]

Esophageal Carcinoma

Pembrolizumab is approved for the treatment of patients with recurrent locally advanced or metastatic squamous cell carcinoma of the esophagus (ESCC), whose tumors express PD-L1 CPS ≥10 with disease progression after one or more prior lines of systemic therapy.[15] The single-arm, Phase 2 KEYNOTE-180 study of pembrolizumab in patients with advanced, metastatic ESCC and adenocarcinoma of the esophagus that progressed after two or more lines of therapy supported the approval of pembrolizumab in this setting.[69] Tumors with a CPS ≥10 (per PD-L1 IHC 22C3) were considered positive for PD-L1 expression. Response to pembrolizumab was enriched in patients with PD-L1–positive tumors; however, durable antitumor activity was observed regardless of PD-L1 status.[69] In the randomized, open-label, Phase 3 KEYNOTE-181 study,[70] pembrolizumab significantly improved OS versus chemotherapy as second-line therapy for advanced esophageal cancer with PD-L1 CPS ≥10. Lastly, in the Phase 3 randomized KEYNOTE-590 study in patients with untreated, advanced esophageal, and esophagogastric junction cancer, pembrolizumab plus chemotherapy was superior to chemotherapy in the overall population, patients with PD-L1 CPS ≥10, and patients with ESCC PD-L1 CPS ≥10.[71]

Cervical Cancer

Pembrolizumab is approved for the treatment of patients with recurrent or metastatic cervical cancer with disease progression on or after chemotherapy whose tumors express PD-L1 CPS ≥1.[15] The Phase 2 KEYNOTE-158 study of pembrolizumab monotherapy demonstrated antitumor activity in patients with PD-L1–positive (CPS ≥1 per PD-L1 IHC 22C3 pharmDx) advanced cervical cancer.[72]

Archived Versus New Samples

Studies in NSCLC have demonstrated that PD-L1 expression can be determined in archival or newly collected tumor samples. For example, a post hoc analysis from KEYNOTE-010 demonstrated that ICI therapy prolonged OS versus docetaxel in patients with PD-L1–positive tumors regardless of whether newly collected or archival samples were used to determine PD-L1 expression.[41] In patients with TPS ≥1%, PFS hazard ratios were similar across archival (0.82 [95% CI, 0.66, 1.02]) and newly collected (0.83 [95% CI, 0.68, 1.02]) samples. In addition, low intrapatient heterogeneity of PD-L1 expression determined in fresh or archival samples was previously demonstrated in an unrelated clinical study of NSCLC tumor specimens from patients receiving open-label atezolizumab.[73] Unfortunately, such data are lacking for other tumor types.

Future Treatments

A number of anti–PD-1 monoclonal antibodies are also approved or under clinical development, including cemiplimab, which has been approved for cutaneous squamous cell carcinoma, and dostarlimab, which has demonstrated efficacy in endometrial cancer.[74,75] Other anti–PD-1 antibodies undergoing clinical development for solid and hematologic tumors that have already received approval outside the United States include tiselizumab, spartalizumab, sintilimab, and toripalimab.[76–78]

MICROSATELLITE INSTABILITY

Hereditary cancers were first described in the early 1900s, followed by the discovery of Lynch syndrome by Henry Lynch in the 1960s.[79] Lynch syndrome-associated cancers arise from germline or somatic loss of function mutations in genes of the MMR pathway,[79] which is responsible for the restoration of DNA integrity after the occurrence of single-base mismatches or short insertions and deletions during replication of small repeat sequences.[80,81] Inactivation of MMR genes through mutation or epigenetic silencing leads to the accumulation of errors in the DNA, resulting in MSI.[79,81] Microsatellites are short repetitive sequences of DNA, and MSI typically presents as repeat length alterations.[79,80] Mutations in the *MLH1, MSH2, MSH6,* or *PSM2* genes of the MMR pathway lead to MSI and the genetic predisposition to cancer observed in Lynch syndrome.[80,82] The four homonym proteins codified by these genes function in heterodimers, namely MLH1-PMS2 and MSH2-MSH6, which identify errors and recruit DNA repair machinery in normal cells or TCs that are microsatellite stable (MSS).[79,80]

MSI was first discovered in colorectal carcinoma (CRC) and accounts for approximately 15% of CRC cases.[83,84] MSI has since been shown to occur in a variety of additional tumor types, including gastric and endometrial, with lower frequency in other cancers.[81,84] The prevalence of high MSI varies across cancer types, but is generally observed at low frequency, with 1.5% of all solid and hematopoietic tumors identified as MSI-H in a real-world cohort.[81,84,85] MSI-H designation is most commonly observed in endometrial (20%), CRC (17%), gastroesophageal (13%), and small intestine (8%) cancers. Prostate and cervical carcinomas, NSCLC, and HNSCC typically have an MSI-H prevalence of ≤4%.[80,86]

Assessment of Microsatellite Instability

Evidence of a genetic basis of predisposition to cancer in Lynch syndrome was provided in 1993 and the identification of mutations in MMR genes shortly followed.[79] These discoveries and technological advances over the years led to the development of guidelines that promote the universal testing of CRCs for Lynch syndrome and dMMR/MSI, including the NCCN and U.S. Multi-Society Task Force on Colorectal Cancer guidelines.[87,88] MSI or dMMR is tested using immunohistochemistry or molecular tests including classic polymerase chain reaction (PCR)-based microsatellite testing and next-generation sequencing (NGS) approaches. The European Society for Medical Oncology (ESMO) Translational Research and Precision Medicine Working Group and the NCCN provide guidance on MSI testing.[80,88] For dMMR testing, immunohistochemistry and/or MSI testing via PCR are recommended as the primary approach for universal screening, although immunohistochemistry is preferred as the initial test by the ESMO Working Group.[80,88] Immunohistochemistry is performed using antibodies that recognize the four MMR proteins: MLH1, MSH2, MSH6, and PMS2.[80,88] MSI testing using PCR is performed with two possible panels: (a) a panel with two mononucleotide (BAT-25 and BAT-26) and three dinucleotide (D5S346, D2S123, and D17S250) repeats and (b) a panel with five poly-A mononucleotide repeats (BAT-25, BAT-26, NR-21, NR-24, MONO-27).[80,88] Both panels are being used to assess MSI in clinical trials, although the poly-A panel offers higher specificity and sensitivity.[80,89]

NGS offers the ability to detect MSI in a sample while concurrently facilitating the detection of other relevant mutations that may guide treatment selection and germline testing for patients with an increased risk of Lynch syndrome.[85,90] NGS can analyze dozens to hundreds of microsatellite loci compared with the five to eight standard loci tested using PCR.[88] Although there are no standard panels established for MSI, there are a number of Comprehensive Genomic Panels (CGP) available that test for more than one gene associated with multiple cancers or multiple cancer syndromes and can provide MSI status.[88] Panels are based on microsatellite sequencing data derived from whole genome sequencing (WGS), whole exome sequencing (WES), or third-generation sequencing (TGS) platforms. Recently, panels specifically designed for the detection of MSI in cancer have been developed and have shown either comparable or better results than the poly-A panel.

Predictive Role of Mismatch Repair/Microsatellite Instability

MSI status can be utilized to identify a unique patient population with highly immunogenic tumors that may respond to ICI therapy.[86] Tumors with dMMR/MSI-H have increased mutation rates that promote antitumor IC recognition and increased TILs, thus making these tumors more likely to respond to anti–PD-1/PD-L1 therapy.[91,92] In addition, MSI-H status appears to confer a survival advantage in CRC that is dependent on stage of disease.[93] MSI-H tumors also appear to be more responsive to immunotherapy-based treatments.[20,83] In a Phase 2 study of 41 pembrolizumab-treated patients with progressive metastatic carcinoma with or without dMMR, immune-related ORR and immune-related PFS rate were substantially higher in patients with dMMR CRC (40% and 78% vs. 0% and 11%, respectively).[20] Interestingly, patients with dMMR non-CRC demonstrated comparable responses to patients with dMMR CRC (immune-related ORR: 71% vs. 67%).[20]

The importance of MSI as a biomarker for predicting response to ICI therapy was emphasized with the FDA accelerated approval of pembrolizumab for patients who have MSI-H or dMMR solid tumors that have progressed following prior treatment and who have no satisfactory alternative treatments.[15] This was the first tissue-agnostic approval for a cancer therapeutic based on a common biomarker rather than a specific tumor type or location.[94] The pan-cancer approval of pembrolizumab based on biomarker status represented a novel treatment strategy wherein treatment is selected on the basis of the genomic profile of the tumor,[94] as opposed to the standardly used approach based on tumor origin, with the ultimate aim of enhancing clinical outcomes and minimizing treatment-related toxicity. Pembrolizumab was also recently approved in the first-line setting for patients with unresectable or metastatic MSI-H or dMMR CRC. This approval was based on results from the Phase 3, randomized open-label KEYNOTE-177 study that evaluated pembrolizumab versus standard of care chemotherapy plus bevacizumab or cetuximab.[95] Tumors were classified as MSI-H when at least two allelic shifts among the three to five analyzed microsatellite markers were detected via PCR or at least one of the four MMR proteins were absent via immunohistochemistry. In KEYNOTE-177, patients demonstrated significantly longer PFS (per RECIST v1.1 by central imaging vendor review; primary

end point) and fewer treatment-related adverse events than with chemotherapy (with or without cetuximab or bevacizumab).[95]

Nivolumab is also approved by the FDA for the treatment of adult and pediatric patients with MSI-H or dMMR metastatic CRC that has progressed with fluoropyrimidine, oxaliplatin, and irinotecan, as a single agent or in combination with ipilimumab.[31] This approval was granted based on outcomes from the Phase 2, open-label CheckMate 142 study (primary end point investigator-assessed ORR) in which a high proportion of patients responded to therapy (nivolumab ORR, 31%; nivolumab plus ipilimumab ORR, 55%), and many of these responses were durable.[96,97] The efficacy and safety of the anti–PD-1 antibody dostarlimab is also being investigated in patients with MSI-H or dMMR and MSS advanced endometrial cancer after demonstrating modest efficacy in the Phase 1/2 GARNET study.[98]

TUMOR MUTATIONAL BURDEN

Tumor antigens were first identified in animal models, including mice with chemically induced tumors, and were referred to as rejection antigens.[99–101] Subsequently, cytotoxic T cells were shown to respond to these tumor-specific antigens and the process of tumor immune surveillance was identified in humans.[13,101,102] Neoantigens are non-self-antigens that may form as a result of the transcription, translation, processing, and presentation of nonsynonymous mutations acquired by proliferating TCs; these neoantigens may be recognized as foreign by the immune system when presented on the TC surface.[13,103–105] TMB is the total number of somatic, nonsynonymous mutations within the tumor exome, which may be a surrogate biomarker for neoantigen burden.[1] The prevalence of somatic mutations varies across tumor types, with TMB being highest in cancers related to chronic exposure to ultraviolet light or mutagens (e.g., tobacco), such as melanoma and lung cancer.[106] Tumors with high neoantigen load have a higher likelihood of eliciting an antitumor immune response, and therefore are more likely to show benefit from ICI therapies that disinhibit immune responses directed at TCs.[8,103,104,107,108] For that reason, TMB has been suggested as a potential predictive biomarker for ICI therapies. The relationship between mutational load and response to ICI therapy has been established in studies of CTLA-4 antibodies in patients with melanoma.[16,103] In retrospective studies, TMB has been shown to be associated with improved responses to PD-1/PD-L1 blockade in melanoma, lung, bladder, and other cancers.[8,16,19,63] Likewise, the principle of high TMB as a biomarker of response to ICI therapies would, in theory, apply to all tumor types, regardless of location or histology.

Defining and Measuring Tumor Mutational Burden

Tumors with a higher mutational burden, such as melanoma and lung cancers, are more immunogenic and generally respond better to immunotherapy, compared with nonimmunogenic tumors, such as hematologic malignancies.[1,109] Median and range of mutational load has been shown to vary across tumor types.[108] TMB is measured using high-throughput sequencing techniques, such as targeted NGS panels or WES. Tumor DNA is extracted from tumor tissue or blood and is processed for sequencing via a series of molecular biologic steps.[110,111] Bioinformatic analysis is then applied to align the raw sequenced data and identify specific genetic alterations. TMB is reported as either mutations/exome (mut/exome) when measured by WES, or as mutations per megabase (mut/Mb) when measured by CGP on a targeted panel of genes.[112]

Whole Exome Sequencing

WES is a comprehensive sequencing method that provides coverage of approximately 26.6 Mb (78% of genes) across the entire exome.[113] A true estimate of mutation burden along with the comprehensive identification of all somatic mutations (coding errors, base substitutions, and short insertions/deletions) present in a patient's tumor exome can only be truly assessed by WES.[114] However, use of WES in clinical practice has been challenging; it incurs a higher cost and a longer turnaround time to align and interpret the raw data, and due to the thousands of genes being assayed, it is not well suited to gene-by-gene validation. In addition, it is difficult to

provide consistent performance and standardize WES analysis. Therefore, for cost-effectiveness, expedience, and ease of implementation in clinical practice, CGP is the preferred diagnostic method of choice.[112,114]

Targeted Next-Generation Sequencing

To date, the FoundationOne®CDx test is the only FDA-approved targeted NGS panel (class III device) for patients with cancer.[112] Two additional NGS panels—namely the Memorial Sloan Kettering-Integrated Mutation Profiling of Actionable Cancer Targets (MSK-IMPACT) and Personal Genome Diagnostics elio (PGDx elio tissue complete) panels—have received FDA clearance (class II device) for use in cancer (Table 45.2).[114–122]

FoundationOne CDx

FoundationOne CDx is an NGS-based companion diagnostic to aid in the identification of patients who may benefit from certain anticancer therapies. This test can measure and report alterations in 324 key cancer genes in FFPE solid tumor samples.[115] The FoundationOne CDx test measures and reports on two biomarkers related to cancer immunotherapy, MSI and TMB. FoundationOne CDx defines TMB as the number of somatic mutations (coding, base substitutions [synonymous and nonsynonymous], and short insertions and deletions) per Mb of tumor genome examined.[115] The test utilizes a computational methodology to distinguish somatic from germline alterations by modeling the alteration's allele frequency.[123] Because no matched normal is used, germline mutations that are not accounted for may skew

Table 45.2 Currently Available Assays to Assess Tumor Mutational Burden in FFPE Tumor Tissue

COMPANY	PANEL NAME	GERMLINE SAMPLES ANALYZED	PANEL SIZE (GENES)	COVERAGE (Mb)	HIGH TMB LEVEL
FDA-approved diagnostic assays					
Foundation Medicine[114,115]	FoundationOne CDx	No	324	0.8	≥10 mut/Mb
FDA-cleared diagnostic assays					
Memorial Sloan Kettering[116,117]	MSK-IMPACT	Yes	468	1.5	Unspecified
Personal Genome Diagnostics[118,119]	PGDx elio	No	507	2.2	Unspecified
Commercial assays/research use only					
Caris Life Sciences[114,120]	Molecular Intelligence Profile	No	592	1.4	≥10 mut/Mb
Illumina[114,121]	TruSight Tumor 170	No	170	0.5	Unspecified
ThermoFisher[114,122]	Oncomine Tumor Mutation Load	No	409	1.7	Unspecified

FDA, U.S. Food and Drug Administration; FFPE, formalin-fixed paraffin-embedded; Mb, megabase; MSK-IMPACT, Memorial Sloan Kettering-Integrated Mutation Profiling of Actionable Cancer Targets; mut, mutation; TMB, tumor mutational burden.

TMB to higher values, particularly in ethnicities with less representation in germline variant databases.[124] The FoundationOne CDx test is the only FDA-approved test to measure and report TMB in patients for treatment with pembrolizumab.

MSK-IMPACT

MSK-IMPACT is a custom hybridization capture panel for the targeted sequencing of all exons and selected introns of 468 key cancer genes in FFPE solid tumors.[116,117,125] MSI status is defined by comparing microsatellites present in tumor samples against matched normal DNA extracted from patient's tissue or peripheral blood.[116,117]

PGDx elio Tissue Complete

PGDx elio tissue complete has been cleared by the FDA for assessing actionable mutations of 507 genes in tumor tissue, as well as assessing MSI and TMB.[118,119]

Use of Matched Normal Samples

MSK-IMPACT is the only NGS panel that uses a matched normal tissue sample (typically a blood sample) to assess TMB.[116,117] Directly comparing the tumor genome to the genome in normal blood ensures that the mutations detected by the MSK-IMPACT are specific to the cancer cells. In addition, looking at normal genomes can show whether there are any inherited genetic mutations associated with an increased risk of cancer. Both FoundationOne CDx and PGDx elio use proprietary reference databases to determine and subtract germline alterations in TMB assessments.

Other Panels

A number of other NGS panels are available for TMB assessment, although they are not standardized and may differ in terms of methodology, gene number, and sample analysis (Table 45.2).[114] When investigated using in silico techniques, variability has been reported between NGS panels, both in terms of over- and underestimation of TMB, highlighting some of the challenges in applying NGS assessment of TMB in clinical practice.[112] The complexity of these biomarkers also highlights the importance of regulatory oversight in the development of these tests for use in treatment decisions for patients. Friends of Cancer Research TMB Harmonization Project was developed to ensure consistency across values from various TMB tests and improve the reliability of using NGS panels for evaluating TMB.[112] These collaborative efforts have resulted in preliminary recommendations and will focus on feasibility of external reference standards in the future.[112]

Blood-based sampling ideally avoids many of the shortcomings of tissue-based testing, including sample accessibility and tumor heterogeneity.[126] However, due to the variable rate of shedding of circulating tumor DNA (ctDNA) into the circulation, depending on location, size, stage, and vascularity of the tumor, it is unknown at this time if blood-based TMB (bTMB) will prove predictive for clinical benefit in tumors. So far, exploratory analyses have suggested that bTMB may be predictive of overall survival in patients with metastatic NSCLC and recurrent HNSCC administered the PD-L1 inhibitor durvalumab, with or without the CTLA-4 inhibitor tremelimumab.[127,128] In a retrospective analysis of the POPLAR and OAK trials, bTMB was well correlated with tissue TMB and was a predictor of improved PFS with the PD-L1 inhibitor atezolizumab.[126,129] The B-F1RST study showed the clinical utility of bTMB (cutoff of ≥16) as a predictive biomarker for PFS and OS in patients with advanced NSCLC receiving first-line atezolizumab.

Tumor Mutational Burden by Whole Exome Sequencing Versus FoundationOne CDx

A comprehensive analysis of 100,000 cancer genomes confirmed that the FoundationOne CDx assay targeting ~1.1 Mb of coding genome correlates with TMB measured by whole exome ($R^2 = 0.74$).[1] This concordance was further validated in a cohort of patients with NSCLC, which revealed a correlation between WES-based TMB and FoundationOne CDx ($R^2 = 0.96$).[130] Using WES and FoundationOne CDx, high concordance was observed in the pan-tumor assessment of tissue TMB (tTMB; Spearman correlation, 0.7; $n = 413$).[131] When individual indications were considered, the concordance was further improved for indications with higher median TMB. tTMB concordance was higher when restricted to NSCLC (Spearman correlation, 0.8; $n = 38$).

Tumor Mutational Burden as a Clinical Biomarker

Emerging evidence in multiple tumor types, including urothelial, anal, biliary, cervical, endometrial, salivary, thyroid, and vulvar carcinoma, as well as mesothelioma, neuroendocrine tumors, and small cell lung cancer, has demonstrated that tumors with high TMB can help predict response to ICI therapy, which may provide an alternative biomarker beyond PD-L1 expression.[8,16,132,133]

Pembrolizumab was approved on June 16, 2020, for the treatment of adult and pediatric patients with unresectable or metastatic solid tumors with tissue TMB-H (≥10 mut/Mb).[15] This is a tissue-agnostic approval for patients who have disease progression following prior treatment and who have no satisfactory alternative treatment options. Traditionally, therapeutic standards are dictated by tissue of disease origin.[15] Like the pan-cancer MSI-H indication, this is an example of a drug approval that is based on the biology of disease as opposed to tissue of disease origin. The approval of pembrolizumab in patients with TMB-H tumors was based on the results from KEYNOTE-158, a nonrandomized, open-label trial evaluating predictive biomarkers in patients with advanced solid tumors.[133]

In this study, 790 patients had tissue evaluable for TMB and 102 patients (13%) were TMB-H. TMB-H was associated with an increased response rate compared with non-TMB-H (29% vs. 6%, respectively).[133] Data across multiple tumor types indicate that TMB, as assessed by WES, can enable patient stratification according to clinical response to pembrolizumab.

To date, TMB testing has only been approved as a companion diagnostic for pembrolizumab monotherapy, where TMB has been shown to be predictive of response across a range of tumors (Table 45.3).[9,41,132–142]

The association between TMB and clinical response to ICI therapy has been investigated in multiple tumor types. In NSCLC, higher TMB levels are correlated with improved outcomes to pembrolizumab, atezolizumab, and durvalumab, with or without tremelimumab.[126,135,143,144] However, in an exploratory analysis of the KEYNOTE-021, KEYNOTE-189, and KEYNOTE-407 trials, tTMB was not significantly associated with efficacy of pembrolizumab plus platinum-based chemotherapy or chemotherapy alone as first-line therapy for metastatic NSCLC, regardless of histology.[143] Collectively, these results indicate that

Table 45.3 Outcomes by Tumor Mutational Burden Status in Patients Receiving Immunotherapy

STUDY/POPULATION	SAMPLE EVALUABLE FOR TMB (n)	REGIMEN	SEQUENCING METHOD	OUTCOMES
NSCLC				
KEYNOTE-010 / KEYNOTE-042[41] Advanced NSCLC PD-L1 TPS ≥1%	KEYNOTE-010: 253 KEYNOTE-042: 793	KEYNOTE-010: Pembrolizumab 200 mg Q3W vs. platinum-based chemotherapy KEYNOTE-042: Pembrolizumab 200 mg Q3W vs. docetaxel 75 mg/m² Q3W	WES (cutpoint ≥175 mut/exome)	Pembrolizumab vs. chemotherapy for tTMB ≥175 mut/exome: Median OS, mo (−010: 14.1 vs. 7.6 mo; −042: 21.9 vs. 11.6 mo) Median PFS, mo (−010: 4.2 vs. 2.4; −042: 6.3 vs. 6.5) ORR (−010: 23.5% vs. 9.8%; −042: 34.4% vs. 30.9%)
CheckMate 227[134] Advanced/recurrent NSCLC PD-L1 expression ≥1%	299	Nivolumab 3 mg/kg Q2W + ipilimumab 1 mg/kg Q6W vs. nivolumab 240 mg Q2W vs. platinum-doublet chemotherapy	FoundationOne CDx assay (cutpoint ≥10 mut/Mb)	Nivolumab + ipilimumab vs. chemotherapy for TMB ≥10 mut/Mb: Median PFS, mo (7.2 vs. 5.5)
IMpower110[135] Chemotherapy-naïve, stage IV NSCLC	389	Atezolizumab 1,200 mg Q3W vs. platinum-based chemotherapy	bTMB score cutoffs of ≥10, ≥16, and ≥20	Atezolizumab vs. chemotherapy bTMB ≥10: median OS, mo (11.2 vs. 10.3); median PFS, mo (5.5 vs. 4.3) bTMB ≥16: median OS, mo (13.9 vs. 8.5); median PFS, mo (6.8 vs. 4.4) bTMB ≥20: median OS, mo (17.2 vs. 10.5); median PFS, mo (6.8 vs. 5.2)
Gastric Cancer				
KEYNOTE-059 (Cohort 1)[136] Recurrent/metastatic gastric/GEJ adenocarcinoma	85	Pembrolizumab 200 mg Q3W	WES	Mutational load significantly associated with response after adjusting for GEP or PD-L1
KEYNOTE-061 Advanced gastric/GEJ adenocarcinoma[137,138]	204	Pembrolizumab 200 mg Q3W	FoundationOne CDx assay (cutpoint ≥10 mut/Mb)	tTMB significantly associated with ORR (p <.001), PFS (p <.001), and OS (p = .003) after adjusting for MSI
	420		WES	tTMB significantly associated with ORR, PFS, and OS (one-sided p <.001 for all) after adjusting for PD-L1
Melanoma				
KEYNOTE-006[139] Unresectable stage III or IV melanoma; enrollment stratified by PD-L1 expression	216	Pembrolizumab 10 mg/kg Q2W or Q3W vs. ipilimumab 3 mg/kg Q3W	WES	tTMB significantly associated with BOR, PFS, and OS (p <.05) in the pembrolizumab arm

(continued)

Table 45.3 Outcomes by Tumor Mutational Burden Status in Patients Receiving Immunotherapy (*continued*)

STUDY/POPULATION	SAMPLE EVALUABLE FOR TMB (N)	REGIMEN	SEQUENCING METHOD	OUTCOMES
Hamid et al[140] Unresectable/metastatic melanoma	23	Atezolizumab 0.1 to 20 mg/kg or ≥10 mg/kg Q3W	FoundationOne CDx assay (cutpoint ≥16 mut/Mb)	tTMB high vs. tTMB low: ORR (50% vs. 0%) Median PFS, mo (20 vs. 1) Median OS, mo (NR vs. 7)
HNSCC				
KEYNOTE-012 (Cohort B/B2)/ KEYNOTE-055[141] Recurrent/metastatic HNSCC resistant to platinum and cetuximab therapies	258	Pembrolizumab 200 mg Q3W	WES	tTMB significantly associated with BOR (*p* <.001), regardless of HPV status
Urothelial Carcinoma				
IMvigor210[142] Metastatic urothelial carcinoma	298	Atezolizumab 1,200 mg Q3W	FoundationOne CDx assay	tTMB significantly associated with response
IMvigor211[132] Metastatic urothelial carcinoma, progressing after platinum-based chemotherapy, PD-L1 ≥5%	544	Atezolizumab 1,200 mg Q3W vs. chemotherapy	FoundationOne CDx assay (cutoff, median 9.65 mut/Mb)	Atezolizumab vs. chemotherapy: Median OS, mo, in high tTMB group (11.3 vs. 8.3) Median OS, mo, in low tTMB group (8.3 vs. 8.1)
IMvigor210[9] Locally advanced/ metastatic urothelial carcinoma, progressing following platinum-based chemotherapy	150	Atezolizumab 1,200 mg Q3W	FoundationOne CDx assay	Median mutational load higher in responders vs. nonresponders (12.4 mut/Mb vs. 6.4 mut/mb; *p* <.0001)
Pan Tumor				
KEYNOTE-158[133] Advanced solid tumors	790	Pembrolizumab 200 mg Q3W	FoundationOne CDx assay (cutpoint ≥10 mut/Mb)	tTMB-high vs. non-tTMB-high: ORR (29% vs. 6%) Median PFS, mo (2.1 vs. 2.1) Median OS, mo (11.7 vs. 12.8)

BOR, best overall response; bTMB, blood-based TMB; CPS, combined positive score; GEJ, gastroesophageal junction; GEP, gene expression profile; HNSCC, head and neck squamous cell carcinoma; HPV, human papillomavirus; IC, immune cell; mo, month; MSI, microsatellite instability; mut/exome, mutations/exome; mut/Mb, mutations per megabase; NR, not reached; NSCLC, non-small cell lung cancer; ORR, objective response rate; OS, overall survival; PD-L1, programmed death ligand 1; PFS, progression-free survival; Q2W, every 2 weeks; Q3W, every 3 weeks; Q6W, every 6 weeks; TC, tumor cells; TMB, tumor mutational burden; TPS, tumor proportion score; tTMB, tissue tumor mutational burden; UC, urothelial carcinoma; WES, whole exome sequencing.

tTMB is predictive of clinical benefit for ICI monotherapy but not in combination with chemotherapy.

In contrast to a combination of ICI and chemotherapy, it is unclear whether TMB-H is associated with increased benefit with combination therapies of PD-1/PD-L1 plus CTLA-4 antibodies. In CheckMate 227, nivolumab plus ipilimumab was associated with a longer PFS and increased response rate, compared with chemotherapy in patients with TMB-H tumors; however, the hazard ratio for survival was not improved in the TMB-H group relative to the non-TMB-H group despite absolute differences in OS in each.[134] In an exploratory analysis of the MYSTIC trial, bTMB ≥20 was associated with an OS and PFS benefit with durvalumab plus tremelimumab compared with chemotherapy; however, the Phase 3 NEPTUNE study

of durvalumab plus tremelimumab versus chemotherapy did not meet its primary end point of OS in TMB-H tumors.[144,145] In KEYNOTE-059 and KEYNOTE-061, mutational load was independently predictive of response to pembrolizumab monotherapy in gastric/GEJ cancer.[136–138] Melanoma, which is noted to have the highest median TMB across solid tumors,[1] showed statistically significant and independent associations with ORR, PFS, and OS in pembrolizumab-treated patients with advanced melanoma in KEYNOTE-006 (Table 45.2).[139] Higher response rates and survival outcomes have also been reported among patients with high TMB with atezolimab.[140] In HNSCC, TMB was independently predictive of response to pembrolizumab in patients with HNSCC, regardless of human papillomavirus status.[141]

Interaction Between Programmed Death Ligand 1 and Tumor Mutational Burden

In advanced UC, an association has been documented between PD-L1 inhibition with atezolizumab and mutation load, as assessed by molecular TCGA (The Cancer Genome Atlas) subtypes.[9] In this study, adding mutation load into a model based on PD-L1 IC staining improved the association with response to atezolizumab, indicating that these two biomarkers are independent and potentially complementary. In KEYNOTE-006, tTMB showed a low but statistically significant correlation with PD-L1 (0.22; p = .001) in patients with advanced melanoma (Table 45.3).[139]

The low but significant association between these two biomarkers highlights the complex biology and influence of TC intrinsic and extrinsic signaling mechanisms that ultimately define these tumors and their response to ICI therapy.[146] Whether high TMB and high PD-L1 represent independent mechanisms or whether they represent different stages of a single cascade must be further investigated.

CONCLUSION

ICIs are the dominant class of immunotherapy agents with robust clinical association of biomarkers with patient outcomes. The clinical development field has rapidly evolved from signal generation for monotherapy agents to signal generation in combination with standard of care (e.g., chemotherapy, vascular endothelial growth factor-targeted therapies) and/or other classes of immunotherapy agents (e.g., immune modulators, cytokines, neoantigen vaccines). There are presently thousands of combinations of checkpoint inhibitor therapies being tested across a large number of cancer types in both solid and hematologic malignancies. The future for clinical development and patient care will depend on expanding benefiting patients with combination therapies, and properly identifying those patients most likely to benefit from a given therapy alone or in combination. Having access to and publication of monotherapy data across diseases has thus been a cornerstone in the design of next-generation trials for combinations. Thus, the validation and refinement of biomarkers that optimize ICI therapy have been increasingly important to enable rational and biology-driven personalization of specific treatment regimens. Future research will focus on identifying biomarkers of acquired resistance to ICIs, which will hopefully fuel the next generation of targets and inform combination strategies in patients.

ACKNOWLEDGMENTS

Funding for this review was provided by Merck Sharp and Dohme Corp., a subsidary of Merck & Co., Inc., Kenilworth, NJ, USA. Medical writing and/or editorial assistance was provided by Kathleen Richards, PhD, Holly C. Cappelli, PhD, CMPP, and Dana Francis, PhD, of ApotheCom (Yardley, PA, USA). This assistance was funded by Merck Sharp & Dohme Corp, a subsidiary of Merck & Co., Inc., Kenilworth, NJ, USA.

KEY REFERENCES

Only key references appear in the print edition. The full reference list appears in the digital product on Springer Publishing Connect: connect.springerpub.com/content/book/978-0-8261-3743-2/part/part03/chapter/ch45

5. Taube JM, Klein A, Brahmer JR, et al. Association of PD-1, PD-1 ligands, and other features of the tumor immune microenvironment with response to anti-PD-1 therapy. *Clin Cancer Res.* 2014;20(19):5064–5074. doi:10.1158/1078-0432.CCR-13-3271

19. Cristescu R, Mogg R, Ayers M, et al. Pan-tumor genomic biomarkers for PD-1 checkpoint blockade-based immunotherapy. *Science.* 2018;362(6411):362. doi:10.1126/science.aar3593

32. Tsao MS, Kerr KM, Kockx M, et al. PD-L1 immunohistochemistry comparability study in real-life clinical samples: results of blueprint Phase 2 project. *J Thorac Oncol.* 2018;13(9):1302–1311. doi:10.1016/j.jtho.2018.05.013

86. Le DT, Durham JN, Smith KN, et al. Mismatch repair deficiency predicts response of solid tumors to PD-1 blockade. *Science.* 2017;357(6349):409–413. doi:10.1126/science.aan6733

106. Alexandrov LB, Nik-Zainal S, Wedge DC, et al. Signatures of mutational processes in human cancer. *Nature.* 2013;500(7463):415–421. doi:10.1038/nature12477

127. Rizvi NA, Cho BC, Reinmuth N, et al. Durvalumab with or without tremelimumab vs standard chemotherapy in first-line treatment of metastatic non-small cell lung cancer: the MYSTIC Phase 3 randomized clinical trial. *JAMA Oncol.* 2020;6(5):661–674. doi:10.1001/jamaoncol.2020.0237

133. Marabelle A, Fakih M, Lopez J, et al. Association of tumour mutational burden with outcomes in patients with advanced solid tumours treated with pembrolizumab: prospective biomarker analysis of the multicohort, open-label, Phase 2 KEYNOTE-158 study. *Lancet Oncol.* 2020;21(10):1353–1365. doi:10.1016/S1470-2045(20)30445-9

46

Tumor Microenvironment Metabolism as a Primordial Checkpoint in Antitumor T Cell Immunity

Greg M. Delgoffe

KEY POINTS

- Tumor cells become metabolically deregulated to support their unrestrained proliferation.

- The type and degree of metabolic deregulation can be variable between patients and cancer types.

- T cells have considerable metabolic needs for activation and persistence.

- The metabolic landscape of the tumor microenvironment is detrimental to immune function.

- Different subsets of T cells have distinct metabolic requirements.

- Alterations of T cell and tumor cell metabolism can modulate immune activity and enhance immunotherapeutic response.

INTRODUCTION

It is now clear that the immune system is not oblivious to the initiation and progression of cancer and, in fact, can stimulate T cells with very high affinity for tumor-associated antigens. These T cells are capable of being re-invigorated through exogenous manipulations, such as blockade of co-inhibitory "checkpoint" molecules (like programmed death 1/PD-1), cytokine administration, oncolytic viruses, and vaccination, resulting in durable antitumor immunity and regression. However, the fact remains that the majority of patients that receive immunotherapies do not respond or receive little benefit.

The heterogeneity of patient responses and current lack of true predictive biomarkers, while frustrating, suggest that the resistance to immunotherapies like PD-1 blockade may not be due to alterations in treatment efficacy. These resistances may be due to patient-specific variabilities like single nucleotide polymorphisms (SNPs) in immune, inflammatory, or chemotactic genes or environmental-specific factors like obesity, age, or, more likely, tumor-specific variabilities.

The ability of tumor cells to continuously mutate and evolve in a Darwinian fashion underlies many of their more insidious traits: metastasis, altered differentiation of stromal tissue, and, indeed, immune evasion. As tumor cells evolve they can produce antigen-loss variants, become defective in antigen presentation, upregulate ligands for co-inhibitory receptors, secrete immunosuppressive cytokines like TGF-β and IL-10, induce T cell death, and recruit regulatory populations like regulatory T cells and myeloid-derived suppressor cells.[1] Many of these evolved traits are even further enhanced by contact with the immune system, for instance, the upregulation of PD-L1 in response to interferons.[2] However, none of these potential immune escape mechanisms fully explain the heterogeneity of patient responses, suggesting that other, more nonimmunologic mechanisms may be at play.

DEREGULATED METABOLISM AS A KEY HALLMARK OF TUMOR CELLS

Otto Heinrich Warburg was a German biochemist who made a number of seminal discoveries regarding carbohydrate metabolism in malignancy.[3] The one with which he is perhaps most well known was the demonstration that tumor cells fermented a heightened level of imported glucose into lactic acid rather than oxidize it in the mitochondria.[3] Lactic acid production in mammalian cells is generally a feedback effect, induced when oxygen is limited in the environment, but tumor cells were discovered to do this even in the presence of oxygen. This phenomenon was thus termed "aerobic glycolysis" or the "Warburg effect" and has been the subject of much study for several decades.[4] Respiration, the process by which pyruvate is converted into acetyl-CoA, driving the TCA cycle to produce reducing intermediates for oxidative phosphorylation (OXPHOS)-mediated production of ATP, is commonly considered to be much more bioenergetically favorable as more ATP is produced per molecule of pyruvate. This has left many wondering why tumor cells would adapt this seemingly unfavorable metabolic phenotype. However, cytosolic fermentation of lactate through lactate dehydrogenase (LDH) has many considerable advantages, especially in a glucose-rich environment or, in the case of a tumor, a cell that outcompetes others for glucose.[4] First, LDH-mediated conversion of pyruvate to lactate results requires the donation of a proton from nicotinamide adenine dinucleotide hydrogen (NADH) stores, thus regenerating NAD+ in the cytosol. Second, while, indeed, aerobic glycolysis does produce far less ATP per molecule of glucose than OXPHOS, kinetic studies have revealed that the aerobic glycolysis reaction takes place almost 100 times faster than that of TCA coupled to OXPHOS.[5] Third, upregulation of aerobic glycolysis machinery might give the cell an initial competitive advantage if oxygen eventually does become limited, a common occurrence in the tumor microenvironment.[6] Finally, and perhaps most importantly, restricting ATP production to the cytosol allows mitochondrial function to be diverted into a more anabolic state, in which TCA cycle intermediates can be used for the production of biomass like amino acids, lipids, and nucleotides, rather than oxidized for ATP generation.[7] This prevents ROS-mediated mitochondrial damage during periods of intense proliferation, among many other sorts of oxidative damage.[8] Taken together, deregulated carbohydrate metabolism is considered to be a major and common phenotype of cancer cells.

However, this is not to say that mitochondrial activity is *suppressed* in tumor cells. While many studies have focused on the bioenergetic fate of glucose, tumor cells, of course, also upregulate multiple other metabolic pathways to support their unrestrained proliferation. Amino acid uptake is increased; cancer cells upregulate several amino acid transporters and become highly dependent on glutaminolysis.[9,10] Tumor cells also become much more dependent on exogenous fatty acid uptake, as a significant proportion of their lipid metabolism is devoted to generation of new membranes.[11] This process is so highly upregulated that the cell represses activity of several desaturase enyzmes, rendering the cancer cell dependent on unsaturated fatty acids and causing a build-up of saturated fats in tumor cells and their microenvironment.[11]

Taken together, a wide variety of studies suggests that a major component of the phenotype of cancer is metabolic deregulation (Figure 46.1). While this has, of course, important implications for the cancer cells themselves, this metabolic state contributes to the generation of a local area of relatively dearth metabolic conditions and the formation of the tumor microenvironment.

METABOLIC FEATURES OF THE TUMOR MICROENVIRONMENT

As mentioned previously, the altered metabolism of tumor cells benefits the tumor in many ways. Intratumoral metabolic heterogeneity ensures that at least some part of the tumor will be successful and find a fuel source that it can use and deplete, while hypoxic regions can protect cancer stem cells and prevent terminal differentiation.[12,13] However, the local depletion of nutrients can have a wide-reaching effect on the microenvironment, including alterations in stromal cell metabolism, altered angiogenesis, and inhibition of tumor-infiltrating leukocyte function.

Cancer cells upregulate high levels of glucose transporters, especially GLUTs 1 and 3, as well as maintain these transmembrane proteins' trafficking to the cell surface.[13] Most cancer cells also upregulate several key rate-limiting enzymes in the glycolytic pathway, including several isoforms of hexokinase, phosphofructokinase, phosphoglycerate mutase, and pyruvate kinase M2.[12] Cancer cells also utilize glucose metabolites for nucleotide synthesis through the pentose phosphate pathway, as well as utilize glucose-derived carbon for the generation of fatty acids used in membrane synthesis.[4] It is this persistent hunger for glucose that enables the use of the FDG tracer for PET imaging. Thus, among all available fuel sources, glucose remains tumor cells' primary one and as such is present in extraordinarily low concentrations in the tumor microenvironment.

That dependence (and preference) for glucose and subsequent aerobic glycolysis also engender the tumor microenvironment with another metabolic feature. As pyruvate is converted into lactate, NADH is converted to NAD+, which generates a proton. This proton is used to shuttle lactate across the plasma membrane through the monocarboxylate transporter (MCT), secreting the lactate and proton and acidifying the extracellular space.[14] Thus, the tumor microenvironment is markedly acidic. Apart from high levels of lactate ion (nearly 50 mM at tumor cores), studies utilizing pH biosensors or even more direct measurements (pH probes inserted into tumors) reveal, indeed, that the pH of the interstitial space in tumors can be as low as 6.5, endangering a considerable amount of extracellular chemistry and preventing uptake of molecules that are coupled to pH gradients.[15,16]

While tumor cells do perform glycolytic metabolism preferentially, a common myth is that glycolysis occurs at the expense of the mitochondria. However, it is likely more accurate that a heightened proportion of glucose gets fermented to lactate (55%–60%, by most measurements), and in fact, it is quite appropriate to say that tumor cells remain extraordinarily oxidative.[4] Indeed, tumor cells have high mitochondrial mass and perform significant levels of oxidative phosphorylation. Thus,

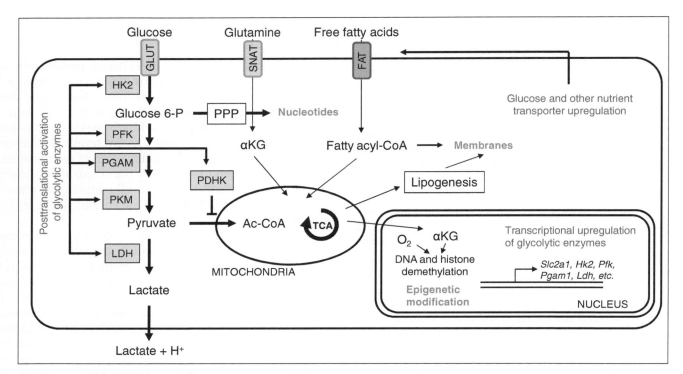

Figure 46.1 Deregulated metabolism as a common phenotype of cancer cells. Cancer cells develop several metabolic adaptations to support their unrestrained proliferation. Aerobic glycolysis is promoted through the transcriptional deregulation of glucose and nutrient transporters and several key glycolytic enzymes as noted. In addition, oncogenic signaling can promote post-translational activation of glycolytic enzymes as well. Tumor cells meet their metabolic needs by utilizing the pentose phosphate pathway (PPP) to generate nucleotides, generating membranes through lipogenesis, and making epigenetic changes like DNA and histone demethylation.

Ac-CoA, acetyl-CoA; aKG, alpha ketogluratate; FAT, fatty acid transporter; HK, hexokinase; LDH, lactate dehydrogenase; PDHK, pyruvate dehydrogenase kinase; PFK, phosphofructokinase; PGAM, phosphoglycerate mutase; PKM, pyruvate kinase M; SNAT, sodium-coupled neutral amino acid transporter; TCA, tricarboxylic acid cycle.

it is becoming clearer that oxygen, too, is an essential metabolite that is outcompeted by tumor cells. That, coupled to deregulated and tortuous angiogenesis, induced through aberrant VEGF signaling, results in areas of extreme hypoxia (1%–2% O_2),[17] far lower than typical hypoxia seen in other inflamed tissues, or in regions that have local hypoxia-like kidneys or bone marrow.

Amino acids represent another pool of essential metabolites that have altered levels in the tumor microenvironment. Glutamine, essential for tumor cell metabolism, is heavily depleted in the tumor microenvironment, whereas glutamate is observed at higher levels in the tumor.[18] Tryptophan and arginine are also depleted actively by both tumor cells and certain suppressive myeloid cell populations through indoleamine 2,3-dioxygenase (IDO) and arginase activity, respectively.[19] Importantly, not only do these suppressive enzymes deplete these critical amino acids from the environment, but the reaction products (tryptophan catabolites like kynurenine and arginine metabolites ornithine and urea) can be heavily immunosuppressive on their own.

T CELL ACTIVATION AND METABOLISM

Prior to recognition of their cognate antigen, naïve T cells must persist for a lifetime in a state of relative quiescence, really only dividing homeostatically when stroma-derived IL-7 signals build-up in the secondary lymphoid organs. These cells are small, having very little cytoplasm, extraordinarily condensed chromatin, and having no discernible function other than simply surviving. However, once a naïve T cell's TCR recognizes its antigen in the context of co-stimulation, a number of very important changes take place. Calcium and lipid-based second messengers activate nuclear factor of activated T cells (NFAT) and AP-1 to initiate transcription of activation-induced genes.[20] The cell rapidly enters a growth phase, synthesizing new membranes, organelles, and nucleotides to prepare for cell division.[7] Chromatin remodeling is initiated, allowing for rapid transcription and DNA replication.[21] And, after a period of around 24 hours, the cell begins undergoing extremely rapid proliferation, averaging cell cycles of around 4 to 6 hours.[22] After a number of divisions, the cell also begins secreting cytokines and, in the case of CD8+ T cells, forming cytotoxic granules that will be used to induce cell death in target cells.

This rapid shift in cellular functionality, from extreme quiescence to extreme activity, is not without cost. Synthesis of membranes requires new fatty acid synthesis. DNA replication requires nucleotide synthesis. Chromatin modification requires post-translational histone and DNA modifications by acetyl groups and other short-carbon chains. Cytokine and granule genes must be transcribed and translated. Cellular motility requires dynamic actin reorganization. Central to all of these processes is metabolism. As such, the bioenergetic demands of an activated, effector T cell are extraordinarily high.[7,22,23]

It was noted, before the cloning of the T cell receptor or MHC restriction, that phytohemaglutanin-stimulated lymphocytes changed the way they metabolized sugars. Even in cell culture with abundant oxygen, the lymphocytes would ferment glucose into lactic acid rather than oxidize it in the mitochondria.[24] While the importance of these pathways in cellular fate and function would not be fully recognized for another 30 years, this initial discovery, that T lymphocytes also performed Warburg metabolism upon activation, paved the way for an entire field of "immunometabolism" research.

METABOLIC REGULATION OF T CELL EFFECTOR FUNCTION AND FATE

Not long after the discovery of T cell glycolysis, several studies utilized the newly developed chromium release assay to measure metabolic control of T cell function, which revealed that while glucose was important for T cell proliferation, it was largely dispensable for T cell cytolysis.[25] However, the exploration of metabolism as a mediator of immune cell activity sat relatively dormant until advances in genetic and flow cytometric analysis would be able to answer some of these questions. Activated T cells upregulate glucose transporters, ensure surface trafficking of said transporters, and upregulate much of the glycolytic machinery, much of this through Akt activation.[26-30] Recent studies utilizing extracellular flux analysis have revealed just how important glycolysis is and that T cells begin diverting glucose to lactic acid production very rapidly upon activation.[31-33] The so-called switch to glycolysis is a multi-step process, orchestrated by molecules like Myc, HIF1a, Akt, mTOR, and the pyruvate carrier inhibitor PDHK1.[8]

Glycolysis in T cells has been shown to be important for many important T cell functions, not merely proliferation. T cells require glycolysis for calcium flux, effector T cell expansion, glycosylation of several signaling intermediates, and the avoidance of tolerogenic programs like anergy.[22,34] The notion that the "moonlighting" functions of many glycolytic enzymes as RNA binding

proteins, known for many years in the cancer field, has important roles in the elaboration of effector cytokines has brought this metabolic pathway to the front and center of much of the focus in T cell biology.[35] Indeed, the dehydrogenase enzymes GAPDH and LDH have been shown to bind the 3' UTR of cytokine mRNA and inhibit translation when metabolically inactive.[33,35] In this way, glycolysis enables the translation and synthesis of cytokine upon T cell activation.

Importantly, as in all cells that perform Warburg metabolism, it is important to remember that glycolysis does not proceed at the expense of mitochondrial metabolism, and, in fact, T cells upregulate OXPHOS pathways after activation as well. More recently, mitochondria have also been studied as not only energy producers but key nodes in cellular fate and function in lymphocytes. Mitochondrial metabolism is sufficient to maintain the survival of quiescent cells, a key point for naïve T cells, which prefer these pathways for their minimal activity and occasional homeostatic division.[31] As these naïve cells receive a homeostatic signal, specifically IL-7 stimulation, they upregulate the glucose transporter GLUT1 as a means to fuel that relatively minor expansion.[36,37] However, after an effector response, T cells enter a memory phase, during which they contract back into quiescence, but are prepared, both quantitatively and qualitatively, to respond again with vigor.[31] Interestingly, T cells shift their metabolic preferences during this memory phase, back from aerobic glycolysis to more OXPHOS-mediated events.[7] Importantly, during the memory transition, T cells also upregulate mitochondrial capacity, such that memory T cells have more and "better" mitochondria.[31] This is thought to bioenergetically "prime" them for reactivation such that they are ready to enter the effector phase upon re-exposure to antigen. This also confers longevity and stemness to this memory T cell. Thus, both mitochondrial and nonmitochondrial energy production are inherently important to all phases of the T cell immune response.

NUTRIENT SENSING IN CONTROL OF T CELL FATE AND FUNCTION

Every somatic cell has some form of nutrient-sensing mechanism. This is important for almost all cellular activity: a cell does not want to translate protein, replicate DNA, make membrane, and divide if there are not sufficient nutrients in the environment to do so. However, with a few notable exceptions, most somatic cells can afford to be lost; a fibroblast will be replaced by its neighbor, and a neutrophil has billions of brethren waiting to be deployed. However, even at the naïve state, a T cell represents the product of a number of life or death decisions that have generated a functional T cell receptor that is specific for non-self peptide with self MHC. A lot of energy has gone into making that clone, and the immune system does not want to lose it due to some perturbations in nutrient availability. Thus, during evolution, T cells have conscripted the nutrient-sensing machinery to make more than simply growth and death decisions and instead have utilized nutrient sensors to dictate complex fate decisions.[38]

In addition to the energetic studies of lymphocytes in the 1970s, the discovery of the macrolide antibiotic rapamycin and its pharmacologic target mTOR had a major impact in the field of immunometabolism.[39,40] Mechanistically, rapamycin binding to FKBP12 promotes the dissociation of mTOR and raptor, one of its adaptor proteins. Biochemical analysis of mTOR in rapamycin-treated cells also revealed the existence of a distinct second complex.[41] Thus, mTOR signaling can occur through two protein complexes, mTORC1 and mTORC2. mTOR acts as a nutrient sensor in most cells, tying together signals from a diverse array of extracellular and intracellular signaling pathways, including energy charge, insulin, cytokines, lipid intermediates, and activation signals. mTOR's level of activation then dictates, through downstream substrates, whether cells will translate protein, initiate ribosome biogenesis, engage lipolysis pathways, or activate the autophagic mechanisms of the cell.[38]

Although a poor antifungal agent, it was soon noted after its discovery that rapamycin was a potent immunosuppressive molecule.[42] However, unlike other potent immunosuppressant molecules like cyclosporine A/FK506, the effects of rapamycin were not acute: they did not result in inhibition of T cell activation, but rather promoted a long-term state of tolerance.[43] Thus, rapamycin and its derivatives are now commonly used to promote graft tolerance and have been shown to promote long-term bone marrow chimerism.[44-46]

Inhibition of mTOR by rapamycin during activation results in anergy, a hyporesponsive state induced when T cells see antigen in the absence of co-stimulatory context.[47] This led many to believe that mTOR may function as a signal integrator for co-stimulation. Genetic deletion of mTOR in T cells, however, revealed that T cells require mTOR activation as a third signal to escape from quiescence and acquire an effector phenotype. CD4+ T cells stimulated in the presence of high doses of rapamycin or when mTOR has been deleted acquire a regulatory phenotype, becoming potently suppressive and expressing Foxp3. Thus, mTOR plays a role in acquiring an effector phenotype.[48]

Interestingly, though, is that mTOR inhibition, like most pathways involved in metabolism, is not merely a switch, and since its discovery has been shown to have a complex role in immune cell fate and function. In 2008, Ahmed and colleagues described a role for mTOR in the effector versus memory response of CD8+ T cells.[49] Interestingly, when mice were treated with very low doses of rapamycin during acute infection, they generated a superior memory response. This is consistent with the idea that at these low doses, mTORC1 is targeted, while mTORC2 is spared.[50] However, mTOR must be dynamically regulated to achieve effector fates, as genetic evidence has shown that, indeed, while mTORC1 deletion in CD8+ T cells results in a poor effector response and enhanced memory differentiation, those memory cells require mTOR to re-engage a recall response.[51]

Deletion of the specific mTOR complexes indeed has shown that mTORC1 and mTORC2 have dynamic regulation of CD4+ T cell fate, such that mTORC2 is dispensable for Th1 and Th17 differentiation.[50] mTORC1, required for inflammatory Th1 and Th17 cells, is dispensable for generation of type 2 immunity.[50] Only through inhibition of both complexes does regulatory T cell differentiation occur.[50]

While mTOR is a dominant nutrient-sensing kinase in T cells, other nutrient sensors play important roles in T cell fate and function. Myc, a transcription factor associated with metabolic reprogramming and glycolysis, is dynamically regulated upon T cell activation and licenses glycolysis and glutaminolysis to occur.[52] It coordinates with mTOR and HIF1α to reprogram T cells for that short-lived effector metabolism associated with rapid proliferation.[52] AMPK, a sensor for energy charge (AMP/ATP balance) in cells, acts to negatively regulate the mTOR machinery as well as program mitochondrial biogenesis and oxidative metabolism.[53] AMPK-deficient T cells make poor memory and regulatory cells, suggesting AMPK acts as a balance to mTOR.[53] Taken together, the wealth of immunologic data on these critical kinases suggests that nutrient sensing not only acutely controls activation and metabolism in immunity but can have long-term effects on T cell function.

T CELL HYPORESPONSIVE PHENOTYPES AND THEIR METABOLIC LINKS

There are many ways in which T cells can be rendered hyporesponsive, probably more than we can adequately identify and measure. In many cases, T cell hyporesponsiveness is a desired trait; a T cell that has escaped central tolerance responds to some self-antigen in the periphery. As it avoids deletion, it still may be a useful clone if a pathogen shares that epitope, but the body does not want to risk autoimmune damage, so the T cell has cell-intrinsic programming to self-regulate: this is referred to as anergy.[22]

Clonal anergy was originally described by Jenkins and Schwartz as a means by which T cells might be rendered inert by self-peptide.[54] TCR ligation occurring in the absence of co-stimulation (canonically CD28 signaling) results in a transcriptional program driven, in part, by NFAT in the absence of AP-1.[55] This program activates negative regulators of T cell signaling, represses metabolic machinery, and inhibits IL-2 translation.[56]

Another form of T cell dysfunction is senescence, which can occur from chronic signaling as well as in aging. Senescent T cells lose their reactivity to the TCR, downregulate co-stimulatory molecules, and have short telomeres.[57] Importantly, these T cells do not necessarily fail to function but rather lose sensitivity to the TCR and can secrete low-level cytokines in a more continuous fashion.

Probably the most "pathologic" of these hyporesponsive phenotypes is one driven not by lack of signaling but through persistent inflammatory signaling. Originally described in chronic viral infection,[58] T cell exhaustion results in a failure to secrete cytokines, proliferate effectively, or lyse target cells.[59] Exhaustion has been extensively studied in the mouse in the lymphochloriomeningitis virus model, but it has become increasingly apparent that the persistent activation associated with cancer also promotes an exhausted phenotype.[60] These studies in T cell exhaustion revealed that as T cells become chronically stimulated, they upregulate co-inhibitory checkpoint molecules like PD-1, LAG-3, and TIM-3, which act both as markers of chronic activation and also inhibitors of T cell activation.[59] Blockade of these molecules or their ligands can reinvigorate T cells in cancer and chronic viral infection.[61,62] Importantly, though, these inhibitory receptors do not outright *cause* T cell exhaustion; T cells deficient in PD-1, for example, still develop an exhausted phenotype.[63] Rather, there are basic processes that underlie T cell exhaustion and PD-1, and other co-inhibitory molecules may simply enforce the phenotype.

Interestingly, these phenotypes of T cell hyporesponsiveness, while having alternative initiating events, have similar metabolic characteristics.[22] Anergic T cells, despite being previously activated, fail to upregulate the metabolic machinery associated with effector T cells—glucose, iron, and amino acid transporters—and demonstrate lower glycolytic output.[64] Senescent T cells have low-level glycolysis continuously, consistent with their lack of TCR reactivity and their constant low-level cytokine production.[57,65] This may be induced by mitochondrial dysfunction, as *Tfam* deficiency can promote T cell senescence in mouse models.[66] The metabolic underpinnings of T cell exhaustion have been most heavily studied in recent years. Several groups have shown exhausted T cells have impaired glucose metabolism and oxidative function, and repressed mitochondrial activity and capacity.[67–69] Notably, more recent data suggest that mitochondrial dysfunction, induced through a number of pathologic signals, likely causes the exhausted T cell phenotype.[70,71] Thus,

these data strongly suggest that metabolism plays a key and central role in T cell function and dysfunction. To truly harness the immune response to cancer, we must identify and mitigate these metabolic checkpoints to allow for unrestrained immunity in the tumor microenvironment.

IMPLICATIONS FOR EFFECTIVE ANTITUMOR IMMUNITY AND IMPROVEMENTS IN IMMUNOTHERAPY

Having understood that the metabolism plays a key and central role in T cell fate, function, and dysfunction, how do these pathways intersect when T cells infiltrate the tumor microenvironment and attempt to carry out an antitumor immune response?

A major driver of this type of "metabolic exhaustion" is competition. T cell metabolic uptake and downstream function, while highly upregulated, are not *de*regulated.[72] Tumor cells are larger, express higher levels of most metabolite transporters, and thus, in most competitive assays, will actively sequester most usable carbon sources. Thus, the energetic potential to carry out an immune response represents another, more primordial type of checkpoint that T cells must overcome in order to effectively carry out an immune response. This has been shown in a number of ways, as those interested in T cell metabolism began applying that study to the tumor microenvironment. First, tumors resistant to immunotherapy tend to take up more glucose, while sensitive tumor models are more metabolically quiescent.[73] T cells that infiltrate tumors cannot compete for glucose, and this loss of glycolytic function can inhibit calcium signaling and subsequent effector function.[74] Extracellular flux analysis has enabled these analyses directly from patient samples, identifying that oxidative metabolism and subsequent generation of hypoxia play a critical role in resistance to anti-PD1 immunotherapy.[75] Additionally, anti-PDL1 treatment of responding tumors can also act to alter the glycolytic function of tumor cells, which suggests that PD-1 blockade works, in part, by altering metabolic competition.[73]

However, in addition to metabolic competition in situ, the very nature of T cell dysfunction in tumor responses may also metabolically cripple the T cell. A T cell has no context when it is responding to antigen; it is merely integrating signals from the environment.[76] As such, it has no sense of the duration, scope, or persistence of activation signals. This is thought to be a major driver of T cell exhaustion in chronic viral infections, and similar phenotypes can be found in cancer cells, especially those of high affinity for tumor antigens.[77–79] As activation drives glycolysis, and the cessation of activation signals promotes mitochondrial biogenesis and activation, an antitumor response, by its persistent nature, actively represses mitochondrial function, which could allow for metabolic plasticity in the tumor microenvironment and upregulates the machinery required to use glycolysis, requiring a fuel which is in the lowest supply.[73] It has been shown that this is indeed the case; tumor-specific T cells in the tumor microenvironment actively repress mitochondrial biogenesis and show decreases in mitochondrial activity and mass, creating a dependence on glycolysis.[68] This is dependent on chronic Akt signaling, which drives down the expression of the mitochondrial biogenesis factor PGC1α.[68] Indeed, it is persistent signaling that alters the metabolic plasticity of T cells, which creates metabolic vulnerabilities and the generation of dysfunctional mitochondria that produce ROS.[69–71] Antioxidant approaches can alleviate T cell exhaustion and promote responses to immunotherapy. Similar results have been found in chronic viral infection, suggesting that there are at least two metabolic checkpoints to overcome: competition in the microenvironment as well as T cell-intrinsic metabolic insufficiency (Figure 46.2).[67]

Not all T cells are functionally crippled in the tumor microenvironment, most notably Foxp3-expressing regulatory T cells (T_{reg} cells). T_{reg} cells are extremely active in cancer, being highly overrepresented in tumors but also being highly proliferative. Thus, T_{reg} cells may possess metabolic proclivities that allow them to thrive within tumors. Indeed, T_{reg} cells eschew glucose metabolism in favor of other sources of carbon, rendering them insensitive to the metabolic insufficiencies in the tumor microenvironment.[80,81] T_{reg} cells have been shown to rely both on fatty acid sources as well as metabolic byproducts like lactic acid, which allow them to thrive in the tumor microenvironment.[82,83] In this way, tumors evade immune destruction not only by starving antitumor immunity but also by feeding suppressor populations.

How can we overcome these metabolic checkpoints to improve cancer therapy? Do more precise ways exist to hinder the metabolism of tumor cells or bolster the metabolism of T cells in a specific manner? Can you tip the energetic balance in favor of antitumor immunity?

As one of the major drivers of metabolic inhibition in the tumor microenvironment is competition, one could envision a scenario in which tumor cell metabolism is targeted. Previous clinical attempts at this have not been successful, as many of these metabolic inhibitors also affect other cells: stromal cells, vasculature, and immune cells. Thus, these therapies can sometimes end up being a zero-sum game. However, advances in understanding the pharmacodynamics of certain inhibitors as well as specific tumor cell targeting mechanisms may reinvigorate some of these strategies. First, as the tumor cell outcompetes other cells for nearly every other substrate, any drug that requires transport rather than passive diffusion is likely to affect the tumor cell first as well as more potently. For instance, it has been demonstrated that the mitochondrial complex I inhibitor metformin can synergize and enable checkpoint blockade immunotherapy in murine models.[84] Second, direct targeting to the tumor cell may be a strategy for delivering metabolic inhibition: this could be done through antibody targeting strategies, tumor-specific moieties, or even through more complex approaches like oncolytic, tumor-targeting viruses. Indeed, oncolytic viruses, as they infect tumor cells, can be engineered to deliver genetic cargo (the FDA-approved T-VEC, for instance, also encodes GM-CSF). Indeed, this genetic cargo can be metabolic

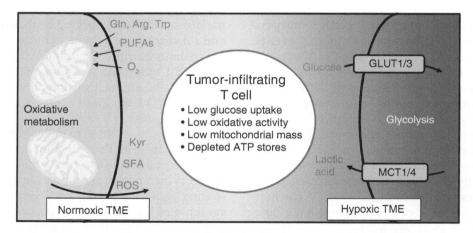

Figure 46.2 **The tumor microenvironment imposes metabolic checkpoints on tumor-infiltrating T cells.** Whether individual areas of a tumor are normoxic (left) or hypoxic (right), the deregulated metabolism of the tumor cells and alterations to surrounding stroma create metabolic competition for the T cell. This can have long-term inhibitory effects on T cell fate, as well as immediately inhibit T cell function.

ATP, adenosine triphosphate; Gln, Arg, Trp, glutamine, arginine, tryptophan; GLUT, glucose transporter; Kyr, kynurenine; MCT, monocarboxylate transporter; PUFAs, polyunsaturated fatty acids; ROS, reactive oxygen species; SFA, saturated fatty acids; TME, tumor microenvironment.

in nature, and encoding the gene for leptin in an oncolytic virus can dramatically reprogram the metabolism of tumor-infiltrating T cells.[85]

Of course, another way to alleviate these metabolic checkpoints would be to metabolically reprogram the T cell itself. This might not only repair cell-intrinsic defects but also arm the T cell to be more metabolically fit in the nutrient-poor microenvironment. Bolstering mitochondrial metabolism through PGC1α-mediated metabolic reprogramming results in superior antitumor function,[68,86] similar to studies using PCK1-mediated reprogramming done by the Kaech group.[74] Chimeric antigen receptor T cells, which are virally redirected to the tumor site, seem like the first and most obvious application of this type of amplification, although drugs designed at bolstering mitochondrial metabolism, in general, might synergize well with other types of immunotherapy in vivo. Further, we have learned that engaging lost co-stimulatory pathways, like the TNFR family member 4-1BB, can promote mitochondrial biogenesis and enable T cell responses.[87,88] Importantly, understanding the defects in these tumor-infiltrating T cells may allow us to also harvest and culture them more effectively ex vivo, resulting in a superior T cell productive for adoptive TIL therapy.

CONCLUSION

The intersection of metabolism and bioenergetics with immunity has garnered much recent interest. It is now clear from work done in metabolic pathway regulation that T cells have extraordinary metabolic needs and utilize nutrient sensors to divert and shape effective immunity for the host. However, these links are not trivial nor academic in nature: T cell function can be inhibited or improved through modulation of metabolism. As T cells enter the tumor microenvironment, chronic activation and inflammation drive them to engage an unsustainable immune response: There is simply not enough fuel in the environment to feed their function, at least with how they are programmed at baseline. Strategies to remodel the environment or bioenergetically arm the T cell have the potential to not only improve existing immunotherapies but to evolve into new therapies for the treatment of cancer.

KEY REFERENCES

Only key references appear in the print edition. The full reference list appears in the digital product on Springer Publishing Connect: connect.springerpub.com/content/book/978-0-8261-3743-2/part/part03/chapter/ch46

7. Pearce EL, Poffenberger MC, Chang CH, Jones RG. Fueling immunity: insights into metabolism and lymphocyte function. *Science*. 2013;342(6155):1242454. doi:10.1126/science.1242454

31. van der Windt GJ, O'Sullivan D, Everts B, et al. CD8 memory T cells have a bioenergetic advantage that underlies their rapid recall ability. *Proc Natl Acad Sci USA*. 2013;110(35):14336–14341. doi:10.1073/pnas.1221740110

38. Pollizzi KN, Powell JD. Integrating canonical and metabolic signalling programmes in the regulation of T cell responses. *Nat Rev Immunol*. 2014;14(7):435–446. doi:10.1038/nri3701

68. Scharping NE, Menk AV, Moreci RS, et al. The tumor microenvironment represses T cell mitochondrial biogenesis to drive intratumoral T cell metabolic insufficiency and dysfunction. *Immunity*. 2016;45(2):374–388. doi:10.1016/j.immuni.2016.07.009

73. Chang CH, Qiu J, O'Sullivan D, et al. Metabolic competition in the tumor microenvironment is a driver of cancer progression. *Cell*. 2015;162(6):1229–1241. doi:10.1016/j.cell.2015.08.016

82. Angelin A, Gil-de-Gómez L, Dahiya S, et al. Foxp3 reprograms T cell metabolism to function in low-glucose, high-lactate environments. *Cell Metab*. 2017;25(6):1282–1293. doi:10.1016/j.cmet.2016.12.018

Age-Related Immune Function Changes as They Relate to Cancer Immunotherapy

Graham Pawelec and Emilie Picard

KEY POINTS

- Increasing evidence suggests that older adult patients with advanced melanoma treated by checkpoint blockade have better response rates and toxicity profiles than younger patients, and the same may be true for other solid cancers as well.

- Response rates to checkpoint blockade are still much less than 100%, and it remains possible that immune aging ("immunosenescence") may contribute to nonresponsiveness in some older adult patients.

- T cell memory responses to shared tumor-associated antigens (TAA) such as NY-ESO-1 and Melan-A are retained in older patients, but responses to neoantigens may be compromised because of the contracted T cell receptor (TCR) repertoire and low numbers of naïve T cells in the older adult.

- Fewer regulatory T cells may infiltrate tumor deposits in older individuals, resulting in less suppression of TAA-specific CD8+ memory T cells.

- When examining parameters of immunity in humans, the effects of age must be distinguished from those of infection with the common β-herpes virus HHV5 (cytomegalovirus [CMV]).

- CMV primarily drives the accumulation of late-differentiated memory cells, especially CD27−CD28−CD57+CD45RA+ T cells, but the loss of naïve cells also occurs in CMV-negative individuals.

- Thus far, however, there is little evidence that CMV infection influences the outcome of cancer immunotherapy.

INTRODUCTION

The efficacy of immunotherapy for multiple solid tumor types using immunomodulatory antibodies for checkpoint blockade depends to a large extent on the freeing of preexisting or newly emerging tumor-specific T cell immunity from the physiological feedback inhibition exploited by cancers to suppress antitumor activity. Evidence that has accumulated over the years strongly suggests that most or all cancer therapies depend for their optimal success on the presence of a functioning immune system to maintain the disease in a chronic state or eliminate it entirely. An important prerequisite for the success of cancer immunotherapy and quite possibly all cancer therapy is the presence in the patient of cells of the adaptive immune arm, primarily T cells, that are able to migrate to, recognize, and control the tumor. Many tumor escape mechanisms have been identified, ranging from downregulation of target antigens to allow cancers to hide from the immune system, to multiple active mechanisms that inhibit local and even systemic immunity. One potential escape mechanism that is now beginning to be considered more widely is whether the perceived waning of immune competence with increasing age (dubbed "immunosenescence")[1] also plays a role in tumor escape.[2] Data from younger immunosuppressed patients suggest that certain tumor types are much more common than in age-matched healthy controls, implying that age-associated immunosuppression might be having a similar negative effect. Data from the small number of animal models tested with the age question in mind are consistent with the notion that the results of cancer immunotherapy protocols in older mice are different, usually worse, than when using the same protocols in younger animals.[3-5] Nonetheless, depending on the model, there may be instances where older animals respond better than young ones.[6] Thus, it will be important to determine the reasons for such discrepant effects of age in animal models and to investigate this issue in humans. It remains possible that immunosenescence might render immunotherapy relying on checkpoint blockade or responsiveness to vaccines less effective in older patients. Additionally, given the recent advances in adoptive T cell therapies,[7] concerns arise as to whether suppressive elements in older individuals may more actively mitigate against successful outcome than in younger patients. With the advent of patient- and tumor-specific neoantigen vaccines and the renewed interest in including vaccination as part of a personalized treatment rationale, the well-accepted view that immunosenescence contributes to poorer responses also comes to the fore.

Even at the time of updating this chapter (April 2020), there still appeared to be no clinical trials of immunotherapy specifically comparing younger and older patients, and there is insufficient data so far on adoptive immunotherapy or cancer vaccination in the older adults to make any kind of statement on results in older adults relative to younger patients. However, much more experience has accumulated in the meantime, including "real-world" experience (i.e., not controlled clinical trials), to encourage the belief that specifically designed trials for the older adult are not really necessary, at least for the treatment of metastatic melanoma where there are the most data. Thus, it seems fairly clear that treatment with anticytotoxic T lymphocyte-associated protein 4 (anti-CTLA-4) antibodies and anti-programmed cell death-1 (PD-1) or programmed cell death-ligand 1 (PD-L1) results in response rates and, importantly, toxicity profiles in older patients that are fairly similar to those of the young, even in patients over 90 years of age.[8,9] There have now been sufficient melanoma patients treated to render this conclusion incontrovertible, as documented by an analysis of nearly 12,000 patients.[10,11] This probably holds not only for melanoma but for other previously intransigent tumors, such as non-small cell lung cancer (NSCLC).[12-14] A study in a real-world setting showed that PD-1/PD-L1 inhibitors were potentially more effective in NSCLC patients over 70 years of age and were associated with a better progression-free survival than in younger patients.[15] There is some evidence that the same may be true for renal cancer.[16] It is intriguing to note that a study of bladder cancer patient responses to immunotherapy with bacillus Calmette-Guerin (BCG) also showed no detrimental effects of age, although the mechanism of action of this agent is very different from checkpoint blockade.[17] It will be crucial to test whether adoptive immunotherapy is less successful in the older adult. Patients older than 65 have been treated with CD19-CAR T cells,[18] but an analysis of the effects of age has not yet appeared.

However, not all patients respond to these immunotherapies, and therefore it remains possible that immunosenescence may be contributing to nonresponsiveness, at least in some older adult individuals. What are the potential mechanisms that could explain changes to immunity with age, either with a positive or negative effect on the outcome of immunotherapy?

IMMUNOSENESCENCE

Detrimental changes to immune function with age are predominantly illustrated by the increased susceptibility of older adults to infectious disease, and the increased severity thereof. This is dramatically documented by the case fatality rate of the newly emerged Coronavirus SARS-CoV-2, which is negligible in the young but up to 20% in the oldest old. The reasons for the increased susceptibility of older adults to many infectious diseases are not exclusively immunological, but it is commonly perceived that dysregulated immunity is primarily responsible for deficient adaptive immune responses and overexuberant innate immune-inflammatory responses in older adults. How can we determine which parameters are important in determining these responses, that is, which biomarkers of immunity reflect "immunological age" rather than chronological age?

To answer this question, many studies over the years have sought to compare immune parameters in people of different ages, usually perforce by means of cross-sectional studies and accessing only peripheral blood. Comparing people currently 20 years of age with those 80 years of age reveals multiple differences in the absolute numbers, frequencies, and functions of essentially every immune parameter measurable in blood. Most susceptible appears to be T cells, especially $CD8^+$ T cells in this respect, but all other parameters have also been noted to be different. These differences are usually referred to as "age-associated changes," but formally this is merely an assumption, and one should only think in terms of differences.[19] Additionally, there are quite disparate data in the literature, which need to be interpreted with caution because of the different cohorts studied and changes to the assay technologies over the years. Given that proviso, despite enormous variation in populations studied, one hallmark feature consistently emerges throughout all studies in different populations at different times, namely, there is a markedly lower number and frequency of naïve $CD8^+$ T cells, and a slightly lower frequency of naïve $CD4^+$ T cells in the peripheral blood of older relatives to younger adults. This is hypothesized to reflect the result of exposures to immune-stimulatory challenges over the life span, mostly by pathogens but also potentially including autoantigens and cancer antigens. These antigens stimulate specific naïve cells to undergo clonal expansion, deal with the challenge, and then revert to memory cells. Because there is little or no replenishment of naïve cells due to the developmentally programmed physiological involution of the thymus starting at puberty, the amount of these naïve T cells decreases over the life span. In certain cases, we may indeed refer to "changes" rather than "differences" in naïve cells because there are instances where the change from naïve to memory can be measured in people following infection or vaccination. Reciprocal to the decrease of naïve cells, most studies have revealed larger numbers of CD8[+] late differentiation-stage memory and effector-memory T cells with age, and the appearance for the first time of CD4[+] T cells of similar late-stage phenotype (CD45RA[+]). It has recently become apparent that the accumulation of the majority of these cells is the result of infection with a single herpesvirus, cytomegalovirus (CMV), with which the majority of older adult people in many countries are infected. One of our own studies in very old breast cancer patients revealed that CMV seropositivity was associated with lower frequencies of naïve and central memory T cells and higher frequencies of effector-memory T cells re-expressing CD45RA (TEMRA) and effector-memory T cells.[20] Other clonal expansions in older people are present, but quantitatively the effect of CMV overrides all others by orders of magnitude. Why this should be the case is still unclear. What is clear is that in developing societies, essentially the whole population is infected with CMV in infancy (with corresponding changes in the peripheral distribution of T cell subsets). In contrast, in the majority of studies of age and immunity (which are of WEIRD populations, that is, Western, Educated, Industrialized, Rich, Democratic), the effect of CMV infection is a confounding factor. This is because only a fraction of the population is infected with CMV at an early age, but this increases with time at a seroconversion rate of 0.5% to 1% per annum (in Germany),[21] with a major variation according to socioeconomic factors (in the United States).[22] Hence, immune phenotyping studies that do not take this major confounding factor into account will end up measuring the effect of CMV, and not of age. The same is true to a lesser degree for assessments of other immune parameters; thus, there are more subtle differences between older and younger people for B cells, dendritic cells, polymorphs, and other innate cells, but many or most of these values are also affected by CMV. It is interesting to note that the effects of infection with CMV appear to be unique to that virus in that other common herpesviruses do not have the same effect.

Here it is important to point out that we are referring strictly to biomarkers. It is obvious that assessing parameters in the blood does not necessarily reflect the state of the entire immune system, but almost all data that we have in humans are restricted to the blood. Such biomarkers are only valuable when they closely correlate with a defined clinical outcome. Efforts to analyze such immune biomarkers and correlate them with clinical outcomes, age-associated diseases, and mortality in longitudinal studies of the same populations over many years will be required to achieve this aim. Obviously, by necessity, these studies are of long duration but are now beginning to yield valuable data; for example, the 9-year follow-up study establishing the "IMM-AGE" score[23] or the much less-sophisticated earlier OCTO/NONA studies.[24]

PERIPHERAL IMMUNE PARAMETERS CORRELATING WITH CANCER PATIENT SURVIVAL

A major hallmark of immunosenescence as previously discussed is thus low levels of naïve-phenotype CD8[+] T cells and potentially high levels of late-differentiated CD8[+] T cells in peripheral blood. However, it must also be borne in mind that these findings may be different for tissue-resident immune cells,[25] or those trafficking through lymphoid organs, but we have insufficient data thus far in humans to make firm conclusions. Nonetheless, in the cancer context, recent data render it likely that T cell clonotypes shared by TILs and peripheral blood T cells reflect the recruitment of effector cells into the tumor, suggesting that parameters measured in blood are directly relevant to immune activity within the tumor.[26] Nonetheless, at the moment, these data obtained from analyzing peripheral blood also need to be considered as biomarkers, and like any other biomarkers, they are only relevant if robustly associated with some clearly defined clinical outcome.

The accumulated high levels of CD8[+] late-differentiated T cells found in many older people do seem to be biomarkers related to mortality, but this is not the case in general for naïve cell levels, possibly because of the reservoir of naïve cells recently found in the lymph nodes. The late-stage differentiated CD8[+] T cells commonly co-express CD57 (HNK-1) as well as CD45RA, but lack or express very low levels of two major co-stimulatory receptors, CD27 and CD28. An accumulation of these cells represents one of the major parameters associated with incipient mortality at 2-, 4-, and 6-year follow-up in a southern Swedish population 85 years of age at baseline (in the OCTO/NONA studies).[24] Merely by virtue of CD28 negativity, and especially if they are also CD57[+], CD8[+] T cells of this phenotype are often referred to in the literature as "senescent." Although some of them may be, one would argue that this phenotype does not indicate senescence, but rather reflects the presence of CMV-specific, highly cytotoxic cells required to maintain essential immunosurveillance against CMV reactivation.[27] As is clear in immunosuppressed patients, the usually relatively innocuous CMV is a powerful pathogen in the absence of constant immune control. The question in the context of cancer immunotherapy then becomes whether these immune parameters, be they referred to in the literature as "senescence" markers or not, are relevant to the clinical outcome of checkpoint blockade. We need to consider not only these phenotypes, of course, but from the point of view of what we know about peripheral diagnostic and predictive biomarkers informative for cancer patient survival, we also need to ask whether all these are sensitive to changes with age and what the impact, if any, of CMV on these might be? Such parameters include T cell repertoire diversity as well as T cell activation and differentiation states, functional measures such as cytokine production, and of course cytotoxicity, the quantity and quality of regulatory T cells (T_{reg} cells), and so-called myeloid-derived suppressor cells (MDSCs). The latter were observed at higher levels in the peripheral blood of older patients with lung or gastric cancer as were T_{reg} cells,[28,29] whereas cytolytic molecules involved in CD8 T cell cytotoxic function were dramatically reduced.[30]

In advanced melanoma, it was found that the presence in the blood of CD4[+] and CD8[+] T cells capable of responding in vitro in an appropriate manner to shared antigens such as NY-ESO-1 and Melan-A is informative for the duration of survival of the individual patient.[31] Combining such functional assays with surface marker phenotyping of peripheral cells identified a composite signature correlating more closely with survival. Although the proportion of T_{reg} cells was higher in patients than controls, the amount of these cells did not contribute to the immune signature associated with survival; rather, the proportion of MDSCs was the crucial factor.[18] It was noted in these patients and in controls that the proportion of T_{reg} cells is higher in the older adult and in patients (and this is the only parameter so far discovered that is not affected by CMV infection). It has been reported that MDSCs increase with age, which may, therefore, have relevance in some older patients,[19] and again CMV affects cells with these phenotypes (monocytic MDSC phenotypes). However, in this experience of treating advanced melanoma patients with ipilimumab, stratifying patients for CMV seropositivity or negativity did not show differences in clinical outcome. Stratifying patients for age less than 50 versus greater than 50, greater than 60, or even greater than 70 years did not impact the clinical outcome of ipilimumab treatment, although numbers of very old patients were low. These results are consistent with those of others.

However, most melanoma patients in our and others studies tend not to be particularly old; therefore, it was asked whether immune signatures as defined earlier would remain informative for the survival of older people (i.e., parameters including T cell functional responses to tumor antigens, and levels of MDSCs). To this end, newly diagnosed breast cancer patients aged 80 years were recruited, to be compared with younger women 40 years of age. It was shown that immune signatures predicting survival in the younger patients were similar to those in melanoma patients: In this case, in vitro T cell responses to the shared antigen Her-2, rather than NY-ESO-1 or Melan-A, together with elevated levels of MDSCs were informative for survival.[20] Moreover, these signatures remained predictive of survival in the very old cohort, suggesting that immunosenescence had no deleterious effects in this context.[21] Because most of these older adult patients were seropositive for CMV, it was also concluded that infection with this persistent virus also did not compromise the antitumor response, as for the melanoma patients.

So does this mean that older CMV-seropositive patients can breathe a sigh of relief in the knowledge that checkpoint blockade therapies are just as likely to be possible for them as for younger patients? Possibly even better: a recent case report described an older adult patient with metastatic bladder cancer initially resistant to treatment with the PD-1/PD-L1 inhibitors atezolizumab/pembrolizumab. This patient developed CMV-gastritis, presumably as a result of latent virus reactivation under checkpoint blockade, but upon treatment with ganciclovir and resumption of anti-PD1/PD-L1 after controlling viremia, the patient then achieved a complete response.[32] But obviously a single case report cannot tell us a great deal and we still have many gaps in our knowledge. The proportion even of younger patients responding to checkpoint blockade can be low, leaving room for some more subtle effects of age and CMV status. Given the low levels of naïve cells in all older people, CMV positive or not, the response to neoantigens may be the most problematic for the aging patient, as described in the following section.

EXPECTED EFFECT OF AGE ON THE RESPONSE TO SHARED ANTIGENS VERSUS NEOANTIGENS, AND REMEDIAL ACTION

Most published trials of active immunotherapy so far have employed shared antigen vaccines, and studies of the results of checkpoint blockade also show that responding T cells in treated patients are often specific for these antigens.[22] As with the examples from our own work given earlier, responses to antigens such as Melan-A and Her-2 are likely to be mediated by memory T cells. Even in the case of "immune privileged" antigens such as NY-ESO-1 that are not normally expressed by somatic tissues, there is evidence for memory responses by T cells from people who do not suffer clinically from cancer. Thus, in all these examples, it is very likely that patients already possess memory against the target antigens. Even in older adult people, immunological memory can be of extremely long duration and not necessarily markedly affected by immunosenescence, consistent with the results referred to previously. However, due to the dearth of naïve T cells in the older adult, the greatest problem affecting immunity in older adults is the difficulty of dealing with new antigens—expressed either by newly emerging pathogens or those to which the person had not been previously exposed. Given the recent realization that potentially the most important target antigens for immunotherapy are those arising as a result of mutations in individual tumors, that is, neoantigens,[23] their recognition could indeed present a problem in the older cancer patient. At least the presence of neoantigens on the tumor is not necessarily reduced in older patients. Thus, for example, the number of neoantigens was higher in gastric cancers of older patients than in their younger counterparts,[33] but this may not be the case for all cancer types.[30] In any case, the question remains whether or not whatever neoantigens are present can be recognized in older adult cancer patients. To the best of our knowledge, only one study has addressed this question so far. Using whole-exome and RNA sequencing, tumor neoantigens that are predicted to bind to major histocompatibility complex class I (MHC-I) were identified in 14 lung cancer patients treated with atezolizumab. Screening for neoantigen-specific T cell responses revealed an enrichment of neoantigen-specific peripheral CD8 T cells in patients responding to atezolizumab, most of whom were over 70 years of age. Neoantigen-specific T cells in atezolizumab-responder patients show a more differentiated effector phenotype than in nonresponders, similar to that of CMV-specific CD8 T cells.[34] Progression of these T cells into a late effector-like phenotype in patients with clinical response suggests that mere presence of neoantigen-specific T cells may not be sufficient, and that their functional quality might be the most important parameter in predicting response to immune checkpoint blockade, in both young and older patients. Given the low number of patients in that study, further investigations will be necessary to fully understand to what extent neoantigens are recognized in older adults. Due to current and expected technological advances in analyzing mutations in individual patients' cancers and in sequencing T cell receptors for antigen, it may become possible to establish whether a particular patient does indeed have a "hole in the repertoire" for potentially crucial neoantigens expressed by the tumor. It could then become theoretically possible to clone the appropriate *TCR* genes and insert them into the patient's T cells for reinfusion. In this scenario, one might be able to turn the large accumulations of CMV-specific memory cells in older patients to advantage by transfecting the appropriate TCRs into these cells, which tend not to proliferate strongly (and therefore would be prevented from reaching the Hayflick limit[24]) but retain potent cytotoxic activity.[25] This approach would still require targeted manipulation of additional tumor escape mechanisms that may be exacerbated in the aged host, for example, the higher levels of MDSCs noted earlier, and possibly T_{reg} cells in some cases, but ways and means to accomplish this are currently under intense investigation.[26]

CONCLUSION

Optimism that cancer immunotherapy for the older adult will prove equally as successful as in the young despite immunosenescence is not misplaced. Memory responses to shared tumor antigens are retained in older adults, but responses to neoantigens may be compromised. We still do not have enough data to determine whether this will be an important issue for some patients, and is an area where research efforts need to be focused. However, relative to the younger patient, this potential problem in the older adult is likely to be quantitative rather than qualitative, and the same solutions to the problem required for younger patients will also apply to older patients. Hence, developments driven by the desire to treat younger patients, and the clinical trials that usually fail to focus on the older patient, will nonetheless be of benefit to the older adult cancer patient as well.

KEY REFERENCES

Only key references appear in the print edition. The full reference list appears in the digital product on Springer Publishing Connect: connect.springerpub.com/content/book/978-0-8261-3743-2/part/part03/chapter/ch47

2. Pawelec G. Does patient age influence anti-cancer immunity? *Semin Immunopathol.* 2019;41(1):125–131. doi:10.1007/s00281-018-0697-6
7. Lynn RC, Weber EW, Sotillo E, et al. c-Jun overexpression in CAR T cells induces exhaustion resistance. *Nature.* 2019;576(7786):293–300. doi:10.1038/s41586-019-1805-z
20. Bailur JK, Pawelec G, Hatse S, et al. Immune profiles of elderly breast cancer patients are altered by chemotherapy and relate to clinical frailty. *Breast Cancer Res.* 2017;19(1):20. doi:10.1186/s13058-017-0813-x
23. Alpert A, Pickman Y, Leipold M, et al. A clinically meaningful metric of immune age derived from high-dimensional longitudinal monitoring. *Nat Med.* 2019;25(3):487–495. doi:10.1038/s41591-019-0381-y
24. Wikby A, Ferguson F, Forsey R, et al. An immune risk phenotype, cognitive impairment, and survival in very late life: impact of allostatic load in Swedish octogenarian and nonagenarian humans. *J Gerontol A Biol Sci Med Sci.* 2005;60(5):556–565. doi:10.1093/gerona/60.5.556
26. Wu TD, Madireddi S, de Almeida PE, et al. Peripheral T cell expansion predicts tumour infiltration and clinical response. *Nature.* 2020;579(7798):274–278. doi:10.1038/s41586-020-2056-8

Clinical Measures: Tumor Response Assessments, Pseudoprogression, and Immunometabolism

Louis F. Chai and Steven C. Katz

KEY POINTS

- Novel responses to immunotherapy are being increasingly appreciated, with pseudoprogression creating an important clinical challenge.

- New imaging criteria are under development to more accurately assess patients receiving immunotherapy in an effort to account for unique findings on diagnostic studies.

- Functional imaging to capture changes in tumor metabolic activity and immune effector cell function may offer enhanced assessment of biologic responses to immunotherapy treatments.

- Exploitations of metabolic pathways may enhance responsiveness to immunotherapy.

- An integrated approach to immunotherapy tumor response assessment incorporating immunotherapy-tailored imaging, laboratory techniques designed to study tumor response, and other clinical data is required for optimal clinical decision making.

INTRODUCTION

Multidisciplinary cancer care has been transformed by the emergence of immuno-oncology (IO) therapies. These changes have required adaptation of clinical management algorithms and response assessments. As the field continues to evolve, clinicians and scientists must continue to build on established knowledge to drive development of systems that accurately define response to treatment. This chapter seeks to provide an overview of tumor response assessments and the need for an integrative, well-rounded approach to accurately capture response patterns to IO therapies with specific emphasis on the integration of conventional imaging techniques with immunometabolic science and tissue-based response assessments.

IMAGING-BASED RESPONSE CRITERIA

The traditional measure of oncologic success was the ability to decrease tumor burden or completely eliminate the cancer altogether as measured by cross-sectional imaging techniques. The main means of achieving such results for solid tumors were primarily through surgical excision, chemotherapy, or radiation. IO therapies are transforming the solid tumor therapeutic landscape and creating the need for new response assessment systems. Cellular therapies such as chimeric antigen receptor T (CAR T) cells and checkpoint inhibitors (CPIs) against cytotoxic T lymphocyte-associated protein 4 (CTLA-4), programmed cell death protein-1 (PD-1), and programmed death ligand 1 (PD-L1) are being integrated into solid tumor care. Starting with approval for ipilimumab (Yervoy) in 2011 for treatment-refractory metastatic melanoma, atezolizumab (Tecentriq), avelumab (Bavencio), cemiplimab (Libtayo), durvalumab (Imfinzi), nivolumab (Opdivo), pembrolizumab (Keytruda), tisagenlecleucel (Kymriah), and axicabtagene ciloleucel (Yescarta) have since been approved for a variety of malignancies.[1] The pace at which IO agents have been introduced and applied for solid tumors has eclipsed the rate at which response assessment methodologies have evolved. This emphasizes the need for novel paradigms for reporting clinical and radiographic responses to therapy.

Traditional Response Criteria

World Health Organization Criteria

The first attempt to develop a standardized framework for monitoring tumor responses to therapy and reporting results were generated by the World Health Organization (WHO).[2,3] The WHO system is based on size measurements and broken into four categories: complete response (CR), partial response (PR), stable disease (SD),

Table 48.1 Traditional Tumor Response Criteria

RESPONSE CRITERIA	CR	PR	SD	PD
WHO	Disappearance of all known disease	≥50% decrease in total tumor size with no new lesions or progression of any lesion(s)	Unable to establish ≥50% decrease in total tumor size, but no increase in total tumor size by ≥25%	≥25% increase in size of lesion(s) with no CR, PR, or SD previously documented
RECIST 1.1	Disappearance of target and non-target lesions	Disappearance of target lesions and PR/SD of non-target lesions with no new lesions **OR** ≥30% decrease in target lesions and non-PD of non-target lesions, with no new lesions	Unable to establish ≥30% decrease in total target lesion size, but no increase in total tumor size by ≥ 20% and non-PD of non-target lesions and no new lesions	≥20% increase in target lesion size with no CR, PR, or SD previously documented **OR** ≥20% increase in non-target lesion size **OR** New lesions detected

Notes: The two widely accepted traditional response criteria are the WHO criteria and RECIST 1.1. Both were designed with the concept of effective therapy resulting in reductions in tumor burden where the main difference between the two is the use of bidimensional tumor measurements with the WHO criteria compared to the unidimensional measurements using RECIST 1.1. Additionally, the WHO criteria accounts for all visible lesions whereas RECIST 1.1 defines 10 target lesions.[4–6]

CR, complete response; PD, progressive disease; PR, partial response; RECIST, Response Evaluation Criteria in Solid Tumors; SD, stable disease; WHO, World Health Organization.

and progressive disease (PD; Table 48.1).[4–6] Importantly, the guidelines for determining sizes relied on the summing of bidimensional measurements of selected lesions, but also left room for unidimensional measurements and "nonmeasurable, evaluable" reporting, adding potential sources of subjectivity to how measurements were performed and reported. However, the WHO criteria did capture the importance of reporting information beyond tumor size such as patient characteristics, specific treatment regimens, and clinical responses to treatment. The WHO criteria was an extraordinary effort that allowed researchers to standardize assessments for the first time and served as the basis of reporting across institutions, therapies, and tumor types for nearly 20 years. However, as therapies and technology advanced, response criteria must adapt.

Response Evaluation Criteria in Solid Tumors (RECIST), RECIST 1.1, and Modified RECIST (mRECIST)

When the WHO criteria were initially introduced, computed tomography (CT) and magnetic resonance imaging (MRI) technology were relatively recent additions to route oncologic care.[4,7] The subsequent improvements in imaging technology, coupled with the lack of strict definitions regarding the number and size of lesions to be monitored by the WHO criteria, led to the development of the Response Evaluation Criteria in Solid Tumors (RECIST 1.0) in 2000.[5] While the response categories remained the same, the critical changes of note were a move away from bidirectional tumor measurements to more consistent unidimensional measurements as well as clearly defining the number and locations of lesions, minimum sizes to be

assessed, and the specifications within each response category. Modifications introduced in RECIST 1.1 included evidence-based changes to the number of lesions requiring monitoring, standardized guidelines for following lymph nodes, and updates to specific response categories (Table 48.1). Crucially, RECIST 1.1 also offered specific imaging modality recommendations including information regarding the use of positron emission tomography (PET) to monitor malignancy response to treatments.[5,8–10]

While response in RECIST 1.1 is based purely on anatomical tumor shrinkage on imaging, this broad concept does not account for tumor viability, where effective therapy may result in massive infiltration of cells, edema, and death of tumor tissue, all of which may be confounders in conventional size measurements.[11] With this concept in mind, modfied RECIST (mRECIST) was created for hepatocellular carcinoma (HCC) with a focus on viable disease burden that was defined by contrast enhancing tumor mass.[12] This distinct criteria proved beneficial, as mRECIST has performed well in defining clinical outcomes accurately in multiple clinical trials as well as an independent prognostic indicator.[11,13–18] The implementation of a disease-specific modification demonstrates that the response criteria should be subject to revisions and innovation as therapeutic landscapes shift.

Positron Emission Tomography Response Criteria in Solid Tumors (PERCIST 1.0)

PERCIST 1.0 provides stringent methods for evaluation of metabolic treatment response and remains the only devoted response criteria for PET imaging.[19–21] Tumor progression correlates with increased activity whereas tumor killing would result in a decrease in detected signal.[21] The guidelines outlined response categories based on PET results and variability in outcomes that may be disease-specific. In applying PERCIST 1.0 for a variety of solid tumors, results suggest that the use of PET/CT for assessment of tumor response may be more appropriate than conventional anatomic imaging such as CT alone with better prediction of outcomes and efficacy of therapy.[22,23] As with all novel imaging response assessment systems, PERCIST 1.0 will be subject to updates. Additionally, even with advanced techniques such as PET/CT, the integration of imaging data with other non-radiographic indicators of response may be required to accurately capture the true biologic activity of IO agents.

Immunotherapy-Specific Response Criteria

The most recent change in the landscape of cancer treatment has come with cellular immunotherapy and the CPIs. Though there remain some barriers with cellular therapies for solid tumors, CPIs have expanded the treatment armamentarium for diseases including metastatic melanoma and carcinomas of the urogenital, pulmonary, and the gastrointestinal (GI) tract.[24–43] However, as the long-term outcomes of these therapies became available, deficiencies in the ability of traditional response criteria to recognize the unexpected responses have been identified. Whereas responses to chemoradiotherapy and surgical resection lead to an expected decrease in measurable tumor burden, immunotherapy functions through an entirely different mechanism by harnessing the native immune system. This creates challenges when applying the WHO or RECIST criteria, indicating that efficacy of new immunotherapy agents may not be accurately captured. Realization of this compelled experts to re-evaluate imaging-based response metrics and develop new criteria.

Immune-Related Response Criteria

Immunotherapy response was first addressed in an effort to develop appropriate response measures in patients receiving immunotherapy.[44] Several important concepts were identified, the most critical of which was the recognition of a potential lag in tumor response by size criteria, where there may be an initial increase in size or appearance of new lesions before a measurable improvement. Additionally, it was noted that even in the setting of stable disease (SD), favorable disease courses were possible given the slowing of progression. Given these observations, efforts were made to provide standardized response criteria that would address the unique biology of immunotherapy leading to the release of the immune-related response criteria (irRC) in 2009 (Table 48.2).[45,46,47]

The irRC modified the WHO criteria based on melanoma IO trial data and updated the categories to be immunotherapy specific with an "immune" prefix

(irCR, irPR, irSD, and irPD). The key change involved the manner in which new lesions were handled. Before irRC, any new lesion seen on posttreatment imaging represented progressive disease (PD), but irRC redefined this by allowing new lesions to be incorporated into the total tumor burden, which is then compared to the index lesions to define response. In this way, if new lesions are identified and total tumor burden is stable, then patients are not classified as PD. Recognizing that supposed tumor enlargement and a new lesion appearing on an imaging study may be reflective of edema rather than disease progression, irRC permits longer-term follow-up to account for novel response kinetics. To this end, comparison of irRC with the WHO criteria showed that 22 of the 57 patients who had PD by the WHO criteria in fact demonstrated irSD or even irPR by irRC.[45] irRC continues to be evaluated as experience grows with immunotherapy and new iterations are likely to be developed.[46] As experience grows, it is becoming clearer that imaging alone may not capture the entirety of clinical response to IO agents and integrating additional response assessments would provide more accurate measurements.

Immune-Related RECIST (irRECIST), Immune RECIST (iRECIST), and Immune-Modified RECIST (imRECIST)

The initial effort in 2013 to update irRC moved from bidimensional to unidimensional tumor measurements for response assessments and was named irRECIST to reflect the use of irRC response categories and RECIST methodologies.[48] With this change, irRECIST was found to have high fidelity in retrospectively matching irRC reporting on the same patients. The main advantage of irRECIST was the higher reproducibility of assessments across multiple evaluators whereas irRC was significantly more variable. Given the importance of reporting standardization, this proved to be a welcome advance, though one that requires more validation in prospective studies with larger cohorts.

RECIST 1.1 was also adapted in 2017 to reflect the changes seen with IO agents and was termed iRECIST (Table 48.2).[49] The goal of a uniform update iRECIST was to provide standardization to the substantial amount of trials that individually modified RECIST 1.1 to fit immunotherapeutics and again restore consistency across outcome reporting. While the majority of iRECIST relies on the RECIST 1.1 backbone, the key change required definitive confirmation of PD in response to the novel response kinetics of IO agents that could appear as PD in the standard assessment time frames (e.g., 6–8 weeks posttreatment), but subsequently be determined to have SD, PR, or CR after longer follow-up. Therefore, they recommended a two-tiered assessment system that classified PD as either unconfirmed (iUPD)

Table 48.2 Immunotherapy-Specific Response Criteria

RESPONSE CRITERIA	IRCR	IRPR	IRSD	IRPD	
irRC	100% size decrease of index lesions **AND** No non-index lesions or new nonmeasurable lesions	100% size decrease of index lesions **AND** Stable or unequivocal progression of non-index lesion and any nonmeasurable lesion changes **OR** ≥50% size decrease in index lesions **AND** Absent, stable, or unequivocal progression of non-index lesions and any non-measurable lesion changes	<50% size decrease or <25% size increase of index lesions **AND** Absent, stable, or unequivocal progression of non-index lesions and any nonmeasurable lesion changes	≥25% size increase of index lesion and any changes of non-index lesions and nonmeasurable lesions	
	iCR	**iPR**	**iSD**	**iUPD**	**iCPD**
iRECIST	Disappearance of target and non-target lesions with no new lesions	≥30% decrease of target lesions with non-iCR/non-iUPD of non-target lesions	<20% increase or <30% decrease of target lesions with non-iCR/non-iUPD of non-target lesions	≥20% increase in target or non-target lesions **OR** Any new lesions on initial response assessment	≥5 millimeter increase in original target or non-target lesions **OR** Increase in number of new lesions from initial response assessment **OR** ≥5 millimeter increase in new target lesions from initial response assessment **OR** Any size increase in new non-target lesions from initial response assessment

Notes: Similar to the traditional response criteria, the two broadly used immune-related response criteria are irRC and iRECIST, which were based on the WHO criteria and RECIST 1.1, respectively. These account for atypical response patterns associated with the use of immunotherapeutic agents in the treatment of solid tumors. Again, as their respective non-immune focused predecessors differed, irRC and iRECIST vary in their tumor measurements (bidimensional vs. unidimensional, respectively). Additionally, iRECIST further specifies progressive disease as unconfirmed (iUPD) or confirmed (iCPD), requiring re-evaluation to ensure true progression based on the mentioned criteria, and if any other response is noted on subsequent assessment, the status is "reset," requiring the two-step iUPD to iCPD diagnosis once again to confirm progression. Confirmation of irPD or iUPD is performed at least 4 weeks after initial diagnosis.[46,47]

iCPD, immune confirmed progressive disease; iCR, immune complete response; iPR, immune partial response; irCR, immune-related complete response; iRECIST, immune response evaluation criteria in solid tumors; irPD, immune-related progressive disease; irPR, immune-related partial response; irRC, immune-related response criteria; irSD. immune-related stable disease; iSD, immune stable disease; iUPD, immune unconfirmed progressive disease.

or confirmed (iCPD), where any iUPD had the opportunity to be "reset" to baseline if any improvement was noted on repeat imaging. Additionally, any new lesions would be assessed as separate entities from the original lesions, giving further flexibility to the definition of PD. While measures such as objective response rate (ORR) and overall survival (OS) remained similar between RECIST 1.1 and iRECIST, the updated response criteria captured long-term stability or eventual response more robustly.[47] However, as iRECIST remains relatively new, direct application and use in clinical trials will be necessary to further elucidate the validity of the criteria; this works in conjunction with multiple assessment parameters. Despite the relatively recent development of

iRECIST, improvements are already being explored. One year after the publication of iRECIST, a separate group sought to further refine response guidelines in the form of imRECIST to expand endpoint metrics beyond ORR and focused on how immunotherapy-specific response patterns contributed to criteria such as progression-free survival (PFS) and OS.[50]

IMAGING MODALITIES AND NOVEL TECHNIQUES

As response criteria and therapeutics for cancer treatment have advanced, so have the imaging techniques in use for diagnosis, staging, and response evaluation of malignancy. While whole body imaging was just becoming widely available when the WHO criteria was released, the anatomy-based CT or MRI modalities are now the two most commonly used techniques for tumor imaging. Furthermore, significant advancements have been made with regards to picture resolution and speed of obtaining images and the potential to combine techniques with sophisticated functional modalities such as PET. New technologies have also reflected the immunotherapy-associated tumor response kinetics where the unique targets and mechanisms of IO agents have paved the way for multiple exciting and novel concepts in the preclinical and clinical space to monitor and track treatment and resulting immunological effects. This progress has allowed for more accurate tumor response assessments, but the multitude of options presents an added variable to reporting, an issue that is addressed in more recent guidelines with great detail. Additionally, novel molecular imaging modalities require further validation before they become the standard in the clinical setting, though preliminary results indicate that they could be an invaluable tool to allow real-time assessment of administered immune cell activity or evaluation of endogenous immune response to immunotherapy.[51,52] To better understand tumor response and the role that each technology plays in assessing response, it is important to understand the function and the applicability of each technique to different scenarios.

Computed Tomography

The CT scan was invented in the early 1970s and advancements in technology have further entrenched it as the gold-standard and ideal modality for diagnosis, staging, and tumor response assessment, a fact that is emphasized by the imaging modality being the recommended technique in all recent response criteria.[3,5,8,12,45,48,49,50,53] One major advantage of the CT scan is the ability to rapidly obtain anatomic information with accurate assessment of lesion size compared to the more time-consuming MRI.[54] The addition of contrast enhancement provides significant benefit where vascular involvement can guide therapy and detection of viable tissues as with mRECIST.[12]

One disadvantage and prevailing concern with CT scans is the radiation exposure, a risk factor for the development of malignancies. However, published data on the low-level radiation from a CT scan and the development of cancer is controversial and the benefits of accurate diagnosis, treatment, and evaluation likely outweigh the risks.[55,56] Furthermore, while CT is excellent for response evaluation when a cytotoxic effect is evaluated, a recent disadvantage may be that anatomic imaging is not sufficient for assessment given delayed antitumor immune responses resulting from IO agents. Utilization of additional response metrics in conjunction is a subject of ongoing research.

Magnetic Resonance Imaging

Although used less frequently than CT, the MRI provides an alternative modality with high resolution and avoidance of radiation. The advancement of MRIs has been similar to CTs, making it another ideal choice for cancer imaging. While not explicitly mentioned in the original WHO criteria, the use of MRI has been incorporated into modern criteria as an acceptable imaging modality though with caveats about significant variability in acquisition and the need to strictly monitor and adjust for such potential inconsistencies.[8]

Beyond the lack of radiation, one recent advantage that has resulted from technological developments is diffusion-weighted imaging (DWI)-MRI. This variant to standard MRIs produces images based on the difference in motion of water molecules in the intracellular, extracellular, and intravascular space with motions being influenced by macromolecules and membrane structures within each compartment. Given that cytotoxic therapy and immunotherapy alter tumor cell membranes, DWI-MRI may be useful as one component of response monitoring, even in light of atypical imaging response patterns seen with IO agents.[57,58]

A second, and perhaps more intriguing, advantage of MRIs is the potential use of alternative contrast agents to label specific cell subtypes and molecules. This would provide a means to track migration, proliferation, and efficacy of adoptively transferred and endogenous immune cells. Among these are gadolinium (Gd), manganese (Mn), superparamagnetic iron oxide (SPIO) particles, perfluorocarbon (PFC) for 19-fluorine (^{19}F) detection, gene alteration with metal-binding reporter genes (e.g. ferritin), and chemical exchange saturation transfer (CEST) agents. Of these, SPIO and PFC have garnered significant attention with clinical trial approvals.[59,60] These techniques have been used to label all cell types and labeling can occur either after ex vivo labeling and adoptive transfer or in vivo labeling of endogenous cells.[51,61–64]

Currently, proof of concept has been suggested in multiple preclinical studies using adoptive cell transfer (ACT) of various immune subsets.[65] In two rodent models, SPIO nanoparticles allowed tracking of DC migration after vaccination and NK cells targeting established tumors after ACT.[64,66] In addition, notable translational work has been studied using PFC-labeled DCs with ^{19}F MRI detection in a Phase 1 clinical trial for stage 4 colorectal cancer.[67] Investigators found that after injection of the labeled DCs, a clear, intense, and localized signal persisted in the tissue for about 24 hours before decreasing by approximately 50% where signal intensity served as a surrogate for cell number. A critical finding was what appeared to be a minimum required dose for detectability using this technique that may be related to cell density and minimum threshold for the MRI. However, despite this limitation, this first-in-human study is a milestone for the future of functional imaging in relation to immunotherapeutics.

Disadvantages of MRIs are the increased length of time needed to acquire images compared with CT scans. This factor is a significant reason patients and providers prefer CT despite the increased radiation exposure. Additionally, differentiation between substances such as air and tissue, and obtaining appropriate three-dimensional spatial resolution, can be problematic with MRI use.[68–70] Finally, due to the use of magnetic fields, hardware such as pacemakers and implantable cardiac devices (ICDs) introduced prior to MRI compatibility standards may limit the population that can obtain such imaging. Despite these limitations, though, MRI still has advantages and are preferred in certain clinical applications such as neurological malignancies. Given the potential functional, cell tracking applications in relation to immunotherapy, MRI may prove to be a powerful tool as one component of tumor response assessment.

Positron Emission Tomography

Initially introduced and standardized for use in 2009 for oncological assessments, PET is a unique imaging modality that has seen rapid development and utilization in diagnosis, staging, and evaluation of therapeutic response.[71] As a functional imaging modality, PET images evaluate the metabolism of different tissues using glycolytic activity as a surrogate. The most commonly used tracer is the fluorine-18 labeled glucose analogue, 2-[18F]-fluoro-2-deoxy-d-glucose (FDG). After injection, the tracer is taken up by cells via cell-membrane glucose transporters and accumulates in the intracellular space.[72,73] This physiology is particularly useful in the setting of cancer due to the increased metabolic activity, and hence, FDG uptake in malignant cells and solid tumors, allowing for simplified differentiation from normal tissue (Figure 48.1). However, this also can be a disadvantage as there is significant variability in sensitivity and specificity for evaluating tumor burden as different tumors demonstrate a wide range of metabolic activity. This activity may not be uniform even when considering a primary tumor and any associated metastases. Finally, the specificity of PET to detect smaller lesions or lymph nodes is restricted.

Many of these limitations can be partially avoided by performing PET in conjunction with CT, which provides functional evaluation with anatomic imaging.[73–76] The combination of PET/CT has been a revolution for diagnosis and treatment response monitoring. Given the advantage of functional and anatomic delineation of disease, it is now consistently used in the management of cancer after the initial recommendation for use was made in RECIST 1.0 followed by specific guidelines in RECIST 1.1.[5,8] One critical response definition that was

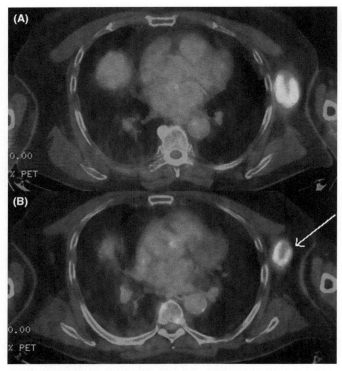

Figure 48.1 PET images pre- and post-checkpoint inhibitor therapy. Patient with melanoma recurrence in the left axilla with increased metabolic activity on PET scan measuring 5.1 x 3.4 centimeters (**A**). Biopsy revealed PD-L1 expression on cells and the patient was treated with combination neoadjuvant ipilimumab and nivolumab, after which repeat imaging was performed, revealing decreased metabolic activity and size at 3.4 x 2.3 centimeters (**B**). ALND revealed replacement lymph node tissue with melanophages within a sclerotic background and areas of necrosis, suggesting complete treatment response.

ALND, axillary lymph node dissection; PD-L1, programmed death-ligand 1; PET, positron emission tomography.

defined was the presence of any positive finding on PET following a negative baseline PET was considered PD.[8,48] However, as the primary imaging modalities recommended were still CT or MRI, those remained the foundation for assessing tumor response.

Currently, the irRC and iRECIST do not comment on the use of PET in monitoring response to immunotherapy, but future iterations may incorporate functional imaging due to the benefits in assessing endogenous immune response to IO agents. Similar to MRI, PET has the capability of tracking activated immune cell subsets, and the opportunity to track specific cells is a distinct advantage for variables such as tumor infiltration of immune cells. Current strategies undergoing investigation include the ImmunoPET, which involves ex vivo labeling of immune cells with radioactive probes, ex vivo gene engineering to express a reporter probe, or in vivo labeling with monoclonal antibodies, all of which allow for immune-specific response assessment.[77,78] Radiolabeling can be accomplished with several compounds including FDG, Gallium-68 (^{68}Ga), Iodine-124([124]I), indium-111 (^{111}In), copper-64 (^{64}Cu), zirconium-89 ([89]Zr), 3'-deoxy-3'-[^{18}F]fluorothymidine (FLT), and 16α-[^{18}F]-fluoro-17β-estradiol (FES), the latter two of which can mimic therapeutic mechanisms of action.[77,79–81]

Ex vivo labeling requires significant work in harvesting the desired population of cells, manipulating and tagging with the radiotracer, expanding, ensuring that viability and functionality is maintained, and reintroducing the cells in vivo prior to imaging.[78] This may be viable in a preclinical model, but in a clinical setting where time to therapy and avoidance of unnecessary procedures is key for patients, this method is less ideal. Hence, the ability to label specified immune cell subsets in vivo for ImmunoPET is appealing. Preclinical data suggests the possibility of this method where a designed, radiolabeled antibody toward a target antigen is introduced in vivo, which then allows monitoring of any cells that express the target antigen via PET scan.[80,82–84] This concept has been applied to specific targets on immune cells such as CD3 for T cells, CD19 for B cells, and CD11b for MDSC, all populations critical in tumor development or response assessment.[85]

This technique may also have a potential role in predicting response to therapies. A growing body of research for biomarkers that could predict responsiveness to specific therapies has yielded potential candidates with perhaps the most prominent being PD-L1 (CD279), a cell surface protein intimately involved in immune regulation and limiting activation of T cells and pro-inflammatory signaling.[86–89] PD-L1 and its receptor PD-1 (CD274) have been the target of many CPI with great success across a spectrum of solid tumors, but not for all patients. Having reliable predictors could help with decision-making regarding with whom to initiate therapy as there are significant costs and risk of immune-related adverse events (irAE) associated with immunotherapy treatment.[90–96] Currently, tumor biopsies followed by immunohistochemistry (IHC) is the standard for determining PD-L1 expression levels, but ImmunoPET may negate the need for such invasive procedures. By tagging an antibody directed against PD-L1, uptake in tumor sites could serve as a surrogate for expression levels and, therefore, treatment responsiveness. Additional markers that have been explored in this arena are CD38 and CTLA-4, among others, but these concepts have only been validated in murine models, requiring further study for use in clinical applications.[97–99]

Finally, utilizing these labeling methods can provide a means to assess trafficking and uptake of antibody therapies after administration. While IO agents are designed as targeted therapies, there remain issues with nonspecific binding, especially with CPIs where CTLA-4, PD-1, and PD-L1 are expressed on healthy tissues to protect against autoimmunity.[100,101] Excessive systemic exposure can result in irAEs that can range from mild to life threatening.[91,94,96] By utilizing ImmunoPET, the degree of nontumor exposure can be better understood and dosage, therapy schedule, and delivery methods can be optimized to gain the maximum benefit while limiting adverse events.[102–105] However, as with other novel imaging technologies, many of these tracking methods are still being developed and optimized. Standardization of these techniques will be required before widespread application and use as a response assessment is possible.

DEFINING AND MANAGING PSEUDOPROGRESSION

When the WHO and RECIST response criteria were designed, the main form of therapies were reductive in nature, where effective treatment resulted in an overall decrease or elimination tumor burden. As such, criteria included discrete categories of response measured by the amount of imaged tumor before and after treatment. However, when immunotherapy was first introduced, the expected radiographic responses were no longer the norm with an unusual rate of what appeared to be progression after therapy. Longer-term follow up using clinical monitoring and survival metrics did not seem to corroborate progression and subsequent imaging confirmed this with findings of delayed responsiveness or SD.[45,106] After the initial report of this phenomenon known as pseudoprogression in melanoma after ipilimumab treatment, it has since been seen with other solid tumors and immunotherapy treatments.[1,45,107–113]

While no standardized definition of pseudoprogression officially exists, the overall concept is intuitive where, after treatment, there is an appearance of PD by the RECIST or WHO criteria, whether it be new lesions or an increase in size or metabolic activity of measurable tumor, followed by SD or some degree of response (Figure 48.2).[35,114] Some reports have also considered worsening of cancer-related physiological changes such as ascites, pleural effusions, organ system failures, or overall clinical deterioration followed by improvement as a component of pseudoprogression, but the majority of cases currently recognize it as a radiographic finding of the primary tumor or lymph nodes.[115–118] The incidence of pseudoprogression has been reported to be up to 14%, though this is variable depending on tumor and treatment types. To account for this phenomenon, the immune-related response criteria were created.[106,107,115,117,119,120] While pseudoprogression may be found in a small fraction of cases, the frequency is not insignificant and may inappropriately influence clinical decision-making. Attempts have been made to better understand the full clinical impact of pseudoprogression by better categorizing the response kinetics into early and late time points, but

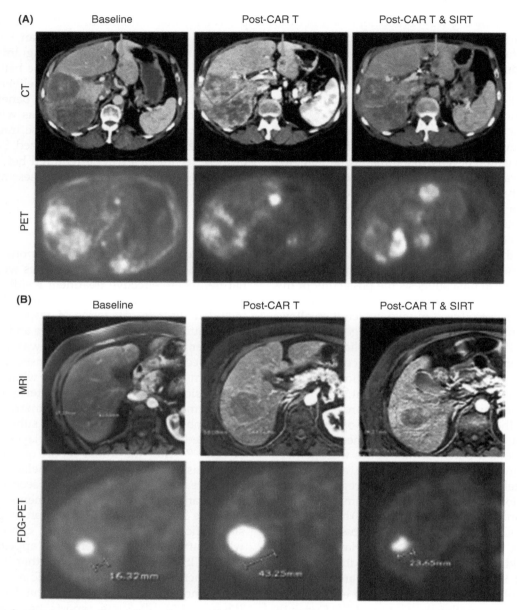

Figure 48.2 Pseudoprogression after cellular immunotherapy on CT and PET. Patients with colorectal liver metastases treated with cellular immunotherapy with imaging pre- and posttreatment. **A:** Representative anatomical CT (top) and functional PET (bottom) imaging from a patient pre- and post-CAR T and SIRT treatments. **B:** Representative anatomical MRI (top) and functional PET (bottom) images of patient pre- and post-CAR T and SIRT treatments. Post-CAR T treatment in both patients, there is a notable flare response on PET imaging and with CT and MRI showing apparent lesion enlargement followed by regression, indicating possible pseudoprogression.

CAR T, chimeric antigen receptor T cell; CT, computed tomography; FDG-PET, fluorodeoxyglucose-positron emission tomography; MRI, magnetic resonance imaging; PET, positron emission tomography; SIRT, selective internal radiation therapy.

Source: Reproduced with permission from Ref. (35). Katz SC, Hardaway J, Prince E, et al. HITM-SIR: phase Ib trial of intraarterial chimeric antigen receptor T-cell therapy and selective internal radiation therapy for CEA⁺ liver metastases. *Cancer Gene Ther.* 2019;27(5):341–355. doi:10.1038/s41417-019-0104-z

overall, individual occurrences should be managed on a case-by-case basis incorporating multiple sources of information including, but not limited to, imaging, laboratory parameters, and clinical correlation.[121]

Mechanisms of Pseudoprogression

Cellular Infiltration

One hypothesis for the development of pseudoprogression is that tumor enlargement is a result of immune cell infiltrate at tumor sites rather than tumor cell proliferation and growth. This strongly correlates with the very mechanism by which various immunotherapy agents are introduced or function. In terms of ACT therapies, cells are expanded significantly ex vivo and reintroduced into the body in addition to the existing endogenous immune cells, leading to an overall increase in circulating antitumor cells and, theoretically, at the tumor site as well. For antibody therapies such as the CPIs, tumor immune-evasive mechanisms are abrogated, allowing the endogenous immune system to activate and respond to tumor antigens, leading to increased trafficking and infiltration of the TME. Suspected new lesions may have been previously too small to be detected until the influx of cells enlarged them to the point of detectability on imaging.[8,119]

This theory has been validated with tissue biopsies of malignant lesions with proven pseudoprogression which revealed an inflammatory milieu including cytotoxic T lymphocytes.[113,122] Further studies in preclinical models and clinical trials to quantify the cellular infiltration after immunotherapy have corroborated these results where up to 12.5-fold increases in cells have been reported with ACT therapies.[123–125] These results provide strong evidence for the increase in cellular tumor penetration as one mechanism for pseudoprogression. Further study of this is warranted as understanding the interaction between immune and tumor cells can help distinguish pseudoprogression from true progression and help correctly categorize responses utilizing multimodality approaches such as ImmunoPET.

Edema and Tumor Necrosis

A second mechanism through which pseudoprogression may develop is the increase in edema and tumor cell necrosis associated with an increased inflammatory response. Many solid tumors already have aberrant vasculature with abnormal endothelial integrity and hydrostatic flow of fluid, and local inflammation generated from tumor response to therapy and increased cellular trafficking further aggravates this, resulting in a large increase in fluid and edema.[126,127] Tumor necrosis contributes to the "enlargement" due to swelling of dying cells as well as propagating the inflammatory response, creating a self-feeding cycle.[106,128] These two factors may contribute to the seeming enlargement of the tumor in the early phase of treatment, followed by clearance of necrotic tissue and resorption of edema whereby the remaining tumor, if any, appears to have shrunken. This process may take place over months, resulting in the abnormal response kinetics seen in relation to immunotherapy.

Clinical Decision-Making With Pseudoprogression

Given this phenomenon has been demonstrated across a variety of solid tumors and IO agents, clinical implications must be considered. While it should be noted pseudoprogression occurs in a minority of patients, treating physicians should recognize that tumor response to immunotherapy is variable and may differ from typical response kinetics. Where a standard clinical algorithm may recommend cessation or changing of therapy in the face of apparent treatment failure, pseudoprogression confounds this decision-making tree. Radiographically, there may appear to be PD, but the patient could be performing well clinically, thus benefiting from treatment regardless of imaging findings. If clinical improvement is seen with paradoxical changes in imaging, a reasonable approach would be to continue treatment with reassessment after 4 to 8 weeks to confirm radiographic changes.[45,49,50] The implications for clinical trial endpoints are also relevant as premature termination from a study may inadvertently bias results and mask potential improvements in outcomes such as ORR, OS, and PFS. Nevertheless, these variables should be considered carefully against clinical deterioration or development of severe irAEs to manage patients. Guidelines for management of adverse events are continuously being refined as are response criteria, but cases should be handled individually, utilizing all information available to inform rational decision-making, always in the interests of the patients' well being.[96] At present, understanding the response to immunotherapy and interpretation of pseudoprogression require a great deal of clinical judgment with integration of a broad range of data inputs. Through exploitation of several unique features of tumor biology, including metabolic programming, we may have opportunities to create novel imaging and response assessment approaches. The overarching goal is to enable more reliable and reproducible response assessments following treatment with IO agents.

IMMUNOMETABOLISM

An important element in the development of effective tumor response imaging is the ability to distinguish normal from malignant tissue. Tumor metabolism is often distinct from that in normal surrounding tissue, providing an opportunity to leverage molecular signatures for more refined imaging approaches in immunotherapy patients. Metabolic pathways serve to produce and consume energy sources utilizing available substrates. These substrates can enter the metabolic pathway at various points, but regardless of input, the goal is the output of adenosine triphosphate (ATP), which drives all cellular energy transfer.[129] The key production pathway of ATP goes through three main processes: glycolysis, the citric acid (CAC) cycle, and oxidative phosphorylation (OXPHOS; Figure 48.3). There are branch points to this sequence that are critical to specific immune functions, notably the pentose phosphate pathway (PPP) and the anaerobic pathway to maintain glycolysis in low oxygen states.[130] To understand immune cellular metabolism in response to malignancy and to utilize components for response assessment, it is critical to understand these basic cellular metabolism pathways.

The close association of immune cell metabolism and activation state is a fairly recent discovery, but the field of immunometabolism is expanding rapidly. One very clear fact is that immune system activation is metabolically demanding. As with normal cell metabolism, all actions of the immune system including development, differentiation, proliferation, activation, migration, effector function, and homeostasis require energy. These are further augmented when there is an activating stimulus for immune function such as tumor development. Immune cells are capable of undergoing glycolysis, the CAC cycle, and OXPHOS to generate energy, but also utilize each component in unique ways for optimal function.

From a cancer treatment perspective, these unique metabolic signatures could make it possible to distinguish antitumor immune cells from malignant cells on imaging. As our understanding of immune cell

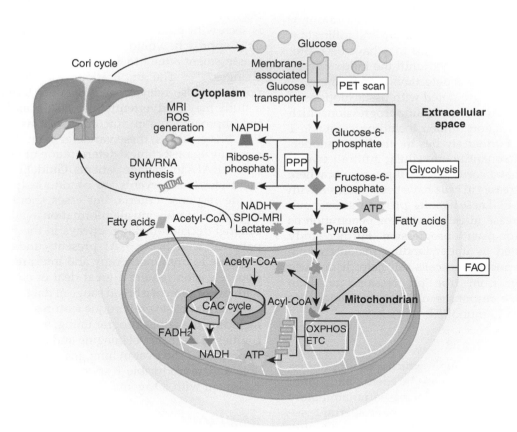

Figure 48.3 **Metabolic pathway.** Under aerobic conditions, cells utilize glucose to generate energy in the form of ATP through glycolysis, the CAC cycle, and OXPHOS. Branches from this main energy pathway provide an alternative route of ATP generation under anaerobic conditions as well as substrates for additional processes such as ribonucleotide production and the antimicrobial respiratory burst functions.

ATP, adenosine triphosphate; CAC, citric acid cycle; CoA, coenzyme A; DNA, deoxyribonucleic acid; ETC, electron transport chain; FADH, flavin adenine dinucleotide hydrogen; FAO, fatty acid oxidation; NADH, nicotinamide adenine dinucleotide hydrogen; NADPH, nicotinamide adenine dinucleotide phosphate hydrogen; OXPHOS, oxidative phosphorylation; PPP, pentose phosphate pathway; RNA, ribonucleic acid; ROS, reactive oxygen species.

metabolic programming is improved, new opportunities to refine response assessments become increasingly available. Tracking of immune cell subsets defined by metabolic configuration could become a method of monitoring the functional and mechanistic impact of immunotherapeutic interventions as with the MRI and PET techniques discussed previously. However, significant work will need to be completed to truly understand individual immune cell biomechanistic function and how to define tumor-specific immune cell signatures for clinical applications.

Metabolism of Innate Immunity

Cells of the innate immune system act as the first line of defense against foreign antigens. Innate immune cells are comprised of macrophages, neutrophils, DCs, and NK cells, among others.[131] Upon introduction of a foreign antigen, activation of the innate immunity is triggered and these cells play a critical role in pathogen clearance through processes such as phagocytosis and microbicidal ROS production. They also trigger the adaptive immune response via antigen presentation and pro-inflammatory cytokine release to generate a more pathogen-specific response. The metabolic requirements of these innate immune cells are unique and correlate with functionality required of each subset.[130]

Neutrophils

The innate immune system relies heavily on neutrophils to provide the initial defense against antigens as they represent the largest fraction of circulating leukocytes and are capable of trafficking readily to the necessary sites.[132] Given their acute response to inflammatory signals, it is unsurprising that neutrophils are highly metabolically active with defense functions including migration, phagocytosis, respiratory burst, cytotoxic granule release, and neutrophil extracellular trap (NET) production.[130,132,133]

Upon arriving to the site of action, neutrophils can engulf invading pathogens through phagocytosis. This is followed by the respiratory burst within the phagosome via initiation of the NADPH oxidase complex. This multicomponent system functions by shuttling electrons provided by NADPH to generate reactive oxygen species (ROS) such as hydrogen peroxide (H_2O_2). Glycolysis is an important step in the metabolic pathway for neutrophils as the conversion of glucose to G6P provides the precursor that can feed into the PPP where consistent reduction of $NADP^+$ to NADPH supplies the fuel for this critical step.[133] In addition to the direct role that ROS play in pathogen destruction, it is likely that ROS also participate in altering the contents of the phagocytic vacuole for efficient protease function, perhaps altering energy requirements for these enzymes.[134,135]

The presence of ROS and critical respiratory burst function can be used as an imaging target as a surrogate for neutrophil expansion. Detection agents that modulate electron spin have been implemented with success in vivo with preclinical models to detect ROS generation, providing a potential means to measure neutrophil activation and metabolic reconfiguration via magnetic resonance technology.[136]

NADPH oxidase also appears to be required for NET formation. NETs are complexes consisting of mitochondrial DNA and neutrophil-derived proteins that neutrophils expel externally to trap microbes and expose them to high concentrations of antimicrobial proteins.[137] Given the use of NADPH for NET production, metabolic requirements are similar to that of ROS generation. Neutrophils that utilize both defense mechanisms have accordingly increased energy needs, again emphasizing the sizeable role that glycolysis plays for this immune subset of cells.

Given the significant amounts of energy required for these functions, neutrophils utilize a unique metabolic profile. Unlike other cells that rely on OXPHOS to generate ATP, neutrophils rely on aerobic glycolysis and glutaminolysis to provide molecules required for ROS generation and NET formation. The preferential utilization of this pathway is hypothesized to allow for continued function even when the cells traffic to inflammatory sites where there may be little oxygen.[130,138] In experimental models, if glycolysis is inhibited in neutrophils, cells are unable to perform phagocytosis, but when excess glutamine is provided, there is increased efficiency of phagocytosis and ROS production.[139,140] Additionally, neutrophils have been shown to have relatively few mitochondria, given their main utilities are for NET production and initiation of neutrophil apoptosis once the initial inflammatory response has subsided.[141] This further emphasizes the minimal role OXPHOS plays in neutrophil metabolism.[138,142] This ability to function in hypoxic environments is key to understanding neutrophil response, with malignancies a prominent feature of TMEs. Understanding the drivers of neutrophil metabolism and function may yield therapeutic options to augment this key participant in the initial inflammatory response and can be leveraged for response imaging to detect increased glycolytic activity or radiolabeled substrates such as glutamine that are important to energy production in neutrophils.

Macrophages

A unique and diverse cell type, macrophages are found in all tissues of the body and provide numerous functions. Along with neutrophils, macrophages participate as a first-line defense against invading antigens in addition to the role they play in tissue repair and homeostasis.[143]

In the context of the immune system, understanding differential macrophage metabolism and function is critical and requires a more specific breakdown of macrophage types where the M1 and M2 macrophages are the key subsets. Likely, this classification oversimplifies the spectrum of macrophage phenotypes in vivo, but the differences in metabolism are distinct and best understood using these designations.

M1 Macrophages (Classically Activated)

Macrophages are influenced to polarize toward defined effector phenotypes by chemocytokine and pathogen exposures. Each phenotype is then characterized by unique cytokine production profiles and transcriptional and translational changes of effector genes and proteins. Broadly speaking, the classically activated, or M1, macrophages are pro-inflammatory in nature and are characteristically activated after exposure to pathogen- or danger-associated molecular patterns (PAMPs, DAMPs) such as lipopolysaccharide (LPS) or inflammatory cytokines such as IFN-γ.[144] M1 macrophages have been shown to participate in the immune response across a broad range of foreign antigens including bacteria, fungi, viruses, and tumor.[145,146]

Activating stimuli trigger M1 macrophage metabolic reprogramming toward pro-inflammatory functions and to fuel activities using aerobic glycolysis and glutaminolysis, which can be monitored using metabolic imaging.[147,148] M1 macrophage reliance on these particular metabolic pathways results from the need for quick surges in energy to feed defensive functions in inflammatory environments that are low in nutrients and oxygen, both of which are necessary for CAC cycle and OXPHOS function.[149] One signal of note is nuclear factor-κB (NF-κB), which is increasingly translocated to the nucleus and is responsible for upregulating synthesis of proteins such as NAPDH oxidase, inducible NO synthase (iNOS), cyclo-oxygenase 2 (COX2), and citrate carrier (CIC), which have roles in producing ROS, nitric oxide (NO), and prostaglandin.[150] Metabolic reconfiguration occurs as early as 20 minutes after stimulation as indicated by increased glucose uptake with full metabolic reprogramming and final effector profile stabilizing within 24 hours.[151] This highlights the rapid first-line defense nature of macrophages. These crucial components of M1 macrophage metabolism represent potential metabolic targets for therapy and immune response monitoring. Clinical trials have shown effective detection of early inflammatory markers such as iNOS using PET scans.[151–153] The ability to track changes in M1 macrophage metabolic profile from initial activation to full reconfiguration could provide critical information early in the treatment course regarding efficacy of immunotherapy.

M2 Macrophages (Alternatively Activated)

Alternatively activated, or M2, macrophages are characterized by activation by IL-4 and are typically considered anti-inflammatory.[144,146] Two of the M2 macrophages' main functions are antiparasitic activity and regulation of inflammation, both of which can be prolonged processes. As such, these cells require long-term energy supplies. Metabolic programming of M2 macrophages favors fatty acid β-oxidation (FAO) and OXPHOS for energy production to reflect this prolonged requirement.[130,154] This is in stark contrast to the requirements for rapid bursts of energy associated with neutrophils and M1 macrophages; this metabolic diversion may also be helpful to distinguish macrophage subtypes on imaging. Detection of fatty acid metabolism using specialized radiotracers such as ^{11}C-palmitate or ^{18}F-FTHA with PET scans has shown some success in liver pathologies, and applying this to malignancy could provide information regarding the metabolic profile of macrophages in TME.[155] Higher iNOS presence would indicate the predominance of M1 macrophages, whereas increased FAO would lean toward M2 expansion. The capability to distinguish between pro- and anti-inflammatory phenotypes on response imaging would be important information to help inform therapeutic efficacy.

At the molecular level, M2 metabolic shifts start with IL-4 stimulation, which triggers recruitment of signal transducer and activator of transcription 6 (STAT6), a key component of M2 metabolic reprogramming. One outcome of STAT6 recruitment and translocation to the nucleus is transcriptional upregulation of genes necessary for β-oxidation of fatty acids and mitochondria biogenesis, providing support for the dependence on OXPHOS.[154] Furthermore, STAT6 has also been found to upregulate PPARγ-coactivator-1β (PGC-1β), which plays a critical role in energy homeostasis and is a necessary component for the induction and stabilization of the M2 metabolic configuration. PGC-1β functions in a positive feedback loop with STAT6, thus perpetuating the M2 metabolic response.[154,156] Apart from STAT6, alternative minor pathways have been described. IL-4 activation also triggers signaling through the Akt–mTORC1 pathway, where Akt and mTORC1 activity level is altered based on the presence or absence of certain amino acids. When nutrients are available, activation of this pathway leads to increased acetyl CoA synthesis, which subsequently increases histone acetylation, leading to significant epigenetic changes that result in enhanced gene transcription related to M2 programming.[146,157] The multiple, independent pathways that lead to stabilization of the M2 phenotype highlights the metabolic importance of FAO and OXPHOS to their immune function. Further elucidation of these pathways may yield more specific targets for monitoring response to immunotherapies.

Dendritic Cells

At the junction of the innate and adaptive arms of the immune system, DCs play a key role as professional antigen-presenting cells (APCs). Functional responsibilities include patrolling tissue for invading microbes, sampling detected microbes for actionable antigens, migrating to lymph nodes and presenting such antigens, and coordinating adaptive immunity activation.[158,159] Given these diverse requirements and the interwoven role in both arms of the immune system, energy requirements are significant. Activating signals, most notably the interaction between PAMPs and TLRs, trigger DC metabolic reprogramming that is underscored by the rapid increase in glycolysis early after activation. This early metabolic reprogramming of DCs is unique in that upregulation of aerobic glycolysis not only facilitates increased ATP production, but also supports glycolytic intermediate entry into the PPP and CAC cycle and de novo fatty acid synthesis for endoplasmic reticulum (ER) and golgi apparatus expansion, both processes required for DC activation.[160,161] The critical nature of this shift is emphasized by the inability for DCs to convert to an activated state if glycolysis is inhibited.[160,162] Furthermore, some DC subsets activate iNOS after prolonged activation, leading to NO production, which inhibits OXPHOS; this further diminishes the mitochondrial role and establishes aerobic glycolysis as the dominant role in the energy-producing pathway.[163] As with neutrophils and macrophages, imaging targeting glycolytic activity or iNOS levels may prove fruitful for tracking DC activation, proliferation, migration, and function in the setting of IO treatment given the dependence on these metabolic pathways.

Several key components of the signaling cascade underlying the metabolic switch in DCs have been studied. The increase in glycolysis appears to be driven by Akt-mediated phosphorylation of hexokinase-II (HK-II), an enzyme that catalyzes the formation of G6P. After TLR stimulation, TANK binding kinase 1 (TBK1) and IκB (IKK) activate Akt, which then phosphorylates HK-II, resulting in increased activity via the glycolytic pathway. Though Akt is similarly active in M2 macrophages, the upregulation of glycolysis in DCs appears to be independent of phosphatidyl inositol 3-kinase (PI3K)/mTORC1, but stabilization of metabolic programing requires induction of HIF-1α, which is mediated by the PI3K/Akt/mTORC1-signaling cascade.[160] As DCs maintain activation and move toward dependence on aerobic glycolysis, upregulation of HIF-1α targets become increasingly important for prolongation of the metabolic structure, and may represent a viable therapeutic target.[160] In addition, given the critical nature of HIF-1α to maintaining DC activation, leveraging it for metabolic imaging as a measure of DC immune response to tumors and treatment may prove fruitful, as has been demonstrated using PET in several preclinical and clinical studies.[164]

Natural Killer Cells

Though NK cells have cytotoxic function and have a lymphoid origin characteristic of the adaptive immune system, they are considered to be a part of the innate immune system, in part due to the ability to activate without antigen sensitization.[165,166] Activation of NK cells instead relies on extracellular signals, though stimulation naturally requires a delicate balance of signals to prevent inappropriate activation of inherent cytotoxic functions.[166] Functionally, NK cells are prominently involved in antiviral and antitumor responses and help to bridge the gap to the adaptive immune response by secreting activating signals such as IFN-γ and TNF-α and increasing the number of DCs.[167] The main activator of NK cells and resultant shift toward a metabolically active state is IL-2, with additional involvement of IL-12 and IL-15.[167–169]

At a baseline, circulating NK cells produce ATP via OXPHOS, and with short bursts of stimulation, this remains the dominant pathway of energy production. However, after prolonged exposure to activating signals, the favored energy pathway shifts toward reliance on glycolysis.[169,170] This metabolic shift from OXPHOS to glycolysis could be an important differentiation point for metabolic imaging that allows monitoring of NK immune activation. Upon stimulation, a number of signaling pathways become activated, most notably involving mTORC1, a molecule involved in multiple immune cell metabolic pathways, as previously described, and critical for NK cell function.[167,168,171] The first step involves phosphorylation and activation of Janus kinases (JAK1 and JAK3), which then diverge down multiple pathways including the PI3K-Akt, ultimately resulting in mTOR activation and transcriptional augmentation of HIF-1α and sterol regulatory element-binding protein 1 and 2 (SREBP1 and SREBP2).[172–174] This signaling cascade results in a number of effects including upregulation of GLUT expression to increase substrates available for energy generation and release of molecules such as IFN-γ and granzyme B.[166,167,175] This intimate link between the NK cell activation and metabolic reprogramming pathways is crucial for proper effector function as evidenced by studies that demonstrate deficiencies from cytokine activation to gene transcription. Furthermore, depletion of required resources can result in attenuation of NK function and metabolism.[168,172,174,176] This knowledge can be leveraged to identify metabolic targets for immune response tracking such as with ImmunoPET for IFN-γ detection or therapeutic targets to stimulate potent antipathogenic NK cell activity.[177]

Metabolism of Adaptive Immunity

While innate immunity provides the initial defense against pathogens, activation of the adaptive immune system provides effector cells designed to target specific antigens and generate immunologic memory for future responses to similar invasions. T and B cells make up the adaptive immune system and provide effector, memory, and regulatory function (Figure 48.3).[130,178] This diverse set of roles played by the adaptive immune cells requires varying energy levels; this is reflected in the metabolic shifts seen upon cellular activation.[167]

T Cells

T cells are a functionally diverse lymphocyte population where activation and polarization is highly contextual. T cells can exist in a resting, homeostatic state; become activated and differentiate into effector cells; and then return to quiescence again as memory T cells. As with innate immune cells, metabolic programming plays an important role in the T cell activity; given the functional diversity, the metabolic demands vary greatly. Given the diversity of these lymphocytes, effector T cell metabolism is discussed here, as this subset is generally the most active against foreign antigens. Many of the current studies evaluating T cell metabolism were performed using $CD4^+$ and $CD8^+$ T cells. B cell metabolism is thought to be similar to that of $CD4^+$ T cells, but active research is ongoing to evaluate for differences.

In the absence of inflammatory stimuli, naïve T cells circulate in the body, awaiting activation. In this state, fuel production is mainly via OXPHOS and FAO and used for migration, maintenance of cellular size, and preventing atrophy and apoptosis. Stabilization of this metabolic conformation requires consistent extracellular signaling through the T cell receptor (TCR) and IL-7. In the absence of these signals, GLUTs are rapidly downregulated, leading to decreased glucose uptake, decreased ATP production, and, ultimately, atrophy and programmed cell death.[179,180]

When naïve T cells encounter DCs in secondary lymphoid organs, antigen-specific T cell activation can occur through parallel signaling with TCRs, major histocompatibility complex (MHC) interaction, and co-stimulatory molecules such as CD28 or 41-BB. This combination of surface receptor activation leads to a cascade of intracellular events including metabolic remodeling. The metabolic demands of activated T cells dramatically increases to support the processes of migration, activation, differentiation, and effector function. As with the cells of innate immunity, activated T cells use aerobic glycolysis and glutaminolysis as the primary source of energy production. In addition to presenting viable means of immune tracking via glycolytic metabolic imaging, the importance of these pathways for proliferation and

activation of T cells is highlighted by the requirement for glutamine regardless of oxygen availability.[181] Activated T cells upregulate GLUTs to mediate increased energy production. This simultaneously provides resources to increase the available intracellular ATP and frees metabolic intermediates for use in anabolic pathways, leading to the synthesis of proteins, lipids, and nucleotides necessary for cellular proliferation and effector functions.[182,183]

The signaling process underlying metabolic reprogramming in an activated T cell is intricate and dynamic with several important intracellular signaling molecules including Akt, AMPK, mTOR, Myc, and HIF-1α.[184] One key regulator is CD28, which facilitates PI3K/Akt activation to act on multiple regulators of glucose uptake and glycolysis.[185] This pathway is stabilized by IL-2 exposure, a cytokine that is strongly associated with T cell activation and proliferation when TCR and CD28 co-stimulation occurs.[186] Another effect of Akt signaling is mTor activation, a central regulator of T cell growth and proliferation, which in turn contributes to the upregulation of Myc and HIF-1α. Myc is important for induction of glycolysis and glutaminolysis; HIF-1α increases glycolysis and acts on a number of genes required for survival and proliferation.[184] Further intricacies contributing to T cell energy production result from input of nutritional molecules into these signaling pathways. For example, mTOR activation is also triggered by levels of intracellular leucine in lymphocytes.[187]

Although these signaling pathways are thought to be shared between most lymphocytes, there are likely unique pathways depending on T cell subset as they serve different functions in the immune response. For example, activated $CD8^+$ T cells differ from $CD4^+$ T cells in that glycolysis is upregulated via augmentation of lactate dehydrogenase rather than mTOR despite both changes being Akt-mediated.[188] Understanding the intricacies involved in T cell activation and metabolism is complicated by the inherent diversity of the population. However, further research in this area is important given the significant role that the adaptive immune system plays in antigen response. The potential to exploit T cell immunometabolism for response monitoring and to distinguish tumor tissue from T cell infiltration would provide critical information regarding immune function and efficacy of immune activation in response to IO agents. Specialized radiolabels or tracers with PET or MRI that are specific for T cells such as CD3 could help overcome the limitation of PET to distinguish between tumor and activated immune cells, both of which are metabolically active.

Malignancy-Related Metabolism

Tumor Cell Metabolism

Like the energetically demanding state of immune cells upon activation, tumor cells require large amounts of energy to sustain rapid cellular proliferation. Tumors classically meet this need with aerobic glycolysis, or Warburg metabolism, and glutaminolysis, despite being oxygen-rich environments. This reliance on the Warburg effect and signaling through molecules such as HIF-1α parallels metabolic reprogramming in some activated immune cells, but in the setting of different nutrient availability. While immune cells typically function in an inflammatory and hypoxic environment that justifies reliance on glycolysis and glutaminolysis, tumor cells typically develop in well-oxygenated tissues before generating their own low-oxygen microenvironment.[189] Thus, the tumor cell dependence on Warburg metabolism is a unique phenomenon and requires further exploration to fully understand tumor development. Targeting these oncogenic metabolic pathways for therapy in combination with treatments that augment the immune system may be of substantial benefit for treatment. Additionally, leveraging unique tumor metabolic signatures and signaling pathways in conjunction with PET or hyperpolarized MRI can help distinguish tumor and immune cells using tumor-specific oxygen levels and metabolic byproduct production such as lactate and LDH.[190]

Myeloid-Derived Suppressor Cell Metabolism

In addition to tumor cells, recruitment and differentiation of MDSC within the TME is influenced by an anti-inflammatory milieu. These suppressor cells negate the activity of the immune system and prevent tumor killing or elimination. They accomplish these functions through mechanisms such as engagement of the PD-1/PD-L1 pathway, induction of immune cell apoptosis, or depletion of nutrients required for immune function.[89,191–194] Because of the rapid expansion and wide array of inhibitory capabilities of MDSC, a significant energy source is required. As with other cell types, recruitment, expansion, and metabolic reprogramming of MDSC are driven by environmental signals such as GM-CSF or CCL2/CCR2 and cellular signaling, including the JAK/STAT3 pathway.[192,195–198] Energy production is dictated by the nutrient availability in the TME, and MDSC can respond accordingly to utilize any component of the metabolic pathway. However, studies demonstrate anti-immune activity may favor utilization of FAO as evidenced by increased cellular accumulation of lipid and mitochondrial mass.[193,198,199] Targeting the lipid metabolism pathway has resulted in decreased immunosuppressive activity and blunted tumor growth and again demonstrates the potential for exploited metabolic pathways to treat or track malignancies and associated cell subtypes.[200–202] Evidence of this has been shown in preclinical models using PET radiolabels to target cell-specific markers to refine response assessment after IO therapy.[203]

Imaging Metabolism

Recognition that tumor and immune cells have unique metabolism has generated interest toward imaging techniques that utilize this distinction. Focus on tumor metabolic profiles could improve early diagnosis as well as increase fidelity of tumor response monitoring in the setting of immunotherapy. As previously detailed, pseudoprogression presents a unique problem and the ability to distinguish tumor cells would undoubtedly clarify treatment response and guide clinical decision-making. Conversely, immunometabolism imaging could provide prognostic information regarding immune system fitness for immunotherapy. Since therapies such as CPIs rely on the endogenous immune system, individuals with weak activation or metabolism may be better suited for therapies such as ACT. In the same vein, the metabolic signature of immune cells could also be used to measure therapeutic efficacy post-intervention. Again, this could clarify abnormal imaging findings as an adequate immune cell response via metabolic imaging techniques would indicate effective therapy rather than treatment failure.

A key imaging modality in this arena is PET. In addition to being a functional scan, PET inherently lends itself to imaging unique cellular signatures as it exploits glycolytic activity to obtain images. Using the previously described novel PET tracers, specific metabolic activity could be monitored.[204] Ongoing work has demonstrated the possibility of imaging activity not only at the cellular level, but for specific metabolic pathways. However, while such advancements in imaging may contribute greatly to understanding tumor response to immunotherapy, a multimodality approach integrating patient observations, laboratory parameters, imaging, and other variables is likely required to truly capture the full scope of therapeutic efficacy in a clinical setting.

TISSUE-BASED IMMUNOMETABOLISM RESPONSE MONITORING

The unique tumor response pattern associated with immunotherapy has required a paradigm shift and a deep understanding of the intricacies of the immune system. Whereas response could be judged solely based on size changes on imaging when therapeutic options were cytoreductive, response to immunotherapy has required the integration of other parameters for a more holistic approach. To meet this need, advances in laboratory and imaging-based technologies have been developed to complement existing assessment parameters such as clinical observations and laboratory panels, some of which were designed with specific attention toward metabolic assessments.

In the field of lab-based methodologies, multiple techniques exist to evaluate the metabolic shifts of endogenous immune response to IO agents. From a cellular perspective, specific populations can be identified with fluorescence activated cell sorting (FACS), or flow cytometry, using unique extra- and intracellular markers. This could be a powerful tool for correlating cell phenotypes to metabolic activity levels and could provide critical information about the metabolic profiles that drive MDSC immunosuppressive mechanisms or changes in pathways that lead to increased exhaustion and apoptosis of immune cells.[58,192,195,196,205] Regarding tumor cells, the presence or absence of certain markers can inform on increases or decreases in metabolic activity, which could serve as a surrogate for therapeutic efficacy. A second method of cell analysis is mass cytometry where ion clouds are quantified by time-of-flight mass spectrometry (TOF-MS), yielding information about transcription factors, cell-specific proteins, and even cell-cell interaction.[206] A powerful method such as this provides granular details of changes in activity and how interactions within a complex environment can alter metabolic profiles in the tumor microenvironment. This highlights the tumor-immune cell interface and could provide invaluable information to the metabolic changes associated with this interaction and potential targets for further analysis or therapy. Finally, biochemical techniques including single-cell RNA sequencing and T cell receptor (TCR) clonotype analysis offer intriguing complementary information where transcriptional and translational changes of metabolism-specific pathways can be paired to determine what is truly biologically relevant.[207,208] For example, single-cell analysis (SCA) can be performed to determine the presence or absence of circulating tumor cells (CTCs) or immune cells based on activation status. This technique allows for identification of important data that informs on tumor cell heterogeneity, the molecular basis of metastasis, and can function as a marker of therapeutic response.[209,210] Data such as these require further validation and study, but could illuminate further mechanisms of tumor development and spread, identify treatment targets, and hold significant promise as a means of therapeutic response parameters.[211–214]

Functionally, the status of immune cells after immunotherapy can be determined using markers to track proliferation such as carboxyfluorescein succinimidyl ester (CFSE) or killing assays such as cytotoxicity or suppression assays. As previously detailed, activation of immune cells results in metabolic shifts that change the profile of activity such as cytokine release, which can be assessed via enzyme-linked immunospot assay (ELISPOT), real-time reverse transcription polymerase chain reaction (RT-PCR), or multiplex platforms such as the Luminex. However, like imaging, these laboratory techniques provide a snapshot of immune activity, whereas the immune activation in response to immunotherapy is a dynamic process. Taking any data point in isolation could result in misinformation, and observing trends in response via serial monitoring would give a more accurate clinical picture. This idea of kinetic analysis complements the necessity for repeat imaging evaluations to account for pseudoprogression and the need for multiple platforms to capture a complete response profile.

The importance of a multimodality approach to evaluate immunotherapy efficacy was emphasized by the recommendations to use a variety of immune-monitoring tools for clinical trials in 2002. At that time, expert groups put forth consensus recommendations to incorporate stringently functional and quantitative studies such as flow cytometry, ELISPOT, and tetramer analysis as valid endpoints to correlate clinical outcomes.[215] Since the release of these recommendations, multiple modalities have been tested and yielded important information, such as metabolic changes that alter cytokine levels and have influenced therapies, such as tocilizumab. The incorporation and validation of these methods provides evidence for standardization of immunotherapy clinical trial execution and endpoints for study.[216] However, just as therapeutics continue to evolve, continued development of alternative methods for monitoring response will be required to capture the complexity of immunotherapy treatment response, especially in relation to the intricate metabolic changes of tumor and immune cells. Currently underway are methods to evaluate changes in specific compartments based on metabolic activity with the ideal outcome being in vivo monitoring given the dynamic state of the TME. The imaging techniques such as ImmunoPET or SPIO-MRI described earlier partially fill this void, but the need for a more global understanding down to the cellular and molecular level will be needed. Greater detail regarding the performance and function of these tissue-based laboratory techniques for other functions are discussed in other chapters of this text.

Taken together, the utilization of multiple modes of analysis would generate data that provides valuable insight into important molecules and pathways that drive response while also guiding clinical decision-making for cancer treatment. For example, an integrative pathway could utilize ImmunoPET to identify tumor targets and TCR clonality followed by single-cell RNA sequencing to confirm immune fitness. Response to therapy is then assessed using a combination of imaging techniques such as SPIO contrast MRI or in vivo labeled immune cells and functional information via mass cytometry and tetramer analysis to produce macro- and microscopic details about metabolic shifts. Cytokine profiles could then be assessed to guide further treatment or to address adverse events. This represents one possibility out of many complementary analytic techniques and demonstrates the comprehensive approach that is required to understand the mechanics of tumor-immune cell interaction and to accurately monitor malignancies treated with IO agents.

CONCLUSION

Standardized and reproducible tumor-response criteria are critical for advancing cancer care and exploring novel therapies. This mentality was adopted when the first criteria was developed in the late 20th century and has evolved to meet modern-day needs when novel kinetics and response patterns such as pseudoprogression have emerged with immunotherapy. This increased understanding of the immune system led to corresponding advances in imaging modalities and laboratory assessments to better understand the effects and responses to immunotherapy. These techniques continue to undergo refinement to suit clinical needs; as more details regarding the intricacy of immune and tumor biology are elucidated, more changes are likely on the horizon whether it be metabolically targeted therapies or more novel response patterns. The rapid rate at which immuno-oncology is developing demand that response criteria, technology, and clinical assessments adjust accordingly. Likely, the optimal approach in clinical care with immunotherapy will require integration of information from the immune-related response criteria, advanced imaging techniques, and biological laboratory assessments to ensure a complete, accurate, and holistic assessment of treatment efficacy.

KEY REFERENCES

Only key references appear in the print edition. The full reference list appears in the digital product on Springer Publishing Connect: connect.springerpub.com/content/book/978-0-8261-3743-2/part/part03/chapter/ch48

1. Chai LF, Prince E, Pillarisetty VG, Katz SC. Challenges in assessing solid tumor responses to immunotherapy. *Cancer Gene Ther.* 2019;27(7–8):528–538. doi:10.1038/s41417-019-0155-1

2. Miller AB, Hoogstraten B, Staquet M, Winkler A. Reporting results of cancer treatment. *Cancer.* 1981;47(1):207–214. doi:10.1002/1097-0142(19810101)47:1<207::AID-CNCR2820470134>3.0.CO;2-6

8. Eisenhauer EA, Therasse P, Bogaerts J, et al. New response evaluation criteria in solid tumours: revised RECIST guideline (version 1.1). *Eur J Cancer.* 2009;45(2):228–247. doi:10.1016/j.ejca.2008.10.026

19. O JH, Lodge MA, Wahl RL. Practical PERCIST: a simplified guide to PET response criteria in solid tumors 1.0. *Radiology.* 2016;280(2):576–584. doi:10.1148/radiol.2016142043

45. Wolchok JD, Hoos A, O'Day S, et al. Guidelines for the evaluation of immune therapy activity in solid tumors: immune-related response criteria. *Clin Cancer Res.* 2009;15(23):7412–7420. doi:10.1158/1078-0432.CCR-09-1624

48. Nishino M, Giobbie-Hurder A, Gargano M, et al. Developing a common language for tumor response to immunotherapy: immune-related response criteria using unidimensional measurements. *Clin Cancer Res.* 2013;19(14):3936–3943. doi:10.1158/1078-0432.CCR-13-0895

49. Seymour L, Bogaerts J, Perrone A, et al. iRECIST: guidelines for response criteria for use in trials testing immunotherapeutics. *Lancet Oncol.* 2017;18(3):e143–e152. doi:10.1016/S1470-2045(17)30074-8

50. Hodi FS, Ballinger M, Lyons B, et al. Immune-modified Response Evaluation Criteria In Solid Tumors (imRECIST): refining guidelines to assess the clinical benefit of cancer immunotherapy. *J Clin Oncol.* 2018;36(9):850–858. doi:10.1200/JCO.2017.75.1644

51. Lee HW, Gangadaran P, Kalimuthu S, Ahn BC. Advances in molecular imaging strategies for in vivo tracking of immune cells. *Biomed Res Int.* 2016;2016:1946585. doi:10.1155/2016/1946585

60. Kim HS, Woo J, Lee JH, et al. In vivo tracking of dendritic cell using MRI reporter gene, ferritin. *PLoS One.* 2015;10(5):e0125291. doi:10.1371/journal.pone.0125291

131. Lérias JR, de Sousa E, Paraschoudi G, et al. Trained immunity for personalized cancer immunotherapy: current knowledge and future opportunities. *Front Microbiol.* 2020;10:2924. doi:10.3389/fmicb.2019.02924

IV

Disease-Specific Treatments and Outcomes

Paolo A. Ascierto

Introduction: General Approach to Cancer Immunotherapy—Lessons Learned From the Past Years

Paolo A. Ascierto

INTRODUCTION

The history of cancer care has witnessed several revolutionary advances in the therapeutic landscape resulting in significantly improved outcomes for patients. These include the introduction of cisplatin in the 1970s for testicular and ovarian cancers, the taxanes in the 1990s for breast and other solid tumors, the advent of anti-HER2 targeted therapy for breast cancer, and c-Kit inhibitors for chronic myeloid leukemia and other cancers at the start of this millennium.

Today, we are witnessing another new era in cancer care—that of immunotherapy. However, the concept of immunotherapy of cancer is nothing new. In the late 19th century, Dr. William Coley, a New York surgeon, injected a mixture of erysipelas toxins and *Bacillus prodigious* to successfully treat unresectable sarcoma. Interestingly, sarcoma represents a tumor that does not appear to respond well to current immunotherapies. The basis for today's new wave of immuno-based treatments is our increasing understanding of molecular pathways involved in the suppression and activation of the immune system. Suppression of T cell activation by programmed cell death 1 (PD-1) protein and/or cytotoxic T lymphocyte antigen-4 (CTLA-4) is one of the major escape mechanisms of cancer cells, and inhibition of these molecules by immune checkpoint inhibitors can successfully activate the immune response to cancer. The importance of the discoveries of PD-1 by Professor Tasuku Honjo and CTLA-4 by Professor James Allison was recognized in their being awarded the Nobel Prize in Physiology or Medicine in 2018.

However, the first new immunotherapy approval was actually the therapeutic vaccine sipuleucel-T, for the treatment of prostate cancer in 2010. This was followed by the first immune checkpoint inhibitor, the anti-CTLA-4 antibody ipilimumab, for the treatment of metastatic melanoma in 2011. These advances represented the first notable successes in this modern era of cancer immunotherapy. In patients with advanced melanoma, ipilimumab was the first treatment to show an improvement in overall survival (OS) for patients with melanoma for more than 30 years.[1] Since then, checkpoint inhibitors, in particular the anti-PD-1 (nivolumab and pembrolizumab) and anti-PD-ligand (L)1 (atezolizumab, avelumab, and durvalumab) antibodies, have revolutionized the treatment of several cancers. In addition to melanoma, these include non-small cell lung cancer (NSCLC), renal cell cancer (RCC), head and neck cancer, urothelial cancer, Hodgkin's lymphoma, and others. Other immunotherapies have also been approved in recent years, including the oncolytic virotherapy talimogene laherparepvec (TVEC) in 2015 for the local treatment of metastatic melanoma, and two CAR T cell therapies in 2017, tisagenlecleucel for the treatment of relapsed or refractory diffuse large B cell lymphoma (DLBCL) and primary mediastinal large B cell lymphoma, and axicabtagene ciloleucel for relapsed or refractory DLBCL and acute lymphoblastic leukemia. However, the immune checkpoint inhibitors will be the focus of this review.

The evidence from modern immunotherapy is that adaptability and memory of the immune system mean long-term survival can be achieved. The potential of long-term benefit with immunotherapy was previously recognized, with durable responses in patients with melanoma treated with high-dose interleukin (IL)-2.[2] With regard to immune checkpoint inhibitor therapy, a meta-analysis of approximately 5,000 patients with advanced melanoma treated with ipilimumab showed that 20% of patients were alive at 10 years (Figure 49.1).[3,4]

Subsequently, the pattern of an extended tail in survival curves seen across several trials has provided evidence of the long-term benefit of checkpoint inhibitors. In melanoma, 3-year OS rates were 51.2% with nivolumab versus 21.6% with dacarbazine in patients with previously

untreated BRAF wild-type advanced melanoma enrolled in the CheckMate 066 trial.[5,6] In updated data, 5-year OS rates were 39% with nivolumab and 17% with dacarbazine.[7] Similarly, in the CheckMate 067 trial, nivolumab plus ipilimumab showed a sustained long-term benefit with 5-year OS of 52%, compared with 44% with nivolumab and 26% with ipilimumab (Figure 49.1).[4,8] In the KEYNOTE-006 trial in patients with advanced melanoma, 5-year OS rates were 39% with pembrolizumab every 2 or 3 weeks and 31% with ipilimumab,[9] while in KEYNOTE-001, the estimated 5-year OS rate with pembrolizumab was 34% in all patients and 41% in treatment-naïve patients.[10] In patients with NSCLC, pooled data from two clinical trials of nivolumab (CheckMate 017 and 057) reported a more than fivefold increase in 5-year OS rate compared with treatment with docetaxel (13.4% vs. 2.6%).[11] In the KEYNOTE-010 trial of patients with previously treated advanced NSCLC with PD-L1 tumor proportion score (TPS) ≥1%, 3-year OS rates were 35% with pembrolizumab and 13% with docetaxel.[12] Among patients who received 35 treatment cycles (~2 years), 3-year OS rate was 99%. In the KEYNOTE-024 study of previously untreated advanced NSCLC patients with PD-L1 TPS expression ≥50%, pembrolizumab monotherapy continued to demonstrate an OS benefit over chemotherapy after long-term median follow-up of 25 months, despite crossover from the control arm to pembrolizumab as subsequent therapy.[13] Anti-PD-1 therapy has also shown a prolonged benefit

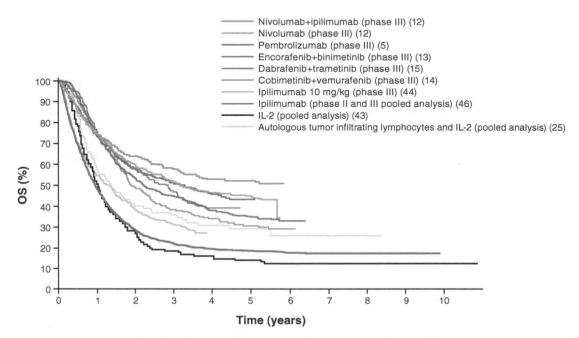

Figure 49.1 Long-term overall survival in clinical trials with immuno-oncology agents and targeted therapies in patients with advanced melanoma.
Source: Reproduced with permission from Michielin O, Atkins MB, Koon HB, et al. Evolving impact of long-term survival results on metastatic melanoma treatment. *J Immunother Cancer.* 2020;8(2):e000948. doi:10.1136/jitc-2020-000948

in recurrent or metastatic squamous cell carcinoma of the head and neck (SCCHN),[14,15] renal cell carcinoma,[16,17] bladder cancer,[18] and Hodgkin's lymphoma.[19]

CHECKPOINT INHIBITORS

Ipilimumab was the first treatment for metastatic melanoma to show an improvement in OS for more than 30 years. Of interest, ipilimumab showed a greater effect on OS than would be expected, given its impact on the surrogate endpoints of overall response rate (ORR) and progression-free survival (PFS). For example, response rates and PFS observed in two pivotal Phase 3 studies with ipilimumab did not correspond with the OS benefit that was achieved.[1,20] This lack of correlation between OS and surrogate endpoints has also been shown with nivolumab in patients with various cancers.[14,21,22] However, anti-PD-1 agents do tend to have an advantage in terms of ORR or PFS, compared with anti-CTLA-4 therapy.[8,23]

One explanation for this apparent inconsistency between ORR/PFS and OS is that the action of immunotherapy is not immediate but rather the effect is somewhat delayed. Another possible explanation is pseudo-progression, in which an increase in the number of immune system cells, rather than tumoral cells, results in the appearance of nodal progression. Such an increase in total tumor burden may be later followed by tumor regression. This appears to be more evident in melanoma than in other tumor types, with around 7% to 12% of melanoma patients having a clinical response after an initial diagnosis of progressive disease according to RECIST criteria, compared with 1% to 2% in some solid tumors.[24] To address this, new immune-related response criteria (irRC) have been developed to assess patients treated with ipilimumab, based on the assessment of total tumoral mass rather than single lesions as is the case with the RECIST and WHO criteria.[25] This allows for the occurrence of new lesions in the context of mixed response (i.e., simultaneous shrinkage of some lesions and increase in others), or a slow increase of existing lesions with the potential of reaching a later response or stable disease. It is also important to consider the irRC for anti-PD-1 agents as well as with anti-CTLA-4 therapy. In studies of nivolumab in patients pretreated with ipilimumab and BRAF inhibitors, 8% of patients had occurrences of new lesions and responded later during the treatment beyond progression (unconventional response).[23,26] Similarly, in the KEYNOTE-001 Phase 1 trial with pembrolizumab, about 15% of patients had an unconventional response.[27] This suggests that the irRC should be considered together with RECIST criteria in order to prevent premature cessation of anti-PD-1 treatment.

Another important characteristic of anti-PD-1 agents is that patients who stop treatment for reasons other than progression, primarily unacceptable toxicity, continue to respond even after therapy is stopped. In the CheckMate 067 trial,[28] 85% of patients who discontinued nivolumab due to drug-related toxicity experienced a complete or partial response and 70% continued to respond despite stopping treatment. Moreover, survival outcomes at 5 years were similar between patients who discontinued nivolumab plus ipilimumab because of treatment-related adverse events during the induction phase and the overall population.[8] Similarly, in the KEYNOTE-001 study of pembrolizumab, 59 of 61 patients (97%) with a complete response (after a median time on treatment of 23 months) maintained their response after stopping treatment.[29] This finding of durable responses after treatment discontinuation raises important questions regarding the most appropriate duration of treatment, and further studies are necessary.

DIFFERENTIAL EFFECT ON THE BASIS OF BIOLOGY

A lesson that we have learned in recent years is that the efficacy of immunotherapy is largely independent of tumor histology and mutational status. For example, in melanoma, ipilimumab has shown efficacy not only in the cutaneous form but also in ocular and mucosal melanoma, tumors with a different biology. Even though results have shown less activity in these melanomas than in the cutaneous form, the possibility of long-term benefit has been observed in both ocular and mucosal lesions, with 1-year OS rates of 27% to 34% in patients with uveal melanoma,[30–32] and 35% in patients with mucosal melanoma.[33]

However, it should be noted that the combination of nivolumab and ipilimumab has been shown to have a greater impact in BRAF-mutated patients compared with BRAF wild-type.[34] Previous reports have also suggested that immunotherapy might be more effective in NRAS-mutated compared with BRAF-mutated or BRAF/NRAS wild-type melanoma.[35] Patients with BRAF V600K-mutant melanoma appear to benefit less from targeted therapy with a BRAF inhibitor with or without MEK inhibitor than patients with V600E-mutant melanoma, potentially due to less reliance on ERK pathway activation and greater use of alternative pathways.[36] In contrast, BRAF V600K melanoma is associated with higher mutational load and better response to immunotherapy.

In patients with NSCLC, epidermal growth factor receptor (EGFR) wild-type tumors are associated with improved survival benefit from immunotherapy compared with EGFR-mutant tumors.[37] It has been suggested that this could be related to increased expression of the immunosuppressive molecule CD73 in EGFR-mutated NSCLC.[38] KRAS-mutated tumors have also been associated with improved response to PD-1 inhibitors.[39]

BIOMARKERS

In recent years, research efforts have focused on trying to identify biomarkers predicting a clinical response to checkpoint inhibitors. In particular, the expression of PD-L1 has been widely evaluated. This was, in part, based on the Phase 1 CheckMate 003 study that enrolled patients with melanoma, kidney cancer, or NSCLC,[40] in which no responses to nivolumab were observed in PD-L1-negative patients. However, subsequent data have contradicted this finding, showing that patients without PD-L1 expression may benefit from treatment with anti-PD-1 treatment. In tumors such as lung cancer, tumor expression of PD-L1 has shown a positive correlation with response. PD-L1 biomarker evaluation has several challenges, including that PD-L1 is an immunological marker and so may be dynamic and inducible. Moreover, since the expression of PD-L1 is not homogeneous within the tumor, the sample selection is complex. There is not yet a definitive assay for PD-L1, and a clear cut-off threshold for PD-L1-positive status has not been established. In addition, the type of cells on which PD-L1 expression is most relevant is not yet clear, with immune infiltrate cells and tumor cells both being used.

Increasing evidence supports high tumor mutational burden (TMB) as predictive of response to PD-1/PD-L1 blockade independent of PD-L1 expression. In the CheckMate 227 study, treatment with nivolumab plus ipilimumab significantly prolonged PFS versus platinum-doublet chemotherapy in patients with advanced NSCLC and TMB (≥ 10 mutations/Mb) independent of PD-L1 expression.[41] Similarly, in the CheckMate 568 trial, TMB was associated with improved response and prolonged PFS in NSCLC patients with or without PD-L1 expression $\geq 1\%$ treated with nivolumab and low-dose ipilimumab.[42] TMB may also be a relevant biomarker in patients with SCLC; patients with high TMB treated with either nivolumab monotherapy or nivolumab plus ipilimumab had improved efficacy compared with those with medium or low TMB.[43]

Immune checkpoint inhibitors have been shown to benefit patients with DNA mismatch repair deficiency (dMMR) or high microsatellite instability (MSI-H), which had led to the first tissue agnostic approval of pembrolizumab in MSI-H cancers. In metastatic colorectal cancer, immunotherapy has shown activity in dMMR/MSI-H tumors but no significant clinical activity in the treatment of patients with mismatch repair proficient/non-MSI-H disease has yet been shown.[44–46] TMB has also been reported to be an independent biomarker within patients with MSI-H metastatic colorectal cancer.[47]

The assessment of biomarkers correlated to TMB such as genomic alterations in DNA damage response (DDR) genes has also been suggested.[48] In addition, liquid biopsies with cell-free DNA or circulating tumor cells to assess DDR genes could help overcome problems with tissue availability.

UNIQUE SAFETY PROFILE

Another important characteristic is that the safety profiles of checkpoint inhibitors differ from those seen with chemotherapy or targeted therapy. Immuno-related adverse events (irAEs) are due to hyperactivation of the immune system subsequent to checkpoint inhibitor stimulation. These include a range of mainly dermatologic, gastrointestinal, endocrine, and hepatic toxicities, as well as several other less frequent inflammatory events. These events have variable times of onset and need careful monitoring, follow-up, and management.

Initial experience obtained with checkpoint inhibitors resulted in the development of algorithms for the treatment of irAEs,[49] and two important points to consider are early recognition of these toxicities and early treatment with steroids. With ipilimumab, the most frequent side effects mainly affect the skin (pruritus and cutaneous rash), gastrointestinal tract (colitis and diarrhea), liver (autoimmune hepatitis), and endocrinopathies (hypothyroiditis, hyperthyroiditis, hypophysis). Other irAEs, such as neuropathy or uveitis, can also occur but are less frequent. The safety profile of anti-PD-1/PD-L1 therapy is similar to that of ipilimumab with the addition of pneumonitis. However, in the majority of cases, pneumonitis is grade 1 to grade 2 and is not a cause for discontinuation of treatment. The incidence of grade 3 to grade 4 irAEs with nivolumab and pembrolizumab is generally lower than with ipilimumab but the same algorithms for their management are still applicable. The combination of ipilimumab plus nivolumab has a higher incidence of grade 3 to grade 4 irAEs than either treatment alone but is not associated with novel immune-related safety signals. Another difference with combination therapy is the possibility of two, three, or more different side effects in the same patient; however, the algorithm for the management of the immune-related toxicity is still valid.

With appropriate and timely treatment, these toxicities are generally manageable but can become severe if not recognized. Indeed, these events can be fatal, with 613 fatal checkpoint inhibitor-related toxic events reported from 2009 through January 2018 in the World Health Organization (WHO) pharmacovigilance database.[50] Fatal toxic effects typically occurred early after therapy initiation. Anti-CTLA-4-related deaths were mostly from colitis (70%), whereas anti-PD-1/PD-L1-related deaths were most often related to pneumonitis (35%), hepatitis (22%), and neurotoxic effects (15%). The highest mortality rate was associated with myocarditis. In another analysis of the WHO database, use of checkpoint inhibitors was associated with an increased risk of myocarditis, as well as pericardial disease and vasculitis.[51] These cardiovascular irAEs were usually severe in the majority of cases, with death occurring in 50% of patients with myocarditis and 21% of patients with pericardial disease.

Several studies have reported a potential association between the occurrence of irAEs during immunotherapy and treatment efficacy, including in patients with melanoma,[52] NSCLC,[53] and renal cell carcinoma.[54] These findings suggest a possible mechanistic association between irAEs and immunotherapy efficacy, but this remains to be proven.

Combination Strategies

Dual Checkpoint Inhibition

Anti-CTLA-4 and anti-PD-1 treatment enhance antitumor immunity through distinct but complementary mechanisms, and preclinical models have shown that blocking both receptors, as compared with blockade of either alone, significantly improves antitumor responses.[55] Several trials have now provided evidence that combined CTLA-4 and PD-1 blockade offers improved outcomes versus either as monotherapy, primarily in advanced melanoma but also in other solid tumors.

Ipilimumab plus nivolumab showed very interesting results in Phase 1/2 melanoma studies,[56,57] which were confirmed in a Phase 3 trial in patients with untreated melanoma[28] that showed improved results with the combination versus monotherapy. Unfortunately, combination therapy was associated with a higher incidence of grade 3 to grade 4 treatment-related AEs in this Phase 3 study; 55% in the nivolumab plus ipilimumab group compared with 16.3% in the nivolumab group, and 27.3% in the ipilimumab group. No new safety signals or additional treatment-related deaths were reported after a follow-up of 5 years.[8] Moreover, OS and PFS among patients who discontinued nivolumab plus ipilimumab due to a treatment-related adverse event during the induction phase were similar to the respective survival rates in the overall population, indicating that early discontinuation due to an adverse event does not reduce long-term survival. However, in the future, it will be important to have a treatment plan that can provide the same improved benefit but with less toxicity, and this is being explored with various dose regimens. In the CheckMate 511 trial, the incidence of grade 3 to grade 5 treatment-related adverse events was significantly lower with nivolumab 3 mg/kg plus ipilimumab 1 mg/kg, compared with nivolumab 1 mg/kg plus ipilimumab 3 mg/kg (34% vs. 48%).[58] Efficacy was generally comparable between groups, suggesting this alternative dosing regimen may be a therapeutic option to reduce adverse events. In addition, the KEYNOTE-029 trial of pembrolizumab 2 mg/kg with ipilimumab 1 mg/kg every 3 weeks for four cycles in advanced melanoma achieved an ORR

of 57% but with a slightly lower incidence of grade 3 to grade 4 AEs (42%).[59,60]

As well as melanoma, combined CTLA-4 and PD-1 blockade has been shown to be effective in other solid tumors, including urothelial cancer, renal cancer, small-cell lung cancer (SCLC), and NSCLC.

In the Phase 1/2 CheckMate 032 study, patients with platinum-pretreated advanced urothelial carcinoma received nivolumab alone, nivolumab 3 mg/kg plus ipilimumab 1 mg/kg every 3 weeks for four doses followed by nivolumab monotherapy, or nivolumab 1 mg/kg plus ipilimumab 3 mg/kg every 3 weeks for four doses followed by nivolumab monotherapy until disease progression or unacceptable toxicity.[61] ORR was 25.6%, 26.9%, and 38.0% in the three treatment arms, respectively, and median duration of response was more than 22 months in all arms. Grade 3 to grade 4 treatment-related adverse events occurred in 26.9%, 30.8%, and 39.1% of patients, respectively.

In advanced RCC, ORR and OS were significantly higher with nivolumab plus ipilimumab than with sunitinib among intermediate-risk and poor-risk patients with previously untreated advanced-stage disease enrolled in the CheckMate-214 trial.[62] The 18-month OS rate was 75% (95% CI: 70–78) with nivolumab plus ipilimumab and 60% (95% CI: 55–65) with sunitinib. Median OS was not reached with nivolumab plus ipilimumab versus 26.0 months with sunitinib (HR for death, 0.63; p <.001). ORR was 42% versus 27% (p <.001). The greater efficacy of nivolumab plus ipilimumab over sunitinib was maintained after extended follow-up (median 32 months), with median OS (median not reached vs. 26.6 months, HR 0.66; p <.0001), median PFS (8.2 vs. 8.3 months, HR 0.77; p = .0014), and ORR (42% vs. 29%; p = .0001), all favoring combined checkpoint inhibition.[63]

Combined immunotherapy may also have a role in the treatment of lung cancer. In the Phase 1/2 open-label CheckMate 032 trial, 216 patients with limited- or extensive-stage SCLC after progression on platinum-based chemotherapy were randomized to nivolumab of three different nivolumab plus ipilimumab dose regimens.[64] ORR rate was 10% in patients receiving nivolumab monotherapy versus 19% to 33% in patients receiving combined nivolumab plus ipilimumab. The combination had a manageable safety profile. Whole-exome sequencing showed that the efficacy of nivolumab plus ipilimumab was enhanced in patients with high TMB, suggesting that this may be a potential biomarker to help identify patients most likely to benefit from combination immunotherapy.[65]

In NSCLC, the combination of tremelimumab plus durvalumab did not improve OS or PFS, compared with chemotherapy.[66] However, nivolumab plus ipilimumab as first-line treatment for advanced NSCLC had a manageable safety profile and showed encouraging clinical activity with a high response rate and durable response in the CheckMate 012 study.[43] In the Phase 3 CheckMate 227 trial, patients with stage IV or recurrent NSCLC not previously treated with chemotherapy and a high TMB were randomized to nivolumab plus ipilimumab, nivolumab monotherapy, or chemotherapy if PD-L1 expression ≥1%, or to nivolumab plus ipilimumab, nivolumab plus chemotherapy, or chemotherapy if PD-L1 expression <1%.[43] PFS was significantly longer with nivolumab plus ipilimumab than with chemotherapy. One-year PFS rate was 42.6% with nivolumab plus ipilimumab versus 13.2% with chemotherapy, and median PFS was 7.2 months (95% CI: 5.5–13.2) versus 5.5 months (95% CI: 4.4–5.8; HR for disease progression or death, 0.58; p <.001). ORR was 45.3% with nivolumab plus ipilimumab and 26.9% with chemotherapy. The benefit of nivolumab plus ipilimumab over chemotherapy was broadly consistent irrespective of PD-L1 expression. In an updated analysis, median OS was significantly longer with nivolumab plus ipilimumab compared with chemotherapy (17.1 vs. 14.9 months, HR 0.79; p = .007) in patients with PD-L1 expression ≥1%; median OS with nivolumab alone was 15.7 months.[67] Median OS was also improved with the combination in patients with PD-L1 <1% (17.1 vs. 13.9 months with chemotherapy and 15.2 months with nivolumab plus chemotherapy).

Checkpoint Inhibition Combined With Other Immunotherapies

In addition to the checkpoint inhibitors, numerous other potential immuno-strategies are being explored to overcome tumor immune evasion mechanisms, such as the promotion of T cell activation pathways, enhancing innate immune function, and the potentiation of immune effector function. Importantly, the development of varied immunotherapeutic approaches with distinct modes of action offers the potential for various combination strategies.

Lymphocyte activation gene-3 (LAG-3; CD223) is a type I transmembrane protein expressed on activated CD4+ and CD8+ T cells and subsets of natural killer (NK) and dendritic cells (DCs) that has an important role in promoting regulatory T cell (T$_{reg}$ cell) activity and suppressing T cell activation and proliferation. In preliminary data, treatment with the anti-LAG-3 agent relatlimab, in combination with nivolumab, resulted in an ORR of 11.5% in patients with advanced melanoma that progressed on prior anti-PD-1/PD-L1 therapy.[68] Responses were more likely in patients with LAG expression ≥1%, irrespective of PD-L1 expression. Another anti-LAG-3 agent in development, MK4280, was well tolerated in combination with pembrolizumab in a first-in-human Phase 1/2 trial in patients with advanced solid tumors,

with a similar adverse event profile as pembrolizumab monotherapy. Partial responses were achieved in four of 15 patients (27%).[69] Several other anti-LAG-3 antibodies are also in development and are being assessed in combination with various anti-PD-1 agents.

Toll-like receptors (TLRs) may serve as important regulators in the development of a variety of cancers. CMP-001 is a CpG-A oligodeoxynucleotide TLR-9 antagonist that activates tumor-associated DCs to produce interferon and induce antitumor systemic immunity. In combination with pembrolizumab, treatment with CMP-001 resulted in a 25% ORR, including six complete responses and 15 partial responses, in patients with anti-PD-1 refractory melanoma.[70] Four patients who continued study therapy beyond initial disease progression achieved a response, and treatment was well tolerated. In another trial, preliminary data reported that neoadjuvant CMP-001, in combination with nivolumab, in PD-1 naïve patients was generally well tolerated with no dose-limiting toxicities or surgery delays related to treatment. A major pathologic response rate of 71% was reported in 21 evaluable patients to date and, of 15 responding patients, 13 had a pathologic complete response.[71] Another TLR-9 agonist, tilsotolimod (IMO-2125), which is administered intratumorally, was well tolerated and showed durable responses when given in combination with ipilimumab in patients with advanced melanoma who had progressed on or after anti-PD-1 therapy.[72]

Bempegaldesleukin (NKTR-214) is a CD122-preferential IL-2 pathway agonist shown to increase tumor-infiltrating lymphocytes, T cell clonality, and PD-L1 expression. In the PIVOT-02 study of 41 melanoma patients treated with at least one dose of bempegaldesleukin plus nivolumab, ORR was 53% with 42% of patients having 100% reduction in target lesions and 34% complete responses.[73] Another trial, the Phase 1/2 PROPEL study, is evaluating NKTR-214 in combination with atezolizumab and pembrolizumab.

Entinostat is an oral class I-selective histone deacetylase (HDAC) inhibitor that leads to downregulation of immunosuppressive cell types in the TME. In the ENCORE-601 trial, 53 patients with advanced melanoma who experienced progression on or after anti-PD-1 therapy received open-label treatment with entinostat plus pembrolizumab.[74,75] Confirmed ORR was 19% (one complete and nine partial responses) and the median duration of response was 12.5 months (range 4–18 months), with four ongoing. An additional nine patients had stable disease for more than 6 months. Median PFS was 4.2 months and safety was acceptable.

CD73 is a catabolic enzyme that dephosphorylates extracellular adenosine monophosphate, leading to an extracellular adenosine increase that stimulates the dysregulation of immune cell infiltrates and a protumorigenic abnormal vascularization, promoting the onset and progression of tumors. In a Phase 1 trial in 59 patients with advanced solid tumors, the CD73 antibody BMS-986179 in combination with nivolumab was well tolerated with a safety profile similar to nivolumab monotherapy.[76] The combination showed preliminary antitumor activity, with CD73 enzyme activity in the tumor vasculature and tumor cells inhibited. Seven patients achieved a confirmed partial response and 10 patients had stable disease. Another anti-CD73 antibody, oleclumab, had a manageable safety profile and encouraging clinical activity in combination with the anti-PD-L1 antibody durvalumab in patients with advanced pancreatic or colorectal cancer.[77]

Checkpoint Inhibition Combined With Other Treatment Modalities

Another important development is the potential to combine immunotherapy with other treatment modalities, such as targeted therapy, chemotherapy, and radiotherapy. Existing treatment modalities cause tumor reduction, not only through cytotoxic/cytostatic effects but also through mechanisms that may potentiate immune activity, including modification of the TME and release of tumor antigens. This activity may be complementary, or even synergistic, to the immunotherapies designed to support an antitumor immune response. Combination approaches may thus increase the long-term benefit for patients, and so increase the proportion of patients who achieve a chronic disease state.

One particular area of focus is the combination of immunotherapy with other treatments, especially targeted therapy. This approach represents a rational combination, given that targeted agents induce a higher rate of response, which is more rapid but shorter in duration, while immunotherapy results in a lower initial response with a slower onset of action but provides a more durable longer-term effect. Initial investigations into combining ipilimumab with the BRAF inhibitor vemurafenib were disappointing, with a Phase 1 study of these two drugs in combination showing an increase in hepatotoxicity that precluded adequate dosing in patients with melanoma.[78] However, subsequent data have shown that combinations of another BRAF inhibitor, dabrafenib, plus ipilimumab with or without trametinib are not associated with hepatotoxicity, although the triple combination was not feasible due to a high risk of bowel perforation.[79] Concerns over the toxicity of ipilimumab in combination has largely shifted focus toward the use of anti-PD-1/PD-L1 agents, which appear to offer better tolerability.

Since the superiority of combined BRAF plus MEK inhibition, compared with BRAF inhibitor monotherapy, has been widely demonstrated, most studies in melanoma have evaluated a triple combination of BRAK and MEK inhibitors plus a PD-1/PD-L1 inhibitor. In the KEYNOTE-022 study, median PFS was 16.0 months with pembrolizumab plus dabrafenib and trametinib compared with 10.3 months with dabrafenib plus trametinib; this difference (hazard ratio [HR] 0.66; $p = .042870$) was nonsignificant because it did not meet the prespecified significance parameter of an HR of ≤0.62.[68] With longer-term follow-up, the triple combination continued to show numerically higher 2-year rates of PFS (41% vs. 16%) and OS (63% vs. 52%).[80] However, these improvements were accompanied by a higher incidence of grade 3 to grade 5 adverse events (58% vs. 25%) and a higher incidence of discontinuation of at least one study drug because of adverse events (43% vs. 18%). In preliminary data from another study (IMPemBra), pembrolizumab plus intermittent dabrafenib plus trametinib appears to be a promising combination in terms of safety and feasibility.[81] At 18 weeks, grade 3 to grade 4 adverse events occurred in 12% of patients receiving pembrolizumab alone and 12% receiving pembrolizumab plus two 1-week courses of dabrafenib plus trametinib; rates were higher in patients receiving pembrolizumab with dabrafenib plus trametinib for two intermittent periods of 2 weeks or 6 continuous weeks (50% and 62%, respectively).[82] ORRs were generally similar across all treatment arms (50%–75%).[83] The BRAF/MEK inhibitor combination of vemurafenib plus cobimetinib has also been assessed in combination with the PD-L1 inhibitor atezolizumab. Triple combination therapy after a 28-day run-in period with cobimetinib plus vemurafenib resulted in substantial but manageable toxicity and a confirmed ORR of 71.8%. Responses were ongoing in 39.3% of patients after 29.9 months of follow-up.[74,75] However, such triple combinations are not currently used outside of a clinical trial setting.

In the IMblaze370 trial in patients with primarily microsatellite-stable locally advanced or metastatic colorectal cancer, atezolizumab plus cobimetinib or atezolizumab alone did not improve OS versus regorafenib.[84] Median OS was 8.87 months (95% CI 7.00–10.61) with atezolizumab plus cobimetinib, 7.10 months (6.05–10.05) with atezolizumab, and 8.51 months (6.41–10.71) with regorafenib. The combination of atezolizumab and cobimetinib also failed to improve PFS, compared with pembrolizumab monotherapy, in patients with previously untreated BRAF V600 wild-type melanoma, missing the primary endpoint of the Phase 3 IMspire170 trial.[85]

An alternative strategy to combine concurrent treatment is sequential therapy. Studies have confirmed that sequential treatment with ipilimumab and vemurafenib results in greater efficacy, compared with treatment with either drug alone. However, the sequence in which to use these treatments remains an important question. Approximately 40% to 50% of patients progressing after BRAF inhibitor treatment have a rapidly progressive disease with death occurring within 1 to 2 months. For these patients, subsequent treatment with ipilimumab may not be optimal, since there is evidence that the full four cycles of ipilimumab treatment are necessary to obtain a meaningful benefit. This can be explained by the immunological mechanism of action of ipilimumab, which means it requires a certain period of time before becoming effective. In data from the Italian expanded access program for ipilimumab, median OS among patients treated with a BRAF inhibitor first was 1.2 months from the end of BRAF inhibition for those who did not complete ipilimumab treatment, compared with 12.7 months for those who did.[49] Similarly, outcomes for patients treated with ipilimumab following BRAF inhibitor discontinuation in a recent trial were poor, with only half able to complete four cycles of ipilimumab and median OS of 5.0 months.[86] However, treatment with ipilimumab (or IL-2) did not appear to negatively influence subsequent response to BRAF inhibitor therapy. Metastases in three or more organ sites and higher baseline lactate dehydrogenase have been shown to be prognostic for worse survival in BRAF-mutated melanoma patients treated with dabrafenib plus trametinib,[59,60] and it has been suggested that patients with these risk factors may benefit more from treatment with a BRAF inhibitor before immunotherapy.[87]

Ongoing studies will further help identify the optimal sequential approach. These include the SECOMBIT trial, a three-arm noncomparative randomized study, which will explore combination immunotherapy (ipilimumab plus nivolumab), followed by combination-targeted therapy (encorafenib plus binimetinib) or vice versa in patients with BRAF-mutated metastatic melanoma. The third arm will involve an 8-week induction period with the combination-targeted therapy, switching at the best response (not at disease progression) to the combination immunotherapy, and then back to the targeted combination at disease progression (NCT02631447). Another study, the Phase 2 EBIN trial (NCT03235245), will compare encorafenib plus binimetinib, followed by nivolumab plus ipilimumab versus nivolumab plus ipilimumab. The ECOG 6134 DREAMseq trial is a randomized Phase 3 study to compare ipilimumab plus nivolumab, followed by dabrafenib plus trametinib versus dabrafenib plus trametinib, followed by ipilimumab and nivolumab in patients with advanced melanoma (NCT02224781).

Immunotherapy has also been combined with other treatment modalities. In NSCLC, pembrolizumab plus chemotherapy with pemetrexed and a platinum-based drug significantly prolonged OS versus chemotherapy alone in patients with nonsquamous NSCLC.[88] The addition of pembrolizumab to carboplatin plus paclitaxel or nab-paclitaxel also resulted in significantly longer OS and PFS than chemotherapy alone in patients with previously untreated squamous NSCLC.[89] In advanced triple-negative breast cancer, the addition of atezolizumab to nab-paclitaxel chemotherapy resulted in significant increases in median PFS in the overall population versus chemotherapy alone (7.2 versus 5.5 months; HR 0.80, $p = .002$) as well as in patients with PD-L1-positive tumors (7.5 versus 5.0 months, HR 0.62; $p < .001$).[90] Median OS was also longer in the immunotherapy group than in the placebo group among patients with PD-L1-positive tumors. Among PD-L1-negative patients, the addition of atezolizumab to nab-paclitaxel failed to extend PFS or OS. Adverse events were consistent with the known safety profiles of each single-agent.

In a trial of 30 patients with hepatocellular carcinoma, treatment with pembrolizumab plus lenvatinib resulted in an ORR of 37% by investigator assessment using mRECIST criteria.[91] By independent imaging review, ORRs of 50% using mRECIST criteria and 37% using RECIST 1.1 criteria were achieved. In renal cell carcinoma, pembrolizumab plus the VEGF inhibitor, axitinib, resulted in significantly improved OS and PFS versus sunitinib as first-line therapy in the KEYNOTE-426 trial.[92] Axitinib has also been evaluated in combination with avelumab in the JAVELIN renal 100 trial, with manageable toxicity and promising antitumor activity in preliminary analysis.[93]

Radiotherapy also has a synergism of action with immunotherapy.[94] Patients with NSCLC who received pembrolizumab after radiotherapy had a significantly better response versus patients receiving pembrolizumab alone (41% vs. 19%).[95] Activity and safety of radiotherapy with anti-PD-1 drug therapy has also been shown in patients with metastatic melanoma.[96;97] However, there are several unanswered questions about this combination with regard to patient selection; the correct sequencing of treatment, radiotherapy dose, and fractionation; and the optimal site to irradiate in metastatic disease.

FROM METASTATIC DISEASE TO ADJUVANT THERAPY

Across studies in melanoma, the best outcomes have generally been observed in patients with favorable prognostic factors, particularly a normal or low lactate dehydrogenase (LDH) level and/or a low disease burden. For example, in the CheckMate 067 trial, there was a trend for improved OS in patients with favorable prognostic factors, with the highest 5-year survival rates with nivolumab plus ipilimumab in patients with normal LDH with or without fewer than three sites of disease.[8] This may also suggest a potential role for immunotherapy at an earlier disease stage and use in the adjuvant setting (Figure 49.2).[4]

Ipilimumab was the first successful checkpoint inhibitor in metastatic melanoma and has also been shown to be effective in the adjuvant setting.[98] However, adjuvant

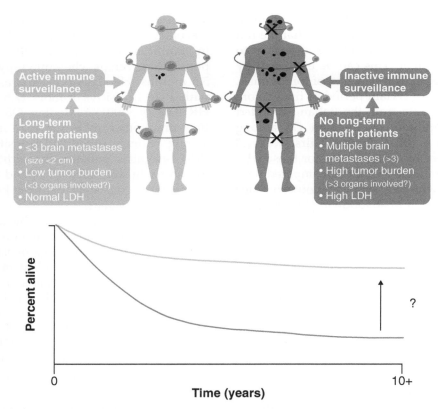

Figure 49.2 Long-term survival and risk factors in patients with metastatic melanoma.

LDH, lactate dehydrogenase.

Source: Reproduced with permission from Michielin O, Atkins MB, Koon HB, et al. Evolving impact of long-term survival results on metastatic melanoma treatment. *J Immunother Cancer.* 2020;8(2):e000948. doi:10.1136/jitc-2020-000948

treatment with ipilimumab is associated with significant toxicity, and means nivolumab and pembrolizumab may be preferred as adjuvant treatment. In the CheckMate 238 trial, the 1-year rate of recurrence-free survival (RFS) was 70.5% with nivolumab versus 60.8% with ipilimumab (HR for disease recurrence or death, 0.65; 97.56% CI: 0.51–0.83; *p* <.001).[99] Treatment-related grade 3 to grade 4 adverse events were reported in 14% of patients treated with nivolumab versus 46% of patients treated with ipilimumab. The estimated cure rate was 55% with nivolumab.[100] Similarly, pembrolizumab significantly increased the 1-year rate of RFS versus placebo (HR for recurrence or death, 0.57; 98.4% CI:0.43–0.74; *p* <.001) in the KEYNOTE-054 trial, with 15% of pembrolizumab patients experiencing treatment-related grade 3 to grade 5 adverse events.[101] The benefit with immunotherapy was consistent across mutational status and PD-L1 expression subgroups. In a secondary analysis of this trial, occurrence of immune-related adverse events was associated with a longer RFS in the pembrolizumab arm.[102]

In NSCLC, the PACIFIC trial compared the anti-PD-L1 antibody durvalumab with placebo as maintenance treatment after two or more cycles of platinum-based chemoradiotherapy in patients with stage III disease without progression. Median PFS from randomization was 16.8 months (95% CI 13.0–18.1) with durvalumab versus 5.6 months (95% CI, 4.6–7.8) with placebo (stratified hazard ratio for disease progression or death, 0.52; 95% CI, 0.42–0.65; *p* <.001).[103] PFS survival rate at 18 months was 44.2% with pembrolizumab versus 27.0% with placebo. Durvalumab therapy also resulted in significantly longer OS than placebo (stratified hazard ratio for death, 0.68; 99.73% CI, 0.47–0.997; *p* = .0025).[104] The 2-year OS rate was 66.3% (95% [CI], 61.7–70.4) with durvalumab versus 55.6% (95% CI, 48.9–61.8) with placebo (*p* = .005). Durvalumab was well tolerated and safety was generally similar between groups.

Several adjuvant trials in melanoma, NSCLC, and other cancers are ongoing with their results eagerly anticipated.

NEOADJUVANT THERAPY: THE NEXT STEP

The next stage in the development of cancer immunotherapy may be a move into the neoadjuvant setting.

Neoadjuvant immunotherapy may allow the tumor burden to be reduced before surgery and induce stronger tumor-specific T cell responses. The efficacy of subsequent adjuvant therapy may also be better predicted, and pathologic response rates can be utilized as surrogate outcome markers for RFS and OS.

In melanoma, neoadjuvant ipilimumab plus nivolumab did not delay surgery and was superior to adjuvant therapy in expanding tumor-resident T cell receptor clones in the OpACIN study.[105] Pathologic response rate was high (78%) but treatment was highly toxic with 90% grade 3 to grade 4 adverse events. In the subsequent Phase 2 OpACIN-neo trial to identify the optimal neoadjuvant ipilimumab and nivolumab combination regimen, two cycles of ipilimumab 1 mg/kg plus nivolumab 3 mg/kg was tolerable, with grade 3 to grade 4 immune-related adverse events observed in one-fifth of patients, and induced a pathologic response in 77% of patients.[82] This dosing schedule might be considered for clinical use but should be compared with standard-of-care adjuvant therapies.

In a randomized Phase 2 study of neoadjuvant nivolumab versus combined ipilimumab with nivolumab in 23 patients with high-risk resectable melanoma, treatment with nivolumab alone resulted in lower responses than the combination (ORR 25% vs. 73%, pathologic complete response 25% vs. 45%).[106] However, nivolumab monotherapy was associated with substantially lower toxicity (treatment-related adverse events grade $\geq$3 in 8% vs. 73% of patients). In a pooled analysis from the International Neoadjuvant Melanoma Consortium, neoadjuvant immunotherapy (nivolumab as monotherapy or in combination with ipilimumab, pembrolizumab) and targeted therapy (dabrafenib plus trametinib) were active in resectable clinical stage III melanoma patients and a pathologic complete response rate was observed in 41% of patients, with 38% receiving immunotherapy and 47% receiving targeted therapy.[107] Recurrence occurred in 14% of patients after immunotherapy (median follow-up 10 months) and 51% after targeted therapy (median follow-up of 22 months). 12-month RFS was improved with IT versus TT (83% vs. 65%, p <.001). Pathologic complete response was correlated with a favorable RFS, with 1-year RFS significantly better in those with versus without pathologic complete response (95% vs. 62%, p <.001), suggesting its potential as a surrogate for long-term benefit.

Neoadjuvant immunotherapy has also shown promise in other cancers. In the CheckMate 358 trial, neoadjuvant nivolumab was well tolerated and induced a major pathologic response in 65% of patients with resectable Merkel cell carcinoma, including 47% complete responses.[108] Among 21 patients followed after surgery, all were progression-free at 6 months and two had relapsed at 1 year. In a different cohort in the same trial,

neoadjuvant nivolumab resulted in presurgery tumor reduction in 11 of 23 (48%) patients with SCCHN.[109] Nivolumab was also well tolerated, with no delays to surgery due to adverse events.

In patients with advanced resectable NSCLC, neoadjuvant nivolumab had an acceptable side-effect profile and was not associated with delays in surgery.[110] A major pathologic response occurred in 45% of resected tumors (45%) and occurred in both PD-L1-positive and PD-L1-negative tumors. In early stage dMMR and MMR-proficient colorectal cancer, neoadjuvant ipilimumab plus nivolumab resulted in major pathologic responses in all of seven dMMR tumors and did not delay surgery.[111] No major pathologic responses were seen in MMR-proficient tumors, although significant increases in T cell infiltration were seen post-treatment. In glioblastoma, neoadjuvant nivolumab resulted in increased chemokine transcripts, higher immune cell infiltration, and augmented T cell receptor clonal diversity among tumor-infiltrating lymphocytes, indicating a local immunomodulatory effect.[112]

EFFICACY IN BRAIN METASTASES

Anti-PD-1/anti-CTLA-4 combination therapy is also being assessed in patients with melanoma metastatic to the brain. In the Phase 2 CheckMate 204 study, nivolumab plus ipilimumab resulted in an intracranial clinical benefit rate of 57% after a median follow-up of 14.0 months, with no unexpected neurologic safety signals in asymptomatic patients with untreated brain metastases.[113] This clinical benefit rate was durable and was maintained at 58% after median follow-up of 21 months.[114] In a separate cohort of patients in the same trial who had neurologic symptoms with or without steroid therapy, clinical benefit rate after a median of 5 months was 22.2% and intracranial ORR was 16.7%.[114]

Similarly, in a Phase 2 trial in patients with asymptomatic melanoma brain metastases and no previous local brain therapy, intracranial ORR was 46% with nivolumab plus ipilimumab versus 20% with nivolumab alone.[115] At median follow-up of 34 months, these responses were maintained with 2-year intracranial PFS rates of 49% with the combination and 15% with nivolumab alone.[116] Patients with brain metastases in whom local therapy had failed or who had neurological symptoms or leptomeningeal disease responded poorly to nivolumab alone, with an intracranial ORR of 6%. Nivolumab plus ipilimumab also improved OS in patients with asymptomatic or symptomatic melanoma brain metastases, especially combined with stereotactic radiosurgery or surgery.[117] Pembrolizumab has also shown intracranial activity with durable responses and an acceptable safety profile in melanoma and NSCLC patients with untreated brain metastases.[118]

CONCLUSION

Immunotherapy in cancer is rapidly evolving, with various treatments being investigated for their potential to provide long-term survival across a broad range of tumor types, and for their synergistic activity when combined with other treatment modalities. It is important now to determine how to advance this field and how to use these new immunotherapies most effectively to achieve the best patient outcomes. Areas of investigation are broad, and include combining or sequencing immunotherapies that target distinct immune pathways, combining or sequencing an immunotherapeutic agent with existing treatment modalities, and determining the optimal schedule of therapies in combination regimens. At present, it is difficult to identify the best combination approaches to pursue, given the limited data and the somewhat unpredictable occurrence of toxicity with some combinations.

Combining immunotherapies that target distinct immune pathways has the potential to overcome more than one of the barriers that tumor cells develop to evade the immune system, and may provide an OS benefit in a greater portion of patients, compared with either agent alone. However, the ideal sequence, schedule, and combination of immunotherapies need to be determined. Likewise, it is important to determine optimal dose, schedule, and sequence when combining an immunotherapy with radiotherapy, chemotherapy, or targeted agents, as these therapies all have different mechanisms of action. A final consideration for combining immunotherapies will be to identify the regimens with the best risk-benefit profile. We can expect improvements in overall clinical efficacy as new agents targeting alternative or overlapping tumor-associated immunosuppressive mechanisms are developed and used in combination or sequentially.

Immuno-oncology therapies have already resulted in significant improvements in survival for patients with cancer. In particular, combined use of these new agents with other treatment modalities may represent a significant new option in the future treatment of melanoma and cancer in general.

KEY REFERENCES

Only key references appear in the print edition. The full reference list appears in the digital product on Springer Publishing Connect: connect.springerpub.com/content/book/978-0-8261-3743-2/part/part04/chapter/ch49

5. Ascierto PA, Ferrucci PF, Fisher R, et al. Dabrafenib, trametinib and pembrolizumab or placebo in BRAF-mutant melanoma. *Nat Med*. 2019;25(6):941–946. doi:10.1038/s41591-019-0448-9
8. Larkin J, Chiarion-Sileni V, Gonzalez R, et al. Five-year survival with combined nivolumab and ipilimumab in advanced melanoma. *N Engl J Med*. 2019;381(16):1535–1546. doi:10.1056/NEJMoa1910836
41. Hellmann MD, Paz-Ares L, Bernabe Caro R, et al. Nivolumab plus ipilimumab in advanced non-small-cell lung cancer. *N Engl J Med*. 2019;381(21):2020–2031. doi:10.1056/NEJMoa1910231
62. Motzer RJ, Tannir NM, Mcdermott DF, et al. Nivolumab plus ipilimumab versus sunitinib in advanced renal-cell carcinoma. *N Engl J Med*. 2018;378(14):1277–1290. doi:10.1056/NEJMoa1712126
89. Paz-Ares L, Luft A, Vicente D, et al. Pembrolizumab plus chemotherapy for squamous non-small-cell lung cancer. *N Engl J Med*. 2018;379(21):2040–2051. doi:10.1056/NEJMoa1810865
90. Schmid P, Adams S, Rugo HS, et al. Atezolizumab and nab-paclitaxel in advanced triple-negative breast cancer. *N Engl J Med*. 2018;379(22):2108–2121. doi:10.1056/NEJMoa1809615
94. Demaria S, Golden EB, Formenti SC. Role of local radiation therapy in cancer immunotherapy. *JAMA Oncol*. 2015;1(9):1325–1332. doi:10.1001/jamaoncol.2015.2756
107. Menzies AM, Rozeman EA, Amaria RN, et al. Pathological response and survival with neoadjuvant therapy in melanoma: a pooled analysis from the International Neoadjuvant Melanoma Consortium (INMC). *J Clin Oncol*. 2019;37(15 suppl):9503. doi:10.1200/JCO.2019.37.15_suppl.9503

Immunotherapy in Melanoma

Antonio Maria Grimaldi, Igor Puzanov, and Paolo A. Ascierto

KEY POINTS

- The immune system plays an important role in melanoma, promoting both tumor progression and regression.

- In the past, cytokines (interferon-α [IFN-α], interleukin-2 [IL-2]) and vaccines were used to treat patients with melanoma. IL-2 showed low response rates; however, 5% to 8% of patients achieved confirmed objective response rate (ORR) and had long-term survival. Melanoma vaccines were generally safe and showed evidence of immunity but had low response rates and no overall survival (OS).

- The development of checkpoint inhibitors (anti-CTLA-4 and anti-PD-1/PDL-1) revolutionized the treatment and long-term survival of melanoma patients, being effective in both metastatic and adjuvant settings regardless of BRAF status.

- Anti-PD-1 (pembrolizumab or nivolumab) adjuvant therapy improved the 4-year relapse-free survival by more than 50%.

- Combination anti-CTLA-4 and anti-PD-1 (ipilimumab/nivolumab) achieved 5-year OS of 53%. However, there is an important unmet need to find an effective treatment for melanoma patients with primary and acquired resistance to immunotherapy.

- Immune checkpoint inhibitors (ICIs) can be combined safely and effectively with other treatments: immunotherapy, chemotherapy, and targeted therapy. Several promising combinations are currently in clinical trials. The optimal sequencing of targeted therapies and ICIs in patients with BRAF-mutation-positive melanoma is under investigation. Biomarker development to enable personalized immunotherapy will be critically important in furthering our progress.

INTRODUCTION

Historically, immunotherapy had been considered one of the most promising therapeutic options for the treatment of melanoma, but it was not until recently that this promise has been truly achieved. Evidence of cancer immunosurveillance that supposedly involved the immune system in tumor growth control mechanisms has long been known: patients with severe and persistent immune system deficiency (e.g., AIDS, patients undergoing organ transplants) develop cancers at rates higher than healthy subjects; T cells infiltrate tumors and have been found to be independent prognostic factors for better outcomes; and some tumors spontaneously regress, likely in response to an immunologic tumor-specific reaction.[1]

Despite considerable progress in understanding the immunological mechanisms and in the possibility of manipulating many aspects of the immune system, clinical results have unfortunately been disappointing for decades. Gradually, a lot of evidence has been accumulated that immunotherapy failures were mainly related to mechanisms of the host's tolerance to tumor antigens and the tumor's capacity to act with a series of escape mechanisms (downregulation of melanoma-associated antigens); inhibition of the maturation of antigen-presenting cells (APCs); instability/loss of antigen expression; and local immunosuppression operated by different cell types, such as myeloid-derived suppressor cells, regulatory T cells (T_{reg} cells), and M2 macrophages, as well as from several soluble substances (e.g., transforming growth factor-β [TGF-β], interleukin-4 [IL-4], IL-6, IL-10, indoleamine 2,3-dioxygenase [IDO], arginase).

The first attempts to use the immune system against cancer may date back to 1890 when William Coley, using live bacteria (Coley's toxin) administered to patients with advanced cancer, observed occasional but significant reductions of the tumor. After a long period of stagnation, interest in cancer immunotherapy had a new revival in 1960, with the observation that the administration of irradiated tumor cells in combination with immunological adjuvants such as Calmette–Guerin Bacille, *Corynebacterium parvum*, or attenuated virus in animal models induced regression of some types of cancer.

Another milestone in the history of immunotherapy was laid in 1988 when Dariavach and colleagues identified and cloned the human gene coding for a molecule that plays a key role in regulating the immune response, the cytotoxic T lymphocyte-associated antigen-4 (CTLA-4) gene.[2]

MELANOMA AND IMMUNE SYSTEM

Cutaneous melanoma has always been an immunosensitive cancer, evidenced by the huge number of scientific papers of immunotherapy, both in the adjuvant and in the metastatic setting. Unfortunately, initial vaccine studies showed low response rates and no clear overall survival (OS) benefits. However, how were these failures explained? The melanoma cells, such as cancer cells, in general, can evade the common mechanisms of an immune response.

In particular, the crucial moments for the activation of the immune system include antigen exposure and then recognition and presentation of these antigens, in the appropriate context, to T and B lymphocytes. T cells are activated when the T cell receptor (TCR) binds to the antigen presented by the major histocompatibility complex (MHC). The T cells then proliferate and migrate into the tumor site, where they carry out their anticancer activity. The activation of T cells during antigen presentation is a tightly regulated process mediated by co-stimulatory and co-inhibitory receptors to maintain immunologic homeostasis. Often these receptors are called "immune checkpoints." An example of the role of co-stimulation in mediating immunity is the link between CD28 on the T cell and B7 on the APC. Binding between CD28 and B7 induces a co-stimulation signal (commonly called the "second signal") required for final T cell activation after binding of TCR with MHC—antigen complex (commonly called the "first signal"). The tumor cells can inhibit T cell responses through the expression of various ligands that interact with inhibitory receptors, such as CTLA-4 and programmed cell death 1 (PD-1) on T cells. To counter these mechanisms, monoclonal antibodies that antagonize these receptors for therapeutic purposes have been developed.[3]

CYTOKINES

Interferon-α

Interferon-α (IFN-α) was perhaps the first cytokine shown to improve outcomes for patients with cancer. Specifically, in the 1980s, IFN demonstrated significant benefit in patients with hairy cell leukemia, enough to obtain U.S. Food and Drug Administration (FDA) approval for this indication. IFN exerts its activity through a series of partially known mechanisms: antiproliferative effects on tumor cells directly, increased expression of tumor antigens, enhancement of innate and adaptive immunity, and antiangiogenic effects. Recent studies have shown that IFN is also an important regulator of cell growth and differentiation and can influence different transduction

pathway signals that directly lead to apoptosis of the cancer cell. In addition, IFN affects different phases of the cell cycle by inducing overexpression of inhibitors of cyclin-dependent kinases. Given these properties, IFN has been used directly and in combination with vaccines for the treatment of patients with cancer.

Numerous studies conducted in the 1990s have explored the efficacy of high-dose IFN therapy as a treatment for patients with metastatic melanoma, predominantly in the adjuvant setting. IFN at high doses as adjuvant therapy has reliably been shown to improve recurrence-free survival. The effect of IFN on improving OS in randomized studies is less clear as OS improvement has been shown in some, but not all, studies. The Eastern Cooperative Oncology Group (ECOG) trial (EST 1684) randomized 287 patients with surgically resected stage III melanoma to IFN-α–2b administered at a maximum tolerated doses of 20 MU/m²/d intravenously (IV) 5 days a week for 1 month and 10 MU/m² three times per week subcutaneously (SC) for 48 weeks, or to observation. At a median follow-up of 6.9 years, IFN-α-2b demonstrated an increment in median disease-free survival (DFS) from 1 to 1.7 years and OS from 2.8 to 3.8 years as compared with observation. Moreover, IFN-α-2b therapy was associated with a 42% improvement in the fraction of patients who were continuously disease-free after treatment (26%–37%) in comparison to observation.[4] However, the use of IFN has been limited by the considerable effort that this treatment requires, both in terms of side effects and the intended duration of the treatment period (1 year).

Meanwhile, the European Organization for Research and Treatment of Cancer (EORTC) developed the use of intermediate doses and PEGylated forms of IFN. Other formulations of IFN, such as PEGylated IFN, have not been more widely used, likely because no OS benefit was seen with this approach. Patients with ulcerated primary melanoma and microscopic lymph node involvement may have the greatest benefit from PEGylated IFN, and this is being studied prospectively.[5]

Many attempts have been made to identify the best responders to IFN, to avoid unnecessary treatments in unresponsive patients. An interesting finding, also seen in patients with metastatic disease, is that the development of autoimmunity appeared to be associated with better outcomes. Gogas et al. published a trial that evaluated 200 patients with stage IIb–III resected melanoma treated with high doses of IFN. In this study, serum levels of a panel of autoantibodies (antithyroid, antinuclear, anti-DNA, anticardiolipin), the development of vitiligo, and the manifestations of autoimmune side effects were analyzed.

In a multivariate analysis, autoimmunity turned out to be an independent prognostic factor for both DFS and OS.[6] However, subsequent studies reported contrasting data.[7] Therefore, at present, it is not possible to discriminate IFN responders from nonresponders based on simple clinical and/or biochemical parameters. Nevertheless, the presence of autoimmunity remains of interest in future studies of immunotherapies in the adjuvant setting.

High doses of IFN have also been tested as a neoadjuvant therapy to increase the surgical resectability of otherwise inoperable lesions and establish increased antitumor immunity to treat microscopic metastatic disease. Moschos et al. reported the results obtained in patients with palpable locoregional adenopathy treated with high-dose IFN. In 11/20 patients enrolled, a response rate of 51% was seen, including three complete pathological responses and two patients with only microscopic residual disease at the time of surgery.

At a follow-up of 15 months, six patients had died of melanoma, and of the 14 alive, 11 did not progress. The immunohistochemical study on biopsies performed before and after treatment highlighted the presence of increased intratumoral CD11[+] and CD3[+] lymphocytes and significantly greater decreases in intratumoral CD83[+] cells in responders as compared with nonresponders. These data support the immunologic mechanisms mediated by IFN that play a role in anticancer responses.[8] IFN in metastatic melanoma has been primarily tested in combination with other drugs, such as chemotherapy. The results of these studies have been modest and contradictory.[9]

Interleukin-2

In addition to IFN, cytokine therapy with IL-2 has also been explored in patients with melanoma and other cancers since the 1980s. In 1992, IL-2 was approved in the United States for the treatment of advanced kidney cancer, and in 1998 IL-2 was approved for metastatic melanoma.

The approval in metastatic melanoma was based on a response rate of approximately 15%, with durable responses in approximately 5% of treated patients.[10–12]

A retrospective analysis of the main trials conducted with the use of high doses of IL-2 between 1985 and 1993, and which involved 270 patients, demonstrated an objective response rate (ORR) of 16%, with persistent and long-lasting responses in 4% of treated patients.[10] Moreover, several Phase 3 studies evaluated whether the addition of IFN-α or mono/poly-chemotherapy to IL-2 resulted in superior responses compared with IL-2 alone. Despite higher response rates, however, these studies have failed to provide evidence of superiority in terms of survival.[13]

However, despite the many limitations, IL-2 was an immunotherapy milestone for metastatic melanoma and represented one of the most convincing "proof of principle" concepts that immunotherapy was able to produce complete and durable responses. IL-2 has also been used in combination with immune-manipulated cells (adoptive immunotherapy) including lymphokine-activated killer (LAK) cells, tumor-infiltrating lymphocytes (TIL), and lymphocytes from peripheral blood, resulting in high response rates, and, in some patients, very long-term responses. It is conceivable that combining IL-2 with vaccines may increase the efficacy of IL-2 as suggested by one study.[14] A Phase 3 multicenter study enrolled 185 patients with metastatic melanoma treated with the combination of gp100 peptide vaccination and high doses of IL-2 versus IL-2 alone. Despite the long period of accrual and difficulties to complete the study because of problems related to high doses of IL-2 used, outcomes including ORR and progression-free survival (PFS) were significantly higher in the combination arm.[14] OS was longer in the combination group as well, but this was not statistically significant.

Vaccines

The administration of substances capable of inducing an immunologic antineoplastic specific response in the host (that can recognize the tumor and put in place specific anticancer activity) that is effective (i.e., capable of destroying and removing the tumor) has been a fascinating objective for many years, but effective clinical results have been difficult to achieve.[15]

It has long been demonstrated by several groups of researchers that many vaccine approaches can induce an increase in the frequency and power of cancer-specific T cells, but often the immunologic response is not associated with tumor regression.[16] Another aspect that has gradually emerged is that the polarization and the maturation status of both APCs and T cells were crucial in the development of programs of vaccine therapy. In addition, the idea that patients with low tumor burden might be the most suitable to this approach encouraged the implementation of numerous trials of adjuvant vaccine therapy.

Over the years, a series of vaccines were tested in melanoma (i.e., peptides, gangliosides, manipulated tumor cells, viral vaccines, DNA plasmids), as well as numerous adjuvants. There has been some association with vaccination and improved immune responses, but Phase 1 to 2 trials, as well as large Phase 3 trials, have been disappointing. The role of vaccines, however, may merit discussion since they have taught us about tumor immunology and may find new clinical utility as adjuncts to the more recently approved immunotherapy regimens.

Peptide Vaccines

An interesting attempt has used multipeptide vaccines, based on their ability to expand and enhance specific immune responses. This approach has been evaluated in several cancers resulting in an acceptable safety profile and data demonstrating the induction of powerful specific CD8+ and CD4+ T cell responses. Slingluff[17] evaluated a vaccine consisting of 12 MHC class I-restricted peptides capable of stimulating the CD8+ T cell response, in combination with an HLA-DR-restricted tetanus-derived peptide in order to also stimulate CD4+ T helper cells. The peptides were emulsified in Freund's incomplete adjuvant and administered with or without granulocyte-macrophage colony-stimulating factor (GM-CSF). In 121 melanoma stage IIB–IV resected patients, a powerful response in both CD8+ and CD4+ T cells was reported.[17] Surprisingly, this immunologic response was almost doubled in patients who had not received GM-CSF, and this profoundly put into question the role of GM-CSF as an adjuvant to peptide vaccines.

For the entire group of patients, the OS and DFS at 3 years were 76% and 52%, respectively. These data were received with great enthusiasm because they showed the ability to induce potent immune responses and the ability to manipulate different aspects of the immune response induced by multipeptide vaccines. Many questions, however, remained about the type of peptides to use and their length, as well as optimizing the use of adjuvants including GM-CSF, Toll-like receptor agonists, and so on.

Another strategy followed by the most recent vaccination approaches has been based on the use of peptides, expressed on the tumor cells of patients in order to obtain more relevant tumor-specific immune responses. After promising results had been obtained from Phase 1 and 2 studies, Phase 3 studies have been performed over large, selected patient populations. However, all of the vaccine therapy studies that have used this approach, involving patients with different disease stages, reported negative results.[18]

One example was represented by peptide vaccine MAGE-A3, an antigen belonging to the class of cancer-testis antigens not expressed by normal adult cells but expressed by many types of cancers and approximately 50% of melanomas. After several clinical studies documented the favorable toxicity profile of this vaccine (fever, fatigue, and local skin reactions), some Phase 2 trials reported interesting results, especially in patients with low tumor burden (unresectable stage III and stage IV M1a). In the Phase 2 "PREDICT" trial, 123 patients with MAGE-A3-positive unresectable stage IIIB-C/IVM1a melanomas received the MAGE-A3 vaccine. Treatment of patients with MAGEA-3 positive unresectable stage IIIB-C/IVM1a melanoma with the MAGE-A3 vaccine demonstrated an overall 1-year OS rate of 83.5%. There was one complete response and two partial responses. In this study, prognostic gene signatures were not predictive of the outcome because positive and negative

patients had similar 1-year OS rates.[19] These studies, therefore, represented the proof of concept for the large Phase 3 studies in both melanoma and lung cancer.

The DERMA study (adjuvant immunotherapy with MAGE-A3 in melanoma), conducted in patients with surgically resected stage III disease and expressing MAGE-A3 on their melanoma, enrolled 1,300 patients worldwide with huge economic and organizational efforts. Unfortunately, in September 2014, the results were announced, and the study did not meet its primary endpoint of demonstrating a superior DFS compared with placebo. Even the attempt to identify subgroups of responder patients using molecular or immunological gene signature was unsuccessful.[20]

The human tumor antigen Preferentially Expressed Antigen of Melanoma (PRAME) is expressed at low levels in normal ovary, endometrium, kidney, and adrenal tissues, and overexpressed in a range of cancers, including 95% of metastatic melanoma tumors.[21] PRAME has been considered a potential candidate for cancer immunotherapy because it is expressed by a variety of tumors and can induce T cell immune responses.

A dose-escalation Phase 1 study was designed to determine the adequate dose of a recombinant PRAME protein (recPRAME, Glaxo-Smith-Kline [GSK], Belgium) administered with GSK's proprietary immunostimulant AS15, through evaluation of the safety and immunogenicity of the PRAME immunotherapeutic in patients with PRAME positive metastatic melanoma. Sixty-six patients with stage IV PRAME-positive melanoma were treated in three consecutive cohorts to receive up to 24 intramuscular injections of the PRAME immunotherapeutic. All patients had detectable anti-PRAME antibodies after four immunizations. The percentage of patients with predefined PRAME-specific CD4+ T cell responses after four immunizations was similar in each cohort. No CD8+ T cell responses were detected. A Phase 2 study is ongoing to further evaluate the 500-μg PRAME immunotherapeutic dose.[22]

Another peptide widely used in clinical trials was gp100, a melanoma-associated antigen expressed in normal melanocytes and melanoma cells. The first pilot studies which tested gp100 with the anti-CTLA-4 antibody ipilimumab in patients with metastatic melanoma have reported interesting results and a relationship between autoimmunity and tumor regression.[23] However, when added to ipilimumab, no survival advantage was reported in the Phase 3 study as a second-line treatment for patients with metastatic melanoma.[24]

Cellular Vaccines

A vaccine made from vaccinia viral lysates of an allogeneic melanoma cell (VMCL), following surgical removal of lymph node metastases, has been tested in Phase 2 and

3 clinical trials. In a Phase 2 study, the administration of the vaccine was associated with depression of natural killer (NK) cell activity against melanoma and K562 target cells in the first 3 to 6 months of treatment. Leucocyte-dependent antibody (LDA) activity against melanoma cells was induced or increased in titer in approximately half of the patients studied. For this reason, vaccines prepared from VMCL were considered a favorable method for increasing immune responses against melanoma.[25]

A prospective, randomized, multicenter trial was then conducted to determine whether immunotherapy with the vaccine over a 2-year period after definitive surgery would improve relapse-free survival (RFS) and OS in patients with stage IIB and III melanoma, compared with a control group treated only with surgery. Seven hundred patients were randomized: 353 to VMCL and 347 to no immunotherapy. Five- and 10-year survival rates for the control and treatment arm were 54.8% versus 60.6% and 41% versus 53.4%, respectively. The median RFS was 43 months in the control group, compared with 83 months in the vaccine group (hazard ratio [HR], 0.86; 95% confidence interval [CI], 0.7–1.07; $p = .17$). Five-year RFS was 50.9% for the treated group and 46.8% for the control group. Unfortunately, adjuvant therapy with vaccine prepared from VMCL for surgically resected melanoma patients was not associated with a statistically significant improvement in OS or RFS.[26] Canvaxin™ (CancerVax Corp., Carlsbad, CA), a therapeutic polyvalent cancer vaccine based on an allogeneic whole-cell formulation, was developed in 1984 and comprised 25 million irradiated melanoma cells derived from three melanoma cell lines. Canvaxin has become one of the most extensively studied melanoma vaccines to date.[27] This formulation contains more than 20 immunogenic melanoma-associated and tumor-associated antigens. At least one of these antigens has been found in every melanoma tumor specimen, and some of the antigens are naturally immunogenic in the absence of an immunotherapeutic stimulus.[26] Phase 2 clinical data indicated improved survival when used as a postsurgical adjuvant treatment in stage III and IV melanoma versus matched pair controls and 11% complete response rate in in-transit melanoma metastases.[28] Considering the encouraging results from Phase 2 trials, two multicenter Phase 3 randomized trials (MMAIT III and IV) of Canvaxin vaccine were conducted in 1998. These trials enrolled patients who had undergone complete resection of regional (stage III) or distant (stage IV) metastatic melanoma to receive postoperative adjuvant treatment with either vaccine plus BCG or placebo plus BCG. The primary endpoint of these trials was OS. In both the studies, Canvaxin was well tolerated, but it failed to demonstrate an advantage in OS as compared with placebo. However, it must be considered that the survival observed in the Canvaxin arm of MMAIT III and IV are similar or slightly better than prior Phase 2 studies, but the placebo arm survival was higher than expected.[29] Another tumor-associated peptide, Melan A/MART1, was used to pulse dendritic cells (DCs) that were then administered to patients with metastatic melanoma in combination with anti-CTLA-4 antibody tremelimumab. Among 16 patients, there were four responses, two of which were partial and two of which were complete and long lasting. Even with the modest number of patients enrolled in the study (due to limitations), the authors concluded that the combination proved to be particularly effective and that the role of the CTLA-4 blockade in maintaining an immune response initiated by the vaccine was crucial.[30]

Intralesional Therapies

Oncolytic Viruses

Another interesting and more recent therapeutic approach consists of oncolytic viruses (OVs). These are emerging as important agents in cancer treatment. OVs offer the attractive therapeutic combination of tumor-specific cell lysis together with immune stimulation, therefore acting as potential in situ tumor vaccines. Talimogene laherparepvec (T-VEC) consists of an OV of the family of herpes simplex virus, type 1 (HSV-1) manipulated and engineered to have a tropism for cancer cells and also encodes GM-CSF. As of November 2016, T-VEC remains the only FDA-approved OV. T-VEC is administered intralesionally and is associated with a favorable toxicity profile. In a Phase 3 randomized trial (2:1 ratio), patients received intratumoral T-VEC or subcutaneous recombinant GM-CSF. Of 436 patients, 295 were allocated to T-VEC and 141 to GM-CSF. At a median follow-up of 49 months, median OS was 23.3 months and 18.9 months (95% CI, 16.0–23.7) in the T-VEC and GM-CSF arms, respectively. DRR was 19.0 and 1.4% and ORR was 31.5 and 6.4%. 50 (16.9%) and 1 (0.7%) patients in the T-VEC and GM-CSF arms, respectively, achieved confirmed ORR. In T-VEC-treated patients, median time to confirmed ORR was 8.6 months and median confirmed ORR duration was not reached. Among patients with a confirmed ORR, 88.5% were estimated to survive at a 5-year landmark analysis. T-VEC efficacy was more pronounced in stage IIIB-IVM1a melanoma as already described in the primary analysis.[31]

Moreover, the favorable safety profile was confirmed with the only side effect of grade 3/4 in more than 2% of patients represented by cellulitis (2.1%).[32] According to these results, this vaccine has been approved by the FDA, Australia, and EMA.

The coxsackievirus CVA21 has the potential to directly target, infect, multiply within, and destroy a wide range of cancer cells, both at the tumor site and throughout the body. CVA21 acts by searching and attaching itself to the surface intercellular adhesion molecule-1 (ICAM-1).

ICAM-1 is upregulated in melanoma and some other cancers (e.g., prostate, bladder, breast, non-small cell lung). Once attached to this protein, the virus is then able to insert itself into the cancer cell, replicate, and burst the cancer cell apart, a process known as lysis, inducing a secondary systemic host-generated antitumor immune response. In the Phase 2 CALM trial,[33] 57 patients with unresectable melanoma and at least one injectable lesion received 10 series of multi-intratumoral CVA21 injections. irPFS rate, the primary endpoint of the study, was 38.6% (22/57) and an ORR was 28.1% (16/57), with eight CRs and eight PRs. Median OS was 26 months (95% CI, 16.7 months—not reached), and the 1-year survival rate was 75.4% (43/57). Tumor responses were observed in injected lesions, non-injected cutaneous lesions, and non-injected visceral lesions. Treatment was well tolerated and no grade 3 or grade 4 treatment-related adverse events (AEs) were observed. CVA21-injected lesions demonstrated an increase of immune cell infiltrates in patients who progressed after immune checkpoint inhibitors. According to this observation, the Melanoma Intratumoral CAVATAK and Ipilimumab (MITCI) study[34] was designed, in which CVA21, in combination with systemic administration of ipilimumab, will be evaluated in patients with unresectable melanoma. The Phase 1b MITCI study (NCT02307149) is investigating the efficacy and safety of IT-administered CVA21 and IV-administered ipilimumab in up to 50 patients with treated or untreated unresectable stage IIIC-IVM1c melanoma. Patients received up to 3 x 108 TCID50 CVA21 IT on study days 1, 3, 5, 8, and 22, and then q3w for a further series of six injections. Ipilimumab (3 mg/kg) q3w was given as four IV infusions starting at Day 22. Combination treatment has been generally well tolerated with surprisingly only one Gr 3 or higher treatment-related AE being ipilimumab-related fatigue. The study met its primary statistical futility endpoint of achieving four or more confirmed objective responses (confirmed ORR or PR) in the first 12 patients enrolled. Of the first 18 patients eligible for investigator response assessment, the confirmed ORR for the ITT population is 50.0% (9/18), with the ORR for immune checkpoint-naïve patients being 60% (6/10) and previous immune checkpoint therapy patients being 38% (3/8). Of note is the encouraging ORR of 57.1% (4/7 patients) in patients with stage IVm1c disease. The DCR (confirmed ORR+PR+SD) on the ITT population is currently 78% (14/18), of which 66% of patients have been administered prior systemic therapy with DCR of 100% (7/7) in patients with stage IVm1c disease. All responses were observed by 3.5 months with complete tumor responses being observed in individual injected and non-injected lesions. Preliminary immune monitoring has indicated that CVA21 plus ipilimumab increases the percentage of activated CD8 and CD4 T cells with effector and memory phenotypes in the peripheral blood. The greatest increases in activated T cells in the peripheral blood occurred after the third ipilimumab dose. The preliminary ORR rate for the ITT population of 50.0% is higher than published rates for either agent used alone (CVA21: ~28% and ipilimumab: ~15%–20%) in advanced melanoma patients.

Allovectin-7

Another treatment administered via intralesional delivery is Allovectin-7. It is a plasmid DNA coding for the human *HLA-B7* gene and β2-microglobulin, complexed with a lipid mixture. In a Phase 2 study, 52 patients with metastatic melanoma were enrolled. The treatment was well tolerated and capable of producing responses, although higher responses were seen in injected lesions than in distant lesions, 18% and 4%, respectively. In another more recent study of 127 pretreated patients, an 11.8% response rate was reported with a median duration of 13.8 months.[35]

LTX-315

LTX-315 is a cationic amphiphilic peptide derivative that permeabilizes inner mitochondrial membranes and induces necrosis.[36] It is a strong inducer of anticancer immune responses if injected into tumors developing in immunocompetent mice.[37] In B16 melanomas in syngenic mice, intratumoral administration of LTX-315 resulted in tumor necrosis and the infiltration of immune cells into the tumor parenchyma, followed by complete regression of the tumor in the majority of the animals. LTX-315 induced the release of danger-associated molecular pattern molecules such as the high mobility group box-1 protein in vitro and the subsequent upregulation of pro-inflammatory cytokines, such as IL-1β, IL-6, and IL-18 in vivo. Animals cured by LTX-315 treatment were protected against a rechallenge with live B16 tumor cells both intradermally and IV.[38] In a Phase 1 dose-escalation study of intratumoral LTX-315 as monotherapy or in combination with either ipilimumab or pembrolizumab in patients with transdermally accessible tumors, 59 patients were treated. Eleven experienced LTX-315-related grade 3/4 adverse events, mainly allergic/anaphylaxis, all resolving without sequelae. Out of 36 patients treated with LTX-315 monotherapy, best overall response of SD at 2 months was seen in 28%. Six melanoma patients received LTX-315 plus ipilimumab; of those, SD was observed in 33%. LTX-315 monotherapy resulted in an increased number of CD8+ T cells in treated lesions in 89% of evaluable biopsied patients. TCR sequencing revealed clonal expansion of T cells in blood after LTX-315 monotherapy, and 50% of these clones were detected in posttreatment biopsied tumors. LTX-315 promotes TILs in all evaluable melanoma patients, converting "cold" tumors to "hot" as demonstrated by gene expression analysis. Moreover, LTX-315 promotes significant expansion of T cell clones in blood, of which several are novel and present in tumor post-treatment, suggesting generation of a de novo antitumor T cell response.[39]

PV-10 (Rose Bengal)

Rose bengal disodium is a water-soluble xanthene dye used in the past as an IV-administered liver function diagnostic agent and currently used by ophthalmologists topically as a diagnostic aid (i.e., for diagnosis of kera-toconjunctivitis sicca, keratitis, abrasions, or corrosions, as well as the detection of foreign bodies).[40] A formulation of rose bengal, as a 10% sterile, nonpyrogenic saline solution (PV–10), has been developed appropriately for intralesional injection to induce chemical tumor ablation. Preclinical in vitro and in vivo studies with melanoma cell lines were performed with promising results,[41] which led to a Phase 1 trial in patients with melanoma metasta-ses accessible for direct intralesional injection. In a Phase 2 study, 62 patients with stage III and 18 with stage IV refractory melanoma were enrolled. The best ORR was 51%, and the complete response rate was 26% for tar-get lesions. The median duration of response was 4.0 months, with 8% of patients, having no evidence of dis-ease after 52 weeks. The toxicity was predominantly mild to moderate and localized to the treatment site, with no treatment-associated grade 4 or 5 AEs. It is hypothesized that the primary ablative effect of PV-10 reduced the size of injected tumors quickly, while regression of uninjected bystander lesions is consistent with a secondary immune response.[42] A Phase 3 study of PV-10 is ongoing to assess PV-10 monotherapy versus systemic chemotherapy with dacarbazine or temozolomide or T-VEC for the treatment of locally advanced cutaneous melanoma in patients who are BRAF V600 wild type and have failed or are not candidates for at least one ICI (NCT02288897). The good toxicity profile and the evidence of activity of PV-10 opens new opportunities for combinations with the ICIs. A Phase 1b–2 study of intratumoral PV-10 in combination with pembrolizumab for the treatment of metastatic mel-anoma is currently enrolling participants (NCT02557321).

Checkpoint Inhibitors

Since 2010, the development of new drugs has revolu-tionized the prognosis of patients with metastatic mel-anoma. Currently, there are two important classes of drugs as mainstays of frontline treatment for metastatic melanoma: inhibitors of small molecules (targeted ther-apy) and monoclonal antibodies directed against specific receptors on cells of the immune system (immunomod-ulatory antibodies). Both groups of drugs were able to improve both PFS and OS. Therefore, the use of chemo-therapy has been replaced by targeted therapies, which include BRAF/MEK inhibitors, for the 40% to 50% of patients (i.e., those with activating mutations of the BRAF gene), and the monoclonal immunomodulatory antibodies (such as the anti-CTLA-4 and anti-PD-1), for all patients with metastatic melanoma, regardless of the mutational status.[43] Immune checkpoint inhibitors are monoclonal antibodies that unleash an immune system attack on cancer cells by blocking immune-modulatory receptors on the surface of immune cells (often T cells). Immunomodulatory antibodies potentiate the antitumor response activating receptors that increase the activity of immune cells (i.e., CD28, OX40, CD137) or blocking receptors that inhibit the activity of immune response (CTLA-4, PD-1, LAG-3).[44]

Today's challenge is to combine or adequately sequence these new drugs to further improve the sur-vival of patients while avoiding intolerable toxicity. A fundamental chapter in the history of immunotherapy of melanoma was written in 1996 when CTLA-4 block-ade induced tumor regression in mouse models.[45] Subsequently, numerous trials with anti-CTLA-4 anti-bodies have been initiated, alone or in combination with melanoma-associated peptides. Thus, modern immuno-therapy was born.[46]

Anti-Cytotoxic T Lymphocyte-Associated Protein 4

Tremelimumab

Tremelimumab is an anti-CTLA-4 human IgG2 monoclo-nal antibody. A Phase 1/2 study established the dosage to be used in later stages of development as 15 mg/kg every 3 months.[47] This schedule of administration differs from that of ipilimumab because of the prolonged plasma half-life of tremelimumab. Tremelimumab resulted in an ORR of 6.6% and a 1- and 2-year survival of 40.3% and 22%, respectively, in a Phase 2 study of 246 patients with pre-treated metastatic melanoma.[48] A Phase 3, randomized, open-label trial in patients with nonpretreated advanced melanoma compared tremelimumab with chemotherapy (dacarbazine or temozolomide by investigator's choice). No statistically significant difference was observed in terms of OS between the two treatment groups (12.6 months vs. 10.7; HR 0.88; $p = .127$). However, the dura-tion of the responses with tremelimumab was signifi-cantly longer than chemotherapy (35.8 months vs. 13.7; $p = .0011$). Several factors, such as the treatment schedule, which provided for an infusion every 3 months and the use of ipilimumab after progression in patients in the che-motherapy group, may have contributed to the lack of an OS benefit of tremelimumab.[49] There are several expla-nations for the failure to reach the main OS endpoint in the Phase 3 trial of tremelimumab: the good unexpected result of the control arm, possibly due to the inclusion of patients with a more favorable prognosis and use of ipili-mumab in a certain proportion of them, and the use of a potentially suboptimal schedule of 90 days for treatment in the tremelimumab arm. However, even despite these factors, the achievement of a median OS of 13 months was considerable, and on the whole, these data support the possibility that tremelimumab may have a role not only in the treatment of melanoma but of cancer in general both as monotherapy and in combination.[50] Similarly, to ipilimumab, immune-related adverse reactions, such as diarrhea and dermatitis, are also common to tremelimumab. Phase 1 to 2 have the recommended dose of 15 mg/kg every 3 months as compared with 10 mg/kg every month, reflecting the greater frequency of grade 3 and grade 4 events with the monthly schedule. The Phase 3 study additionally showed the occurrence of endocrine disorders such as thyroiditis and hypophysitis in 7% of patients.

Recently, Eroglu et al. published the pooled long-term survival data of patients treated within Phase 1 and 2 trials of tremelimumab. The median OS was 13 months (95% CI: 10–16.6). An ORR of 15.6% with a median duration of response of 6.5 years (range of 3–136 + months) was also seen. The median OS rate at 5 years was 20% (95% CI: 13%–26%), while the 10 and 12.5 years was 16% (95% CI: 9%–23%). These long-term data support efficacy of CTLA-4 blockade with tremelimumab and many ongoing studies of tremelimumab in patients with various tumors are ongoing.[51]

Ipilimumab

Single Agent

In recent years, the introduction of immunological checkpoint inhibitor drugs has been a major turning point in melanoma immunotherapy.

The first drug that became available in the clinic was ipilimumab, a monoclonal antibody directed against the CTLA-4 receptor, present on activated T lymphocytes and that physiologically regulates the immune response.[52] In fact, the binding of CTLA-4 with its ligand B7 (CD86) generates a negative signal that induces an anergy state in the lymphocytes. The binding of the anti-CTLA-4 antibody to the molecule, preventing the initiation of these inhibitory signals, results in an increase in antitumor lymphocyte T activity (Figure 50.1). The approval of ipilimumab was based on a randomized three-arms Phase 3 study[23] performed on 676 pretreated patients. Patients received ipilimumab together with a peptide vaccine (gp100), or ipilimumab + placebo, or gp100 + placebo in a ratio of 3:1:1. Overall survival was significantly longer with ipilimumab alone or in combination with the vaccine (10.1 months) compared with the vaccine alone (6.4 months). The antibody was administered intravenously at a dose of 3 mg/kg every 3 weeks for four cycles. Patients whose disease progressed at least 3 months after the last administration of ipilimumab

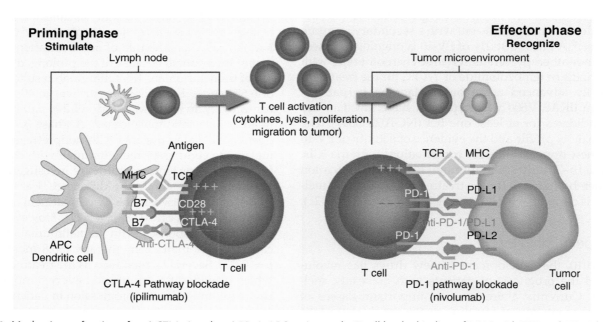

Figure 50.1 Mechanisms of action of anti-CTLA-4 and anti-PD-1. APC activates the T cell by the binding of MHC with TCR and B7 with CD28. After the activation, the system limits itself with the binding B7 with CTLA-4, which gives an inhibiting signal to the T cell. Anti-CTLA-4 blocks the inhibiting signals induced by the binding of B7 with CTLA-4, with consequent T cell potentiation. Anti-PD-1/PDL-1, blocking the binding with PD-1/PDL-1 in the tumor microenvironment, unleashes the immune response against melanoma cells.

APC, antigen-presenting cell; CTLA-4, cytotoxic T lymphocyte-associated protein 4; MHC, major histocompatibility complex; PD-1, programmed cell death protein 1; PD-L1, programmed death ligand 1; TCR, T cell receptor.

or from week 12 (disease stability lasting more than 6 months, or recovery of disease after RP or RC) could receive a similar re-induction to the previous scheme. It should be noted that 15 out of 23 patients achieved partial responses or stability after re-induction.

Ipilimumab is associated with the risk of immune-related side effects. Sixty percent of the immune-related adverse events were recorded in the study population. Approximately 15% of patients experienced grade 3 or grade 4 adverse events. Dermatitis was the most frequent immune-related event, and diarrhea was the most dangerous (perforation risk if not promptly treated). According to recent indications, severe cases should be treated with high-dose corticosteroids. Immune-related toxicity can be fatal if left untreated, and seven deaths were recorded in the Phase 3 study.

A second Phase 3 (double-blind) study was conducted on 502 patients with previously untreated metastatic melanoma. Patients were randomized to receive dacarbazine + ipilimumab [with a dose schedule of 10 mg/kg every 3 weeks for four cycles (induction phase) and then 10 mg/kg every 3 months until progression (maintenance phase)] or dacarbazine + placebo.

The primary endpoint was achieved in the ipilimumab arm, demonstrating better overall survival compared with dacarbazine alone (11.2 months vs. 9.1 months). The 3-year survival was 20.8% and 12.2% for patients who received ipilimumab and placebo, respectively (HR = 0.72; p <.001).

The incidence of grade 3 and grade 4 AEs was 56% in the ipilimumab arm; there was evidence of an increase in liver toxicity, as expected in relation to the potential hepatotoxicity of each therapeutic agent, and a lower incidence of diarrhea. Despite the higher incidence of grade 3 to grade 4 AEs, no toxic death was recorded, as evidence of the effectiveness of the application of the algorithms for the treatment of immune-related-toxicity.[53] A pooled analysis of 1,861 patients with advanced melanoma treated with ipilimumab from 10 prospective studies and two retrospective studies demonstrated a 21% survival rate from the third year after the treatment, lasting in the following years,[54] demonstrating the long duration of the response induced by ipilimumab.

Ipilimumab was approved by the FDA, and later by EMA, at 3 mg/kg because the data from the studies MDX-020 (ipi 3 mg/kg) and CA184-024 (ipi 10 mg/kg) showed similar results in terms of ORR, PFS, and OS while a higher G3/4 toxicity was associated with ipilimumab at 10 mg/kg. Moreover, the benefit was reached with only four injections; indeed, in the study CA184-024 only 92 patients (36.8%) of patients treated with ipilimumab plus dacarbazine received all four cycles of the induction phase. At least one maintenance dose was administered in 43 patients in the ipilimumab-dacarbazine group (17.2%). For these reasons, the FDA approved the schedule of ipilimumab at 3

mg/kg for four cycles and asked Bristol Myers Squibb for a clinical trial comparing the two dosages of ipilimumab.

According to what was requested, the FDA designed the trial CA194-169, a randomized Phase 3 study, comparing treatment with ipilimumab 3 mg/kg for four doses versus ipilimumab 10 mg/kg for four doses in 727 patients with metastatic melanoma. The primary endpoint was the OS. The higher-dose treatment arm showed an advantage in terms of median OS (15.7 months vs. 11.5 months (HR = 0.84, 95% CI 0.70–0.99; p =.04), and a higher incidence of immune-mediated toxicity, in particular diarrhea, colitis, hepatitis, and hypophysitis.[55] The update of this trial with a median follow-up of 61 months showed a statistically significant improvement in 5-year overall survival with ipilimumab 10 mg/kg versus 3 mg/kg in patients with metastatic melanoma who had not received a prior BRAF or checkpoint inhibitor (25% vs. 19%). Ipilimumab demonstrated equal efficacy in both BRAF-mutated and wild-type patients. These results suggest the emergence of a plateau in the OS curve, consistent with previous ipilimumab studies. Safety was similar to the previous analysis in which ipilimumab at 10 mg/kg was associated with higher rates of treatment-related AEs.[56]

The kinetics of the response to treatment with ipilimumab may have a pattern characterized by an initial increase of the tumor burden and only then a reduction of the disease. For this reason, specific criteria for the evaluation of the antitumor activity of immunotherapy, the Immune-Related Response Criteria (IRRC), have been formulated to identify the patients achieving a late benefit from treatment with immunotherapy.[57]

Combination Treatments With Ipilimumab

Chemotherapy

Attempts to further improve results with ipilimumab therapy by combining with other treatment modalities (e.g., chemotherapy, RT, or other procedures such as electrochemotherapy [ECT]) have also been explored. In a Phase 3 study, ipilimumab in combination with dacarbazine was compared with dacarbazine alone. OS was significantly longer in the group receiving combined ipilimumab plus dacarbazine (11.2 vs. 9.1 months), with higher survival rates in the ipilimumab plus dacarbazine group at 1 year (47.3% vs. 36.3%), 2 years (28.5% vs. 17.9%), and 3 years (20.8% vs. 12.2%). Grade 3 to grade 4 AEs occurred in 56.3% of patients treated with the combination, as compared with 27.5% treated with chemotherapy alone.[53] An update of this trial showed a significant 5-year survival rate of 18.2% for patients treated with ipilimumab plus dacarbazine versus 8.8% for patients treated with dacarbazine, indicating that the long-term survival rate plateaus after 3 years.[58] This trial did not test whether dacarbazine added efficacy to ipilimumab, but it supported the OS benefits of ipilimumab over historical melanoma treatments, such as dacarbazine monotherapy. Due to the AE profile, typically ipilimumab is not administered in combination with dacarbazine.

In a Phase 2 trial, 86 patients with pretreated metastatic melanoma were treated with ipilimumab in combination with fotemustine. At a median follow-up of 39.9 months, median OS was 12.9 months, and the 3-year survival rate was 28.5% for the whole study population, and 12.7 months and 27.8% for patients with brain metastases. Grade 3 to grade 4 treatment-related AEs, secondary to chemotherapy or immunotherapy, were reported by 55% of patients.[59,60]

Anti-Angiogenesis

It has been shown that vascular endothelial growth factor (VEGF) suppresses DC maturation and modulates lymphocyte-endothelial trafficking, with consequent immune suppression. Thus, an anti-VEGF agent should enhance antimelanoma immune responses. Based on this rationale, ipilimumab was combined with bevacizumab in a Phase 1b trial that included different dosing regimens for both drugs. Of the 46 patients enrolled, eight had a partial response and 22 had stable disease, resulting in a disease control rate (DCR) of 67.4%. The median survival was 25.1 months.[61] Eleven study patients (23.9%) had treatment-related, grade 3 events.

Granulocyte-Macrophage Colony-Stimulating Factor

In a Phase 2 randomized trial, 245 metastatic melanoma patients were treated with ipilimumab at 10 mg/kg in combination with sargramostim (recombinant GM-CSF) at 250 µg subcutaneously day 1 to day 14 or ipilimumab alone. At a median follow-up of 13.3 months, median OS for ipilimumab plus sargramostim was 17.5 months, compared with 12.7 months for ipilimumab alone. The 1-year survival rate for the combination was 68.9% versus 52.9% for ipilimumab alone. However, no difference in PFS was observed (3.1 months for both groups). Moreover, the rate of high-grade toxicity was lower in the combination group (44.9% vs. 58.3%) as compared with the ipilimumab arm.[62] Whether GM-CSF adds efficacy to ipilimumab at 3 mg/kg remains unknown.

Talimogene Laherparepvec

There is always more interest in modifying the tumor microenvironment (TME) to enhance immune cell localization and activation, as well as to overcome resistance to anti-PD-1/PD-L1 therapies (programmed cell death protein 1/programmed death ligand 1). These approaches include oncolytic viruses such as T-VEC in combination with checkpoint inhibitors. T-VEC is a herpes simplex virus (HSV)-1-based oncolytic immunotherapy designed to selectively replicate in tumors, produce GM-CSF, and stimulate antitumor immune responses in melanoma. In a Phase 1b study of 19 patients, ORR was 50%, and 44% of patients had a durable response lasting more than 6 months.

Eighteen-month PFS was 50%. Median OS was not reached, but 12- and 18-month survival rates were 72.2% and 67%, respectively.[63] The favorable response rate in this study is intriguing, but this group of patients generally had more favorable disease characteristics than patients treated in prior ipilimumab clinical trials.

A randomized Phase 2 open-label study enrolled melanoma patients, 54% stage IIIB, IVM1a and 45% IVM1b/c, to be treated with the combination ipilimumab + T-VEC or ipilimumab alone.[64] No more than one prior therapy was allowed if patients were BRAF wild-type, and no more than two prior therapies if BRAF mutant. One hundred ninety-eight patients were randomly assigned to T-VEC plus ipilimumab ($n = 98$), or ipilimumab alone ($n = 100$). The ORR was 39% in patients receiving the combination therapy and 18% in patients receiving ipilimumab alone. Responses were not limited to injected lesions; visceral lesion decreases were observed in 52% of patients in the combination arm and 23% of patients in the ipilimumab arm. Median PFS was 8.2 months for the combination and 6.4 for ipilimumab (HR 0.83 [0.56–1.23]), indicating a further activation of the immune response combining anti-CTLA-4 antibody and a locoregional treatment as T-VEC. Despite the advantage of the combination in median PFS, the two curves of PFS were very similar. Toxicity profile was acceptable in the combination arm. Frequently occurring adverse events included fatigue (combination, 59%; ipilimumab alone, 42%); chills (combination, 53%; ipilimumab alone, 3%); and diarrhea (combination, 42%; ipilimumab alone, 35%). Incidence of grade ≥3 AEs was 45% and 35%, respectively. Three patients in the combination arm had fatal AEs, but none were treatment related.

Radiotherapy

Preclinical in vitro and in vivo studies suggest radiotherapy results in immunologic effects that may be beneficial to checkpoint inhibition. However, only case reports and retrospective studies have suggested the potential for some benefit of this approach in patients. In one study,[65] RT performed with palliative intent in patients progressing after ipilimumab demonstrated a systemic effect (abscopal effect). Among 21 ipilimumab-progressing patients, an RT-induced abscopal response was observed in 11 patients (52%), of whom nine had a partial response (43%) and two had stable disease (10%). Median OS was 13 months (range: 6–26) for all 21 patients but increased to 22.4 months when assessed in patients with an abscopal response compared with 8.3 months in patients without a systemic response. Prospective, randomized studies of ipilimumab with or without RT are needed before fully recognizing whether RT adds to the efficacy of checkpoint blockade.

Electrochemotherapy

Ipilimumab has also been combined with locoregional treatment such as ECT. In one study, ipilimumab plus ECT demonstrated a local objective response in 67% of patients, with 27% complete responses and 40% partial responses. According to immune-related response criteria, a systemic response was observed in nine patients (five partial responses and four stable diseases), resulting in a DCR of 60%.[66] The association of ECT combined with ipilimumab or PD-1 inhibition has been investigated in a cohort of 33 patients with unresectable or metastatic melanoma. Twenty-eight patients received ipilimumab, and five patients were treated with a PD-1 inhibitor (three with pembrolizumab and two with nivolumab). The local ORR was 66.7%. The systemic ORR was 19.2% and 40.0% in the ipilimumab and PD-1 cohort, respectively. The median OS was not reached at the time of the analysis in patients with ipilimumab and resulted in 15 months in the PD-1 group. Grade 3 to grade 4 systemic AEs were observed in 25.0% patients in the ipilimumab group.[67]

Another study analyzed clinical data from 127 melanoma patients treated with ipilimumab and local peripheral treatments (LPT), such as radiotherapy or ECT. Eighty-two patients received ipilimumab and 45 ipilimumab and additional LPT if indicated for local tumor control. The addition of LPT to ipilimumab significantly prolonged OS (median OS 93 vs. 42 weeks, unadjusted HR, 0.46; $p = .0028$). Adverse immune-related events were not increased by the combination treatment and LPT-induced local toxicities that were mild in most of the cases. These data suggest that LPT, such as radiotherapy or ECT, modulates systemic immune responses, and that the combination with systemic immune checkpoint blockade might be beneficial.[68]

Targeted Therapy

Combination approaches involving immunotherapy with targeted therapy are also being investigated based somewhat on the demonstration that BRAF inhibitors may have immunogenic effects such as recruitment of cytotoxic lymphocytes into the melanoma TME, increase of tumor-associated antigens, overexpression of the interpheron-g receptor, and reduction of immune-suppressive mechanisms (MDSC, CD73, etc.). However, the first combination experience of vemurafenib plus ipilimumab was stopped early due to hepatotoxicity and rash.[69] This liver toxicity generally appeared after the first administration and resolved after stopping the treatment and with the administration of glucocorticoids. Ipilimumab was also combined with the other BRAF inhibitor, dabrafenib, in a Phase 1

trial, and this combination was shown to be feasible in terms of safety. The same study also assessed the triple association of ipilimumab with dabrafenib and the MEK inhibitor, trametinib; however, this was stopped early because of a high rate of bowel perforation.[70]

However, the combination of an anti-PD-1/PDL-1 agent, rather than ipilimumab, with BRAF and MEK inhibitors seem to be feasible in terms of toxicity and may result in higher frequency of long-lasting responses.

Anti-Programmed Cell Death Protein 1

PD-1 is another inhibitory receptor involved in T cell regulation, constitutively expressed on T cells in the thymus and induced on peripheral T and B cells upon activation.[71] Its physiological role is to downregulate T cell activity upon binding to two receptors, PD-L1 and PD-L2, expressed in normal tissues but constitutively expressed or induced on several tumors.[72] PD-1/PD-L1-dependent immune inhibition is responsible for immune resistance resulting in tumor cell evasion.

Thus, the PD-1/PD-L1 blockade may revert the immunocompromised status of tumor-bearing hosts and activate the host immune system to eradicate tumors (Figure 50.1).[73]

More recently, antibodies against the PD-1 inhibitory checkpoint (nivolumab and pembrolizumab) have been introduced into the clinical practice for the treatment of advanced melanoma (stage III or IV). These immunomodulating antibodies have been shown to be superior in terms of efficacy and tolerability compared with ipilimumab.

Pembrolizumab

The randomized Phase 3 study KEYNOTE-006[74] evaluated superiority of treatment with pembrolizumab 10 mg/kg every 2 or 3 weeks up to a maximum of 2 years or progression of disease versus four cycles of ipilimumab every 3 weeks. The study population consisted of 834 patients with advanced melanoma who had not received more than one line of treatment (patients with BRAF mutation and aggressive disease also had to have received treatment with BRAF inhibitor). The OS and PFS of pembrolizumab versus ipilimumab were the two co-primary endpoints; secondary objectives were the response rate and tolerability of the treatment. At a median follow-up of 60 months, treatment with pembrolizumab was superior to ipilimumab in terms of median PFS (11.6 vs. 3.7 months. HR: 0.54 95% CI:0.43–0.67) and 2-, 3-, and 4-year PFS, respectively (37.3% vs. 17.5%, 33.1% vs. 14.5%, and 26.9% vs. 8%). Treatment with pembrolizumab was also superior in terms of median OS (38.7 months vs. 17.1 months. HR: 0.73. 95% CI: 0.57–0.93) and 2-, 3-, 4-, and 5-year overall survival, compared with ipilimumab (58% vs. 44.7%, 51.2% vs. 40.8%, 44.3% vs. 36.4%, and 43.2% vs. 33.0%, respectively).[75]

In addition, at a median follow-up of 34.2 months after the end of treatment, the 24-month PFS for all 103 patients was 78.4%. Between these progression-free patients, 85.4% had obtained a complete response, 82.3% a partial response, and 39.9% a stable disease.[76]

In terms of tolerability, the arm with ipilimumab had a higher incidence of grade 3-5 AEs (19.9%), compared with the two treatment arms with pembrolizumab (13.1% in q14 and 10.1% in q21). The most frequent toxicities in the pembrolizumab arm were fatigue, cutaneous rash, diarrhea, and pruritus, and among the immune-related toxicities the most frequent was hypothyroidism (10.1% in q14 and 8.7% in q 21). Similarly, grade 3 to grade 4 colitis was higher in the ipilimumab arm (8.2% vs. 1.4%–2.5%). The rate of discontinuation due to adverse events was higher in the ipilimumab arm (9.4%) versus pembrolizumab q14 (4.0%) and q21 (6.9%).

The KEYNOTE-002 study,[77] a randomized Phase 2 trial, evaluated the efficacy of pembrolizumab in patients with advanced melanoma, pretreated with ipilimumab and, if BRAF mutated, with BRAF or MEK inhibitor. The study evaluated two cohorts of patients treated with pembrolizumab (in two different schedules) and one cohort of patients treated with a type of chemotherapy chosen by the investigator. A total of 540 patients were enrolled. At median follow-up of 13.5 months, median OS was 13.4 months for pembrolizumab at 2 mg/kg, 14.7 months for pembrolizumab at 10 mg/kg, and 11.0 months for chemotherapy. The 18-month OS rates were 40%, 44%, and 36%; 24-month rates were 36%, 38%, and 30%. HR for OS was 0.86 (95% CI 0.67–1.10) for 2 mg/kg (p = .1173) and 0.74 (0.57–0.96) for 10 mg/kg (p = .0106), with no difference between doses (0.87 [95% CI 0.67–1.12]). When the 98 (55%) patients in the chemotherapy arm who crossed-over were censored, HR was 0.79 (95% CI 0.58–1.08) for 2 mg/kg (p = .0683) and 0.67 (95% CI 0.49–0.92) for 10 mg/kg (p = .0068), with no difference between doses (0.87 [95% CI 0.67–1.12]).[78]

The primary endpoint of the study at the second interim analysis was PFS, but the sample size was evaluated according to the OS at the final analysis. The 24-month PFS rates were 16% for 2 mg/kg, 22% for 10 mg/kg, and <1% for chemo. ORR was 22%, 28%, and 4%; 73%, 74%, and 13% of responders had no progression at a follow-up of more than 13 months. Grade 3 to grade 5 drug-related AE rates results were lower with pembrolizumab (13% and 17% vs. 26%) than with chemotherapy. The most recent follow-up at 58.5 months confirmed the superiority of pembrolizumab on chemotherapy in terms of OS and PFS. Indeed, 3- and 4-year OS of pembrolizumab were 30.3% and 27.2%, respectively, as 3- and 4-year PFS of pembrolizumab were 16.9% and 15%. Between the patients who achieved a response, median duration of response was more than 50 months. Similarly, 15% grade (G). 3/4 toxicity was confirmed.[79]

Pembrolizumab was approved for metastatic melanoma by the FDA at 2 mg/kg, according to the data of the Phase 1 trial KEYNOTE-001. This study enrolled 655 patients with metastatic melanoma; 151 were treatment naïve and 504 were previously treated. After a median follow-up of 55 months, 5-year PFS rates were 21% in all patients and 29% in treatment-naïve patients; median PFS was 8.3 months (95% CI, 5.8–11.1) and 16.9 months (95% CI, 9.3–35.5) in all patients and treatment-naïve patients, respectively. The 5-year OS rate was 34% in all patients and 41% in treatment-naïve patients, like the 4-year rates of 38% and 48%, respectively. Median OS was 23.8 months (95% CI, 20.2–30.4) in all patients and 38.6 months (95% CI, 27.2–NR) in treatment-naïve patients. Around 17% of the patients (n = 114) experienced grade 3/4 AEs and 7.8% (n = 51) discontinued the treatment because of an AE.[80]

Pembrolizumab is also approved in adjuvant settings for patients with resected melanoma at high risk of recurrence. The EORTC 1325/KEYNOTE-054 study, a randomized Phase 3 clinical trial, enrolled patients with radically resected stage III (AJCC 7) cutaneous melanoma.[81] In the trial, 1,019 patients were randomized with a 1:1 ratio to pembrolizumab 200 mg flat dose every 3 weeks (n = 514) or placebo (n = 505). The two co-primary endpoints were RFS in the overall population and in those with PD-L1–positive tumors. Pembrolizumab compared with placebo resulted in prolonged RFS in the overall population. At a median follow-up of 3.5 years, the RFS rate was 59.8% for pembrolizumab and 41.4% for placebo (HR, 0.59; 95% CI, 0.47–0.68). Pembrolizumab reduced the incidence of distant metastasis at first recurrence (24.9% vs. 39.5% of placebo HR 0.57), and the incidence of locoregional only recurrence (14.0% vs. 18.9% of placebo HR 0.73). Indeed, the 3.5 years DMFS is 65.3 for pembrolizumab and 49.4% for placebo. The impact of pembrolizumab on RFS and DMFS was similar according to AJCC-7 and AJCC-8 staging, as well as BRAF mutation status.[82] Anyway, the overall survival benefit of adjuvant pembrolizumab will be hard to demonstrate due to the design of the study that allowed the crossover to pembrolizumab for patients progressing after adjuvant placebo and due to the effective lines of post-progression treatment.

Nivolumab

The randomized Phase 3 study CheckMate 037[83] evaluated treatment with nivolumab versus the investigator's choice chemotherapy (ICC) (dacarbazine or paclitaxel in combination with carboplatin) in patients with advanced melanoma in progression after previous treatment with ipilimumab and in patients with BRAF mutation, also with BRAF inhibitor. The study was conducted on a sample of 405 patients, 272 treated with nivolumab, and 133 treated with chemotherapy. The primary objective was to evaluate the OS and RR. Secondary objectives were PFS and the evaluation of the predictive role of PD-L1 expression. At a median follow-up of 24 months,[84] treatment with nivolumab was superior to ICC in terms of ORR (27% vs. 10%). In the nivolumab arm, grade 3 to grade 4 adverse events were 14% versus 34% of ICC. Median overall survival was 16 months for nivolumab versus 14 months for ICC and median PFS was 3.1 versus 3.7, respectively. It must be specified that more nivolumab-treated patients had brain metastases (20% vs. 14%) and elevated levels of LDH (52% vs. 38%) at baseline. Furthermore, 41% of the patients treated with ICC received an anti-PD-1 treatment after progression. Moreover, the choice of the evaluation of the response with RECIST criteria (instead of the irRECIST criteria) could also have underestimated the real activity of treatment with nivolumab considering the possible benefit even beyond the progression.

The CheckMate 066 study,[85] a randomized double-blinded Phase 3 study of superiority, evaluated treatment with nivolumab versus dacarbazine in patients with advanced BRAF-wild type melanoma in the first-line treatment. The study was conducted on a population of 418 patients. The primary objective was OS, while secondary objectives were the evaluation of PFS, the rate of objective responses (RR), and the predictive role of PD-L1 expression. Treatment with nivolumab was superior in OS, with a proportion of patients alive at 1 year of 72.9% (95% CI, 65.5–78.9) in the nivolumab arm and 42.1% (95% CI, 33.0–50.9) in the chemotherapy arm. Treatment with nivolumab also showed higher PFS (HR = 0.43; 95% CI, 0.34–0.56) and RR (40.0%, 95% CI 33.3–47.0 vs. 13.9%, 95% CI 9.5–19.4, with a OR = 4.06, p <.001). The incidence of grade 3 to grade 4 AEs was lower in the nivolumab arm (11.7 vs. 17.6%). The study update, with a minimum follow-up of 60 months, reported a 5-year OS of patients who received nivolumab of 39% versus 17% of patients who received dacarbazine. PFS rates were 28% and 3%, respectively, and ORR was 42% with nivolumab and 14% with dacarbazine; among patients alive at 5 years, ORR was 81% and 39%, respectively. Five-year OS was 38% in patients randomly assigned to dacarbazine who had subsequent therapy, including nivolumab. Among 75 nivolumab-treated patients alive and evaluable at the 5-year analysis, 83% had not received subsequent therapy, 23% were still on study treatment, and 60% were treatment free.[86]

The randomized double-blind Phase 3 study CheckMate 067,[87] recently updated,[16] evaluated the superiority of the combination nivolumab + ipilimumab versus ipilimumab and nivolumab versus ipilimumab (1:1:1) in the first-line treatment of patients with advanced melanoma. The study population was 945 patients, of which 31.1% had the BRAF mutation. The primary endpoints were PFS and OS; secondary endpoints were the ORR, tolerability, and the predictive role of the immunohistochemical expression of PD-L1. The study was designed to compare the combination of nivolumab + ipilimumab versus ipilimumab and nivolumab versus ipilimumab. The median PFS in the nivolumab group was 6.9 months versus 2.9 months for patients treated with ipilimumab. The median overall survival was 36.9 months (28.3–NR) in the nivolumab group and 19.9 (16.9–24.6) in the ipilimumab group. At a median follow-up of 60 months, treatment with nivolumab alone demonstrated a statistically superior HR for PFS (HR 0.53, 95% CI 0.44–0.64; p <.0001) and OS (HR 0.65, 95% CI 0.53–0.79; p <.0001) as compared with ipilimumab. The 5-year PFS was 29% and 8%, respectively, and the 5-year OS was 44% with nivolumab and 26% with ipilimumab.[88] As post-progression treatment, 29% of the patients in the nivolumab arm were treated with ipilimumab, while 45% of the patients in the ipilimumab group were treated with anti-PD-1. So, the advantage in terms of survival demonstrated by nivolumab depends on not only the frontline therapy but also post-progression treatment. The tolerability profile was better in the nivolumab than in the ipilimumab arm (G.3 toxicity 22% vs. 28%) with a discontinuation of treatment due to toxicity of 7.7% versus 14.8%, respectively.

Nivolumab is also approved for the adjuvant treatment of radically resected melanoma patients at high risk of recurrence. The CheckMate 238 study, a Phase 3 double-blind clinical trial, enrolled patients with completely resected stage IIIB/C or IV melanoma.[89] Patients were randomized with a 1:1 ratio to receive nivolumab at 3 mg/kg every 2 weeks (n = 453) or ipilimumab at 10 mg/kg every 2 weeks for four doses, and every 12 weeks thereafter (n = 453), for 1 year or until disease recurrence/unacceptable toxicity. RFS was the primary endpoint. At a median follow-up of 48 months,[90] nivolumab showed superior RFS versus ipilimumab with 4-year RFS rates of 52% versus 41% (HR, 0.71–95% CI, 0.60–0.86). The superiority of nivolumab was confirmed both in stage III and stage IV radically resected subgroups and in PDL-1 expression <5% and >5% subgroups, suggesting that PDL-1 expression levels are not specifically predictive of response to anti-PD-1 drugs. Nivolumab confirmed to be superior to ipilimumab for RFS in BRAF-mutant (0.79 95% C.I. 0.60–1.05) and BRAF-wild-type (0.69 95% C.I. 0.53–0.91) subgroups. The 48-month overall survival rates were similar in both treatment groups (NIVO, 78%; IPI, 77%), but more patients treated with IPI received subsequent therapy, including immunotherapy (57% with ipilimumab and 49% with nivolumab among patients with recurrence) and target therapy (25% with ipilimumab and 24% with nivolumab; Table 50.1).

Overall, when considering the significantly improved ORR, PFS, and OS with the PD-1 agents pembrolizumab

Table 50.1 Comparison Between the Data From the Three Phase 3 Clinical Trials in Adjuvant Setting CheckMate 238 (CM-238), KEYNOTE-054 (KN-054), and Combi AD. Treatment With Anti-PD-1 Has a Lower Rate of Grade 3/4 Toxicity. The Difference of RFS Observed at 1 Year Between Target Therapy and Immunotherapy in BRAF-Mutant Melanoma Patients Disappears at 2 and 3 Years, With the Possibility of a Long-Term Benefit for the Treatment With Anti-PD-1. The Patient Population Enrolled in the Trial CheckMate 238 Had a Higher Risk of Relapse as Compared With the KEYNOTE-054 and Combi-AD Clinical Trials and Nivolumab Was Compared With Ipilimumab, While Pembrolizumab and Dabrafenib Plus Trametinib Were Compared With Placebo

	STUDY POPULATION	G.3/4 TRAE (%)	TRAE DISCONT. RATE (%)	HR RFS	1Y-RFS (%)	3Y-RFS (%)	3Y-RFS (BRAFMUT) (%)	4Y-RFS (%)	HR DMFS
Nivolumab *CM-238*	*BRAF mut + wt* Stage III B, C, and IV NED	14	4	0.71	70	58	58	52	0.79
Pembrolizumab *KN-054*	*BRAF mut + wt* Stage III A, B, C	14.7	13.8	0.59	75.3	63.7	62	59 (3.5y)	0.60
Dabrafenib plus Trametinib *Combi AD*	*BRAF mut* Stage III A, B, C	41	26	0.51	88	59	59	54	0.55

BRAFMUT, BRAF mutant; DMFS, distant metastasis free survival; G.3/4 TRAE, Grade 3/4 treatment-related adverse events; HR, hazard ratio; RFS, relapse free survival; TRAE, treatment-related adverse events.

and nivolumab, the PD-1 agents represent a fundamental step forward in the treatment of patients with advanced melanoma. Treatment with anti-PD-1 drugs (pembrolizumab and nivolumab) has an acceptable tolerability profile, better than ipilimumab and clearly different from the chemotherapy. In general, most AEs are immune-mediated, so they can be managed with symptomatic or immunomodulatory therapy (e.g., steroids) depending on the grade and duration of the event. The rate of treatment interruption with anti-PD-1 for toxicity is low (range in studies examined by 3%–8%).

Combination of Anti-Programmed Cell Death 1 Plus Anti-Cytotoxic T Lymphocyte Antigen 4

Ipilimumab Plus Nivolumab

To further improve the efficacy of immunotherapy for the treatment of metastatic melanoma, anti-PD-1 and anti-CTLA-4 have been combined.

The randomized, double-blind Phase 3 study CheckMate 067 randomized 945 patients with unresectable advanced melanoma to the combination of nivolumab + ipilimumab, to ipilimumab, or to nivolumab.[87,91] The primary endpoints were PFS and OS. Secondary endpoints were ORR, tolerability, and the predictive role of the immunohistochemical expression of PD-L1. The study was designed to compare the combination of nivolumab + ipilimumab versus ipilimumab and nivolumab versus ipilimumab. The study was not planned to compare the combination arm with nivolumab alone. Around 32% of the enrolled patients had BRAF[V600] mutation. Median PFS was 11.5 months

(95% CI 8.7–19.3) in the nivolumab + ipilimumab group, 6.9 months (5.1–10.2) in the nivolumab group, and 2.9 months (2.8–3.2) in the ipilimumab group. The HR for PFS for the combination versus ipilimumab was 0.42 (95% CI 0.35–0.51; p <.0001) and for nivolumab versus ipilimumab was 0.53 (0.44–0.64; p <.0001). ORR was 58.3% (95% CI 52.6–63.8) for the combination, 44,6% (95% CI 39.1–50.3) for nivolumab, and 19.0% (95% CI 14.9–23.8) for ipilimumab. Median duration of response was 50.1 months (44.0–NR) in the nivolumab + ipilimumab group, was not reached in the nivolumab group (45.7–NR), and was 14.4 months (8.3–NR) in the ipilimumab group. At a minimum follow-up of 60 months, the median overall survival was more than 60.0 months (median OS was not reached) in the nivolumab + ipilimumab group and 36.9 months in the nivolumab group, as compared with 19.9 months in the ipilimumab group (HR for death with nivolumab + ipilimumab vs. ipilimumab, 0.52; HR for death with nivolumab vs. ipilimumab, 0.63).[88] Overall survival at 5 years was 52% in the nivolumab + ipilimumab group and 44% in the nivolumab group, as compared with 26% in the ipilimumab group. No sustained deterioration of health-related quality of life was observed during or after treatment with nivolumab + ipilimumab or with nivolumab alone. Treatment-related grade 3/4 adverse events were reported in 59% of patients who received nivolumab + ipilimumab, 22% who received nivolumab, and 28% who received ipilimumab. In the study, there were four treatment-related deaths: two in the nivolumab + ipilimumab group (one for cardiomyopathy and one for liver necrosis), one in the nivolumab group for neutropenia, and one in the ipilimumab group for colon perforation.

The predictive role of PD-L1 expression regarding the efficacy of the combination of nivolumab single agent remains to be defined, but nivolumab combined with ipilimumab obtained a higher OS in both PD-L1 positive and negative patients with the cutoff >5%.

Currently, the combination of nivolumab 1 mg/kg and ipilimumab 3 mg/kg has been approved by the FDA and EMA but is not available in European countries.

To determine if a different dosage of nivolumab and ipilimumab improves the safety profile of the combination, the Phase 3b/4 study CheckMate 511 was conducted. This study randomized 358 metastatic melanoma patients to NIVO 3 mg/kg + IPI 1 mg/kg or to NIVO 3 mg/kg + IPI 1 mg/kg. At a minimum follow-up of 12 months, the incidence of treatment-related grade 3 to grade 5 AEs among treated patients was significantly lower with NIVO3 + IPI1 versus NIVO1 + IPI3 (33.9% vs. 48,3%). In terms of efficacy, the two schedules were similar for ORR (45.6% vs. 50.6%), median PFS (9.9 vs. 8.9 months), and 12 months PFS (47.2% vs. 46.4%). Median OS was not reached and 12-month OS was 79.7% and 81.0%, respectively.[92] However, the study was not powered to demonstrate a difference of efficacy between the two arms, but rather to verify if a reduced dose of ipilimumab improves the safety profile of the combination.

The efficacy and safety of nivolumab + ipilimumab were evaluated in patients with melanoma who had untreated brain metastases in an open-label, multicenter, Phase 2 study (CheckMate 204).[93]

Ninety-four patients with metastatic melanoma, non-irradiated brain metastasis, and no neurologic symptoms were enrolled in the trial. At a median follow-up of 14.0 months, the rate of intracranial clinical benefit was 57%, the rate of complete response was 26%, the rate of partial response was 30%, and the rate of stable disease for at least 6 months was 2%. The rate of extracranial clinical benefit was 56%. Treatment-related grade 3 or grade 4 AEs were reported in 55% of patients, including events involving the central nervous system in 7%. One patient died from immune-related myocarditis. The safety profile of the regimen was similar to that reported in patients with melanoma who do not have brain metastases.[94]

The advantage of the combination of nivolumab + ipilimumab seems to be the potential benefit in terms of ORR, long-term PFS, and OS. This advantage has been demonstrated in the comparison with ipilimumab; however, the studies do not allow researchers to establish a statistical comparison between the combination and nivolumab single agent. However, there was an increase in toxicity with the combination compared with single-agent treatments, with a greater frequency of early interruption of treatment (although the interruption due to AEs seems to affect positively the long-term benefit of the treatment received). In this trial, a particular patient population, the metastatic mucosal melanoma, was enrolled. Seventy-nine patients were treated, 28 with nivolumab plus ipilimumab, 23 with nivolumab, and 28 with ipilimumab alone. Mucosal melanoma patients had similar safety outcomes but poorer long-term efficacy versus the ITT population. Indeed, ORR rates for the mucosal and ITT populations were 43% and 58% for nivolumab + ipilimumab, 30% and 45% for nivolumab, and 7% and 19% for ipilimumab, respectively. The 5-year PFS was 29% for nivolumab + ipilimumab, 14% for nivolumab, and 0% for ipilimumab. The 5-year OS was 36%, 17%, and 7%, respectively. Nine of 28 patients in the nivolumab + ipilimumab group (32%) discontinued treatment and remained treatment-free at 60 months from randomization. In the mucosal patient population, PFS appeared to be an appropriate surrogate for OS.[95]

Ipilimumab Plus Pembrolizumab

In order to reduce the toxicity of the combination, several attempts have been performed. The Phase 2 study KEYNOTE-029 combined pembrolizumab with reduced-dose ipilimumab.[96] Fifty-three patients were treated with pembrolizumab at 2 mg/kg plus ipilimumab at 1 mg/kg. At a median follow-up of 36.8 months, ORR in the overall population was 62% with 27% complete remissions, and median duration of response was not reached. Median PFS was not reached at the time of analysis, and 36-month PFS was 59%. Similarly, median OS was not reached, and 36-month OS was 73%. Grade 3/4 toxicity was 47%, and 33% of the patients discontinued therapy for toxicity. No treatment-related deaths were registered. Altogether, 72% of the patients received the four doses of ipilimumab and 31% completed 2 years of treatment. These data are very encouraging, but looking at the baseline characteristics of the study population, 56% were M1C, only 25% had elevated LDH levels, and 83% were PD-L1 positive. These characteristics are not consistent with those of the normal population and are correlated with a better prognosis.

Part 1B was an expansion cohort of the open-label, Phase 1b portion of KEYNOTE-029.[97] A total of 153 patients received at least one dose of pembrolizumab plus ipilimumab. At a median follow-up of 36.8 months, 71.9% had received four doses of ipilimumab and 30.7% had completed 2 years of pembrolizumab; 26.1% completed both treatments. Treatment-related adverse events occurred in 96.1% (47.1% grade 3/4; no deaths), leading to discontinuation of one or both study drugs in 35.9%. ORR was 62.1% with 42 (27.5%) complete and 53 (34.6%) partial responses. Median DOR was not reached; 36-month ongoing response rate was 84.2%. Median PFS and OS were not reached; 36-month rates were 59.1% and 73.4%, respectively.

Other Combinations

The impetus behind the development of novel combinations is to identify regimens that can overcome primary or acquired resistance to anti-PD-1/PD-L1 and/or reduce toxicity, compared with combination therapy with anti-CTLA-4 and anti-PD-1. With the introduction of the combination of two checkpoint inhibitors, more than 50% of the patients are alive at 5 years, but in the same way about 50% have no or very limited benefit. This probably depends on the cancer-immune phenotype that distinguishes inflamed tumors, with the presence of intratumoral CD8+ T cell infiltrate; immune-excluded tumors, with presence of CD8+ T cells that reside solely in the periphery; and immune-desert tumors, with little or no CD8+ T cell infiltration. Only inflamed tumors respond to immunotherapy. This has created an unmet need to make tumors that are not sensitive to immunotherapy become sensitive ("to make a cold tumor hot"). A strategy to make this is the combination of immunotherapy with other treatments, so the potential of anti-PD-1s in combination with other novel agents is also being explored (Figure 50.2).[98]

Anti-Programmed Cell Death 1 Plus Target Therapy

In BRAF-mutated melanoma, the "ideal therapy" should have the rapid kinetics of response of the target therapy and the long-lasting duration of response of the immunotherapy; for this reason, several clinical trials have been conducted trying to combine both of these characteristics. The combination of anti-BRAF target therapy with anti-CTLA-4 proved to be toxic,[69] but the BRAF and MEK inhibitors combo has shown good possibilities of combination with anti-PD-1/PD-L1 antibodies. Moreover, BRAF plus MEK inhibitors induce important changes in the TME with an increase in MHC expression, improved IFNAR and tumor-associated antigens, and reduction of CD73. With all these effects, TME becomes much more immunogenic due to the reduction of adenosine, T_{reg} cell, and MDSC levels, and for the increased activity of CD4-CD8+ lymphocytes (Figure 50.3).[99]

Until now, at least four "triple combinations" of anti-PD(L)1 plus BRAF/MEK inhibitors have been designed: durvalumab + dabrafenib and trametinib, atezolizumab + vemurafenib and cobimetinib, pembrolizumab + dabrafenib and trametinib, and spartalizumab + dabrafenib and trametinib. The combination pembrolizumab + dabrafenib and trametinib has been compared in a Phase 2 study versus the anti-BRAF/MEK target therapy. The KEYNOTE-022.[100] is a randomized, placebo-controlled, Phase 2 trial, which randomized 120 untreated metastatic BRAF-mutated patients to pembrolizumab + dabrafenib and trametinib or to placebo plus dabrafenib and trametinib. Median PFS was 16.0 months (95% CI 8.6–21.5) with the triple combination versus 10.3 months (95% CI 7.0–15.6) with dabrafenib + trametinib (HR, 0.66; $p = .04287$). Twelve-month PFS rates were 59% versus 45%. ORR was 63% versus 72%; confirmed ORR rates were 18% versus 13%. There was no difference observed in terms of time to response. Median DOR was 18.7 months (range 1.9+ to 22.1) versus 12.5 (2.1–19.5+). More patients (60%) on pembrolizumab + dabrafenib and trametinib had responses lasting more than 18 months versus dabrafenib + trametinib (28%). OS rates at 12 months were 79% versus 73%. Despite these data, PFS, the primary endpoint, did not reach the statistical significance threshold per study design because it required a HR per significance <0.62.

An updated analysis of KEYNOTE-022 took place after a median follow-up of 28.0 months. Median PFS by investigator review was 16.9 (95% confidence interval [CI], 11.3–27.9) months with pembrolizumab and 10.7 months with placebo (HR, 0.53; 95% CI, 0.34–0.83). Rates of PFS at 24 months were 41.0% with pembrolizumab versus 16.3% with placebo. Median overall survival was not reached at the time of the analysis with pembrolizumab and was 26.3 months with placebo (HR 0.64). Rates of overall survival at 24 months were 63.0% versus 51.7%. The ORR was 63.3% with pembrolizumab and 71.7% with placebo, with a median duration of response of 25.1 months and 12.1 months with pembrolizumab and placebo, respectively (HR, 0.32). Rates of duration of response after 24 months were 54.9% and 15.9% with pembrolizumab and placebo, respectively. Grade 3 to grade 5 treatment-emergent adverse events occurred in 35 (58.3%) patients in the pembrolizumab and 15 (25.0%) patients in the placebo arm. One patient died of pembrolizumab-related pneumonitis.[100]

Other combinations of target therapy plus immunotherapy have been tested in clinical trials. A Phase 1 study (NCT02027961) showed that 10 mg/kg of the PD-L1 inhibitor durvalumab every 2 weeks in combination with dabrafenib and trametinib had a manageable safety profile and evidence of clinical activity in patients with stage IIIC/IV melanoma. Patients with BRAF mutation treated with a combination of BRAF and MEK inhibition exhibited the greatest immune activation as well as the greatest clinical activity.[32] In cohort A (combination of durvalumab + dabrafenib + trametinib) on 26 patients treated, ORR was 69% and DCR was 100%. Grade 3/4 AEs was 39%.[101]

Another triplet combination being assessed in patients with metastatic BRAF-mutant melanoma is the anti-PD-L1 inhibitor atezolizumab in combination with the BRAF inhibitor vemurafenib plus the MEK inhibitor cobimetinib. In a Phase 1B dose escalation and expansion cohort study, patients received a 28-day lead in of cobimetinib + vemurafenib followed by a triple combination of 720 mg of vemurafenib, 60 mg of cobimetinib, and 800 mg of atezolizumab. Preliminary data from 34 patients suggest that this triple combination has a manageable

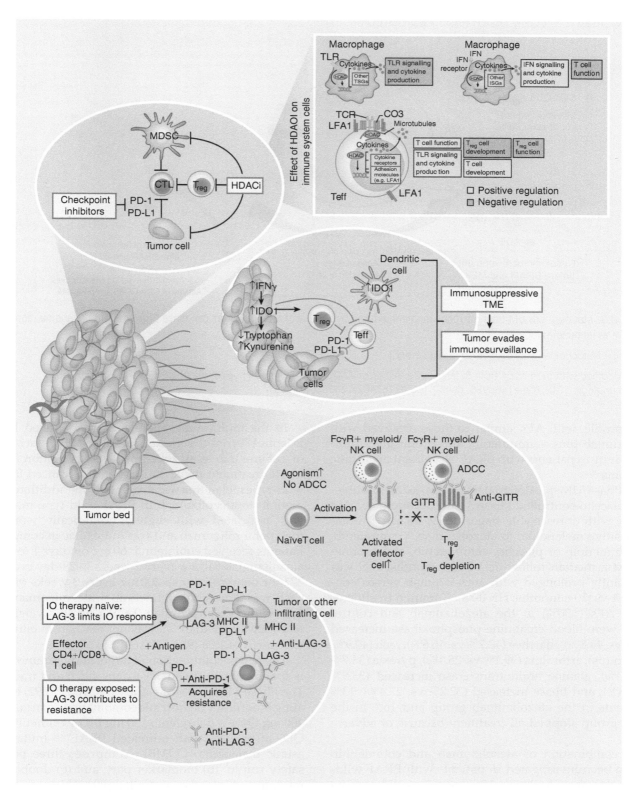

Figure 50.2 New emerging pathways for combinations with anti-PD-1/PD-L1 compounds. From top, the rationale to combine HDAC inhibitors (e.g., entinostat, domatinostat), IDO1 inhibitors (e.g., epacadostat), anti-GITR (e.g., BMS-986156), anti-LAG-3 (e.g., relatlimab) with anti-PD-1/PDL-1.

ADCC, antibody-dependent cellular cytotoxicity; IDO, indoleamine 2,3-dioxygenase; IFN, interferon; MDSC, myeloid-derived suppressor cell; MHC, major histocompatibility complex; NK, natural killer; PD-1, programmed cell death 1; PD-L1, programmed cell death ligand 1; Teff, effector T cells; TLR, Toll-like receptors; TME, tumor microenvironment; T$_{reg}$, regulatory T.

Source: Reproduced with permission from Reference 98: Ascierto PA, McArthur GA. Checkpoint inhibitors in melanoma and early phase development in solid tumors: what's the future? *J Transl Med.* 2017;15(1):173. https://doi.org/10.1186/s12967-017-1278-5

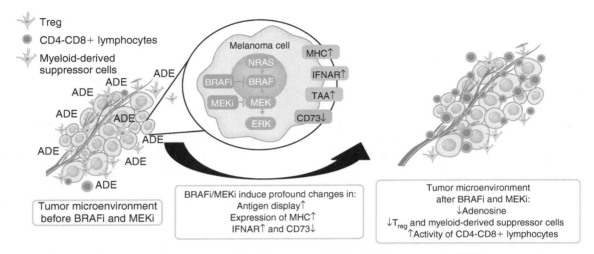

Figure 50.3 Modifications of tumor microenvironment induced by BRAF and MEK inhibitors can make BRAF-mutant melanoma more responsive to immunotherapy.

MHC, major histocompatibility complex; T_{reg}, regulatory T.

Source: Modified with permission from Reference 99: Ascierto PA, Dummer R. Immunological effects of BRAF+MEK inhibition. *Oncoimmunology.* 2018;7(9):e1468955. doi:10.1080/2162402X.2018.1468955

safety profile, with AEs similar to those observed with atezolizumab plus vemurafenib, and promising antitumor activity in patients with BRAF^{V600}–mutant metastatic melanoma.[102]

The Phase 3 IMspire150 trial (NCT02908672), a double-blind, placebo-controlled Phase 3 study, randomized 514 patients with unresectable stage IIIc-IV, BRAF^{V600} mutation-positive melanoma, to atezolizumab, vemurafenib, and cobimetinib or placebo, vemurafenib, and cobimetinib. At a median follow-up of 18·9 months, PFS was significantly prolonged with atezolizumab versus control (15·1 vs. 10·6 months; HR 0·78). Common treatment-related AEs (>30%) in the atezolizumab and control groups were blood creatinine phosphokinase increased (51.3% vs. 44.8%), diarrhea (42.2% vs. 46.6%), rash (40.9%, both groups), arthralgia (39.1% vs. 28.1%), pyrexia (38.7% vs. 26.0%), alanine aminotransferase increased (33.9% vs. 22.8%), and lipase increased (32.2% vs. 27.4%); 13% of patients in the atezolizumab group and 16% in the control group stopped all treatment because of adverse events.[103]

The combination of atezolizumab and cobimetinib has also been investigated in patients with BRAF wild-type melanoma. A Phase 1B study in solid tumors included 20 patients with metastatic melanoma, 10 of whom had BRAF wild-type tumors.[34] A clinical benefit of the combination was observed regardless of BRAF status (BRAF-mutant: ORR, 40%; median PFS, 11.9 months; BRAF wild type: ORR, 50%; median PFS, 15.7 months). Atezolizumab and cobimetinib also had a manageable safety profile, like that observed with atezolizumab alone or cobimetinib plus vemurafenib.

In the multicenter, open-label, randomized Phase 3 IMspire170 trial, the efficacy, safety, and pharmacokinetics of cobimetinib + atezolizumab versus pembrolizumab in 446 treatment-naïve patients with advanced BRAF^{V600} wild-type melanoma was evaluated. The addition of cobimetinib to atezolizumab in BRAF wild-type melanoma was associated with slightly numerically worse PFS than pembrolizumab and was quite toxic in comparison. Patients received cobimetinib 60 mg on days 1 to 21 plus atezolizumab 840 mg every 2 weeks in 28-day cycles (*n* = 222) or pembrolizumab 200 mg every 3 weeks (*n* = 224). ORR was 26% with cobimetinib + atezolizumab versus 32% with pembrolizumab. DCR was 46% versus 44%, respectively. Median OS was not reached in either arm, with a HR of 1.06 (95% CI 0.69–1.61).[104]

The newer combination of target and immunotherapy is spartalizumab (PDR001) + dabrafenib and trametinib. The Phase 1 to 3 COMBI-i study (NCT02967692) is evaluating the efficacy of the triple combination (spartalizumab 400 mg Q4W + dabrafenib 150 mg BID + trametinib 2 mg QD) in patients with untreated BRAF^{V600}–mutant metastatic melanoma. COMBI-i comprises three parts: (a) safety run-in; (b) biomarker part; and (c) double-blind, randomized, placebo-controlled part. Thirty-six patients were enrolled (nine in part 1 and 27 in part 2); 50% had stage IV M1c and 42% had elevated LDH levels. At a median follow-up of 15.2 months, the treatment was ongoing in 17 patients (47%). The ORR was 75%, with 33% complete responses. The 12-month DOR rate was 71.4%, and 12-month PFS and OS rates were 65.3% and 85.9%, respectively. In patients with high baseline LDH: ORR was 67%, with three CRs (20%), median

PFS was 10.7 months, and median OS was not reached. All patients had ≥1 AE; 27 (75%) had grade ≥3 AEs. Six patients (17%) had AEs leading to discontinuation of all three study drugs. Any-grade AEs in ≥40% of patients included pyrexia, chills, fatigue, cough, and arthralgia. Grade ≥3 AEs in >3 patients were neutropenia, pyrexia, and increased lipase. These encouraging results led to tpart III of this study.[105] The Phase 3 COMBI-i trial evaluated the investigational immunotherapy spartalizumab (PDR001) in combination with dabrafenib and trametinib, compared with dabrafenib and trametinib alone among treatment-naïve patients with advanced BRAF[V600] mutation-positive cutaneous melanoma. The trial did not meet its primary endpoint of investigator-assessed PFS because mPFS was 16.2 months for the triple combination and 12 months for dabrafenib + trametinib. The 1- and 2-year PFS were 58% and 44% for spartalizumab + dabrafenib and trametinib versus 50% and 35% for the control arm. Median DOR was not reached in the experimental arm and was 20.7 months for dabrafenib + trametinib. The 1- and 2-year DOR were 66% and 55% for spartalizumab + dabrafenib + trametinib versus 61% and 48% of the control arm. A higher number of toxicity-related dose modifications/interruptions was detected in the spartalizumab + dabrafenib + trametinib arm (19%) than in the control arm (8.7%), while the rate of the patients that discontinued treatment for progression of disease in the dabrafenib + trametinib arm (48.3%) was higher as compared with the spartalizumab + dabrafenib + trametinib arm (37.1%). Indeed, G3/4 adverse events were more frequent with the experimental arm (54.7%) than with the control arm (33.3%). Considering the biomarker analysis, a strong correlation between PFS and tumor mutational burden (TMB) emerged. A cutoff of 10 mut/MB was used to identify high and low TMB patients. Patients with low TMB had median PFS, and 1- and 2-year PFS were very similar in both the experimental and the control arm (mPFS 12.8 months vs. 12 months—HR 0.907). Patients with high TMB (>10 mut/MB) treated with spartalizumab + dabrafenib + trametinib had a mPFS of 23.9 months versus 11.8 months of dabrafenib + trametinib (hazard ratio 0.703). See Table 50.2.[106]

Anti-Programmed Cell Death 1 Plus Anti-Indoleamine 2,3-Dioxygenase

Indoleamine 2,3-dioxygenase (IDO1) is an intracellular enzyme induced by interferon-gamma that catalyzes the first and rate-limiting step in the kynurenine pathway, the O_2-dependent oxidation of L-tryptophan to N-formylkynurenine.[107] In tumors, depletion of tryptophan and production of kynurenine makes the TME immunosuppressive with a resulting help to immunosurveillance evasion of tumor cells.

Epacadostat is a potent and selective IDO-1 inhibitor[108] that has been evaluated in combination with both pembrolizumab and nivolumab.

In an open-label Phase 1/2 trial enrolling patients with multiple tumor types (ECHO-202/KEYNOTE-037), epacadostat in association with pembrolizumab showed promising antitumor activity in patients with advanced melanoma.[109] In 63 evaluable patients with melanoma, the ORR was 56% (complete response 14%), and the disease control rate was 71%. Median PFS was 12.4 months, and 18-month PFS was 49%.

Among treatment-naïve patients with advanced disease treated with 100 mg of epacadostat (38 patients), ORR was 58% (confirmed ORR, 8%), the disease control rate was 74%, and median PFS was 22.8 months. Epacadostat + pembrolizumab showed a favorable safety profile, with an incidence of grade 3/4 toxicity of 20%.

This combination has been further evaluated versus pembrolizumab monotherapy in a Phase 3 study of 706 patients with advanced melanoma (ECHO-301/KEYNOTE-252). In this randomized, double-blind Phase 3 trial.[110] the addition of epacadostat to pembrolizumab did not result in greater clinical benefit over anti-PD-1 alone. At a median follow-up of 14 months, the combination of epacadostat + pembrolizumab did not result in a significantly longer PFS as compared with placebo + pembrolizumab (median 4.7 vs. 4.9 months) and 12-month PFS rate was 37% in both groups (hazard ratio: 1.00; 95% CI: 0.83–1.21). Similarly, the 12-month OS rate was 74% in both groups (hazard ratio: 1.13; 95% CI: 0.86–1.49). ORR was 34.2% and 31.5% in the epacadostat + pembrolizumab and placebo + pembrolizumab groups, respectively. The trial was stopped after the combination failed the study's first primary goal.

A similar combination, epacadostat + nivolumab, was studied in the open-label Phase 1/2 ECHO-204 trial of patients with advanced solid tumors. The combination was generally well tolerated and showed promising antitumor activity.[111] In 40 patients with metastatic melanoma not previously treated with IDO inhibitors or checkpoint inhibitors (except for anti–CTLA-4), ORR was 63% with 5% confirmed ORR, and the disease control rate was 88%. Responses were obtained regardless of PD-L1 expression. The toxicity of the combination was manageable, and directly proportional to the dose of epacadostat.

Another selective IDO-1 inhibitor, BMS-986205, has been studied in combination with nivolumab. In a Phase 1/2A trial, in 289 heavily pretreated patients with advanced solid tumors (CA017-003), BMS-986205 (linrodostat) + nivolumab showed antitumor activity and had a favorable safety profile, with grade 3/4 TRAEs in 11% of patients and no treatment-related deaths.[112] The Phase 3 randomized, double-blind study of BMS-986205 + nivolumab versus nivolumab alone in patients with

Table 50.2 Comparison Between the Data of Clinical Trials KEYNOTE-022, IMspire 150, and Combi-I. Only the Triple Combination of Vemurafenib, Cobimetinib, and Atezolizumab (IMspire 150) Achieved Statistical Significance for Primary Endpoint

	ORR (%)	MOS (MONTHS)	1-Y OS (%)	2-Y OS (%)	MPFS (MONTHS)	1-Y PFS (%)	2-Y PFS (%)	G.3/4TRAE (%)
KEYNOTE-022 *Dab + Tra + Pem*	63.3	NR	79	63	16	62	41	57
IMSPIRE 150 *Vem + Cobi + Atz*	66.3	28.8	76.7	60.4	15.1	54	38	79
COMBI-I *Dab + Tra + Spa*	68.5	NR	84	68	16.2	58	44	54.7

1-Y OS, 1 year overall survival; 2-Y OS, 2 year overall survival; 1-Y PFS, 1 year progression free survival; 2-Y PFS, 2 years progression free survival; Atz, atezolizumab; Cobi, cobimetinib; Dab, dabrafenib; G.3/4 TRAE, Grade 3/4 treatment-related adverse events; IPI, ipilimumab; MOS, median overall survival; MPFS, median progression free survival; NIVO, nivolumab; NR, not reached; ORR, objective response rate; Pem, pembrolizumab; Tra, trametinib; Vem, vemurafenib.

untreated advanced melanoma will demonstrate if the combination of linrodostat + nivolumab is superior to monotherapy.

Anti-Programmed Cell Death 1 Plus Histone Deacetylase Inhibitors

Histone deacetylase (HDAC) is a class of enzymes that remove acetyl groups from an ε-N-acetyl lysine amino acid on a histone, allowing the histones to wrap the DNA more tightly. This is important because DNA is wrapped around histones, and DNA expression is regulated by acetylation and deacetylation. HDAC inhibitors (HDACis) are compounds that act on nonhistone proteins that are related to acetylation. HDACis can alter the degree of acetylation of these molecules and, therefore, increase or repress their activity. Entinostat is an oral, class I selective histone deacetylase inhibitor that has shown preclinically to enhance the activity of immune checkpoint blockade through the reduction of functionally immunosuppressive myeloid-derived suppressor cells (MDSCs) and regulatory T cells (T_{reg} cells). The trial ENCORE-601[113] enrolled patients refractory to previous treatment with checkpoint inhibitors to be treated with entinostat in combination with pembrolizumab. Between the 53 patients, refractory to prior PD-(L)1 therapy, 36% had elevated LDH, 70% had prior ipilimumab, and 23% had prior BRAF/MEK inhibitors. With the combination entinostat + pembrolizumab, the confirmed objective response with entinostat + pembrolizumab was 19% (1 confirmed ORR and 9 PRs), the median duration of response was 12.5 months (range 4–18 months) with five responders ongoing at the time of data cutoff. Seven patients have had stable disease for more than 6 months, resulting in a clinical benefit rate (confirmed ORR, PR, SD >6 months) of 32% (95% CI: 20%–46%). The median PFS was 4.2 months. Five patients (9%) experienced a grade 3/4 immune-related AE (two events of rash, one

each of colitis, pneumonitis, and autoimmune hepatitis). Preliminary biomarker analysis supports the hypothesis that the addition of entinostat to anti-PD-1 restores inflammation in the TME necessary for successful re-treatment with an anti–PD-(L)1 monoclonal antibody.[114]

Domatinostat is another inhibitor of the enzymes HDAC 1, 2, and 3, which are believed to play important roles in the regulation of aberrant cancer signaling. This compound is a small molecule, orally administered for the treatment of cancer. The SENSITIZE study (NCT03278665) is an open-label, multicenter, Phase 1b/2 study designed to evaluate the combination treatment of domatinostat with pembrolizumab in patients with metastatic melanoma who are refractory to prior treatment with anti-PD-1 antibodies.[115] Twenty-three patients were enrolled into the study. The safety profile indicates that domatinostat-specific adverse events add to the known safety profile of pembrolizumab, but no exacerbation of immune-related adverse events in rate and severity has been observed so far. Domatinostat alone and in combination was considered safe. First signs of efficacy have been observed, including one patient with a partial response and two with stable disease per irRECIST 1.1. Tumor biopsies at baseline showed a domatinostat-induced alteration of the TME including infiltration of CD8+ T cells, the presence of PD-1/PD-L1 positive cells, and changes on gene expression levels.

Anti-Programmed Cell Death 1 Plus Anti-Lymphocyte Activation Gene-3

Signaling via T cell inhibitory receptors (e.g., PD-1, CTLA-4, lymphocyte activation gene-3 [LAG-3]) can lead to T cell dysfunction and consequent tumor immune escape. Simultaneous blockade of two immune checkpoints as LAG-3 and PD-1 may synergistically restore T cell antitumor activity. Relatlimab (BMS-986016) is a monoclonal antibody directed against the inhibitor receptor LAG-3, with potential immune checkpoint inhibitory and antineoplastic activities. Relatlimab has been investigated in combination with nivolumab. In a Phase 1/2a study of 55 heavily pretreated patients with advanced melanoma refractory to or relapsed on anti–PD-1/PD-L1 therapy, 67% of patients had M1c disease, 38% had elevated LDH, and 15% had very elevated LDH; 76% were heavily pretreated with more than two previous therapies and 40% had progressive disease as best response to previous anti-PD-1 treatment. In this challenging cohort, ORR was 13%, with a 20% response rate in patients with LAG-3 expression ≥1% versus only 7% in LAG-3⁻ (<1%) patients. Also, 45% of the LAG-3 positive patients experienced a reduction of tumor burden with durable responses. Expression of PD-L1 had no impact on response. Among six partial responses, three were in resistant patients and two were in refractory patients. The safety profile was comparable to that of nivolumab monotherapy.[116] A randomized Phase 2/3 trial of nivolumab + relatlimab versus nivolumab monotherapy (CA224-047) as first-line treatment for untreated metastatic melanoma patients is now ongoing (NCT03470922).

In preclinical models, a triple combination of anti-PD-1, HDAC inhibitors and anti-LAG-3 has already shown impressive efficacy. Considering the safety profile of the single drugs and the potential efficacy of this combination, a first-in-human trial has already been designed.

Anti-Programmed Cell Death 1 Plus Lenvatinib

Lenvatinib is a small-molecule tyrosine kinase inhibitor that inhibits vascular endothelial growth factor receptor (VEGFR1-3), fibroblast growth factor receptor (FGFR1-4), platelet-derived growth factor receptor-α (PDGFR-α), stem cell factor receptor (KIT), and rearranged during transfection (RET). These receptors are important for tumor angiogenesis, and lenvatinib inhibits tumor angiogenesis by inhibiting functions of these receptors. In preclinical studies, lenvatinib decreased tumor-associated macrophage populations, increased CD8⁺ T cell infiltration, and augmented PD-1 inhibitor activity; thus, lenvatinib was considered a rational combination partner for anti-PD-1.[117]

The combination of lenvatinib + pembrolizumab was tested in patients with melanoma that progressed on anti-PD-1 therapy, a challenging population. In a Phase 1b/2 study, the combination of lenvatinib + pembrolizumab was used to treat 21 patients with metastatic melanoma progressing after two or more lines of therapy. At a median follow-up of 16 months, the ORR was 47.6%, the median PFS was 5.5 months, and the 12-month PFS was 34.7%. According to these results, the Phase 2

open-label LEAP-004 study for patients with melanoma was conducted that progressed on anti-PD-1 therapy, including that which progressed on anti-PD-1 + anti-CTLA-4 therapy.[118] There were 103 patients enrolled in this study; 67.0% had stage M1c/M1d disease, 55.3% had LDH >ULN (20.4% ≥2 × ULN), and 36.9% had BRAFⱽ⁶⁰⁰ mutation. In addition, 61.2% received ≥2 prior therapies for metastatic melanoma, 32.0% received prior BRAF ± MEK inhibition, and 28.2% had PD on prior anti-PD-1/ L1 + anti-CTLA-4. At a median follow-up of 12.0 months, confirmed ORR was 21.4% (2 confirmed ORR, 20 PR) overall and 31.0% (1 confirmed ORR, 8 PR) for patients with progression on prior anti-PD-1/L1 + anti-CTLA-4. DCR was 65.0%. Median DOR was 6.3 months and 6-month DOR was 72.6%. Median PFS and OS were 4.2 months (3.5–6.3) and 13.9 months (95% CI 10.8–NR). The most common treatment-related AEs were hypertension (56.3%), diarrhea (35.9%), and nausea (34.0%). TRAEs were grade 3 to grade 4 in 44.7%, grade 5 in 1.0%, and led to discontinuation of lenvatinib and/or pembrolizumab in 7.8%. These data support lenvatinib + pembrolizumab as a potential regimen for this challenging population and need confirmation in the Phase 3 randomized trial.

The ongoing Phase 3 randomized trial LEAP-003 is designed to compare the efficacy and safety of pembrolizumab ± lenvatinib in untreated advanced melanoma (NCT03820986). Patients will be randomized 1:1 to pembrolizumab 200 mg every 3 weeks plus lenvatinib 20 mg or placebo plus pembrolizumab.

Anti-Programmed Cell Death 1 Plus Anti-Toll-Like Receptor9

Toll-like receptor 9 (TLR9) is an important receptor expressed on immune-system cells including DCs, macrophages, NK cells, and other APCs.[119] TLR9 preferentially triggers signaling cascades that lead to a pro-inflammatory cytokine response. TLR9 agonists directly induce activation and maturation of plasmacytoid DCs and enhance differentiation of B cells into antibody-secreting plasma cells. Preclinical and early clinical data support the use of TLR9 agonists in patients with solid tumors and hematologic malignancies. In preclinical studies, TLR9 agonists have shown activity not only as monotherapy but also in combination with multiple other therapies, as immunotherapies and other agents. Tilsotolimod (IMO-2125) is a synthetic oligonucleotide that binds to TLR9, altering TME by improving antigen presentation of DCs and macrophages with subsequent proliferation of antigen-specific cytotoxic T lymphocytes (CD8⁺ T cells). Tilsotolimod is administered by intratumoral injection, and the induced immune activation has been evidenced in both injected and uninjected tumors. In the Phase 1/2 trial ILLUMINATE-204,[120] tilsotolimod has been combined with ipilimumab to assess clinical activity of the combination in patients resistant or refractory to anti-PD-(L)1 therapy. Tilsotolimod was administered to a single tumor injection during weeks 1, 2, 3, 5, 8, and 11 and ipilimumab was administered at 3 mg/kg from week 2 as per the product label. Sixty-two patients were treated with tilsotolimod in combination with ipilimumab. Of these, 52 received the recommended Phase 2 dose (RP2D) of 8 mg, and 49 were evaluable for efficacy. The median OS was 21.0 months (95% CI: 9.8–not reached [NR]), and the ORR per RECIST v1.1 was 22.4% (95% CI: 11.8–36.6), including two complete responses. Median duration of response was 11.4 months (95% CI: 3.3–NR) with 7/11 responses lasting ≥6 months. The disease control rate was 71.4% (95% CI: 56.7–83.4). Tumor reduction was observed in injected and non-injected lesions. Analysis of biopsies showed rapid local IFN-α gene expression, DC maturation, and expansion of shared CD8$^+$ T cell clones in injected and non-injected tumors. Grade ≥3 AEs were observed in 48% (30/62) of patients, most commonly increased ALT and AST and colitis, and 26% experienced immune-related AEs. No AEs led to treatment discontinuation or death. However, 11 patients (42.3%) had grade 3 side effects, and two subjects (7.7%) had grade 4 AEs. A Phase 3 trial ILLUMINATE-301, comparing ipilimumab + tilsotolimod versus ipilimumab alone in patients progressing after anti-PD-1 therapy is now ongoing (NCT03445533).

SD-101 is a synthetic class-C CpG-oligodeoxynucleotide that stimulates plasmacytoid DCs through engagement of TLR9.[39] This TLR9 agonist was tested in a Phase 1b/2 study,[48] in combination with pembrolizumab at 200 mg every 3 weeks for the treatment of patients with advanced melanoma naïve to anti-PD-1 therapy.[121] Eighty-six patients have been enrolled, 45 with SD-101 at 2 mg in up to four lesions and 41 with SD-101 at 8 mg in a single lesion. Both the arms had similar baseline characteristics. At a median follow-up of 8.1 months in the 2 mg group and 8.3 months in the 8 mg group, ORR in the 2 mg group was 71%, with 13% confirmed ORR, and in the 8 mg group was 49% with 7% confirmed ORR. Responses were observed in both injected and non-injected lesions, including visceral. The median DOR was not reached in either group. In the 2-mg arm, ORR was about the same in PD-L1 positive and negative patients (80%/79%), while in the 8-mg arm ORR was higher in PD-L1 positive patients (62%/40%). The median PFS in the 2-mg group was not reached, and in 8 mg was 10.4 months. Six-month PFS rate in 2 mg was 81% and in 8 mg was 60%. The 2-mg dose of SD-101 can be considered the optimal dose based on these efficacy, safety, and biomarker data, showing increased immune activation consistent with the biology of TLR9

activation. The SD-101 safety profile consists of transient flu-like symptoms. Frequently observed grade 3/4 treatment-related AEs were myalgia, headache, fatigue, and chills. The combination of SD-101 and pembrolizumab shows promising response rates compared with those expected with pembrolizumab alone, even if the data must be confirmed in a randomized Phase 3 trial. The combination is well tolerated with no evidence of an increased rate of irAEs. These data will be considered in further studies comparing the combination of SD-101 + pembrolizumab to pembrolizumab alone.

Talimogene Laherperepvec Plus Anti-Programmed Cell Death 1

The oncolytic virus T-VEC combined with ipilimumab has been demonstrated to be effective.[122] Considering this synergism, it was hypothesized that the combination of T-VEC + anti-PD-1 could have been more effective. In the MASTERKEY-265 Phase 1b/3 study, which combined T-VEC + pembrolizumab for the treatment of unresectable stage IIIB-IV melanoma (NCT02263508), 21 patients were enrolled, 48% with IIIB-IVM1a, 52% with IVM1b/c disease, and 19% with BRAF mutation. Grade 3/4 toxicity was 33%, and the most common AEs were fatigue, pyrexia, and chills. Per immune-related response criteria, confirmed ORR was 48% and confirmed ORR rate was 14%. The randomized, placebo-controlled Phase 3 of this study, now ongoing, is comparing the combination T-VEC + pembrolizumab to pembrolizumab alone.[123]

Several other Phase 1 and 2 studies with intralesional treatments combined with checkpoint inhibitors (e.g., PV10, CVA21, LTX-315, STING agonists) are ongoing to define the activity of these compounds in combination with ICIs in patients progressing on anti-PD-1/PD-L1 treatment.

Anti-Programmed Cell Death 1 Plus NKTR-214

NKTR-214 (bempegaldesleukin) is a CD122-biased agonist, which stimulates CD8$^+$ effector T cells and NK cells in the body by targeting CD122 specific receptors found on the surface of these immune cells. CD122 is also known as the interleukin-2 receptor beta subunit, a key signaling receptor that is known to increase proliferation of these effector T cells.[124] In clinical and preclinical studies, treatment with NKTR-214 resulted in expansion of these immune cells and mobilization into the TME, creating a favorable condition for an antitumor immune response. Moreover, NKTR-214 has been shown to convert baseline PD-L1$^-$ in PD-L1$^+$.[125] In a Phase 1/2 study (PIVOT-02 trial) NKTR-214 was combined with nivolumab for the treatment of several tumors. Thirty-eight patients with untreated advanced melanoma were enrolled in the trial. ORR was 53% with 34% complete remissions (13/38). Disease control rate was 74% and median time to response was 2 months. The grade 3/4 treatment-related adverse events rate was 19.5%. The combined treatment demonstrated T cell infiltration and activation in the TME and induced an increase in absolute lymphocyte count with activated and proliferating CD4, CD8, and NK cells in peripheral blood, providing clear activation of the interleukin-2 pathway.[126]

A Phase 3 trial evaluating bempegaldesleukin in combination with nivolumab versus nivolumab alone in first-line advanced melanoma patients is currently ongoing (NCT03635983).

Anti-Programmed Cell Death 1 Plus Glucocorticoid-Induced Tumor Necrosis Factor Receptor-Related Gene Agonists

Nivolumab has also been assessed in combination with the glucocorticoid-induced tumor necrosis factor receptor-related gene (GITR) agonist, BMS-986156. GITR is a co-stimulatory activating receptor that is upregulated upon T cell activation. Antitumor activity of GITR agonists may be via increased T effector cell survival and function, reduced T_{reg}-mediated suppression of T effector cells, and T_{reg} cell reduction through conversion to effector cells. In a Phase 1/2a study of in-patients with advanced solid tumors to date 29 patients have received BMS-986156 alone and 37 have received BMS-986156 + nivolumab. No dose-limiting toxicities have been

reported, and the most common treatment-related AEs have included pyrexia, chills, and fatigue, with all grade 1/2 except in four patients. The safety profile of the combination was similar to monotherapy. The combination showed antitumor activity in several patients, increasing proliferating (Ki67+) NK and CD8 cells in peripheral blood and increasing the activation and proliferation of CD8 memory cells. Patients who responded included heavily pretreated patients with metastatic melanoma progressed on anti-PD-1 therapy, cervical cancer, adenocarcinoma of the ampulla of Vater, nasopharyngeal cancer, and so on.[127]

CONCLUSION

Over recent years, major advances in the treatment of melanoma have been achieved. However, additional improvements are still required, and several combining strategies are in development. Combined immunotherapies (ipilimumab with nivolumab) and combined anti-BRAF and MEK target therapies (dabrafenib with trametinib, vemurafenib with cobimetinib, and encorafenib with binimetinib) were the first combinations to show significant benefit in overall survival in melanoma beyond what has been observed with monotherapy. Target therapy has higher response rates, but these may be limited in duration. Conversely, immunotherapy may have lower response rates, but more durable responses (Figure 50.4). The next step will be the right sequencing of these combinations in BRAF-mutant patients, to improve their outcome. One strategy could be a short course of

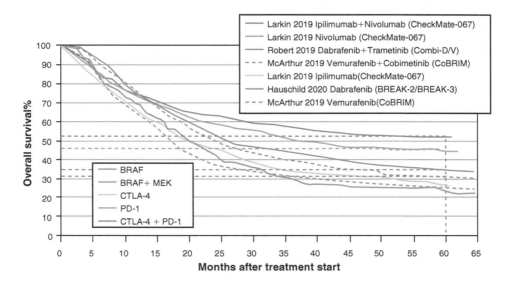

Figure 50.4 OS Kaplan-Meier survival curves of melanoma patients treated in selected clinical trials with published 5-year follow-up data.

Source: Reproduced with permission from Reference 46: Ugurel S, Röhmel J, Ascierto PA, et al. Survival of patients with advanced metastatic melanoma: the impact of MAP kinase pathway inhibition and immune checkpoint inhibition—update 2019. *Eur J Cancer.* 2020;130:126–138. https://doi.org/10.1016/j.ejca.2020.02.021

target therapy, switched to combo immunotherapy prior to progression of the disease. In order to answer this question there is the ongoing SECOMBIT study,[128] a randomized three-arms Phase 2 study (NCT02631447). Two hundred and fifty-one patients with untreated, metastatic BRAF[V600]-mutated melanoma were randomized with a 1:1:1 ratio to Arm A starting with encorafenib + binimetinib until progression of disease, followed by ipilimumab + nivolumab, or Arm B starting with the immunotherapy until progression of disease, followed by target therapy, or Arm C starting with encorafenib + binimetinib for 8 weeks, followed by ipilimumab + nivolumab until progression of disease, followed by target therapy. Sixty-nine patients were treated in arm A, 71 in arm B, and 69 in arm C. At a median follow-up of 17.5 months, mPFS was 15.8 months in arm A, 7.2 months in arm B, and 11.4 months in arm C. In the three arms, 1-year PFS was 60%, 43%, and 46%, and 2-year PFS was 35%, 38%, and 39%, respectively. ORR was 82.6% (confirmed ORR 21.7%) in arm A, 45.1% (confirmed ORR 15.5%) in arm B, and 78.3% (confirmed ORR 29.0%) in arm C. G3/4 toxicity was 49% in arm A, 73% in arm B, and 51% in arm C, while grade 3/4 treatment-related AEs were 28%, 54%, and 32%. Despite the difference in terms of mPFS, the 2-year PFS rate is similar among the different arms. The study is still ongoing.

The continuous identification of novel therapeutic targets and combinations offers opportunities to improve the prognosis of metastatic melanoma patients by overcoming de novo and acquired resistance to immune and target therapy. Overall, these new combinatorial approaches offer further potential to improve long-term survival for patients with metastatic melanoma.

KEY REFERENCES

Only key references appear in the print edition. The full reference list appears in the digital product on Springer Publishing Connect: connect.springerpub.com/content/book/978-0-8261-3743-2/part/part04/chapter/ch50

23. Hodi FS, O'Day SJ, Mcdermott DF, et al. Improved survival with ipilimumab in patients with metastatic melanoma. *N Engl J Med*. 2010;363(8):711–723. doi:10.1056/NEJMoa1003466

57. Wolchok JD, Hoos A, O'Day S, et al. Guidelines for the evaluation of immune therapy activity in solid tumors: immune-related response criteria. *Clin Cancer Res*. 2009;15(23):7412–7420. doi:10.1158/1078-0432.CCR-09-1624

75. Robert C, Ribas A, Schachter J, et al. Pembrolizumab versus ipilimumab in advanced melanoma (KEYNOTE-006): post-hoc 5-year results from an open-label, multicentre, randomised, controlled, Phase 3 study. *Lancet Oncol*. 2019;20(9):1239–1251. doi:10.1016/S1470-2045(19)30388-2

82. Eggermont AMM, Blank CU, Mandala' M, et al. LBA46 pembrolizumab versus placebo after complete resection of high-risk stage III melanoma: final results regarding distant metastasis-free survival from the EORTC 1325-MG/KEYNOTE 054 double-blinded Phase III trial. *Ann Oncol*. 2020;31:S1175. doi:10.1016/j.annonc.2020.08.2276

88. Larkin J, Chiarion-Sileni V, Gonzalez R, et al. Five-year survival with combined nivolumab and ipilimumab in advanced melanoma. *N Engl J Med*. 2019;381(16):1535–1546. doi:10.1056/NEJMoa1910836

90. Ascierto PA, del Vecchio M, Mandalá M, et al. Adjuvant nivolumab versus ipilimumab in resected stage IIIB-C and stage IV melanoma (CheckMate 238): 4-year results from a multicentre, double-blind, randomised, controlled, Phase 3 trial. *Lancet Oncol*. 2020;21(11):1465–1477. doi:10.1016/S1470-2045(20)30494-0

128. Ascierto PA, Mandala M, Ferrucci PF, et al. LBA45 first report of efficacy and safety from the Phase II study SECOMBIT (SEquential COMBo Immuno and Targeted therapy study). *Ann Oncol*. 2020;31:S1173–S1174. doi:10.1016/j.annonc.2020.08.2275

51

Other Cutaneous Tumors: Basal Cell Carcinoma, Cutaneous Squamous Cell Carcinoma, Merkel Cell Carcinoma, and Cutaneous Sarcomas

Jürgen C. Becker, Shailender Bhatia, Alexander Guminski, and Selma Ugurel

KEY POINTS

- Nonmelanoma skin cancers (NMSCs) represent a heterogeneous group of diseases including basal cell carcinoma (BCC), cutaneous squamous cell carcinoma (cSCC), and Merkel cell carcinoma (MCC), among others. As a group, NMSCs are the most commonly diagnosed malignancies in the world with an estimated incidence of 7.7 million cases in 2017, representing more than 30% of all cancer diagnoses.

- The central role of the sonic hedgehog (SHH)/patched 1 (PTCH1)/smoothened (SMO) pathway in both hereditary and sporadic BCC has been identified; thus, SMO inhibition has become a therapeutic strategy for advanced BCC not amendable by surgery or radiation. However, the impact of SMO inhibition on the tumor microenvironment is not completely understood; a notion of particular importance for possible combination or sequential immunotherapies.

- Pharmacologic activation of Toll-like receptor (TLR) on myeloid components of the immune system such as macrophages and dendritic cells represents an efficient strategy for boosting anticancer immunity. The TLR 7 agonist imiquimod induced clinical and histological clearance rates of up to 75% in superficial BCC.

- The extraordinarily high mutational burden in both BCC and cSCC resulting in numerous neoantigens possibly recognized by the host immune system suggests a strong immunogenicity of these UV-associated tumors.

- The immune response is known to play a crucial role in the development and prognosis of BCC, cSCC, and MCC; immune escape mechanisms usually observed in immunogenic tumors—for example, infiltration by regulatory T cells (T_{reg} cells) or expression of programmed death-ligand 1 (PD-L1)—are frequently observed.

- Clinical data clearly demonstrate that blockade of the programmed cell death 1 (PD-1)/PD-L1 pathway induces durable, therapeutic immune responses against BCC and cSCC in a large proportion of patients with advanced disease. PD-1 inhibition has replaced chemotherapy as the standard of care for patients requiring systemic therapy for cSCC, with the exception of immune suppressed solid organ transplant patients who remain a difficult-to-treat subgroup. Similar data in MCC are emerging.

- Viral carcinogenesis of MCC and the oncogenic addiction to continuous expression of virally encoded transforming early genes explain the exquisite immunogenicity of the majority of MCCs (virus-positive MCC or VP-MCC); the remaining tumors (virus-negative MCC or VN-MCC) are characterized by a high mutational burden with an ultraviolet (UV)-signature, resulting in numerous neoantigens.

- Adaptive immune response to MCC induces PD-L1 expression leading to exhaustion of tumor-specific T cells. Reversal of this immune evasion mechanism through PD-1/PD-L1 blocking antibodies has proven to be highly efficacious in advanced MCC, regardless of its viral status.

- The value of immunotherapy in cutaneous soft tissue sarcoma is still controversial. However, early data suggest clinical activity of PD-1 blockade in classic and endemic Kaposi's sarcoma (KS).

INTRODUCTION

Until recently, most of the attention with respect to tumor immunology and immunotherapy of skin cancer was focused on melanoma. This is based on the fact that the mutational landscape and high frequency of mutations present in melanoma exceed those of other solid tumors. This high mutational load provides the basis for a variety of neoantigens presented by this cancer entity, resulting in an exquisite immunogenicity and explaining the particular success of immunotherapies in the treatment of melanoma.[1] This high frequency of mutations is due to the etiologic role of ultraviolet (UV) radiation exposure and typically constitute single-base alterations, that is, cytidine to thymidine (C to T) substitutions.[1] However, the etiologic role of UV radiation is equally or even better established in other skin cancers such as basal cell carcinoma (BCC), cutaneous squamous cell carcinoma (cSCC), and Merkel cell carcinoma (MCC; Figure 51.1A–51.1C).[2] Those skin cancers in which UV-associated mutations are rare such as Merkel cell polyomavirus (MCPyV)-positive MCCs (VP-MCC) are critically dependent on the constitutive expression of the MCPyV-encoded transforming early genes, which as foreign antigens are probably even more immunogenic. Similarly, Kaposi's sarcoma (KS) is causally associated with KS herpesvirus (KSHV) infection (Figure 51.1D). Due to KSHV's reliance on modifying immune responses to efficiently infect its host, immunotherapy is an attractive option for treating KSHV-associated malignancies.

Notwithstanding the fact that immunotherapy has not been tested to the same extent in BCC, cSCC, and MCC, the link between immunosuppression and these cancer entities has been well described.[3,4] Indeed, the hazard ratios for immunosuppressed patients to develop BCC, cSCC, or MCC dramatically exceed those for the risk to develop melanoma. Moreover, these skin cancers are characterized by an increased aggressiveness in immunosuppressed patients, that is, higher recurrence rates, increased rate of regional metastasis, impaired response to therapy, and higher mortality by skin cancer metastasis.[5] The fact that even metastatic lesions may regress upon cessation of immunosuppression strongly supports its causative role and suggests the likelihood of success of immunotherapeutic strategies in these skin cancers.[6]

BASAL CELL CARCINOMA

There are 2.8 million new cases of BCC diagnosed each year in the United States, and 700,000 new cases annually

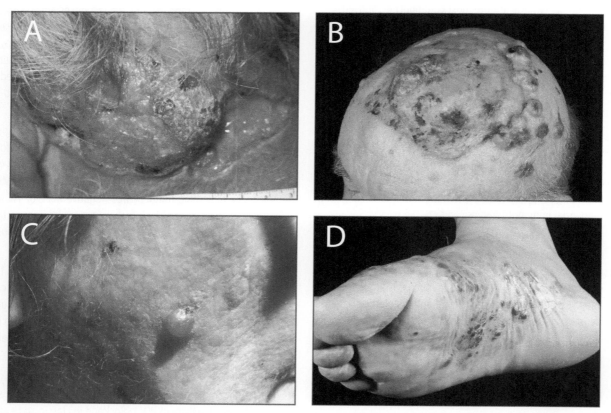

Figure 51.1 Nonmelanoma skin cancer. Clinical appearance of (**A**) a locally advanced basal cell carcinoma (BCC), (**B**) local relapse with satellite and in transit metastases of a cutaneous squamous cell carcinoma (cSCC), (**C**) a primary Merkel cell carcinoma (MCC) on chronically UV-damaged skin, and (**D**) a classical Kaposi's sarcoma (KS).

in Europe.[7] Thus, BCC is the most common tumor in humans and its incidence is still increasing. Notably, the incidence of BCC is rising, particularly in younger individuals and in women. BCC accounts for 80% to 90% of all primary skin cancers. The clinical appearance of BCCs is characterized by their translucency, ulceration, telangiectasias, and the presence of a rolled border. However, these features vary by clinical subtype, which includes nodular, pigmented, morpheaform, and superficial BCCs, as well as fibroepithelioma of Pinkus.

Although most BCCs are indolent, slowly growing tumors, they may manifest aggressive behavior such as perineural invasion and metastatic spread (Figure 51.1A). According to the National Comprehensive Cancer Network (NCCN), BCCs should be stratified into low- and high-risk subtypes.[7] This stratification is based on location, size, border, pathological subtype, perineural involvement, recurrence, prior radiation treatment, or immunosuppression. Fortunately, the metastatic potential of BCC is extremely low, with metastases seen in only 0.0028% to 0.1% of cases. For patients with distant metastases, multidisciplinary consultation is recommended to consider systemic therapy options discussed in the text that follows. However, even locally advanced and destructive tumors, which are encountered more often than metastatic BCC and are typically associated with a long history of the disease, may pose a significant therapeutic dilemma. Although surgery and radiation therapy remain the criterion standard of therapy, curative treatment may be associated with substantial morbidity. Thus, in these cases systemic therapy as for metastatic BCC may be indicated.

UV exposure is the most important risk factor in basal cell carcinogenesis. Indeed, the characterization of the genetic landscape of sporadic BCCs using whole-exome sequencing revealed that BCCs carry a higher mutational burden than any other known human cancer, and the majority of these mutations were C to T transitions.[8] Moreover, tumors from anatomic regions with chronic UV exposure were shown to harbor higher mutational rates than those with intermittent UV exposure.

Genetic workup of patients with Gorlin syndrome, an autosomal dominant disorder predisposing to multiple BCCs, identified a central role of the sonic hedgehog (SHH)/patched 1 (PTCH1)/smoothened (SMO) pathway in familiar BCCs, which could be subsequently extended to sporadic BCCs. Binding of SHH to the extracellular domain of PTCH1 revokes SMO inhibition, thereby activating the transcription factor GLI, which regulates the transcription of hedgehog target genes. Thus, SMO inhibition became an effective therapeutic strategy with introduction of the SMO small-molecule inhibitors vismodegib and sonidegib.[9]

Standard excision with a 4-mm margin is the mainstay of treatment for primary BCCs with nonaggressive histology, occurring on low-risk sites, where tissue conservation is not imperative.[10] If tissue conservation is a key issue, particularly in the face, Mohs micrographic surgery facilitates optimal margin control. In cases in which surgery is not indicated or feasible, radiation therapy, including external beam radiation, superficial x-ray therapy (XRT), and brachytherapy, have all been used and proven to be effective in the treatment of BCC.[10] Alternative treatment options for low-risk BCC, particularly superficial BCC, include cryosurgery with liquid nitrogen, curettage and electrodesiccation, photodynamic therapy, topically applied pyrimidine analog 5-fluorouracil (5-FU), or topical immunotherapy by application of the Toll-like receptor (TLR) 7 agonist imiquimod.[10]

The human genome encodes ten TLRs, each of which exhibits a particular pattern of expression and responds to specific signals. Roughly, TLRs can be subdivided depending on their endosomal (TLR 3, 7, 8, 9, and 10) or plasma membraneous (TLR 1, 2, 4, 5, and 6) localization.[11] TLRs constitute the initial defense responding to danger signals (be they of microbial or endogenous origin) by promoting immune effector functions. Pharmacologic activation of TLRs on myeloid components of the immune system such as macrophages and dendritic cells represents an efficient strategy for boosting anticancer immunity.[11] Imiquimod is capable of enhancing both innate and adaptive immune responses. The stimulation of TLRs results in the activation of a signaling cascade that recruits protein kinases and transcription factors, ultimately promoting maturation and the secretion of interleukins 12 and 18 and type I interferons by target cells. The secretion of these cytokines induces the secretion of type II interferons by infiltrating T cells promoting the development of Th1 lymphocyte-mediated immune responses.

In clinical trials testing the efficacy of imiquimod for superficial BCC, clinical and histological clearance rates of up to 75% were observed.[12] Based on these data in 2004, the U.S. Food and Drug Administration (FDA) approved imiquimod in a 5% cream formulation for the treatment of biopsy-confirmed, primary superficial BCCs of size less than 2 cm in diameter. Bath-Hextall et al. reported their multicenter trial in which 501 participants with nodular or superficial BCCs were randomly assigned to either daily imiquimod for 6 weeks or surgical excision.[13] Localization of tumors on the nose, temple, eyelids, and ears was an exclusion criterion. To confirm the rate of durable responses, patients were followed for 3 years. At that time point, 84% of patients in the imiquimod group were free of local relapse compared to 98% of those who underwent excisions. Notably, there was no difference between groups with respect to the patient-assessed cosmetic outcomes. Topical imiquimod cream may be considered for patients with small superficial BCCs in low-risk anatomic locations who are unable or unwilling to undergo destructive or surgical treatments.[14]

Before the advent of the small-molecule smoothened inhibitors, treatment options for advanced and metastatic BCC included surgery, radiation, and cisplatin-based chemotherapy regimens.[7,10] All of these were employed despite no clear evidence of efficacy, largely due to the lack of clinical trials. The first prospective clinical trial conducted in advanced BCC was testing the SMO inhibitor vismodegib, resulting in an objective response rate of 30% in metastatic BCC. After 12 months of additional follow-up, the objective response rate increased to 33%.[15] Although all the responses were partial, the majority of patients (73%) experienced tumor shrinkage, with a median duration of objective response of 7.6 months. Similar findings were reported in the SafeTy Events in VIsmodEgib (STEVIE) trial, in which an overall response rate of 37.9% was found among 29 patients with metastatic BCC.[16] In locally advanced BCC inappropriate for surgery or radiotherapy, the objective response rate was 43%, with complete responses in 13 patients (21%) and a median duration of response of 7.6 months. After 12 months of additional follow-up, the objective response rate increased to nearly 48%, with a median duration of response of 9.5 months. Higher response rates among 453 patients with locally advanced BCC were reported in the STEVIE trial, with an overall response rate of 66.7%.[16] Comparable findings were more recently reported with use of another SMO inhibitor, sonidegib, in patients with locally advanced BCC.[9,17,18] The side effects of the smoothened inhibitors include muscle spasms, taste disturbance, alopecia, nausea, and fatigue, leading to frequent discontinuations of therapy in almost half of the treated patients.[9] In 2012 and 2015, vismodegib and sonidegib gained FDA approval, respectively.

Tissue PD-L1 expression has been associated with response to anti-PD-1 antibodies in many tumor types. In a study analyzing 40 BCCs, PD-L1 expression on tumor cells was observed in 22%, but in 82% on tumor-infiltrating immune cells.[19] PD-L1 was observed in close geographic association to PD-1+ tumor-infiltrating lymphocytes. Furthermore, the incidence of BCC in patients treated with immune checkpoint inhibitors for melanoma was substantially lower than in patients receiving targeted therapy.[20] Thus, it is not surprising that an increasing number of reports strongly suggest that advanced BCC can also be successfully treated with immune checkpoint inhibitors such as the anti-PD-1 antibodies pembrolizumab, nivolumab, or cemiplimab.[21–25] The results of the primary analysis of a single-arm, Phase 2 trial (NCT03132636) testing the therapeutic effect of cemiplimab in patients with advanced BCC either not tolerating or whose tumors were resistant to hedgehog inhibitors have been reported at the virtual 2020 ESMO congress.[26] About one-third of the 84 enrolled patients were intolerant, and in two-thirds the tumor were resistant to hedgehog inhibition. Age and sex distribution as well as localization of the tumor was as expected for a cohort with locally advanced BCC. The overall response rate was 31% with five complete and 21 partial responses; notably, an additional 41 patients experienced a stabilization of the disease. The estimated progression-free survival time was 19.3 months. Exploratory biomarker analyses of pretreatment samples identifies MHC class I downregulation as a potential mechanism of immune evasion. Interestingly, in a recent study using paired single-cell RNA and TCR sequencing on site-matched tumors from patients with basal or squamous cell carcinoma before and after anti-PD-1 therapy revealed the coupling of tumor recognition, clonal expansion, and T cell dysfunction marked by clonal expansion of CD8+CD39+ T cells, which co-expressed markers of chronic T cell activation and exhaustion.[27]

It is increasingly recognized that several molecular targeted agents also exert noncanonical functions; such effects have been particularly described with respect to immunomodulation. However, the detailed underlying mechanisms are only partly understood. These notions raise the question of which would be the best sequencing of these two different therapeutic approaches or if even an initial combination of hedgehog inhibition and immunotherapy would yield the best benefit for the patients. The currently available literature addressing this question is limited and conflicting. Analysis of BCC samples before and 4 weeks after hedgehog inhibitor therapy revealed an influx of immune cells and an upregulation of PD-L1 expression on tumor cells, thus suggesting a synergistic effect of hedgehog pathway and PD-1 inhibition.[28] However, treatment of pembrolizumab resulted in responses in four out of nine patients (i.e., a response rate of 44%), whereas the combination of vismodegib and pembrolizumab achieved a response rate of only 29%.[29]

CUTANEOUS SQUAMOUS CELL CARCINOMA

cSCC is a common skin cancer, with rising incidence rates particularly in Western countries. However, despite the high incidence, population-based data on cSCC incidence, survival, and mortality are rather sparse.[30,31] Population-based studies on incidence performed in Northern Europe demonstrated that age-standardized incidence rates are rapidly increasing. Results from a national survey in Australia in 2002 showed that 118,000 new cSCC cases were diagnosed among the 21 million inhabitants. According to estimates from medical claims data in the United States, 450,000 persons of the 298 million inhabitants were treated for cSCC in 2006. Recent estimates of changing SCC incidence and mortality across the United States, Germany, and Australia have been reported.[32] Clinically, cSCC presents initially as an asymptomatic plaque or nodule that enlarges over time; it then becomes crateriform ("keratoacanthoma like"), botryomycotic, or ulcerated.[30] Patients may also present with a flat ulcer segregated by a raised border. Predilection sites of cSCC are the chronically UV-exposed areas, that is, the lower lip, ear, nose, cheek, and the dorsum of the hands. Tumor margins may extend beyond the visible borders of the lesion. cSCCs can infiltrate through fascia, periostea, perichondria, and neural sheaths. Gene expression profiling has been used to improve the identification, beyond current clinicopathological features, of patients at higher risk of relapse.[33]

Efforts to identify genetic driver mutations in cSCC have been hampered by the very high frequency of mutations associated with UV damage, which can be 5 to 15 times higher than what is found in other solid cancers, only exceeded by BCC.[34,35] This extraordinarily high mutation rate not only makes it difficult to identify driver mutations from passengers, but also underscores the high mutational burden, which subsequently gives rise to numerous neoantigens, potentially recognized by the host immune system resulting in the immunogenicity of cSCC. Comparison of matched primaries and nodal metastases using a custom gene panel has identified epidermal growth factor receptor (EGFR) aberrations prominent in localized disease, whereas CDH1 and Wnt pathway activation was noted in metastases only.[36] RTK/RAS, TP53, TGF-β, NOTCH1, PI3K, and cell cycle pathways were activated, indicating the complex genetic landscape of cSCC.

Although its general prognosis is excellent with a cure rate of primary cSCC by surgery exceeding 95%, approximately 4% of cases develop nodal or loco-regional metastases and 1.5% die from the disease, which corresponds to about 6,750 annual deaths from cSCC in the United States (Figure 51.1B).[37] Risk factors for an aggressive clinical course are tumor diameters larger than 2 cm, invasion depth beyond the dermis, immunosuppression, poor differentiation, and perineural invasion of nerves >0.1 mm.[30,31] Notably, local recurrence is associated with a worse prognosis, that is, recurrent cSCC is characterized by an increased rate of metastasis as high as 30%. Notably, a substantial proportion of deaths occur due to local progression in the absence of metastatic disease.

Prior to the recent clinical studies of PD-1 inhibitors there was limited published evidence to guide systemic therapy, especially chemotherapy, in cSCC. Even a comprehensive literature search only retrieves very few reports that provided conclusive information for the treatment of advanced metastatic cSCC (stage III/IV).[30,31] Most published reports represent small case series or isolated observational studies. A pooled analysis of 28 observational studies involving 119 patients with advanced cSCC using diverse treatment modalities reported a surprisingly high overall response rate.

However, such retrospective analyses are intrinsically hampered by a strong publication bias toward positive reports of responding patients, and, more importantly, no data on overall survival benefits have been reported.[30,31] Still, stage III and IV cSCC can be responsive to various therapeutics apart from immunotherapy; a notion to bear in mind for patients resistant to immunotherapy.

EGFR signaling in tumorigenesis has been demonstrated in a variety of human cancers. Activation of EGFR has been observed in cSCC, while its overexpression has been associated with worse outcome. Consequently, inhibition of EGFR signaling has been tested as treatment for metastatic cSCCs. Most reports, however, were on studies performed in head and neck mucosal SCC (HNSCC) and not in cSCC.[38,39] Given some similarities between mucosal and cutaneous SCC, clinicians have extrapolated treatment strategies shown effective in mucosal head and neck SCC to cutaneous origin SCC. Since EGFR inhibitors, either as monoclonal antibodies (cetuximab, panitumumab) or as small-molecule kinase inhibitors (erlotinib, gefitinib), have been approved for the treatment of advanced HNSCC, and the chimeric monoclonal antibody (mAb) cetuximab demonstrated encouraging results in the treatment of cSCC in anecdotal case reports, a number of investigator-initiated trials have been performed in advanced cSCC. In the largest Phase I2 study of 36 patients with unresectable cSCC, cetuximab at an initial dose of 400 mg/m^2 body surface followed by weekly doses of 250 mg/m^2 for at least 6 weeks achieved an objective response rate of 25% (3% complete and 22% partial responses) and disease stabilization in 42%.[40] Of note, it appears that the therapeutic effect of EGFR targeting agents largely depends on their capacity to activate the host's immune system rather than blocking EGFR signaling.[38,39] For patients with cSCC not amenable to curative therapy, gefitinib achieved a response rate of 16% with only partial responses seen, and stable disease in 35% among 37 evaluable patients. Median duration of response was 31.4 months and the progression-free survival for the overall group was 3.8 months.[41] Gefitinib was tested as a neoadjuvant therapy with an 18.2% complete response rate and 27.3% having partial responses in 23 patients.[42] The largest retrospective series of cSCC patients treated with systemic chemotherapy or anti-EGFR therapy identified 82 patients with median overall survivals of 16.2 and 15.3 months for locally advanced and metastatic disease, respectively. Of note, only 29% of patients received second-line therapy.[43]

Recent reports have revealed the therapeutic potential of cell-mediated immunity in cSCC. The immune response is known to play a crucial role in the development and prognosis of cSCC. This notion is supported by the observations that (a) cSCC are more frequent and more aggressive in immune-compromised individuals, (b) a CD8$^+$ T cell infiltrate is associated with an improved prognosis even in advanced stages, (c) there are anecdotal reports on immune-modulating interventions in advanced cSCC patients, and finally (d) anti-EGFR antibodies but not small-molecule inhibitors improve overall survival in metastatic cSCC patients.[30,31] Indeed, expression of PD-L1 in human cSCC tissue samples has been reported across multiple primary sites. These studies revealed high levels of PD-L1 expression in the majority of tumors. Variability in expression rates between studies is likely due to different antibodies employed for staining, the use of fresh or paraffin-embedded samples, and potential site-specific differences in expression. Moreover, PD-L1 expression is not restricted to the cancerous cells, but is also observed on myeloid cells such as macrophages and dendritic cell (DC) subpopulations in cSCC.[44]

Preclinical data clearly demonstrate that blockade of the PD-1/PD-L1 pathway augments immune responses to HNSCC, which led to phase 3 clinical trials showing a clear benefit from checkpoint inhibitor therapy and thus led to FDA approval of anti-PD-1 agents and ongoing trials in recurrent/metastatic HNSCC patients.[45] The encouraging clinical responses observed in blocking the PD-L1 immune checkpoint in mucosal HNSCC together with the high immunogenicity of cSCC, the expression of PD-L1 on cSCC tumor cells, the promising safety profile, and the strong medical need in metastatic cSCC provided the rationale for clinical trials testing immunotherapy by immune checkpoint blockade in cSCC. A prospective Phase 2 trial of the IgG4 anti-PD-1 inhibitor cemiplimab in unresectable, locally advanced cSCC not amenable to further radiotherapy or metastatic disease reported response rates of 50% in a Phase 1 expansion cohort of locally advanced and metastatic patients and 47% in a Phase 2 cohort of metastatic patients treated at 3 mg/kg every 2 weeks.[46] Further follow-up has documented an improvement in response rates over time, such that complete responses in patients with metastatic cSCC increased from 6.8% at 9.4 months follow-up to 16.9% after approximately 1 year and to 20.3% at a median follow-up of 15.7 months.[47] Toxicity was consistent with other studies of single-agent anti-PD-1. Most common, any grade toxicities and percentage of patients affected were fatigue (34.7%), diarrhea (27.5%), nausea (23.8%), and pruritus (21.2%). Grade 3 or above immune-related toxicities included pneumonitis in 2.6%, autoimmune hepatitis in 1.6%, and anemia, colitis, and diarrhea in 1% each. Quality of life measures confirmed an improvement for patients on treatment. Response rates were lower for patients having received prior chemotherapy. An analysis of biomarkers has not yet revealed clear predictors of response or resistance. The approved dose of cemiplimab is 350 mg flat dose administered every 3 weeks. Pembrolizumab in chemotherapy-naïve, predominantly older adult patients has been reported in the

CARSKIN trial with a response rate of 39.5% in 39 subjects.[48] A pilot study of cemiplimab prior to surgery in 20 patients with locally advanced cSCC reported an objective response rate of 30%; however, pathology at surgery showed a complete pathological response (i.e., no tumor cells present) in 55%.[49]

A number of ongoing trials are assessing the role of PD-1 inhibitors in additional clinical situations and in combinations (Table 51.1). Two large randomized Phase 3 trials are examining the value of adding anti-PD-1 versus placebo following surgery and adjuvant radiotherapy for resected high-risk cSCC (Keynote 630, REGN 1788). The combination of the anti-PD-L1 antibody avelumab and the anti-EGFR-antibody cetuximab is currently tested in anti-PD-1 refractory cSCC (AliCe). Another approach is preoperative or neoadjuvant treatment of locally advanced cSCC either with anti-PD-1 alone (REGN 1901) or in combination with a direct intratumoral injection of the cytolytic virus RP1. Definitive treatment of locally advanced cSCC with pembrolizumab and radiotherapy has been reported.[51] Solid organ transplant recipients have a high risk of lethal disease courses of cSCC; however, treatment with PD-1 inhibitors risks inducing tumor rejection. A notable case report describes complete eradication of metastatic cSCC from pembrolizumab treatment in a patient with a renal transplant who also had rejection of the transplanted kidney necessitating a return to dialysis. Four and a half years later the patient had another transplant and resumed immune suppression, and after a further 10 and a half months later remained in remission from cSCC.[52]

Anti-PD-1 therapy has become the new standard of care for patients with advanced or metastatic cSCC, with the exception of solid organ transplant recipients (Figure 51.2).[7] Important further areas of study include treatment of patients with primary or acquired resistance to checkpoint inhibitors, prospective studies in patients with conditions such as CLL, and more profound immune suppression such as solid organ transplant recipients and potential use to reduce invasive cSCC in patients with field cancerization and multiple primary lesions.

MERKEL CELL CARCINOMA

MCC is a highly aggressive neuroendocrine carcinoma of the skin, demonstrating a high rate of recurrence and metastasis.[53] MCC is a rare tumor, with age-adjusted annual incidence rates of 0.18 to 0.41 per 100,000 persons in the United States and Europe, and almost 1 per 100,000 persons in Australia.[54,55] However, the age-adapted incidence appears to have tripled from 1986 to 2001, with a statistically significant annual increase of 8%. For example, in the Netherlands, the annual age-standardized incidence rate per million increased from 1.7 in 1993 to

Table 51.1 Important Completed and Ongoing Immunotherapy Trials in Cutaneous Squamous Cell Carcinoma

TRIAL	DESIGN	POPULATION	# OF PATIENTS	ARMS	PROGRESS	PRIMARY ENDPOINT	RESULTS	REFERENCE
REGN/Sanofi	Phase 1/2 single arm	Unresectable locally advanced or metastatic, prior systemic treatment allowed	193	Cemiplimab	Completed	ORR	Updated ORR 54%, mDOR not reached, mOS not reached, estimated 24 months OS 73%, 76% of responses ongoing at 24 m	Migden et al.[46] Rischin et al.[47]
Keynote 629	Phase 2 single arm	Unresectable locally advanced or metastatic, prior systemic treatment allowed	105	Pembrolizumab	Completed	ORR	Response rate 34%, disease control rate 52.4%, mPFS 6.9 m, mOS not reached, 12-month OS 60.3%	Grob et al.[50]
Carskin	Phase 2 single arm	Unresectable, no prior systemic treatment	39	Pembrolizumab	Completed	ORR	Response rate 41% at week 15, , PFS 6.7 m, mOS 25.3 m, no responding patient progressing over 22.4 m median follow-up	Maubec et al.[48]
C-POST REGN 1788	Randomized Phase 3	Resected high-risk, post adjuvant radiotherapy	412	Cemiplimab vs. Placebo	Recruiting	DFS	N/A Estimated completion Q1 2026	NCT03969004
Keynote 630	Randomized Phase 3	Resected high-risk, post adjuvant radiotherapy	570	Pembrolizumab vs. Placebo	Recruiting	RFS	N/A Estimated completion Q3 2027	NCT03833167
REGN 1901	Phase 2 single arm	Locally advanced, stage II–IV M0, preoperative	76	Cemiplimab 350 mg q3w x4 then surgery +/- 9 months adjuvant Cemiplimab	Recruiting	pCR	N/A Estimated completion Q4 2024	NCT04154943
CARPASS	Phase 3	Unresectable locally advanced or metastatic	240	Cemiplimab vs Cemiplimab + directly injected oncolytic HSV1 virus (RP1)	Recruiting	ORR	N/A Estimated completion Q1 2024	NCT04050436
CONTRAC	Phase 1/2	Advanced cSCC in renal transplant or allogeneic haematopoietic stem cell transplant	12	Cemiplimab for Allo HSCT For renal transplant patients: Cemiplimab + Everolimus vs. Cemiplimab + Sirolimus vs. Cemiplimab + Prednisone	Recruiting	DLT	N/A Estimated completion Q3 2022	NCT04339062
ALiCe	Phase 2 single arm	Unresectable stage III or IV	52	Avelumab + Cetuximab	Recruiting	ORR	N/A Estimated completion Q1 2021	Eudract 2018-001708-12

DFS, Disease-free survival; DLT, dose limiting toxicity; mDOR, median duration of response; mOS, median overall survival; ORR, objective response rate; OS, overall survival; REGN, regeneron; RFS, relapse-free survival.

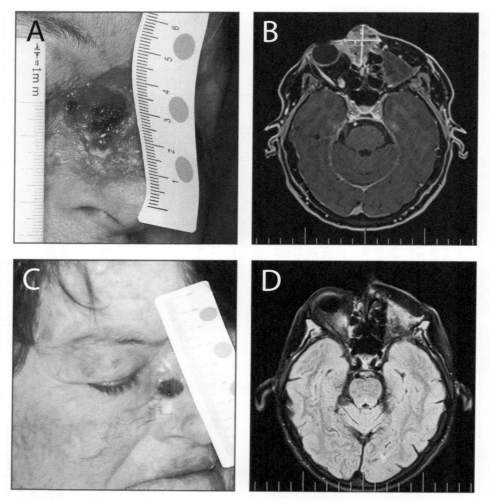

Figure 51.2 Clinical response of an advanced cutaneous squamous cell carcinoma (cSCC) to PD-1 blockade cemiplimab. Patient with previous left orbital exenteration for cSCC with subsequent recurrence in right side of nose involving right eye socket (**A**, **B**). Since the patient declined a right orbital exenteration, systemic treatment with cemiplimab was started resulting in a complete remission (**C**, **D**). The residual abnormality in clinical picture corresponds to a histology confirmed fibrotic reaction without any signs of active cancer.

1997 to 3.5 in 2003 to 2007.[56] The rising incidence of MCC (and other NMSCs) is most likely related to the aging population trends, which reflect increasing cumulative UV exposure over a lifetime and decreasing protection due to immunosenescence.[57]

MCC is a fast-growing, asymptomatic, solitary, firm, nonsensitive, flesh to red to violaceous nodule with a smooth, shiny surface. MCC characteristically develops and grows rapidly over weeks to months on chronically sun-damaged skin (Figure 51.1C).[53] Thus, the predominant sites are head and neck (more than half of cases) and extremities (one-third of cases), whereas trunk as well as oral and genital mucosa are involved in less than 10% of cases.

The identification of a polyomavirus, the Merkel cell polyomavirus (MCPyV), which is clonally integrated in the majority of MCC cases, together with the observation that MCPyV-positive MCC (VP-MCC) cell lines critically depend on the continuous expression of the virally encoded transforming early genes (i.e., small and large T antigen), strongly suggests a viral carcinogenesis of MCC.[58,59] The integrated viral genomes are characterized by an individual, that is, tumor-specific pattern of large T antigen gene mutations that incapacitate viral DNA replication. Both humoral and cellular immune responses have been demonstrated against virally encoded proteins.[60–62] VP-MCCs are characterized by high expression of retinoblastoma 1 protein and low expression of p53, that is, two of the interaction partners of the large T antigen. Notably, while immune responses against MCPyV capsid proteins can be readily detected in the general population, responses against the transforming early genes are restricted to MCC patients. The presence of the MCPyV in about 80% of MCC cases has been confirmed in several studies. However, in about 20% of cases, MCPyV cannot be detected, and this percentage is higher for MCCs located in chronically UV-exposed skin.[63] Most MCCs are located in the dermis; less frequently, an intraepidermal component is reported. Notably, MCCs with an intraepidermal component are frequently admixed with an SCC (collision tumors).[64] Interestingly, combined cSCC and MCC are consistently negative for MCPyV and are characterized by a high mutational load, which is comparable to that observed in cSCC. Several recent reports taking advantage of high-throughput sequencing support the paradigm of two distinct disease etiologies for MCC: one driven by MCPyV integration and seemingly requiring few additional mutations, and the other driven by UV-associated activating and tumor-suppressing mutations.[53] The latter share genetic similarities to SCC including a UV mutation profile and recurrent mutations in NOTCH1, TP53, and HRAS.

Most patients are diagnosed with localized disease (stage I and II), but at least one-third suffer from either microscopic or macroscopic lymph node involvement (stage III). Up to 5% are diagnosed with advanced metastatic disease (stage IV); a similar number of patients may present with isolated metastases from an unknown primary. For those with stage IV disease, common sites of metastases include distant lymph nodes, distant skin, lung, central nervous system, and bone.

While surgery and radiotherapy can achieve high rates of locoregional control, MCC has a propensity for early systemic dissemination. The 5-year survival rate for stage I and II is up to 60%, which is reduced to about 40% for stage III and less than 20% for stage IV disease.[65] Until recently, MCC was treated like other high-grade small cell neuroendocrine cancers with chemotherapy such as cisplatin and etoposide. MCC has a high rate of initial response to chemotherapy (~65%), but the responses are seldom durable and average overall survival was less than 1 year for metastatic disease.

The recent advances in our understanding of the immune biology of MCC, including the discovery of MCPyV and of the immune exhaustion mechanisms prevalent in MCC tumors, led to a clinical trial using PD-L1 inhibitor avelumab in patients who had previously progressed after chemotherapy. After at least 1 year of follow-up, the response rate with avelumab treatment was 33%, and the 1-year overall survival was 52%.[66,67] The impressive therapeutic effect of inhibiting the PD-1/PD-L1 checkpoint axis in MCC was further confirmed with the PD-1 inhibitor pembrolizumab in a trial conducted by the National Cancer Institute Cancer Immunotherapy Trial Network (NCI CITN).[68,69] The response rate was 56% in a treatment-naïve study population, including 24% complete responders. Avelumab was subsequently tested in treatment-naïve patients.[70] The response rate was 62%, markedly higher than the

trial in patients whose disease had progressed on/after chemotherapy. The fact that PD-L1 inhibition was less effective when used after chemotherapy suggests that the cytotoxic agents may be harmful to immune effector cells and blunt response to subsequent immunotherapy. Importantly, the responses to immunotherapy are frequent, rapid-onset (days to weeks), and durable (Figure 51.3). Due to these characteristics, pembrolizumab and avelumab are now considered the current standard of care for first-line MCC; up to now these drugs have not been directly compared against each other.

The avelumab and pembrolizumab studies have also examined tumor tissue PD-L1 expression and T cell infiltrate as potential biomarkers, but neither was predictive of response. However, conclusions are limited by underpowered analyses in these small studies. The co-localization of PD-L1 and PD-1 in the tumor microenvironment may have higher utility in predicting response, as this metric was significantly higher in responders than in nonresponders.[71]

The revolutionary success of immunotherapy in metastatic MCC has spurred several ongoing randomized trials of immune checkpoint inhibitor therapy in the adjuvant space, including trials using avelumab (NCT03271372), pembrolizumab (NCT03712605), and nivolumab (NCT02196961). Nivolumab has also been investigated in the neoadjuvant setting in a small study.[72] Patients with advanced but resectable MCC were treated with two doses of nivolumab (days 1 and 15) followed by surgery. Among 36 patients who underwent surgery, 17 (47.2%) achieved a pathologic complete response (pCR). Among 33 radiographically evaluable patients who underwent surgery, 18 (54.5%) had tumor reductions ≥30%.

While the efficacy of immune checkpoint inhibitors in advanced MCC is impressive, a significant proportion of patients still do not respond at all (primary resistance) or progress after initial clinical benefit (secondary resistance).[73] While possible biomarkers predicting resistance are emerging, they still have not been validated in prospective cohorts.[74] Thus, there still is a significant unmet need for these patients. Emerging clinical data suggest that alternate checkpoint inhibitors (e.g., CTLA-4 antibodies) can result in therapeutic benefit in some patients who do not respond to PD-1 or PDL-1 blockade.[75] Multiple clinical trials are investigating radiation therapy, other checkpoint inhibitors, oncolytic viruses, Toll-like receptor agonists, cytokine therapy, vaccines, adoptive T cell therapy, inhibition of the MDM2 protein, or epigenetic modifiers.

CUTANEOUS SARCOMAS

Malignant fibrohistiocytic tumors are a heterogeneous group of mesenchymal neoplasms that may occur in the

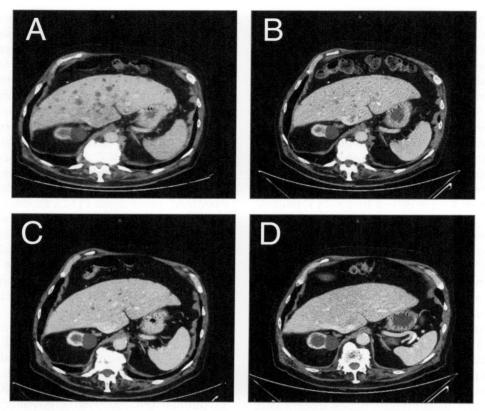

Figure 51.3 **Clinical response of liver metastases of a Merkel cell carcinoma (MCC) to PD-L1 blockade with avelumab.** CT scan of rapidly progressing multiple bilobar liver metastases from MCC before start of immunotherapy with avelumab (**A**), and after 2 (**B**) and 4 months (**C**) of therapy, resulting in a complete response still ongoing at 3 years (**D**).

skin and subcutaneous tissues.[76,77] Diagnosis of these tumors may be difficult, as they are rare, and a wide morphological diversity of types and subtypes has been described. The most frequent cutaneous sarcoma is dermatofibrosarcoma protuberans, followed by atypical fibroxanthoma, cutaneous undifferentiated pleomorphic sarcoma, leiomyosarcoma, liposarcoma, and angiosarcoma. The typical clinical feature of these tumors is their mostly asymptomatic appearance. For diagnosis, the histologic workup is therefore the key feature, but immunohistochemistry as well as molecular diagnostics is becoming increasingly important—particularly with respect to therapeutic decisions. The primary treatment for locally resectable tumors is complete surgical removal. First-line systemic therapy with an anthracycline remains the standard of care for advanced sarcomas. However, choice of subsequent therapy beyond anthracyclines remains challenging.[78,79] Novel systemic therapies using molecular findings to direct therapy in subtype-specific trials are ongoing, but hampered by the low incidence of the respective subtypes. Thus, experience from real-world retrospective data is important for improving outcomes in patients with advanced disease.

The value of immunotherapy in soft tissue sarcoma in general is still controversial. Responses to both pembrolizumab and nivolumab have been reported in varying frequencies and durations.[80–83] The most promising results were observed in the SARC028 Phase 2 study, in which pembrolizumab as a single agent showed activity in unselected soft tissue sarcoma of all types with an ORR of 17.5%. The 3-month PFS was observed in only half of the patients.[82]

Kaposi sarcoma (KS) was first reported by Moritz Kaposi as a multifocal pigmented sarcoma of the skin in older adult men of Mediterranean or Jewish ancestry.[84] However, KS gained public attention as an AIDS-defining malignancy. Kaposi sarcoma (KS) is an endothelial cell tumor with an inflammatory component and highly heterogenous histopathology. Cutaneous KS may occur in multiple forms, such as localized or disseminated purple-blue plaques or nodules of the skin, which are often associated with lymphedema (Figure 51.1D). KS encompasses the following four clinical variants: classic (aka, sporadic), AIDS-related (aka, epidemic), endemic (in sub-Saharan Africa), and iatrogenic (in transplant recipients). KS is causally associated with KSHV infection, but the viral carcinogenesis is still not completely understood. It involves a balance between immune activating and suppressing mechanisms allowing a latent infection that lasts for the entire life of the infected host. For example, KSHV infection induces an increased PD-L1 expression in monocytes and could contribute to immune evasion.[84] Adaptive immune responses to KSHV are evident, as reflected by the higher incidence of KSHV infection and KSHV-associated malignancies in patients with immunodeficiencies. This notion also reflects the fact that one therapeutic approach for KS patients with a reversible immunosuppression is to alleviate this suppression (e.g., treatment of HIV patients with cART or reducing the level of iatrogenic immunosuppression). Immunomodulating—and antiviral—agents, including interferons, lenalidomide, and bortezomib, have been used with variable efficacy, but a retrospective chart review revealed that PD-1 blocking antibodies demonstrated significant antitumor effects in a group of patients with HIV-associated KS.[85] Consequently, the safety and efficacy of anti-PD-1 antibodies were prospectively tested in patients with HIV and advanced cancer.[86] This study demonstrated that although anti-PD-1 therapy shows promising activity in KSHV-associated cancers, a previously undescribed KSHV-associated B-cell lymphoproliferation was observed. The activity of an immune checkpoint blockade in classic and endemic KS was reported at the virtual 2020 ESMO congress.[87] Eight patients with classic and nine with endemic KS received pembrolizumab every 3 weeks over 6 months, resulting in two complete and 10 partial responses for a best overall response rate of 71%. Toxicity was tolerable and KSHV-associated B cell lymphoproliferation was observed.

CONCLUSION

Based on either their high mutational loads caused by an UV carcinogenesis or the expression of foreign antigens associated with a viral carcinogenesis, NMSCs are highly immunogenic cancers. Immunotherapy trials with PD-1/PD-L1 blocking antibodies have shown impressive efficacy to date. However, not all patients respond to immunotherapy, and some develop secondary resistance. In addition to the search for predictive biomarkers, there is a dire unmet need for finding effective therapies in immune competent patients who do not respond to PD-1/PD-L1 blockade. Mechanistic studies to understand both intrinsic and acquired mechanisms of resistance are critical to uncover new rational therapies to overcome these. Fortunately, there are a variety of investigational immunotherapy approaches currently underway to help improve upon the initial results of checkpoint inhibitor immunotherapy.

KEY REFERENCES

Only key references appear in the print edition. The full reference list appears in the digital product on Springer Publishing Connect: connect.springerpub.com/content/book/978-0-8261-3743-2/part/part04/chapter/ch51

19. Lipson EJ, Lilo MT, Ogurtsova A, et al. Basal cell carcinoma: PD-L1/PD-1 checkpoint expression and tumor regression after PD-1 blockade. *J Immunother Cancer.* 2017;5:1–5. doi:10.1186/s40425-017-0228-3
47. Rischin D, Migden MR, Lim AM, et al. Phase 2 study of cemiplimab in patients with metastatic cutaneous squamous cell carcinoma: primary analysis of fixed-dosing, long-term outcome of weight-based dosing. *J Immunother Cancer.* 2020;8(1):e000775–e000778. doi:10.1136/jitc-2020-000775
48. Maubec E, Boubaya M, Petrow P, et al. Phase II study of pembrolizumab as first-line, single-drug therapy for patients with unresectable cutaneous squamous cell carcinomas. *J Clin Oncol.* 2020;38(26):3051–3061. doi:10.1200/JCO.19.03357.
68. Nghiem PT, Bhatia S, Lipson EJ, et al. PD-1 blockade with pembrolizumab in advanced Merkel-cell carcinoma. *N Engl J Med.* 2016;374(26):2542–2552. doi:10.1056/NEJMoa1603702
74. Spassova I, Ugurel S, Terheyden P, et al. Predominance of central memory T cells with high T-cell receptor repertoire diversity is associated with response to PD-1/PD-L1 inhibition in Merkel cell carcinoma. *Clin Cancer Res.* 2020;26(9):2257–2267. doi:10.1158/1078-0432.CCR-19-2244
80. D'Angelo SP, Mahoney MR, van Tine BA, et al. Nivolumab with or without ipilimumab treatment for metastatic sarcoma (Alliance A091401): two open-label, non-comparative, randomised, Phase 2 trials. *Lancet Oncol.* 2018;19(3):416–426. doi:10.1016/S1470-2045(18)30006-8
85. Galanina N, Goodman AM, Cohen PR, et al. Successful treatment of HIV-associated Kaposi sarcoma with immune checkpoint blockade. *Cancer Immunol Res.* 2018;6(10):1129–1135. doi:10.1158/2326-6066.CIR-18-0121

Immunotherapy in Genitourinary Malignancies

Moshe C. Ornstein and Brian I. Rini

KEY POINTS

- Novel immunotherapy-based combinations have changed the landscape of therapy in genitourinary (GU) malignancies.

- Approved immunotherapeutic agents in metastatic renal cell carcinoma (mRCC) are interleukin-2 (IL-2), interferon-alpha (IFN-α), nivolumab, ipilimumab/nivolumab, axitinib/pembrolizumab, and axitinib/avelumab.

- In urothelial carcinoma (UC), bacillus Calmette–Guérin (BCG) is approved for local therapy. In metastatic UC, five checkpoint inhibitors (atezolizumab, avelumab, pembrolizumab, durvalumab, and nivolumab) are approved in various settings.

- The only approved prostate cancer-specific immunotherapy is sipuleucel-T, which is approved in the metastatic castration-resistant prostate cancer (mCRPC) setting. Pembrolizumab can be used in prostate cancer in patients with microsatellite instability-high (MSI-H), mismatch repair deficient (dMMR), or with a tumor mutational burden (TMB) of $\geq$ 10 m/MB.

- Multiple Phase 3 trials are ongoing which will likely shift the treatment paradigm over the next few years.

- Key challenges with immunotherapy in GU malignancies include toxicity management, duration of therapy, and sequencing of therapies.

INTRODUCTION

The genitourinary (GU) malignancies, particularly renal cell carcinoma (RCC), bladder cancer (henceforth, urothelial carcinoma or UC), and prostate cancer, have been at the forefront of immuno-oncology for decades. Although comprehensive overviews of immunotherapeutic concepts and mechanisms are detailed elsewhere in this book, the general objective of cancer immunotherapy is to alert, activate, and enhance the innate immune response to cancer. In GU oncology, immunotherapy continues to be a cornerstone of therapy, particularly in the treatment of metastatic disease.[1-4] In this chapter, a general overview of the history of immunotherapy in GU malignancies is described with a particular focus on those agents that are currently approved in each malignancy. Additionally, future directions in each section highlight forthcoming prospects for immunotherapy in GU oncology.

RENAL CELL CARCINOMA

RCC is at the forefront of immunotherapy in oncology in general and in GU malignancies in particular. For decades, high-dose interleukin-2 (HD IL-2) has been an effective therapy in a subset of RCC patients despite the high rates of toxicity. More recently, checkpoint inhibitors (CPIs) have begun to rapidly change the immunotherapeutic landscape in RCC. Similarly, given the sensitivity of RCC to immunotherapy, a number of clinical trials involving cancer vaccines have been conducted, although thus far no vaccines have been approved for the treatment of RCC. A brief overview of the history of immunotherapy in RCC is discussed.

Interleukin-2

Recombinant HD IL-2 was one of the first immunotherapies used in oncology. Early studies of intravenous HD IL-2 in RCC used doses ranging from 600,000 to 720,000 IU/kg every 8 hours for 5 consecutive days for up to 14 doses. One course of therapy consisted of two 5-day cycles given on days 1 and 15 with a maximum of three courses of therapy given to patients who tolerated therapy and had either stable disease (SD) or a response to therapy.[5,6]

The decision to treat mRCC patients with IL-2 needs to be made cautiously with careful patient selection. HD IL-2 is associated with high rates of toxicity including hypotension (71%), diarrhea (67%), and chills (52%), which are a likely result of the IL-2-mediated release of pro-inflammatory cytokines.[7,8] In the Cytokine Working Group prospective "SELECT" trial of 120 mRCC patients treated with IL-2, two patients (1.7%) suffered treatment-related deaths.[3] However, despite the high rates of adverse events (AEs), the rationale for the continued use of HD IL-2 is that it produces a durable complete response in 5% to 7% of patients.[5,6]

Given the high rates of toxicity, it is critical to identify those patients most likely to respond to therapy and those who may develop a sustained response. Retrospective studies have demonstrated that a good performance status and no bone metastases are associated with a favorable prognosis,[9] whereas high tumor burden (e.g., multiple metastatic sites) and aggressive disease course (progression-free survival [PFS] <1 year, IL-2 treatment within 6 months of therapy, etc.) are associated with poorer outcomes.[10,11] Carbonic anhydrase IX (CAIX) has also been used as a biomarker for response to IL-2, with retrospective studies noting that high CAIX expression by immunohistochemistry (IHC) is associated with improved response rates and survival.[12,13] Based on these findings, Atkins et al. developed a model that combines histology and CAIX IHC expression to stratify mRCC patients receiving IL-2 into "good" and "poor" risk categories based on their likelihood of response to IL-2.[12] Other similar retrospective models have been developed as well.[14,15]

The previously mentioned SELECT trial of 120 patients with mRCC treated with IL-2 was conducted to validate predictors of response to therapy.[3] The overall response rate (ORR) was 25%, complete response rate (CRR) was 2.5%, and 11% of patients had a durable remission for at least 3 years. Only patients with clear cell histology responded to IL-2 therapy although no validation of CAIX staining or other pathological predictive models was established.[3] Although clinical outcomes are encouraging, additional prospective data are needed to identify those patients most likely to benefit from therapy.

In summary, HD IL-2 remains an effective immunotherapy in mRCC and produces durable responses in a small subset of patients. Given the lack of prospective predictive models as well as the high rates of toxicity associated with IL-2, the treatment is currently restricted to patients with clear cell pathology, good performance status, and minimal comorbidities. The role of IL-2 in the context of newly approved immunotherapy regimens listed in the text that follows is less certain. A small series of mRCC patients treated with IL-2 after CPIs demonstrated a 24% ORR with two complete responses and expected toxicity. Further prospective investigation is required.[16]

Interferon-α

IFN-α is a cytokine with proven efficacy in RCC at a variety of doses and schedules.[12,17] The ORR for IFN-α

as monotherapy in clinical trials is approximately 7% to 10% with a median survival of approximately 11 to 13 months.[17] However, compared to monotherapy, IFN-α is more effective in combination with bevacizumab, a vascular endothelial growth factor (VEGF) antibody. As such, there is no current role for the use of IFN-α as monotherapy in RCC. In the Phase 3 CALGB 90206 trial, 732 patients with previously untreated mRCC were randomized to receive IFN-α monotherapy or IFN-α plus bevacizumab.[18,19] The median progression-free survival (mPFS) was significantly longer in the combination arm (8.5 months) compared to the IFN-α monotherapy arm (5.2 months; p <.0001). The ORR was also higher in the IFN-α plus bevacizumab arm compared to the IFN-α monotherapy cohort (25.5% vs. 13.1; p <.0001).[18] However, the study's primary endpoint of overall survival (OS) was subsequently reported and there was no statistical difference between the combination arm and the IFN-α monotherapy cohort (median overall survival [mOS]: 18.3 vs. 17.4 months; hazard ratio [HR]: 0.86, 95% confidence interval [CI]: 0.73–1.01; p = .069).[19]

Similar findings were noted in the Phase 3 AVastin fOr RENal cell cancer (AVOREN) trial. A total of 649 patients previously untreated with mRCC were randomized to receive IFN-α plus placebo or IFN-α combined with bevacizumab.[20,21] The primary end-point was OS with secondary endpoints of PFS and safety. Data regarding PFS were first published with a mPFS of 10.2 months in the IFN-α/bevacizumab group compared to 5.4 months in the IFN-α/placebo cohort (HR: 0.63, 95% CI 0.52–0.75; p = .0001).[21] Similar to the CALGB 90206 trial, mOS was similar between IFN-α/bevacizumab and IFN-α/placebo groups (23.3 vs. 21.3 months, HR 0.86; 95% CI 0.72–1.04; p = .1291).[20] These data highlight the effect of bevacizumab when added to IFN-α. The role of bevacizumab as monotherapy, however, remains unclear.[22–24] With current changes in the therapeutic landscape of mRCC, it is unlikely that studies to further define the role of single-agent IFN in mRCC will be conducted.

Checkpoint Inhibitors

Treatment-Refractory Metastatic Cell Renal Carcinoma

Nivolumab is a fully human immunoglobulin G4 (IgG4) monoclonal antibody inhibitor of programmed death-1 (PD-1). It is approved in intravenous form at a dose of 3 mg/kg every 2 weeks for the treatment of mRCC that has previously been treated with VEGF-directed therapy.[4] The ORR for mRCC patients treated with nivolumab in Phase 1 and 2 trials was between 20% and 27% with a manageable toxicity profile that included fatigue, rash, diarrhea, and pruritus as some of the more common AEs.[25,26] Importantly, the mOS in the Phase 2 trial that investigated nivolumab at various doses in mRCC was 18.2 to 25.5 months, which led to OS as a primary endpoint in the Phase 3 trial.[4,26]

The Phase 3 CheckMate 025 study compared nivolumab 3 mg/kg every 2 weeks or everolimus 10 mg orally daily for the treatment of patients with previously treated advanced RCC.[4] A total of 821 patients were randomized, and 803 patients were treated (406 with nivolumab; 397 with everolimus). Median age was 62 years, with males representing 75% of patients. Most patients (72%) had only been treated with one prior antiangiogenic therapy. At the time of the study analysis, mOS was 25.0 months in the nivolumab patients compared to 19.6 months in the patients treated with everolimus (HR: 0.73, 98.5% CI 0.57–0.93; p = .002).[4]

The final analysis of a minimum follow-up of >5 years (minimum 64 months) was recently presented.[27] The mOS was sustained for nivolumab versus everolimus (25.8 vs. 19.7 months; HR 0.73 95% CI 0.62–0.85) with number of patients alive at 5 years favoring nivolumab as well (26% vs. 18%). Nivolumab also had a superior ORR (23% vs. 4%), CR rate (4% vs. 2%), and median duration of response (18.2% vs. 14%).[27] These data provide important support for the long-term durability of CPI in treatment-refractory mRCC.

Long-term survival data from the Phase 1 and 2 trials have subsequently been presented.[28] At a minimum of 50.5 months of follow-up, the 3- and 5-year OS rates for the 34 patients in the Phase 1 trial were 41% and 34%, respectively. Similarly, for the 167 patients treated in the Phase 2 trial, the 3-year OS rate was 35% with a minimum follow-up of 38 months. Interestingly, of the 48 patients in the Phase 2 trial who were still alive at a minimum of 4 years follow-up, 19 patients had a best overall response of PD, suggesting that even patients who do not appear to respond to conventional response evaluation criteria in solid tumors (RECIST) criteria can experience a durable benefit from nivolumab. Moreover, 15 patients (31%) who were alive at 4 years of follow-up did not require subsequent therapy.[28] The appeal of nivolumab, therefore, in addition to its tolerability, is the long-term responses that occur in a subset of patients including those who develop an initial PD.

Most patients (79%) treated with nivolumab in the CheckMate 025 trial experienced treatment-related AEs. The most common AEs of any grade that occurred in at least 10% of patients were fatigue, rash, decreased appetite, diarrhea, and pruritus. Only 77 patients (19%) experienced a grade 3 or 4 AE with fatigue being the most common grade 3/4 AE (2%). Thirty-one patients (8%) treated with nivolumab discontinued therapy secondary to AEs, and no treatment-related deaths were reported.[4]

Treatment-Naïve Metastatic Renal Cell Carcinoma

As noted, the first U.S. Food and Drug Administration (FDA)-approved CPI for the treatment of RCC was nivolumab in patients with mRCC who had received prior angiogenic therapy. Over the last few years, however, significant progress has been made with a variety of other CPIs investigated as single-agent therapy, in combination with other CPIs, and in combination with tyrosine kinase inhibitors (TKIs).

The first CPI-based combination therapy to achieve FDA approval was ipilimumab in combination with nivolumab in patients with treatment-naïve mRCC. Ipilimumab is a humanized monoclonal anticytotoxic T-lymphocyte antigen-4 (CTLA-4) described in detail elsewhere in this book. Ipilimumab was combined with nivolumab in the Phase 1 CheckMate 016 trial in patients with previously treated or treatment-naïve advanced RCC.[29] In the expanded cohort, 94 patients were randomized to receive either nivolumab 1 mg/kg combined with ipilimumab 3 mg/kg (N1 + I3) or nivolumab 3 mg/kg plus ipilimumab 1 mg/kg (N3 + I1) every 3 weeks for four doses followed by nivolumab 3 mg/kg every 2 weeks until disease progression or toxicity. ORR and mPFS were 38% and 30.3 months in the N3 + I1 arm and 43% and 36.0 months in the N1 + I3 arm.[29]

There were similar AEs between the two arms, and the toxicity profile was similar to the nivolumab monotherapy overall. However, 64% of patients in the N1 + I3 arm and 34% of patients in the N3 + I1 arm experienced grade 3 and 4 AEs.[29] For these reasons, the N3 + I1 combination was chosen as the dose for further studies in mRCC.

The Phase 3 Checkmate 214 trial investigated the use of nivolumab plus ipilimumab versus sunitinib in treatment-naïve mRCC.[30] The co-primary endpoints of the trial were OS, ORR, and PFS in the IMDC intermediate- and poor-risk populations. A total of 425 intermediate/poor risk patients were randomized to ipilimumab/nivolumab and 422 patients to sunitinib. With a median follow-up of 25.2 months, the median OS in the intermediate/poor patients favored ipilimumab/nivolumab (NR vs. 26.0 months; HR 0.63; p <.001). The ORR (42% vs. 27%; p <.001), and CR rate (9% vs. 1%) were also higher in the ipilimumab/nivolumab patients. Although the mPFS was numerically higher in ipilimumab/nivolumab versus sunitinib (11.6 vs. 8.4 months; HR 0.82; p = .03), it did not meet the prespecified 0.009 threshold. In the initial analysis of the favorable-risk patients, the ORR was higher for sunitinib versus ipilimumab/nivolumab (52% vs. 29%) and the HR for death was 1.45 (99.8% CI 0.51–4.12; p = .27) in favor of sunitinib, although only 37 total deaths had occurred in this group. There was a higher CR rate with ipilimumab/nivolumab versus sunitinib (11% vs. 6%) in the favorable-risk patients as well.[30]

Treatment-related AEs (TRAEs) of any grade (93% vs. 97%) and grade ≥3 (46% vs. 63%) were lower with ipilimumab/nivolumab. However, given immune-related AE (irAE), 35% of patients treated with ipilimumab/nivolumab required high doses of steroids defined as at least 40 mg of a prednisone equivalent per day.[30] Quality of life data also favored the ipilimumab/nivolumab arm.[30,31] On April 16, 2018, the FDA approved the use of ipilimumab/nivolumab as a treatment for treatment-naïve intermediate and poor risk mRCC.

Extended follow-up from this trial was subsequently presented.[32] With a minimum follow-up of 42 months, in the ITT population the OS (HR 0.72; 95% CI 0.61–0.86) and ORR (39.1% vs. 32.6%) favored ipilimumab/nivolumab versus sunitinib. In the favorable-risk population, the ORR was higher for sunitinib (54.0% vs. 28.8%) and the hazard ratio for death was 1.19 (95% CI 0.77–1.85). In the intermediate/poor risk cohort, the benefit was in favor of ipilimumab/nivolumab in terms of ORR (42.1% vs. 26.3%), PFS (HR 0.75; 95% CI 0.62–0.90), and OS (HR 0.66; 95% CI 0.55–0.80). The CR rate favored ipilimumab/nivolumab in the favorable (12.8% vs. 5.6%), intermediate/poor (10.1% vs. 1.4%), and ITT (10.7% vs. 2.4%) cohorts. These sustained responses to therapy at a minimum of 42 months of follow-up further support the use of ipilimumab/nivolumab in intermediate/poor risk treatment-naïve mRCC.[32]

Importantly, the use of ipilimumab/nivolumab in mRCC should be limited to its regimen as per the Checkmate 214 trial in which ipilimumab/nivolumab was given as a combination therapy upfront for up to four cycles followed by maintenance nivolumab. Trials that have attempted to give nivolumab monotherapy for all patients with the addition of ipilimumab as "salvage" therapy in patients with a suboptimal response to nivolumab monotherapy have reported inferior outcomes compared to those trials in which ipilimumab/nivolumab is given in combination upfront.[30,33–35] For example, the ORR with ipilimumab/nivolumab is 42% when given in combination in the frontline setting and only 4% to 13% with a salvage approach. Similarly, CR rates are superior when given in combination per Checkmate 214 (11%) compared to adding ipilimumab following treatment with nivolumab monotherapy (0%–3%).[33–36]

The rationale for the combination of CPI and VEGF-directed therapy in mRCC is the potential for anti-VEGF therapy to create a more immunopermissive tumor microenvironment, thus enhancing the efficacy of immunotherapy.[37] KEYNOTE-426 was a randomized Phase 3 trial in which 861 patients with ccRCC were randomized to receive pembrolizumab (anti PD-1) and axitinib versus sunitinib.[38] The primary endpoint was OS and PFS in the intent-to-treat ITT population. With an initial median follow-up of 12.8 months, there was a OS benefit favoring axitinib/pembrolizumab with a higher percentage of patients still alive at 12 months (89.9% vs. 78.3%; HR 0.53; 95% CI 0.38–0.74; p <.0001). The mPFS of axitinib/pembrolizumab and sunitinib were 15.1 and 11.1 months, respectively (HR 0.69; 95% CI 0.57–0.84; p <.001). The

secondary endpoint of ORR also favored the combination arm of axitinib/pembrolizumab as well (59.3% vs. 39.7%; 95% CI, 31.1–40.4; p <.001).[38]

Based on these data, the FDA approved the combination of pembrolizumab and axitinib in previously untreated ccRCC on April 19, 2019. In an updated analysis with a median follow-up of 30.6 months, the efficacy of this combination was maintained.[39] The mOS still favored axitinib/pembrolizumab (NR vs. 35.7; HR 0.68, 95% CI 0.55–0.85, p = .0003) as did the mPFS (15.4 vs. 11.1 months; 0.71, p <.0001). The ORR (60% vs. 40%) and the CR rates (9% vs. 3%) were also sustained in favor of axitinib/pembrolizumab. There were no additional safety concerns. These data further supported the role of axitinib and pembrolizumab in treatment-naïve mRCC.

The combination of avelumab (anti-PD-L1) and axitinib versus sunitinib was studied in the Phase 3 JAVELIN Renal 101 study. A total of 886 patients were randomized in this trial with primary endpoints of PFS and OS in the PD-L1-positive patients.[40] In the 560 PD-L1-positive patients, the mPFS favored axitinib/avelumab (13.8 vs. 7.2 months; HR 0.61; 95% CI 0.47–0.79; p <.001) as did the ORR (55.2% vs. 25.5%). Rates of any grade AE (99.3% and 99.3%) and grade ≥3 (71.2% and 71.5%) were similar among the axitinib/avelumab and sunitinib cohorts, respectively.[40] The FDA approved this combination for use in previously untreated mRCC on May 14, 2019.

An updated efficacy analysis of this trial (minimum follow-up of 13 months) was subsequently published.[41] Median PFS favored axitinib/avelumab in the PD-L1-positive patients (13.8 vs. 7.0 months; HR 0.62; 95% CI 0.490–0.777; p <.0001) and in the overall population (13.3 vs. 8.0 months; HR 0.69; p <.0001). Although OS data numerically favored axitinib and avelumab in both the PD-L1-positive (HR 0.828; 95% CI 0.596–1.151; p = .1301) and overall populations (HR 0.796; 95% CI 0.616–1.027; one-sided p = .0392) they did not reach statistical significance.[41] This regimen is used less in mRCC due to the lack of OS benefit.

The last of the Phase 3 IO-TKI combinations presented was the CHECKMATE-9ER trial, in which 651 patients with treatment-naïve ccRCR were randomized to receive cabozantinib/nivolumab versus sunitinib.[27] The primary endpoint in this trial was PFS per blinded independent central review (BICR) and key secondary endpoints were OS, ORR by BICR, and safety. With a median follow-up of 18.1 months, mPFS (16.6 vs. 8.3 months; HR 0.51; 95% CI 0.41–0.64; p <.0001), OS (HR 0.60; 98.89% CI 0.40–0.89; p = .0010), and ORR (55.7% vs. 27.1%; p <.0001) were all improved in the cabozantinib/nivolumab patients. Rates of any grade treatment-related AE (96.6% and 93.1%) and grade ≥3 (60.6% vs. 50.9%) were slightly higher in the cabozantinib/nivolumab than the sunitinib cohorts.[27] This combination is currently under FDA review for approval.

The previous CPI-based regimen for treatment-naïve mRCC have resulted in important improvements of clinical outcomes for patients with mRCC. A number of trials investigating other combinations such as lenvatinib/pembrolizumab and ipilimumab/nivolumab/cabozantinib are ongoing.[42,43]

In addition to the three previously mentioned IO-TKI trials, the IMMOTION 151 trial of atezolizumab plus bevacizumab (VEGF antibody) versus sunitinib was reported.[44] The primary endpoints of this trial were investigator-assessed PFS in the PD-L1-positive patients and OS in the ITT population. A total of 915 patients were enrolled in the trial. mPFS in the PD-L1-positive patients favored the atezolizumab/bevacizumab cohort (11.2 vs. 7.7 months; HR 0.74; 95% CI 0.57–0.96; $p = .0217$). In the ITT population, the mPFS favored the combination therapy cohort with an HR of 0.93. However, the 95% CI for OS in this cohort was 0.76 to 1.14, and thus did not meet statistical significance for OS. This combination is not approved for use in mRCC.

Currently, however, with the approvals of combination ipilimumab/nivolumab as well as two IO-TKI combinations (axitinib/pembrolizumab and axitinib/avelumab), the choices for frontline therapy in mRCC are plentiful. Deciding on which regimen to choose is more nuanced. Both ipilimumab/nivolumab and axitinib/pembrolizumab have demonstrated statistically significant improvements in OS and as such have become commonly used standard of care treatments in this patient population. The combination of axitinib/avelumab has yet to demonstrate an OS benefit.

The choice between an IO-IO versus IO-TKI regimens is based on multiple considerations. Ipilimumab/nivolumab has the benefit of having the longest clinical trial follow-up, durability of control, treatment-free interval data, and a significantly improved QOL benefit compared to TKI therapy. Conversely, the ORR and PFS are lower with this regimen compared with the IO-TKI regimens and it can have significant toxicity during the induction regimen of ipilimumab and nivolumab. Likewise, its benefit in IMDC favorable-risk patients is unproven.

The IO-TKI regimen of axitinib/pembrolizumab has the advantage of having well-established ORR, PFS, and OS across IMDC subgroups as well as a higher ORR and PFS, which is important in initial tumor burden control. However, with any IO-TKI regimen there is chronic daily therapy with TKI and the durability of response is not as well-established given the shorter duration of follow-up.

There are a host of other clinically relevant issues related to the use of CPI-based therapy in patients with mRCC. Historically, patients with sarcomatoid RCC (sRCC) had a poorer prognosis. However, the outcomes in sRCC with CPI-based regimens has drastically improved. The ORR and CR in the sRCC subgroups in the ipilimumab/nivolumab (60.8% and 18.9%), axitinib/pembrolizumab (58.8% and 11.8%), and bevacizumab/atezolizumab (49% and 10%) trials are all significantly improved compared to historical outcomes and even compared to pure ccRCC histology.[45–47] The mPFS and OS are also improved in sRCC in all three combinations compared to the sunitinib control arm, which thus established CPI-based combination therapy as an important standard of care in patients with sRCC. The biology behind the enhanced sensitivity of sRCC to checkpoint inhibition has not yet been elucidated.

Similarly, although the large Phase 3 CPI-based clinical trials were in clear cell RCC, retrospective data exists to support the use of CPI-based therapy in patients with non-ccRCC as well.[48,49] There are some prospective clinical trials with CPI monotherapy that demonstrate ORR of 10% to 25% and a duration of response of approximately 15 months.[50,51] Additional trials are ongoing to define the role of CPI in nccRCC.[52–54]

The duration of therapy with CPI-based regimens is not clearly defined though the standard of care in most regimens is treatment continuation until disease progression or unacceptable toxicity. Early clinical trials clearly indicate that patients can benefit from CPI therapy even after therapy discontinuation. Likewise, data nivolumab monotherapy in mRCC supports durable responses in patients following therapy discontinuation.[55] Ongoing trials are further investigating the role of discontinuation of CPI based on response to treatment in an attempt to maximize efficacy with shorter durations of treatment.[56,57]

The role of biomarkers in treatment selection in mRCC is also ill-defined. There are no approved biomarkers to guide treatment selection. Specifically, the role of PD-L1 testing mRCC does not have an established role given varying outcomes in clinical trials and data supporting favorable outcomes across PD-L1 levels. It is important to note that genomic subclassifications have identified associations between specific angiogenic and immunomodulatory gene expression signatures and response to CPI therapy.[58,59] With incorporation of such techniques and approaches in future clinical trials, biomarker-based treatment selection may have a future role in mRCC.

While the aforementioned data reviewed the role of CPI-based combination therapy in mRCC, there are data to also support the use of CPI monotherapy in mRCC. For example, data for monotherapy pembrolizumab in treatment-naïve ccRCC demonstrates an ORR of 36.4% and a PFS of 7.2%.[60] Other data with CPI monotherapy in treatment-naïve RCC demonstrate similar outcomes.[33,58] However, the role of such therapy in clinical practice is not established and patients receiving CPI therapy for frontline mRCC should receive combination therapy as previously noted barring contraindications.

Beyond the role of CPI-based therapy in frontline mRCC there are emerging data for the role and activity of CPI therapy in patients with CPI-refractory mRCC. A Phase 2 trial of lenvatinib and pembrolizumab in patients with CPI-refractory mRCC showed an ORR of 55%, mPFS of 11.3 months, and median duration of response of 12 months.[61] Although it is a nonrandomized trial, it supports activity of immunotherapy following CPI failure. Ongoing trials such as the CONTACT-03 trial (atezolizumab/cabozantinib vs. cabozantinib) are investigating the role of CPI therapy in patients whose cancer has progressed on a prior CPI-based regimen.[62]

Perioperative Immunotherapy

Although there are currently no immunotherapies approved in the perioperative setting in patients with local or locally advanced RCC, their robust activity in mRCC suggest a potential role in the neoadjuvant and adjuvant setting. In particular, there is a theoretical benefit to the use of CPI in the neoadjuvant setting since the tumor neoantigens are in place and this may result in an enhanced immune response. However, there are also concerns of the role of immunotherapy in this setting in terms of the potential for treatment-related toxicity that can potentially delay and/or complicate the surgery.

A recent Phase 1b trial investigated the safety of neoadjuvant ± adjuvant durvalumab with or without tremelimumab in 29 patients with high-risk localized RCC (clinical stage T2b-4 and/or N1, M0 disease).[63] Although the maximum tolerated dose was not reached, the study was closed early with a higher than expected number of adverse events. Importantly, however, there were no surgical complications or delays to surgery that were related to therapy.

The ongoing PROSPER study is a Phase 3 randomized trial of patients with locally advanced RCC in which patients are randomized to receive preoperative and postoperative nivolumab versus observation.[64] This biomarker-rich trial will hopefully shed light on the clinical efficacy of perioperative CPI in RCC as well as the biology surrounding its use. A number of trials have investigated the role of immunotherapy following the resection of high-risk RCC. These include trials of monotherapy with pembrolizumab, atezolizumab, nivolumab, or nivolumab/ipilimumab, among others.[65-67] Results from these trials are pending.

Vaccines

AGS-003

AGS-003 is an autologous dendritic cell (DC) vaccine consisting of DCs coelectroporated with the synthetic CD40L RNA and the patient's amplified tumor RNA.[68-70] When injected into patients, CD40 ligation leads to a production of IL-12, thus optimizing CD8$^+$ T cell induction. Additionally, these RNA-containing DCs present patient-specific antigens to T cells, thereby enhancing the immune response.[69,70] Twenty-one patients with intermediate- or poor-risk mRCC who underwent nephrectomy were treated postoperatively with sunitinib and AGS-003 intradermal injections until disease progression.[68] The mPFS was 11 months, and mOS was 30 months. Additionally, CD8$^+$ CD28$^+$ CD45RA$^-$ T cells were increased compared to baseline and correlated with survival.

These findings led to the development of the ADAPT trial, a Phase 3 trial in which patients with mRCC who undergo cytoreductive nephrectomy are randomized to receive standard of care sunitinib with or without AGS-003 (now termed Rocapuldencel-T). Of the 769 patients in this trial, the median OS did not differ between the Rocapuldencel-T/Sunitinib group (27.7 months) and the SOC cohort (32.4 months; HR 1.10; 95% CI 0.83–1.40).[71] The trial was thus terminated early and the development of Rocapuldencel-T in mRCC is unlikely.

IMA901

IMA901 is a cancer vaccine comprised of nine HLA-A*02-restricted tumor-associated peptides (TUMAPs) and one human leukocyte antigen–antigen D-related (HLA-DR)-restricted TUMAP. Phase 1/2 trials with IMA901 plus immunomodulators cyclophosphamide and granulocyte-monocyte colony-stimulating factor (GM-CSF) in patients with mRCC demonstrated an association between OS and responses to multiple TUMAPs. Similarly, specific populations of myeloid-derived suppressor cells (MDSCs) were prognostic for OS.[72] Based on these findings, the Phase 3 IMPRINT trial was conducted in which 339 HLA-A*02-positive patients with mRCC were randomized to receive sunitinib alone or sunitinib and up to 10 intradermal vaccinations of IMA901 plus GM-CSF. Cyclophosphamide was given prior to the first vaccine infusion to reduce regulatory T cells. The mOS (primary endpoint) was 38.1 months in the vaccine arm and not reached in the sunitinib arm (HR: 1.34, $p = .08$). Moreover, unlike the Phase 2 study, there were no correlations between T cell responses and outcomes.[73] IMA901 thus remains under investigation but does not currently have a role in the treatment of RCC.

Future Directions

Immunotherapy in mRCC is dominated by CPI-based therapy, which has revolutionized care in mRCC. Although the first approved CPI was nivolumab for patients with treatment-refractory mRCC, most patients will now receive CPI-based combination therapy as their frontline treatment option for mRCC. The role of immunotherapy in the neoadjuvant and adjuvant settings is not yet defined. Likewise, ongoing clinical trials will determine optimal treatment duration, sequencing, role of CPI in nccRCC, CPI treatment in immunotherapy-refractory disease, and biomarker research to define choice of CPI-CPI versus CPI-TKI therapy. In addition to optimizing therapy with currently approved agents, novel immune agents such as chimeric antigen receptor T cells and T cell agonists are in development and may expand the role of immunotherapy in mRCC (Table 52.1).[82,83]

Table 52.1 Select Pivotal Practice-Changing Trials in Genitourinary Immunotherapy

TRIAL	INTERVENTION	PATIENT POPULATION	PHASE	N	ORR	PFS[a]	OS[a]	CONCLUSIONS/PRACTICE POINTS
RENAL CELL CARCINOMA								
Atkins et al.[74]	IL-2/IFN vs. IL-2	Treatment-naïve mRCC	2[b]	99	11% vs. 17%	N/A	15.5 vs. 16	• 5.6% CR rate in IL-2 cohort • Longer duration of responses in IL-2 cohort • Study prospectively established IL-2 monotherapy as a standard of care in mRCC
Motzer et al. (CheckMate 025)[4]	Nivolumab vs. everolimus	Previously treated mRCC	3	821	25% vs. 5%	4.6 vs. 4.4	25.0 vs. 21.8	• Established nivolumab as a standard of care in patients who received prior antiangiogenic therapy
Motzer et al. (CheckMate 214)[75]	Nivolumab/ Ipilimumab vs. sunitinib	Treatment-naïve mRCC	3[c]	847	42% vs. 27%	11.6 vs. 8.4	NR vs. 26	• First dual-CPI trial in frontline mRCC • Established nivolumab/ ipilimumab as a standard of care for frontline mRCC
Rini et al. (KEYNOTE-426)[38]	Axitinib/ Pembrolizumab vs. sunitinib	Treatment-naïve mRCC	3	861	59.3% vs. 35.7%	15.1 vs. 11.1	NR vs. 35.7[d]	• First CPI-TKI trial in frontline mRCC • Established axitinib/ pembrolizumab as a standard of care for frontline mRCC
BLADDER CANCER								
Rosenberg et al. (IMvigor210)[76]	Atezolizumab	Platinum-refractory metastatic/ unresectable UC[e]	2	310	15%	2.1	11.4	• Trial led to approval of atezolizumab in this setting.
Balar et al. (KEYNOTE-052)[77]	Pembrolizumab	Cisplatin-ineligible metastatic/ unresectable UC	2	370	24%	2.0	6 month OS: 67%	• Trial led to approval of pembrolizumab in this setting.
Powles et al. (JAVELIN Bladder 100)[78]	Avelumab vs. BSC	Maintenance CPI following chemotherapy in metastatic/ unresectable UC	3	700	NA[f]	3.7 vs. 2.0	21.4 vs. 14.3	• Trial led to approval of avelumab as maintenance therapy in patients with mUC whose cancer did not progress following frontline chemotherapy.
Balar et al. (KEYNOTE-057)[79]	Pembrolizumab	BCG-refractory non-muscle invasive UC	2	103	38.8[g]	12-month PFS 82.7%[g]	12-month OS 97.9%[g]	• Established pembrolizumab as a treatment option for patients with BCG-refractory NMIBC who decline or are not candidates for cystectomy

(continued)

Table 52.1 Select Pivotal Practice-Changing Trials in Genitourinary Immunotherapy (*continued*)

TRIAL	INTERVENTION	PATIENT POPULATION	PHASE	N	ORR	PFS[a]	OS[a]	CONCLUSIONS/PRACTICE POINTS
PROSTATE CANCER								
Kantoff et al. IMPACT[80]	Sipuleucel-T vs. placebo	mCRPC	3	512	N/A[h]	3.7 vs. 3.6	25.8 vs. 21.7	• No significant change in PSA with sipuleucel-T so cannot accurately measure response rates[h] • Benefit of therapy is in OS • Approved for mCRPC but role of therapy unclear in setting of novel oral agents

[a]PFS and OS in months unless otherwise noted.

[b]Randomized Phase 2 trial.

[c]Primary endpoint was in intermediate- and poor-risk patients. Those results are reported here.

[d]Median OS was not reached for either arm in initial publication. OS data presented here are from an extended follow-up publication.[39]

[e]Study included two cohorts. Cohort 1 included patients who were platinum ineligible. Cohort 2 included patients refractory to platinum-based therapy. Those results are presented in this table.

[f]Since the trial was maintenance therapy, there was no response rate reported.

[g]Response rate in this trial was complete response rate. Twelve-month PFS and OS were published in an extended follow-up manuscript.[81]

[h]Although no traditional ORR is reported, there were a number of immune responses that were significantly higher in the sipuleucel-T cohort.

BCG, bacillus Calmette-Guerin; Bev, bevacizumab; BSC, best supportive care; CPI, checkpoint inhibitor; CR, complete response; GU, genitourinary; IFN-α, interferon-alpha; IL-2, interleukin-2; mCRPC, metastatic castration-resistant prostate cancer; mRCC, metastatic renal cell carcinoma; NA, not applicable; NMIBC, nonmuscle invasive bladder cancer; NR, not reached; ORR, overall response rate; OS, overall survival; PFS, progression-free survival; PSA, prostate-specific antigen; TKI. tyrosine kinase inhibitor; UC, urothelial carcinoma.

BLADDER CANCER

Historically, immunotherapy in bladder cancer (henceforth, urothelial carcinoma [UC]) was limited to local intravesical therapy with BCG vaccine for patients with nonmuscle invasive bladder cancer (NMIBC).[84] However, with the advent of immune CPIs, systemic immunotherapy is now available for select patients with metastatic UC as well.[76–78,85–87]

Bacillus Calmette–Guérin

BCG is a live attenuated vaccine of *Mycobacterium bovis* that was initially developed in the early 1900s as a vaccine against tuberculosis.[84] It was later observed that patients with tuberculosis actually had lower rates of cancer and subsequently hypothesized that mycobacteria might possess either direct antitumor effects or tumor suppressor properties. This set the stage for preclinical animal models in the 1970s, which demonstrated that a delayed immunologic response in organisms infected with BCG resulted in tumor inhibition.[88] The antitumor effect of BCG is not cytotoxic in nature but rather a multifaceted and sustained activation of the local immune system.[89] BCG was then investigated as a potential immunotherapy in multiple cancers but had not demonstrated consistent results.[84] In UC, however, the role of BCG was confirmed with two early randomized trials demonstrating a decrease in tumor recurrence in patients receiving intravesical BCG.[2,84,90,91]

Intravesical BCG is administered a few weeks after TURBT with an induction period of once weekly injections for 6 weeks. It is currently approved for the use of superficial UC of the bladder (Tis; large, multifocal, recurrent, or high-grade Ta; or T1). The role of maintenance BCG is less clear but generally follows the Southwest Oncology Group (SWOG) regimen of induction for 6 weeks followed by 3 weeks of maintenance every 3 to 6 months for at least 1 year if tolerated by the patient.[92] BCG is given with 50 mL of sterile saline directly into the bladder through a catheter where it is retained for 2 hours.

The most comprehensive analysis of complications and toxicities from BCG is from an analysis of 585 patients treated with BCG on six clinical trials. The most common side effects occurring in at least half the patients were urinary frequency (71%) and cystitis (67%). Other common side effects included fever (25%) and hematuria (23%).[93] As BCG is a live attenuated vaccine, it should not be administered to patients with active urinary infections, traumatic catheterization, bacteriuria, or gross hematuria who can develop systemic infections if they are treated with BCG in these settings.[93]

IFN-α has been extensively studied in combination with BCG for the treatment of superficial bladder cancers.[94,95] As the helper T cell-1 (Th1) response in the bladder is critical to BCG efficacy, the rationale for this combination rests in the enhanced Th1 stimulation with IFN-α, which can augment the immune response to BCG.

In a large Phase 2 trial of more than 1,000 patients with BCG-naïve or BCG-refractory superficial bladder cancer, the combination of BCG and IFN-α demonstrated durable disease-free periods with relatively low toxicity rates.[94] However, there is only one randomized trial of 670 BCG-naïve patients with superficial bladder cancer comparing BCG alone and combined BCG/IFN-α. In this trial, the combination of BCG/IFN-α did not demonstrate a benefit in tumor recurrence in patients compared to BCG alone but did increase constitutional symptoms.[96] As such, there is no documented role for combined IFN-α/BCG in the frontline treatment of NMIBC. Patients with BCG-refractory disease or post-BCG relapse may potentially benefit from the addition of IFN-α to BCG, though many of these patients are considered for cystectomy to prevent progression of the disease.

Checkpoint Inhibitors

Platinum-Refractory Metastatic Urothelial Carcinoma

There are currently five FDA-approved CPIs for the treatment of patients with mUC that has progressed following treatment. They are pembrolizumab, atezolizumab, nivolumab, avelumab, and durvalumab. The most robust data (in the form of Phase 3 trials) exist for pembrolizumab and atezolizumab and an overview of data will thus be reviewed here.

KEYNOTE-045 was a Phase 3 trial in which patients with platinum-refractory mUC were randomized to receive pembrolizumab versus physician-choice of chemotherapy (vinflunine, docetaxel, paclitaxel).[87] The co-primary endpoints were OS and PFS in the overall population and PD-L1-positive patient. PD-L1 positivity was defined as a combined positive score (CPS) of 10% or higher. CPS is further defined as the percentage of PD-L1-positive immune-infiltrating and tumor cells relative to the total number of tumor cells.

In total, 542 patients were randomized. The mOS favored the pembrolizumab group in the overall population (10.3 vs. 7.4 months; HR 0.73; 95% CI 0.59–0.91; $p = .002$) as well as the PD-L1-positive population (8.0 vs. 5.2 months; HR 0.57; 95% CI 0.37–0.88; $p = .005$). Median PFS was similar between pembrolizumab and chemotherapy in the overall population (HR 0.98; 95% CI 0.81–1.19; $p = .42$) and PD-L1-positive cohorts (HR 0.89; 95% CI 0.61–1.28; $p = 0.24$). Rates of any grade AE were 60.9% and 90.2% in the pembrolizumab and chemotherapy cohorts, respectively; and fever grade ≥3 events in patients receiving pembrolizumab compared to chemotherapy (15.0% vs. 49.4%).[88]

Quality of life also favored the pembrolizumab patients with a prolonged time to deterioration and stable/improved global health status and QOL scores compared to patients on chemotherapy.[97] In a subsequent analysis of greater than 2 years of follow-up, the durability of clinical superiority of pembrolizumab was demonstrated. Median duration of response (DOR) for pembrolizumab was not reached (range, 1.6-30.0) compared to a median DOR of 4.4 months (range 1.4–29.9) in patients receiving chemotherapy.[98] Pembrolizumab is thus a standard of care for patients with mUC whose cancer has progressed on platinum-based chemotherapy and was approved by the FDA on May 18, 2017.

Atezolizumab was initially approved on May 18, 2016, on the basis of the results of cohort 2 of the IMvigor210 trial in which 310 patients with inoperable locally advanced or metastatic UC who progressed despite prior treatment with platinum-based therapy were treated with atezolizumab 1,200 mg IV every 3 weeks until loss of clinical benefit.[76] The primary endpoint was an ORR higher than the historical control of 10% ORR in this setting. Biomarker prediction of response was also investigated using the percentage of tumor microenvironment PD-L1-positive IC in the tumor microenvironment (IC0 <1%; IC1 ≥1% but <5%; IC2/3 ≥5%). One hundred and three patients (33%) were IC0, 207 (67%) were IC1/2/3, and 100 (32%) were IC2/3. The ORR for all patients was 15% and significantly greater than historical control of 10% ($p = .0058$). Although responses were noted in patients with any IC score, higher PD-L1 expression was associated with increased ORR compared to the historical control, with ORR of 27% for IC2/3 (95% CI 19–37; $p <.0001$) and 18% for IC1/2/3 (95% CI 13–24; $p = .0004$).[76]

The confirmatory Phase 3 trial for atezolizumab in this setting was the Phase 3 IMvigor211, which randomized patients to receive atezolizumab versus physician choice of chemotherapy (paclitaxel, doccetaxel, or vinflunine).[86] The primary endpoint of the trial was the hierarchical testing in prespecified populations as follows: IC2/3 (per the previously mentioned IMvigor210 trial), followed by IC1/2/3, followed by the ITT population.

A total of 931 patients were randomized. In the 234 patients in the IC2/3 population, the mOS was similar between atezolizumab and chemotherapy (11.1 vs. 10·6 months; HR 0.87, 95% CI 0.63–1.21; $p = .41$). Given the hierarchical testing of the primary endpoint, since the IC/2/3 population did not archive statistical significance, further analysis was precluded. The ORR (23% vs. 22%) and the duration of response (15.9 vs. 8·3 months; HR 0.57, 95% CI 0.26–1.26) were numerically higher in the pembrolizumab vs. the chemotherapy arms. An exploratory analysis of the ITT, however, did reveal a longer DOR in those receiving atezolizumab (21.7 vs. 7.4 months) as well as improved mOS (8.6 vs. 8.0 months; HR 0.85; 95% CI 0.73–0.99).[86] Given these findings and the lack of additional safety findings in this trial, atezolizumab remains an option for mUC patients with platinum-refractory mUC.

In 2017, nivolumab, durvalumab, and avelumab were all approved for use in platinum refractory mUC on the bases of either Phase 1 and/or Phase 2 trials.[85,99,100] The approval of these agents in the absence of Phase 3 clinical trial data highlights the prior unmet meet for viable therapies in this setting. In addition, the combination of ipilimumab and nivolumab in this setting is under investigation.[101]

Platinum Ineligible Metastatic Urothelial Carcinoma

The initial approval of atezolizumab in patients with cisplatin-ineligible mUC was based on Cohort 1 of the IMvigor210 trial.[102] This was a single-arm Phase 2 trial in which patients were treated with atezolizumab 1,200 mg IV every 3 weeks until disease progression. Of the 119 evaluable patients (with a median follow-up of 17/2 months), the ORR and CR were 23.9% and 9%, respectively, with responses occurring across PD-L1 groups. The mOS was 15.9 months (10.4-NE). The rates of any grade and grade ≥3 TRAEs were 66% and 16%, respectively, with irAEs occurring in 12% of patients. The FDA-approved atezolizumab in this setting on April 17, 2017.

Pembrolizumab is also approved (FDA approval date: May 18, 2017) as frontline treatment for cisplatin-ineligible mUC patients. Similar to atezolizumab, its approval is based on a single-arm Phase 2 trial with a primary endpoint of ORR in all patients and those with positive PD-L1 expression in tumor and inflammatory cells.[77] A total of 370 patients with treatment-naïve cisplatin-inelolgble mUC received pembrolizumab. With a median follow-up of 5 months, the ORR was 24% in all patients and 38% in those with CPS ≥ 10%. AEs were typical of CPI in mUC studies with no new safety signals noted.

In an updated analysis with a minimum follow-up of 2 years, the median DOR was 30.1 months (95% CI, 18.1-NR), with responses of ≥12 in 67% of patients and ≥24 months in 52% of responders. The mOS was 11.3 months (95% CI 9.7–13.1 months) with a 24-month OS rate of 31/2%. Responses to treatment and their durability was improved in patients with CPS ≥ 10, with an ORR of 47.3% and mOS of 18.5 months.[102]

Given the previous data, the only CPI agents currently approved in the cisplatin-ineligible mUC population are atezolizumab and pembrolizumab. A variety of other trials in frontline mUC are ongoing. Recently, the DANUBE trial in which patients with treatment-naïve mUC were randomized to receive durvalumab versus durvalumab/tremelimumab versus chemotherapy failed to demonstrate a statistically significant OS benefit.[103] Additional CPI trials are ongoing including the investigation of ipilimumab/nivolumab and the combination of CPI agents with other non-IO agents.[104,105]

It is important to note that in July 2018, the FDA updated the labels of atezolizumab and pembrolizumab for use in frontline treatment of mUC with platinum-ineligible UC. Patients ineligible for any platinum-based chemotherapy may receive pembrolizumab or atezolizumab regardless of PD-L1 status. However, patients who are cisplatin-ineligible but still meet criteria for other platinum-based regimens (e.g., carboplatin) may only receive frontline CPI if they are PD-L1 positive. PD-L1 positive is defined as CPS ≥ 10% for pembrolizumab and PD-L1-positive stating of ≥5% of tumor-infiltrating immune cells.[106]

Maintenance Checkpoint Inhibitors in Metastatic Urothelial Carcinoma

The JAVELIN Bladder 100 trial investigated the role of maintenance avelumab in mUC. In this randomized Phase 3 trial, 700 patients with mUC who received front-line treatment with gemcitabine/cisplatin or gemcitabine/carboplatin and did not experience disease progression after four to six cycles were randomized to receive avelumab versus best supportive care (BSC). The primary endpoints in the trial were OS in the ITT and PD-L1-positive populations.[78]

In the ITT population, the mOS was 21.4 months with avelumab versus 14.3 months with BSC alone (HR 0.69; 95% CI 0.56–0.86; $p = 0.001$). The 1-year OS was 71.3% and 58.4% in the avelumab and BSC arms, respectively. The 1-year OS was also improved with avelumab maintenance therapy in the PD-L1-positive population (79.1% vs. 60.4%; HR 0.56; 95% CI 0.40–0.79; $p < .001$). The rate of all grade AEs (98% vs. 77.7%) and grade ≥3 AEs (47.4% vs. 25.2) was higher in the avelumab-treated patients.[78] On the basis of the OS benefit, on June 30, 2020, the FDA approved the use of maintenance avelumab in patients with mUC whose cancer did not progress on front-line platinum-based chemotherapy, and this is the standard of care approach.

Galsky et al. published a similar randomized Phase 2 trial of maintenance pembrolizumab in the setting that also showed improved PFS with maintenance therapy. However, mOS has yet to be demonstrated.[107] As such, avelumab remains the only approved therapy for maintenance treatment following front-line chemotherapy in mUC.

Checkpoint Inhibitor + Chemotherapy in Metastatic Urothelial Carcinoma

Given the efficacy of chemotherapy and CPI as monotherapies in mUC as well as efficacy of combined chemotherapy and CPI in other malignancies, the combination of CPI and chemotherapy was investigated in mUC. The IMvigor130 study was a Phase 3 trial in which 1,213 patients with treatment-naïve metastatic UC were randomized to receive atezolizumab with platinum-chemotherapy (group A) versus atezolizumab (group B) versus platinum-chemotherapy plus placebo (group C). The study primary endpoint was

PFS and OS in group A versus group C, with a co-primary endpoint of OS in group B versus group C only if the OS favored group A versus group C.[108]

With a median follow-up for survival of 11.8 months, the mPFS favored group A versus group C (8.2 vs. 6.3 months; 0.82, 95% CI 0.70–0.96; p = .007) as did mOS (group A: 16.0 months; group C: 13.4 months; HR 0.83, 0.69–1.00; p = .027). Median OS for group B and group C was 15.7 and 13.1 months, respectively.[108] The Phase 3 KEYNOTE-361 trial of pembrolizumab with chemotherapy versus chemotherapy alone in mUC was likewise negative for an OS benefit.[109] Given the lack of OS benefit with the addition of CPI to chemotherapy monotherapy in frontline mUC, the combination of chemotherapy and CPI is not yet recommended in mUC.

Neoadjuvant and Adjuvant Checkpoint Indicators in Urothelial Carcinoma

The standard of care for patients with muscle-invasive bladder cancer (MIBC) is cisplatin-based neoadjuvant chemotherapy (NAC) followed by surgery.[110] Patients who are ineligible for cisplatin chemotherapy should not receive carboplatin-based chemotherapy as no survival benefit has been demonstrated with this regimen in the neoadjuvant setting. Given the efficacy of CPI in mUC, its role in the neoadjuvant setting for patients with MIBC is under investigation.

The PURE-01 was a single-arm Phase 2 trial of neoadjuvant pembrolizumab (three cycles) in patients with MIBC regardless of whether they were cisplatin eligible.[111] The primary endpoint was pathological response (pT0) in the ITT population. A total of 50 patients were enrolled: 54% had cT3 tumor, 42% had cT2, and 4% had cT2-3N1. Only one patient had to discontinue therapy prior to surgery because of AEs (grade 3 elevated transaminase). All patients successfully underwent a radical cystectomy with 21 (42%) patients achieving pT0. In the 35 patients with PD-L1 CPS ≥ 10%, the pT0 rate was 54.3%.[111] Despite limitations of a single-arm Phase 2 trial, these data suggest a role for CPI therapy as neoadjuvant therapy in MIBC.

Powles et al. published a similar single-arm Phase 2 trial of atezolizumab (two cycles) in MIBC patients who were ineligible or refused cisplatin-based NAC.[112] This was the ABACUS trial with a primary endpoint of pathological complete response (pCR) and secondary endpoints related to safety, biomarker analyses, and recurrence-free relapse. Of the 95 patients enrolled, the pCR rate was 31%. Importantly, there were no unexpected surgical complications attributed to therapy. Baseline higher than expected preexisting activated T cells correlated with outcome. Tissue analyses of tumors that responded to therapy demonstrated predominantly gene expressions related to tissue repair, which made biomarker analyses

and interpretation challenging.[112] Similar to the PURE-01 trial, these data support the further investigation of CPI in the neoadjuvant setting for MIBC.

More recently, two trials of combined anti-CTLA-4 and anti-PD-(L)1 as neoadjuvant therapy in MIBC were reported. The NABUCCO trial was a Phase 2 trial to assess the feasibility of two doses of ipilimumab and nivolumab in patients with stage III MIBC.[113] Of the 24 patients enrolled, all patients were able to undergo a cystectomy and rates of grade ≥3 irAEs were 55%. In total, 11 patients (54%) achieved a pCR. Baseline CD8+ presence or T-effector signatures did not correlate with response to treatment.

In a similar single arm, Phase 2 study, Gao et al. treated cisplatin-ineligible MIBC patients who had high-risk features (e.g., bulky tumors, variant histology, hydronephrosis, etc.) with two cycles of neoadjuvant durvalumab (anti-PD-L1) and tremelimumab (anti-CTLA-4).[114] Of the 28 patients enrolled, 37.5% achieved a pCR and only 21% of patients developed a grade ≥3 irAE. The 1-year relapse-free survival was 82.8%. Genomic analyses did not confirm gene signatures associated with responses in prior CPI trials in MIBC. Furthermore, there was no correlation between PD-L1 status and response to therapy.

Taken together, these trials demonstrate the relative safety and efficacy of CPI therapy prior to surgery in MIBC with no consistent biomarkers to predict for pCR. Whereas the aforementioned trials investigated the role of CPI therapy alone as a neoadjuvant option in MIBC, additional trials have published results of combination CPI and chemotherapy prior to cystectomy in patients with MIBC.

The BLASST-1 (Bladder Cancer Signal Seeking Trial) trial was a Phase 2 single-arm trial in which patients with MIBC (cT2-T4a, N ≤ 1, M0) who were cisplatin-eligible were treated with neoadjvuant gemcitabine, cisplatin, and nivolumab for four cycles.[115] The primary endpoint of the study was a pathological response (PaR) defined and ≤pT1N0 and secondary endpoints included safety and 2-year PFS. A total of 41 patients were enrolled and the PaR rate was 65.8%. There were no delays to surgery or surgical complications related to surgery. Roughly 25% of patients had grade ≥3 AE.[115] PFS and correlative work are ongoing but early signals highlight the safety and efficacy of combined CPI and chemotherapy in MIBC.

More recently, interim results from cohort 2 of the GU14-188 trial were presented.[116] In this cohort, patients with cisplatin-ineligible MIBC were treated with the combination of gemcitabine and pembrolizumab preoperatively. The primary endpoint was pathological response (PaR; ≤pT1N0). Of the 32 patients enrolled in this cohort, the PaIR was 51.6%, with 45.2% achieving a pCR (pT0N0). The adverse event profile was similar to other trials using CPI in this setting. Taken together, BLASST-1 and GU14-188 trials demonstrate a need for further investigation of the combination of CPI and chemotherapy as neoadjuvant therapy in MIBC.

With multiple Phase 2 trials demonstrating safety and efficacy of CPI-based preoperative therapy in MIBC, a host of Phase 3 trials are ongoing to definitively determine its role in this setting. These trials are investigating the role of CPI alone or in combination with chemotherapy in patients with cisplatin-eligible and cisplatin-ineligible MIBC, and their results, if positive, will shift the standard of care for neoadjuvant therapy in MIBC.[117-121]

With CPI activity in MIBC and in mUC, the IMvigor010 trial investigated the role of atezolizumab in patients with MIBC following cystectomy.[122] In this Phase 3 trial, patients with MIBC (either ypT2-4a or ypN+ if they had NAC or pT3-4a or pN+ for those who did not receive NAC) were randomized postcystectomy to receive either atezolizumab or observation for 1 year. The primary endpoint was disease-free survival (DFS). A total of 809 patients were enrolled and with a median follow-up of 21.9 months, the mDFS for atezolizumab was 19.4 months and 16.6 months for those in observation (HR 0.89; 95% CI 0.74–1.08; $p = 0.2446$). PD-L1 status did not influence outcome. Likewise, at the first interim analysis, the mOS was not reached in either arm but with approximately 120 events occurring in each arm, the hazard ration for OS was 0.85 (95% CI 0.66–1.09; $p = 0.1951$).[122] There is therefore currently no role for adjuvant immunotherapy in MIBC. However, a recent press release noted that the double-blind Phase 3 CheckMate-274 trial of adjuvant nivolumab versus placebo demonstrated a disease-free survival benefit for nivolumab.[123,124] Additional data are pending. Similarly, the Phase 3 AMBASSADOR trial (pembrolizumab vs. observation as adjuvant therapy in UC) is ongoing.[125]

Nonmuscle Invasive Urothelial Carcinoma

As previously mentioned, the treatment of NMIBC is generally limited to treatment with intravesical therapy such as BCG to decrease disease recurrence.[1,2,89,93] However, given the role of CPI in mUC and the evolving understanding of its use in MIBC, investigations of its use in NMIBC were investigated.

The KEYNOTE-057 trial was a single-arm Phase 2 trial of pembrolizumab in patients with BCG-refractory NMIBC with carcinoma in situ (CIS) with or without papillary features. The study's primary endpoint was CRR with secondary endpoints including safety and durability of response. Of the 103 patients who were enrolled, the CRR at 3 months was 38.8%, and 72.5% of patients who achieved a 3-month CR had a sustained response with a median follow-up of 14.0 months. Although the median duration of CR was not reached, 80.2% had a sustained response of ≥6 months. Treatment-related AEs were consistent with pembrolizumab monotherapy in

other trials.[79] Given these data on January 8, 2020, the FDA approved pembrolizumab in patients with BCG-refractory NMIBC who refuse or are not a candidate for cystectomy.

Additional follow-up of KEYNOTE-057 were presented post-FDA approval. With a median follow-up of 284 months, the CRR was 40.6%, median DOR was 16.2 months, and 46.2% had a DOR ≥12 months. The 12-month PFS and OS were 82.7% and OS 97.9%, respectively, further supporting the use of pembrolizumab in patients with BCG-refractory high-risk NMIBC.[80] Other CPIs are also under investigation in this setting.[126]

Future Directions

Until the advent of CPIs, immunotherapy with UC was limited to BCG and IFN-α in localized disease. Over the last 5 years, CPI monotherapy has been approved in NMIBC, cisplatin-ineligible mUC, platinum-refractory mUC, and as maintenance therapy after platinum-based chemotherapy in mUC. The next rational approval for CPI in UC based on the previously mentioned data is for MIBC in the neoadjuvant setting either for patients who are not cisplatin candidates or in combination with cisplatin-based NAC. The role of CPI in adjuvant UC is less certain. In addition to the expanded use of CPI monotherapy in mUC, the next few years will see an evolution in the combination of CPI with novel agents such as antibody drug conjugates.[105] Additionally, the biomarker-based research beyond PD-L1 will hopefully redefine the use of CPI in mUC. Lastly, novel therapies with vaccines, monoclonal antibodies, and adoptive T cell therapies[127,128] are being developed in metastatic and unresectable UC to improve outcomes in this setting, which is an otherwise poor outcome (Table 52.2).

PROSTATE CANCER

Of the GU malignancies, prostate cancer has the fewest approved immunotherapies despite a variety of prostate cancer-specific antigens that are potential natural targets for immunotherapy. Although numerous clinical trials have been conducted investigating the role of various immunotherapeutics in prostate cancer, there is currently only one FDA-approved immunotherapy specifically for prostate cancer.[128,129] Immunotherapy for prostate cancer primarily revolves around prostate cancer vaccines and CPIs.

Prostate Cancer Vaccines

Sipuleucel-T

Sipuleucel-T is an autologous DC vaccine that expresses a fusion protein of prostatic acid phosphatase (PAP) and GM-CSF. It is approved for the treatment of nonvisceral

Table 52.2 Select Ongoing Phase 3 Clinical Trials in Genitourinary Oncology

TRIAL REGISTRATION	TITLE
RENAL CELL CARCINOMA	
NCT03793166	Immunotherapy With Nivolumab and Ipilimumab Followed by Nivolumab or Nivolumab With Cabozantinib for Patients With Advanced Kidney Cancer, The PDIGREE Study
NCT03937219	Study of Cabozantinib in Combination With Nivolumab and Ipilimumab in Patients With Previously Untreated Advanced or Metastatic Renal Cell Carcinoma
NCT02811861	Lenvatinib/Pembrolizumab Versus Sunitinib Alone as Treatment of Advanced Renal Cell Carcinoma
NCT03055013	PROSPER: A Phase 3 Randomized Study Comparing Perioperative Nivolumab (nivo) Versus Observation in Patients With Renal Cell Carcinoma (RCC) Undergoing Nephrectomy (ECOG-ACRIN 8143).
BLADDER CANCER	
NCT03036098	Study of Nivolumab in Combination With Ipilimumab or Standard of Care Chemotherapy Compared to the Standard of Care Chemotherapy Alone in Treatment of Participants With Untreated Inoperable or Metastatic Urothelial Cancer
NCT04223856	Enfortumab Vedotin and Pembrolizumab vs. Chemotherapy Alone in Untreated Locally Advanced or Metastatic Urothelial Cancer
NCT03661320	ENERGIZE: A Phase 3 Study of Neoadjuvant Chemotherapy Alone or With Nivolumab With/Without Linrodostat Mesylate for Muscle-Invasive Bladder Cancer
NCT03924856	Perioperative Pembrolizumab (MK-3475) Plus Neoadjuvant Chemotherapy Versus Perioperative Placebo Plus Neoadjuvant Chemotherapy for Cisplatin-Eligible Muscle-Invasive Bladder Cancer (MIBC; MK-3475-866/KEYNOTE-866)
NCT03924895	Perioperative Pembrolizumab (MK-3475) Plus Cystectomy or Perioperative Pembrolizumab Plus Enfortumab Vedotin Plus Cystectomy Versus Cystectomy Alone in Cisplatin-Ineligible Participants With Muscle-Invasive Bladder Cancer (MK-3475-905/KEYNOTE-905/EV-303)
PROSTATE CANCER	
NCT03061539 (Phase 2)	Nivolumab and Ipilimumab Treatment in Prostate Cancer With an Immunogenic Signature (NEPTUNES)

(continued)

Table 52.2 Select Ongoing Phase 3 Clinical Trials in Genitourinary Oncology (*continued*)

TRIAL REGISTRATION	TITLE
PROSTATE CANCER	
NCT02601014 (Phase 2)	Biomarker-Driven Therapy With Nivolumab and Ipilimumab in Treating Patients With Metastatic Hormone-Resistant Prostate Cancer Expressing AR-V7 (STARVE-PC)
NCT03834493	Study of Pembrolizumab (MK-3475) Plus Enzalutamide Versus Placebo Plus Enzalutamide in Participants With Metastatic Castration-Resistant Prostate Cancer (mCRPC; MK-3475-641/KEYNOTE-641)

mCRPC in asymptomatic or minimally symptomatic patients on the basis of clinical trials demonstrating an OS benefit compared to placebo.[80]

The process of developing and administering sipuleucel-T is complex. Briefly, a patient's peripheral blood mononuclear cells are extracted via leukapheresis, and CD54+ antigen-presenting cells (APCs) including DCs are isolated and exposed in vitro to a recombinant immunogenic fusion protein, PA2024, consisting of the PAP–GM-CSF fusion protein. These activated cells are subsequently infused into the patients approximately 3 days after being extracted with the goal of using the GM-CSF immune activation to stimulate the T cell immune response to the PAP antigen. The process is repeated every 2 weeks for a total of three treatments.

Phase 1 and 2 clinical trials demonstrated the safety of and objective responses to sipuleucel-T.[130,131] Subsequently, two small Phase 3 trials, D9901 ($n = 127$) and D9902A ($n = 98$), were conducted in which patients were randomized in 2:1 ratio to receive sipuleucel-T or placebo.[128,131] Both trials enrolled patients with mCRPC who were on continuous androgen deprivation therapy (ADT) and only if they had already undergone bilateral orchiectomy, and excluded patients with cancer-related bone pain and those who had visceral metastases. The primary endpoint for both studies was time to progression (TTP) as defined by PD on serial imaging, new pain that correlated with radiographic finding, or clinical events associated with PD such as pathological fracture, cord compression, and so on.

A combined analysis from D9901 and D9902A (which was prematurely terminated when TTP results from D9901 became available) was conducted.[128] In the combined analysis, 147 patients received sipuleucel-T and 78 received placebo. The median TTP did not significantly differ between the sipuleucel-T and the placebo cohorts

(11.1 vs. 9.7 months; HR 1.26, 95% CI 0.95–1.68, log-rank $p = .111$) although the exploratory OS analysis statistically favored the patients (23.2 vs. 18.9 months; 95% HR 1.50, CI 1.10–2.05, $p = .011$).

Given these findings, the Immunotherapy for Prostate Adenocarcinoma Treatment (IMPACT) multicenter, double-blind, placebo-controlled, Phase 3 trial enrolled 512 mCRPC patients to receive sipuleucel-T or placebo in a 2:1 ratio with OS as the primary endpoint.[80] The inclusion criteria and treatment plan (every 2 weeks for three treatments) were similar to the earlier studies. Median OS was 25.8 months in the sipuleucel-T group compared to 21.7 months in the patients receiving placebo for a relative risk reduction for the death of 22% (HR 0.78, 95% CI 0.61–0.98, $p = .03$). The OS differences between the cohorts were significant regardless of subsequent therapy. Similar to the D9901 and D9902A studies, the TTP was similar between the two cohorts.[80] Based on these trials, sipuleucel-T received FDA approval on April 29, 2010, for the treatment of minimally symptomatic or asymptomatic nonvisceral mCRPC.

There are a number of factors to be considered with the use of sipuleucel-T. First, there are a number of toxicities associated with this therapy; more than 95% of patients will experience an AE, although most are low grade. In a combined review of 601 patients treated with sipuleucel-T, the most common AEs of any grade occurring in more than 20% of patients were chills (51%), fatigue (41%), fever (31%), back pain (30%), and nausea (22%). The most common AEs of grade 3 or higher were back pain (3%) and chills (2.2%).[132] Also of importance is that despite the survival advantage with sipuleucel-T, the clinical trials did not indicate a benefit with regard to progression as determined by prostate-specific antigen (PSA) levels or radiographic findings. This presents a challenge to patients and clinicians alike as there is no objective measure by which to monitor the impact of therapy on individual patients. Additionally, the use of sipuleucel-T and its appropriate timing in the sequence of multiple approved therapies for mCRPC including oral agents such as enzalutamide and abiraterone remains ill defined. Regardless of the limitations, sipuleucel-T remains the only FDA-approved immunotherapy for prostate cancer.

PSA-TRICOM (PROSTVAC-VF)

PSA-TRICOM is a vaccine that consists of fowlpox and vaccinia virus vectors containing the *PSA* gene and three co-stimulatory transgenes (leukocyte function-associated antigen 3, B7-1, and intracellular adhesion molecule 1). The hypothesis is that the PSA serves as an antigen, which in combination with co-stimulatory molecules can enhance the T cell cytotoxic response to prostate cancer.

A randomized Phase 2 trial was conducted in which 125 patients with minimally symptomatic mCRPC were randomized in 2:1 ratio to receive PROSTVAC-VF and GM-CSF or to receive empty vectors plus placebo GM-CSF.[129] PFS was the primary endpoint of the study with no significant difference between the mPFS of 3.8 months in the PROSTVAC-VF patients and 3.7 months in the placebo arm (HR:0.88, 95% CI 0.57–1.38, $p = .6$). However, the secondary endpoint of OS did achieve statistical significance with a longer mOS in patients treated with PROSTVAC-VF compared to placebo (25.1 vs. 16.6 months; HR 0.56, 95% CI 0.37–0.85, $p = .0061$). The toxicity profile was notable for injection site reactions, fatigue, fever, and nausea.

A Phase 3 trial comparing PROSTVAC-VF and GM-CSF (arm VG), PROSTVAC-VF plus saline injection (arm VG), and a vaccine placebo (arm P) was subsequently conducted.[133] Each arm had over 430 patients and the primary endpoint was OS. The key secondary endpoint was patients alive without events (AWE, defined as pain or radiographic progression, initiation of chemotherapy, or death). The trial was stopped early because futility criteria were reached at the third interim analysis. There was no difference in mOS among the three arms (VG: 33.2 months; V: 34.4 months; P: 34.3 months). Likewise, AWE at 6 months was similar among the groups (VG: 28.0%; V: 29.4%; P: 30.3). As such, this treatment regimen is not likely to be approved as monotherapy.

GVAX

GVAX is a prostate cancer vaccine that is comprised of two irradiated prostate cancer cell lines (LNCaP and PC-3) genetically engineered to express GM-CSF. Phase 1 and 2 trials demonstrated safety and efficacy in patients with mCRPC.[134,135] Subsequently, two Phase 3 trials were conducted investigating the role of GVAX in advanced prostate cancer. In 2004, the Vaccine Immunotherapy With Allogenic Prostate Cancer Cell Lines 1 (VITAL-1) trial was initiated in which patients with asymptomatic chemotherapy-naïve mCRPC were randomized to receive either GVAX or docetaxel and prednisone.[136] In 2005, the VITAL-2 trial opened in which patients with symptomatic mCRPC were randomized to receive GVAX and docetaxel versus standard docetaxel and prednisone.[137]

Both trials were prematurely terminated. The VITAL-1 trial was closed when in August 2008 an independent safety monitoring committee noted 67 deaths in the GVAX and docetaxel arm compared to only 47 deaths in the docetaxel/prednisone cohort. In October 2008, VITAL-2 was terminated when investigators declared that the study was unlikely to meet its primary endpoint.[136–138] There are a variety of explanations for the results of these trials including no placebo arm in VITAL-1 and a lack of optimal data for the combination of GVAX and chemotherapy in VITAL-2.[138] Regardless of the rationale, GVAX is not approved as a vaccine, highlighting the complexity of vaccine development and approval in advanced prostate cancer.

Checkpoint Inhibitors

Ipilimumab has been investigated as a potential immunotherapy for prostate cancer. The use of ipilimumab in this setting was based on studies that noted significant T cell infiltration in prostate cancer tissue, suggesting that enhancement of the T cell response with CPIs could lead to improved outcomes.[139] Indeed, early preclinical models investigating ipilimumab were conducted in prostate cancer.[140] A Phase 1/2 dose-escalation study of ipilimumab in chemotherapy-treated and chemotherapy-naïve patients with mCRPC demonstrated safety and efficacy.[141]

As such, the CA 184-043, Phase 3, randomized, double-blind, multicenter study was conducted. This study enrolled patients with mCRPC who had at least one site of bone metastases and had progressed on docetaxel therapy. Seven hundred and ninety-nine patients were randomized to receive 8 Gy of radiation to at least one bone site, followed by either ipilimumab 10 mg/kg or placebo once every 3 weeks for a maximum of four doses with an option for maintenance ipilimumab or placebo every 3 months in nonprogressing patients who were tolerating therapy well.[142] The decision to use ipilimumab postradiotherapy was based on data that the immune system activity is enhanced by radiotherapy, and is thus potentially primed for anti-CTLA agents.[143] The primary endpoint was OS.[142]

The toxicity profile from ipilimumab in this study was similar to other ipilimumab clinical trials with diarrhea (51%), fatigue (38%), and nausea (32%) the most common AEs in the treatment group. There were also four treatment-related deaths (1%) in ipilimumab-treated patients. The primary endpoint of mOS did not statistically differ between the ipilimumab and placebo groups (11.2 vs. 10.0 months; HR 0.85, 95% CI 0.72–1.00, $p = 0.053$).[142] It should be noted, however, that a secondary analysis of OS revealed high numbers of early deaths in the ipilimumab cohort. As a result, the HR for deaths for ipilimumab versus placebo favored the ipilimumab cohort from 5 to 12 months (HR 0.65, 95% CI 0.50–0.85) and beyond 12 months (HR 0.60, 95% CI 0.43–0.86).[142] Additionally, there was an improvement in the secondary endpoint of PFS and exploratory endpoint of PSA response favoring the ipilimumab patients. Although no definitive conclusions can be drawn from this secondary OS analysis and secondary endpoints, these data may suggest enough clinical activity and benefit for investigation in future studies.

A second study of ipilimumab in chemotherapy-naïve mCRPC patients was subsequently conducted in which close to 600 patients were randomized to receive ipilimumab or placebo with a primary endpoint of OS.[144] The median OS did not significantly differ between the ipilimumab (mOS 28.7 months) and placebo (29.7 months) arms. The mPFS favored ipilimumab (5.6 vs. 3.8 months; HR 0.67; 95.87% CI 0.55–0.81). However, given the lack of OS benefit, ipilimumab is not approved as monotherapy in mCRPC.

In addition to the clinical activity of ipilimumab monotherapy, there is some activity for pembrolizumab in patients with mCRPC. However, ORR (5%–37%) and mOS (7.9–14.1 months) are modest.[145,146] As such, CPI monotherapy is not approved for patients with metastatic prostate cancer. Importantly, however, pembrolizumab monotherapy may be used based on the tumor agnostic approval in patients with microsatellite instability-high (MSI-H), mismatch repair deficient (dMMR), or with a tumor mutational burden (TMB) of ≥10 m/MB.

Given the clinical activity—despite negative OS results—in ipilimumab monotherapy trials in mCRPC, investigation into the combination of ipilimumab and nivolumab in mCRPC. The Checkmate 650 trial was a Phase 2 trial that enrolled two cohorts of mCRPC patients: those who had not received prior chemotherapy (Cohort 1; $n = 45$) and patients who had received prior chemotherapy (Cohort 2; $n = 45$).[147] The median follow-up for cohort 1 was 11.9 months and for cohort 2 13.5 months. The ORR and OS were higher in cohort 1 (25%, 19 months) than cohort 2 (10%, 15.2 months). The regimen was relatively well tolerated with Gr ≥ 3 TRAEs 42.2% and 53.3% in cohorts 1 and 2, respectively.

Interestingly, patients with tumoral PD-L1 ≥ 1 had higher ORR, PSA response, radiographic PFS, and OS compared with those patients whose PD-L1 <1. Similar findings were noted when comparing patients with TMB above the median with those whose tumor had TMB below the median. As such, although the clinical activity is relatively modest on the overall population, a subset of patients based on PD-L1 expression and PD-L1 positivity may have improved responses. Other trials of ipilimumab and nivolumab in mCRPC include STARVE-PC and NEPTUNES.[148,149] Results are pending.

In addition to the combination of two CPIs, other agents are being investigated in combination with CPI with the hypothesis that alternative agents can serve as improved partners for checkpoint blockade. For example, the androgen receptor inhibitor enzalutamide has the potential to enhance IFN-γ signaling which can produce a more immunopermissive tumor microenvironment, thereby sensitizing tumors to immunotherapy. As such, the Phase 3 IMbassador250 trial was conducted in which patients with mCRPC were randomized to receive atezolizumab plus enzalutamide versus atezolizumab alone. The primary endpoint was OS. Key secondary endpoints were ORR, rPFS, PSA response rate, and safety.[150]

A total of 759 patients were randomized. There was no difference in OS between the atezolizumab/enzalutamide and enzalutamide groups (15.2 vs. 16.6 months;

HR 1.12, 95% CI 0.91–1.37; p = 0.28. All grade TRAEs (77.8% vs. 51.1%) and those grade ≥3 (30.2% vs. 9.9%) were generally consistent with the atezolizumab and enzalutamide.[150] Although this combination is safe, the role of CPI and novel hormonal agents in mCRPC is unclear. KEYNOTE-641 comparing pembrolizumab/enzalutamide versus pembrolizumab alone is ongoing.[151]

Future Directions

Given the multiple inherent antigens in prostate cancer, it is hypothesized that immunotherapy would be a natural treatment option for these patients. As such, although the only currently approved immunotherapy is sipuleucel-T, additional studies are being conducted to further define the role of immunotherapy in prostate cancer. One particular challenge with immunotherapy in advanced prostate cancer is the recent approval of oral therapies that are easily administered, have minimal side effects, and have demonstrated a survival benefit in clinical trials.[152,153] The benefit of immunotherapy is often in low volume and low PSA prostate cancer,[80] and these patients already have a variety of treatment options in the mCRPC state. The multiple unimpressive results listed previously such as ipilimumab/nivolumab and atezolizumab/enzalutamide in mCRPC underscore the challenge of immunotherapy in this setting. The question of whether the lack of benefit is a result of an inherently immunotherapy-resistant tumor or simply that the appropriate immunotherapy/androgen-directed partnership has not yet been defined will be answered with further clinical trials. However, despite challenges in the development of immunotherapy in this setting, further advances with CPIs, vaccines, and other immune modulators are ongoing. With the recent approval of oral agents, clinical trials for immunotherapy in prostate cancer will need to incorporate the timing and combinations of immunotherapies with novel antiandrogens to optimize durable responses for patients.

CONCLUSION

The dampening of the immune system in the setting of malignancy is a primary mechanism of cancer growth and proliferation. The goal of immunotherapy is to stimulate and enhance the innate immune system to control and eradicate cancer. In GU oncology, immunotherapy has been a focus of treatment and research for decades. Bladder, prostate, and renal cancers all have immunotherapeutic agents approved to treat metastatic disease including cytokine therapy, vaccines, and immune CPIs. Similarly, bladder cancer has a local immunotherapy (BCG) approved for the treatment and prevention of localized disease and recurrence.

Despite recent advances in GU immunotherapy, there are a number of important considerations in the discovery and development of novel immunotherapeutics. Most of these malignancies have proven chemotherapies and targeted agents with acceptable toxicities that have clear clinical benefit. The timing, sequencing, combinations, and new immunotherapies in the context of multiple lines of established therapies need to be optimized. Biomarkers are also critically needed to identify those patients likely to benefit from immunotherapy versus cytotoxic agents. Although there are limitations in current GU malignancy immunotherapies, the success of the last few years produces great optimism for the future.

KEY REFERENCES

Only key references appear in the print edition. The full reference list appears in the digital product on Springer Publishing Connect: connect.springerpub.com/content/book/978-0-8261-3743-2/part/part04/chapter/ch52

30. Motzer RJ, Tannir NM, Mcdermott DF, et al. Nivolumab plus ipilimumab versus sunitinib in advanced renal-cell carcinoma. *N Engl J Med Overseas Ed.* 2018;378(14):1277–1290. doi:10.1056/NEJMoa1712126
38. Rini BI, Plimack ER, Stus V, et al. Pembrolizumab plus axitinib versus sunitinib for advanced renal-cell carcinoma. *N Engl J Med.* 2019;380(12):1116–1127. doi:10.1056/NEJMoa1816714
77. Balar AV, Castellano D, O'Donnell PH, et al. First-line pembrolizumab in cisplatin-ineligible patients with locally advanced and unresectable or metastatic urothelial cancer (keynote-052): a multicentre, single-arm, Phase 2 study. *Lancet Oncol.* 2017;18(11):1483–1492. doi:10.1016/S1470-2045(17)30616-2
78. Powles T, Park SH, Voog E, et al. Avelumab maintenance therapy for advanced or metastatic urothelial carcinoma. *N Engl J Med.* 2020;383(13):1218–1230. doi:10.1056/NEJMoa2002788
80. Kantoff PW, Higano CS, Shore ND, et al. Sipuleucel-T immunotherapy for castration-resistant prostate cancer. *N Engl J Med.* 2010;363(5):411–422. doi:10.1056/NEJMoa1001294
87. Bellmunt J, de Wit R, Vaughn DJ, et al. Pembrolizumab as second-line therapy for advanced urothelial carcinoma. *N Engl J Med.* 2017;376(11):1015–1026. doi:10.1056/NEJMoa1613683

Immunotherapy in Gastrointestinal Malignancies

Dave R. Gupta, Usha Malhotra, and Mihir M. Shah

KEY POINTS

- Comprehensive genomic evaluation of colon and gastric cancers has characterized distinct molecular subtypes with potential therapeutic consequences.

- Multiple trials are ongoing to establish the role of checkpoint inhibitors as monotherapy as well as in combination with other agents in gastric, esophageal, and colon cancers.

- Programmed cell death protein 1 (PD-1) and programmed death ligand 1 (PD-L1)-directed therapy has shown a response in the refractory gastric cancer population. Ongoing trials will establish the role of these agents in molecularly predefined gastric cancer subtypes.

- Checkpoint inhibition has shown promising results in microsatellite instability-high (MSI-H) colorectal cancer. Studies are ongoing to define the appropriate timing and combination strategy with these agents.

- Checkpoint inhibition has demonstrated significant survival benefit in second-line locally advanced, unresectable, and metastatic esophageal and GE-junction cancers with PD-L1 expression or squamous cell histology. Ongoing studies aim to define optimal timing and therapy combinations.

- MSI, PD-1/PD-L1 expression, and Epstein–Barr virus (EBV) status are potential biomarkers predictive of response to immune checkpoint inhibitors (ICIs) in gastrointestinal cancers.

INTRODUCTION

Immunotherapy refers to therapeutic management that targets elements of the immune system to enhance eradication of cancer cells. Various immunological approaches, such as vaccines, cytokines, adoptive cell therapy, and so on, have been evaluated as possible therapy options in cancer. Mechanism of immune evasion and generation of immune tolerance by tumor cells has been an area of active research over the past several decades. Immune activation in response to foreign antigens and immune cell downregulation to prevent the destruction of normal tissues is achieved by a complex network of signaling cascades with inhibitory checkpoints like cytotoxic T lymphocyte antigen 4 (CTLA-4) and programmed cell death protein 1 (PD-1).[1] The main downstream effectors of immune response are T lymphocytes that harbor the checkpoint receptors. Cancer cells escape immune detection and eradication by modulating membrane-bound ligands which interact with these checkpoint receptors.[2] Checkpoint inhibitors restore T cell activity against tumor cells by blocking the interaction between these receptors and ligands. Three major classes of checkpoint inhibitors used in cancer therapy are the antibodies directed to CTLA-4, PD-1, and programmed death ligand 1 (PD-L1). Clinical benefit of this class of agents in melanoma[3] and lung cancer,[4] among others, has led to the active investigation of PD-1-directed therapy as a therapeutic tool in gastrointestinal cancers. In this chapter, we aim to review the emerging role of the PD-L1/PD-1 blockade in gastric cancer (GC) and the impact of immunotherapy on microsatellite instability-high (MSI-H) colorectal carcinoma (CRC).

IMMUNE-MODULATORY TARGETS IN GASTRIC CANCER MOLECULAR SUBTYPES

GC is the fifth most common malignancy in the world, with almost 1 million new cases annually. It is the third leading cause of cancer death worldwide, with around 723,000 deaths each year.[5] Extensive regional variation is observed in the incidence of GC, with a predominance of the disease in Asia, Eastern Europe, and South America

Author's Disclosure: Dr. Usha Malhotra is the clinical director at Merck & Co. (the pharmaceutical company that developed pembrolizumab) since December 2018.

Table 53.1 Molecular Subtypes of Gastric Cancer

MOLECULAR SUBTYPE	PERCENTAGE (%)	PREDOMINANT HISTOLOGICAL PHENOTYPE	MOLECULAR CHARACTERISTICS
EBV	9	Medullary features, nest of tumors, no clear gland formation	PIK3CA mutation, JAK 2 amplification, POL1/2 overexpression, EBV-CIMP, CDKN2A silencing, immune cell signaling
CIN	50	Intestinal, proximal predominance	TP53 mutation, RTK-RAS activation, HER2 amplification
GS	20	Diffuse	CDH1, RHOA mutations, CLDN18-APHGAP fusion, cell adhesion
MSI	22	Distal predominance, intestinal	Hypermutation, gastric CIMP, MLH1 silencing, mitotic pathways

CIMP, CpG island methylator phenotype; CIN, chromosomal instability; EBV, Epstein–Barr virus; GS, genomically stable; HER, human epidermal growth factor receptor; MSI, microsatellite instability; RTK-RAS, receptor tyrosine kinase/Ras GTPase.

that has been attributed to various environmental and genetic factors.

In recent years, with the advent of next-generation sequencing and advanced bioinformatics algorithms, the molecular basis of gastric carcinogenesis and its correlation with pathological phenotype have been better elucidated. Under The Cancer Genome Atlas (TCGA) project, a comprehensive molecular evaluation of 295 therapy-naïve fresh frozen primary gastric adenocarcinoma samples was performed. Based on this data, GC has been classified into four distinct molecular phenotypes: EBV[+], MSI, genomically stable, and chromosomal instability (see Table 53.1).[6] The EBV subtype represented 9% of the patients in this cohort. The EBV subtype demonstrated extreme DNA hypermethylation, recurrent PIK3CA mutations, and amplification of Janus kinase 2 (JAK 2), CD 274 (PD-L1), and PDCD1LG2 (PD-L2). The MSI subtype accounted for 22% of the patients and harbored high tumor mutational burden, including mutations involving targetable signals.[6] The genomically stable variant has a predominance of diffuse histology and mutations involving *RHOA* and *CDH1* genes. Chromosomal instability subtype display marked aneuploidy and receptor tyrosine kinase amplifications. The EBV and MSI subtypes have been of great interest due to the potentially therapeutic efficacy of PD-1/PD-L1-directed agents. In addition to EBV and MSI status, expression of PD-1/PD-L1 has also been proposed as a predictive biomarker of response to checkpoint inhibition. In KEYNOTE-012, a pivotal trial showing the activity of PD-1–directed therapy in GC, 40% of the patients screened were found to be PD-L1[+], and 17% of the analyzed samples had MSI. The EBV status was not collected in this study.[7] This is consistent with other studies, where PD-1/PD-L1 positivity is reported to be as high as 40% in GC.[8–12] Rich lymphocytic infiltrate is found in tumor stroma of GC associated with EBV[+] or MSI.[13] The lymphoid stroma has abundant CD8[+] T cells that can mount a strong antitumor immune response.[14–16] A study from the department of pathology at the University of Pittsburgh Medical Center concluded

that EBV[+] or MSI GCs are more likely to express PD-L1 and have increased CD8[+] T cells at the invasive tumor front (ITF) compared to EBV[-]/microsatellite stable (MSS) cancers. In the same study, PD-L1 expression was not associated with depth of invasion or nodal metastasis. On multivariate analysis, although MSI was an independent predictor of disease-free survival, PD-L1 was not found to be associated with the clinical outcome.[17] PD-L1 expression in tumor results in an increase in apoptosis of antigen-specific T cells in vitro.[18] An increase in antitumor immunity and inhibition of tumor growth has been noted in vivo with PD-L1 blockade.[19–21] PD-L1 is expressed on T cells, B cells, natural killer (NK) cells, dendritic cells (DCs), monocytes/macrophages, mast cells, and various tumor types, where it may play a potential role in tumor immune escape.[22] Hence, the PD-1 blockade may enhance the NK cell activity in tumors and may increase the antibody production due to its effect on the PD-1[+] B cells.[23] A state of exhaustion or energy among cognate antigen-specific T cells induced by elevated levels of persistent PD-1 expression can occur from chronic antigen exposure (viral or tumoral). It seems this state is partially reversible by blockade of the PD-1 pathway.[24] These observations provide a rationale for antitumor activity of checkpoint inhibitors.

EARLY CLINICAL DATA WITH CHECKPOINT INHIBITORS IN GASTRIC CANCER

Agents directed against CTLA-4 and PD-1 are under active clinical investigation for GC. The first agent evaluated in this class was tremelimumab, an anti-CTLA-4 antibody, as a second-line therapy for advanced gastroesophageal cancer (GEC) in a Phase 2 trial.[25] This trial enrolled 18 patients, and although it failed to meet its primary efficacy endpoint, one patient had a durable partial response and remained on the study for 32 months, prompting additional evaluation of these agents. Another study was presented at the American Society of Clinical Oncology Annual Meeting (ASCO 2016). This Phase 2 trial compared the efficacy of sequential ipilimumab, another anti-CTLA-4 antibody, versus best supportive care following first-line chemotherapy in advanced GC (NCT01585987). Patients with advanced GC were randomized to best supportive care or ipilimumab for up to 3 years after completion of first-line chemotherapy. The primary endpoint of this study was immune-related progression-free survival (PFS). After enrolling 114 patients and performing the first interim analysis, the study was closed and data were analyzed. The authors concluded that there was no improvement in immune-related PFS or overall survival (OS) with ipilimumab. The toxicity profile was similar to other studies using ipilimumab.[26] A Phase 1b/2 study evaluating tremelimumab and durvalumab, an anti-PD-L1 antibody, as single agents and in combination revealed similarly low response and survival rates in advanced GC.

Pembrolizumab is the first PD-1 blocking antibody, which has shown efficacy in a large cohort of GEC patients. KEYNOTE-012 was a Phase 1b study with a cohort of PD-L1+ advanced GC refractory to standard of care therapies.[7] The PD-L1 assessment was based on immunohistochemistry (IHC) and was considered positive if at least 1% of cells expressed PD-L1 (which included tumor cells and contiguous inflammatory cells) or if a distinctive interface pattern was detected. A total of 162 patients with refractory advanced GC were screened, and 65 patients (40%) were found to be positive for PD-L1. Thirty-nine patients were enrolled to receive single-agent pembrolizumab at a dose of 10 mg/kg intravenously every 2 weeks. An ORR of 22.2% by central review and 33.0% by investigator review was reported in this refractory patient population. In patients who had at least one post-baseline tumor assessment, 53% (17/32) showed a decrease in target lesions. No complete responses were observed. Median time to response was 8 weeks based on the central review. Eighty-five percent of the enrolled patients discontinued pembrolizumab, almost all due to disease progression. A PFS of 1.9 months and an OS of 11.4 months with a manageable safety profile were reported.

KEYNOTE-028, another Phase 1b study, evaluated single-agent pembrolizumab in PD-L1+ advanced solid tumors. In the GEC cohort, a total of 90 patients who experienced disease progression on standard-of-care therapy were screened and 37 patients (41%) were found to be positive for PD-L1. Twenty-three patients were enrolled and treated with pembrolizumab 10 mg/kg every 2 weeks for up to 2 years. Seventy-seven percent of the patients had squamous cell carcinoma, 18% adenocarcinoma, and 5% mucoepidermoid histology. Four patients (7.4%) experienced grade 3 adverse events (AEs) related to the study drug. Total treatment-related adverse events (TRAEs) of all grades were reported in nine patients (39.1%). The toxicity profile was considered to be manageable. An ORR of 30% and stable disease rate of 13% was observed. The median duration of response was 40 weeks (24.1–46.1), with five of the seven responses maintained at the time of data cutoff.[27]

In addition to pembrolizumab, nivolumab, a human IgG4 anti-PD-1 monoclonal antibody, has also been evaluated for GC. CheckMate-032, a Phase 1/2 trial, enrolled patients with stage IV GC or GEC into three arms: nivolumab monotherapy 3 mg/kg IV (NIVO3) every 2 weeks, combination therapy of nivolumab 1 mg/kg plus ipilimumab 3 mg/kg IV (NIVO1 + IPI3) every 3 weeks for four cycles, or nivolumab 3 mg/kg with ipilimumab 1 mg/kg IV (NIVO3 + IPI1) every 3 weeks for four cycles. Both combination therapy arms were followed by nivolumab monotherapy (NIVO3) every 2 weeks. Respectively, each arm resulted in a median OS of 6.2 versus 6.9 versus 4.8 months, and 1-year-survival of 39% versus 35% versus 24% (NIVO3 vs. NIVO1 + IPI3 vs. NIVO3 + IPI1). Combination therapies did report higher severe TRAEs, occurring in 10% versus 43% versus 25% of patients in these respective arms, which were largely manageable and reversible. The NIVO1 + IPI3 regimen has been selected to be further evaluated in a Phase 3 clinical trial for GEC.[28]

In another Phase 1b study, JAVELIN, patients with advanced GC or GEC received avelumab (anti-PD-L1 antibody) 10 mg/kg every 2 weeks as maintenance therapy after induction with cytotoxic chemotherapy. Twelve percent of the patients had grade 3 or higher treatment-related or treatment-emergent AEs. In the chemotherapy refractory group, the median PFS was 36 weeks, and 11.6 weeks for PD-L1+ and PD-L1– patients, respectively. In the group that did not progress on first-line chemotherapy, median PFS values were 17.6 and 11.6 weeks, for the PDL-1+ and PD-1– cohorts, respectively. The median PFS was longer in PD-L1+ patients, although objective responses and disease stabilization were noted in both groups.[29]

OTHER IMMUNE-MODULATORY APPROACHES IN GASTRIC CANCER

Bacterial Agents

The role of immunomodulation and utilization of innate immune response as a therapeutic approach for cancer has been studied over many decades. Bacillus Calmette–Guérin (BCG) was evaluated as early as the 1960s as a potential anticancer agent.[30] In a study for stage I to IV GC, 140 patients underwent gastrectomy followed by adjuvant chemotherapy with 5-fluorouracil (5-FU), cytosine arabinoside, and mitomycin C (FAM: 10 weekly doses) with or without BCG vaccine weekly for 2 months. Improved survival was noted in patients who received both in comparison to patients who did not receive adjuvant therapy, suggesting a possible role of immuno-therapy.[31] A similar study in stage III to IV GC patients randomized 156 patients to receive immunochemother-apy [FAM + BCG], chemotherapy, or observation after curative-intent surgery. This study showed that patients who received immunochemotherapy had an improved 10-year survival of 47%, compared with 30% in patients who received adjuvant chemotherapy alone. Survival was poor (15.2%) in patients in the observation arm with no adjuvant therapy after surgery.[32]

OK-432, a lyophilized mixture of group A *Streptococcus pyogenes* Su strain treated with benzylpenicillin, was also evaluated in GC. In this study, 287 patients were random-ized to doxifluridine (5'-DFUR) or combination therapy of 5'-DFUR and OK-432 after gastric resection with cura-tive intent. Combination therapy did not improve 5-year survival in locally advanced GC patients.[33]

Toll-Like Receptor Agonists

Toll-like receptors (TLRs) have an established role in recognition of invading microbial pathogens and gener-ation of an immune response. Their potential utility as modulators of innate immune response against cancer cells is still not clearly elucidated. TLR agonists have been evaluated in the treatment of GC. Polyadenylic-polyuridylic acid (pA-pU), a synthetic double-stranded complex of polyribonucleotides, is a TL3-agonist. In a Phase 3 trial for localized GC, immunochemotherapy (5-FU, adriamycin, and pA-pU) was associated with sig-nificantly improved 15-year survival of 50.1% compared with 38.1% for chemotherapy alone (5-FU and adria-mycin). Locally advanced GC patients or patients with increased lymph node (LN) disease burden had the most survival benefit on subset analysis.[34]

Adoptive Cell Therapy

Adoptive cell therapy involves expansion of tumor-spe-cific T cells ex vivo followed by infusion into patients for a more robust anticancer T cell response. Multiple techniques based on adoptive cells are currently under evaluation. In a study evaluating this approach in patients with advanced GC, the combination of chemo-therapy (5-FU + cisplatin + doxifluridine) and adoptive cell therapy with tumor-associated lymphocytes (TALs) improved the survival to 11.5 months compared with 8.3 months with chemotherapy alone. In this study, all patients underwent surgery, and tumor-associated lym-phocytes were obtained from the surgical specimen. After ex vivo expansion, TALs were administered to autolo-gous donors. The survival benefit was not influenced by clinical or pathological factors.[35] In another study, when autologous cytokine-induced killer (CIK) cells were administered to locally advanced GC patients after gas-trectomy and adjuvant 5-FU–based chemotherapy, the

median OS was higher at 48.1 months compared to 42.1 months with observation after surgery and 5-FU-based chemotherapy. Subset analysis showed that immuno-therapy was beneficial particularly for intestinal-type GC and not advantageous for diffuse or mixed-type GC.[36]

Vaccines

Vaccines stimulate the immune system to generate a humoral/cellular response. Protein-bound polysaccha-ride K (PSK), derived from the CM-101 strain of the fun-gus *Coriolus versicolor*, was used as a tumor vaccine in GC. It was administered to patients after gastrectomy for stage II/III GC. Two hundred and fifty-four patients received adjuvant oral fluoropyrimidine chemother-apy or immunochemotherapy (chemotherapy + PSK). Though the 5-year survival rates were equivalent in both arms, the patients with LN disease had an improved 5-year OS of 47.8% with immunochemotherapy com-pared to 22.8% with chemotherapy.[37]

In a later Phase 2 multicenter study, patients with metastatic or unresectable GC or GEC received G17DT (nine-amino acid epitope derived from gastrin-17) with chemotherapy (cisplatin/5-FU). Sixty-nine percent of the patients who developed an immune response (respond-ers) had a longer time to progression, with median OS of 10.3 months compared to 3.8 months for nonresponders.[38] In another Phase 1/2 trial, 22 patients with advanced GC, HLA-A24-restricted vascular endothelial growth factor receptor (VEGFR)-1, and VEGFR-2 vaccines were admin-istered with S1 and cisplatin chemotherapy. The partial response rate was 55%, with median time to progression of 9.6 months and median OS of 14.2 months. Better response rates were documented in patients who showed increased cytotoxic T lymphocytes in response to the vaccine.[39]

ROLE OF PROGRAMMED CELL DEATH 1/ PROGRAMMED DEATH LIGAND 1 INHIBITION IN GASTRIC CANCER

Although multiple approaches to modulate and activate immune pathways have been evaluated, checkpoint inhi-bition with PD-1/PD-L1-directed therapy has shown the most promising results that appear to be clinically relevant. As detailed earlier, Phase 1 trials using pembrolizumab monotherapy have shown response rates of 20% to 30% in refractory GC after failure of standard-of-care therapy. Available studies report PD-L1 expression in about 40% of GCs.[8-12] Based on the TCGA analysis, two potential molec-ular subtypes that may derive benefit from immune-di-rected therapy (EBV+ and MSI subtype) account for 30% of the GCs. Hence, based on available data, there are a substantial proportion of patients that can potentially benefit from PD-1/PD-L1-directed therapy. This has led to considerable interest in evaluating this class of agents in GC, and a number of studies are ongoing.

Preclinical and mechanistic data support a possible synergistic effect in combination with chemotherapy and radiation. Although the primary mechanism of radiation is DNA damage and cell death, it has been shown that radiation has an immunomodulatory effect, with increased expression of immunogenic antigens on tumor cells and alterations in the tumor microenvironment (TME).[40–42] Studies have also reported direct and indirect utilization of innate and adaptive immune systems in addition to direct cell injury by cytotoxic chemotherapy agents.[43,44] This data has provided the scientific basis on which to evaluate PD-1/PD-L1-directed therapy in combination with chemotherapy. Most of the published and ongoing studies have evaluated checkpoint inhibitors for advanced GC. The majority of GC patients treated with curative intent have a relapse within the first 3 years and succumb to the disease. It is hypothesized that metastases occur early in the course and can evade immune surveillance. Hence, early immune system modulation may potentiate eradication of disseminated cancer cells and improve clinical outcome. Thus, it may be more consequential to evaluate this modality in the adjuvant setting.

While the early data are exciting, there are a number of challenges in defining the optimal niche of immunotherapy in the treatment algorithm of GC. Unanswered questions include establishing validated biomarkers available and feasible for general clinical practice outside of research institutions; understanding the interaction between chemotherapy, other targeted therapies, and immunotherapy; and the optimal timing and sequence of different therapeutic options. At this time, the use of checkpoint inhibitors for GC remains limited to use in a clinical trial setting, but the results of ongoing studies are awaited.

ROLE OF IMMUNE MODULATION IN COLORECTAL CANCER

CRC remains a major cause of morbidity and mortality worldwide. Globally, CRC incidence is 1.4 million with a mortality of 700,000 annually.[5] Treatment has evolved over the past several decades with the availability of newer agents, including VEGF- and endothelial growth factor receptor-targeted therapy. Although some progress has been made in improving outcomes, the results are not optimal, emphasizing the need for novel approaches. The Society for Immunotherapy of Cancer (SITC) led an international consortium to evaluate the prognostic role of an Immunoscore (IM), a systematic scoring system developed by Galon et al., based on presence of CD8 positive cytotoxic T cells and CD45RO memory T cells at the tumor center and invasive margin.[45] To evaluate this tool in a routine clinical setting, analysis of 1,336 therapy-naïve stage I to III colon cancer patients was conducted by the international SITC consortium. Using

standard immunohistochemistry protocols for CD3 and CD8 detection and quantification using digital pathology, the IM was established for each patient specimen. Time to recurrence was significantly longer in stage I/II/III colon cancer patients with high IMs versus those with low IMs. The relapse rate was decreased by 50% in the presence of high IMs. Low IMs identified a high-risk subset of patients with stage II colon cancer.[46] These studies demonstrated the impact of immunomodulation on prognostic outcomes of patients with colon cancer. The impact of the Immunoscore as a predictive marker for response to immunotherapy in CRC remains undefined. However, immunotherapy presents an attractive option for CRC patients, especially those with a high IM; a variety of approaches, including vaccines, cytokines, adoptive cell therapy, and checkpoint inhibition, are currently in clinical trials.

Antitumor Vaccines

In a multicenter study of patients with metastatic CRC, 77 patients received a synthetic vaccine targeting beta-human chorionic gonadotropin (β-HCG). The vaccine contained a COOH-terminal peptide of the β-HCG (CTP37) conjugated with diphtheria toxoid (DT). The median survival for patients who demonstrated anti-HCG antibody levels greater than or equal to the median value was 45 weeks, compared with 24 weeks for patients with antibody levels lower than the median value. DT antibody levels did not have an impact on survival.[47] In a Phase 2 multicenter study, G17DT, a human immunogen that stimulates antibody production against the growth factor gastrin 17 was administered in combination with irinotecan to patients with metastatic CRC refractory to irinotecan. Survival for anti-G17 responders (based on antibody titers) was 9 months, significantly longer than 5.6 months for nonresponders.[48] In a Phase 3 prospective randomized trial, 80 eligible patients with CRC were treated with either resection and autologous tumor cell-BCG vaccine or resection alone. A significant survival benefit was noted in colon cancer patients who received BCG, but not in rectal cancer patients who received BCG.[49] A Phase 3 trial using ATV-NDV (Newcastle disease virus-infected intact autologous tumor cell vaccine) in patients after complete resection of colorectal liver metastases demonstrated that ATV-NDV was beneficial in prolonging overall and metastasis-free survival in colon cancer patients, but not in rectal cancer patients.[50]

Adoptive T Cell Therapy

A pilot study involving the use of autologous in vitro expanded lymphocytes isolated from the tumor-draining sentinel lymph node enrolled 16 patients with disseminated or locally advanced high-risk CRC. Complete tumor regression was noted in four out of nine stage IV patients. Two years and 6 months was the median survival time in stage IV patients, compared with 0.8 years in conventionally treated controls.[51] Although many of these studies have substantiated the proof of concept for immunotherapy in CRC patients, the results have not panned out in larger cohorts. In the past few years, checkpoint inhibition has shown favorable outcomes in MSI-H CRC, leading to increasing interest in this approach.

Molecular and Clinical Characteristics of Microsatellite Instability High Colorectal Cancer

Tumor transcriptome, phenotype, and clinical behavior are intimately related, as evident from multiple gene-expression studies. Increasing knowledge and understanding of molecular mechanisms and genomic alterations involved in the pathogenesis of CRC has led to the delineation of four distinct subtypes: MSI-H, canonical, metabolic, and mesenchymal (see Table 53.2).[52] MSI-H subtype accounts for 15% of early stage and 5% of advanced CRCs.[53,54] The main pathogenic mechanism in MSI-H is a deficiency in one of the mismatch repair (MMR) proteins.[55] MMR proteins involved in DNA repair include MLH1, MSH2, MSH6, and PMS2. Germline mutations or epigenetic silencing of encoding genes can result in MMR protein deficiency (dMMR). In sporadic cases of CRC with dMMR, the most common inciting event is MLH1 promoter hypermethylation, although a mutation in genes encoding for MSH2, MSH6, MLH3, PMS2, and EXO1 can also occur.[56] In contrast, Lynch syndrome (hereditary nonpolyposis colon cancer

[HNPCC]) phenotype is associated with germline mutations in non-MLH1 genes.[57,58] MMR deficiency results in accumulation of errors in repetitive DNA sequences (microsatellites); hence, MSI-H is a functional outcome of MMR deficiency. Growing literature on MSI in colon cancer and its association with Lynch syndrome highlighted the need for consensus guidelines. In 1997, a National Cancer Institute (NCI) workshop was organized to develop uniform criteria for detection and definition of MSI status, as well as to elucidate the implications of MSI status on clinical outcome and research. A set of five microsatellites was recommended as a reference panel for measuring MSI. The MSI-H was defined as instability in two or more of these markers.[59] The number of somatic mutations in dMMR CRC is 10 to 100 times the number in MMR-proficient CRC.[60-62] The MSI-H CRCs have a distinct clinical profile characterized by expansive right-sided tumors with likely mucinous differentiation and extensive infiltration with lymphocytes (TILs).[63]

It appears that patients with MSI-H early stage CRC had a favorable prognosis and a decreased risk of distant metastases.[64,65] but were not responsive to standard 5-FU-based adjuvant chemotherapy regimens.[66,67] Improved survival of MSI-H CRC and weakened response to cytotoxic chemotherapy has been attributed to heightened immune response by tumor-infiltrating T cell subsets (CD3+, CD8+, CD45RO+, and Foxp3+).[68] Immune infiltrates are reported to be a better predictor of survival in CRC compared with TNM classification.[69] On the contrary, in the metastatic setting MSI-H status has been associated with worse clinical outcome. In a pooled

Table 53.2 Consensus Molecular Subtypes (CMS) of Colon Cancer

CONSENSUS MOLECULAR SUBTYPE (CMS)	PERCENTAGE (EARLY STAGE)	PREDOMINANT HISTOLOGICAL PHENOTYPE	MOLECULAR CHARACTERISTICS	CLINICAL CHARACTERISTICS
CMS1 MSI immune	14	Solid and/or trabecular or mucinous features	High mutation burden, hypermethylation, MSI-H, BRAF mutation, immune infiltration, SCNAs low	More frequent in females; right-sided lesions, high histological grade, poor survival after relapse
CMS 2 canonical	37	Complex tubular structure	Epithelial, *WNT* and *MYC* activation, SCNAs high	Left-sided, superior survival after relapse
CMS3 metabolic	13	Papillary morphology	Epithelial, mixed MSI SCNAs low, KRAS mutations, metabolic deregulation	
CMS4 mesenchymal	23	Desmoplastic reaction with high stroma	SCNAs high, stromal infiltration, TGF activation, angiogenesis	Diagnosed at more advanced stages; worse relapse-free and overall survival
Mixed	13	Overlapping characteristics of different subtypes	Transition phenotype or intratumoral heterogeneity	

CMS, consensus molecular subtype; MSI, microsatellite instability; MSI-H, microsatellite instability high; SCNAs, somatic copy number alterations; TGF, transforming growth factor.

analysis from four Phase 3 studies for metastatic CRC (CAIRO, CAIRO2, COIN, and FOCUS), patients with MSI-H CRC were seen to have worse median PFS (6.2 vs. 7.6 months) and OS (13.6 vs. 16.8 months) compared to patients with MSS CRC.[70]

SCIENTIFIC RATIONALE AND CLINICAL DATA FOR IMMUNOTHERAPY IN MICROSATELLITE INSTABILITY HIGH COLORECTAL CANCER

MSI-H CRC has been proposed to exhibit increased immunogenicity, which has been the basis for evaluation of various immune-based therapies in this subgroup. MSI-H CRCs are prone to accumulate frameshift mutations due to dMMR proteins. These frameshift mutations lead to the production of tumor-specific peptides referred to as "neoantigens." Neoantigens have been shown to elicit a robust immune response, presumably through uptake by macrophages and DCs and subsequent priming of cytotoxic T lymphocytes.[71–74] Despite higher immunogenicity and more robust immune responses, MSI-H CRC can evade immune clearance. Mechanisms of immune evasion are proposed to be related to loss of HLA class I expression and subsequent disruption of antigen presentation and immune recognition.[75] Multiple immune checkpoints like PD-1, PD-L1, CTLA-4, and lymphocyte activation gene-3 (LAG-3), as well as metabolic immune inhibitors, such as indoleamine 2,3-dioxygenase (IDO), are shown to be significantly upregulated in MSI-H CRC, which leads to inhibition of effector T cell function and hence immune evasion.[76] Thus, the use of checkpoint blockade or IDO inhibitors is expected to restore T cell function and lead to cancer cell destruction. Thus, various immunomodulatory approaches are being evaluated in MSI-H CRC. Immune-based therapeutic options include vaccines, CTLA-4-directed therapy, or checkpoint (PD-1 and PD-L1) inhibitors and IDO inhibitors. Many trials have been conducted to evaluate the therapeutic efficacy of vaccines in CRC, although not specifically in MSI-H CRC, but results have been inconclusive.[50,77,78] The role of anti-CTLA-4 antibodies is also not clearly defined. A Phase 2 study evaluating tremelimumab in metastatic CRC reported response rates of 2%.[79] Though PD-1 inhibitors have shown encouraging results, responses have been largely restricted to MSI-H subtype. In a Phase 1 study evaluating safety and toxicity of nivolumab in advanced solid tumors, no objective responses were seen in the CRC cohort.[80]

In a Phase 2 study where 41 patients with progressive metastatic cancer received pembrolizumab monotherapy, the ORR and PFS rate were 40% and 78%, respectively, for dMMR CRC, compared to 0% and 11%, respectively, for MMR-proficient CRC.[81] Among the 10 patients with dMMR CRC, 90% had stable disease or objective response (95% confidence intervals [CIs]: 55,

100). In patients whose carcinoembrionic antigen (CEA) level could be assessed, substantial decreases in CEA levels were noted in dMMR CRC (7/10 patients) compared with MMR-proficient CRC (0/19), and the degree of reduction in CEA levels after one dose of pembrolizumab was predictive of both PFS ($p = 0.01$) and OS ($p = 0.02$). Somatic mutations per tumor were significantly higher in dMMR when compared with MMR-proficient tumors (1,782 and 73, respectively), and somatic mutation burden was positively correlated with PFS. Toxicities were manageable and similar to other studies using pembrolizumab. Most frequent toxicities included rash or pruritus (24%); thyroiditis, hypothyroidism, or hypophysitis (10%); and asymptomatic pancreatitis (15%).

In a subsequent large Phase II study called CheckMate-142, 119 patients with dMMR/MSI-H metastatic CRC with at least two prior chemotherapy regimens received combination therapy with nivolumab and ipilimumab, followed by nivolumab maintenance therapy.[82] The ORR was 54.6% with a 3.4% complete response rate. The 12-month PFS and OS rates were 71% and 87%, respectively. There was no comparison arm; however, this efficacy data compares favorably to historical controls for nivolumab monotherapy in a similar population. While the aforementioned pembrolizumab monotherapy trial featured a higher PFS, this cross-trial comparison is limited by its much smaller sample size and its high prevalence of Lynch syndrome. Safety data was similar to other studies using combination immunotherapy in solid tumors, with a 32% rate of grade 3 to 4 TRAEs including transaminitis (11%), pancreatitis (4%), anemia (3%), and colitis (3%), ultimately leading to a 13% rate of discontinuation. Interestingly, patients who discontinued treatment due to TRAEs still had favorable efficacy data, with an ORRresponse rate of 63%.

Pembrolizumab monotherapy has recently demonstrated efficacy in the first-line setting in metastatic dMMR/MSI-H CRC in the Phase 3 KEYNOTE-177 clinical trial. In the trial, 307 patients were randomized to pembrolizumab monotherapy for up to 2 years versus standard of care chemotherapy, with investigator choice of FOLFOX or FOLFIRI +/− bevacizumab or cetuximab. Pembrolizumab monotherapy demonstrated superior PFS to chemotherapy, with median PFS at 16.5 months versus 8.2 months (HR 0.60, $p=0.0002$), 12-month PFS at 55.3% versus 37.3%, and 24-month PFS at 48.3% versus 18.6%, respectively. Patients assigned to pembrolizumab experienced higher ORR, 43.8% versus 33.1%, with median DOR not reached in the pembrolizumab arm versus 10.6 months with chemotherapy. Importantly, rates of grade 3 to 5 TRAEs were also much lower in the upfront pembrolizumab arm, 22% versus 66% for chemotherapy, with 0 versus 1 treatment-related deaths.[83]

The role of neoadjuvant combination immune checkpoint inhibitor (ICI) therapy has been evaluated in a recent exploratory study in stage I to III CRC.[84] Patients with MSI CRC were given one dose of ipilimumab and two doses of nivolumab prior to surgery. Patients with MSS CRC were randomized to the same regimen with or without celecoxib. Among the patients, 35 were evaluable for treatment response. In the MSI group, 100% of patients experienced a pathologic response, with 60% experiencing a pathologic complete response (pCR). By comparison, patients with MSS CRC who received neoadjuvant combination therapy experienced a 27% rate of pathologic response, with a 13% pCR rate. Those with MSS CRC randomized to combination therapy alone experienced a 25% pathologic response rate, each of these being pCR, and those with the addition of celecoxib had a 29% pathologic response rate, with no instances of pCR. In total, 13% of patients experienced grade 3 to 4 TRAEs, which were generally manageable, with no deaths.

Multiple studies are ongoing to further evaluate the role of checkpoint inhibitors such as pembrolizumab, nivolumab, durvalumab, and atezolizumab in monotherapy or immune combination therapy in front-line, neoadjuvant, and non-metastatic CRC.

IMPACT OF IMMUNOTHERAPY ON MICROSATELLITE INSTABILITY HIGH COLORECTAL CANCER

To date, ICIs have been the only class of immunotherapeutic agents that have shown activity in MSI-H colon cancers. The basis of this activity is believed to be a high burden of tumor neoantigens, profuse infiltration by lymphocytes, and generation of an immune-responsive environment by increased expression of PD-1/PD-L1. Clinical data suggests benefit of PD-1/PD-L1 monotherapy or combination therapy with CTLA-4 blockade in select patients with CRC. Careful assessment of predictive biomarkers is necessary to optimize patient selection for these therapies. Late-stage data now strongly supports the use of ICI monotherapy in first-line metastatic dMMR/MSI-H CRC based on substantially improved PFS and decreased toxicity. Early phase data suggests a potential role for combination immune checkpoint therapy in later lines of therapy for metastatic dMMR/MSI-H CRC as well as in the neoadjuvant setting for non-metastatic dMMR/MSI-H CRC. The high expression of other ICIs in MSI-H CRC[76] further supports the potential utility of alternate immunotherapy agents in addition to PD-1/PD-L1-directed therapy. Although, based on current evidence, the target population for checkpoint-directed therapy is limited to metastatic dMMR/MSI-H CRC, future studies are needed to identify other biomarkers that may predict clinical benefit in CRC, as well as further clarify the role of immune therapies in front-line settings, in early stage disease, and in the adjuvant setting.

RATIONALE FOR IMMUNE CHECKPOINT THERAPY IN ESOPHAGEAL AND ESOPHAGOGASTRIC JUNCTION CANCERS

As with other gastrointestinal tumors, there is a scientific rationale to predict that patients whose tumors express PD-L1 and those whose tumors are MSI-H are more likely to benefit from the use of immunotherapy, especially ICIs. Increased PD-L1 expression suggests subversion of the host immune checkpoint system in the TME as a means of escaping immunologic detection. MSI-H tumors have increased neoantigen expression, which provide a structural basis for immunologic detection, and are also commonly associated with other mechanisms of immune evasion, both of which support the theory for identifying patients with tumor characteristics that suggest enhanced benefit from immunotherapy.

The benefit of ICIs in PD-L1 expressing and MSI-H tumors have now been validated in the clinical context for a variety of solid tumors, including esophageal cancer (EC) and esophagogastric junction (EGJ) cancers. U.S. Food and Drug Administration (FDA) approval and National Comprehensive Cancer Network (NCCN) guidelines support the use of pembrolizumab in second-line esophageal squamous cell cancer (ESCC) with PD-L1 expression or MSI-H, and third-line EC and EGJ adenocarcinoma are supported by data directly from clinical trials in EC as well as by inference from data in other solid tumors.

CLINICAL DATA FOR IMMUNE CHECKPOINT THERAPY IN ESOPHAGEAL AND ESOPHAGOGASTRIC JUNCTION CANCERS

The landmark clinical trials for immunotherapy in second-line EC and EGJ cancers are large Phase 3 trials called KEYNOTE-181 for pembrolizumab and ATTRACTION-3 for nivolumab.

In KEYNOTE-181, 628 patients with advanced or metastatic esophageal cancer refractory to first-line therapy were randomized to receive either pembrolizumab or investigator's choice of chemotherapy.[85] Patients were included with squamous cell carcinoma or adenocarcinoma, with EC or EGJ cancer. The overall population of patients did not experience a significant OS benefit with pembrolizumab. However, the pre-specified co-primary outcome of OS in the 222 PD-L1 expressing patients (CPS ≥10) did show significant OS benefit for pembrolizumab use in this subpopulation, with median OS of 9.3 months versus 6.7 months (p = 0.0074) and 12-month OS rate of 43% versus 20%. Importantly, this was accomplished with fewer drug-related AEs (64% vs. 86%) and fewer severe drug-related AEs (18% vs. 41%). This was the first large randomized trial to demonstrate a survival benefit for an ICI in EC, supporting its use in the second-line setting.

This data was further supported by the ATTRACTION-3 trial[86] evaluating nivolumab. This Phase 3 trial consisted of 419 patients with at least second-line unresectable or advanced EC who were refractory or intolerant to fluoropyrimidine-based or platinum-based chemotherapy. This trial was limited to patients with squamous cell histology. No PD-L1 expression cut-off was specified for trial inclusion. Patients were randomized to nivolumab or investigator's choice of taxol chemotherapy. Patients who were randomized to the nivolumab arm experienced a significant improvement in median OS, 10.9 months versus 8.4 months ($p = 0.019$), with significantly fewer grade 3 or 4 TRAEs, 18% versus 63%, respectively. This data supports the use of ICI therapy in the second-line setting for unresectable or advanced esophageal squamous cell carcinoma (ESCC).

Further studies are needed to expand and refine the use of ICI therapy in patients with EC, including examining the possible benefits as a first-line therapy, as an adjuvant therapy, in combination with other treatments, or in other subpopulations of patients. An ongoing Phase 3 trial called KEYNOTE-590 is evaluating the use of pembrolizumab compared to conventional chemotherapy in first-line advanced or metastatic ESCC with positive PD-L1 expression (CPS ≥10). CheckMate 577 is a Phase 3 randomized trial examining OS benefit of adjuvant nivolumab with resected EC or EGJ cancer. CheckMate 648 and CheckMate 649 aim to explore other combinations of checkpoint inhibitor therapy, such as PD-L1 therapy combined with chemotherapy, as well as the role for combination checkpoint immunotherapy targeting both PD-L1 and CTLA-4.

There are also ongoing early clinical and preclinical trials examining the potential roles of other immune therapies for EC, including adoptive T cell therapy, cancer vaccines, and oncolytic virus therapy (OBP-301), which each have the potential to alter the landscape of immunotherapy treatment in gastrointestinal malignancies.

CONCLUSION

As emerging oncologic immunotherapy candidates stream forward, great changes are being made in the landscape of potential treatments for gastrointestinal cancers. Strong preclinical data have predicted esophageal, gastric, and colorectal cancer vulnerability to immunotherapy. Based on site of disease, subgroups have been identified based on their microsatellite instability (MSI), PD-L1 expression, and histology that demonstrate a significant survival benefit from checkpoint inhibitor therapy, prompting FDA label expansion and inclusion into national treatment guidelines. These strategies have shown benefit in the refractory setting for gastroesophageal cancers. The recent pivotal data demonstrating clinical benefit in first-line metastatic MSI-H colorectal cancer is promising. Ongoing clinical trials aim to expand the identified subsets of patients who would benefit from checkpoint inhibitor therapies, and to identify novel immunotherapeutic agents and approaches that can further expand the toolkit for the treatment of gastrointestinal cancers.

KEY REFERENCES

Only key references appear in the print edition. The full reference list appears in the digital product on Springer Publishing Connect: connect.springerpub.com/content/book/978-0-8261-3743-2/part/part04/chapter/ch53

27. Doi T, Piha-Paul SA, Jalal SI, et al. Updated results for the advanced esophageal carcinoma cohort of the Phase Ib KEYNOTE-028 study of pembrolizumab (MK-3475). *J Clin Oncol.* 2016;34(4 suppl):7. doi:10.1200/jco.2016.34.4_suppl.7
32. Popiela T, Kulig J, Czupryna A, et al. Efficiency of adjuvant immunochemotherapy following curative resection in patients with locally advanced gastric cancer. *Gastric Cancer.* 2004;7(4):240–245. doi:10.1007/s10120-004-0299-y
83. Andre T, Shiu K-K, Kim TW, et al. Pembrolizumab versus chemotherapy for microsatellite instability-high/mismatch repair deficient metastatic colorectal cancer: the Phase 3 KEYNOTE-177 study. *J Clin Oncol.* 2020;38(18 suppl):LBA4. doi:10.1200/JCO.2020.38.18_suppl.LBA4
85. Kojima T, Muro K, Francois E, et al. Pembrolizumab versus chemotherapy as second-line therapy for advanced esophageal cancer: Phase III KEYNOTE-181 study. *J Clin Oncol.* 2019;37(4 suppl):2. doi:10.1200/JCO.2019.37.4_suppl.2
86. Kato K, Cho BC, Takahashi M, et al. Nivolumab versus chemotherapy in patients with advanced oesophageal squamous cell carcinoma refractory or intolerant to previous chemotherapy (ATTRACTION-3): a multicentre, randomised, open-label, Phase 3 trial. *Lancet Oncol.* 2019;20(11):1506–1517. doi:10.1016/S1470-2045(19)30626-6

54

Immunotherapy of Hepatocellular Carcinoma

Piera Federico, Margaret Ottaviano, and Bruno Daniele

KEY POINTS

- Hepatocellular carcinoma (HCC) mostly develops in the background of a cirrhotic liver. In addition, the liver is distinct as a tolerogenic organ, and hepatic inflammatory conditions can often influence the immune response against HCC.

- Several immunological features, including the density of immune infiltrates and the expression of receptors involved in exhaustion of the T cell response, are related to the prognosis of HCC patients undergoing liver resection.

- Until recently, different strategies aimed at enhancing the immune response against HCC have been tested in the setting of clinical trials with only minor therapeutic results; tested agents included cytokines, active immunization using peptide or dendritic cell platforms, and genetically modified viruses.

- More recently, antibodies that interact with immune checkpoint molecules to stimulate T cell response and prevent T cell exhaustion have shown encouraging activity against this tumor. A pilot clinical trial first showed that tremelimumab, an anticytotoxic T lymphocyte-associated antigen 4 (CTLA-4) antibody, induced objective tumor responses and durable disease stabilization with a favorable safety profile.

- A large trial has recently shown that the combination of atezolizumab, a programmed death ligand 1 (PD-L1)-blocking antibody, and bevacizumab (an anti-VEGF MoAb) significantly increase overall survival and progression-free survival (PFS) in patients with unresectable HCC, compared to sorafenib.

- A number of ongoing clinical trials compare a variety of combinations with the standard of care in first- or second-line therapy of patients with advanced HCC. Other trials have been testing the role of immunotherapy as adjuvant therapy after resection or percutaneous ablation or in association of intrarterial treatments.

BACKGROUND, EPIDEMIOLOGY, AND RISK FACTORS

Several research studies have been carried out to understand how cancer evades the immune system and thus to identify therapies that could directly act on a patient's immune system in a way that restores or induces a response to cancer. Immunotherapy in cancer was defined as 2013's Breakthrough of the Year by *Science magazine*[1] and currently plays a major role in the modern fight against cancer. The clinical success of immune checkpoint inhibitors (ICIs) has boosted interest in the field of immuno-oncology, leading to regulatory approvals of several agents for the treatment of a variety of malignancies. The first to be approved in 2011 was the anti-CTLA-4 antibody ipilimumab for the treatment of unresectable or metastatic melanoma.[2] Subsequently, the anti-programmed cell death 1 (anti-PD-1s), nivolumab and pembrolizumab, received regulatory approvals for the treatment of melanoma and several other cancers. More recently, three anti-programmed death ligand 1 (anti-PD-L1) antibodies have received approval: atezolizumab and durvalumab, for locally advanced or metastatic urothelial carcinoma, metastatic non-small cell lung cancer (NSCLC), and triple-negative breast cancer (TNBC), and avelumab, for the treatment of locally advanced or metastatic urothelial carcinoma and metastatic Merkel cell carcinoma (Figure 54.1).[3] Moreover, in the last years, the peculiar immunogenic microenvironment of hepatocellular carcinoma (HCC) has restored interest in the systemic therapies for HCC, opening the way for introducing ICIs for HCC treatment.

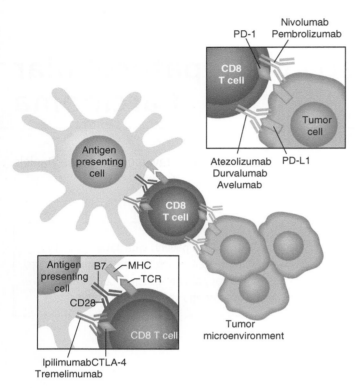

Figure 54.1 Mechanisms of action of immune checkpoint inhibitors anti-CTLA4 and anti-PD(L)1. CTLA-4 (a B7/CD28 family member) and PD-1 are co-inhibitory receptors expressed on the cell surface of T cells which bind to their corresponding ligands (CD80/86 and PD-L1/-L2, respectively) to render T cells anergic. The blocking of these mechanisms can restore an antitumor immune response.

CTLA-4, cytotoxic T lymphocyte associated antigen 4; MHC, major histocompatibility complex; PD-1, programmed death 1; PD-L1, programmed death ligand 1; TCR, T cell receptor.

HCC, which accounts for about 80% of primary liver cancers worldwide, is a leading cause of cancer-related death in many parts of the world. Over the past few decades, notable progress has been made in understanding the epidemiology, risk factors, and biology of HCC. In addition, several approaches to prevention, surveillance, early detection, diagnosis, and treatment have been developed. Where these approaches have been applied in comprehensive programs in high-incidence populations, they have shown their efficacy in preventing HCC and in controlling overall mortality from the disease. However, incidence and cancer-specific mortality still continue to increase in many countries, and the majority of HCC patients still present at an advanced stage in many parts of the world; as a result, HCC is estimated to be the fourth most common cause of cancer-related death overall worldwide.[4,5] Between 2005 and 2015, following lung cancer, liver cancer was the second leading cause of years of life lost from cancer worldwide, with a 4.6%

increase in absolute years of life lost.[6,7] To date, overall survival of HCC patients is substantially different across the world.[8-11] Median survival in Taiwan and Japan is significantly higher than in sub-Saharan Africa, where the median survival is only 2.5 months, probably due to the dramatic effects of the absence of surveillance programs and effective available treatments. Taiwan and Japan, differently, have the best clinical outcomes of patients with HCC, likely because both countries have comprehensive and intensive liver cancer surveillance programs, by using multiple tumor biomarkers [alpha-fetoprotein (AFP), the Lens culinaris agglutinin-reactive glycoform (AFP-L3), and des-gamma-carboxy prothrombin (DCP)] and liver ultrasonography reflexing to cross-sectional imaging in high-risk individuals presenting with new or suspicious liver nodules.[12] Consequently, more than 70% of HCCs are diagnosed at very early stages, and therapies with curative intent may be delivered. HCC clinical outcomes in Korea, China, North America, and Europe are not comparable to those of Taiwan or Japan, where more than 60% of patients present with intermediate-stage or advanced-stage HCC at diagnosis.[7]

In the majority of cases, particularly in high-resource countries, HCC develops as a sequel of chronic hepatitis, mostly in patients with liver cirrhosis from hepatitis B virus (HBV) or hepatitis C virus (HCV) infection. The annual incidence of HCC is 2% to 5% in patients with cirrhosis from chronic HBV or HCV infection.[13] Frequently, HBV-related HCC may occur in the absence of cirrhotic liver disease, accounting for 30% to 50% of HCC in HBV endemic areas such as Eastern Asia and most African countries.[11] Differently, in studies from the United States where HBV is not endemic, more than 90% of patients with HBV-related HCC have cirrhotic liver disease.[14] Differences in HBV transmission, age and duration of infection, and environmental exposures may explain the higher frequency of HCC in patients with HBV without cirrhosis in HBV endemic areas. Globally, chronic HBV infection is the leading cause of HCC in Eastern Asian countries and most African countries, except for northern Africa where the prevalence of HCV is highest,[8,9] while HCV is the leading virus-related cause of HCC in North America, Europe, Japan, parts of central Asia including Mongolia, and northern Africa and the Middle East, particularly Egypt.[8,11] In most developed countries, non-alcoholic fatty liver disease (NAFLD) is now the most common liver disease and a major risk factor for HCC. It is estimated that between 10% and 20% of HCC cases in the United States are due to NAFLD, and NAFLD-associated HCC occurs frequently in the absence of cirrhosis.[15-20] More recently, special attention is focused on association between diabetes mellitus and HCC risk, since insulin resistance and consequent production of reactive oxygen species that trigger hepatic inflammation are thought to have a role in hepatocarcinogenesis.[21-23]

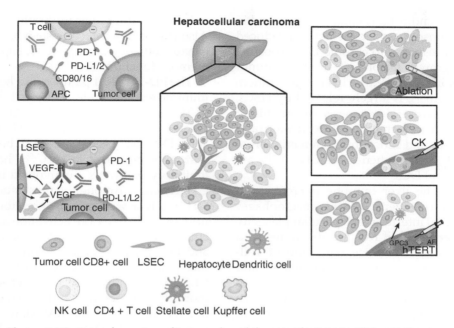

Figure 54.2 General overview of immune-based therapies for hepatocellular carcinoma.

HEPATOCELLULAR CARCINOMA TREATMENTS

Treatments of HCC include liver transplantation, surgical resection, targeted therapy, radiotherapy, interventional therapy (transarterial chemoembolization [TACE], radiofrequency ablation [RFA]) and systemic therapy, including immunotherapy (Figure 54.2). The evidence supporting the use of immunotherapy in HCC will be discussed in the following paragraphs.

THE IMMUNOLOGICAL ENVIRONMENT IN HEPATOCELLULAR CARCINOMA

The liver is a "tolerogenic" organ that can stimulate its immune responses to prevent undesirable pathogen attack and tumor initiation. However, as a typical inflammation-linked tumorigenesis, immune evasion is one of the processes occurring during the initiation and evolution of HCC.[24] A number of immune suppressor mechanisms, including intratumoral inclusion of immunosuppressive cell populations, defective antigen presentation, and activation of multiple inhibitory receptor-ligand pathways, promote tolerance over immunity, and favor progression of HCC.[25,26] The level of immune suppression in the tumor microenvironment (TME) is directly correlated with poor prognosis in HCC patients. As a consequence, to better stimulate antitumor immunity, more details about the suppressed immune landscape of HCC are subsequently elucidated. The HCC TME is a dynamic system, which comprises cancer cells, cytokine environment, extracellular matrix, immune cell subsets, and other components.[27,28] Here, starting from the HCC TME description, we discuss new advances in the immunological landscape of HCC.

HEPATIC IMMUNE TOLEROGENESIS

The functional junction between portal and arterial inflow in the liver represents a primary anatomical site of immune recognition.[29] To protect the liver parenchyma from tissue injury, several mechanisms contribute to prevent exposure to microbial antigens and conserved molecular motifs known as danger- or pathogen-associated molecular patterns (DAMPs/PAMPs), making the liver a largely immunosuppressive microenvironment. The functional heterogeneity of the liver immunological landscape is evidenced by the different nature of stromal cells including liver sinusoidal endothelial cells (LSECs), hepatic stellate cells (HSCs), and liver resident macrophages or Kupffer cells (KCs), as well as cells of the adaptive immune response including CD4+, CD8+ T lymphocytes, and natural killer (NK) cells.[30] LSECs have antigen-presenting capacity, thus activating antigen-specific CD4+ T cell responses.[31] LSECs regulate immune cell recruitment through specific integrins (αLβ2, α4β1, α4β7) that facilitate lymphocyte capture and subsequent chemotaxis mediated by pathways such as CXCL9-11/CXCR3, CXCL16/CXCR6, and CX3CL1/CX3CR1.[32] In response to lipopolysaccharide, the antigen-presentation capacity of LSECs is inhibited by downregulation of constitutively expressed major histocompatibility complex (MHC) class II, CD80 and CD86 molecules.[33] A key role of this immune-tolerogenic state is played by abundance of prostaglandin E2 (PGE2) and interleukin 10 (IL-10), two immunosuppressive mediators produced by KC and LSECs in response to chronic LPS exposure. Also, transforming growth factor-β (TGF-β), an immunosuppressive cytokine involved in liver regeneration, inflammation, and fibrosis, is largely released by HSCs, which contribute to liver tolerogenesis by inhibiting lymphocyte infiltration, inducing PD-L1 expression, and facilitating recruitment and functional differentiation of regulatory T cells (T$_{reg}$ cells) when naïve CD4$^+$ cells are recruited to professional DCs.[34-38]

KCs contribute to the liver immune microenvironment as nonmigratory liver resident macrophages located in the sinusoidal interface with peculiar plasticity in response to danger signals.[39] KCs are able to respond to injury via expression of a large repertoire of Toll-like receptors, scavenger receptors, complement, and Fc-gamma receptors.[40] Normally, KC-mediated antigen presentation induces tolerogenic immunity by reduction of CD4$^+$ T cell responses and T$_{reg}$ cell expansion.[41] In response to LPS, KCs promote immunosuppression by IL-6 downregulation and IL-10 release.[42-44]

PATHOGENESIS AND PROGRESSION OF HEPATOCELLULAR CARCINOMA: IMMUNE-MEDIATED MECHANISMS

It is widely acknowledged that increased T lymphocyte infiltrate is associated with improved survival outcomes in HCC.[45] Cytotoxic CD8$^+$ T cells (CTLs) play a pivotal role in the HCC antitumor immunity.[46] CTLs promote T cell receptor (TCR)-mediated, antigen-dependent cytotoxicity against tumors, directly inducing cell death via membrane-bound FAS-ligand and inhibiting tumor proliferation via IFN-γ secretion.[47] As CD8$^+$ T cells, as well as CD4$^+$ T helper (Th) cells, play a crucial role in the HCC antitumor immunity: when activated in the presence of DC-derived type-1 interferon and IL-12, they release several pro-inflammatory (Th1) cytokines, which induce CTL proliferation and thus antitumor immunity.[48] Higher levels of Th1 cytokines (IFN-γ, IL-2, IL-1α, IL-1β) are, in fact, associated with favorable prognosis.[49] When T cell exhaustion occurs, it is characterized by impaired pro-inflammatory responses upon stimulation, reduced cytokine production, impaired proliferation, and reduced cytotoxicity and over-expression of co-inhibitory receptors including CTLA-4, PD-1, LAG-3, and TIM-3. Intratumoral and circulating exhausted CD8$^+$ T cells are associated with poor prognostic trait in HCC.[50,51] Exhaustion within the TME is multifactorial and dominated by a cytokine pathway featuring IL-10 and TGF-β, which prohibits activation of CTLs and Th1 CD4$^+$ T cells.[52,53] Single cell analysis of TCR sequences has recently confirmed clonal expansion of exhausted CD8$^+$ T cell clusters in HCC, indicating that CTL clones expand

within the tumor after infiltration, becoming exhausted. Also transcription factors such as TOX, linked to T cell exhaustion, are overexpressed, suppressing effector and memory function.[54,55]

The PD-1/PD-L1 pathway is a key actionable driver of immune exhaustion in HCC, and works by suppression of TCR signaling via the PI3K/AKT pathway, inhibiting T cell survival and growth.[56,57] High expression of PD-1 and PD-L1 has been reported to be generally associated with poor prognosis in HCC;[58,59] however, several other inhibitory pathways are involved in blocking antitumor CTL function. Among the most studied in the last years, CTLA-4 is a well-known inhibitory receptor, which is upregulated after T cell activation and acts competitively, antagonizing CD80 and CD86 co-stimulatory molecules and by downstream inhibition of AKT.[60] Other inhibitory pathways are: TIM-3, which is expressed on CD4$^+$, CD8$^+$ tumor-infiltrating leukocytes (TILs), and intratumoral T$_{reg}$ cells in HCC and linked to HCC susceptibility in HBV-carriers;[61-64] and LAG-3, which is associated with hypofunctional CD8$^+$ responses in HCC TILs.[65,66] Special attention is due to T$_{reg}$ cells, which are CD4$^+$/CD25$^+$/ Foxp3$^+$ immune-suppressive T cells whose higher levels in HCC are associated with disease progression[67] and reduced survival.[68] They are recruited intratumorally via CCL17/CCL22 secretion by tumor-associated macrophages (TAMs).[69,70] In addition, T$_{reg}$ cell differentiation is promoted by the production of TGF-β, IL-10, and other mediators including COX-2 and indoleamine 2,3-dioxygenase (IDO) by stromal and tumor cells.[71]

T$_{reg}$ cells enhance antigen presentation by downregulation of DC expression of CD80 and CD86.[72] They can directly inhibit the cytotoxic capacity of CTLs realizing suppressive cytokines like TGF-β and IL-10 and antagonizing the effect of IL-2. T$_{reg}$ cells can also directly lyse antigen-presenting cells (APCs) via granzyme-mediated cytolysis.[73] Moreover, HCC TME is characterized by other identified suppressive lymphocyte populations such as Th2 CD4$^+$ Th cells, which are activated in the presence of IL-10 derived from intratumoral myeloid cells;[74] and Tr1 cells, which are induced in HCC by interaction with plasmacytoid dendritic cells via ligation of ICOS.[75] Higher expression of Th2 cytokines (IL-4, IL-5, and IL-10) is associated with disease progression and metastasis in HCC as a likely consequence of IL-4-mediated recruitment of TAM, which produce TGF-β and vascular endothelial growth factor (VEGF). IL-17 producing Th17 subsets have also been reported in HCC. Th17 intratumoral accumulations are linked to poor survival promoting angiogenesis.[76] NK cells are innate lymphoid cells that represent more than 30% of liver resident lymphocytes[77] and are a homogeneous population identified by the abundance of specific cell receptors (CD56, CD16). Liver resident NK cells (lrNK) are mostly CD56^{bright} CD16^{dim} that reside in the thin-walled sinusoids along Kupffer cells.[78,79] Circulating

NK cells (CD56^{dim} CD16^{bright}) are being recruited to the inflamed liver and, next to lrNK cells, are activated by cytokines such as IL-2, IL-12, IL-18, and IL-15, secreted by hepatocytes and Kupffer cells.[80] Once activated, NK cells act rapidly, without the requirement for antigen presentation, by producing cytokines (mainly IFN-γ, TNF-α) and chemokines, and inducing target cell apoptosis via death-inducing molecules—the FAS receptor and the TNF-Related Apoptosis Inducing Ligand (TRAIL)—and via the release of cytotoxic granules.[81–83] Dysfunctional NK cells have been described in settings of chronic inflammation such as NASH,[84] viral hepatitis,[85] and the TME.[86] Reduced membrane expression of certain NK-activating ligands (NKG2D) in HCC patients correlate with disease progression and early recurrence.[87,88] TGF-β downregulates NKG2D receptors and upregulates inhibitory receptors such as TIGIT and CD96 on NK cells[89,90] and CD94/NKG2A on NK and T cells.[91] In HCC patients, intra-tumoral NK cells with a high level of CD96 were functionally exhausted with reduced production of IFN-γ and TNF-α and correlate with shorter disease-free survival and overall survival times.[92] The two main myeloid cell populations characterizing the TME are TAMs and myeloid-derived suppressor cells (MDSCs). MDSCs are a more immature myeloid population found in both the peripheral circulation and intratumors, while TAMs are tissue-resident only. Endothelial and HSC production of CXCL12 promotes intratumoral myeloid cell recruitment via chemokine receptor CXCR4.[93] Infiltrating MDSCs elicit tumor progression,[94] and higher circulating MDSCs increase the risk of HCC recurrence after ablative therapy.[95] MDSCs produce arginase, thus reducing arginine in the TME and suppressing T cell proliferation. In addition, they promote T$_{reg}$ cell expansion due to the production of IL-10 and TGF-β and promote inhibitory signaling in effector T cells through surface expression of PD-L1.[96] TAMs are the predominant TIL population, associated with poor prognosis in HCC.[97] In fact, TAMs produce growth factors including TGF-β and VEGF to promote tumor growth and development, promote cancer cell stemness through activation of NF-κB, and promote metastasis through the production of matrix metalloproteinases.[97] TAMs can also directly inhibit antitumor cytotoxic T cell proliferation and stimulate regulatory CD4$^+$ T cell expansion via surface expression of PD-L1, secretion of IL-10 and TGF-β, and through the production of nitric oxide and arginase in the same manner as MDSCs.

IMMUNOTHERAPEUTIC APPROACHES

Several recent studies have suggested that tumor antigen-specific immunotherapy and other approaches modulating immunogenicity have become attractive strategies for HCC treatment. Generally, these immunotherapeutic approaches for HCC could be mainly divided into cell-based (mainly refers to DCs)/non-cell based vaccines, adoptive cell transfer (ACT), cytokine/antibody-based immune regimens, immune-checkpoint blockade (ICB), and combination of immunotherapeutic agents with other drugs.

VACCINES

The investigation of antitumor vaccine has been promptly addressed against immune-dominant peptides of oncofetal proteins such as alpha-fetoprotein (AFP), glypican-3 (GPC3), telomerase reverse transcriptase, and many others such as MAGE-A1 and NY-ESO-1.[98] However, the coexistence of multiple inhibitory mechanisms and the accumulation of infiltrating T$_{reg}$ cells constitute a barrier to the effective development of vaccines as therapies for HCC.[98] Therefore, approaches including preconditioning with low-dose cyclophosphamide (a T$_{reg}$ cell depleting agent) and stimulation with colony-stimulating factors have been pursued,[99] with no successes in terms of long-term, clinically meaningful antitumor responses. Ex vivo stimulation of DCs, to overcome cancer immune evasion by promoting effective antigen presentation and inducing immunological memory, have showed mixed results limited to disease stabilization in most studies.[100–102] Heterogeneity in DC vaccination manufacturing and the need for dedicated facilities for apheresis and re-infusion of DCs makes this approach difficult to adopt in the absence of more convincing evidence of efficacy.[103] The identification of new tumor-associated antigens (TAAs) based on analysis of the mutanome and peptidome of HCC patients is the basis of the HEPAVAC project. The resulting HLA-A2$^-$ and HLA-A28$^-$restricted peptides are administered together with a strong RNA-based adjuvant to patients with HCC effectively treated by resection, ablation, or locoregional therapies; results are waited.[104]

ADOPTIVE TRANSFER OF GENETICALLY MODIFIED LYMPHOCYTES

ACT is predominantly conquering the modern scenario of tumor immunotherapy, and it consists of cytolytic activity against tumor cells thanks to the transfer of lymphocytes from the patients themselves or from donors. Before the emergence of chimeric antigen receptor T cells (CAR T cells), adoptive transfer therapy in HCC mainly focused on TILs and cytokine-induced killer cells.[105–107] With the recent discovery of CAR T cells and their surprising therapeutic effect on hematological tumors,[108] the effect of CAR T cell therapy in solid malignancies, including HCC, has attracted attention. Currently, at present, the most used CAR structure consists of a single-chain antibody extracellular domain that recognizes and binds specific antigens, an extracellular hinge region, a transmembrane region, and an intracellular domain that provides proliferation and activation signals. Multiple studies have showed that GPC3 is an attractive liver cancer-specific target, because its expression is high in HCC tissues but limited in normal tissues.[109] GPC3-specific CAR T cell therapy for HCC shows a strong killing effect on GPC3+ HCC cells both in vivo and in vitro.[110] Moreover, a relevant Phase 1 clinical trial study (ClinicalTrials.gov identifier: NCT02395250) demonstrated that autologous T cells allowing GPC3-specific CARs were safe and effective in patients with relapsed or refractory HCC, and another Phase 1 clinical trial (ClinicalTrials.gov identifier: NCT02541370) involving CD133-directed CAR T cells for advanced HCC demonstrated controllable toxicities and effectiveness.[111] However, immunosuppressive microenvironments can block the infiltration of CAR T cells into tumor tissues, thus reducing CAR T cell-mediated antitumor effects.[112] Of note, a recent study showed that the inhibition of PD-1 expression in GPC3-specific CAR T cells can enhance the killing effect of CAR T cells on HCC cells.[113]

TREATMENT OF HEPATOCELLULAR CARCINOMA BASED ON NATURAL KILLER CELLS

Similar to T cells, NK cells can be modified with CARs that recognize antigens expressed by tumors and combine with signaling components that enhance NK cell activity. Currently, only a few studies regarding the treatment of solid tumors such as HCC are available. A recent study demonstrated that GPC3-specific CAR NK cells constructed with NK-92 cells could effectively inhibit proliferation and promote apoptosis in HCC cells.[114] Furthermore, CAR NK cells have lower toxicity than CAR T cells and do not need patient matching, which makes CAR NK cells more promising for cancer treatment.[115]

TOLL-LIKE RECEPTOR AGONISTS

Recently, particular attention has been dedicated to the role of TLR agonists as a vaccine adjuvant and tumor immunotherapeutic agent.[116-118] As a vaccine adjuvant, TLR agonists elicit antigen presentation by promoting the maturation of DCs. Multiple TLRs, such as TLR3 and TLR9, have been expressed on HCC cells.[119-121] The TLR2/4 agonist OM-174 has potential roles in the prevention of invasion and metastasis in HCC.[122] TLR agonists can also work as adjuvants to stimulate the immune system during tumor treatment, but their effects on tumor cells cannot be ignored.

PREDICTIVE BIOMARKERS

There is an urgent need to find clinically available predictive biomarkers of response and survival to soon identify patients who may benefit from immunotherapies avoiding life-threatening immunotoxicity.

PROGRAMMED DEATH LIGAND 1 EXPRESSION

Immunohistochemical detection of PD-L1 has been recognized as a potential predictor of response to anti-PD-1/PD-L1 differently across the variety of malignancies. Assessment of PD-L1 expression is challenged and a clear role as a predictive biomarker in HCC has not yet been highlighted. In KEYNOTE-224, assessment of PD-L1 expression by a 22c3 PharmDx companion diagnostic assay was available from 52 out of 104 participants. Combined tumoral and stromal PD-L1 expression was associated with higher ORR ($p = 0.021$) and PFS ($p = 0.026$) to pembrolizumab, whereas tumor cell staining alone was not ($p = 0.088$ and 0.096, respectively). In CheckMate 040, PD-L1 expression in tumor cells was assessed using the 28-8 PharmDx assay. In the expansion cohort ($n = 174$), 9/34 patients with PD-L1 >1% achieved an objective response (26%) compared with 26 out of 140 (19%) with PD-L1 <1%, highlighting the great deal of analytical heterogeneity of PD-L1 assay that may explain the scarce performance of PD-L1 as biomarker.

TUMOR MUTATIONAL BURDEN

Tumor mutational burden (TMB) measures the number of somatic nonsynonymous mutations per mega-base (Mut/Mb) in the coding genome of a tumor cell.[123] It is assumed that tumors with high TMB (>10 mut/Mb) are richer in neoantigens and therefore intrinsically immunogenic. Compared with other tumors, HCC is characterized by a median number of 5 Mut/Mb, ranging from 0.5 to 10 Mut/Mb.[124-127] Alteration of mismatch repair mechanisms, which contribute to a hypermutated phenotype, may also occur in HCC.[128] Analyses of genomic databases confirmed the low prevalence of TMB-high HCC (median 4 Mut/Mb) and limited evidence for a predictive role of TMB.[129]

THE GUT MICROBIOTA AS POTENTIAL BIOMARKER

Microbial proteins are able to prime T cell responses[130] and are deeply involved in the induction, training, and function of the host immune system.[131,132] It has been demonstrated that the gut microbiome may induce resistance to ICPI in a number of tumors treated with anti-PD1,[133-135] as well as play a pivotal role in liver inflammation, chronic fibrosis, liver cirrhosis, and HCC development via the gut–liver axis.[136-138] A small study of eight HCC patients treated with anti-PD1 has showed taxonomic diversity and enrichment in 20 species comprising Akkermansia and Ruminococcaceae to predict for response,[139] highlighting that also in HCC patients the gut microbioma may influence the clinical outcomes of ICIs. Further studies are warranted to better elucidate the implied action mechanism.

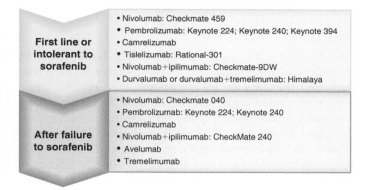

First line or intolerant to sorafenib	• Nivolumab: Checkmate 459 • Pembrolizumab: Keynote 224; Keynote 240; Keynote 394 • Camrelizumab • Tislelizumab: Rational-301 • Nivolumab+ipilimumab: Checkmate-9DW • Durvalumab or durvalumab+tremelimumab: Himalaya
After failure to sorafenib	• Nivolumab: Checkmate 040 • Pembrolizumab: Keynote 224; Keynote 240 • Camrelizumab • Nivolumab+ipilimumab: CheckMate 240 • Avelumab • Tremelimumab

Figure 54.3 Completed or ongoing trials of immune checkpoint inhibitors in advanced hepatocellular carcinoma.

SYSTEMIC THERAPY IN ADVANCED HEPATOCELLULAR CARCINOMA

Since the publication of the SHARP trial in 1998[140] and for almost a decade, the tyrosine kinase inhibitor (TKI) sorafenib was the only drug effective for the treatment of patients with advanced HCC. In the past few years, new TKIs proved to be effective both in first- (lenvatinib)[141] and second-line (regorafenib, cabozantinib) treatment.[142,143] In addition, the anti-VEGFR MoAb Ramucirumab improved OS of patients with HCC and high (≥ 400 ng/mL) alphafetoprotein (AFP) levels.[144] In HCC, ICIs have been used as monotherapy or in combination (with chemotherapy or other immunotherapy or biological agents). Among different ICIs, we can distinguish three subgroups: anti-PD-1, anti-PD-L1, and anti-CTLA-4 agents. Well-known combinations include two types of ICIs: anti-PD-1/PD-L1 and anti-CTLA-4 antibodies. Figure 54.3 summarizes the drugs and the major trials in this setting.

ANTI-PROGRAMMED CELL DEATH PROTEIN 1 ANTIBODIES

Nivolumab, pembrolizumab, Camrelizumab, and tislelizumab are the most relevant anti-PD-1 agents investigated in the field of HCC.

Nivolumab is the first antibody approved by the U.S. Food and Drug Administration (FDA) for the treatment of patients with HCC after sorafenib treatment failure. The Phase 1/2 CheckMate 040 study[145] showed an objective response rate (ORR) of 15% with a median overall survival (OS) of 15 months in patients with advanced HCC receiving nivolumab. The study revealed the therapeutic potential of nivolumab with a good safety profile in patients with HCC who have few treatment options. Additionally, nivolumab proved safe in patients with HBV or HCV infections, where no increase in hepatitis

reactivation was observed. Based on the previous results, the CheckMate 459 trial evaluated the clinical efficacy and safety of nivolumab versus sorafenib as first-line therapy in patients with unresectable HCC. The primary endpoint of the study was not reached (OS: 16.4 vs. 14.7 months in the experimental and standard arm, respectively).[146] Clinical benefit was observed across all the predefined subgroups and ORR was 15% in patients treated with nivolumab and 7% in those who received sorafenib. Of note, 140 patients (38%) in the experimental arm and 170 patients (46%) in the control arm received subsequent treatments.

Pembrolizumab is the other anti-PD1 antibody approved through an acceleration process by the FDA for the treatment of patients with HCC who have been previously treated with sorafenib. In the Phase 2 study KEYNOTE-224,[147] pembrolizumab (200 mg intravenously every 3 weeks for about 2 years or until disease progression, unacceptable toxicity, patient withdrawal, or investigator decision) was tested in 104 Child–Pugh class A sorafenib-refractory (80%) or intolerant (20%) patients with advanced HCC. Drug-related adverse events of grade 3–4 were reported in 26 patients (25%); the most frequent was hypertransaminasemia (6%). The encouraging efficacy of pembrolizumab was demonstrated by the ORR of 17%; 14 of the 18 patients who responded maintained the response for over 9 months. Median PFS and OS were 4.9 months and 12.9 months, respectively. Additionally, the trial evaluated the relationship between PD-L1 expression and response to treatment by using two indices of PD-L1 expression. The first was the combined positive score (CPS), which was defined as the number of PD-L1+ cells (tumor cells, lymphocytes, and macrophages), divided by the total number of viable tumor cells and multiplied by 100; the second was the tumor proportion score (TPS), defined as the number of tumor cells that express PD-L1 (either partial or complete staining) divided by the total number of viable tumor cells and multiplied by 100. The higher response rate was recorded in CPS positive tumors. In the Phase 3 trial KEYNOTE-240[148], 413 patients with advanced HCC, Child–Pugh class A and good performance status, who were intolerant or progressing to sorafenib, were randomized to receive pembrolizumab plus best supportive care (BSC) or placebo plus BSC. The trial showed a median OS of 13.9 months in the pembrolizumab arm and 10.6 months in the placebo arm. The benefit, however, did not reach the prespecified endpoint of statistical significance. Another Phase 3 trial, the KEYNOTE-394, is currently testing the efficacy of pembrolizumab versus placebo in Asian patients with advanced HCC as second-line therapy.

Camrelizumab and tislelizumab are the other anti-PD-1 agents investigated in HCC. A Phase 2/3 trial is enrolling patients with advanced HCC who had failure or intolerance to prior systemic treatment. Patients receive camrelizumab 3 mg/kg every 2 or 3 weeks.[149] Tislelizumab is being tested in the Phase 3 RATIONALE-301 trial versus sorafenib as a first-line treatment.[150]

In November 2019, based on the data from the Phase 1/2 CheckMate 040 study,[151] the FDA granted breakthrough therapy designation to nivolumab in combination with ipilimumab for patients with advanced HCC who had been treated with sorafenib. The trial showed that nivolumab plus ipilimumab achieved clinically meaningful responses and had an acceptable safety profile compared to nivolumab monotherapy (ORR: 31% and 14%, respectively) with a median OS of 22.8 months in the nivolumab + ipilimumab group. On March 10, 2020, the FDA granted accelerated approval to the combination of nivolumab and ipilimumab for patients with HCC who had been previously treated with sorafenib, according to the following schedule: nivolumab 1 mg/kg followed by ipilimumab 3 mg/kg on the same day every 3 weeks for 4 doses, then nivolumab 240 mg every 2 weeks or 480 mg every 4 weeks. Finally, the CheckMate 9DW trial, evaluating nivolumab + ipilimumab versus standard care (sorafenib or lenvatinib) in patients with advanced HCC who have received no prior systemic therapy, is currently ongoing (NCT04039707).

ANTI-PROGRAMMED DEATH LIGAND 1 ANTIBODIES

Durvalumab and avelumab are the anti-PD-L1 agents investigated in HCC. A Phase 1/2 trial of durvalumab monotherapy for solid cancers, including HCC, showed a 10% response rate and a median survival time of 13.2 months in a cohort of 40 patients with HCC.[152]

Avelumab is currently being tested in both monotherapy and combination therapy for advanced HCC.[153] A Phase 2 study of avelumab is ongoing in HCC patients previously treated with sorafenib (NCT03389126).

Durvalumab has been tested in combination with tremelimumab in a Phase 1/2 study of 40 patients with advanced HCC. The ORR was 15%, disease-control rates at 16 weeks was 57%, and all the confirmed responses were observed in uninfected patients.[154] The encouraging results of this study led to the inception of the randomized Phase 3 HIMALAYA trial (NCT03298451) that is currently evaluating the efficacy and safety of the combination of durvalumab + tremelimumab or durvalumab monotherapy versus sorafenib as first-line treatment for patients with unresectable HCC and no prior systemic therapy.

In January 2020, the FDA granted the combination of durvalumab and tremelimumab the orphan drug designation for treating patients affected by HCC.[155]

ANTI-CYTOTOXIC T LYMPHOCYTE-ASSOCIATED PROTEIN 4 ANTIBODIES

The first anti-CTLA-4 antibody investigated in the field of HCC was tremelimumab. In particular, a Phase 2 trial reported the data on HCC patients with chronic HCV infection treated with tremelimumab at 15 mg/kg intravenously administered every 90 days until tumor progression or severe toxicity.[156] Partial response rate was 17.6%, disease control rate was 76.4%, and time to progression was 6.48 months (95% CI, 3.95–9.14 months). Although a significant proportion of patients in Child–Pugh stage B were included in the study (42.9%), the safety profile of the treatment was acceptable.

COMBINATION THERAPIES BETWEEN IMMUNE CHECKPOINT INHIBITORS AND OTHER DRUGS

Targeted therapies have played a pivotal role in the medical management of HCC. Sorafenib was the first and, for nearly a decade, the only drug to demonstrate a significant OS benefit in treatment-naïve, advanced HCC patients.[140] Combination therapy with ICIs and targeted agents is not only justified by evidence of single-agent activity, but also by the complex bidirectional relationship existing between angiogenesis and immunity.[157] In fact, resistance to anti-angiogenic therapy is determined, at least in part, by an immunosuppressive microenvironment characterized by higher T_{reg} cell infiltration and stronger PD-L1 expression.[158] The expression of PD-L1 itself is strongly placed under the transcriptional regulation of hypoxia inducible factor 1-alpha.[159] In HCC, sorafenib therapy induces PD-L1 overexpression[160] and preclinical evidence in mouse models suggests a correlation with T_{reg} cell accumulation and M2-macrophage polarization, which is a process by which macrophages adopt a tumor supportive phenotype through hypoxia. These data present an appealing rationale for combination therapy.[161] Inhibition of tumor angiogenesis, and in particular VEGF, contributes to the normalization of the endothelial barrier by regulating key adhesion molecules for immune cell homing to the tumor.[162]

Atezolizumab (anti-PD-L1) plus bevacizumab, pembrolizumab + lenvatinib, camrelizumab + apatinib, and avelumab + axitinib are the combinations of ICIs and angiogenesis inhibitors that have been tested in HCC up to date.

KEYNOTE-524 is a Phase 1b study that tested the safety of pembrolizumab and lenvatinib in patients with unresectable HCC that was not amenable to locoregional treatment.[163] This study showed ORR of 36.7% by RECIST 1.1 criteria. increasing to 50% when modified RECIST criteria were used. Based on the promising initial results, the FDA approved the combination. A Phase 3 study (LEAP-002 study-NCT03713593) evaluating lenvatinib +

pembrolizumab versus lenvatinib and placebo as first-line therapy for patients with advanced HCC is currently ongoing.[164]

In July 2018, the FDA granted breakthrough therapy designation to atezolizumab (1,200 mg fixed dose) in combination with bevacizumab (15 mg/kg every 3 weeks) in advanced HCC, based on the results of the Phase 1b GO30140 Study.[165] The Phase 3 IMbrave150 trial demonstrated that atezolizumab in combination with bevacizumab reduced the risk of death by 42% and the risk of disease progression by 41% if compared with sorafenib.[166] The median OS was not reached in the combination arm and was 13.2 months in patients treated with sorafenib. The median PFS in patients who received atezolizumab + bevacizumab was 6.8 months versus 4.3 months in the sorafenib group. Decline in physical functioning and role functioning was also delayed with the combination treatment.[167]

The Phase 1b VEGF Liver 100 study investigated the safety of avelumab coadministered with the VEGF receptor kinase 1, 2, 3 inhibitor axitinib. The study has demonstrated an ORR of 13.6% based on RECIST 1.1 and 31.8% when responses were evaluated by mRECIST criteria. Median PFS was 5.5 and 3.8 months, based on RECIST 1.1 and mRECIST, respectively. Despite fairly high levels of grade 3 TKI-TRAEs, including hypertension (50%) and hand–foot syndrome (22.7%), no grade ≥3 immune-related adverse events (irAEs) were reported.[168]

Atezolizumab + cabozantinib, sintilimab (anti-PD-1) + bevacizumab biosimilar. and spartalizumab plus other agents are the most important combinations that are currently being tested in clinical trials in addition to the others mentioned previously. Several other studies are ongoing with combinations of ICIs and molecular targeted agents,[169] such as nivolumab + lenvatinib (NCT03418922), nivolumab + cabozantinib (NCT03299946), nivolumab + bevacizumab (NCT03382886), pembrolizumab + regorafenib (NCT03347292), and pembrolizumab + sorafenib (NCT03211416).[170]

IMMUNOTHERAPY IN LOCALIZED DISEASE

Locoregional therapies, TACE, RFA, or radiation therapy have traditionally played a major role in the treatment of liver-confined HCC. Evidence suggests that locoregional therapies can produce quantifiable changes in immune cell subsets, leading to the premise that the local ischemic and cytotoxic effects caused by these procedures lead to the release of neoantigens, promoting immunogenic cell death.[171] To date, the pilot study of tremelimumab combined with ablation/TACE is the most comprehensive prospective study that looked at the synergistic effect of local and systemic therapy.[172] It showed favorable outcomes, including a partial response rate of 26%, time to

tumor progression of 7.4 months, and OS of 12.3 months. In addition, ICIs are potentially beneficial in both neoadjuvant and adjuvant therapy—after resection or ablation—and in combination with TACE, cytotoxic chemotherapy, or radiotherapy. In fact, recurrence rates after curative therapy (resection or ablation) in early stage HCC are particularly high (about 70% at 5 years). This is mainly related to the presence of extremely small microsatellite metastatic lesions that are undetectable by imaging even at the time of resection or ablation. Theoretically, microsatellite lesions and intrahepatic metastases may be suppressed by the administration of anti-PD-1 antibody after recruitment of cytotoxic T lymphocytes to the microsatellite lesions upon release of tumor antigens by TACE or RFA.[173] Mizukoshi et al.[174] observed a significant increase in tumor-specific T cells, which is indicative of posttreatment tumor antigen release, after RFA in 62% of patients and a significant correlation between tumor-specific T cells and recurrence-free survival.

Several studies are currently ongoing in HCC in order to evaluate the safety and efficacy of adjuvant treatments in patients who have high risk of recurrence after curative hepatic resection or ablation. In particular, the CheckMate 9DX (NCT03383458) and the KEYNOTE-937 (NCT03867084) are ongoing studies evaluating the effect of nivolumab or pembrolizumab; EMERALD-2 (NCT03847428) is assessing the efficacy and safety of durvalumab in combination with bevacizumab versus durvalumab monotherapy or placebo; IMbrave050 (NCT04102098) is a Phase 3 study currently comparing atezolizumab + bevacizumab with active surveillance.

Recently, the neoadjuvant setting has been receiving increasing attention for emerging applications of anti-CTLA-4 and PD-1 monoclonal antibodies: ipilimumab + nivolumab (NCT03682276; NCT03510871) and cabozantinib + nivolumab (NCT03299946).

For patients with intermediate stage HCC, all the studies that evaluated the combination of sorafenib and TACE failed to show an improvement in OS as compared with sorafenib or TACE monotherapy.[175–177] In particular, the TACTICS study comparing TACE + sorafenib versus TACE alone in unresectable HCC showed an improved PFS (25.2 vs. 13.5 months), but the OS data were immature at the data cutoff.[178]

Combining ICI to TACE may improve *the efficacy of TACE*, because it has been shown to be associated with enhanced tumor-associated antigens spread along with an increase in VEGF levels. The Phase 1/2 PETAL clinical trial, which evaluated the safety and activity of pembrolizumab administered every 3 weeks for a maximum of 1 year after conventional TACE, reported no evidence of synergistic toxicity with TACE.[36] Additionally, clinical trials testing TACE + nivolumab (NCT03143270) and durvalumab + tremelimumab following TACE (NCT03638141) are ongoing.

A more complex approach has recently been proposed by the combination of TACE with both ICI and a molecular-target agent with an anti-VEGF effect. Some examples are the ongoing LEAP-012 study (combination of TACE with pembrolizumab and lenvatinib, NCT04246177) and the EMERALD-1 study (combination of TACE with durvalumab and bevacizumab, NCT03778957).

Lastly, transarterial radioembolization promotes radiation-induced tumor damage similar to that induced by stereotactic radiation therapy. Based on this concept, several early phase studies (Phase 1 and 2), by combining this locoregional approach to ICIs, are recruiting patients (NCT02837029; NCT03033446; NCT03099564; NCT03380130; NCT03316872).

CONCLUSION

HCC is characterized by immune tolerance and the infiltration of a variety of immune cells, a great number of suppressive molecules, complex pro-inflammatory/immune-regulatory signaling, and intricate interactions between different pathways. The HCC TME plays a crucial role in HCC survival outcomes, which are deeply influenced by the exhaustion phenomenon of TILs, induced by transcriptional and epigenetical alterations, metabolic reprogramming, and lack of co-stimulatory signals. Furthermore, the benefit of current predictive biomarkers (e.g., PD-L1 expression level and TMB) in HCC patients receiving ICIs are still limited. The cellular or molecular mechanisms of immune evasion in HCC still need to be investigated in depth and are crucial to better understand the immunological landscape of HCC. Immunotherapy brings great promises and new opportunities for HCC therapeutics, although some patients do not respond to this treatment. In addition to the current combination regimens of ICIs with TKIs, or individualized cell therapeutic approaches, more effective ways to reinforce antitumor responses are urgently warranted.

KEY REFERENCES

Only key references appear in the print edition. The full reference list appears in the digital product on Springer Publishing Connect: connect.springerpub.com/content/book/978-0-8261-3743-2/part/part04/chapter/ch54

43. Varol C, Mildner A, Jung S. Macrophages: development and tissue specialization. *Annu Rev Immunol*. 2015;33:643–675. doi:10.1146/annurev-immunol-032414-112220
70. Langhans B, Nischalke HD, Krämer B, et al. Role of regulatory T cells and checkpoint inhibition in hepatocellular carcinoma. *Cancer Immunol Immunother*. 2019;68(12):2055–2066. doi:10.1007/s00262-019-02427-4
125. Totoki Y, Tatsuno K, Covington KR, et al. Trans-ancestry mutational landscape of hepatocellular carcinoma genomes. *Nat Genet*. 2014;46(12):1267–1273. doi:10.1038/ng.3126

Immunotherapy for Gynecologic Malignancies

Kunle Odunsi, Thinle Chodon, and Cornelia L. Trimble

KEY POINTS

- Human papillomavirus (HPV) infections are very common. In the setting of a natural infection, both humoral and adaptive immune responses to viral antigens required for disease initiation and persistence are weak. Persistent infection is the clinical setting for developing disease.

- It is possible to elicit an HPV-specific T cell immune response with peripheral vaccination, in patients with established CIN2/3. After vaccination, the magnitude and quality of the tissue-localized immune response change drastically.

- Adoptive T cell immunotherapy using tumor-infiltrating lymphocytes or T cell receptor (TCR) E6/E7 engineered T cells is showing promise of clinical benefit.

- Ovarian cancer patients with high tumor infiltration by CD8+ T cells have improved survival compared to patients without infiltration, but several mechanisms of immunosuppression exist within the ovarian cancer microenvironment. These include the role of immune inhibitor receptors and their ligands, indoleamine 2,3-dioxygenase (IDO), transforming growth factor-beta (TGF-β), and other mechanisms.

- The most promising tumor antigens (TAs) in ovarian cancer are the cancer-testis (CT) family of antigens, such as NY-ESO-1. The role of mutational antigens is yet to be defined.

- Combinational immunotherapy strategies that continually enhance antitumor immunity and counteract immune suppression will be required for durable tumor control.

INTRODUCTION

The development of strategies for actively stimulating immunological rejection of tumors, previously an elusive goal, has been accelerated by recent improved understanding of the molecular basis of immune recognition and immune regulation of cancer cells. This led to the concept of "cancer immunoediting,"[1–3] which holds that the immune system not only protects the host against development of primary cancers but also sculpts tumor immunogenicity.[3] In gynecological malignancies, support for the concept comes from correlative human studies demonstrating that tumor infiltration by lymphocytes is a reflection of a tumor-related immune response. Data from these studies indicate that the presence of tumor-infiltrating lymphocytes (TILs) is associated with improved clinical outcome in ovarian, uterine, and cervical cancers.[4–7] A meta-analysis of 10 studies with 1,815 ovarian cancer patients confirmed the observation that a lack of intraepithelial lymphocytes (i.e., TILs) is significantly associated with a worse survival among ovarian cancer patients.[8] Recently, a large study of more than 5,500 epithelial ovarian cancer (EOC) patients by the Ovarian Tumor Tissue Analysis consortium confirmed the observation that CD8+ TILs were significantly associated with longer overall survival (OS) (2.8, 3.0, 3.8, and 5.1 years for patients with no, low, moderate, or high levels of CD8+ TIL, respectively).[9]

The major criteria for the immunological destruction of tumors include generation of sufficient numbers of effector T cells with high avidity recognition of tumor antigens (TAs) in vivo, trafficking and infiltration into the tumor, overcoming of inhibitory networks in the tumor microenvironment (TME), and persistence of the antitumor T cells. In the past decade, although several immune-based interventions have gained regulatory approval in many solid tumors, none has been approved for gynecologic malignancies. These interventions include cancer vaccines, cell-based therapy, immune checkpoint blockade, and oncolytic virus-based therapy. Here, we briefly review the current understanding of the host immune responses to ovarian, uterine, and cervical cancers; progress in immunotherapies; and future directions to the pathway for cure.

OVARIAN CANCER

In 2020, more than 300,000 new cases of EOC are expected worldwide, with more than 190,000 expected deaths.[10] Although significant advances have been made in the surgical management and in systemic therapeutic approaches, currently, the 5-year relative survival is 47.6% for all types of EOC,[11] only a modest improvement over the past 30 years. The recent introduction of poly (ADP-Ribose) polymerases (PARP) inhibitors has renewed opportunities for making a significant impact on EOC outcomes, both for BRCA-mutant and BRCA wild-type tumors.[12] Approximately 70% of EOC patients present with advanced disease,[13] and although the majority will respond to surgery and first-line chemotherapy, most of these responses are not durable: more than 90% of suboptimally surgically debulked patients and 70% of optimally debulked patients will relapse in 18–24 months.[14] The prognosis is poorest for (a) patients whose disease progresses while on first-line chemotherapy regimens without sustaining a clinical benefit (refractory disease) and (b) those whose disease recurs in less than 6 months (platinum-resistant disease). The major subtypes of ovarian carcinomas include high-grade serous carcinoma, endometrioid carcinoma (EC), clear cell carcinoma, low-grade serous carcinoma (LGSC), and mucinous carcinoma (MC). More recently, four molecular subtypes (C1/mesenchymal, C2/immune, C4/differentiated, and C5/proliferative) have been identified in HGSC and validated by gene expression profiling,[15,16] and these are associated with differential clinical outcomes. To date, immunotherapy approaches in ovarian cancer have not taken these molecular features or the tumor "immunoscore" into account.[17]

Immune Inhibitory Network and Immune Checkpoint Inhibitors in Ovarian Cancer

Traditional chemotherapy and newer targeted therapies appear to have reached a plateau in terms of the improvement in clinical outcomes and survival in ovarian cancer patients. An advantage of immunotherapy is the potential to treat ovarian cancer regardless of its state of drug resistance. A major barrier to successful cancer immunotherapy is the immunosuppressive microenvironment in which the tumor cells are located. Even if large numbers of tumor-specific T cells are generated in patients by active immunization or adoptive transfer, these T cells may not readily destroy tumor targets in vivo. In ovarian cancer, some of the major mechanisms that subvert antitumor immunity in the TME include suppressor immune cells such as regulatory T cells (T_{reg} cells),[5,18] myeloid-derived suppressor cells,[19–21] and tumor-associated macrophages (TAM), inhibitory cytokines such as transforming growth factor-beta (TGF-β) and IL-10,[21] immune checkpoint receptors,[22–24] and anomalous vessel formation in a network of cancer cells, pericytes, stromal cells, and inhibitory molecules expressed by the

extracellular matrix.[5,25,26] In addition, hypoxia, oxidative stress, mitochondrial DNA, and aberrant metabolism, such as indoleamine-2,3-dioxygenase (IDO)-mediated tryptophan catabolism leading to nutrient depletion, are prevalent within this hostile TME.[27,28] Moreover, tumor cell plasticity leads to antigen loss variants, heterogeneous expression of TAs, and very few unique TAs. This redundant immunosuppressive network may pose an impediment to efficacious immunotherapy, thus facilitating tumor progression.

Emerging evidence suggests that the elevated expression of inhibitory receptors on TA-specific T cells is one of the mechanisms by which tumors evade host immune surveillance.[29] Although blockade of the inhibitory receptors with specific antibodies has shown significant promise in overcoming immune suppression and mediating tumor regression,[30,31] multiple inhibitory receptors (including CD160, killer cell lectin-like receptor G1 [KLRG-1], T cell immunoglobulin, and mucin domain-containing 3 [TIM-3], 2B4, B- and T-lymphocyte attenuator [BTLA], and lymphocyte activation gene 3 protein [LAG-3]) are often co-expressed on tumor-antigen specific CD8[+] T cells.[32] In human ovarian cancer, a subset of TA-specific CD8[+] T cells that co-express programmed death-ligand 1 (PD-L1) and LAG-3 have been described and are impaired in interferon-gamma (IFN-γ) and cytokines, such as tumor necrosis factor-alpha (TNF-α) production compared with PD-1 or LAG-3 single-positive cells.[25] Simultaneous blockade of PD-1 or LAG-3 ex vivo restored the effector function of the human ovarian TA-specific T cells to a level that is higher than the additive effects of single blockade of PD-1 or LAG-3 alone.[24] In a mouse model of ovarian cancer, blockade of LAG-3 synergized with PD-1 blockade to enhance CD8[+] TIL function and promoted better control of transplanted ovarian tumors, whereas single-agent blockade had little or no effect.[33] The combinatorial blockade of LAG-3 and PD-1 with antibodies significantly increased the number of T cells in the TME, enhanced CD8[+] T cell function, and reduced CD4[+]CD25[+]forkhead box p3 (Foxp3[+]) T_{reg} cells. The collaboration between PD-1 and LAG-3 appeared to involve enhanced recruitment of Src homology region 2 domain-containing phosphatase-1 (SHP1) or SHP2 to the T cell receptor (TCR) complex, thereby negatively co-regulating T cell signaling and function.[33,34]

Immune modulation is designed to reinstate an existing anticancer immune response or elicit novel responses as a result of antigen spreading. This has been achieved through four general strategies: (a) the inhibition of immunosuppressive receptors expressed by activated T lymphocytes, such as cytotoxic T lymphocyte-associated protein 4 (CTLA-4) and PD-1; (b) the inhibition of the principal ligands of these receptors, such as the PD-1 ligand CD274 (PD-L1 or B7-H1); (c) the activation of co-stimulatory receptors expressed on the surface of immune effector cells, such as TNF receptor superfamily, member 4 (TNFRSF4 or OX40), TNFRSF9 (CD137 or 4-1BB), and TNFRSF18 (GITR); and (d) the neutralization of immunosuppressive factors released in the TME, such as TGF-β1 or IDO. Inhibition of immunosuppressive receptors expressed by activated T lymphocytes is commonly referred to as *checkpoint blockade*. In ovarian cancer, patients with higher tumoral expression levels of PD-L1 exhibited significantly shorter OS when compared with patients with lower expression levels.[35] More recent evidence indicates that within-patient spatial immune microenvironment variation shapes intraperitoneal malignant spread in high grade serous ovarian cancer.[36]

Therapies for blocking two inhibitory checkpoint receptors, PD-1 and CTLA-4, have been approved by the U.S. Food and Drug Administration (FDA) for overcoming this tumor evasion mechanism in many solid cancers including melanoma.[37–39] The first published data supporting immune checkpoint inhibitors as a potentially valuable therapeutic approach in ovarian cancer were observed in trials of the anti-PD-1 antibody nivolumab, and the anti-PD-L1 antibody BMS-93655, resulting in complete or partial responses in 6% of patients with advanced stage ovarian cancer.[30] Subsequently, another Phase 1 trial using nivolumab demonstrated objective response rates (ORRs) as high as 15% and 45% with stable disease in patients with platinum-resistant ovarian cancer.[40] Unfortunately, we have yet to achieve dramatic antitumor responses (similar to melanoma patients) through blocking immune checkpoint targets in ovarian cancer patients.

The challenges faced by checkpoint inhibitor monotherapy may be attributed to redundant aspects of the ovarian cancer TME. These mechanisms include (a) low intrinsic immunogenicity as a result of relatively low mutational/neo-antigen burden, (b) compensatory upregulation of alternate immune checkpoints following monotherapy,[34] and (c) TIL expression of multiple co-inhibitory receptors.[24,33] Further evidence for the limitations of immune checkpoint inhibition therapy was revealed in recent Phase 1b trials. Monotherapy using either the anti-PD-L1 antibody, avelumab[41] or anti-PD-1 antibody, pembrolizumab[42] showed similar results to the initial studies where few or no patients had a complete response but the majority of patients had partial responses and stable disease.

The potential for checkpoint inhibition to control disease progression has led to significant interest in using a combination of inhibitors or combination therapy with traditional chemotherapy or maintenance regimens. The combination of nivolumab and ipilimumab has been tested in various trials (NCT03342417, NCT02498600, NCT03355976), and reported to produce statistically higher response rates (31.4%) than nivolumab alone (12.2%) in a Phase 2 study of 100 patients with persistent or recurrent OC. The median progression-free survival (PFS) was 2 and 3.9 months in the nivolumab and nivolumab plus ipilimumab groups, respectively, with a PFI-stratified hazard ratio of 0.53 (95% CI: 0.34–0.82); the respective hazard ratio for death was 0.79 (95% CI: 0.44–1.42).[43]

Several PARP inhibitors (PARPi) have been approved as maintenance therapy in ovarian cancer.[44–46] By blocking DNA repair in tumor cells, PARPi increase tumor mutational load and potentiate response to ICI.[47] In addition, PARPi activate IFN signaling via the cGAS/STING pathway in BRCA-deficient tumors, and synergize with PD-1 or CTLA-4 blockade in the mouse models.[48–50] There are a number of clinical trials investigating PARPi therapies in combination with immune checkpoint inhibition.[51–54] The recently published TOPACIO/KEYNOTE-162 trial is a Phase 1/2 study of patients with platinum-resistant ovarian cancer or triple negative breast cancer who were treated with the PARPi, niraparib, and pembrolizumab.[55] Of the pooled 62 ovarian cancer patients, 48% had platinum-resistant status, 35% were homologous recombination (HR) deficient and 79% had BRCA^wt tumors. During the median follow-up of 12.4 months, 47% of ovarian cancer patients had stable disease, 13% had partial response, and 5% had a complete response. The median PFS interval was 3.4 months and overall survival is not yet available.[55] Additional ongoing studies in ovarian cancer patients include a Phase 1b/2 trial of avelumab in combination with the PARPi, talazoparib (NCT03330405), the JAVELIN Medley trial of avelumab with immune modulators, 4-1BB and OX40 (NCT02554812), and two trials using another anti-PD-L1 antibody, MEDI4736 (durvalumab), in combination with olaparib and either Bevacizumab (MENDIOLA, NCT02734004) or cediranib (NCT02484404).

Regarding combination of checkpoint inhibition with chemotherapy, the Phase 3 JAVELIN Ovarian 200 study, which compared pegylated liposomal doxorubicin (PLD) to the combination of PLD and anti-PD-L1 antibody avelumab,[56] did not show a statistically significant difference for the combination when compared with PLD alone, neither in PFS (HR: 0.78, repeated confidence interval [RCI], 0.587–1.244; one-sided p value = .0301), nor in OS (HR: 0.89; RCI: 0.744–1.241; one-sided p value = .2082). In this study, ORR was 13.3% (95% CI: 8.8%–19.0%) for the combination, 3.7% (95% CI: 1.5%–7.5%) for single-agent avelumab, and 4.2% (95% CI: 1.8%–8.1%) for the PLD alone.[57] Two ongoing Phase 3 trials are investigating a combination of atezolizumab and platinum chemotherapy plus bevacizumab as second/third-line therapy and/or maintenance therapy in patients with platinum-sensitive recurrent ovarian cancer (NCT02891824,

NCT03598270). Of interest, pembrolizumab combined with Mirvetuximab soravtansine (a folate receptor alpha [ADC], comprising an FRα-binding antibody linked to the tubulin-disrupting maytansinoid DM4) has also shown preliminary signs of efficacy in a heavily pretreated population of FRα-positive PREOC patients in the Phase 1b/2 FORWARD II trial (NCT02606305).[58] Finally, the combination of oral metronomic cyclophosphamide with bevacizumab and pembrolizumab produced an ORR of 37.5% (all partial responses) and PFS was overall 70% at 6 months (59% in the platinum-resistant population).[59]

Planned and ongoing clinical trials to investigate the efficacy of combinations of checkpoint inhibition include with: TIL therapy (NCT03287674), intraperitoneal chemotherapy (NCT03734692), doxorubicin and motolimod, a TLR 8 agonist (NCT02431559), immune-modulation (NCT03267589), and autologous engineered tumor cells expressing immune stimulatory, GM-CSF, and shRNA for downregulation of furin, a critical enzyme in TGF-β production (NCT03073525). A summary of selected combination studies is presented in Table 55.1.

Inhibition of Indoleamine 2,3 Dioxygenase

Another critical tolerogenic mechanism in ovarian cancer is mediated by IDO, an immunoregulatory enzyme that contributes to profound immune suppression in ovarian cancer.[60] IDO catalyzes the rate-limiting step of tryptophan (Trp) degradation along the kynurenine pathway. Both the reduction in local Trp levels and the production of Trp catabolites that are inhibitory to cells contribute to the immunosuppressive effects,[61] culminating in multipronged negative effects on T lymphocytes (notably on proliferation, function, and survival). IDO activity also promotes the differentiation of naïve T cells to cells with a regulatory phenotype (T_{reg} cell).[62] As increased T_{reg} cell activity has been shown to promote tumor growth and T_{reg} cell depletion has been shown to allow an otherwise ineffectual antitumor immune response to occur,[18] IDO expansion of T_{reg} cells may provide an additional mechanism whereby IDO could promote an immunosuppressive environment.

Interestingly, clinical trials in which platinum-resistant ovarian cancer patients received monotherapy with IDO inhibitors yielded little clinical benefit (SEASCAPE trial, NCT02575807). Ongoing clinical studies are exploring combination therapy with IDO and (a) traditional chemotherapy and T cell activation via PDX-Survivac (NCT02785250) and (b) checkpoint inhibitors and dendritic cell (DC) vaccines (NCT02432378). Furthermore, one multimodal strategy involves vaccine-induced tumor-specific T cells within a TME deficient in IDO activity. Currently a Phase 1/2b clinical trial is investigating the effect of an IDO inhibitor, epacadostat, combined with a DEC205mAb/NY-ESO-1 fusion protein and poly ICLC adjuvant therapy in ovarian cancer patients in remission (NCT02166905). If these approaches are successful, they will highlight a valuable tool for preventing recurrence and prolonging remission in ovarian cancer.

Tumor Antigens and Vaccine Therapy for Ovarian Cancer

The development of approaches for analyzing humoral[63] and cellular[64] immune reactivity to cancer in the context of the autologous host led to the molecular characterization of TAs recognized by autologous CD8+ T cells[65] and/or antibodies.[66] Some of these approaches include *serological analysis of recombinant cDNA expression libraries* (SEREX);[67] differential gene expression analysis, T cell epitope cloning;[68] and bioinformatics.[69] As a consequence of these advances, human TAs defined to date can be classified into one or more of the following categories: (a) differentiation antigens (that are restricted to defined tissues), for example, tyrosinase,[70] Melan-A/MART-1,[71] and gp 100;[72] (b) mutational antigens (that are altered forms of proteins); (c) amplification antigens, for example, HER2/neu;[73] (d) splice variant antigens, for example, NY-CO-37/PDZ-45[58] and ING1;[74] (e) glycolipid antigens, for example, MUC1;[75] (f) viral antigens, for example, HPV and Epstein–Barr virus; and (g) CT antigens (that are restricted in expression to the germ line and tumors), for example, MAGE,[76] NY-ESO-1,[67] and LAGE-1.[77]

Although there are several options in deciding which antigen to target, the fundamental requirements of the ideal TAs include: (a) limited or no expression in normal tissues, but aberrant expression at high frequencies in tumor; (b) immunogenicity; and (c) a role in tumor progression. Although none of the current TAs completely meet all of these criteria, the family of CT antigens are the closest. CT antigens are a subclass of TAs encoded by approximately 140 genes. CT genes or gene families have been found with the following two distinguishing features: (a) mRNA expression in testis and cancer cells and (b) no or highly restricted mRNA expression in normal adult somatic cells. Among CT antigens, NY-ESO-1, initially defined by SEREX in esophageal cancer,[67] has been analyzed extensively in several malignancies, including ovarian cancer. The antigen elicits both cellular and humoral immune responses in a high proportion of patients with advanced NY-ESO-1-expressing tumors, including ovarian cancer.[78,79]

A number of NY-ESO-1-based clinical trials have been conducted in ovarian cancer patients, and additional trials are ongoing. Details of some of the studies are as follows.

Table 55.1 Select Combination Studies of Immune Checkpoint Inhibitors in Ovarian Cancer

Study TITLE	TRIAL IDENTIFIER	PRIMARY ENDPOINTS	RESULTS
A Phase II Study of Pembrolizumab with Cisplatin and Gemcitabine Treatment in Patients With Recurrent Platinum-Resistant Ovarian Cancer	NCT02608684	ORR by RECIST	CR: 5.6% PR: 55.6% SD: 27.8% PD: 11:1%
A Phase II Study of Pembrolizumab Combined With Pegylated Liposomal Doxorubicin for Recurrent Platinum Resistant Ovarian, Fallopian Tube or Peritoneal Cancer	NCT02865811	CBR	ORR: 11.5%
Phase 3 Study to Evaluate the Efficacy and Safety of Avelumab (MSB0010718C) in Combination With and/or Following Chemotherapy in Patients With Previously Untreated Epithelial Ovarian Cancer JAVELIN OVARIAN 100	NCT02718417	PFS	Arm 1: N/A Arm 2: PFS: 16.8 months Arm 3: PFS: 18.1 months
Phase 3 Study of Avelumab Alone or in Combination With Pegylated Liposomal Doxorubicin Alone in Patients With Platinum-Resistant/Refractory Ovarian Cancer	NCT02580058	OS; PFS	PFS: 1.9 months vs. PFS: 3.7 months vs. PFS: 3.5 months
A Phase II Study of Nivolumab in Combination With Bevacizumab or in Combination With Bevacizumab and Rucaparib for the Treatment of Relapsed Epithelial Ovarian, Fallopian Tube, or Peritoneal Cancer	NCT02873962	ORR by RECIST	ORR: 28.9% (40% platinum-sensitive 16.7% platinum-resistant)
A Phase 1/1b, Multiple Dose, Dose Escalation and Expansion Study to Investigate the Safety, Pharmacokinetics and Antitumor Activity of the Anti-PD-1 Monoclonal Antibody BGB-A317 in Combination With the PARP Inhibitor BGB-290 in Subjects With Advanced Solid Tumors	NCT02660034	Phase 1: AEs; DLT; MTD Phase 1b: ORR, PFS, DOR, DCR, CBR, OS	PR: 7(5 EOC)/38 patients CR:1(EOC)/38 patients
Phase I/II Study of antiPD1 Antibody MEDI4736 in Combination With Olaparib and/or Cediranib for Advanced Solid Tumors and Advanced or Recurrent Ovarian, Triple Negative Breast, Lung, Prostate, and Colorectal Cancers	NCT02484404	Phase 1: RP2D Phase 2: ORR	DCR: 53%
Phase 1/2 Study of Niraparib in Combination With Pembrolizumab in Patients With Advanced or Metastatic Triple-Negative Breast Cancer and in Patients With Recurrent Ovarian Cancer	NCT02657889	Phase 1: DLT, AEs Phase 2: ORR	ORR:25%
A Phase I/II Study of MEDI4736 in Combination With Olaparib (PARP Inhibitor) in Patients With Advanced Solid Tumors	NCT02734004	DCR, Safety and Tolerability, ORR	DCR: 81% ORR: 63%
Phase II Randomized Trial of Nivolumab With or Without Ipilimumab in Patients With Persistent or Recurrent Epithelial Ovarian, Primary Peritoneal, or Fallopian Tube Cancer	NCT02498600	ORR	ORR: 12.2% (Arm 1), 31.4% (Arm 2) PFS: 2 mo. (Arm 1), 3.9 mo. (Arm 2)
A Phase I Study of Concomitant WT1 Analog Peptide Vaccine With Montanide and GM-CSF in Combination With Nivolumab in Patients With Recurrent Ovarian Cancer Who Are in Second or Greater Remission	NCT02737787	DLT	1-year PFS: 64.0%
A Randomized, Placebo-Controlled, Double-Blind, Multicenter Phase 1b/2 Study of Avelumab With or Without Entinostat in Patients With Advanced Epithelial Ovarian Cancer Which Has Progressed or Recurred After First-Line Platinum-Based Chemotherapy and at Least Two Subsequent Lines of Treatment With a Safety Lead-In	NCT02915523	AEs; DLT; MTD /RP2D	PFS: 1.64 mo. (Arm 1) 1.51 mo. (Arm 2)

AE, adverse event; CBR, clinical benefit rate; DCR, disease control rate; DLT, dose limiting toxicity; DOR, duration of response; MTD, maximum tolerated dose; ORR, objective response rate; OS, overall survival; PFS, progression-free survival; RECIST, Response Evaluation Criteria in Solid Tumors; RP2D, recommended Phase II dose

A pilot clinical trial of NY-ESO-1DP4 p157–170 (NY-ESO-1DP4), a peptide of potentially dual major histocompatibility complex (MHC) class I and class II specificities, in patients with epithelial ovarian, fallopian tube, or primary peritoneal carcinoma whose tumors express NY-ESO-1 or LAGE-1: In this trial, 18 ovarian cancer patients who were no evidence of disease (NED) after therapy for primary or recurrent disease were vaccinated with an NY-ESO-1 epitope, $ESO_{157-170}$, a naturally processed helper epitope that is recognized by CD4$^+$ T cells in the context of human leukocyte antigen (HLA)-DP4 (i.e., HLA-DPB1*0401 and *0402).[80] This NY-ESO-1 epitope has HLA-A2 ($ESO_{157-165}$) and HLA-A24 ($ESO_{158-166}$) motifs embedded in its natural sequence. The study tested whether active immunization with $ESO_{157-170}$ would elicit NY-ESO-1-specific CD4$^+$ and CD8$^+$ T cell responses in ovarian cancer patients with minimal disease burden. The peptide SLLMWITQC (100 µg) was mixed with 0.5 mL of montanide ISA-51, given by subcutaneous injection once every 3 weeks for a total of five to 15 doses. There was induction of CD4$^+$ T cell responses in 83% of patients, and CD8$^+$ T cell responses in 60% of HLA-A2$^+$ patients, but in none of the five HLA-A24$^+$ patients. Although the majority of patients were heavily pretreated, the median time to disease progression/recurrence from the start of vaccination was 19.0 months.[81]

Phase 1 study of NY-ESO-1b peptide and montanide ISA-51 vaccination of patients with EOC in high-risk first remission: This study enrolled nine patients to assess the primary and secondary endpoints of toxicity and immunogenicity. Eligible patients were those with high-risk EOC (defined by suboptimal initial debulking surgery, failure to normalize CA-125 after three cycles of chemotherapy, or positive second-look surgery) in complete clinical response (cCR), as documented by CT scan and CA-125 levels after completion of primary surgery and chemotherapy. The HLA-A*0201–specific NY-ESO-1b peptide SLLMWITQC (position 157–165; 100 µg) mixed with 0.5 mL of montanide ISA-51 was given by subcutaneous injection once every 3 weeks for a total of five doses (weeks 1, 4, 7, 10, and 13). Three of four patients (75%) with NY-ESO-1–positive tumor showed T cell immunity by tetramer and ELISPOT. Four of five patients (80%) with NY-ESO-1–negative tumor showed T cell immunity by tetramer and/or ELISPOT. The median PFS was 13 months.[82]

Phase 2 study of recombinant vaccinia-NY-ESO-1 (rV-NY-ESO-1) and recombinant fowlpox-NY-ESO-1 (rF-NY-ESO-1) in patients with epithelial ovarian, fallopian tube, or primary peritoneal carcinoma whose tumors express NY-ESO-1 or LAGE-1 antigen: This is the only reported Phase 2 clinical trial of NY-ESO-1 vaccine therapy in ovarian cancer.[83] The objective of the study was to test whether a priming immunization strategy with recombinant vaccinia-NY-ESO-1 (rV-NY-ESO-1), followed by booster vaccinations with recombinant fowlpox-NY-ESO-1 (rF-NY-ESO-1), would minimize the risk of progressive disease in advanced ovarian cancer patients, following first-line therapy. Integrated NY-ESO-1-specific antibody and CD4$^+$ and CD8$^+$ T cells were induced in a high proportion of the patients. The clinical results showed that (a) seronegative patients who remained seronegative but developed CD4$^+$ and/or CD8$^+$ T cell responses, and (b) seronegative patients who seroconverted and developed CD4$^+$ and/or CD8$^+$ T cell responses demonstrated improved OS (median, 52.4 and 48.4 months, respectively) compared with other categories of patients (median, 14.5 months; $p < .0001$).

Clinical trials to enhance NY-ESO-1 vaccine efficacy (http://www.clinicaltrials.gov): In an effort to enhance NY-ESO-1 vaccine efficacy, a number of novel approaches are undergoing clinical evaluation. These include:

1. *The use of pox viral vectors expressing NY-ESO-1 and TRICOM, TRIad of COstimulatory Molecules (B7-1, ICAM-1, and ligand leukocyte function-associated antigen [LFA-3])*: These three molecules are found on antigen-presenting cells (APCs). B7.1 (CD80) is a protein that interacts with T cell ligand CD28 resulting in T cell stimulation. ICAM-1 (CD56) is an adhesion molecule found on the surface of APCs that binds to the T cell LFA-1. LFA-3 (human CD58) is a surface protein that binds to CD2 expressed on T cells, resulting in T cell stimulation and priming.[84] Together, the use of TRICOM in pox viral constructs has been shown to expand antigen-specific CD8$^+$ T cells with superior functional avidity,[74–76] leading to better tumor control.

2. *The use of novel adjuvant formulations to enhance magnitude of immune response (study of NY-ESO-1 overlapping peptides and immunoadjuvants montanide and poly-inosinic and poly-cytidylic acids, poly-lysine also known as Hiltonol [Poly-ICLC], NCT00616941)*: In this study, ovarian cancer patients in second or third remission were immunized with NY-ESO-1 peptides and a novel adjuvant, poly-ICLC. Polyriboinosinic–polyribocytoidylic acid (poly I:C), a synthetic double-stranded RNA (dsRNA), is recognized by Toll-like receptor 3 (TLR3) and other intracellular receptors. This approach generated robust effector T cell responses with significant potential for tumor control.[85]

3. *Combination of NY-ESO-1 vaccination with a strategy to counteract immune escape due to antigen or MHC downregulation (NCT0088779)*: In a completed protocol, the demethylating agent decitabine was combined with chemotherapy and vaccine therapy in order to induce MHC and TA expression in tumors, and promote "antigenic" dose to effector T cells.[86] The regimen was safe, with limited and clinically manageable toxicities.

Both global and promoter-specific DNA hypomethylation occurred in blood and circulating DNAs, the latter of which probably reflects tumor cell responses. Increased NY-ESO-1 serum antibodies and T cell responses were observed in the majority of patients, and antibody spreading to additional TAs was also observed. Disease stabilization or partial clinical response occurred in 60% of evaluable patients.

4. *Combination of NY-ESO-1 vaccination with rapamycin as a strategy to generate memory T cells for durable tumor protection (NCT01536054):* In this study, vaccination is combined with rapamycin in various doses and schedules, in order to determine a regimen that best generates memory T cell responses. The induction of memory T cell responses is a key to prevent tumor recurrence, but has been a major challenge for all tumor immunotherapy approaches. Recent studies indicate that inhibition of mammalian target of rapamycin (mTOR) activity switches T-bet for eomesodermin expression and slants CD8$^+$ effector cells for memory precursor-like phenotype.[87,88] Moreover, in vivo murine studies have shown that sirolimus augments antigen-specific vaccination by inducing a long-lasting, tumor-protective memory T cell response. Therefore, this trial will test whether mTOR inhibition will condition vaccine-induced T cells for enhanced persistence, antigen recall, and tumor efficacy in ovarian cancer.

5. *Combination of NY-ESO-1 vaccination with an inhibitor of IDO as a strategy to counteract IDO-mediated resistance to immunotherapy (NCT02166905):* IDO is an important resistance mechanism that allows ovarian cancer to escape immune attack. This clinical trial tests a novel strategy of selectively breaking IDO-mediated immune tolerance and simultaneously promoting the generation of TA-specific T cells via vaccination against NY-ESO-1. The NY-ESO-1 vaccine in this trial vaccine is composed of DEC205mAb-NY-ESO-1 fusion protein (CDX-1401) with adjuvant poly-ICLC. The DEC-205 receptor has been shown to be an efficient monoclonal antibody (mAb)-based target to enhance the induction of strong antigen-specific immune responses and cross-presentation in mice[89] and humans.[90] The receptor is also expressed on human monocyte-derived DCs along with other endocytic receptors, such as the mannose receptor/CD206 and DC-SIGN/CD209.[91] In preclinical studies, full-length NY-ESO-1 was fused to the C-terminus of human anti-DEC-205 (DEC205mAb-NY-ESO-1 fusion protein). Although nontargeted and antibody-targeted NY-ESO-1 proteins similarly activated CD4$^+$ T cells, cross-presentation to CD8$^+$ T cells was only efficiently induced by antibody-targeted NY-ESO-1.[92] Therefore, in this clinical trial, the DEC-205 mAb-NY-ESO-1 fusion protein was directly injected subcutaneously in an effort to prime endogenous DCs with full-length NY-ESO-1 protein and thereby prime specific CD4$^+$ and CD8$^+$ T cells to NY-ESO-1. The trial is focused on ovarian cancer patients in first or subsequent remission. The success of the trial could lead to the development of a novel strategy to lengthen remission rates in ovarian cancer patients and minimize the risk of relapse.

Whole Tumor Vaccines in Ovarian Cancer

A pilot study at the University of Pennsylvania is testing administration of partially mature DCs pulsed with autologous tumor cell lysate to subjects with recurrent ovarian cancer in combination with immunomodulation using oral metronomic cyclophosphamide (to deplete T$_{reg}$ cells)[93] and bevacizumab (to disrupt the blood-tumor endothelial barrier).[94] Although whole tumor vaccines offer distinct advantages, some drawbacks warrant consideration. First, surgical procurement of a large number of autologous tumor cells may not be possible in many patients. Alternatives to this limitation exist, including use of allogeneic cell lines or the use of tumor mRNA. RNA electroporation of DCs is a convenient approach to generate a potent tumor vaccine.[95] An additional concern with whole tumor vaccination relates to the inclusion of a large number of "self" antigens, which could potentially drive tolerogenic responses, that is, expand T$_{reg}$ cells rather than cytotoxic lymphocyte responses. Other work has demonstrated that DCs can be polarized ex vivo with the use of IFNs, TLR agonists, or p38 mitogen-activated protein kinase inhibitors to drive cytotoxic lymphocytes and Th17 effector cells at the expense of T$_{reg}$ cell activity.[96] However, if immunization is successful, there may be increased concern for breaking tolerance to "self" antigens, leading to immunopathology. To date, pilot studies with whole tumor cell vaccines have reported no autoimmunity in patients with ovarian cancer. Furthermore, depletion of T$_{reg}$ cells is a likewise critical maneuver to enhance vaccine therapy.

Neoantigen Vaccines

Advances in next-generation sequencing and epitope prediction now permit the rapid identification of mutant tumor neoantigens. This has led to efforts to use these mutant tumor neoantigens for personalizing cancer immunotherapies. Indirect support for this approach comes from studies demonstrating (a) that infusion of autologous ex vivo expanded TILs can induce objective clinical responses in metastatic melanoma,[97] and (b) the relationship between pretherapy CD8$^+$ T cell infiltrates and response to checkpoint blockade in melanoma.[98] Deep-sequencing technologies permit easy identification of the mutations present within the protein-encoding part of the genome (the exome) of an individual tumor, allowing for prediction of potential neoantigens. Several preclinical and clinical studies have now confirmed the possibility of identifying neoantigens on the basis of cancer exome data.[99,100] Although there are limitations on probing the mutational profile of a tumor in a single biopsy, it is evident that the vast majority of neoantigens occur within exonic sequences and do not lead to the formation of neoantigens that are recognized by autologous T cells. Consequently, a robust pipeline for filtering the cancer exome data is essential. Epitope presentation of neoantigens by MHC class I molecules may be predicted using previously established algorithms that analyze critical features, such as the likelihood of proteasomal processing, transport into the endoplasmic reticulum, and affinity for the relevant MHC class I alleles. In order to predict epitope abundance, gene and/or protein expression levels can also be integrated into the analysis. Based on these considerations, it becomes of interest to stimulate neoantigen-specific T cell responses in cancer patients using two possible approaches. The first is to synthesize long peptide vaccines that encode a set of predicted neoantigens. The second approach is to identify and expand preexisting neoantigen-specific T cell populations to create either bulk neoantigen-specific T cell products or TCR-engineered T cells for adoptive therapy. Although these approaches have not yet been reported in ovarian cancer clinical trials, it is anticipated that such clinical trials will be undertaken in the near future.

Adoptive T Cell Therapy

Adoptive cell transfer (ACT) is an approach that involves: (a) the collection of circulating or tumor-infiltrating T cells;[101] (b) modification and/or expansion and activation ex vivo; and (c) their reinfusion into patients, usually after lymphodepleting preconditioning chemotherapy. Initial studies demonstrating the potential of T cell immunotherapy to eradicate solid tumors came from the National Cancer Institute (NCI) in studies of adoptive transfer of in vitro selected TILs.[102] Unfortunately, methods of isolating and manufacturing TILs are labor intensive and only successful in a subset of patients.[101,103] In order to improve the therapeutic potential of transferred cells, peripheral blood lymphocytes (PBLs) with unique antigen specificity can be genetically modified to express: (a) a TA-specific TCR or (b) a chimeric antigen receptor (CAR), that is, a transmembrane protein comprising the tumor-associated antigen (TAA)-binding domain of an immunoglobulin linked to one or more co-stimulatory molecules. ACT using TCR-engineered T cells has resulted in objective responses in the majority of treated melanoma patients,[104] but the efficacy is still limited in several solid tumors, including ovarian cancer. CD19-specific CAR T cells have also demonstrated encouraging results of inducing complete response in

70% to 90% of patients with relapsed or refractory B cell acute lymphoblastic leukemia.[105] Despite these spectacular results, the majority of clinical responses are short-lived with ultimate tumor relapse. A major explanation for this suboptimal outcome is the relatively limited long-term survival and effect or function due to suppression or exhaustion of infused engineered T cells. No ACT protocol is currently approved by the FDA for use in gynecologic cancer patients.

Interestingly, a recent experimental mouse model supports the efficacy of CD4+ T helper lymphocytes in adoptive immunotherapy. Mice with established tumors were treated with adoptive transfer using in vitro activated T lymphocytes harvested from tumor-draining lymph nodes. The results demonstrated that expanded sorted CD4+ T helper lymphocytes from the tumor-draining lymph node have therapeutic efficacy on their own, and a synergistic effect was found when CD4+ T helper lymphocytes were used in combination with expanded cytotoxic CD8+ T lymphocytes.[106] In addition, adoptive transfer of a TA-specific CD4+ T cell clone to one patient with metastatic malignant melanoma was reported to have allowed that patient to remain disease free 2 years later.[107]

For ovarian cancer, there are a number of ongoing trials evaluating the efficacy of TILs (NCT02482090, NCT01883297). In addition, Phase 1 studies of engineered T cells targeting MUC16 (NCT02498912), mesothelin (NCT01583686), and NY-ESO-1 (NCT01567891, NCT02457650) are ongoing. In preparation for ACT, patients usually receive lymphodepleting conditioning chemotherapy, and low- or high-dose interleukin-2 (IL-2) is administered after the transfer for T cell expansion. As ACT becomes more common, it becomes very important that all centers performing this procedure be familiar with potential adverse events that may occur and management of those events. Cytokine release syndrome, typically occurring between postinfusion days 2 and 10, manifests as fever, hypotension, and respiratory insufficiency, and can be managed with tocilizumab (an IL-6-receptor antagonist) and general supportive treatment in an intensive care unit setting. High-dose corticosteroids are administered in life-threatening cases. Patients who have undergone multiple cycles of chemotherapy in the past may end up with persistent pancytopenia, and therefore it is advisable to decrease the dose of conditioning chemotherapy and cryopreserve stem cell reserves for backup.

Increasing evidence indicates that T cells that are expanded ex vivo, to maintain more stem-like T cell populations known as T stem cell memory (Tscm) cells, are capable of a more sustained response by replenishing effectors.[108] A clear benefit of transferring less mature, more stem-like cells is likely due to increased persistence and replenishing capability of these cells in vivo.

Conceptually, starting with hematopoietic stem/progenitor cells (HSCs), there is potential to further augment persistence of engineered T cells. This is because the regenerative nature of HSCs may provide a long-lasting, potentially lifelong supply of effector T cells engineered against TAs by TCR genes. This approach is currently being tested in an ongoing clinical trial in ovarian cancer patients at Roswell Park Comprehensive Cancer Center (NCT03691376).

ENDOMETRIAL (UTERINE) CANCER

Endometrial cancer is the most common gynecologic malignancy in developed countries. Preclinical and clinical investigation of immunotherapy for endometrial cancer is not as advanced as for ovarian or cervical cancer. This is probably because the majority of the patients present with grades 1 and 2, low-stage endometrioid tumors, and surgical resection with hysterectomy alone results in cure for these patients. However, for patients with advanced-stage disease and/or high-risk histological subtypes, the prognosis remains poor. Interestingly, approximately 20% to 30% of endometrial cancers are characterized by high microsatellite instability (MSI-H) due to genetic or epigenetic defects in components of the DNA mismatch repair pathway. These patients have high somatic mutation and neo-antigen load, and potentially high infiltration by T cells. Based on data from colon cancer indicating that patients with MSI-H tumors show improved ORR and PFS[109] to checkpoint blockade, MSI-H endometrial cancer patients were tested in multiple studies. In May 2017, pembrolizumab as a single agent received accelerated approval for refractory MSI-H solid tumors, including endometrial carcinoma, in which it demonstrated a 36% ORR and durations of response ongoing with a range of 4 to 17 months.[110] Subsequently, in September 2019, the FDA granted accelerated approval to pembrolizumab plus lenvatinib for the treatment of patients with advanced endometrial carcinoma regardless of MSI or mismatch repair status and who have disease progression following prior systemic therapy. The approval was based on a KEYNOTE-146 trial that demonstrated ORR of 38.3% (95% CI, 28.5%–48.9%) with 10 complete responses (10.6%) in patients with previously treated metastatic endometrial cancer whose tumors were not MSI-H/dMMR.[111]

Another subset of highly immunogenic endometrial cancers is characterized by ultra-high somatic mutation rates resulting from defects in the proofreading function of the replicative DNA polymerase epsilon (POLE).[112] These tumors are predominantly endometrioid, grade III, associated with peritumoral and TILs, and reported to have the highest number of predicted neoantigens per tumor sample.[112] Collectively, these results provide a rationale for the use of checkpoint inhibitors in endometrial cancers harboring the POLE ultramutated phenotype and MSI-H. Other cancer immunotherapy strategies, such as cancer vaccines and ACTs, that are applicable to ovarian cancer may also be relevant for advanced, recurrent, or metastatic endometrial cancers.

CERVICAL CANCER

On a global scale, approximately one in six new cancer diagnoses is attributable to an infectious pathogen. HPVs cause approximately 30% of malignancies attributable to specific infections, including cancers of the cervix, vagina, vulva, anus, and oropharynx.[113] Despite the existence of preventive HPV vaccines and screening methods to detect HPV, cervical cancer remains the second largest cause of cancer mortality in women in low-resource settings.

HPV infects cervical epithelium shortly after sexual debut,[114,115] and can be detected in up to 50% of young women who have initiated sexual intercourse in the preceding 36 months.[115,116] Infections are asymptomatic, and although most are transient, resolution can take 1 to 2 years.[117,118] Older women take longer to clear infections, as do smokers and women with underlying immunosuppression.[118] The clinically silent nature of these infections facilitates maintenance of a large herd burden of transmissible HPV. Moreover, rates of preventive vaccination in eligible U.S. cohorts, young people age 9 to 26, have been suboptimal; in 2010, less than half of adolescent girls aged 13 to 17 years had initiated vaccination.[119] Among vaccine initiators, less than one-third complete all three vaccinations in the three-vaccination regimen. The incidence of HPV-associated cancers in anatomic sites for which screening algorithms have not yet been validated, particularly in the oropharynx, is increasing steadily, and will likely bypass that of cervical cancer in the near future. The existing prophylactic vaccines, Gardasil© and Cervarix©, have no therapeutic effect.

Biology of HPV Infection

HPVs are non-enveloped, double-stranded DNA viruses, which are tropic for mucosal tissues. The genome consists of three functionally divided regions: (a) a noncoding regulatory region; (b) an early proteins region, which encodes for six early proteins (E1, E2, E4-E7); and (c) a late region, which encodes for the viral capsid proteins L1 and L2.[120] HPVs infect basal epithelial (skin or mucosal) cells. More than 200 HPV genotypes have been identified. Oncogenic genotypes include HPV 16, 18, 31, 33, 35, 39, 45, 51, 52, 56, 58, 59, and 66.

The development of squamous cervical cancer, other anogenital cancers, and head and neck cancers occurs in the setting of a persistent infection with an oncogenic HPV. Virtually all squamous cancers of the cervix (SCCx) and its precursor, HGSILs/CIN2/3, are caused by HPV, most commonly HPV16. The development of both cervical cancer and HGSIL/CIN2/3 is associated with the integration of the HPV genome into the host genome and subsequent expression of two HPV early gene products, E6 and E7, which inactivate p53 and pRb, respectively.[121] Viral integration sites, though randomly distributed within the human genome,[122] occur principally at sites where human DNA is prone to breakage (e.g., fragile sites), and appear to affect only the expression of the HPV genome itself. Specifically, E1 and/or E2 are most frequently disrupted in integration, whereas the E6 and E7 viral oncogenes are retained, resulting in constitutive expression. Expression of both E6 and E7 is functionally required to initiate and maintain neoplastic transformation.[123,124] Morphologically at the cellular level, high-grade intraepithelial lesions are characterized by a high nuclear-to-cytoplasmic ratio. Histologically, high-grade lesions display full-thickness lack of cell maturation, and are mitotically active.

Immune Responses in Natural Infection

In the setting of a natural HPV infection, both humoral and adaptive systemic immune responses are weak. Antibody titers after viral clearance are detectable in 50% to 70% of persons.[125] Although the quality of the humoral response to natural infection appears to have interpersonal variation, most B memory cells elicited by natural infection generate antibodies that have low avidity and are nonneutralizing.[126,127] Similarly, T cell responses to viral antigens are marginal, require ex vivo stimulation to be detectable, and do not reliably distinguish persons whose lesions will regress from those whose lesions will not.[120,128] In point of fact, persistent HPV infections and preinvasive HPV lesions are limited to the squamous mucosa, and are presented in a noninflammatory context without systemic viremia. Infections are anatomically restricted to the mucosal epithelium and do not elicit systemic symptoms.[115,118] Using ex vivo stimulation, HPV16 E7-specific cytotoxic T cells have been detected in women with CIN3[120,129] and cervical cancer;[130,131] however, to date, no clear association has been made between the magnitude of response in the blood and clinical outcomes. Peripheral blood cytotoxic T cell responses to HPV16-E6, in contrast, have been linked to clinical outcomes. In particular, a CD4+ T cell response to E6 is associated with better clinical outcomes.[132] Conversely, functionally impaired E6-specific CD4+ T cell responses have been associated with cervical cancers.[133] Despite the rarity of HPV-specific memory T cells in the blood, a subset of persons with CIN2/3 do mount an effective response; not all CIN2/3 lesions progress to invasive cancer. We,

and others, have reported that in a time frame of 4 to 6 months, about 35% of CIN2/3 lesions undergo spontaneous regression.[134] Lesions resulting from mono-infection with HPV16 are less likely to undergo regression than lesions caused by other HPV genotypes: in this time frame, about 20% to 25% of HPV16-associated CIN2/3 lesions regressed.

The fact that neither the magnitude nor the breadth of naturally occurring T cell responses detected in the blood are robust predictors of regression of preinvasive HPV disease of the cervix raises the question of whether it is possible to identify factors in the target lesion that could predict disease outcome, or characteristics of the immune response that eliminate either infection, incipient malignancy, or cancer. Tissue-based studies of HPV lesions are revealing factors associated with clinical outcomes. In CIN2/3 lesions that do not regress, although CD8+ T cell infiltrates in the mucosa are increased, they are largely restricted to the stroma, failing to access the lesional epithelium.[135] The presence of intraepithelial CD8+ T cells, in contrast, is associated with subsequent regression. Similarly, in HPV-associated cancers of the cervix and oropharynx, the presence of intratumoral CD8+ T cells is associated with better prognosis.[130,136,137] In the end, systemic immune responses to viral proteins required for disease are weak, and do not reliably predict clinical behavior, underscoring the need for a better understanding of the mucosal microenvironment. Quantitative methods, including image analysis-directed rapid immune-laser capture microdissection, will make it possible to analyze specific cell subsets isolated from specific histologic contexts.[117]

Preventative Vaccines

Current methods for preventing HPV disease include screening, using either cytology or HPV testing, or a combination of both. Prophylactic vaccines that protect against infection with oncogenic HPV genotypes are comprised of noninfective recombinant virus-like particles (VLPs) of L1, one of the two HPV capsid proteins. These VLPs do not contain viral DNA, and thus are completely noninfectious and nononcogenic. Currently, three constructs are available: Cervarix©, which targets HPV types 16 and 18 (bHPV); Gardasil4©, which targets HPV types 6, 11, 16, and 18 (qHPV); and Gardasil9©, which targets HPV types 6, 11, 16, 18, 31, 33, 45, 52, and 58 (nHPV). All are highly effective against HPV infections not only in the cervix, but also other anatomical sites, in both sexes. These vaccines elicit robust antibody responses that are 1 to 2 logs greater than those elicited by natural infection.[126] In persons known to have been previously exposed to HPV, a single vaccination with qHPV drastically enhanced both the magnitude and the quality of the antibody response. In contrast to the nonneutralizing antibodies generated by natural infections, antibodies elicited by vaccination were neutralizing.[126] Emerging evidence suggests that vaccination with a preventative vaccine after excisional treatment of CIN2/3 significantly decreases the likelihood of disease recurrence.[138]

Therapeutic Vaccines

In contrast to the prophylactic vaccines, the development of new therapeutic vaccines is focused on targeting E6 and E7. Effector T cell responses to these viral, non-self oncoproteins, which are constitutively expressed by transformed cells, are likely to play a role in mediating lesion regression. Persons with preinvasive disease present an unparalleled opportunity to determine proof-of-principle for immunotherapeutic strategies. These lesions are directly accessible and clinically indolent, providing an opportunity to assess the relevant tissue before and after intervention. Moreover, a subset of patients does respond, thereby making it possible to determine either pretreatment characteristics that predict therapeutic effect, or characteristics of induced immune responses that predict therapeutic benefit. Tissue studies will also afford the ability to determine mechanisms of immune suppression mediated by different stages of HPV disease.

Several vaccine platforms have been evaluated, including naked DNA; DNA administered with electroporation; viral vectors, including modified vaccinia Ankara (MVA) and vaccinia virus; peptides administered with adjuvant; and bacterial constructs, such as *Listeria monocytogenes*. Despite promising data derived from preclinical models, translation to humans has been modest. To date, vaccine-induced immune responses in humans with any stage of HPV disease have been minimal. In retrospect, this apparent discrepancy may be in part a consequence of trial design. Most trials administered immunotherapeutics peripherally, and most trials were designed to evaluate conventional endpoints, including immune responses in the blood, and lesion regression versus persistence. In fact, postvaccination tissue resection specimens in persons with HPV16+ CIN2/3 who had received heterologous DNA-prime, recombinant vaccinia (TA-HPV) boost vaccination before resection showed drastic changes in the target lesions.[139] These included robust immune cell infiltrates in both the stromal and epithelial compartments, which were restricted to residual CIN2/3, and did not involve adjacent normal mucosa. These infiltrates contained clonally expanded populations of TCRs, which were in many cases organized into tertiary lymphoid structures or outright germinal centers and had a Th1 phenotype. This study established two critical points: that it was possible to elicit an effector response to antigens that had been present in a chronic fashion, and that T

cells generated by peripheral, intramuscular vaccination could traffic to the relevant immunologic target. In resections that had residual CIN2/3, these lesions were heavily infiltrated with CD8+ T cells that were colocalized with apoptotic lesional squamous epithelial cells. This finding suggested that a planned resection proximate to vaccination essentially censored the endpoint. By conventional measures, that is, peripheral blood T cell responses to vaccine antigens, and complete histologic regression, this regimen was a failure. However, there was no way to conclude that vaccination had "failed," given the findings in the target tissue. This insight has informed the design of subsequent clinical trials in persons with preinvasive HPV disease: tissue endpoints are obtained at a longer interval after therapeutic interventions, and although peripheral blood T cell responses are measured, quantitative measures in the lesion microenvironment are included.

A subsequent Phase 2 trial testing therapeutic vaccination for HPV16 or 18+ CIN2/3 reported a 49% rate of histologic regression. Although a subset of subjects who received placebo also had histologic regression, HPV became undetectable in 80% of vaccinated subjects who had histologic regression, in contrast to 30% of spontaneous regressions. The concomitant clearance of detectable virus in vaccinated subjects suggests that rates of recurrence may be lower in vaccinated subjects compared with those who received placebo; persistent HPV infection after resection of a preinvasive lesion is the most predictive risk for recurrence.[140]

Recently, the efficacy of therapeutic vaccination with human papillomavirus type 16 synthetic long peptides (HPV16-SLPs) in combination with standard carboplatin and paclitaxel chemotherapy was demonstrated in patients with HPV16-positive cervical cancer.[141] Treatment efficacy was directly related to a chemotherapy-mediated altered composition of the myeloid cell population in the blood and tumor, an effect that was most pronounced starting 2 weeks after the second cycle of chemotherapy.

Manipulating the Tumor Microenvironment

Like many other solid tumors, HPV-associated malignancies establish an immune-suppressive local microenvironment. The HPV life cycle is not cytolytic, and replication and assembly are temporally linked with cellular differentiation of squamous epithelial cells, absent pro-inflammatory signals. Virus is shed in terminally differentiated squamous cells. The initial exposure to HPV antigens is minimal, and may not prompt activation of the immune response. E6 and E7 inhibit both IFN receptor signaling and activation of the IFN response genes.[142] E7 also further impairs the innate response by downregulating TLR9 transcription. HPV downregulates cell surface MHC class I expression,[143] and inhibits the production of pro-inflammatory cytokines.[144]

Macrophage infiltration in both the stromal and epithelial compartments increases with the severity of HPV lesions, from HPV-infected cells to CIN2/3 to squamous cancers.[145,146] These macrophages are derived from circulating peripheral blood monocytes, which migrate to the tumor site, where they differentiate into macrophages and DCs.[147] Their functional polarization is mediated by tumor-secreted TGF-β and IL-10.[148] As early in disease development as CIN2, the intensity of macrophage infiltrates correlates directly with the number of lymphatic vessels.[146] Epithelial expression of COX-2 increases with disease severity, which in turn inhibits DC maturation, reduces the ability of DCs to stimulate T cell proliferation, and increases production of IL-10.[149] HPVs have also been shown to suppress maturation and function of Langerhans cells, which are epithelial-resident APCs.[150–152] However, this suppressive phenotype can be reversed in the presence of TLR3 agonists.[153] Similarly, the tissue microenvironment induces and maintains tissue-specific gene expression and function of resident and recruited macrophages.[154–156] A growing body of evidence demonstrates functional plasticity in tissue macrophages; an induced suppressive or tolerizing phenotype can be reeducated by CD4+ Th1 T cells, to an activated, effector phenotype, with cell surface expression of co-stimulatory molecules.[157]

Finally, different cell subsets in HPV-associated malignancies, including tumor epithelium, TAMs, and CD8+ T cells, frequently express PD-L1.[158,159] Although the presence of PD-L1 expression is associated with impaired cell-mediated immunity in HPV disease,[159] tumor expression in and of itself is not a reliable biomarker for likelihood of response to PD-1 blockade.[160] The presence of a gene signature of IFN-γ-inducible genes, however, is somewhat associated with response to PD-1 blockade. This finding is consistent with what has been observed in other solid tumors: namely, that clinical benefit from PD-1 blockade is more likely to occur in the setting of a preexisting host tumor-specific immune response. Therefore, it is possible that an indirect measure, such as Ki67, which is upregulated after activation via engagement of cognate antigen with the TCR, may be more predictive of response.

Immune Checkpoint Inhibitors

Several studies of ICIs alone or in combination in recurrent cervical cancer were recently completed or ongoing. In a Phase 2 evaluation of nivolumab in the treatment of persistent or recurrent cervical cancer (NCT02257528/NRG-GY002), the response rate was 4% (1/25; 90% CI, 0.4%–22.9%), and 36% of patients had stable disease (9/25; 90% CI: 20.2%–54.4%), with a median duration of SD of 5.7 months (range, 3.5–12.7).[161] In contrast, in the Phase 1/2 CheckMate 358 Trial (NCT02488759), nivolumab resulted in ORR of 26.3% (95% CI, 9.1–51.2) in patients with metastatic cervical cancer.[162] In the KEYNOTE-158 study of pembrolizumab, the response rate was 14.3%, and 91% of the patients studied had a duration of response of at least 6 months, and the OS was 9.4 months. Despite the relatively low response rates, the durable antitumor activity and safe profile led the FDA to grant approval of pembrolizumab in June 2018. Of note, all patients who responded were positive for PD-L1, and none without PD-L1 responded.

Immunomodulatory Effects of Conventional Cancer Treatment Modalities

Conventional anticancer treatment modalities, such as chemotherapy and radiation, have immunomodulatory effects. Metronomic cyclophosphamide, for example, depletes circulating T_{reg} cells.[93] In the case of cervical cancer, no effective therapies exist for metastatic or recurrent disease. The treatment options for inoperable primary tumors, and recurrent and metastatic disease, include a combination of platinum-based chemotherapy and radiation, both of which are known to enhance susceptibility of cervical cancers to cytotoxic T cells, in addition to their direct cytotoxic effect. Alkylating agents, including cisplatin, induce a high rate of genomic mutations.[163] Some of the immunomodulatory effects of radiation include upregulated expression of TAAs[164] and upregulation of MHC class I expression on tumor cells. Ionizing radiation enhances epitope spreading.[165] An example of how these different attributes could be leveraged in persons with metastatic or recurrent disease might be to deplete T_{reg} cells with low-dose cyclophosphamide; prime initially with a therapeutic vaccine, or infusion of tumor-specific CTL; followed by chemoradiation. This is illustrated by the report of the effect of a combination of carboplatin and paclitaxel (CarboTaxol) in patients with advanced cervical cancers; this regimen was followed by a significant decrease in the frequency of circulating myeloid cells, which reached nadir at 1 to 2 weeks after two cycles.[141] A second cohort then received a therapeutic vaccination 2 weeks after the last cycle of CarboTaxol. None of the patients had an endogenous, preexisting response to HPV16. These responses were of greater magnitude than those observed in a previous trial in which patients were vaccinated 1 month after chemotherapy.[166] However, no clinical responses were reported.

In sum, although much is known about the immunobiology of HPV-associated malignancies, there is much to learn about the timing and sequence of anticancer treatment modalities. HPV-associated lesions are relatively accessible, and viral antigens provide targets for both immunotherapy as well as for monitoring, and so it becomes possible to dissect out mechanisms of action in the lesion microenvironment, as well as to identify proof-of-principle of therapeutic approaches.

Adoptive T Cell Therapy

So far, no viable therapies have been identified for either metastatic or recurrent cancers. One approach that shows promise in patients with metastatic HPV disease involves identifying tumor-specific T cells from the endogenous response, namely, from TILs. A recent report of HPV-targeted TILs in persons with pretreated, metastatic cervical cancer describes tumor responses in three of nine women: two complete responses and one partial response.[167] In a follow-up Phase 2 trial, objective tumor responses occurred in five of 18 (28%) patients with cervical cancer.[168] Two of the responses in cervical cancer were complete and ongoing 67 and 53 months after treatment. These outcomes are significant because there are no effective therapies for recurrent or metastatic cervical cancer.

Approaches to identify endogenous responses to HPV include either ex vivo stimulation of PBLs, or isolation from TILs. Although some of the T cells in the tumor bed may be nonspecific, recruited by a chemokine gradient, in some solid tumors, many of the tumor T cells express activation markers that are upregulated when the cell is activated by engagement of the TCR with its cognate antigen. Two markers that have been investigated are PD-1 and CD137. Several groups have reported that activated T cells in the TME are enriched for clonally expanded populations of tumor-reactive T cells.[169,170] The ability to isolate autologous HPV-specific TILs will provide the opportunity to assess the TCR repertoire and the functional polarization of relevant cells. Identification of TCRs with high avidity for tumor epitopes could pave the way for generation of TCR libraries across HLA phenotypes. Autologous T cells genetically engineered to express HLA-matched HPV-specific TCRs are also being used as individualized treatment for HPV-associated cervical cancer.[171,172]

CONCLUSION

Cancer immunotherapy is evolving quickly and understanding the dynamics of the response to this therapy in gynecologic malignancies in order to find ways to overcome immune suppression and counterregulation should lead to the development of effective personalized approaches. Immunotherapy is expected to mediate tumor destruction and drive local inflammation in the TME, but also trigger coordinated induction of multiple counterregulatory and suppressive pathways like IDO, TGF-β, PD-L1, and T_{reg} cells. Concomitant blockade of these suppressive pathways at the time of vaccination or T cell transfer will allow inflammation-induced transformation of the tumor milieu from a tolerogenic to an immunogenic signature. Based on the limited results of blockade of the PD-1/PD-L1 pathway in ovarian and other gynecologic cancers, it is important to consider opportunities for combination therapies. These include dual checkpoint blockade; for example, the combination of CTLA-4 and PD-1 blockade or combination with ACT. Ipilimumab removes a physiologic brake on T cells during activation, whereas anti–PD-1 removes a brake on activation during T cell effector function. This combination may also overcome resistance to CTLA-4 blockade mediated by tumor PD-L1 expression or resistance to PD-1 blockade mediated by T cell downregulation through the co-expression of CTLA-4. Another potential checkpoint combination therapy is blockade of PD-1 and LAG-3, an approach that has demonstrated excellent results in preclinical models of ovarian cancer. Additional potential combinations include combinations with targeted agents such as bevacizumab, chemotherapies with potential to cause immunogenic cell death, and vaccine combinations.

KEY REFERENCES

Only key references appear in the print edition. The full reference list appears in the digital product on Springer Publishing Connect: connect.springerpub.com/content/book/978-0-8261-3743-2/part/part04/chapter/ch55

5. Sato E, Olson SH, Ahn J, et al. Intraepithelial CD8⁺ tumor-infiltrating lymphocytes and a high CD8⁺/regulatory T cell ratio are associated with favorable prognosis in ovarian cancer. *Proc Natl Acad Sci USA*. 2005;102(51):18538–18543. doi:10.1073/pnas.0509182102

7. Zhang L, Conejo-Garcia JR, Katsaros D, et al. Intratumoral T cells, recurrence, and survival in epithelial ovarian cancer. *N Engl J Med*. 2003;348:203–213. doi:10.1056/NEJMoa020177

24. Matsuzaki J, Gnjatic S, Mhawech-Fauceglia P, et al. Tumor-infiltrating NY-ESO-1-specific CD8⁺ T cells are negatively regulated by LAG-3 and PD-1 in human ovarian cancer. *Proc Natl Acad Sci USA*. 2010;107(17):7875–7880. doi:10.1073/pnas.1003345107

43. Zamarin D, Burger RA, Sill MW, et al. Randomized Phase II trial of nivolumab versus nivolumab and ipilimumab for recurrent or persistent ovarian cancer: an NRG oncology study. *J Clin Oncol*. 2020;38(16):1814–1823. doi:10.1200/JCO.19.02059

55. Konstantinopoulos PA, Waggoner S, Vidal GA, et al. Single-arm Phases 1 and 2 trial of niraparib in combination with pembrolizumab in patients with recurrent platinum-resistant ovarian carcinoma. *JAMA Oncol*. 2019;5(8):1141–1149. doi:10.1001/jamaoncol.2019.1048

109. Le DT, Uram JN, Wang H, et al. PD-1 blockade in tumors with mismatch-repair deficiency. *N Engl J Med*. 2015;372(26):2509–2520. doi:10.1056/NEJMoa1500596

167. Stevanovic S, Draper LM, Langhan MM, et al. Complete regression of metastatic cervical cancer after treatment with human papillomavirus-targeted tumor-infiltrating T cells. *J Clin Oncol*. 2015;33(14):1543–1550. doi:10.1200/JCO.2014.58.9093

Breast Cancer Immunotherapy

Leisha A. Emens and Rita Nanda

KEY POINTS

- Breast cancer is a heterogeneous disease.

- Immunity plays a dual role in breast cancer, promoting both tumor elimination and disease progression.

- Tumor-infiltrating lymphocytes are prognostic and predictive in human epidermal growth factor receptor (HER2[+]) and triple-negative breast cancer (TNBC).

- Programmed cell death 1/programmed cell death ligand 1 (PD-1/PD-L1) antagonists alone and with chemotherapy have clear clinical activity in PD-L1 immune cell (IC) + patients with metastatic TNBC.

- Adding PD-1/PD-L1 antagonists to standard neoadjuvant chemotherapy for early TNBC improves the rate of pathologic complete response (pCR) regardless of PD-L1 status.

- Antagonists of cytotoxic T lymphocytic antigen-4 (CTLA-4) and lymphocyte antigen gene-3 (LAG-3) show early evidence of immunologic and clinical activity in breast cancer.

- PD-1/PD-L1 antagonists combined with precision medicines (such as inhibitors of PARP, PIK3CA, MEK) show promising clinical activity in early trials.

- Therapeutic breast cancer vaccines are safe and immunologically active.

- Vaccines have potential for the primary and secondary prevention of breast cancer.

- Combination strategies are the future of breast cancer immunotherapy.

INTRODUCTION

Breast cancer is the most common malignancy in women worldwide, with almost 2.1 million new cases in 2018.[1] In the United States alone, breast cancer causes more than 42,000 deaths annually.[2] Optimizing standard treatments for breast cancer has improved overall survival (OS) over the last 40 years,[3–5] and newer precision medicines, including immunotherapies, have further improved clinical outcomes. Monoclonal antibodies specific for the programmed death-1 (PD-1) pathway have now demonstrated clinical benefit in patients with triple-negative breast cancer (TNBC), with emerging evidence for clinical activity in human epidermal growth factor receptor (HER2[+]) and hormone receptor-positive (HR[+]) breast cancer.[6,7] This chapter provides an overview of recent advances and ongoing investigations in immune-based treatment strategies.

BREAST CANCER IS A HETEROGENEOUS DISEASE

Breast cancer is not one disease, but rather a diverse group of malignancies with distinct clinical behavior. Systemic breast cancer therapy has historically been based on estrogen receptor (ER), progesterone receptor (PR), and HER2 expression. Breast cancers that are HR[+] are eligible for treatment with endocrine therapy, tumors that are HER2[+] can benefit from HER2-directed therapy, and all forms of breast cancer—including TNBC—are candidates for chemotherapy.[8] In the past few years, a number of targeted therapies have gained regulatory approval for all forms of breast cancer, including three distinct classes of agents for advanced TNBC.[9] It is critical to consider this basic clinical framework as immuno-oncology approaches are implemented for breast cancer therapy.

MOLECULAR TARGETS FOR BREAST CANCER THERAPY

Endocrine therapy for HR[+] breast cancer continues to be refined. The selective ER destroyer (SERD) fulvestrant combined with the aromatase inhibitor letrozole improves clinical outcomes in patients with metastatic disease.[10] Targeted inhibitors of cyclin-dependent kinases 4 and 6 (CDK4/6; palbociclib, ribociclib, or abemaciclib) added to either an aromatase inhibitor or fulvestrant have clear survival benefit in metastatic disease,[11–14] and emerging data suggest activity in early breast cancer.

HER2-targeted therapy has been transformational for HER2[+] breast cancer patients. The combination of trastuzumab, pertuzumab, and chemotherapy improves OS in advanced breast cancer,[15] and in early breast cancer trastuzumab-based chemotherapy reduces the risk of relapse by approximately 50%.[16,17] The judicious use of sequential HER2-directed therapy enhances quality of life and prolongs survival in patients with metastatic HER2[+] disease.[18] This includes switching chemotherapies on a trastuzumab backbone, and also integrating the HER2 tyrosine kinase inhibitor lapatinib in combination with capecitabine or trastuzumab (particularly when brain metastases are present). Trastuzumab-emtansine (T-DM1) is an antibody drug conjugate (ADC) that improves PFS and OS relative to lapatinib plus capecitabine in patients with HER2[+] metastatic breast cancer.[19] More recently, adding the HER2 kinase inhibitor tucatinib to capecitabine and trastuzumab further extended both PFS and OS, even in patients with brain metastases, who historically have poor outcomes.[20] A new ADC, trastuzumab deruxtecan (DS-8201), has demonstrated durable clinical activity in patients with heavily treated HER2[+] metastatic disease.[21] Pertuzumab, a monoclonal antibody that recognizes a distinct epitope of HER2, added to trastuzumab and docetaxel for the first-line therapy of relapsed HER2[+] disease improves both PFS and OS.[22,23] In the neoadjuvant setting, adding pertuzumab to trastuzumab, carboplatin, and docetaxel (TCHP) improved the pathologic complete response (pCR) rate to 66%.[24] Moreover, T-DM1 further decreases the risk of relapse in patients with residual disease after neoadjuvant trastuzumab-based therapy by 50%.[25] Extended adjuvant therapy with neratinib after trastuzumab-based chemotherapy has also been shown to improve clinical outcomes.[26]

Until recently, chemotherapy was the only U.S. Food and Drug Administration (FDA)–approved treatment for TNBC in the United States. Now, two poly (ADP-ribose) polymerase (PARP) inhibitors (olaparib and talazoparib) have regulatory approval in advanced HER2-negative breast cancer patients with a germline mutation in BRCA1/2 (gBRCA1/2).[27] Also, the ADC sacituzumab govitecan-hziy, specific for the human trophoblast cell-surface antigen-2 (Trop-2), is available for patients with treatment-refractory advanced TNBC.[28] Finally, the first immunotherapy-based regimen, *nab*-paclitaxel plus the PD-L1 inhibitor atezolizumab, is approved for advanced programmed death ligand-1[+] (PD-L1[+]) TNBC.[29]

HOST–TUMOR INTERACTIONS AND BREAST CANCER IMMUNOTHERAPY

The immune system plays a dual role in breast cancer development and progression. This is best explained by selective immune pressure that first promotes tumor elimination, then immune-editing, and ultimately immune escape.[30,31] Early in tumor development, an acute inflammatory response triggered by stromal remodeling and angiogenesis initiates recruitment of innate immune effectors (macrophages, dendritic cells [DCs], natural killer [NK] cells), resulting in the production of interleukin-12 (IL-12) and interferon gamma (IFN-γ), resulting in tumor cell death. Here, DCs mature, process tumor-associated antigens, and migrate to tumor-draining lymph nodes to present antigen and activate naïve T cells. These activated T cells expand and traffic to the tumor microenvironment (TME), where they lyse tumor cells. This immune response either results in tumor eradication, or in the selection of tumor cell escape variants with defects in antigen processing and presentation, antigen mutation or loss, defects in T cell signaling, imbalances in immune checkpoint activity, or defects in IFN signaling. The tumor evolves to a state of equilibrium, with tumor eradication balanced by immune escape (Figure 56.1). In this phase, inflammation shifts from acute to chronic, with suppressive macrophages, regulatory T cells (T_{regs} cells), myeloid-derived suppressor cells (MDSCs), regulatory B cells, and tumor-associated fibroblasts dominating. Ultimately, a T helper type 2 (Th2) cytokine profile results,[32] and adaptive immune resistance is established.[33] At this stage, tumors escape immune surveillance to grow and metastasize unchecked. A better understanding of this process should inform the development of effective immunotherapies that tip the balance back toward tumor elimination. From a clinical perspective, it is now clear that some breast tumors naturally induce an adaptive immune response, contain tumor-infiltrating T cells (TILs) at diagnosis, and may also express PD-L1.[34] Lymphocyte predominant breast cancers have stromal or intratumoral lymphocytes accounting for over 50 to 60% of tumor tissue,[35] with a linear (not dichotomous) relationship between TIL and clinical outcomes. The presence of TILs at diagnosis is both prognostic and predictive.[36]

IMMUNE CHECKPOINT MODULATION FOR METASTATIC BREAST CANCER

Programmed Cell Death 1/Programmed Cell Death Ligand 1 Blockade

Early trials of PD-1/PD-L1 antagonists demonstrated their safety in breast cancer, with clinical activity varying with breast cancer subtype. Data across early trials and antibodies are consistent, regardless of the antibody tested (Table 56.1). TNBC uniquely presented both high unmet clinical need and evidence of preexisting immunity in some patients. Most randomized Phase 2 and 3 clinical trials have thus focused on TNBC, with some work in HER2[+] breast cancer (Table 56.2).

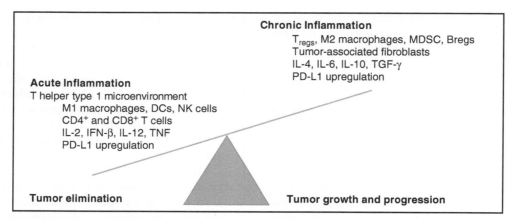

Figure 56.1 The immune system plays a role in breast tumor growth and progression, and also in breast tumor elimination. Early in the process of tumor development, the production of IL-12 and IFN-γ as a result of the acute inflammatory response establishes a T helper type 1 environment. During this phase, DCs mature, process tumor-associated antigens, and migrate to the tumor-draining lymph nodes to present antigen and activate naïve CD4+ and CD8+ T cells, which lyse tumor cells. This immune response initially results in complete tumor eradication, and the pressure it imposes ultimately results in the selection of tumor cell variants that escape the immune response. As inflammation shifts from acute to chronic, the TME evolves to a T helper type 2 profile. Adaptive immune resistance is established, and breast tumors grow unchecked.

DC, dendritic cell; IFN, interferon; IL, interleukin; MDSC, myeloid-derived suppressor cell; NK, natural killer; PD-L1, programmed cell death protein ligand-1; TGF, transforming growth factor; T_{reg}, regulatory T.

Table 56.1 Early Nonrandomized Clinical Trials of Programmed Cell Death Protein 1/Programmed Cell Death Protein Ligand-1 Blockade in Advanced Breast Cancer

TRIAL	SAMPLE SIZE	PATIENT POPULATION	PD-L1 STATUS	ORR	DCR	MEDIAN DOR	MEDIAN PFS	MEDIAN OS	REF
JAVELIN Avelumab monotherapy	n = 168 n = 58	All breast cancers mTNBC any line	Not PD-L1 selected	3.0% 5.2%	28% 31%	Not reached	5.9 weeks 5.9 weeks	8.1 months 9.2 months	37
Atezolizumab monotherapy	n = 115	mTNBC any line	n = 91 PD-L1+ n = 21 PD-L1-	10%	13%	21.0 months	1.4 months	8.9 months	38
Atezolizumab + *nab*-paclitaxel	n = 33	mTNBC any line	Not PD-L1 selected	39.4%	51.5%	9.1 months	5.5 months	14.7 months	39
KEYNOTE-012 Pembrolizumab monotherapy	n = 32	mTNBC any line	PD-L1 selected	18.5%	25.9%	Not reached	1.9 months	11.2 months	40
KEYNOTE-086 Pembrolizumab monotherapy Cohort A	n = 170	mTNBC ≥2nd line	Not PD-L1 selected n = 105 PD-L1+ n = 64 PD-L1-	5.3% 5.7% 4.7%	7.6% 9.5% 4.7%	Not reached Not reached 4.4 months	2.0 months 2.0 months 1.9 months	9.0 months 8.8 months 9.7 months	41
KEYNOTE-086 Pembrolizumab monotherapy Cohort B	n = 84	mTNBC 1st line	PD-L1 selected	21.4%	23.8%	10.4 months	2.1 months	18.0 months	42
PANACEA Pembrolizumab + Trastuzumab	n = 58	mHER2+ Trastuzumab^R	n = 46 PD-L1+ n = 18 PD-L1-	15% 0%	23.9% 0%	3.5 months 0 months	2.7 months 2.5 months	Not reached 7.0 months	7

DCR, disease control rate; DOR, duration of response; mTNBC, metastatic triple-negative breast cancer; mHER2+, metastatic human epidermal growth factor-2+; PD-1, programmed death protein-1; PD-L1, programmed death protein ligand-1; ORR, objective response rate; OS, overall survival; PFS, progression-free survival; Ref, reference; trastuzumab^R, trastuzumab resistant.

IMpassion130

Atezolizumab was evaluated in IMpassion130, a global, randomized, double-blind, placebo-controlled clinical trial based on early data demonstrating its safety and clinical activity as monotherapy and combined with *nab*-paclitaxel.[29] A Phase 1a monotherapy study evaluated atezolizumab in 115 patients with advanced TNBC.[38]

PD-L1 IC+ patients were initially enrolled, and eligibility was later expanded to include PD-L1 IC- TNBC patients; 69% of prescreened patients had PD-L1 IC+ tumors. The objective response rate (ORR) in 112 patients evaluable for efficacy was 10%, with an ORR of 24% first line, and 6% later line (Table 56.1). The median duration of response (DOR) was 21 months, and the median progression-free

Table 56.2 Randomized Phase 2 and 3 Clinical Trials of Immunotherapy in Advanced Breast Cancer

TRIAL	SAMPLE SIZE	KEY ELIGIBILITY	INTERVENTIONAL ARMS	ORR	MEDIAN PFS	MEDIAN OS	REF
IMpassion130 Phase 3 randomized 1:1 double-blind placebo-controlled	n = 902	1st line mTNBC TFI ≥12 months Any PD-L1 status	Atezolizumab + *nab*-paclitaxel vs. placebo + *nab*-paclitaxel	ITT 56% vs. 46% PD-L1 IC+ 59% vs. 43%	ITT 7.2 months vs. 5.5 months PD-L1 IC+ 7.5 months vs. 5.0 months	ITT 21.0 months vs. 18.7 months PD-L1 IC+ 25.0 months vs. 18.0 months	29, 43–46
IMpassion131 Phase 3 randomized 2:1 double-blind placebo-controlled	n = 943	1st line mTNBC TFI ≥12 months Any PD-L1 status	Atezolizumab + paclitaxel vs. placebo + paclitaxel	PD-L1 IC+ 63.4% vs. 55.4% ITT 53.6% vs. 47.5%	PD-L1 IC+ 6.0 months vs. 5.7 months ITT 5.7 months vs. 5.6 months	PD-L1 IC+ 28.3 months vs. 22.1 months ITT 22.8 months vs. 19.2 months	47
KEYNOTE 119 Phase 3 randomized 1:1 open-label	n = 622	mTNBC 2nd or 3rd line Prior A and T Any PD-L1 status	Pembrolizumab monotherapy vs. chemotherapy of physician's choice*	ITT 9.6% vs. 10.6% CPS ≥ 1 12.3% vs. 9.4% CPS ≥ 10 17.7% vs. 9.2% CPS ≥ 20† 26.3% vs. 11.5%	ITT 2.1 vs. 3.3 months CPS ≥ 1 2.1 vs. 3.1 months CPS ≥ 10 2.1 vs. 3.4 months CPS ≥ 20† 3.4 vs. 2.4 months	ITT 9.9 vs. 10.8 months CPS ≥ 1 10.7 vs. 10.2 months CPS ≥ 10 12.7 vs. 11.6 months CPS ≥ 20† 14.9 vs. 12.5 months	48
KEYNOTE 355 Phase 3 randomized 2:1 double-blind placebo-controlled	n = 847	1st line mTNBC TFI ≥ 6 months Any PD-L1 status	Pembrolizumab + chemotherapy‡ vs. placebo + chemotherapy	NR	ITT 7.5 vs. 5.6 months CPS ≥ 1 7.6 vs. 5.6 months CPS ≥ 10 9.7 vs. 5.6 months	NR	49

(continued)

Table 56.2 Randomized Phase 2 and 3 Clinical Trials of Immunotherapy in Advanced Breast Cancer (*continued*)

TRIAL	SAMPLE SIZE	KEY ELIGIBILITY	INTERVENTIONAL ARMS	ORR	MEDIAN PFS	MEDIAN OS	REF
KATE2 Phase 2 randomized 2:1 double-blind placebo-controlled	*n* = 202	mHER2+ BC Prior trastuzumab Prior taxane Any PD-L1 status	Atezolizumab + T-DM1 vs. placebo + T-DM1	ITT 45% vs. 43% PD-L1 IC+ 59% vs. 43%	ITT 8.2 months vs. 6.8 months PD-L1 IC+ 8.5 months vs. 4.1 months	NR 1-year OS ITT 89% vs. 89% 1-year OS PD-L1 IC+ 94.3% vs. 87.9% 1-year OS PD-L1 IC- 85.1% vs. 89.7%	50
Phase 2 randomized 1:1 open-label	*n* = 88	mER + HER2neg BC ≥2 lines prior endocrine therapy 0–2 lines prior chemotherapy	Eribulin + pembrolizumab vs. eribulin	ORR 27% vs. 34%	4.1 months vs. 4.2 months	ITT 13.4 vs. 12.5 months PD-L1+ 10.4 vs. 13.1 months	51

A, anthracycline; CPS, combined positive score; IC, immune cells; ITT, intention-to-treat; mER+HER2neg BC, metastatic estrogen receptor+ human epidermal growth factor-2+ breast cancer; mHER2+ BC, metastatic human epidermal growth factor-2+ breast cancer; mTNBC, metastatic triple-negative breast cancer; NR, not reported; ORR, overall response rate; OS, overall survival; PD-L1, programmed death ligand-1; PFS, progression-free survival; T, taxane; T-DM1, ado-trastuzumab emtansine; TFI, treatment-free interval.

*KEYNOTE-119: chemotherapy of physician's choice could be capecitabine, eribulin, gemcitabine, eribulin.

†Exploratory endpoint.

‡KEYNOTE-355: chemotherapy of physician's choice could be paclitaxel, *nab*-paclitaxel, or gemicitabine + carboplatin.

survival (PFS) and OS were 1.4 and 8.9 months. The median OS for first-line patients was 17.6 months compared to 7.3 months for patients treated beyond first line. Only patients with PD-L1+ immune cells (IC) occupying 1% or more of the tumor area-derived clinical benefit. This data, together with data from a small Phase 1b trial of atezolizumab with *nab*-paclitaxel in patients with advanced TNBC,[39] established the foundation for IMpassion130.

IMpassion130 randomized 902 patients 1:1 to *nab*-paclitaxel with either atezolizumab or placebo (Table 56.2).[29] Key eligibility criteria included incurable TNBC of any PD-L1 status relapsed ≥12 months from prior adjuvant chemotherapy, allowed adjuvant taxane, and not yet treated in the advanced disease setting. Stratification factors included liver metastases, prior taxane use, and PD-L1 IC expression. The study had four co-primary endpoints: PFS in the ITT and PD-L1 IC+ population (tested in parallel), and OS in the ITT and PD-L1 IC+ population (tested hierarchically). There was a statistically significant improvement in PFS in both the ITT and PD-L1 IC+ population, which was clinically meaningful in PD-L1 IC+ patients. Across the first, second, and final analyses, OS was not statistically significant in the ITT population, but there was a consistent and clinically meaningful improvement in OS in the PD-L1 IC+ population.[29,43,44] The final analysis showed an OS improvement of 7.5 months.[44] The combination was well-tolerated, with thyroid dysfunction and rash as the most common immune-related adverse events. Patient-reported outcomes and health-related quality of life were similar between arms.[45] Exploratory biomarker analyses evaluating stromal TILs, CD8+ T cells, PD-L1 expression in breast tumor cells, and the presence of a BRCA mutation revealed that these biomarkers were associated with clinical benefit only if the patient was also PD-L1 IC+.[46] The combination of atezolizumab and *nab*-paclitaxel is approved for the treatment of advanced PD-L1 IC+ TNBC by multiple health authorities. It is the first immunotherapy approved for breast cancer.

IMpassion131

IMPassion131 is a global, randomized, double-blind, placebo-controlled Phase 3 clinical trial that randomized 651 patients 2:1 to paclitaxel plus either atezolizumab or placebo (Table 56.2).[47] Key eligibility criteria included incurable TNBC of any PD-L1 status with a treatment-free interval from therapy (that may have included a taxane) with curative intent of 12 months or more, and no prior treatment for advanced TNBC. Stratification factors included liver metastases, prior taxane use, PD-L1 IC expression, and world region. The primary endpoint of the study was investigator-assessed PFS, hierarchically tested first in the PD-L1 IC⁺ population, and then, if significant, in the ITT population. In contrast to IMpassion131, there was no significant difference in PFS in either the PD-L1 IC⁺ or ITT populations with the addition of atezolizumab to paclitaxel. There was also no significant difference in OS (a secondary endpoint). Further exploration is required to understand potential reasons for the different results observed with IMpassion130 and IMpassion131.

KATE2

KATE2 is a global, randomized, double-blind, placebo-controlled Phase 2 clinical trial that tested T-DM1 with atezolizumab or placebo in patients with metastatic HER2⁺ breast cancer previously treated with trastuzumab and a taxane (Table 56.2).[50] Patients were randomized 2:1 to receive atezolizumab (133 patients) or placebo (69 patients) with T-DM1, and PFS was the primary endpoint; 42% of patients were PD-L1 IC⁺. The addition of atezolizumab to T-DM1 improved median PFS from 6.8 to 8.2 months in the ITT patient population (HR: 0.82, 95% CI: 0.55–1.23), and from 4.1 to 8.5 months in the PD-L1 IC+ population (HR: 0.60, 95% CI: 0.32–1.11). An exploratory analysis suggested a possible OS benefit in patients with PD-L1 IC⁺ disease. This combination will be definitively evaluated in KATE3, a randomized Phase 3 trial of PD-L1 IC⁺ patients with metastatic HER2⁺ breast cancer.

KEYNOTE-119

Two randomized Phase 3 trials evaluating pembrolizumab in advanced TNBC have been reported (Table 56.2). A two-arm Phase 2 monotherapy trial, KEYNOTE-086, set the stage for KEYNOTE 119.[41,42] KEYNOTE-086 enrolled patients with advanced TNBC into one of two cohorts (Table 56.1). Cohort A enrolled patients (n = 170) who had previously received at least one prior therapy for metastatic disease, regardless of PD-L1 expression, and cohort B enrolled PD-L1⁺ patients (n = 84) who had not yet been treated for advanced TNBC. In cohort A the entire group had an ORR of 5.3%, and the PD-L1⁺ group (61.8% of patients) had an ORR of 5.7%. In cohort B, the ORR was 21.4%; median PFS and OS were 2.1 months and 18.0 months, respectively. KEYNOTE-119 evaluated pembrolizumab monotherapy relative to single agent chemotherapy (capecitabine, gemcitabine, eribulin, and vinorelbine), randomizing 622 patients with recurrent TNBC treated with one to two prior therapies for metastatic disease 1:1 to pembrolizumab or chemotherapy (Table 56.2).[48] The study had three co-primary endpoints of OS in participants with disease having a combined positive score (CPS) ≥10, CPS ≥1, and any CPS. The

prevalence of PD-L1⁺ disease in the study was ~65% for CPS ≥1, ~31% for CPS ≥10, and ~17% for CPS ≥ 20. The study did not show a difference in PFS and OS at a CPS of ≥10 or ≥1; however, an exploratory analysis revealed improved PFS and OS with pembrolizumab at a CPS ≥ 20, with HRs of 0.76 (95% CI: 0.49–1.18) and 0.58 (95% CI: 0.38–0.88), respectively. The ORRs and DORs at a CPS ≥ 20 were 26.3% and 11.5%, and not reached and 7.1 months for pembrolizumab and chemotherapy, respectively.

KEYNOTE-355

KEYNOTE-355 is a randomized, double-blind, placebo-controlled Phase 3 study that evaluated pembrolizumab combined with chemotherapy relative to placebo with chemotherapy as first-line therapy for advanced TNBC; chemotherapy options included *nab*-paclitaxel, paclitaxel, and gemcitabine plus carboplatin (Table 56.2).[49] The study enrolled 847 patients of any PD-L1 status who had completed treatment with curative intent at least 6 months prior, and randomized them 2:1 to receive pembrolizumab or placebo with chemotherapy. The study had multiple co-primary endpoints: PFS in the ITT, CPS ≥ 1, and CPS ≥ 10 populations, and OS in the ITT, CPS ≥ 1, and CPS ≥ 10 populations; secondary endpoints included ORR, DOR, DCR, and safety. This study demonstrated an improvement in PFS with pembrolizumab and chemotherapy relative to chemotherapy with placebo in patients with PD-L1⁺ CPS ≥ 10 metastatic TNBC (9.7 vs. 5.6 months, HR: 0.65 [95% CI 0.49-0.86], *p* = .0012) but not for patients with lower levels of PD-L1 expression. OS has not been reported, and safety was consistent with the known toxicity profiles of each regimen.

The TONIC Trial

The adaptive, Phase 2 TONIC trial evaluated nivolumab alone or preceded by a 2-week induction with radiation (3x8Gy), low-dose cyclophosphamide, cisplatin, or doxorubicin in patients with metastatic TNBC.[52] The ORR was 20%, and most responses were observed in the cisplatin (ORR 23%) and doxorubicin (ORR 35%) cohorts. Doxorubicin priming was associated with the highest ORR and the greatest change in immunoregulatory genes related to inflammation, JAK/STAT, TNF-α, and PD-1/PD-L1 signaling, and T cell cytotoxicity pathways. These findings require confirmation in a prospective, controlled clinical trial.

Eribulin + Pembrolizumab

Very few ER⁺ HER2-negative metastatic breast cancer patients are PD-L1⁺ and have the potential to respond to monotherapy with PD-1/PD-L1 inhibitors, and combination therapies may enhance the likelihood of clinical benefit in these patients. A multicenter, randomized

Phase 2 clinical trial evaluated eribulin combined with pembrolizumab relative to eribulin alone in 88 patients with ER+ HER2-negative metastatic breast cancer who had received at least two lines of prior hormonal therapy and up to two lines of chemotherapy.[51] Patients were equally randomized between the arms, and patients assigned to eribulin monotherapy were allowed to crossover to eribulin plus pembrolizumab at disease progression. The primary endpoint was PFS, with secondary endpoints of ORR and OS. There was no difference in any of these three clinical endpoints between the arms.

LAG-3 Modulation

The soluble recombinant dimeric lymphocyte antigen gene-3 (LAG-3)-Ig fusion protein IMP321 binds with high avidity to major histocompatibility complex (MHC) class II proteins, resulting in DC maturation and durable CD8+ T cell responses. It was tested with weekly paclitaxel as first-line therapy in 30 patients with metastatic breast cancer.[53] The combination was safe, with an ORR of 50%, and a 6-month PFS rate of 90%. Biomarker analyses revealed a sustained increase in activated antigen-presenting cells, NK cells and CD8+ T effector memory cells (Table 56.3). A press release about the follow-up Phase 2b randomized, double-blind, placebo-controlled study in metastatic HR+ breast cancer patients revealed that there was no difference in 6-month PFS (p = .341).[54]

However, there was a trend toward clinical benefit with IMP321 in luminal B breast cancer patients (HR: 0.65), and in those with low monocytes at baseline (HR: 0.65). These data are not yet published, and the observations require testing in prospective clinical trials.

Cytotoxic T Lymphocytic Antigen 4 Blockade

Cytotoxic T lymphocytic antigen 4 (CTLA-4) is upregulated after T cell activation, where binding to its ligands CD80/CD86 sends a negative signal to downregulate T cell activation. Ipilimumab and tremelimumab, antagonists of CTLA-4, have been tested in breast cancer (Table 56.3). Tremelimumab (3 and 10 mg/kg every 28 or 90 days) was evaluated with concurrent exemestane in a Phase I trial of 26 patients with metastatic HR+ breast cancer.[55] Five patients had dose-limiting toxicity, four with diarrhea and one with transaminitis. The maximum tolerated dose was 6 mg/kg every 90 days. The best response was SD for ≥12 weeks or in 42% (11/26) of patients. Most patients developed increased peripheral ICOS+ CD4+ and CD8+ T cells, and a marked increase in the ratio of ICOS+/Foxp3+ T cells. Ipilimumab was tested preoperatively in 19 early stage breast cancer patients.[57] Patients received preoperative cryoablation (n = 7), single-dose 10 mg/kg ipilimumab (n = 6), or both (n = 6). No surgical delays occurred, and one grade 3 rash was noted. Combination therapy was associated with durable

Table 56.3 Clinical Trials Targeting LAG-3 and CTLA-4 in Breast Cancer

AGENT	BREAST CANCER TYPE	TRIAL PHASE	COMBINATION THERAPY	CLINICAL BENEFIT	REF
IMP-321 (LAG-3Ig)	Luminal breast cancer and TNBC	1/2	Paclitaxel 80 mg/m² weekly	ORR: 50% 6-month PFS: 90%	53
IMP-321 (eftilagimod-alpha)	Luminal breast cancer (ER + HER2neg)	2b	Paclitaxel 80 mg/m² weekly + eftilagimod-alpha for 6 months, followed by eftilagimod-alpha alone vs. Paclitaxel 80 mg/m² weekly + placebo for 6 months, followed by placebo alone	6-month PFS 63% vs. 54% HR: 0.93, p = .341 ORR = 48.3% with eftilagimod-alpha with paclitaxel vs. 38.4% with placebo with paclitaxel	54
Tremelimumab	Luminal breast cancer	1	Exemestane 25 mg daily	12-week SD: 42%	55
Tremelimumab	Luminal breast cancer and TNBC	1	Durvalumab	ORR 17% ITT ORR 43% TNBC	56
Ipilimumab	Early breast cancer (neoadjuvant)	1	Cryoablation	N/A	57,58

Ig, immunoglobulin; LAG-3, lymphocyte activation globulin-3; N/A, not applicable; ORR, overall response rate; PFS, progression-free survival; SD, stable disease; TNBC, triple negative breast cancer.

elevations in circulating T helper type 1 cytokines, CD4+ and CD8+ T cells expressing ICOS and Ki67, and an increased ratio of effector/T_{regs} cells within the tumor. Deep sequencing of T cell receptor DNA revealed clonally expanded TILs that correlated with the TIL score.[58]

Another single-arm pilot study evaluated tremelimumab with durvalumab in 18 patients with HER2- breast cancer, 11 with HR+ breast cancer and 7 with TNBC.[56] All responses occurred in TNBC patients, with ORRs of 17% and 43% in the ITT group and in TNBC patients, respectively. Responders had upregulation of immune gene expression and higher mutational loads.

IMMUNE CHECKPOINT MODULATION FOR EARLY BREAST CANCER

Neoadjuvant Trials

Clinical trials of immune checkpoint blockade in advanced breast cancer demonstrated that response rates are highest when used frontline, and in combination with chemotherapy. This led to great interest in evaluating immune checkpoint modulation for early breast cancer. Several neoadjuvant PD-1/PD-L1 blockade trials have been reported (Table 56.4).

Table 56.4 Randomized Phase 2 and 3 Clinical Trials Evaluating Immunotherapy in Early Breast Cancer

TRIAL	PATIENT POPULATION	SAMPLE SIZE	INTERVENTIONAL ARMS	PCR RATE* IMMUNOTHERAPY VS. CONTROL	REF
I-SPY2 Phase 2	HER2-	n = 201 n = 69	Paclitaxel x 4 → AC x 4 vs. paclitaxel + pembrolizumab x 4 → AC x 4	HR+: 30% vs. 13% TNBC: 60% vs. 22%	59, 60
	HER2-	n = 295 n = 73	Paclitaxel x 4 → AC x 4 vs. paclitaxel + pembrolizumab x 4 → pembrolizumab x 4	HR+: 15% vs. 15% TNBC: 27% vs. 27%	61
	HER2-	n = 299 n = 74	Paclitaxel x 4 → AC x 4 vs. olaparib + durvalumab + paclitaxel x 4 → AC x 4	HR+: 28% vs. 14% TNBC: 47% vs. 27%	62
KEYNOTE-522 Phase 3	TNBC	n = 390 n = 784	Paclitaxel + carbo + placebo → AC/EC + placebo x 4 → surgery → placebo vs. paclitaxel + carbo + pembrolizumab → AC/EC + pembrolizumab x 4 → surgery → pembrolizumab	ITT: 64.8% vs. 51.2% LN-: 64.9% vs. 58.6% LN+: 64.8% vs. 44.1%	63
GeparNuevo Phase 2	TNBC	n = 86 n = 88	Nab-paclitaxel + placebo x 4 → EC + placebo x 4 → surgery vs. nab-paclitaxel + durvalumab x 4 → EC + durvalumab x 4 → surgery	Window: 61.0% vs. 41.4% Concurrent: 53.4% vs. 44.2%	64, 65
NeoTripaPD-L1 Phase 3	TNBC	n = 42 n = 138	Nab-paclitaxel + carboplatin x 8 → surgery → AC/EC/FEC x 4 vs. nab-paclitaxel + carboplatin + atezolizumab x 8 → surgery → AC/EC/FEC x 4	ITT: 43.5% vs. 40.8% PD-L1+: 51.9% vs. 48.0% PD-L1-: 32.2% vs. 32.3%	66
IMpassion031 Phase 3	TNBC	n = 165 n = 168	Nab-paclitaxel + atezolizumab x 4 → AC + atezolizumab x 4 → surgery → atezolizumab vs. nab-paclitaxel + placebo x 4 → AC + placebo x 4 → surgery → observation	ITT: 57.6% vs. 41.4% PD-L1+: 68.8% vs. 49.3% PD-L1-: 47.7% vs. 34.4%	67

AC, doxorubicin + cyclophosphamide; carbo, carboplatin; EC, epirubicin + cyclophosphamide; EFS, event-free survival; FEC, 5-fluorouracil + epirubicin + cyclophosphamide; HER2, human epidermal growth factor receptor-2; HR, hormone receptor; ITT, intent-to-treat; LN, lymph node; NR, not reported; pCR, pathologic complete response; PD-L1, programmed death protein ligand-1; TNBC, triple-negative breast cancer.

*pCR rates in the I-SPY2 trials are estimated rates given the adaptive trial design.

I-SPY2

I-SPY2 is an adaptively randomized, Phase 2 multi-center neoadjuvant platform trial designed to accelerate drug development for early breast cancer. It evaluates multiple investigational agents concurrently against a common control arm (weekly paclitaxel for 12 weeks followed by doxorubicin plus cyclophosphamide every 2 to 3 weeks for four cycles).[68,69] The primary endpoint is pCR rate, defined as the absence of invasive cancer in the breast and regional lymph nodes at surgery. Graduation for efficacy occurs if the predefined efficacy threshold of 85% probability of success in a subtype-specific, hypothetical 300 patient Phase 3 trial is met. Investigational arms may be discontinued for lack of efficacy, futility, or toxicity.

Three arms of I-SPY2 evaluating immune checkpoint modulation have been reported; all enrolled patients with HR+/HER2- breast cancer or TNBC. The first investigated four cycles of pembrolizumab added to paclitaxel followed by AC (pembro4).[59] Pembro4 graduated for both HR+/HER2- and TNBC after 69 patients were randomized to pembrolizumab (40 HR+/HER2- and 29 TNBC) relative to 201 control patients. The estimated pCR rates were 30% versus 13% and 60% versus 22% for pembrolizumab versus control in the HR+/HER2- breast cancer and TNBC cohorts, respectively. The most common immune-related adverse events were pruritis and thyroid dysfunction in 31.9% and 13.0% of patients, respectively. Unexpectedly, irreversible adrenal insufficiency (AI) occurred at a rate of 8.7% (6/69) patients randomized to pembrolizumab; in metastatic disease the rate of AI is <1%. Exploratory immune biomarker analyses showed differences between HR+/HER2- disease and TNBC, where IC infiltrates (CD3+ T cells, CD8+ T cells, T$_{regs}$ cells, and PD-1+ T cells) were associated with pCR in HR+/HER2- tumors but not in TNBC.[60] PD-L1 expression (stromal and combined) was associated with pCR for both HR+/HER2- tumors and TNBC.

A second arm investigated eight cycles of pembrolizumab;[61] patients received paclitaxel plus pembrolizumab for four cycles followed by four cycles of pembrolizumab alone (pembro8-noAC). Seventy-three patients were treated, three of whom progressed on pembrolizumab alone. This arm was terminated, and investigators given the option to administer AC with pembrolizumab or proceed to definitive surgery following paclitaxel and pembrolizumab. The estimated pCR rates for the HR+/HER2- and TNBC tumors were identical for pembrolizumab versus control therapy, at 15% versus 15% and 27% versus 27%, respectively. AEs were as expected for the drug class.

I-SPY2 also evaluated the PARP inhibitor olaparib and the PD-L1 inhibitor durvalumab added to paclitaxel followed by AC.[62] After 73 patients were randomized (52 HR+/HER2-; 21 TNBC), this arm graduated in both patient groups. Estimated pCR rates were 28% versus 14% and 47% versus 27% for olaparib plus durvalumab versus control in the HR+/HER2- and TNBC cohorts, respectively. No unexpected adverse events emerged. Based on the success of these arms, I-SPY2 is investigating innovative combinations, including pembrolizumab plus SD-101 (a Toll-like receptor 9 agonist), cemiplimab (anti-PD-1) with paclitaxel, and cemiplimab plus REGN3767 (a LAG-3 antagonist).

KEYNOTE-522

KEYNOTE-522 is a global, randomized, double-blind, placebo-controlled Phase 3 trial of pembrolizumab for early-stage TNBC (Table 56.4).[63] Previously untreated stage II-III TNBC patients were randomized 2:1 to neoadjuvant pembrolizumab or placebo plus paclitaxel and carboplatin followed by AC; a total of 1,174 patients were enrolled. Following definitive surgery, patients received nine cycles of adjuvant pembrolizumab or placebo consistent with their assigned treatment arm. The primary endpoints were pCR and event-free survival (EFS) in the ITT population. At first analysis (conducted on the first 602 patients randomized), the pCR rate was 64.8% with pembrolizumab plus chemotherapy versus 51.2% with chemotherapy alone (p <.001). Patients with lymph node-positive disease had a greater improvement in the rate of pCR with the addition of pembrolizumab to standard chemotherapy (20.6% absolute improvement: 44.1% to 64.8%), relative to those with node-negative disease (6.3% absolute improvement: 58.6% to 64.9%). Benefit was observed regardless of PD-L1 status, though there was a trend toward greater improvement in PD-L1+ patients. At first analysis (104 events), a trend to improvement in 18-month EFS favored pembrolizumab (91.3% vs. 85.3%; HR: 0.63). AI occurred in 4.5% of patients randomized to pembrolizumab, half the rate observed in the I-SPY2 pembro4 arm (8.7%); no unexpected safety signals emerged. These positive findings from KEYNOTE-522 represent an elegant validation of the I-SPY2 adaptively randomized Phase 2 trial strategy, which aims to efficiently identify promising regimens to move forward to Phase 3 registrational trials. The ongoing KEYNOTE-756 trial will further address the role of PD-1 blockade plus chemotherapy in early-stage, high-risk HR+/HER2- breast cancer.

GeparNuevo

GeparNuevo is a randomized Phase 2 trial that investigated the addition of durvalumab to neoadjuvant taxane and anthracycline-based therapy for early TNBC (Table 56.4)[64] Participants were randomized to receive one dose of durvalumab or placebo 2 weeks prior to starting chemotherapy (window-phase), and then combined with weekly *nab*-paclitaxel for 12 weeks, followed by four cycles of EC with durvalumab or placebo. Due to concern about chemotherapy delays, the study was amended to eliminate the window-phase after 117 patients were enrolled. The primary endpoint was pCR, defined as the absence of both invasive and in situ residual disease in the breast and axilla at surgery. A total of 174 TNBC patients were enrolled. In the ITT population, pCR rates with durvalumab versus placebo were 53.4% versus 44.3% ($p = .287$). In the window cohort, the pCR rates with durvalumab versus placebo were 61.0% and 41.4%, respectively ($p = .035$). There was a trend to improve pCR rates with higher levels of stromal tumor-infiltrating lymphocytes (sTIL) and in PD-L1$^+$ versus PD-L1$^-$ tumors in all patients, regardless of arm (54.3% versus 30.0%; $p = .048$). Additional analyses showed that tumor mutational burden and immune gene expression profile added independent value for pCR prediction.[67]

NeoTRIPaPDL1

The NeoTRIPaPDL1 Michelangelo trial is a randomized Phase 3 trial of eight cycles of neoadjuvant carboplatin and *nab*-paclitaxel with or without atezolizumab, followed by surgery and adjuvant anthracycline-based treatment (Table 56.4).[66] This trial enrolled 280 patients with previously untreated TNBC. The primary endpoint was 5-year EFS; secondary endpoints were pCR (defined as the absence of invasive cancer in the breast and lymph nodes at surgery) and safety. There was no significant difference in the pCR rate for the atezolizumab arm compared to the control arm for the overall population (43.5% vs. 40.8%), those with PD-L1 IC$^+$ disease (51.9% vs. 48.0%), or those with PD-L1 IC$^-$ disease (32.2% vs. 32.3%). No unexpected adverse events emerged.

IMpassion031

IMpassion031 is a global, randomized, double-blind, placebo-controlled Phase 3 trial of neoadjuvant atezolizumab for early stage TNBC (Table 56.4).[67] Previously untreated stage II to III TNBC patients were randomized 1:1 to neoadjuvant atezolizumab or placebo plus weekly *nab*-paclitaxel followed by AC. Following definitive surgery, patients received 11 doses of adjuvant atezolizumab or observation consistent with their assigned treatment arm. Co-primary endpoints included pCR rates in the ITT and PD-L1 IC$^+$ patient populations, and secondary endpoints included EFS, DFS, and OS in the ITT and PD-L1 IC$^+$ patient groups. Stratification factors included disease stage and PD-L1 IC status. In 333 patients enrolled, the pCR rates were 57.6% and 41.1% in the atezolizumab/chemotherapy and placebo/chemotherapy groups, respectively ($p = .0044$). There was a numerical difference in pCR rates between PD-L1 IC$^+$ and PD-L1 IC$^-$ patients that favored the addition of atezolizumab, with point differences of 19.5% and 13.3%, respectively. Although

these secondary endpoints are premature, they support the pCR benefit observed for atezolizumab/chemotherapy. These data are consistent with the data generated by KEYNOTE 522.

Multiple trials are investigating adjuvant immunotherapy either in combination with standard of care chemotherapy or as monotherapy in those who are at high risk of recurrence, including those with large tumors, multiple positive lymph nodes, and those who fail to achieve a pCR with neoadjuvant chemotherapy. None have yet been reported.

BREAST CANCER VACCINES FOR THERAPY AND PREVENTION

Breast cancer vaccines are designed to induce and/or amplify tumor-specific T cells that recognize and lyse tumor cells.[70,71] The development of effective antigen-specific vaccines depends in part on the identification of breast tumor antigens that are potent tumor rejection targets. Although cancer vaccines induce antigen-specific immune responses, these responses historically do not often correlate with clinical benefit. This lack of clinical activity is probably multifactorial, resulting from immune checkpoints and other suppressive factors in the TME; alterations in tumor antigen expression, processing, and presentation; and lack of knowledge of the most effective tumor rejection antigens. Recent data correlating the response to immune checkpoint blockade with mutational load and a higher density of neo-antigens have stimulated increasing interest in personalized vaccine strategies.[72,73]

Several vaccine platforms have been tested in breast cancer (Table 56.5). Initial trials used MHC class I-binding short peptides with adjuvants, with the induction of modest, short-lived CD8$^+$ T cell responses. To provide T cell help, second generation peptide vaccines included a heterologous CD4$^+$ T helper peptide epitope or long peptides that deliver both CD4$^+$ and CD8$^+$ T cell epitopes. Alternatively, peptides or proteins loaded onto DCs may more optimally prime the immune response. Whole tumor cells or tumor cell lysates loaded onto DCs as multiantigen vaccine strategies increase the likelihood of including critical tumor rejection targets and decrease the risk of immune escape due to antigen loss variants. Notably, the safety of breast cancer vaccines is quite favorable, with side effects limited to local injection site reactions, fever, myalgias, and sometimes rash. Clinical activity is typically low.

Therapeutic Breast Cancer Vaccines for Metastatic Disease

Most breast cancer vaccines have been tested in the setting of advanced disease (Table 56.6). Breast cancer

Table 56.5 Breast Cancer Vaccine Platforms

PLATFORM	REQUIREMENT FOR MHC MATCH	RELATIVE IMMUNOGENICITY
ANTIGEN-BASED		
Peptide adjuvant	Yes	Low
Protein + adjuvant	No	Low
Carbohydrate + adjuvant	No	Low
GENETICALLY ENGINEERED		
Plasmid DNA	No	Low
Recombinant virus	No	Medium
Recombinant bacteria	No	Medium
CELL-BASED		
Whole tumor cell	No	Low
Dendritic cell	No	Medium

MHC, major histocompatibility complex.

vaccines that target mucin-1 (MUC-1) and other carbohydrate antigens have been tested in metastatic breast cancer. MUC-1 is an aberrantly glycosylated protein expressed in transformed cells of secretory origin with altered epitopes at carbohydrate residues and peptide sequences unmasked by altered glycosylation. Early trials demonstrated the induction of antibody but not T cells.[71]

A multicenter Phase 3 clinical study randomized 1,028 patients with metastatic breast cancer to receive low-dose cyclophosphamide (CY) with a MUC-1 epitope conjugated to keyhole limpet hemocyanin (KLH; experimental arm) or CY with unmodified KLH (control arm).[75] No survival benefit emerged, but patients on concomitant endocrine therapy tended to have longer time to disease progression and OS. A smaller trial tested the GLOBO-H-KLH carbohydrate vaccine with the QS-21 adjuvant in 27 patients with metastatic breast cancer. IgM antibody and new complement-dependent cytotoxicity (CDC)/antibody-dependent cellular cytotoxicity (ADCC) were detected, and the 2-year disease-free survival (DFS) rate was 56%.[74] A more recent Phase 2 randomized, placebo-controlled study of Globo H-KLH vaccine adagloxad simolenin (OBI-821/OBI-822) in patients with previously treated metastatic breast cancer showed that the vaccine did not improve PFS.[87] However, an association between the humoral immune response and PFS was observed, and treatment was well-tolerated.

PANVAC is a viral-based vaccine that delivers MUC-1, carcinoembryonic antigen (CEA), and three co-stimulatory molecules (B7.1, ICAM-1, and LFA-3). Early trials demonstrated safety, immune responses, and possible clinical activity.[86] PANVAC was tested with docetaxel in 25 patients relative to docetaxel alone in 23 patients. PFS was 7.9 months with the combination, and 3.9 months with docetaxel alone. Immune responses to MUC-1 and CEA were detected in both groups, and immunity and PFS benefit were not associated.

HER2 peptide and protein vaccines given with adjuvant granulocyte-macrophage colony-stimulating factor (GM-CSF) in metastatic breast cancer patients have been tested in multiple trials. Whereas short HER2 peptides induced transient CD8+ T cell responses,[88] long peptides containing both CD4+ and CD8+ T cell epitopes induced new delayed type hypersensitivity (DTH—a biomarker of CD4+ T cell-dependent immunity), and durable HER2-specific CD8+ T cell responses characterized by epitope spreading within and beyond HER2.[89–91] Vaccination with a HER2 intracellular domain (ICD) protein induced similar immunity.[92] Clinical responses and survival have not been reported on these studies. A HER2 peptide vaccine was also tested with standard trastuzumab in 22 HER2+ metastatic breast cancer patients.[85] HER2-specific immunity was enhanced, and there was an inverse correlation between survival and serum transforming growth factor-β (TGF-β). The OS endpoint was not reached at a median follow-up of 3 years. The HER2-specific DC vaccine sipuleucel-T was tested in 18 HER2+ metastatic breast cancer patients, with new HER2-specific T cell proliferation; clinical activity reflected one partial response and three patients with stable disease ≥12 months.[93] A HER2-specific viral particle vaccine with adjuvant montanide was tested in ~100 advanced HER2+ breast cancer patients,[80,81] with evidence of vaccine-induced antibodies and clinical benefit in some patients. Other vaccines tested in small numbers of metastatic breast cancer patients targeted telomerase, survivin, p53, and mammoglobin.[71]

An allogeneic GM-CSF-secreting breast cancer vaccine that delivers multiple antigens (including HER2) has been tested with chemotherapy and trastuzumab. The paracrine secretion of GM-CSF results in a large influx of DCs at the vaccine site, which process and present antigens to CD4+ and CD8+ T cells and cross-prime the antitumor immune response. This vaccine was tested in sequence with immune-modulating doses of CY and doxorubicin (DOX), with HER2-specific DTH induced and antibody responses maximized at the lowest dose of CY and the highest dose of DOX tested.[82] The most active dose of CY induced apoptosis in T_{regs} cells while sparing effector T cells, creating a window for effective vaccination.[83] This vaccine was also tested with low-dose CY and trastuzumab in 20 patients with HER2+ metastatic breast

Table 56.6 Selected Breast Cancer Vaccine Trials

VACCINE	PATIENT POPULATION	ANTIGEN-SPECIFIC IMMUNE RESPONSE	CLINICAL BENEFIT	REF
CY-placebo vs. CY-GLOBO H-KLH	MBC n = 348	New GLOBO H-specific Ig	No difference	74
CY-KLH vs. CY + STn + KLH	MBC n = 1,028	New STn-specific Ig	No difference	75
HER2 peptide E75 + GM-CSF	EBC n = 187	Augmented HER2-specific T cell responses	Possible 10% improvement in OS	76
Placebo + GM-CSF vs. HER2 peptide E75 + GM-CSF (nelipepimut-S)	EBC n = 758	NR	No difference	77
HER2 peptide AE37 + GM-CSF	EBC n = 298	Augmented HER2-specific T cell responses	No difference	78
HER2 peptide GP2 + GM-CSF	EBC n = 98	Augmented HER2-specific T cell responses	No difference	79
NeuGcGM3 VSSP + montanide	MBC n = 79	Augmented HER2-specific antibody responses	Trend toward survival improvement	80, 81
GVAX CY and DOX	MBC n = 28	Enhanced HER2-specific antibody and DTH in about 1/3 of patients	NR	82, 83
GVAX Trastuzumab and CY	HER2+ MBC n = 20	Enhanced HER2-specific DTH and T cell responses	Trend toward longer PFS and OS	84
HER2 peptide Trastuzumab	HER2+ MBC n = 22	Augmented HER2-specific immunity	NR	85
PANVAC + docetaxel vs. docetaxel	MBC n = 48	Induction of immunity to CEA and MUC-1	Possible PFS benefit (7.9 vs. 3.9 months)	86

CEA, carcinoembryonic antigen; CY, cyclophosphamide; DOX, doxorubicin; DTH, delayed type hypersensitivity; EBC, early breast cancer; GM-CSF, granulocyte-macrophage colony-stimulating factor; HER2, human epidermal growth factor receptor-2; Ig, immunoglobulin; KLH, keyhole limpet hemocyanin; MBC, metastatic breast cancer; MUC-1, mucin-1; NR, not reported; OS, overall survival; PFS, progression-free survival; STn, clustered sialoglycoprotein; VSSP, very small size proteoliposomes.

cancer.[84] Polyfunctional HER2-specific CD8+ T cells expanded across the vaccination cycles, with increased HER2-specific DTH in 35% of patients. A trend toward longer PFS and OS was observed in DTH responders. CD80-modified whole cell vaccines and DC: autologous breast tumor cell fusions have also been tested.[71]

Vaccines for Secondary Prevention

Vaccines have also been tested in early breast cancer as a consolidation strategy after standard local and systemic therapy has been completed (Table 56.6). The HER2-derived peptide vaccine E75 (nelipepimut-S) with GM-CSF adjuvant has been extensively studied in the adjuvant setting for the prevention of relapse. Two trials enrolled 187 patients with any level of HER2 expression,

where 108 HLA-A2/A3+ patients were vaccinated, and 108 HLA-A2/A3− patients were followed as controls (the E75 peptide will not bind to other HLA molecules).[76] The groups were well balanced except that vaccinated patients were more likely to be ER/PR negative. The 5-year OS rates were 90% and 80% in vaccinated and control patients, respectively ($p = .08$), though optimally vaccinated patients had a 95% DFS rate ($p = .05$). Immune analyses revealed HER2 epitope spreading. The randomized, double-blind Phase 3 PRESENT trial enrolled 758 patients with early stage, lymph node-positive breast cancer with low-to-intermediate levels of HER2 expression, randomizing them 1:1 to receive nelipepimut-S (E75) or placebo with adjuvant GM-CSF.[77] This level of HER2 expression was specified based on early trials that demonstrated more robust immunity in patients with lower levels of HER2 expression than high levels of HER2 expression,[94] possibly due to greater immune tolerance with high HER2 expression. The vaccine was well-tolerated, but there was no difference in DFS. A more recent randomized clinical trial tested nelipepimut-S with GM-CSF plus trastuzumab versus GM-CSF alone plus trastuzumab in 276 patients with high-risk early breast cancer expressing low levels of HER2 after definitive standard therapy.[95] No difference in DFS between the groups emerged, but an exploratory analysis suggested clinical benefit in patients with early TNBC.

Another vaccine tested for secondary breast cancer prevention is the MHC class II epitope vaccine AE37, which is the HER2 AE36 epitope covalently linked to the Ii-Key peptide LRMK to enhance epitope charging and augment antigen presentation.[78] This hybrid peptide AE37 induces HER2-specific CD4[+] T cells better than the native peptide AE36. The AE37 peptide vaccine was tested in a randomized Phase 2 trial that enrolled 298 early breast cancer patients with any HER2 expression to receive AE37 with GM-CSF or GM-CSF alone. There was no difference in recurrence rates (12.4% vs. 13.8% [p = .70]). A third study evaluated a distinct HER2 peptide vaccine, GP2, in 98 patients with early HER2[+] breast cancer, randomizing them to GP2 with GM-CSF or GM-CSF alone after the completion of all adjuvant therapy, including trastuzumab.[79] The DFS rates at 34 months for vaccinated and control patients were 100% and 89% (p = .08). Finally, a prospective, randomized, single-blind Phase 2 trial evaluated GP2 (to induce CD8[+] T cells) or AE37 (to induce CD4[+] T cells) in high-risk HER2-expressing breast cancer patients; no difference in 5-year DFS was found.[96]

Breast Cancer Vaccines for Primary Prevention

Vaccines for the primary prevention of breast cancer would be ideal. Ductal carcinoma in situ (DCIS) is a premalignant precursor to invasive breast cancer typically managed with surgery, and endocrine therapy if ER[+] is a platform for evaluating primary prevention strategies. The intranodal injection of DCs loaded with HER2 peptides was evaluated in 27 DCIS patients,[97] with the induction of high numbers of HER2-specific T cells. At surgery, 5/27 vaccinated patients (18.5%) had no evidence of DCIS, and another 11/22 patients (50%) had eradication of HER2 expression in their residual DCIS, likely reflecting immune-editing. A follow-up randomized selection evaluated three different administration routes (intralesional, intranodal, or both) in patients with DCIS (n = 42) or early invasive breast cancer (n = 12).[98] Similar levels of peripheral immunity were induced with all routes, and pCR was higher in DCIS patients (28.6%) than in patients with invasive disease (8.3%). In DCIS patients, immunity in the sentinel lymph node but not the peripheral blood was associated with pCR. Applying

breast cancer vaccine strategies in individuals without breast lesions but at high risk of developing invasive disease due to family history or a known germline mutation in BRCA1/2 or other inherited breast genes will require well-designed clinical trials.

CONCLUSION

There is a complex interplay between breast cancer and the immune system. Randomized clinical trials have now demonstrated the clinical activity of PD-1/PD-L1 antagonists combined with chemotherapy in both early and metastatic TNBC, and also combined with a HER2-specific monoclonal antibody-based therapeutic in HER2[+] metastatic breast cancer. The potential for clinical benefit is restricted to patients with PD-L1[+] disease for both metastatic TNBC and advanced HER2[+] breast cancer, representing about 40% of patients in both groups. Notably, the combination of atezolizumab and *nab*-paclitaxel is approved by health authorities and endorsed by multiple international guidelines as a standard of care for the first-line treatment of PD-L1[+] advanced TNBC. Although atezolizumab with *nab*-paclitaxel resulted in a significant improvement in PFS and a clinically meaningful OS benefit in IMpassion130, there was no treatment effect associated with the combination of atezolizumab and paclitaxel in IMpassion131. Given that the trials enrolled patient populations with very similar eligibility criteria, the reason for this difference is unclear. Possibilities include subtle differences in the chemotherapy agent itself; the differential use of steroids in the two trials (used as premedication for paclitaxel in IMpassion131 but not for *nab*-paclitaxel in IMpassion130); unrecognized heterogeneity in the patient populations due to disease biology, geography, or other factors; and study design differences. The impact of these variables on the trial results requires further exploration.

The KEYNOTE-522 trial demonstrated a significant improvement in pCR with the addition of the PD-1 inhibitor pembrolizumab to standard neoadjuvant chemotherapy. In contrast, the GeparNuevo and NeoTRIPaPDL1 trials failed to demonstrate significant improvements in pCR with the addition of a PD-L1 antagonist. Several variables could account for this difference. First, in KEYNOTE-522 greater benefit from pembrolizumab was associated with lymph node-positive disease. GeparNuevo included lower risk TNBC patients, including those with T1c, lymph node-negative tumors. The lack of improvement in pCR in GeparNuevo may be related to the inclusion of these lower risk patients who are less likely to benefit from PD-1/PD-L1 blockade. Second, patients who received a single dose of durvalumab 2 weeks prior to chemotherapy appeared to have a greater improvement in pCR. In addition, NeoTRIPaPDL1 and I-SPY2 pembro8-noAC failed to demonstrate a significant improvement in pCR. Coupled with the results of the TONIC trial, these data suggest that the anthracyclines may be more synergistic than other chemotherapies with PD-1/PD-L1 inhibitors. These first neoadjuvant trials thus highlight several important variables for optimizing neoadjuvant immunotherapy: the chemotherapy partner, treatment sequence and duration, and predictive clinico-pathologic characteristics and biomarkers for selecting patients for neoadjuvant immunotherapy. Identifying patients most likely to derive clinical benefit or experience irAEs will improve the therapeutic index of immunotherapy for early breast cancer, which is crucial for patients with curable disease.

Interestingly, whereas in metastatic breast cancer clinical benefit is associated with PD-L1 expression in the TME, in early breast cancer the clinical benefit of adding PD-1/PD-L1 blockade to standard therapy appears to be independent of PD-L1 expression. These findings imply an evolution in the immunobiology of breast cancer with disease progression that has implications for the use of immunotherapy in the clinic, and detailed investigation of the host/tumor interaction with disease initiation and progression as it impacts clinical benefit from immunotherapy is needed.

Beyond PD-1/PD-L1 modulators, breast cancer vaccines have been tested for many years, and have particular promise as primary and secondary prevention strategies. Other immuno-oncology agents are under investigation for breast cancer therapy, including other immune checkpoint modulators (LAG-3, TIM-3, OX-40, TIGIT), macrophage modulators, inhibitors of amino acid and nucleic acid metabolism, and adoptive T cell therapies. Early trials of immunotherapies combined with precision medicines, such as those that target PARP, phosphatidylinositol-4,5-bisphosphate-3 kinase catalytic subunit alpha (PIK3CA), and mitogen-activated protein kinase kinase (MEK), have also shown promise in the clinic. The future for breast cancer patients is bright, as immune-based therapies that enter clinical practice establish durable responses that translate into long-term survival benefit.

KEY REFERENCES

Only key references appear in the print edition. The full reference list appears in the digital product on Springer Publishing Connect: connect.springerpub.com/content/book/978-0-8261-3743-2/part/part04/chapter/ch56

43. Schmid P, Rugo HS, Adams S, et al. Atezolizumab plus *nab*-paclitaxel as first-line treatment for unresectable, locally advanced or metastatic triple-negative breast cancer (IMpassion130): updated efficacy results from a randomized, double-blind, placebo-controlled, Phase 3 trial. *Lancet Oncol.* 2020;21:44–59. doi:10.1016/S1470-2045(19)30689-8

47. Miles DW, Gligorov J, Andre F, et al. LBA15 primary results from IMpassion131, a double-blind placebo-controlled randomised Phase 3 trial of first-line paclitaxel +/- atezolizumab for unresectable locally-advanced/metastatic triple-negative breast cancer. *ESMO Virtual Congress.* 2020;31(suppl 4):S1147–S1148. doi:10.1016/j.annonc.2020.08.2243

49. Cortes J, Cescon DW, Rugo HS, et al. KEYNOTE-355: randomized, double-blind, Phase III study of pembrolizumab + chemotherapy versus placebo + chemotherapy for previously untreated locally recurrent inoperable or metastatic triple-negative breast cancer. *J Clin Oncol.* 2020;38;(15 suppl):1000. doi:10.1200/JCO.2020.38.15_suppl.1000

50. Emens LA, Esteva FJ, Beresford M, et al. Atezolizumab plus trastuzumab emtansine (T-DM1) versus T-DM1 plus placebo in previously treated, HER2-positive advanced breast cancer: results from KATE2, a randomized, double-blind, Phase 2 trial. *Lancet Oncol.* 2020;21(10):1283–1295. doi:10.1016/S1470-2045(20)30465-4

59. Nanda R, Liu MC, Yau C, et al. Effect of pembrolizumab plus neoadjuvant chemotherapy on pathologic complete response in women with early-stage breast cancer: an analysis of the ongoing Phase 2 adaptively randomized I-SPY2 trial. *JAMA Oncol.* 2020;6:1–9. doi:10.1001/jamaoncol.2019.6650

62. Pusztai L, Han HS, Yau C, et al. Evaluation of durvalumab in combination with olaparib and paclitaxel in high-risk HER2-negative stage II/III breast cancer: results from the I-SPY2 trial [abstract CT011]. *Cancer Res.* 2020;80(4 Suppl): abstract nr CT011. doi:10.1158/1538-7445.AM2020-CT011

63. Schmid P, Cortes J, Pusztai L, et al. Pembrolizumab for early triple-negative breast cancer. *N Engl J Med.* 2020;382:810–821. doi:10.1056/NEJMoa1910549

67. Mittendorf EA, Zhang H, Barrios CH, et al. Neoadjuvant atezolizumab in combination with sequential *nab*-paclitaxel and anthracycline-based chemotherapy versus placebo and chemotherapy in patients with early-stage triple-negative breast cancer (IMpassion 031): a randomised, double-blind, Phase 3 trial. *Lancet Oncol.* 2020;396(10257):1090–1100. doi:10.1016/ S0140-6736(20)31953-X

Immunotherapy for Lung Cancer and Malignant Pleural Mesothelioma

Paola Ghanem and Julie R. Brahmer

KEY POINTS

- Immune checkpoint inhibitors (ICIs) alone or in combination with or without chemotherapy have changed the treatment landscape for patients with advanced non-small cell lung cancer (NSCLC).

- Patients with locally advanced NSCLC have improved survival when given consolidation durvalumab after concurrent chemotherapy and radiation.

- ICIs in combination with chemotherapy improve survival in patients with metastatic small cell lung cancer (SCLC).

- Combination of ICIs improved survival in patients with unresectable malignant pleural mesothelioma.

INTRODUCTION

Lung cancer remains the leading cause of death worldwide with a 5-year survival rate of 19.6%.[1] Lung cancer also remains the second most common cancer across all genders, while being more common in males than females.[2] For every 100,000 individuals, 55 are newly diagnosed with lung cancer and 37 die.[3,4] Although the annual rates of new lung cancer cases might have decreased from 1999 to 2017, the annual number of new cases is on the rise.[3,4] To date, the best cytotoxic regimens only infrequently cure late-stage lung cancer and aim to gain control over the progression of the disease rather than complete remission.

Histologically, there exists two main categories of lung cancer: 80% are non-small cell lung cancer (NSCLC) and 15% are small cell lung cancer (SCLC), while the remaining types constitute 5% of all lung cancer. NSCLC can further be specified by type: 40% are adenocarcinoma, 30% are squamous cell carcinoma, and 10% are large cell carcinoma.[5]

Identification of driver mutations is paramount for selecting the most appropriate treatment in patients with NSCLC, particularly adenocarcinoma. These driver mutations have mainly been identified over the years for NSCLC and can be treated with targeted therapy for that specific mutation. For example, epidermal growth factor receptor (EGFR) mutation has high prevalence in females, nonsmokers, and in the adenocarcinoma subtype. In fact, this subgroup of population responds well to receptor tyrosine kinase inhibitors (RTKIs).[6-8] and poorly to checkpoint inhibitors with no apparent benefit on overall survival (OS) and progression-free survival (PFS).[9-11] Other known mutations or gene fusions for adenocarcinoma that have specific targeted therapies approved for treatment of advanced disease include: ALK fusion, BRAF^{V600e} mutation, MET exon 14 skipping mutation, RET fusions, and ROS-1 fusions. Approximately 31% of adenocarcinoma have unidentified mutations.[12] Loss of function (phosphatase and tensin homolog [PTEN]) and gain of function (PIK3CA) appear to be more common mutations in squamous cell lung carcinoma.[13]

As for SCLC, p53 mutation is identified in 75% to 98% of all cases.[14] However, targeted therapy is nonexistent in SCLC; therefore, identification of driver mutations does not offer additional information in the choice of treatment. Chemoimmunotherapy regimens are now the best treatment for patients with extensive-disease SCLC.

For patients with advanced NSCLC and no driver mutation or fusion, immunotherapy has become routinely part of the treatment options. In fact, studies have shown that the tumor microenvironment (TME) of lung cancer is rich in immune suppressive cells, which is a nidus for tumor-promoting factors.[15,16] These studies have proven that lung cancer is immunogenic and is able to evade the immune system via numerous mechanisms: secretion of immunosuppressive cytokines such as interleukin 10 (IL-10) and transforming growth factor-beta (TGF-β).[17] High concentration of regulatory T cells (T$_{reg}$ cells)[18] and dysfunction of the antigen-presentation complex.[19] Antigen-specific immunotherapy CIMAvax-EGF is the first therapeutic cancer vaccine with promising results for advanced NSCLC.[20] However, while vaccine immunotherapy has not led to significant advancement in the management of lung cancer, immune checkpoint inhibitors (ICIs) have offered important progress by targeting immune evasive mechanisms effectively. In 2015, nivolumab was approved for advanced stage non-squamous and squamous NSCLC for patients who progressed on platinum doublet chemotherapy.[9,21] Nivolumab not only significantly increased the response rate (RR) but also prolonged median OS compared to docetaxel. This encouraged a series of new trials to study nivolumab as well as other checkpoint inhibitors as second- and first-line therapy for chemotherapy-naïve patients with advanced NSCLC.

This chapter will review the common types of ICIs and their mechanisms of action. The most updated guidelines of first- and second-line therapy for both NSCLC and SCLC, along with the advances in treatment strategies in malignant pleural mesothelioma, will be presented. The chapter will also cover the rationale for the use of the programmed death ligand 1 (PD-L1), tumor proportion score (TPS), and tumor mutational burden (TMB) as predictive biomarkers in the clinical setting.

LUNG CANCER VACCINE

In an attempt to induce antigen-specific immune response and enhance tumor rejection, therapeutic vaccines have been developed and tested in clinical trials. These vaccines aim at boosting the immune system to recognize and destroy cancer antigens.[22] Many Phase 3 trials testing the BLP25 vaccine and the melanoma antigen encoding gene A3 (MAGE-A3) vaccine have failed to meet their primary endpoints.[23,24] Among all vaccines studied, CIMAvax-EGF has demonstrated a survival advantage in patients with advanced NSCLC. This vaccine is made up of the EGF protein, conjugated to the p64 protein from the meningitis B bacteria with Montanide ISA 51 used as an adjuvant.[25] Although EGFR is not exclusively found on cancer cells, this vaccine would allow the immune system to form antibodies against EGF. This prevents cells, whose cell cycle regulation is dependent on EGF-EGFR interaction, from growing.[26] For that reason, patients with advanced NSCLC are candidates for this therapeutic vaccine though this is only approved for use in select countries and not in the United States. In 2016, the Cuban vaccine CIMAvax-EGF was approved for maintenance treatment for patients with advanced NSCLC, after first-line chemotherapy[27] in select countries. The Phase 3 open-label trial recruited 405 patients with stage IIIB/IV NSCLC after having received upfront chemotherapy. All patients had achieved either stable disease, partial response, or complete response after chemotherapy. Patients received either the vaccine with best supportive care or best supportive care alone. CIMAvax-EGF has shown significant increase in OS.[27] Median OS was 10.83 months versus 8.86 months ($p = 0.04$). Additionally, high EGF baseline concentration was shown to be a good predictive marker as it was associated with longer OS in patients who have received the vaccine; median OS was 14.66 months.[27] In a follow-up study, the vaccine has proved to be immunogenic.[20] Anti-EGF titers have reached a plateau of 1:10,000 sera dilution with no clonal exhaustion after 2 years of monthly vaccination.[20] After CIMAvax-EGF's approval in Cuba and additional countries, in late 2016, the U.S. Food and Drug Administration (FDA) has authorized the study of CIMAvax in the United States by the Roswell Park Cancer Institute to pursue a Phase 1/2 clinical trial.[28] This Phase 1 trial studied the combination of nivolumab and CIMAvax-EGF as second-line therapy in advanced NSCLC.[28] This combination was shown to be safe and demonstrated an ORR was 44%.[28] In March 2019, the final results of the Phase 1 trial aligned with the interim analysis and showed an objective response rate (ORR) of 31%.[29] The Phase 2 trial is still ongoing. Additional National Cancer Institute (NCI)-supported Phase 1/2 clinical trials of the vaccine are also currently being investigated.[30,31]

IMMUNE CHECKPOINT INHIBITORS

Basic Principles of Immune Checkpoint Blockade

Several mechanisms allow tumor cells to evade the immune system and avoid tumor rejection.[32] The understanding of the concept of immunosurveillance has allowed the development of checkpoint inhibitors. These checkpoint inhibitors block inhibitory pathways that control T cell response in the host, thus resulting in enhancing the antitumor T cell response.[33] Two main therapeutic strategies, mainly programmed cell death 1 (PD-1) pathway targeting antibodies and cytotoxic T lymphocyte-associated antigen 4 (CTLA-4) antibodies, have emanated over the past decade and allowed the FDA's approval of several agents.

Programmed Cell Death 1 Inhibitors

The PD-1 is a transmembrane protein receptor present on immune cells such as activated T lymphocytes, T_{reg} cells, and natural killer (NK) cells.[33] This glycoprotein binds to its ligand (PD-L1), which can be present on the tumor cells. This interaction triggers an inhibitory signaling cascade that allows tumor cells to evade the immune system and recognition.[34] PD-1 inhibitors are monoclonal antibodies that prevent this interaction and allow the T cell population to exert its antitumor function.[35,36] Pembrolizumab, nivolumab, and cemiplimab are all monoclonal antibodies that inhibit PD-1.

Similarly, monoclonal antibodies inhibiting PD-L1 will also prevent the escape of tumor cells from the immune system. Atezolizumab, durvalumab, and avelumab are monoclonal antibodies against PD-L1.

Cytotoxic T Lymphocyte-Associated Antigen 4 Inhibitors

A second adopted mechanism for tumor cells to evade the immune system is through the interaction of CTLA-4 with its ligand CD28.[32] CTLA-4 is present on the surface of T lymphocytes. It competes with CD28 present on T cells, to interact with the B7 protein present on the antigen-presenting cells (APCs) and prevent CD28's interaction with ligand B7, a necessary co-stimulatory signal that leads to T cell activation.[37] By inhibiting CTLA-4, the T cell population is free to exert its antitumor effect and reject the tumor.[37] Ipilimumab and tremilimumab are monoclonal antibodies against CTLA-4.

TREATMENT

Non-Small Cell Lung Cancer

For patients with stage I to III resectable NSCLC, surgery accompanied with neoadjuvant or adjuvant chemotherapy remains the gold standard.[38] Patients with unresectable stage III disease will undergo concurrent chemotherapy and radiation therapy followed by durvalumab.[39] Prior to the approval of PD-1 ICI, platinum (cisplatin or carboplatin)-based chemotherapy has been the standard of care for advanced disease NSCLC.[40] Carboplatin or cisplatin are usually combined with either docetaxel, gemcitabine, paclitaxel, pemetrexed, or vinorelbine.[41] In a randomized control trial, the comparison of four chemotherapy regimens did not demonstrate superiority of any of the regimens.[41] PD-1 checkpoint blockade has led to significant changes in standard of care for patients with advanced NSCLC without driver mutations. The studies that have led to these changes are discussed in the text that follows and are summarized in Table 57.1.[9,11,21,42–53]

Second-Line Therapy

In 2015, nivolumab, a PD-1 inhibitor, was studied in a Phase 2 trial (CheckMate 063) for advanced refractory squamous NSCLC.[54] The lack of effective standard therapy for refractory squamous NSCLC was urgently needed. CheckMate 063 was the first Phase 2 trial to study the activity of PD-1 inhibitor for advanced NSCLC. The ORR was 14.5% with 77% of responses ongoing at the time of analysis, while 26% had stable disease. Together, these findings demonstrate significant clinical benefit and supported the Phase 3 study of nivolumab in the squamous NSCLC patient population.[54] In 2015, two separate Phase

3 trials compared nivolumab in advanced squamous NSCLC[21] and nonsquamous NSCLC with docetaxel in patients who have progressed on platinum-based chemotherapy.[9] The median OS with nivolumab was 9.2 months, 3.2 months longer than that with docetaxel in squamous subtype.[21] A similar 2.8 months increase in OS was seen in nonsquamous subtype ($p = .002$).[9] The risk of death was 41% lower with nivolumab with squamous histology ($p < .001$) and median PFS was 3.5 months with nivolumab versus 2.8 months with docetaxel ($p < .001$).[21] At 1 year, the OS was 18% higher in squamous type and 12% higher in the nonsquamous histology[9,21] with nivolumab treatment. The 1-year PFS was 19% for nonsquamous NSCLC versus 8% with docetaxel. This clinical benefit was consistently seen across all PD-L1 expression categories ($\geq 1\%$, $\geq 5\%$, $\geq 10\%$).[9,21] Continuous benefit from nivolumab-based therapy was demonstrated recently whereby the 5-year pooled OS for both trials (CheckMate 017 and CheckMate 057) proved to be higher in the nivolumab-treated group versus docetaxel (13.4% vs. 2.6%). This translates into impressive clinical benefit as patients who did not progress at 3 years were shown to have 78.3% chance of remaining progression-free at 5 years.[55] Importantly, the consistent benefit of nivolumab as second-line monotherapy in patients with advanced NSCLC was not accompanied with an increase in frequency of grade 3 to 4 adverse events (AEs) compared to docetaxel.[9] The successful use of nivolumab monotherapy in NSCLC has allowed a series of trials to test the efficacy of other ICIs. In 2016, pembrolizumab was studied in an open label Phase 2/3 trial as second-line therapy for patients with positive PD-L1 expression $\geq 1\%$ (KEYNOTE-010). In the total population, the median OS increased by at least 1.9 months depending on the dose of pembrolizumab used (2 or 10 mg/kg). However, the median PFS with pembrolizumab (independent of the dose) was not shown to be higher than with docetaxel.[53] However, in patients with PD-L1 $\geq 50\%$, both OS and PFS appeared to be longer with pembrolizumab.[53] These findings align with the KEYNOTE-001 Phase 1 trial, whereby pembrolizumab's efficacy was higher in patients with PD-L1 expression $\geq 50\%$.[56,57] This unprecedented benefit for refractory NSCLC was accompanied with lower grade 3 to 4 AEs with pembrolizumab than with docetaxel.[53] The OAK trial was the first Phase 3 randomized trial to study the PD-L1 inhibitor, atezolizumab, in advanced NSCLC in patients who have progressed after first-line therapy.[11] The OAK trial included patients with advanced NSCLC and any PD-L1 expression and demonstrated prolonged median OS of 13.8 months with atezolizumab versus 9.6 months with docetaxel ($p = .0003$) in the ITT population. Patients with low or absent PD-L1 expression also benefited from atezolizumab (12.6 months vs. 8.9 months), although a lower ORR was observed. The median OS increase of 3.7 months was similar in both

Table 57.1 Immune Checkpoint Inhibitor Phase 3 Trials in Advanced NSCLC

AUTHOR AND YEAR	TRIAL NAME N	HISTOLOGY	AGENT	RESULTS	PD-L1 EXPRESSION	AE OF GRADE 3 OR MORE
				First-Line Single Agent		
Reck et al. (2016)[42]	KEYNOTE-024 N = 305 2016	Squamous and nonsquamous	Pembrolizumab vs. chemotherapy	ORR 44.8% vs. 27.8% Median PFS 10.3 vs. 6 months 6-month OS 80.2% vs. 72.4%	≥50%	26.6% vs. 53.3%
Sezer et al. (2020)[43]	EMPOWER-Lung 1 N = 563 2020	Squamous and nonsquamous	Cemiplimab vs. chemotherapy	Median PFS 8.2 vs. 5.7 months Median OS not reached vs. 14.2 months	≥50%	37.2% vs. 48.5%
Mok et al. (2019)[44]	KEYNOTE-042 N = 1,274	Squamous and nonsquamous	Pembrolizumab vs. chemotherapy	OS 16.7 vs. 12.1 months OS 20.2 vs. 12.2 months No significant change in PFS	PD-L1 ≥1% PD-L1≥ 50%	18% vs. 41%
Herbst et al. (2020)[45]	IMpower110 N = 572	Squamous and nonsquamous	Atezolizumab vs. chemotherapy	Median OS 20.2 vs. 13.1 months	PD-L1≥ 50%	N/A
				Combination of ICI and Chemotherapy		
Gandhi et al. (2018)[46]	KEYNOTE-189 N = 616	Nonsquamous	Pembrolizumab with chemotherapy	1-year OS 69.2% vs. 49.4% Median PFS 8.8 vs. 4.9 months	PD-L1 <1% and ≥1%	67.2% vs. 65.8%
Paz-Ares et al. (2018)[47]	KEYNOTE-407 N = 559	Squamous	Pembrolizumab with chemotherapy	Median OS 15.9 vs. 11.3 months Median PFS 6.4 vs. 4.8 months	PD-L1 <1% and ≥1%	69.8% vs. 68.2%
Socinski et al. (2018)[48]	IMpower150 N = 692	Nonsquamous	Atezolizumab with chemotherapy and bevacizumab vs. bevacizumab and chemotherapy	Median PFS 8.3 vs. 6.8 months Median OS 19.2 months vs. 14.7 months	PD-L1 <1% and ≥1%	55.7% vs. 47.7 %
				Combination of ICI with ICI		
Hellmann et al. (2018)[49,50]	CheckMate227 N = 1,739	Squamous and nonsquamous	Nivolumab and ipilimumab vs. chemotherapy	ORR 45.3% vs. 26.9% 1-year PFS 42.6% vs. 13.2% Median PFS 7.2 vs. 5.5 months	PD-L1 <1% and ≥1% And high TMB	31.2% vs. 36.1%
Ramalingam et al. (2020)[51]	CheckMate 227 3-year survival data	Squamous and nonsquamous	Nivolumab and ipilimumab vs. chemotherapy	3-year OS 33% vs. 22% 3-year PFS 18% vs. 4% 3-year OS 34% vs. 15% 3-year PFS 13% vs. 2%	PD-L1 ≥1% PD-L1<1%	N/A

(continued)

			Combination of Two ICI and Chemotherapy			
Reck et al. (2020)[52]	CheckMate 9LA N = 719	Squamous and nonsquamous	Nivolumab and ipilimumab and chemotherapy vs. chemotherapy alone	Median OS 15.6 vs. 10.9 months	PD-L1 <1% and ≥1%	47% vs. 38%
			Second-Line Single Agent			
Brahmer et al. (2015)[21]	CheckMate 017 N = 272	Squamous	Nivolumab vs. docetaxel	RR 20% vs. 9% Median OS 9.2 vs. 6 months Median PFS 3.5 vs. 2.8 months	PD-L1≥1%	7% vs. 55%
Borghaei et al. (2015)[9]	CheckMate 057 N = 582	Nonsquamous	Nivolumab vs. docetaxel	RR 19% vs. 12% Median OS 12.2 vs. 9.4 months Median PFS 2.3 vs. 4.2 months 1-year PFS 19% vs. 8%	PD-L1≥1%	10% vs. 54%
Herbst et al. (2016)[53]	KEYNOTE-010 N = 1,034	Squamous and nonsquamous	Pembrolizumab (2 mg/kg) vs. docetaxel	Median OS 10.4 vs. 8.5 months Median PFS 3.9 vs. 4 months (not significant) Median OS 14.9 vs. 8.2 months Median PFS 5 vs. 4.1 months	PD-L1 ≥1% PD-L1 ≥50%	13% vs. 35%
Rittmeyer et al. (2017)[11]	OAK N = 850	Squamous and nonsquamous	Atezolizumab vs. chemotherapy	Median OS 13.8 vs. 9.6 months Median OS 12.6 vs. 8.9 months	PD-L1≥1% PD-L1 <1%	15% vs. 43%

All results are statistically significant unless mentioned otherwise.

AE, adverse events; ICI, immune checkpoint inhibitor; NSCLC, non-small cell lung cancer; ORR, objective response rate; OS, overall survival; PD-L1, programmed cell death-ligand 1; PFS, progression free survival; RR, response rate; TMB, tumor mutational burden.

squamous and nonsquamous histology. Similar to previous studies, the frequency of grade 3 to 4 AEs was lower with atezolizumab[11] compared with docetaxel. While pembrolizumab, nivolumab, and atezolizumab offered survival benefit to patients with NSCLC, the median OS with avelumab, a PD-L1 inhibitor, did not differ compared to docetaxel ($p = 0.16$). However, exploratory analyses done on patients with high PD-L1 ≥50% and PD-L1 ≥80% demonstrated longer OS and PFS ($p = 0.0052$, $p = 0.0023$ respectively) irrespective of tumor histology.[12]

In summary, PD-1 blockade has shown consistent activity in the second-line treatment for advanced NSCLC compared to docetaxel. While response rates (RR) are similar, the prolonged duration of response, improved survival, and less high-grade toxicities compared with docetaxel have led to nivolumab and atezolizumab's approval regardless of the PD-L1 expression and pembrolizumab's approval in patients with PD-L1 tumor expression of ≥1%.

First-Line Therapy

Single Agent

Both trials CheckMate 057 and CheckMate 017 have demonstrated successful clinical benefit for the use of ICIs in the second-line treatment for patients with advanced NSCLC.[9,21] These findings encouraged researchers to study ICIs as upfront therapy for patients newly diagnosed with NSCLC. In the KEYNOTE-001 Phase 1 trial, PD-1 inhibitor pembrolizumab's efficacy and safety were studied. The median PFS was 3.6 months and median OS 12 months in the total population,[56] which included patients treated in the first-line treatment setting as well as those with heavily pretreated NSCLC. In this trial, a PD-L1 expression cutoff of 50% was used to identify patients' cancers that had high PD-L1 expression. In patients with tumors with PD-L1 expression of greater than or equal to 50%, the ORR was 45.2% and median PFS was 6.3 months, significantly higher than in the total population.[56] This trial has shown an association between high PD-L1 expression (≥ 50%) and improved efficacy,[56] particularly in the first-line treatment setting. In 2016, the KEYNOTE-024 trial studied upfront treatment with pembrolizumab compared with platinum-based chemotherapy for advanced NSCLC in patients with no driver mutations and with PD-L1 expression ≥50%.[42] The cutoff of 50% was selected based on the results of the Phase 1 KEYNOTE-001 study and Phase 3 KEYNOTE-010 trial where tumors with PD-L1 expression ≥50% were more likely to respond to PD-1 inhibitors such as pembrolizumab.[42,56] The KEYNOTE-024 trial showed the superiority of pembrolizumab compared with traditional chemotherapy as the RR was 44.8% compared with 27.8% in the platinum-based chemotherapy group, with an increase in PFS by more than 4 months (10.3 months

versus 6 months).[42] Pembrolizumab was associated with longer OS at 6 months (80.2% vs. 72.4%, $p = 0.005$), demonstrating significant clinical benefit.[42] Five-year survival improvement was also reported as 32% in the pembrolizumab-treated group, effectively doubling the 5-year survival from 16%.[58] More recently, cemiplimab, a PD-1 inhibitor, demonstrated a similar significant increase in PFS in patients with PD-L1 ≥50% compared with standard chemotherapy (8.2 months vs. 5.7 months, $p < 0.0001$). Median OS was not reached with the cemiplimab group compared with the platinum-based chemotherapy group of 14.2 months ($p = 0.0002$).[59]

However, the lack of effective novel upfront therapy for patients with PD-L1 expression <50% prompted in 2018 the first-line treatment study of pembrolizumab monotherapy in NSCLC patients with PD-L1 expression ≥1%[44] based on the success of pembrolizumab (KEYNOTE-010 trial) in the second-line setting. In the KEYNOTE-042 trial, the OS was significantly longer in the pembrolizumab group for any PD-L1 positive expression compared with chemotherapy, with OS of 20 months versus 12.2 months for PD-L1 ≥50% and 16.7 months versus 12.1 months for PD-L1 ≥1%. While treatment-related death was similar across both arms (2%), treatment-related grade 3 to 4 AEs were lower with pembrolizumab (18% vs. 41%). While the effect on OS was greater in PD-L1 expression ≥50%, the clinical benefit remained significant in those with PD-L1 expression of ≥1%. The findings strongly encourage the use of pembrolizumab monotherapy in PD-L1-positive NSCLC.[44] On the other hand, single-agent atezolizumab was also studied against first-line chemotherapy for PD-L1 ≥1%.[53] Patients with high PD-L1 expression and treated with the ICI achieved a longer OS (20.2 months vs. 13.1 months).[45] This study led to the FDA approval of atezolizumab in the first-line treatment setting for advanced NSCLC patients with PD-L1 TPS of 50% or greater or IC ≥10%.

In summary, first-line single-agent PD-1 blockade improves survival in NSCLC patients with PD-L1 TPS of ≥1%. In patients with PD-L1 TPS of at least 50%, PD-1 blockade can provide significant improvement in 5-year survival. Thus, immunotherapy pembrolizumab can provide NSCLC patients with PD-L1 high cancer long-term disease control, effectively making lung cancer a chronic disease or potentially curing patients. Other PD-1 checkpoint inhibitors, like atezolizumab, also have demonstrated improvement in survival in patients with high PD-L1 expression as well as cemiplimab.

First-Line Therapy

Combination of Immune Checkpoint Inhibitor and Chemotherapy

In order to maximize control over the progression of the disease, the combination of pembrolizumab and chemotherapy as first-line therapy was shown to be superior to standard chemotherapy in patients with advanced NSCLC, regardless of the PD-L1 expression.[46,47] This combination improved median OS by 4.6 months, median PFS by 1.6 months (p <0.001) in squamous NSCLC,[47] and median PFS increased by 3.9 months in nonsquamous NSCLC (p <0.001).[46] The 1-year OS in nonsquamous histology was 69.2% in the pembrolizumab combination group versus 49.4% in the placebo combination group.[46] The increase in OS was shown to be consistent across all categories of PD-L1 expression (<1%, 1% to 49%, and ≥50%) for all histologic types of advanced NSCLC.[46,47] These two studies demonstrated the superiority of combination therapy for those whose PD-L1 expression <50%. Importantly, the combination therapy did not increase the frequency of AEs associated with chemotherapy. Similarly, the addition of pembrolizumab to chemotherapy did not increase the immunotoxicities compared with pembrolizumab monotherapy.[42,53] However, to date no direct comparison has been made between pembrolizumab monotherapy and combination therapy with chemotherapy in patients with advanced NSCLC and PD-L1 expression ≥50%. Consideration of patient-specific factors should drive decision-making as to the best treatment.[53] Nonetheless, the successful combination of pembrolizumab with chemotherapy was not replicated with the CTLA-4 inhibitor, ipilimumab. In 2017, in patients with advanced squamous NSCLC, the median OS was 13.4 months in the ipilimumab/chemotherapy group compared with 12.4 months in the chemotherapy alone group (p = 0.25). The PFS was similar across both groups (5.6 months). An increase in frequency of grade 3 and 4 AEs was additionally observed in the combination group.[60] One possible explanation would be that by inhibiting CTLA-4, ipilimumab stimulates early stage T cell activation. However, this response may not be strong enough as the lymphoid TME may not present enough effector T cells.[34] Although this was primarily hypothesized in SCLC, similar tumor behavior could exist in NSCLC and therefore would explain the previously noted observations.[34]

With the aim to maximize control over the disease and augment clinical benefit, combination therapy of atezolizumab with chemotherapy and vascular endothelial growth factor (VEGF) inhibitor bevacizumab was studied in advanced nonsquamous NSCLC.[48] In fact, bevacizumab was shown to decrease the activity of immunosuppressive cells such as myeloid-derived suppressor cells (MDSC) and T_{reg} cells.[48] This restores the anticancer immunity, which is enhanced through VEGF-mediated immunomodulatory effects.[61,62] In this trial, one arm received atezolizumab with carboplatin and paclitaxel (ACP), the second arm received bevacizumab and CP (BCP), and the third arm received the combination of bevacizumab, atezolizumab, and CP

(ABCP). Combination therapy (ABCP) did not result in new AEs than those associated with each individual drug. The median OS and PFS were prolonged in ABCP compared with BCP (19.2 months vs. 14.7 months, p = 0.02, and 8.3 vs. 6.8 months, p <0.001, respectively). These observations were similar regardless of the presence of driving mutations, PD-L1 expression, and Teff gene signature expression. This study was particularly relevant as it included individuals with any PD-L1 expression, with or without EGFR mutations and ALK translocations.[48] This is of importance since previous studies have failed to demonstrate significant changes in OS and PFS in patients with EGFR or ALK mutations with the use of PD-1 or PD-L1 inhibitors.[11,53]

In summary, pembrolizumab in combination with platinum-based chemotherapy improves survival in patients with advanced NSCLC regardless of PD-L1 expression. No trial has yet to compare single-agent PD-1 blockade in patients with PD-L1 high tumors (≥50%) with the combination with chemotherapy. Thus, decisions on whether to use single-agent PD-1 blockade or in combination with chemotherapy depends on patients' bulk of disease and possible tolerance of chemotherapy.

First-Line Therapy

Combination of Two Immune Checkpoint Inhibitors

While the addition of PD-1/PD-L1 inhibitors to chemotherapy appeared to be effective, interest was rising on the combination of two ICIs for which mechanisms of action differ (i.e., PD-1 and CTLA-4 blockade). In CheckMate 227, the combination of nivolumab (3 mg/kg every 2 weeks) and ipilimumab (1 mg/kg every 6 weeks) was compared with standard platinum-based chemotherapy as well as compared to nivolumab monotherapy (240 mg every 2 weeks). In an early phase analysis, the 1-year PFS rate was 42.6% with nivolumab + ipilimumab versus 13.2% with chemotherapy, and the median PFS was 7.2 months versus 5.5 months with chemotherapy (p <0.001). This observation was consistent across all PDL-1 expression categories. The ORR increased with combination of ICIs by 18.4% compared with chemotherapy alone. These observations were significantly prolonged for patients with high TMB (≥10 mutations per megabase) receiving combination therapy.[50] In the second part of the analysis, OS with the combination of nivolumab and ipilimumab was compared with standard chemotherapy. Contrary to studies where ICI monotherapy appears to be primarily effective when PD-L1 expression is above 50%, the OS was 17.2 months, an increase of 5 months in the combination arm in patients whose PD-L1 expression <1%. In patients whose PD-L1 ≥1% the OS was 17.1 months, an increase of 2.2 months from the chemotherapy group (p = .007). The median duration of response was 23.3 months in the combination group versus 6.2 in the chemotherapy group. Less frequent grade 3 or 4 AEs occurred with the combination group (32.8% vs. 36%), which reinforces the added benefit of combining two ICIs.[63] While the combination of chemotherapy and CTLA-4 did not provide added clinical benefit in patients with advanced NSCLC,[60] the combination of a CTLA-4 and PD-1 inhibitor proved to be successful. A 3-year survival analysis of this clinical trial has demonstrated the long-lasting effect of combination immunotherapy. In fact, the RR of patients on combination therapy who express PD-L1 is 38% compared with 4% in the chemotherapy group. This continued survival benefit was seen at 3 years despite having administered the combination therapy for a maximum of 2 years. The PFS with combination of ICIs was 4.5 times that of the chemotherapy arm. In those with no expression of PD-L1, the OS of the combination of ipilimumab and nivolumab was more than twice that of the standard therapy. The ipilimumab and nivolumab combination also provided continuous benefit 3 years after the onset of response in 34% of these individuals with no PD-L1 expression.[51] Multiple immunotherapy combinations have been studied to date. However, few have resulted in improvement in both PFS and RR.

Recently, a Phase 2 trial investigated the combination of atezolizumab with tiragolumab, a monoclonal antibody against T cell immunoreceptor with Ig and ITIM domains (anti-TIGIT antibody), versus atezolizumab in the first-line treatment setting.[64] TIGIT is an inhibitory checkpoint expressed on T cells and NK cells. TIGIT expression is associated with PD-L1 expression.[65] Blockade of TIGIT blocks its effector poliovirus receptor (PVR) present on tumor cells and APCs. Thus, blockade of both TIGIT and PD-L1 may be complementary in antitumor activity. Patients diagnosed with NSCLC and PD-L1 ≥1% demonstrated improved clinical outcomes with the combination therapy. The atezolizumab and tiragolumab combination demonstrated improved median OS (5.6 months vs. 3.9 months), PFS (5.55 months vs. 3.88 months), and ORR (37.3% vs. 20.6%).[64] In subgroup analyses, patients with PD-L1 expression ≥50% demonstrated improved ORR of 66% and PFS (median PFS not reached), compared with patients with PD-L1 expression of 1% to 49% (ORR of 16%, median PFS of 4.04 months). Phase 3 trial investigating atezolizumab and tiragolumab combination therapy in patients with PD-L1 expression ≥50% is currently ongoing (NCT04294810).

First-Line Therapy

Combination of Two Immune Checkpoint Inhibitors and Chemotherapy

While both the combination of PD-1 inhibitor with chemotherapy on one hand[46,47] and PD-1 inhibitor with CTLA-4 inhibitor on the other[63] demonstrated prolonged PFS and

OS compared with standard therapy, the hypothesis that four drug combination therapies with two checkpoint inhibitors and a short course of platinum-based combination chemotherapy (two cycles) could provide additional benefit regardless of PD-L1 expression is currently being studied.[52] This study increased OS in the treatment group compared with the standard chemotherapy group (four cycles), with median OS 15.6 versus 10.9 months (p = 0.0006). The clinical benefit seen on OS and PFS was consistent across all PD-L1 categories. However, grades 3 and 4 AEs appeared to be higher in the combination group versus standard therapy (47% vs. 38%).[52]

In summary, combination immunotherapy, combining nivolumab and ipilimumab, has demonstrated a significant improvement in survival in patients with PD-L1+ NSCLC and also an improvement in survival in patients with PD-L1- disease. Combining chemotherapy for two cycles with nivolumab and ipilimumab demonstrated a significant improvement in survival in patients with NSCLC regardless of PD-L1 expression level. Nivolumab and ipilimumab have complementary mechanisms of action which can increase the risk of immune-related side effects. These side effects are manageable.

Special Lung Cancer Subpopulations

Epidermal Growth Factor Receptor and ALK Mutant

Despite the clinical benefit of ICIs in NSCLC with no driver mutations, PD-1 immune checkpoint blockade (ICB) did not prove to be as effective in tumors with driver mutations such as EGFR and ALK mutations. In the second-line treatment setting, OS did not improve on nivolumab nor atezolizumab compared with chemotherapy in patients with EGFR mutations.[9,11] Although the results from the previous studies were exploratory analyses, one Phase 2 trial studied pembrolizumab in patients with driver mutations, no prior RTKI therapy, and positive PD-L1 expression.[66] This trial was interrupted due to the lack of efficacy, as an objective response was not achieved in any patient. Two deaths occurred over 6 months with many treatment discontinuations due to drug side effects (adrenal insufficiency, pneumonitis etc.).[66] One hypothesis to the lack of efficacy of checkpoint inhibitors in the EGFR mutant is the low mutational heterogeneity of the tumors. However, additional studies are required to answer this question.[67] Due to data from the second-line setting studies (CheckMate 057, KEYNOTE-010, and OAK trials), nearly all first-line studies did not include patients with EGFR mutations or ALK translocations except for the IMpower 150 study of atezolizumab, bevacizumab + paclitaxel, and carboplatin. In a subset analysis, patients with EGFR mutations and ALK translocations did benefit from the four-drug regimen compared with combination chemotherapy in the first-line setting (PFS of 9.7 vs. 6.1 months, HR:0.59).[48]

Consolidation Therapy With Durvalumab in Unresectable Stage 3 Non-Small Cell Lung Cancer

Single-agent immunotherapy has proved to be successful in prolonging OS in metastatic disease. In 2018, the addition of maintenance therapy with durvalumab, given once every 2 weeks for 1 year after disease was stable or responsive to concurrent chemotherapy and radiation, also proved to be successful in stage III unresectable NSCLC in controlling the progression of disease. The 36-month OS with durvalumab was 57% versus 43.5% in the placebo group. The median PFS was 17.2 months versus 5.6 months.[39] This prolonged PFS was accompanied with an increase in time to death and time to distant metastasis of 12.1 months. Durvalumab significantly increased the 4-year OS compared with placebo (49.6% vs. 36.3%). Similarly, 4-year PFS were 35.3% and 19.5% favoring durvalumab.[68] This improvement in survival was seen in all groups except in an unplanned subset analysis by PD-L1 where patients with PD-L1⁻ disease were less likely to benefit from durvalumab. This led to differences in approval in the European Union, where durvalumab is only approved in patients who have PD-L1+ disease where it is approved in the United States regardless of PD-L1 expression.[69,70]

Neoadjuvant and Adjuvant Immunotherapy

As the role of ICI therapy has become fundamental in the advanced stage setting, recent studies have investigated the role of ICI in patients with curative intent in resectable NSCLC in both the neoadjuvant and adjuvant setting. The CheckMate 159 study was the first Phase 1 trial studying the feasibility of nivolumab therapy in the neoadjuvant setting in 22 patients with stage I to IIIA NSCLC.[71] Major pathologic response (MPR) was achieved in 45% of cases. The safety and feasibility of ICI-based therapy observed in this trial has allowed numerous subsequent trials to investigate additional novel neoadjuvant-based therapies. In the LCMC3 Phase 2 trial, atezolizumab monotherapy was also investigated in 101 patients. MPR was achieved in 19.5% of cases independent of PD-L1 status and TMB.[72] The combination of immunotherapy with nivolumab and chemotherapy,[73] atezolizumab with chemotherapy,[74] and nivolumab with ipilimumab[75,76] were further investigated in Phase 2 trials. As the majority of the designed Phase 2 trials were encouraging, Phase 3 trials have been developed to confirm previous observations. Recently, the CheckMate 816 investigating nivolumab and platinum-based doublet combination therapy was the first Phase 3 trial to confirm and demonstrate superior pathologic complete response (pCR) with combination therapy versus chemotherapy in the neoadjuvant setting of patients with resectable NSCLC.[77] Ongoing Phase 3 trials investigating

Table 57.2 Ongoing Phase 3 Trials Investigating Immune Checkpoint Inhibitor in the Neoadjuvant/Adjuvant Setting

CLINICAL TRIAL NCT IDENTIFIER	DISEASE STAGE	INTERVENTION
Neoadjuvant		
IMPower030 NCT03456063	II-IIIB	Atezolizumab + chemotherapy vs. chemotherapy
CheckMate 816 NCT02998528	IB-IIA	Nivolumab + chemotherapy vs. chemotherapy
KEYNOTE-671 NCT03425643	II-IIIB	Pembrolizumab + chemotherapy vs. chemotherapy
AEGEAN NCT03800134	IIA-IIIB	Durvalumab + chemotherapy vs. chemotherapy
NCT02904954	II-III	Durvalumab +/− radiotherapy
Adjuvant		
ANVIL NCT02595944	IB-IIIA	Nivolumab vs. observation +/− adjuvant chemotherapy
PEARLS/ KEYNOTE-091	IB-IIIA	Pembrolizumab vs. placebo +/− adjuvant chemotherapy
IMpower010 NCT02486718	IB-IIIA	Atezolizumab + chemotherapy vs. best supportive care + chemotherapy
BR31 NCT02273375	IB-IIIB	Durvalumab vs. placebo +/− adjuvant chemotherapy

anti-PD-1/PD-L1 agents in the adjuvant and neoadjuvant setting are currently taking place and are summarized in Table 57.2.

Small Cell Lung Cancer

SCLC is an aggressive disease. Patients with limited stage SCLC undergo thoracic radiotherapy concurrently with chemotherapy.[78] However, no treatment option produces a consistent long-term durable response in patients with extensive disease SCLC (ED-SCLC). Relapse is common and median survival time is 1 to 2 years from diagnosis.[79] Table 57.3[80-85] summarizes the immune-related Phase 3 trials in SCLC.

Second-Line Therapy

Prior to the start of immunotherapy, patients with ED-SCLC who have relapsed were considered for best supportive care with hospice, additional cycles of chemotherapy, or clinical trials. Some reports have shown

Table 57.3 Immune Checkpoint Inhibitor Phase 3 Trials in ED-SCLC

AUTHOR YEAR	TRIAL NAME N	AGENT	RESULTS	PD-L1 EXPRESSION	AE OF GRADE 3 OR MORE
First Line					
Horn et al. (2018)[80]	IMpower133 N = 201	Atezolizumab with carboplatin and etoposide	RR 60.2% vs. 64.4% (not significant) Median OS 12.3 vs. 10.3 months Median PFS 5.2 vs. 4.3 months	N/A	56.6% vs. 56.1 %
Paz-Ares et al. (2019)[81,82]	CASPAIN trial N = 537	Durvalumab with etoposide and platinum-chemotherapy	Median OS 13 months vs. 10.3 months	N/A	62% in both
Rudin et al. (2020)[83]	KEYNOTE-604 N = 453	Pembrolizumab with etoposide	ORR 70.6% vs. 61.8% 2-year OS 22.5% vs. 11.2% 1-year PFS 13.6% vs. 3.1%	PD-L1 expression not a prognostic factor	76.7% vs. 74.9%
Second Line					
Ready et al. (2019)[84]	CheckMate 032 N = 109	Nivolumab monotherapy No comparison group	ORR 11.9% 1-year OS 28.3%	PD-L1 expression not a prognostic factor	11.9%
Ready et al. (2020)[85]	CheckMate 032 N = 243	Nivolumab with ipilimumab vs. nivolumab monotherapy	ORR 21.9% vs. 11.6% Median OS 5.7 vs. 4.7 months, not significant Median PFS 1.4 vs. 1.5 months, not significant		37.5% vs. 12.9%

All results are statistically significant unless mentioned otherwise.

AE, adverse events; ED-SCLC, extensive-disease small cell lung cancer; ICI, immune checkpoint inhibitor; ORR, objective response rate; OS, overall survival; PD-L1, programmed cell death ligand 1; PFS, progression-free survival.

that among those who have received first-line chemotherapy, 10% to 20% will require third-line therapy in their lifetime. This observation was critical and highlighted the need to find new therapeutic options.[86,87] In 2006, oral topotecan demonstrated clinical benefit with a median OS of 25.9 weeks compared with 13.9 weeks with best supportive care (BSC). Importantly, quality of life was more commonly maintained in patients receiving oral topotecan with good partial and stable disease responses.[88] For several years, oral or IV topotecan was the standard drug for patients with recurrent or metastatic SCLC.[88] To date, patients with recurrent and metastatic SCLC, previously heavily treated, have a number of immunotherapy-related treatments. Recently, pembrolizumab was FDA approved for this category of patients. Pembrolizumab has demonstrated a median OS of 7.7 months and an ORR of 19.3%. Two patients had achieved a complete response and 14 achieved a partial response. In addition, 61% of those responders had responses lasting more than 18 months. Over a median follow-up duration of 7.7 months, the median duration of response was not achieved. Pembrolizumab was well

tolerated with a rate of 9.6% of grade 3 to 4 AEs. These observations were consistent across all PD-L1 categories.[89] Although this study lacked a comparison group, the median OS was 7.7 months compared with 4.4 months in other studies.[90] This trial highlights the clinical benefit of pembrolizumab as a third-line therapy.[89] Initial Phase 1/2 trials on patients with recurrent SCLC who have failed previous chemotherapy have shown the effective antitumor activity of nivolumab monotherapy and nivolumab and ipilimumab combination therapy.[91] The CheckMate 032 trial is a Phase 3 clinical trial that compared nivolumab monotherapy to nivolumab + ipilimumab as a third-line therapy from pooled nonrandomized and randomized cohorts of patients with recurrent SCLC. In the initial report assessing the efficacy and safety of nivolumab monotherapy, the ORR of patients who have received nivolumab monotherapy was 11.9% and the median duration of response was 17.9 months.[84] Nivolumab achieved durable responses with a 1-year OS of 28.3%. Nivolumab was well tolerated and caused 11.9% of grade 3 or 4 AEs. Based on these findings, the FDA has recently approved nivolumab for patients with recurrent or metastatic SCLC who have progressed after more than two lines of chemotherapy.[84] In 2019, the final findings of the combination of nivolumab and ipilimumab have shown significantly improved ORR of 21.9% in the combination group versus 11.6% with nivolumab monotherapy ($p = 0.03$).[85] However, the increase in ORR did not translate into increased OS or PFS for the combination group. The 2-year OS was similar across both arms (17.9% for nivolumab and 16.9% for nivolumab and ipilimumab. Grade 3 and 4 AEs were significantly more frequent with the combination of ICIs. The lack of tolerability of the nivolumab/ipilimumab combination therapy could explain the discrepancy between the ORR and the PFS/OS, as most patients would discontinue treatment.[85]

In summary, single-agent PD-1 blockade has shown efficacy in the third-line treatment setting. Immunotherapy is now a treatment option for previously treated patients who have not yet received PD-1/PD-L1 blockade. PD-L1 has not proven to be a biomarker for response in SCLC.

First-Line Therapy

In 2013, preclinical studies have shown a synergistic effect with ipilimumab and platinum/etoposide.[92] A Phase 2 trial has also shown the clinical benefit of ipilimumab/carboplatin/paclitaxel's combination in ED-SCLC.[93] This prompted the study of ipilimumab and etoposide/platinum in a Phase 3 trial in ED-SCLC.[94] In this Phase 3 trial, the addition of ipilimumab to etoposide and cisplatin or carboplatin did not prolong OS (11 months for the combination and 10.9 months for the chemotherapy/placebo group, $p = 0.3775$). Increased frequency of diarrhea, rash, and colitis were more frequent in the combination group. The treatment arm also observed higher rates of treatment discontinuation (18% vs. 2%) and treatment-related deaths (five vs. two deaths).[94] In the IMpower133 trial, atezolizumab added to carboplatin and etoposide has demonstrated a significant 2-month increase in median OS (12.3 months, $p = 0.007$). The median PFS was also significantly longer in the treatment arm with 5.2 months versus 4.3 months ($p = 0.02$). Although ORR and median duration of response were similar across both groups, the 1-year OS was 13% higher in the atezolizumab group (51.7% vs. 38.2%).[80] The clinical benefit of adding atezolizumab to chemotherapy did not increase the frequency of hematologic nor immune-related AEs compared with chemotherapy and atezolizumab monotherapy, respectively.[11] In the CASPIAN trial, durvalumab's addition to etoposide and platinum therapy in the first-line setting prolonged OS significantly by 3 months when compared with chemotherapy alone (13 months vs. 10.3 months).[81] At 18 months, more patients were alive in the durvalumab + platinum/etoposide group

than in the standard chemotherapy group (34% vs. 25%). Grade 3 to 4 AEs as well as treatment-related deaths were shown to be similar across both groups (34% vs. 25% and 5% vs. 6%, respectively).[81] These findings align with the ones observed in the IMpower133 trial using atezolizumab with chemotherapy.[80] More recently, in the KEYNOTE-604 trial, the combination of pembrolizumab and etoposide has significantly prolonged PFS ($p = 0.0023$), with a 1-year PFS rate of 13.6% in the combination group and 3.1% in the standard therapy.[83] However, the median OS was not significantly improved. The 2-year OS was 22.5% and 11.2% with ORR of 70.6% and 61.8% in the combination treatment and control group, respectively. The addition of pembrolizumab to etoposide did not result in an increase in frequency of grade 3 to 4 AEs, although discontinuation was more frequent in the combination group (14.8% vs. 6.3%). The hematologic AEs related to cytotoxic agents did not appear to be increased by the addition of pembrolizumab, while the immune-related AEs appeared to be similar to those of the pembrolizumab monotherapy.[83] Death-related AEs were similar across both arms.[83] Interestingly and similar to NSCLC,[46,47] PD-L1 expression did not appear to be a prognostic factor; regardless of the PD-L1 expression, the combination therapy was consistently superior to standard therapy in ED-SCLC. Patients with brain metastasis did not appear to benefit from the combination of pembrolizumab with chemotherapy. However, the sample size for this category was small and therefore results should be interpreted with caution.[83] Together, these trials (IMpower133, CASPIAN trial, and KEYNOTE-604), have revolutionized the first-line treatment options of ED-SCLC. The combination of ICIs (atezolizumab, durvalumab, and pembrolizumab) with chemotherapy (platinum and etoposide) have contributed to significant progress in the clinical outcomes of ED-SCLC.

Maintenance Therapy

With the rising role of ICIs in ED-SCLC, the CheckMate 451 Phase 3 trial, aimed to investigate the role of nivolumab and ipilimumab or nivolumab monotherapy versus placebo as maintenance therapy in patients who had responded to first-line platinum-based chemotherapy. However, this trial failed to meet its primary endpoints. The OS of patients treated with nivolumab and ipilimumab or nivolumab alone did not improve when compared to placebo.[95]

EVALUATION OF TISSUE BIOPSY AT THE TIME OF DIAGNOSIS

Predictive Value of Genomic Alterations

Identification of driver mutations is particularly important in determining the prognosis of patients with advanced NSCLC. Patients with the mutant form of EGFR appear to have longer PFS compared to those with wild type EGFR (9.1 months versus 4 months, $p = 0.001$) in advanced NSCLC receiving first line chemotherapy with/without EGFR-RTKI.[96] To note, EGFR mutation is rare in SCLC.[97] Interestingly, never smoker patients with EGFR mutation positive cancer show better response to RTKIs than patients with a heavy smoking history.[98] Female patients also have greater response to RTKIs than male patients.[98] However, as previously mentioned, EGFR mutant disease responds weakly to immunotherapies when compared to wild type, possibly due to low TMB.

Predictive Value of PD-L1 Expression

Defining and identifying biomarkers are important steps in patient care in order to optimize their immunotherapy treatment. The TPS is one of the biomarkers. TPS is equal to the percentage of tumor cells staining positive for PD-L1 over the total tumor size. This score is most commonly used in NSCLC. Several studies have supported the use of PD-L1 expression as a prognostic factor. According to several studies, higher PD-L1 expression leads to longer OS and PFS in patients receiving PD-1 or PD-L1 inhibitors.[42,44,53,56] High expression of PD-L1 is defined as expression higher than or equal to 50%.[56] For patients with advanced NSCLC and high PD-L1 ≥50%, single-agent pembrolizumab has shown to prolong OS and PFS in patients with lower TPS scores.[44] The CheckMate 057 trial also demonstrated improved OS and PFS in patients with greater PD-L1 expression receiving nivolumab for nonsquamous NSCLC.[9] However, in squamous NSCLC, nivolumab improved OS and PFS independent of PD-L1 expression.[21] Similarly, the addition of pembrolizumab to chemotherapy improved OS and PFS consistently across all PD-L1 categories for squamous NSCLC.[47] PD-L1 has not been associated with improvement in survival with PD-1 checkpoint blockade in SCLC.[49,82,99–101]

Predictive Value of Intratumoral Lymphoid Infiltrates

Preclinical and clinical studies have shown that the density of tumor-infiltrating lymphocytes (TILs) was positively associated with prognosis and survival.[102] A meta-analysis evaluating the presence of TILs and clinical outcomes was performed. High levels of CD8+ T cell, CD3+ and CD4+, had a positive prognostic effect and improved OS (hazard ratio [HR] 0.91, 0.77, 0.78, respectively).[103] In patients with NSCLC who received atezolizumab first in human Phase 1 study, the response to the ICI was significantly associated with the tumor-infiltrating immune cells' PD-L1 expression ($p = 0.015$),

in addition to the tumor cell PD-L1 expression compared with those with a negative TIL PD-L1 expression. For patients with tumor-infiltrating immune cells (IC) and IHC score of 3, 83% of patients responded to anti-PD-L1 therapy. In patients with an IC IHC score of 2, 43% of patients had limited response to therapy with stable disease. However, this association was not as strong between tumor response and tumor cell PD-L1 expression.[104] This study resulted in a different scoring system for the use of atezolizumab for NSCLC. In SCLC, atezolizumab was shown to improve OS compared with docetaxel independent of the tumor cell PD-L1 expression and IC status.[11] Based on the IMpower133 trial, combination of atezolizumab with chemotherapy (etoposide and carboplatin) yielded a higher proportion of long-term survivors. This association was seen independent of PD-L1 expression.[100]

Predictive Value of Tumor Mutational Burden

One other predictive biomarker is TMB, defined as the number of mutations over megabases. Although not yet standardized, high TMB is defined as 10 mutations per megabase.[50] In advanced NSCLC, the combination of ICIs nivolumab and ipilimumab in the first-line setting has decreased the risk of death by 42% rather than with chemotherapy in patients with high TMB.[50] The benefit was significantly greater in the combination group, demonstrating longer PFS, whereas in patients with low TMB, the combination therapy did not prove to be superior to chemotherapy alone.[50] Even in patients with negative PD-L1 expression, high TMB was associated with longer PFS in patients receiving nivolumab with chemotherapy.[52] On the other hand, in the IMpower133 trial, the combination of atezolizumab and chemotherapy in ED-SCLC demonstrated greater OS and PFS than chemotherapy alone. However, TMB at either cutoff of 10 or 16 mutations per megabase did not help predict a potential survival benefit for patients with high TMB.[80]

MESOTHELIOMA

Mesothelioma is a locally invasive and rapidly progressive disease with a poor prognosis; median OS is 13 months.[105] Surgical resection is amenable in a minority of patients with a 5-year survival close to 20%.[106] Conventional treatment for unresectable mesothelioma has been unchanged for many years. Pemetrexed and cisplatin combination therapy was approved for unresectable mesothelioma in 2004.[107] With the rise in immunologic-based therapies in the clinical setting, several trials have investigated the use of ICIs in malignant pleural mesothelioma (MPM). This has led to the recent FDA approval of ipilimumab and nivolumab combination therapy as first-line treatment in patients diagnosed with unresectable MPM. In this randomized Phase 3 trial (CheckMate 743), combination of ICIs significantly improved OS compared with chemotherapy (18.1 months vs. 14.1 months).[108] At 2 years, 41% of patients remained alive in the ICI combination group versus 27% in the chemotherapy group.[108] In a subset analysis, the magnitude of clinical benefit was higher in patients with sarcomatoid and mixed histology versus patients with epithelioid histology (HR 0.46 vs. 0.86).[108] However, median OS with ICIs was similar between the different histology (18.1 months for non-epithelioid and 18.7 months for epithelioid), while median OS with chemotherapy was superior in the epithelioid subtype versus non-epithelioid (16.5 months vs. 8.8 months),[10] which is typical of the lack of benefit of chemotherapy in the non-epithelioid subtype of mesothelioma.

This breakthrough in malignant pleural mesothelioma comes after several efforts have been made to investigate the role of ICI as salvage therapy. Despite the lack of improvement in OS in a double-blind Phase 2b trial investigating single-agent tremelimumab versus placebo in recurrent MPM,[109] further trials with PD-1 and PD-L1 inhibitors were more promising. In 2018, a Phase 2 trial investigated the use of nivolumab as second-line therapy in patients with MPM.[110] Single-agent nivolumab demonstrated improved clinical outcomes; 24% of patients had a partial response and 24% had stable disease at 12 weeks of therapy.[110] The clinical benefit was also seen at 6 months, with 29% of patients being free of progression and 74% of patients having survived.[110] In a Phase 1b trial, avelumab was investigated in recurrent MPM and demonstrated clinical benefit.[111] Median PFS was 4.2 months and median OS was 10.7 months. The disease control rate was observed in 58% of patients. The 1-year OS was seen in 48.3% of patients.[111] In the KEYNOTE-028, Phase 1b trial, pembrolizumab demonstrated an ORR of 72% in the second-line setting of patients with recurrent MPM and PD-L1 ≥1% with a median duration of response of 12 months.[112] Pembrolizumab also demonstrated robust antitumor activity in a Phase 2 trial with an ORR of 66% and median PFS and OS of 4.5 months and 11.5 months, respectively.[113] However, in the PROMISE-meso randomized Phase 3 trial, pembrolizumab did not improve PFS nor OS in recurrent MPM.[114] The combination with nivolumab and ipilimumab has also demonstrated a disease control rate of 68% in the INITIATE Phase 2 trial in patients diagnosed with recurrent MPM.[115] To date, several trials investigating combination therapy of ICI with chemotherapy in the frontline setting are ongoing.

IMMUNE-RELATED TOXICITIES

General Overview of Immune-Related Adverse Events

Despite the success of ICI in prolonging OS, ICIs often result in AEs.[116] These immune-related AEs (irAEs) are unique to ICIs and can affect any organ system. Contrarily to chemotherapy, which results in acute-onset myelosuppressive and emetic side effects, ICIs produce delayed onset side effects mimicking autoimmune and inflammatory diseases.[117,118] These AEs can further be divided into early onset and late-onset AEs. Early onset irAEs often present as epithelial inflammation such as skin rashes, pneumonitis, and colitis, while delayed onset irAEs are more organ-specific reactions and could take the form of neurologic events and hypophysitis.[119] Their underlying pathophysiology is not yet fully elucidated. However, the understanding of the pathophysiology of autoimmune diseases can be extrapolated to explain irAEs. Autoimmune diseases result from the failure of T lymphocytes to tolerate self-antigens, which results in the development of a pro-inflammatory response.[120,121] In fact, studies have shown that mutations in the genes coding for CTLA-4 and PD-1 protein could result in autoimmune diseases such as celiac, diabetes mellitus, rheumatoid arthritis, and others.[120,121]

Incidence and Prevalence

Due to inconsistency in the reporting of irAEs, no comprehensive data on the incidence of irAEs has yet been officially reported. In fact, the incidence varies widely depending on each trial; it is said that the incidence of irAEs with the use of a single agent could range from 15% to 90%[122,123] and differ based on the type of ICI administered.[124] PD-1/PD-L1 inhibitors appear to result in a lower incidence in irAEs than CTLA-4 inhibitor ipilimumab. The overall incidence of any grade irAEs across all PD-1/PD-L1 inhibitors is 26.8% and 6.1% of high grade irAEs,[125] while for CTLA-4 inhibitor, overall incidence is reported to be 72% while 24% is for high grade irAEs.[126] Significantly higher rates of fatal irAEs were reported with CTLA-4 monotherapy than PD-1 inhibitor (1.08% vs. 0.36%).[127] It is also no surprise that, despite the gained survival advantage from the combination of two checkpoint inhibitors, the incidence of irAEs of such combination is greater than each monotherapy.[127,128]

Grading

Since management of irAEs depends on the severity of the ICIs' related toxicity, a specific grading was developed.[129] Table 57.4 illustrates each grade's severity with its respective general management.

Management

Rapid identification and grading of irAEs is crucial in the management of ICI-related toxicity. Holding immunotherapy and permanent discontinuation are often

Table 57.4 Grading and Management of Immune-Related Adverse Events

GRADE	SEVERITY	MANAGEMENT
Grade 1	Mild, asymptomatic	Observation, intervention not needed
Grade 2	Moderate	Low dose steroid +/– hold immunotherapy
Grade 3	Severe	High dose steroids, stop immunotherapy, hospitalization indicated, consider intensive care unit
Grade 4	Life threatening	High dose steroids, permanently stop immunotherapy, hospitalization indicated
Grade 5	Death	

essential. Since irAEs could be seen as flare-ups of the pro-inflammatory state, immunosuppression remains the mainstay of treatment for most high-grade AEs.[119] Short-term use of corticosteroid with adequate tapering is paramount. Response to steroids should be monitored over the following 48 to 72 hours and escalation to additional immunosuppressants may be necessary in steroid-refractory cases.[130] Detailed algorithms have been elaborated for the management of irAEs based on each organ system.[130]

Special Consideration

Several reports have hypothesized that the development of irAEs could present a positive prognostic factor and be used as a biomarker of treatment response. In a retrospective analysis, in patients with advanced malignancies, the development of gastrointestinal irAEs was found to be an independent predictor for survival.[131] Similarly, in a prospective cohort, patients who developed rheumatologic irAEs were found to have improved RR.[132]

CONCLUSION

ICB has dramatically changed the treatment landscape of lung cancer. Dramatic long-term survival has been seen in some patients with previously felt incurable disease. Single-agent PD-1 and PD-L1 blocking antibodies first demonstrated significant survival improvements with long-term disease response and control in the second-line treatment setting in metastatic NSCLC and then rapidly was translated into improvement in survival in the first line treatment setting in PD-L1 TPS positive disease. When combined with chemotherapy as in the case of pembrolizumab or chemotherapy and anti-VEGF therapy as in the case of atezolizumab, these combinations showed dramatic improvement in

survival regardless of PD-L1 TPS. Combination immunotherapy with nivolumab and ipilimumab dramatically improved survival in patients with PD-L1 positive disease and in combination with chemotherapy regardless of PD-L1 status. These various combinations are available for the treatment of advanced disease. One year of durvalumab after response or stabilization with concurrent chemotherapy has significantly reduced disease recurrence and improved survival in patients with unresectable stage 3 disease. SCLC has not been left out of this dramatic change in treatment options, where the addition of PD-L1 blocking antibodies in combination with standard chemotherapy for extensive stage disease has improved the survival of these patients who had not seen an improvement in frontline therapy options for decades. Additional advances in the field of immunotherapy are ongoing. Recent approval for combination of ipilimumab and nivolumab has revolutionized upfront therapy for patients with unresectable malignant pleural mesothelioma. Continued work on mechanisms of resistance in order to tailor therapy for those patients' disease that either doesn't respond to immunotherapy or whose disease becomes resistant to this therapy is ongoing and key to the future of immunotherapy's success for patients with lung cancer and malignant pleural mesothelioma.

KEY REFERENCES

Only key references appear in the print edition. The full reference list appears in the digital product on Springer Publishing Connect: connect.springerpub.com/content/book/978-0-8261-3743-2/part/part04/chapter/ch57

27. Rodriguez PC, Popa X, Martínez O, et al. A Phase III clinical trial of the epidermal growth factor vaccine CIMAvax-EGF as switch maintenance therapy in advanced non-small cell lung cancer patients. *Clin Cancer Res.* 2016;22(15):3782–3790. doi:10.1158/1078-0432.CCR-15-0855
46. Gandhi L, Rodríguez-Abreu D, Gadgeel S, et al. Pembrolizumab plus chemotherapy in metastatic non-small-cell lung cancer. *N Engl J Med.* 2018;378(22):2078–2092. doi:10.1056/NEJMoa1801005
47. Paz-Ares L, Luft A, Vicente D, et al. Pembrolizumab plus chemotherapy for squamous non-small-cell lung cancer. *N Engl J Med.* 2018;379(21):2040–2051. doi:10.1056/NEJMoa1810865
48. Socinski MA, Jotte RM, Cappuzzo F, et al. Atezolizumab for first-line treatment of metastatic nonsquamous NSCLC. *N Engl J Med.* 2018;378(24):2288–2301. doi:10.1056/NEJMoa1716948
56. Garon EB, Rizvi NA, Hui R, et al. Pembrolizumab for the treatment of non-small-cell lung cancer. *N Engl J Med.* 2015;372(21):2018–2028. doi:10.1056/NEJMoa1501824
58. Brahmer JR, Rodriguez-Abreu D, Robinson AG, et al. LBA51 KEYNOTE-024 5-year OS update: first-line (1L) pembrolizumab (pembro) vs platinum-based chemotherapy (chemo) in patients (pts) with metastatic NSCLC and PD-L1 tumour proportion score (TPS) ≥50%. *Ann Oncol.* 2020;31(suppl 4):S1181–S1182. doi:10.1016/j.annonc.2020.08.2284
63. Hellmann MD, Paz-Ares L, Bernabe Caro R, et al. Nivolumab plus ipilimumab in advanced non-small-cell lung cancer. *N Engl J Med.* 2019;381(21):2020–2031. doi:10.1056/NEJMoa1910231

70. Gray JE, Villegas A, Daniel D, et al. Three-year overall survival with durvalumab after chemoradiotherapy in Stage III NSCLC-update from PACIFIC. *J Thorac Oncol*. 2020;15(2):288–293. doi:10.1016/j.jtho.2019.10.002

81. Paz-Ares L, Dvorkin M, Chen Y, et al. Durvalumab plus platinum-etoposide versus platinum-etoposide in first-line treatment of extensive-stage small-cell lung cancer (CASPIAN): a randomised, controlled, open-label, Phase 3 trial. *Lancet*. 2019;394(10212):1929–1939. doi:10.1016/S0140-6736(19)32222-6

100. Liu S. V, Horn L, Mok T, et al. 1781MO IMpower133: characterisation of long-term survivors treated first-line with chemotherapy ± atezolizumab in extensive-stage small cell lung cancer. *Ann Oncol*. 2020;31(suppl 4):S1032–S1033. doi:10.1016/j.annonc.2020.08.1543

58

Head and Neck Cancer

Nicole C. Schmitt and Robert L. Ferris

KEY POINTS

- Head and neck squamous cell carcinomas (HNSCC) are relatively immunogenic due to a high number of genomic alterations compared with other tumor types; however, these tumors have developed numerous ways to evade immune surveillance.

- A growing proportion of HNSCC is related to human papillomavirus (HPV), and these HPV-associated tumors evade antiviral and antitumor immunity via resistance to interferons and increased expression of coinhibitory immune checkpoints.

- Targeted monoclonal antibodies (moAbs) to HNSCC tumor antigens may work in part by stimulating immune responses, including antibody-dependent cellular cytotoxicity (ADCC). Cetuximab, a chimeric anti-epidermal growth factor receptor (EGFR) mAb, is U.S. Food and Drug Administration (FDA) approved for treatment of HNSCC.

- Inhibitors of immune checkpoints have shown activity in recurrent/metastatic HNSCC and are currently under study for previously untreated, locally advanced disease.

- Preventive vaccines are useful for the prevention of future HPV infection but are not useful for treatment of preexisting HPV-related oropharyngeal carcinoma. Therapeutic vaccines for HPV-related HNSCC are under study, and some immune and/or clinical responses to vaccination have been reported.

- Multiple Phase 1 clinical studies involving adoptive transfer of antigen-specific or chimeric antigen receptor (CAR) T cells are currently recruiting patients with HNSCC.

- Combinations of multiple immunotherapies, or of immunotherapy plus standard therapy, have shown promise for HNSCC and will likely play a major role in the future treatment of this disease.

INTRODUCTION

Head and neck squamous cell carcinoma (HNSCC), the sixth most common cancer type worldwide,[1] involves multiple sites in the upper aerodigestive tract including the oral cavity, oropharynx, larynx, and hypopharynx. Risk factors include carcinogens (tobacco and alcohol) and high-risk subtypes of the human papillomavirus (HPV). While patients who present with early stage disease have reasonable survival rates, most patients present with advanced disease.[1] Patients with HPV-negative disease continue to have a poor prognosis, with little improvement in survival rates over the past two decades. Patients with HPV-related disease have a better prognosis, but these patients are often diagnosed at a younger age and must live for decades with the sequelae of treatment including difficulty with speech and swallowing. Thus, recent studies have aimed at improving survival for patients with HPV-negative disease and maintaining survival rates for HPV-positive patients while reducing long-term treatment-related toxicities.[2]

Analysis of HNSCC specimens by the Cancer Genome Atlas research network demonstrated that this tumor type has a high level of genomic alterations compared with other tumor types,[3] suggesting HNSCC patients may respond relatively well to immunotherapy. While study of HNSCC tumors has shown evidence of immune responses,[2] these tumors have developed several methods of evading the immune system. Patients with HIV and low CD4 counts who develop HNSCC have a worse prognosis,[4,5] underscoring the importance of the immune system in the development and progression of this disease. In this chapter we describe the ways by which HNSCC may evade the immune response, followed by a summary of preclinical and clinical studies of immunotherapy.

IMMUNE ESCAPE IN HEAD AND NECK CANCER

Head and neck tumors have a high level of genomic alterations leading to an abundance of tumor antigens, and in the case of HPV-related disease, the presence of

Table 58.1 Mechanisms of Immune Escape in Head and Neck Squamous Cell Carcinomas. These Mechanisms Include Intrinsic Changes in the Tumor Cells and Aberrant Immune Responses

TUMOR CELL INTRINSIC MECHANISMS
Decreased expression or mutation of MHC class I and other APM components
Secretion of immunosuppressive factors and cytokines by tumor cells (TGF-β, PGE2, IL-10)
Increased expression of PD-L1
ABERRANT IMMUNE RESPONSES
Decrease in circulating CTLs and other immune effector cells
Dysfunction of effector T cells, NK cells, and dendritic cells
Increased numbers of T$_{reg}$ cells, M2 macrophages, and MDSCs in the tumor microenvironment and circulation
Dominance of Th2 cytokine response
Decreased expression of T cell receptor zeta chain
Increased expression of coinhibitory checkpoint receptors and decreased expression of co-stimulatory checkpoint receptors on antigen-presenting cells and T cells

APM, antigen processing machinery; CTL, cytotoxic T lymphocyte; IL-1, interleukin 1; MDSC, myeloid-derived suppressor cell; mHC, major histocompatibility complex; NK, natural killer; PD-L1, programmed death ligand 1; PGE2, prostaglandin E2; PD-L1, programmed death ligand 1; TGF-β, transforming growth factor beta; T$_{reg}$, regulatory T.

viral antigens. Multiple mechanisms of immune escape are thus involved in the formation of these tumors. These mechanisms, including features intrinsic to the tumor cells as well as dysfunction of specific components of the immune response, are summarized in Table 58.1.

As explained in earlier chapters of this book, immune cells must process and present tumor antigens in order to induce an antitumor immune response. A number of candidate tumor antigens in HNSCC have been identified.[6] In HNSCC, tumor cells often evade the resulting immune response by downregulating major histocompatibility complex (MHC) class I,[7–10] which renders the tumor cells more susceptible to killing by natural killer (NK) cells but less likely to induce adaptive immunity and killing by cytotoxic T lymphocytes (CTLs). Multiple studies suggest that absence of MHC class I in HNSCC may be an indicator of poor prognosis.[8,10] Head and neck tumor cells have also been found to have downregulation of other components of the antigen processing machinery (APM), including transporter associated with antigen processing 1/2 (TAP1/2), tapasin, and LMP2.[9,11,12] These low levels of APM components may be increased

by treating HNSCC cells with interferon-gamma (IFN-γ), suggesting that they are suppressed rather than genetically absent.[9,12] Low levels of APM components in HNSCC have been linked to aberrant levels of signal transduction and activator of transcription (STAT) proteins: increased activity of STAT3 and the phosphatase SHP2 lead to decreased phospho-STAT1 signaling, which is critical for transcription of IFN-γ-dependent genes including those coding for APM components.[13–15] Polymorphisms in the genes coding for these APM components may also be important. A study of HNSCC patients showed that human leukocyte antigen (HLA) types DRB1*03 and DRB1*08/*13 were associated with lower stage disease, while type DRB1*04 was associated with a lower risk of disease recurrence.[16]

In addition to downregulation of APM components, HNSCC tumor cells may secrete factors and cytokines that inhibit the immune response, such as transforming growth factor beta (TGF-β), interleukin 10 (IL-10), granulocyte-macrophage colony-stimulating factor (GM-CSF), and prostaglandin E2 (PGE2).[17,18] Immune cells in the circulation and tumor microenvironment (TME) also tend to secrete these immunosuppressive cytokines, promoting an immunosuppressive T helper (Th2) cytokine milieu.[19] Analyses of serum from HNSCC patients have shown increased levels of immunosuppressive/Th2 cytokines and decreased levels of immunostimulatory/Th1 cytokines.[20,21]

Aberrant responses of immune cells also contribute to the pathogenesis of HNSCC. Circulating CTLs from HNSCC patients may be more susceptible to apoptosis, and thus their numbers in the circulation are decreased. Numbers of effector T cells, NK cells, and antigen-presenting cells (APCs) may be decreased in the circulation and TME.[18,22–24] Conversely, numbers of immunosuppressive regulatory T cells (T$_{reg}$ cells), M2 macrophages, and myeloid-derived suppressor cells (MDSCs) may be increased both peripherally and in the TME.[7,19,22,24,25]

Inherent dysfunction of immune cells has also been noted, including effector T cells, NK cells, and dendritic cells (DCs). T cells may express decreased levels of the zeta chain of the T cell receptor (TCR), decreased levels of co-stimulatory receptors such as CD137, OX40, and 41BB, and increased levels of coinhibitory checkpoint receptors such as programmed death 1 (PD-1) and cytotoxic T lymphocyte-associated protein 4 (CTLA-4).[26,27] The relevance and implications of PD-1 expressing tumor-infiltrating lymphocytes (TILs) and programmed death ligand 1 (PD-L1) expression by head and neck tumor cells are under study and are further discussed next.

Mechanisms Specific to Human Papillomavirus-Related Disease

HPV is a non-enveloped, double-stranded DNA virus that infects squamous epithelial cells.[28] The HPV genome includes early genes *E1* and *E2*, involved in replication; *E5*, *E6*, and *E7*, which are oncoproteins that alter cell cycle regulation of host cells; and *E4*, an additional early gene that has not been well characterized. The late genes *L1* and *L2* encode for the viral capsid.[28,29] The oncoproteins E6 and E7 functionally inactivate the p53 and Rb tumor suppressors, leading to oncogenesis. High-risk subtypes of HPV have been linked to oropharyngeal and anogenital malignancy; in these subtypes, E6 and E7 bind p53 and Rb with greater affinity than with lower-risk subtypes.[16,18,30–33] The vast majority of oropharyngeal carcinoma cases linked to HPV involve the HPV-16 subtype.[30] Most individuals who encounter these viruses will mount an antibody response and clear the infection within 12 to 18 months.[28] For reasons that are not entirely understood, some individuals will fail to clear the infection, instead harboring the virus in the cryptic lymphoid tissue within the palatine and lingual tonsils of the oropharynx. Decades later, HPV oncogenes may lead to malignant transformation of the oropharyngeal epithelial cells.[31] In order for HPV to persist and cause malignant transformation, it must evade antiviral immunity. The incidence of HPV-related malignancies is higher in immunosuppressed individuals, including patients with HIV, congenital immunodeficiency, autoimmunity, and iatrogenic immunosuppression following solid organ transplantation.[31–34] In addition, it has been found that patients with HPV-related oropharyngeal carcinoma with high numbers of TILs may have better outcomes than patients with low numbers of TIL.[35] These findings suggest that aberrant immune responses play a critical role in the pathogenesis of HPV-related epithelial cancers.

The Human Papillomavirus Life Cycle and Immune Evasion

The human papillomaviridae have evolved several ways of evading antiviral immunity, which are summarized in Table 58.2. One important strategy for immune evasion by HPV involves its life cycle (Figure 58.1).[36] HPV infection occurs in the basal layers of epithelia, where early gene products are at low copy numbers. After low-level replication in these basal layers, the viral DNA is then incorporated as an intracellular episome, with the oncoproteins E6 and E7 kept at low expression levels.[37] As the host cells in the basal layer began to differentiate into keratinocytes and approach the surface epithelium, viral replication and E6/E7 levels increase. Production of the capsid proteins and viral assembly then occur just before mature keratinocytes are shed from the epithelium.[38] During this life cycle, the HPV virus spends most of its time in the basal layers, where immune cells are scarce, and then quickly passes through the more superficial layers where immune cells are more abundant.[28,38] The L1 capsid protein, which is the most immunogenic

Table 58.2 Mechanisms of Immune Escape Specific to HPV-Related Head and Neck Squamous Cell Carcinomas

Viral life cycle that minimizes exposure of immunogenic viral components to host immune cells
Decreased production and function of interferons and interferon-responsive genes
Impaired host cell lysis by NK cells
Downregulation of Toll-like receptor 9
E6/E7-mediated inhibition of inflammatory responses
E5/E7-mediated decreases in expression of MHC class I and other APM components
Increased intratumoral expression of PD-L1 and PD-1
Development of T cell tolerance to persistent HPV infection

APM, antigen processing machinery; HPV, human papillomavirus; NK, natural killer; PD-1, programmed cell death 1; PD-L1, programmed death ligand 1.

component of the virus, is expressed late and briefly during the viral life cycle.[32] By shedding along with desquamated keratinocytes in the superficial epithelium, the virus does not require host cell lysis for release, and it thus avoids causing an inflammatory reaction that would stimulate an adaptive immune response.[28,38–41] Furthermore, the virus has very limited exposure to the bloodstream or lymphatic channels, minimizing its detection by immune cells.[38–40]

It has been suggested that the tonsillar crypts of the oropharynx provide an ideal location for prolonged HPV infection. In the squamous epithelium of these tonsillar crypts, the basement membrane is disrupted, which may facilitate the entry of HPV.[42] There may also be enriched expression of the immune checkpoint ligand programmed death ligand 1 (PD-L1) within these tonsillar crypts.[43] Immune checkpoints are further discussed next.

Modulation of Innate Immunity by Human Papillomavirus

Innate antiviral immunity involves the production of inflammatory cytokines and the killing of infected cells by NK cells. Type I interferons, produced by infected cells, have antiviral and immunostimulatory effects. Type II interferon (IFN-γ), produced by NK and T cells, plays important roles in leukocyte migration, inflammation, and stimulation of the adaptive immune response. In the literature regarding HPV, there are numerous examples of the viral oncogenes disrupting production of interferons or downstream interferon-responsive genes.[32,37–39,44,45] Human papillomaviridae can also interfere with the production or function of other immunostimulatory cytokines

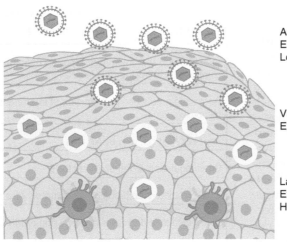

Figure 58.1 Life cycle of the human papillomavirus.

Source: Adapted with permission from Reference 36: Schmitt NC, Ferris RL, Kim S. The role of immune modulation in the carcinogenesis and treatment of HPV associated oropharyngeal cancer. In: Miller DL, Stack MS, eds. *Human Papillomavirus (HPV)-Associated Oropharyngeal Cancer.* Springer; 2015:291–306. Illustration created with Biorender.com.

and chemokines, such as IL-18, monocyte chemoattractant protein 1 (MCP-1), and IL-8.[32,38,39,46,47] Levels of the proinflammatory cytokines IL-1, IL-6, and tumor necrosis factor alpha may also be downregulated in HPV-positive versus HPV-negative tumor cells.[28,33,48] In addition, whole exome sequencing of HNSCC tumors in The Cancer Genome Atlas (TCGA) showed that a high proportion of HPV-positive tumors (20%) had inactivating mutations of TNF receptor-associated factor 3 (TRAF-3), which activates interferons and NF-κB signaling in response to viruses.[49] HPV-related malignancies have also been associated with immunosuppressive Th2 cytokine profiles.[28,33,38,46]

Several other components of innate immunity may also be affected by HPV. Tumor cells from HPV-positive tumors may be resistant to NK-mediated lysis.[33,39] Toll-like receptor (TLR) 9, which plays a major role in the innate immune response to HPV, may be downregulated by E6 and E7 from high-risk HPV subtypes.[46,50]

Modulation of Adaptive Immunity By HPV

In addition to inhibiting innate immunity, human papillomaviridae have developed ways of inhibiting the adaptive immune response, in part by interfering with antigen presentation. As described earlier, HPV infection can inhibit the inflammatory response, which is required for DC maturation and presentation of antigens.[41,47] Furthermore, the HPV oncoproteins E5, E6, and E7 induce decreased levels of various components of the antigen presentation machinery in host cells, including TAP-1, TAP-2, tapasin, MHC class I and II, and the proteasome subunit low molecular mass protein 2 (LMP-2).[11,38,39,46,51,52]

Effector T lymphocytes are critical in the immune response to HPV. The clearance of HPV is mediated in large part by CD4+ and CD8+ T lymphocytes specific for E6 and E7.[33,51] One study of HPV-related oropharyngeal carcinoma demonstrated high levels of TIL, and the levels correlated with patient outcomes.[53] Other studies have corroborated this finding of higher numbers of TIL in HPV-positive oropharyngeal tumors than in HPV-negative HNSCC tumors.[54] However, HPV-positive tumors may also have a higher proportion of immunosuppressive T$_{reg}$ cells, and the high number of CTLs include many that are anergic or "exhausted," as further discussed next.[30,55]

Immune Checkpoint Pathways in Human Papillomavirus-Related Oropharyngeal Carcinoma

The role of immune checkpoint pathways in HPV-related HNSCC is a subject under some debate. As previously described and in earlier chapters of this book, CTLA-4 and PD-1 pathways exist to prevent exaggerated immune responses and autoimmunity. In the first published study on PD-1 in HPV-related oropharyngeal squamous cell carcinoma (OPSCC), PD-1 expression on CTLs was noted to be increased in HPV-positive OPSCC specimens versus normal tonsil tissue, and PD-L1 expression on tumor cells was higher in HPV-positive tumors than in HPV-negative tumors.[43] This was corroborated in a second study showing high levels of PD-1 among TIL from HPV-positive specimens.[55] Paradoxically, patients with HPV-positive tumors and higher levels of PD-1 expression on TIL, but not PD-L1 on tumor cells, had a much improved survival compared with patients with low PD-1 on TIL.[55] The authors speculated that the increased PD-1 expression on TIL was an indication of a more robust underlying immune response, leading to improved survival.[55] A study limited to HPV-negative tumors demonstrated that high PD-1 expression on TIL is not unique to HPV-positive tumors.[56] Two additional studies showed no differences according to HPV status in PD-1 expression among TIL[57] or PD-L1 expression among tumor cells.[58] However, when Kansy and colleagues classified TIL from HNSCC specimens as demonstrating low, intermediate, or high expression of PD-1, they noted that TIL from HPV+ tumors were more likely overall to be PD-1-positive, but PD-1-high TIL were more often seen in HPV-negative tumors and correlated with worse prognosis.[59] These observations provide a rationale for the use of PD-1 pathway blockade for HNSCC, especially for HPV-related disease. Clinical trials of checkpoint inhibitors for HNSCC are summarized next.

IMMUNOTHERAPEUTIC STRATEGIES IN HEAD AND NECK CANCER

The field of immunotherapy for treatment of solid tumors is rapidly expanding. As with other tumor types, several different immunotherapeutic strategies are under investigation for HNSCC, which are summarized in Table 58.3.

Table 58.3 Immunotherapeutic Strategies Under Investigation for Head and Neck Squamous Cell Carcinomas

IMMUNOTHERAPEUTIC STRATEGY	PHASE OF STUDY	EXAMPLE CLINICAL TRIALS
Tumor antigen-targeting moAbs (cetuximab)	FDA approved for R/M and PULA HNSCC	EXTREME/NCT00122460 NCT00004227
Coinhibitory checkpoint inhibitors		
Anti-PD-1/Anti-PD-L1 moAbs (nivolumab, pembrolizumab, durvalumab/MEDI4736)	FDA approved for R/M HNSCC, Phase 3 for PULA HNSCC	CheckMate 141/NCT02105636, KEYNOTE-012/NCT01848834, KEYNOTE-40/NCT02252042, KEYNOTE-048/NCT02358031, KEYNOTE-055/NCT02255097, KEYNOTE-689/NCT03765918, RTOG3504, NCT02253992, NCT02289209, NCT01693562, NCT02291055, NCT02207530, NCT02319044, NCT02369874, NCT02124850
Anti-CTLA-4 moAbs (ipilimumab, tremelimumab)	Phase 2	NCT01860430, NCT02319044, NCT02369874, NCT01935921
Co-Stimulatory checkpoint agonists		
CD137 agonists	Phase 1	NCT02253992, NCT02110082
OX40 agonists	Phase 1	NCT03336606, NCT03894618
Vaccines		
Peptide vaccines	Phase 1	NCT00257738, NCT01462838, NCT02526316
Viral or bacterial (*Listeria*) vector (ADXS11-001)	Phase 1	NCT02002182, NCT02291055
Dendritic cell vaccines	Phase 1	NCT00404339
Adoptive T cell transfer		
Pooled T cells responsive to HPV oncoproteins	Phase 1	NCT01585428, NCT02379520
T cells with engineered TCR	Phase 1	NCT02280811, NCT02858310, NCT02379520, NCT04015336, NCT04044950
Chimeric antigen receptor (CAR) T cells	Phase 1	NCT01818323
Inhibitors of MDSC, T_{reg} cells, or macrophage trafficking/function	Phase 1	NCT03690986, NCT02499328
Toll-like receptor agonists	Phase 2	NCT01836029, NCT01334177, NCT02124850
STING agonists	Phase 1/2	NCT03937141, NCT03010176

FDA, U.S. Food and Drug Administration; HNSCC, head and neck squamous cell carcinoma; HPV, human papillomavirus; MDSC, myeloid-derived suppressor cell; moAbs, monoclonal antibodies; PULA, previously untreated, locally advanced; R/M, recurrent/metastatic; STING, Stimulator of Interferon Genes; TCR, T cell receptor; T_{reg}, regulatory T.

Tumor Antigen-Targeting Monoclonal Antibodies

Monoclonal antibodies (moAbs) targeting specific tumor antigens are frequently used to treat HNSCC. Cetuximab, a chimeric mouse-human immunoglobulin G1 (IgG1) targeting epidermal growth factor receptor (EGFR), is FDA-approved for the treatment of HNSCC. Cetuximab has been shown to increase survival for previously untreated, locoregional disease compared with radiation alone, and it also improves survival of patients with recurrent or metastatic disease when added to standard cytotoxic chemotherapy.[60,61] While EGFR is overexpressed in the vast majority of HNSCC tumors, tumor levels of EGFR do not predict response to cetuximab or other EGFR moAbs, and only a subset of patients respond.[62] Anti-EGFR moAbs induce tumor cell death in part by antibody-dependent cellular cytotoxicity (ADCC), mediated in part by NK cells (Figure 58.2), which may be influenced by Fcγ receptor IIIa polymorphisms.[62,63] The released antibody-coated tumor antigens can then be engulfed by APCs or detected by Fcγ receptors, leading to antigen cross-presentation and activation of tumor antigen-specific CTLs.[2,62,64,65] Such tumor antigen-specific CTLs have been noted in tumor specimens for cetuximab-treated HNSCC patients and appear to correlate with response to cetuximab and clinical outcomes.[65,66] The process of cetuximab-induced ADCC, NK:DC crosstalk, and subsequent adaptive immunity may be enhanced by stimulation of TLR 8[67] and appears to be antibody isotype specific, since panitumumab, a fully humanized IgG2 antibody, inhibits EGFR to the same degree as cetuximab but fails to elicit these immune responses.[68] Cetuximab may further improve adaptive immune responses in HNSCC patients by increasing tumor-cell expression of HLA class I and expanding the variety of T cell receptors in the peripheral blood.[69,70] Cetuximab has also been found to alter levels of immune-suppressive T_{reg} cells and MDSCs to different degrees in responders and nonresponders, which may also help explain why only a subset of HNSCC patients respond.[71,72] In addition to cetuximab and other anti-EGFR moAbs, other moAbs targeting tumor antigens (HER3, IGFR) and cytokines (VEGF, HGF) are under study in clinical trials for HNSCC.[2]

Immune Checkpoints

Coinhibitory Checkpoints

Coinhibitory checkpoint pathways exist to prevent exaggerated immunity, but in the TME they represent a frequent mechanism of immune escape. Several different coinhibitory checkpoints have been identified and studied, and these are detailed extensively elsewhere in this book. As in other tumor types, moAbs targeting PD-1 and CTLA-4 pathways have shown promising results in preclinical studies and clinical trials of HNSCC. As illustrated by the sheer number of clinical trials listed in Table 58.3, coinhibitory checkpoints are the most widely studied immunotherapeutic strategy for HNSCC in ongoing and recently completed clinical trials.

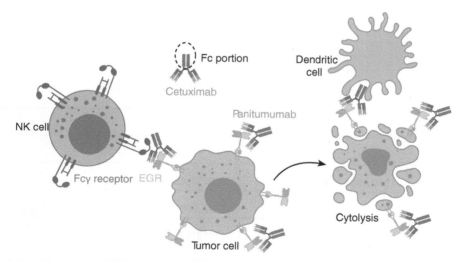

Figure 58.2 Cetuximab-mediated antibody-dependent cellular cytotoxicity (ADCC). Cetuximab binds to EGFR on tumor cells and is detected by immune effector cells, leading to cell lysis. Antibody-coated tumor cell antigens are then recognized or engulfed by dendritic cells, which mature and activate an adaptive immune response. Other anti-EGFR monoclonal antibodies, such as panitumumab, do not induce these immune responses.

EGFR, epidermal growth factor receptor.

Source: Illustration created with Biorender.com.

Programmed Death 1 Pathway

As described earlier, PD-1 and PD-L1 expression have been noted in both HPV-positive and HPV-negative HNSCC, though some studies suggest that PD-1 expression by TIL may be higher in HPV-positive tumors.[2,43,55,56,73] The second ligand of PD-1, PD-L2, has not been extensively studied and may be less important in the pathogenesis of HNSCC.[74] In one of the earliest preclinical studies of PD-L1 inhibition, mice bearing tumors expressing PD-L1 were treated with anti-PD-L1 and adoptive cell transfer (ACT); the majority of the mice were cured.[73] Initial clinical trials of moAbs inhibiting this pathway in HNSCC recruited patients with recurrent or metastatic (R/M) disease that was refractory to standard, first-line therapy. The standard first-line therapy previously consisted of the EXTREME regimen, combining cisplatin, fluorouracil, and cetuximab. Although the median overall survival with the EXTREME regimen is about 10 months,[75] many patients who do not respond demonstrate very poor survival with second-line therapies. The CheckMate-141 trial randomized patients with R/M HNSCC who had failed platinum chemotherapy to receive investigator's choice (cetuximab or cytotoxic chemotherapy) or the anti-PD-1 moAb nivolumab; this trial was stopped early after meeting its primary endpoint of increased overall survival.[76] Median overall survival was 7.5 months with nivolumab and 5.1 months for investigator's choice agents, with a 30% reduction in death (hazard ratio, 0.7); the one-year overall survival more than doubled, from 17% to 36%.[76] Nivolumab was well tolerated, with lower rates of grade 3 to grade 4 toxicities than with investigator's choice second-line therapies. Very few patients demonstrated "pseudoprogression" or mild flare of their tumors. This was the first randomized, Phase 3 immunotherapy study to show an improvement in survival for R/M HNSCC.[76] In a very similar Phase 3 trial of the anti-PD-1 antibody pembrolizumab (KEYNOTE-40), the median overall survival was 8.4 months with pembrolizumab versus 6.9 months with investigator's choice standard therapy.[77] The KEYNOTE-012 trial of pembrolizumab enrolled patients with R/M HNSCC, many of whom had failed to respond to multiple prior therapies, and many of whom did not have PD-L1 positive tumors.[78,79] Overall response rate (ORR) was slightly higher in HPV-positive patients, and approximately one-third of the enrolled patients demonstrated a response or stable disease while on pembrolizumab. The responses were prolonged, with 6-month progression-free survival (PFS) of about 25% and some durable responses of up to 2 years. Grade 3 to grade 4 toxicities occurred in 12% of patients, with no treatment-related deaths.[78,79] Similarly, in a Phase 2 study of pembrolizumab for patients with R/M HNSCC who had failed treatment with platinum and cetuximab (KEYNOTE-055), 18% had a response and 18% had stable disease, for a total of 36%

benefit rate in this heavily pretreated patient population. Similar to KEYNOTE-012, 12% of patients had grade 3 to grade 5 toxicities, with one treatment-related death.[80] Similar response and survival rates were seen in a trial of patients with R/M HNSCC treated with the PD-L1 inhibitor durvalumab (MEDI4736), despite a median of three prior lines of systemic therapy; responses were higher in patients with PD-L1-positive tumors.[81] In sum, a significant proportion of patients with recurrent or metastatic HNSCC appear to benefit from monotherapy with PD-1 moAbs, despite failing multiple prior lines of therapy.

Based on the previously described clinical trials, tumor PD-L1 status is one predictor of responses to anti-PD-1 therapy. The KEYNOTE-012 trial showed a 22% response rate for tumors that were PD-L1 positive, versus 4% response rate for tumors that were PD-L1 negative.[78] In CheckMate 141, patients with PD-L1-positive tumors had a 45% reduction in the risk of death with nivolumab, versus 27% for PD-L1-negative tumors.[82] KEYNOTE-040 established the combined positive score (CPS), defined as the total number of cells (tumor cells, lymphocytes, and macrophages) expressing PD-L1 divided by the total number of tumor cells, then multiplied by 100.[83] The tumor proportion score (TPS) was defined as the proportion of tumor cells expressing membranous PD-L1.[83] The best responses to pembrolizumab were seen in patients with a CPS ≥1 and TPS >50%.[83]

Data regarding responses to anti-PD-1 therapy according to HPV status are mixed. An improved ORR was seen for HPV-positive versus -negative patients in KEYNOTE-012,[78] but not in the CheckMate 141 trial.[82] In the HAWK trial, where the PD-L1 inhibitor durvalumab was used for patients with recurrent/metastatic disease and high PD-L1 expression, the ORR was 16% overall but 29% in HPV-positive patients.[84] Multiple smaller studies have shown that HPV-positive tumors tend to have increased numbers of immune effector cells and may respond better to anti-PD-1/PD-L1 therapy.[59,85]

Prior therapy is another factor influencing responses to anti-PD-1 therapy in HNSCC patients. Most patients in the KEYNOTE-012, KEYNOTE-040, and CheckMate 141 studies had already failed at least two prior lines of therapy for recurrent or metastatic disease.[78,83,86] A subsequent analysis of data from CheckMate 141 showed that patients without prior cetuximab exposure had a greater survival benefit with nivolumab.[87] In KEYNOTE-055, a single-arm study of patients who had failed both platinum-based chemotherapy and cetuximab, the ORR was 16%.[80] The potential mechanisms for overlapping resistance to cetuximab and anti-PD-1 therapy have not yet been fully elucidated.

The KEYNOTE-012 and CheckMate 141 studies led to FDA approval of pembrolizumab and nivolumab, respectively, in 2016 as second-line treatment for patients with recurrent/metastatic HNSCC who had already failed platinum-based chemotherapy. The EXTREME trial had previously established cisplatin, cetuximab, and fluorouracil as the standard first-line therapy for recurrent/metastatic HNSCC.[75] The KEYNOTE-048 trial was designed to establish whether anti-PD-1 therapy would be effective as a first-line therapy. Patients were randomized to receive the EXTREME regimen versus first-line, single-agent pembrolizumab, versus pembrolizumab (instead of cetuximab) in combination with the platinum/fluorouracil doublet. The second interim analysis demonstrated improved overall survival with pembrolizumab alone in patients with a combined positive score (CPS) ≥1, leading to FDA approval for first-line pembrolizumab in 2019. On final analysis, pembrolizumab/chemotherapy was associated with better response rates and improved survival versus cetuximab/chemotherapy (EXTREME), regardless of PD-L1 status.[88] Based on these results from KEYNOTE-048, the current standard of care for first-line treatment of recurrent/metastatic HNSCC is pembrolizumab alone for patients with CPS ≥1 and pembrolizumab plus cisplatin/fluorouracil for CPS <1.

Now established as standard therapy for recurrent/metastatic HNSCC, anti-PD-1/PD-L1 therapy is currently under study in patients with previously untreated, locally advanced disease. Studies of neoadjuvant checkpoint blockade suggest that the responses are much higher than in the recurrent/metastatic setting. As an example, preliminary results from a trial of neoadjuvant pembrolizumab in locally advanced, high-risk HNSCC showed a 43% rate of pathologic response, with some patients showing a complete pathologic response in surgical specimens.[89] Several similar studies are currently underway. The role of anti-PD-1/PD-L1 in patients treated with radiation therapy is discussed in the text that follows (see "Combination Therapies").

Cytotoxic T Lymphocyte-Associated Protein 4

CTLA-4 inhibitors, though well established as effective therapy in melanoma and other tumor types,[90] have been less studied for HNSCC. Clinical trials for HNSCC have consisted of therapeutic combinations including antibodies inhibiting CTLA-4 and other forms of immunotherapy and/or standard therapy, which are discussed later in this chapter (see "Combination Therapies"). In particular, the Phase 2 CONDOR trial randomized HNSCC patients with recurrent/metastatic, platinum-refractory, PD-L1-low tumors to treatment with durvalumab (anti-PD-L1), tremelimumab (anti-CTLA-4), or the combination,[91] based on the rationale that patients with PD-L1 low tumors might benefit from blocking CTLA-4. The ORR to durvalumab was 9.2%, and fewer patients (1.6%) responded to tremelimumab

alone. Adding tremelimumab resulted in a higher incidence of grade 3/4 immune-related adverse events without improving the ORR (7.8%), suggesting that adding an anti-CTLA-4 antibody may not be an ideal strategy for improving responses to anti-PD-1/PD-L1 therapy for PD-L1-low tumors.[91]

Other Coinhibitory Checkpoints

As described in other chapters, the upregulation of other coinhibitory checkpoints, including TIM-3, LAG-3, TIGIT, and IDO1, may increase resistance to anti-PD-1 therapy.[92–96] Interestingly, HPV-positive tumors tend to have higher expression of these T cell exhaustion markers versus HPV-negative tumors.[92,97] Elevated IDO1 gene expression has been described in HNSCC specimens that also expressed PD-L1.[92] Elevated levels of TIGIT on CD4[+] and CD8[+] T cells from HNSCC patients have also been described, and anti-TIGIT therapy led to delayed tumor growth in a murine model, with further delay when anti-PD-1 therapy was added.[93] Tumor specimens from HNSCC patients are also enriched in PD-1[+ and] TIM-3[+] T cells.[98,99] TIM-3 blockade, which has been explored in preclinical studies, is a particularly attractive strategy since TIM-3 is expressed on both exhausted CD8[+] T cells and immunosuppressive T_{reg} cells.[94,95,98] Targeting LAG-3 in addition to PD-1 has also demonstrated effective antitumor activity in preclinical murine studies.[96]

Co-Stimulatory Checkpoints

Another strategy is to use agonist antibodies targeting co-stimulatory receptors, such as OX40, CD137 (also known as 4-1BB), CD40, or their ligands in order to stimulate T cell function. Preclinical studies have shown enhanced antitumor immunity with OX40 agonists, and high levels of intratumoral, OX40-positive T cells exist in HNSCC patients.[100] However, another study showed decreased levels of OX40 and CD137 on T cells from the peripheral blood of HNSCC patients compared with healthy controls, with the lowest levels of these co-stimulatory signals on T cells from patients with advanced stage disease.[26] Despite these mixed preclinical and clinical data, the idea that the balance of co-stimulatory to coinhibitory checkpoints may be shifted in favor of a tumor-permissive microenvironment provides a rationale for the use of co-stimulatory agonists for HNSCC, particularly in combination with coinhibitory checkpoint inhibitors. A Phase 1 trial of a neoadjuvant anti-OX40 antibody for HNSCC and melanoma is recruiting (NCT03336606). A fusion protein targeting both PD-1 and OX40 is also in Phase 1 for lymphoma and solid tumors, including HNSCC (NCT03894618). A preclinical study showed improved tumor control by adding an agonist of CD137 to chemoradiation in a mouse model of HPV-positive HNSCC,[101] and multiple Phase 1 trials of CD137-targeting antibodies for HNSCC and other solid tumors have been completed (NCT02253992, NCT02110082, NCT01471210). Combinations of these agents with other co-stimulatory or coinhibitory checkpoint inhibitors are under study in clinical trials for multiple solid tumor types,[100] as described in other chapters.

Vaccines for Head and Neck Squamous Cell Cancer

Tumor vaccines may consist of peptides, DNA, whole tumor cells, or DCs pulsed or loaded with a tumor antigen. Tumor vaccines can also be delivered by viral or bacterial vectors. Oncolytic viruses preferentially infect and lyse tumor cells more than normal cells.[102] Such viruses can activate interferon responses, TLRs, and other pathways that activate antitumor immunity, in addition to releasing antigenic material from dying tumor cells to the TME.[102] The most successful oncolytic virus thus far is talimogene laherparepvec (T-VEC), an attenuated herpes simplex 1 (HSV-1) virus that also encodes for GM-CSF. As described in other chapters, T-VEC has shown efficacy alone and with anti-PD-1 checkpoint blockade for melanoma.[103] An oncolytic virus similar to T-VEC (HSV-1, encoding GM-CSF) was used in a Phase 1 study to patients with previously untreated, locally advanced HNSCC, in addition to standard chemoradiation. Most patients demonstrated a complete response on posttreatment neck dissection, and the vaccine was well tolerated.[104] More recently, the oncolytic vaccinia virus GL-ONC1 was used in combination with chemoradiation in a Phase 1 study for oropharyngeal carcinoma, with favorable outcomes.[105]

A limited number of trials have used DC vaccines for head and neck cancer. A Phase 1 study of autologous DCs loaded with HLA class I p53 peptides showed modest p53-specific immunity, a decrease in the number of T_{reg} cells, and favorable clinical outcomes in vaccinated patients.[106] Transfection of DCs with lysyl oxidase-like 4 (LOXL4) may be another possible vaccination strategy for HNSCC.[107]

Human Papillomavirus-Specific Therapies

Though patients with HPV-related HNSCC have an improved survival compared with patients who have HPV-negative disease, there is significant enthusiasm for decreasing toxicities in these relatively younger patients with improved prognosis. One such strategy is to use immunotherapy in place of cytotoxic therapy, or in order to reduce radiation doses.[2] Some patients with HPV-related disease will relapse, and these patients with recurrent or metastatic disease may respond better to immunotherapy than patients with recurrent HPV-negative disease.[2] In addition to agents widely studied for all solid tumor types, specific antiviral immune therapies have been designed for patients with HPV-related OPSCC.

Preventive Human Papillomavirus Vaccines

As discussed earlier, most individuals who become exposed to HPV will mount an antibody response and clear the virus. The natural antibody response to the virus is a slow process that occurs in response to the L1 capsid protein, since HPV early genes do not induce an antibody response.[32,108] It is unclear whether antibodies induced by natural infection with HPV will be protective against reinfection.[46]

Preventive vaccines were developed primarily to eradicate cervical cancer and other anogenital malignancies, but these vaccines are likely to dramatically reduce HPV-related oropharyngeal carcinoma as well. The vaccines include virus-like particles (VLPs) resembling the L1 capsid protein, and unlike natural infection, vaccination introduces these VLPs to the lymphatic system.[108] Initially, two preventive vaccines were currently available: a bivalent vaccine that protects against high-risk subtypes 16 and 18 (Gardasil®, Merck and Company, Whitehouse Station, New Jersey) and a quadrivalent vaccine that also protects against the low-risk subtypes 6 and 11 (Cervarix®, GlaxoSmithKline Biologicals, Rixensart, Belgium). In multiple Phase 3, randomized, and double-blinded, controlled trials involving thousands of young women, these vaccines were found to be 90% to 100% effective, leading to public health initiatives to vaccinate preadolescent girls worldwide.[109] More recently, a nonavalent vaccine was introduced, providing immunity against five additional subtypes of HPV for a total of nine subtypes.[110]

While promising, most of these prior studies did not include men, who are more likely to develop HPV-related oropharyngeal carcinoma. More recent studies have examined how these two vaccines affect HPV infection in the oral cavity and in men. A randomized, double-blind controlled trial of over 4,000 young men showed Gardasil to be over 90% effective in preventing HPV-related anogenital lesions.[109,111] The Centers for Disease Control and Prevention currently recommend vaccination for preadolescent boys in addition to girls, which is likely to reduce future rates of oropharyngeal carcinoma. The effects of these vaccines on oropharyngeal malignancy are not yet well known but are currently under study.[50,112] Studies in men do show that antibodies to HPV are present in the oral cavity following vaccination, but oral antibody levels appear to decline over time.[113] The incidence of oral HPV infection is also significantly reduced in young adults who have been previously vaccinated.[114] Despite these promising results on the presence of oral HPV infections and antibodies, the rate of vaccination remains somewhat low, and long-term effects on the incidence of oropharyngeal cancer remain unclear.[112,114]

Therapeutic Human Papillomavirus Vaccines

Multiple types of therapeutic vaccines for HPV-related malignancies are under investigation. Many of these vaccines have been tested in clinical trials for HPV-related cervical cancer and are described elsewhere in this book. For HPV-related OPSCC, a few clinical and preclinical vaccine studies have shown modest results. In one preclinical study, vaccination with synthetic long peptides from HPV 16 induced synergistic tumor cell killing when given with cisplatin chemotherapy.[115] In another preclinical study, intratumoral injection of an HPV-16 E7 peptide vaccine with poly(I:C) adjuvant induced a robust antitumor immune response in the TC-1 syngeneic mouse carcinoma model engineered to express HPV E6 and E7.[116] A peptide vaccine consisting of HLA class I and HLA class II restricted melanoma antigen E (MAGE)-A3 or HPV-16 peptides was designed with a "Trojan" approach, to prevent proteolysis of the antigenic peptides and deliver them directly to the endoplasmic reticulum and Golgi apparatus.[117] In four of the five vaccinated OPSCC patients, antigen-specific peripheral blood responses were noted, and the vaccine was well tolerated. However, none of the patients had a clinical response by Response Evaluation Criteria in Solid Tumors (RECIST) criteria.[117,118] Similarly, a Phase 1 trial of a p16^{INK4A} peptide vaccine, including patients with HPV-related anogenital and head and neck cancer, showed antigen-specific immune responses, but no clinical responses; however, several patients demonstrated stable disease after vaccination.[119] More recently, a DNA vaccine consisting of three plasmids expressing HPV E6 and E7 proteins along with adjuvant IL-12 (MEDI0457/INO-3112) induced E6/E7-specific immune responses and was well-tolerated in a pilot study of HNSCC patients with advanced HPV-related disease.[120]

Vaccines employing viral or bacterial vectors for tumor antigen delivery have also been studied. In a preclinical tumor model, a *Listeria*-based HPV-16 E7 vaccine delayed tumor growth and increased levels of antigen-specific CD8$^+$ T cells in the peripheral blood, spleen, and TME.[121] Following promising results with the *Listeria*-based HPV-16 antigen vaccine ADXS11-001 in cervical cancer patients, a Phase 1 trial was opened for oropharyngeal cancer patients (NCT01598792); however, the trial was terminated after one patient developed systemic listeriosis.[118,122] A Phase 2 window-of-opportunity trial using the ADXS11-001 *Listeria* vaccine prior to transoral robotic surgery for HPV-related OPSCC is currently active, with change in the E6/E7-specific CTL responses and toxicity as the primary endpoints (NCT02002182). A Phase 2 trial comparing ADXS11-001 to the PD-L1 inhibitor MEDI4736 alone or in combination for patients with recurrent or metastatic HPV-related malignancies has completed accrual (NCT02291055). Vaccines using Vaccinia and other viral vectors are under study in cervical cancer and may be applicable to OPSCC as well.[2,118]

Adoptive T Cell Therapy

Another strategy under study for HNSCC is ACT. Much of the work thus far on T cell transfer has focused on HPV-related disease. In a preclinical murine model of cervical cancer, adoptive transfer of HPV E7-specific T cells resulted in synergistic tumor cell killing when given with cisplatin, in part by improving antigen presentation.[123] While ACT is technically challenging and costly, effective methods for harvesting T cells from patients with HPV-related OPSCC and generating HPV E6/E7-specific T cells on a large scale have been developed.[124] The use of HPV E6/E7-specific T cells for patients with HPV-related malignancies has been under study at multiple centers. Some of the cervical cancer patients receiving autologous T cells with engineered HPV 16-specific TCRs at the National Cancer Institute have shown complete responses,[125] and patients with oropharyngeal cancer have also been included. To enhance the efficacy of infused T cells, trials at the National Cancer Institute are using TCRs engineered to specifically recognize HPV-16 E6 or E7 peptides. Infusion of T cells recognizing E6 provided some durable responses, and patients who did not respond demonstrated defects in interferon responses or antigen presentation.[126] Trials involving the infusion of HLA-A2:01-restricted, E7-specific TCR T cells are enrolling for patients with recurrent/metastatic disease (NCT02858310) or previously untreated, locally advanced disease (NCT04015336, NCT04044950).

Chimeric antigen receptor (CAR) T cells have also been engineered for use in HNSCC. T4 immunotherapy consists of the transfer of autologous T cells engineered to express chimeric receptors for ErbB dimers, which are frequently upregulated in HNSCC, and the 4ab receptor, which converts IL-4 into a signal for enrichment and expansion of T cells.[127] This T4 CAR T immunotherapy has shown promising results in preclinical studies of HNSCC[127] and is currently under investigation in a Phase 1 clinical trial (NCT01818323).

Toll-Like Receptor Agonists

TLRs play an integral role in the response to viruses, immunogenic cell death, inflammation, and innate immunity.[128] TLR levels may differ between HPV-positive and HPV-negative HNSCC, and may also correlate with the degree of T cell infiltration and with prognosis.[128,129] In preclinical studies, a TLR 8 (TLR8) agonist, VTX-2337(Motolimod), enhanced the killing of tumor cells by NK cells in combination with cetuximab.[67,130] Another study using syngeneic murine models showed excellent antitumor activity of TLR7/9 agonists, which was further enhanced by anti-PD-1 therapy.[131] A Phase 1b trial of motolimod with cetuximab for recurrent/metastatic HNSCC showed some partial responses, with about half of the patients demonstrating stable disease and NK cells that were more activated.[132] A randomized, controlled clinical trial comparing motolimod versus placebo in combination with the EXTREME regimen (platinum, fluorouracil, and cetuximab) for recurrent or metastatic HNSCC showed no difference in overall survival or PFS.[133] However, patients with HPV-positive disease or who exhibited a reaction at the injection site had improved outcomes.[133]

Stimulator of Interferon Genes Agonists

Cyclic dinucleotides (CDN) activate the STING receptor, leading to the production of interferons and pro-inflammatory cytokines. Preclinical and clinical studies investigating natural and synthetic CDN have shown promising results.[134] In preclinical murine models of HNSCC, intratumoral injection of CDN induced tumor regression and enhanced antitumor immune responses, which were further enhanced with anti-PD-1 therapy.[135,136] A Phase 1 clinical trial involving intratumoral injection of the Stimulator of Interferon Genes (STING) agonist MK-1454 alone or with systemic pembrolizumab for lymphomas and solid tumors, including HSNCC, is recruiting (NCT03010176). Preliminary results from that trial have shown encouraging safety and evidence of immune responses in both arms, but measurable responses were limited to the dual-treatment arm.[137] Another clinical trial combining the STING agonist ADU-S100 (also known as MIW815) with pembrolizumab is currently enrolling patients with PD-L1-positive, recurrent/metastatic HNSCC (NCT03937141). Combinations with anti-CTLA-4 antibodies are also under investigation, including a combination of ADU-S100 plus ipilimumab for solid tumors and lymphomas (NCT02675439).

Inhibition of Myeloid-Derived Suppressor Cells, Regulatory T Cells, and Macrophages

A major cause of resistance to immunotherapy involving T cells or NK cells is the presence of immunosuppressive cells, such as MDSCs, T_{reg} cells, or M2 macrophages. Preclinical studies have shown that responses to immunotherapy can be enhanced by depleting immunosuppressive myeloid cells or by inhibiting the trafficking of these cells to the TME.[138–140] A moAb inhibiting semaphorin4D improved responses to immune checkpoint blockade (ICB) in murine models by inhibiting MDSC trafficking and function,[141] and a window-of-opportunity trial is underway with this agent in combination with ICB for previously-untreated, surgically resectable HNSCC (NCT03690986). Another way of inhibiting

MDSC recruitment to the TME is by blocking the chemokine receptor CXCR2, which is under investigation in a Phase 1/2 study for recurrent/metastatic HNSCC and other solid tumors (NCT02499328). Another strategy for inhibiting MDSC function is by inhibiting intermediates responsible for MDSC production of immunosuppressive metabolites, including IDO and STAT3. Multiple Phase 1 and 2 trials are underway to investigate the use of IDO or STAT3 antagonists either alone or in combination with ICB.[142–144]

Multiple preclinical and clinical studies have attempted to preferentially deplete or inhibit T_{reg} cells by targeting CD25, CCR4, or GITR.[142] As described earlier, targeting particular coinhibitory or co-stimulatory molecules, including TIM-3, OX40, and CTLA-4, may have the added benefit of inhibiting T_{reg} cells in addition to enhancing effector T cell function.[94,95,98,100,142] Blocking of the chemotactic factor colony-stimulating factor 1 (CSF1) or its receptor, CSF1R, may inhibit the recruitment and immunosuppressive M2 polarization of tumor associated macrophages.[145] However, a trial of the CSFR1 inhibitor PLX3397 combined with pembrolizumab for melanoma and other solid tumors, including HNSCC, was closed due to limited evidence of efficacy (NCT02452424). Another trial of a CSF1R inhibitor combined with nivolumab for HNSCC and other advanced solid tumors is active but no longer recruiting (NCT02526017).

Combination Therapies

Similar to other tumor types, resistance to ICB is a major hurdle in HNSCC. Although single-agent immunotherapies have shown activity, response rates may be increased by combining multiple forms of immunotherapy, or by combining immunotherapy with standard or targeted therapy, to achieve additive or synergistic activity. Immunotherapy in combination with cytotoxic chemotherapy and/or radiation is under study, in addition to combinations of cetuximab with other forms of immunotherapy, and the combined use of multiple coinhibitory and/or co-stimulatory checkpoint inhibitors.

Combinations of Immunotherapy

As described earlier, cetuximab enhances multiple aspects of innate and adaptive antitumor immunity in HNSCC, but response may be limited by CTLA-4-expressing T_{reg} cells and other immunosuppressive cells.[63–65,71,72] Thus, combining cetuximab with other forms of immunotherapy is an attractive strategy. In a trial of cetuximab and the anti-CTLA-4 moAb ipilimumab with radiation for patients with previously untreated, locally advanced, HPV-negative or high-risk, HPV-positive HNSCC (NCT01935921), 18 patients were enrolled, and the combination resulted in encouraging response and survival outcomes at 2 years posttreatment, with acceptable toxicity.[146] In a Phase 1b trial (NCT02110082), cetuximab was combined with the CD137 agonist urelumab. This combination was also well tolerated and increased antigen processing machinery (HLA-DR) in peripheral blood DCs.[147]

Other strategies for combining multiple immunotherapy drugs in HNSCC include the use of multiple coinhibitory checkpoint inhibitors, or a coinhibitory checkpoint inhibitor in combination with a co-stimulatory checkpoint agonist. The Phase 2 CONDOR trial showed no benefit from adding anti-CTLA-4 therapy (tremelimumab) to anti-PD-L1 therapy (durvalumab) in patients with PD-L1-low tumors,[84] and similar results were seen in the Phase 3 EAGLE study.[148] Additional trials are underway using the IDO1 inhibitor epacadostat combined with nivolumab (ECHO-204) or with pembrolizumab (ECHO-202/KEYNOTE-037). These combinations have shown encouraging response rates and appear to be well tolerated.[143,144] A Phase 1 trial was recently completed that combined nivolumab (anti-PD-1) and urelumab (CD137 agonist) in multiple tumor types including HNSCC (NCT02253992).

Checkpoint inhibitors have also been combined with vaccines or oncolytic viruses for HNSCC. Several trials combining HPV-specific vaccines with checkpoint inhibitors are underway for HPV-related HNSCC.[2] A Phase 1b study combining pembrolizumab with T-VEC (HSV-1-based oncolytic virus) enrolled 36 patients with recurrent/metastatic HNSCC. The ORR was 16.7% and the disease control rate was 38.9%,[149] suggesting that the addition of T-VEC did not provide any additional benefit versus historical data with anti-PD-1 antibodies alone.

Lastly, the innate immune system can be enlisted by combining TLR and STING agonists with checkpoint inhibitors. A preclinical study using syngeneic murine models of HNSCC showed additive activity with TLR7/9 inhibitors and anti-PD-1.[131] A Phase 1b/2 study for recurrent/metastatic HNSCC is combining pembrolizumab with intratumoral injection of SD-101, a synthetic TLR9 agonist, with a preliminary disease control rate of 48%.[150] A combination of anti-PD-1 therapy and an intratumoral injection of STING agonist showed synergistic activity in a murine model of HNSCC, and preliminary results of a trial combining pembrolizumab with intratumor injection of the STING agonist MK-1454 have been encouraging.[136,137] Another preclinical study showed that STING activation can further enhance cetuximab-induced activation of NK cells and DC maturation,[151] suggesting a rationale for combining cetuximab with STING agonists.

Immunotherapy Combined With Standard Therapy

Similar to other cancer types, especially lung cancer, a growing body of evidence suggests that standard therapies such as radiation and cytotoxic chemotherapy may enhance antitumor immune responses in HNSCC. It has been established in numerous tumor types that radiation and cytotoxic drugs may promote immunogenic cell death, antigen processing/presentation, and adaptive immunity,[152–154] in addition to the release of antigens from dying cells following treatment. In a syngeneic murine model of HPV-positive HNSCC, Rag1 mice lacking functional T and B cells did not respond to cisplatin or radiation, suggesting that adaptive immunity is required for optimal responses to these standard therapies.[155] Other preclinical experiments suggest that cisplatin chemotherapy may increase tumor cell expression of antigen processing machinery components and of PD-L1, and additive antitumor activity was seen when cisplatin was paired with anti-PD-1/PD-L1 in a syngeneic mouse model of HNSCC.[156] Platinum chemotherapy drugs can also induce immunogenic cell death, leading to activation of DCs and enhanced adaptive immunity.[157–160]

Numerous studies have shown that checkpoint inhibitors can enhance the "abscopal" effect of radiation-induced cell death outside of the radiation field.[2,161,162] One observational clinical study showed increases in peripheral blood CD8+ T cells following radiation therapy in HNSCC patients,[163] further suggesting that checkpoint inhibitors may enhance the antitumor immune effects of radiotherapy in HNSCC patients.

Multiple clinical trials combining immunotherapy with standard therapies for HNSCC are underway or were recently completed. One of the most promising strategies involves the use of neoadjuvant ICB prior to surgical resection. These "window of opportunity" trials facilitate comparison of the immune microenvironment in tumor resection specimens to baseline biopsy specimens, offering mechanistic information and estimation of efficacy for novel therapies and combinations.[164] During the current era, when hundreds of novel therapies and combinations are under investigation, window-of-opportunity trials can help inform the design of larger studies.[164] Furthermore, preclinical studies suggest that immunotherapy induces more robust antigen-specific responses and may be most efficacious when delivered prior to surgery rather than afterward.[164,165] Response rates in trials of neoadjuvant ICB have so far been much higher than response rates in heavily pre-treated patients with recurrent/metastatic disease.[89,166] Three different Phase 2 studies have administered pembrolizumab or nivolumab in the neoadjuvant setting and along with postoperative chemoradiation in HNSCC with high-risk disease. Pathologic responses were >40%, with some patients demonstrating a complete pathologic response.[89,166,167] The potential for progressive disease while awaiting surgery, or of delayed surgery due to toxicity, are serious concerns about this approach. However, in the previously described studies, PD-1 blockade was well tolerated and did not usually delay the timing of surgery.[89,166,167] A Phase 3 study investing neoadjuvant and adjuvant pembrolizumab for patients with high-risk, resectable HNSCC (KEYNOTE-689) is currently underway.[168]

Another window-of-opportunity trial combined motolimod (TLR8 agonist) and cetuximab. Preclinical experiments showed that this combination can shift macrophages toward an antitumor M1 phenotype and inhibit the function of MDSCs.[169] In a Phase 1b study of 14 patients, neoadjuvant motolimod plus cetuximab decreased MDSCs, increased M1 macrophages and CD8+ T cells, and decreased coinhibitory checkpoint receptor expression.[169]

ICB has also been used in the adjuvant (postsurgical) setting for high-risk disease. A Phase 1 study showed that pembrolizumab can be safely given with adjuvant cisplatin chemoradiation for high-risk disease.[170] Another Phase 1 study will use durvalumab (anti-PD-L1) and tremelimumab (anti-CTLA-4) instead of cisplatin as systemic adjuvant therapy for intermediate-risk disease.[171] It appears likely that neoadjuvant and adjuvant ICB will soon become integrated into standard treatment regimens for patients with intermediate- or high-risk, surgically resectable HNSCC.

ICB has also been delivered successfully with definitive radiation and chemoradiation. For patients who are not eligible to receive standard cisplatin-based chemoradiation due to the substantial toxicities associated with cisplatin, durvalumab and pembrolizumab have been administered concurrently with radiation, with a favorable toxicity profile.[172,173] Another trial used a nivolumab and ipilimumab with concurrent radiation, which was also well tolerated.[174] Larger studies with long-term follow-up will be needed to compare the efficacy of these regimens to standard chemoradiation.

For patients with high-risk HNSCC who can tolerate cisplatin, ICB has been added to definitive chemoradiation regimens, with the intent of improving survival. One study adding pembrolizumab to radiation and weekly cisplatin showed reasonable safety and feasibility, with all patients receiving the intended 70 Gy dose of radiation and 85% receiving the goal cisplatin dose of ≥ 200 mg/m^2.[175] In RTOG 3504, nivolumab was added to four different regimens for patients with intermediate- or high-risk HNSCC: (a) weekly, low-dose cisplatin with radiation; (b) high-dose cisplatin given every 3 weeks with radiation; (c) cetuximab and radiation; and (d) radiation alone. Concomitant nivolumab was delivered safely with all regimens, but additional nivolumab following radiation was not feasible after high-dose cisplatin or in cisplatin-ineligible patients.[176] Two large randomized, placebo-controlled studies adding anti-PD-1/anti-PD-L1 therapy

to cisplatin-based chemoradiation for patients with high-risk disease are expected to provide further information on efficacy.[177,178]

Immunotherapy Combined With Targeted Therapy

Another treatment option under study is the addition of immunotherapy to targeted therapies with known activity in HNSCC. Studies using syngeneic murine models of HNSCC have shown that drugs antagonizing inhibitor of apoptosis proteins (IAPs) enhance multiple aspects of antitumor immunity, particularly when paired with radiation.[179,180] Furthermore, a window-of-opportunity study using the IAP antagonist Debio 1143 for HNSCC showed increased CD8+ T cells and PD-1/PD-L1 staining in surgical specimens.[181] Inhibitors of WEE1 kinase, which have antitumor activity in HNSCC,[182] have also been shown in preclinical studies to enhance multiple aspects of antitumor immunity. Similarly to IAP antagonists, the immunostimulatory effects of the WEE1 kinase inhibitor AZD1775 are further enhanced by radiation and/or ICB.[183,184] A MEK inhibitor also enhanced response to anti-PD-1 therapy in a syngeneic model of HNSCC, in part via increased PD-L1 and MHC class I expression.[185] PI3K inhibitors, which may inhibit MDSC function, are also under investigation alone or in combination with ICB in multiple trials for HNSCC.[142]

Biomarkers of Response to Immunotherapy in Head and Neck Squamous Cell Cancer

Several markers of response have been noted in trials of immunotherapy for HNSCC. As noted with other tumor types, HNSCC tumors with a higher tumor mutational burden (TMB) tend to respond better to checkpoint blockade. Smoking history, which correlates with a higher TMB, also correlates with improved responses to ICB in HNSCC.[186,187] In addition to overall TMB, mutations in *NOTCH1*, *SMARCA4*, and frameshift mutations in tumor suppressor genes also correlate with responses to anti-PD-1/PD-L1 therapy in HPV-negative HNSCC.[186]

As previously mentioned, patients treated with anti-PD-1 moAbs tend to respond better if their tumors have higher levels of PD-L1; for example, in the CheckMate 141 trial, response rates and survival were greater with PD-L1 expression greater than or equal to 1%.[188] In the KEYNOTE-012 trial, tumors that met a certain threshold score for PD-L1-positivity were associated with improved response rates when inflammatory cells were included in the scoring, but not when tumor cells alone were scored.[189] The combined positive score (CPS) established in the KEYNOTE-040 trial is now used to determine whether patients with recurrent/metastatic disease are likely to respond to anti-PD-1 therapy alone versus in combination with chemotherapy.

The degree of PD-1 expression on TILs may also be important. Kansy and colleagues evaluated PD-1 expression in HNSCC tumor specimens and found that although the proportion of PD-1⁺ TIL was higher in HPV-related tumors, TIL with very high surface levels of PD-1 were found primarily in HPV-negative tumors and predicted poor prognosis.[59] The PD-1-high TIL were less functional, as measured by IFN-γ production, and were depleted in a mouse model of HNSCC upon treatment with anti-PD-1 antibody.[59] These results suggest that high levels of PD-1 in TIL from HNSCC patients may have the opposite effect of high PD-L1 expression in tumor cells.

In addition to PD-1/PD-L1, the expression of other co-stimulatory and coinhibitory checkpoints may also predict immunotherapeutic responses. In a cohort of HNSCC patients treated with anti-PD-1/PD-L1 over 3 years, Hanna and colleagues used flow cytometry and sequencing data to show that TIM-3 and LAG-3 co-expression with PD-1 were higher on TIL from nonresponders.[186] Similarly, further analysis of data from the CheckMate 141 trial showed that responders to nivolumab demonstrated decreases in CTLA-4⁺ T cells and lower numbers of PD-1⁺ CD8⁺ T cells and PD-1⁺ T$_{reg}$ cells at baseline.[190]

As shown in other tumor types, interferon-related genes may also serve as biomarkers of response to immunotherapy in HNSCC. Prat and colleagues profiled the expression of gene expression signatures associated with CD8/CD4⁺ T cell activation, NK cell activity, and IFN activation in tumor samples from patients treated with anti-PD-1 therapy, including many with HNSCC, finding that these gene signatures were significantly associated with stable disease and PFS.[191] A gene expression profile (GEP) containing IFN-γ-related genes important for antigen presentation, adaptive immunity, and chemokine expression has also been created using baseline mRNA samples from patients with melanoma, HNSCC, and several other tumor types treated with pembrolizumab.[192] Most patients demonstrating either stable disease or a response to pembrolizumab had a high IFN-γ signature score, but a subset of patients with a high score had progressive disease. These results suggest that the expression of IFN-γ-related genes is necessary but not sufficient for a good response to pembrolizumab,[192] and additional biomarkers of response to anti-PD-1 therapy are still needed.

In HNSCC patients treated with cetuximab, increased intratumoral T$_{reg}$ cells and peripheral blood monocytic MDSCs may correlate with poor outcomes,[71,72] whereas a decrease in granulocytic MDSCs in the peripheral blood may correlate with favorable outcomes.[72] Despite the increasing data on efficacy and mechanisms of cetuximab and checkpoint inhibitors, only a subset of patients

respond to these drugs. Further studies are needed to better predict which HNSCC patients are most likely to benefit from specific forms of immunotherapy.

CONCLUSION

Immunotherapy for HNSCC has enormous potential, since this disease features a high genomic alteration rate and, in cases of HPV-related disease, the presence of viral antigens. Despite evasion of the immune system by these tumors, multiple forms of immunotherapy have shown promise for HNSCC. The use of immunotherapy in addition to, or instead of, surgery, radiation, and cytotoxic drugs represents the future of standard treatment for head and neck cancer.

KEY REFERENCES

Only key references appear in the print edition. The full reference list appears in the digital product on Springer Publishing Connect: connect.springerpub.com/content/book/978-0-8261-3743-2/part/part04/chapter/ch58

59. Kansy BA, Concha-Benavente F, Srivastava RM, et al. PD-1 status in CD8⁺ T cells associates with survival and anti-PD-1 therapeutic outcomes in head and neck cancer. *Cancer Res.* 2017;77(22):6353–6364. doi:10.1158/0008-5472.CAN-16-3167

76. Ferris RL, Blumenschein G, Jr, Fayette J, et al. Nivolumab for recurrent squamous-cell carcinoma of the head and neck. *N Engl J Med.* 2016;375(19):1856–1867. doi:10.1056/NEJMoa1602252

77. Cohen EEW, Soulières D, Le Tourneau C, et al. Pembrolizumab versus methotrexate, docetaxel, or cetuximab for recurrent or metastatic head-and-neck squamous cell carcinoma (KEYNOTE-040): a randomised, open-label, Phase 3 study. *Lancet.* 2019;393(10167):156–167. doi:10.1016/S0140-6736(18)31999-8

78. Chow LQM, Haddad R, Gupta S, et al. Antitumor activity of pembrolizumab in biomarker-unselected patients with recurrent and/or metastatic head and neck squamous cell carcinoma: results from the Phase Ib KEYNOTE-012 expansion cohort. *J Clin Oncol.* 2016;34(32):3838–3845. doi:10.1200/JCO.2016.68.1478

82. Ferris RL, Blumenschein G, Fayette J, et al. Nivolumab vs investigator's choice in recurrent or metastatic squamous cell carcinoma of the head and neck: 2-year long-term survival update of CheckMate 141 with analyses by tumor PD-L1 expression. *Oral Oncol.* 2018;81:45–51. doi:10.1016/j.oraloncology.2018.04.008

88. Burtness B, Harrington KJ, Greil R, et al. Pembrolizumab alone or with chemotherapy versus cetuximab with chemotherapy for recurrent or metastatic squamous cell carcinoma of the head and neck (KEYNOTE-048): a randomised, open-label, Phase 3 study. *Lancet.* 2019;394(10212):1915–1928. doi:10.1016/S0140-6736(19)32591-7

91. Siu LL, Even C, Mesía R, et al. Safety and efficacy of durvalumab with or without tremelimumab in patients with PD-L1-low/negative recurrent or metastatic HNSCC: the Phase 2 CONDOR randomized clinical trial. *JAMA Oncol.* 2019;5(2):195–203. doi:10.1001/jamaoncol.2018.4628

111. Giuliano AR, Palefsky JM, Goldstone S, et al. Efficacy of quadrivalent HPV vaccine against HPV infection and disease in males. *N Engl J Med.* 2011;364(5):401–411. doi:10.1056/NEJMoa0909537

Immunotherapy of Hematologic Malignancies: Lymphomas, Leukemias, and Myeloma

Adrian Bot, John M. Timmerman, and Patricia A. Young

KEY POINTS

- Hematologic malignancies have long been a proving ground for new immunotherapeutic modalities given their inherent susceptibility to immune attack and well-characterized cell surface targets.

- Blood cancers, especially certain types of leukemias and lymphomas, appear uniquely susceptible to one of the oldest and most profound forms of immunotherapy: allogeneic stem cell transplantation, which depends on the graft-versus-tumor immune response mediated by T and natural killer (NK) cells.

- Anti-CD20 antibodies, including the first monoclonal antibody approved for use in cancer (rituximab), revolutionized the treatment of B cell malignancies, providing major improvements in survival with little added toxicity.

- Antibody-dependent cellular cytotoxicity (ADCC), whereby antibody-coated target cells activate Fc receptors on NK cells, is the principal mechanism of action for most antibodies targeting cell surface differentiation antigens on lymphomas (e.g., CD20) and myelomas (e.g., CD38).

- Hodgkin lymphoma has the highest degree of responsiveness to programmed cell death-1 (PD-1) checkpoint blockade among all human cancers, with more than two-thirds of patients achieving durable remissions. Select non-Hodgkin lymphomas (NHLs) and multiple myeloma are also amenable to successful treatment with PD-1/programmed death ligand 1 (PD-L1) blockade.

- Chimeric antigen receptor (CAR) T cells targeting CD19 have provided robust proof of principle for the promise of CAR T cells and other adoptive T cell therapies for the treatment of cancer, resulting in five products approved to that in lymphomas, leukemias, and multiple myeloma,

and many in various stages of development (Box 59.1). With the majority of treated patients experiencing durable tumor regressions following a single treatment, albeit with significant toxicity risks, immense efforts are underway to bring this complex, personalized form of therapy to large numbers of blood cancer patients. Scaling efforts resulted in >5,000 patients treated, worldwide, with continuous improvement in the management of toxicities supporting an increasing footprint in an outpatient setting.

- Interferon alpha (IFN-α) has clinical activity against multiple hematologic cancers, including several forms of NHL, hairy cell leukemia, chronic myeloid leukemia, and multiple myeloma. New technologies to target IFN-α efficiently to tumors using antibody–IFN fusion proteins or small molecule inducers of IFN-α are being employed to improve their therapeutic index.

- The large number of immunotherapeutic agents with activity against blood cancers offers unprecedented opportunities to develop chemotherapy-free treatment combinatorial regimens for these cancers, and again lead the way toward novel treatment strategies for many cancer types.

IMMUNOTHERAPY OF HEMATOLOGIC MALIGNANCIES: UNIQUE OPPORTUNITIES AND CHALLENGES

Hematologic cancers, including lymphomas (Hodgkin and non-Hodgkin), leukemias (acute lymphoid, acute myeloid, and chronic lymphocytic), and plasma cell cancers (multiple myeloma and Waldenstrom's macro-globulinemia) hold a special place in the history of cancer immunotherapy development. As described in this chapter, they include diseases that can be cured in some instances by stem cell transplantation, were the first

BOX 59.1   FIVE T CELL THERAPY PRODUCTS APPROVED TO DATE: ALL IN B CELL MALIGNANCIES AND ALL TARGET CD19

August 30, 2017–Kymriah® (tisagenlecleucel) for the treatment of patients up to 25 years of age with **B cell precursor acute lymphoblastic leukemia (ALL)** that is refractory or in second or later relapse

October 18, 2017–Yescarta® (axicabtagene ciloleucel) for the treatment of adults with certain types of **relapsed or refractory large B cell lymphoma** after receiving two or more lines of systematic therapy

May 1, 2018–Kymriah® (tisagenlecleucel) for the treatment of adult patients with **relapsed or refractory (r/r) large B cell lymphoma** after two or more lines of systematic therapy

July 24, 2020–Tecartus® (X19) for **relapsed or refractory mantle cell lymphoma**

February 8, 2021–Breyanzi® (lisocabtagene maraleucel) **for adults with relapsed or refractory large B cell lymphoma (R/R LBCL)** after two or more lines of systematic therapy

April 14, 2021–Idecabtagene vicleucel (Abecma) for people with multiple myeloma that has not responded to or has returned after at least four different prior cancer treatments.

---

cancers successfully treated with monoclonal antibodies (B cell lymphomas), can routinely respond to adoptive cellular therapy with chimeric antigen receptor (CAR) T cells (CD19+ lymphomas and leukemias), and can be spectacularly sensitive to programmed cell death 1 (PD-1) blockade (Hodgkin lymphoma). Hematologic malignancies, *as cancers of immune cells themselves*, represent a unique setting and challenge to immunotherapy: we must turn the immune system "on itself" to fight malignant forms of leukocytes. In this lies the challenge to exploit antigenic, genetic, and phenotypic differences between normal and transformed cells, most often pitting effector and target cells of the same lymphoid lineage against each other. The difficulty of this task is further compounded by the fact that hematologic malignancies are not among the most immunogenic of cancers as measured by their mutational loads. In the landmark study of Lawrence et al., analyzing the numbers of mutations present in 27 different cancer types,[1] hematologic cancers rank ninth (diffuse large B cell lymphoma [DLBCL]), 15th (multiple myeloma), 19th (chronic lymphoid leukemia), and 24th (acute myeloid leukemia).

The earliest and arguably most potent form of immunotherapy for hematologic cancers is allogeneic stem cell transplantation, in which hematopoietic stem cells from a human leukocyte antigen (HLA)-matched donor (either peripheral blood stem cells or bone marrow) are transplanted into a cancer-bearing host after lymphodepleting chemotherapy or whole-body radiation, replacing the patient's own immune system with that of the incoming graft.[2] This drastic maneuver serves as a point of reference for adoptive cellular therapy, involving the polyclonal activation of donor-derived effector cells that, if all goes well, can recognize and attack the host's tumor cells to a greater degree than the host's normal tissues. Mechanisms of the hoped-for "graft-versus-tumor" effect include not only CD4+ and CD8+ T cells, but also natural killer (NK) cells if there exists a favorable mismatch in the killer inhibitory receptors (KIRs) between the host and donor marrow graft.[3] However, allogeneic stem cell transplantation remains an imperfect therapy due to the risk of graft-versus-host disease, a common and potentially life-threatening complication of transplantation in which leukocytes from the donor graft attack host tissues, with the most common manifestations being rash, colitis, hepatitis, and less often pulmonary and upper gastrointestinal toxicities. The prevention and treatment of this side effect involves the requirement for strong immune-suppressive medications, which carry the risk of serious and potentially fatal infectious complications in up to 20% of cases. Nonetheless, as allogeneic stem cell transplantation can truly cure some patients with chemotherapy-refractory leukemias and lymphomas, a major goal for the immunotherapy of blood cancers is to obtain this same level of success without having to perform a donor transplant that puts one at risk of graft-versus-host disease.

LYMPHOMAS AND LYMPHOID LEUKEMIAS

Lymphoid malignancies represent the largest class of hematologic cancers, and are highly heterogeneous in their histologic characteristics and clinical behavior. In the latest 2016 World Health Organization (WHO) classification system, they now include more than 40 types of mature B cell neoplasms (non-Hodgkin lymphoma [NHL], chronic lymphocytic leukemia [CLL], and plasma cell neoplasms), 28 forms of T and NK cell neoplasms, and five subtypes of Hodgkin lymphoma.[4] However, most immunotherapy studies focus on the common B cell NHL subtypes, such as DLBCL (the most common NHL), or slower-growing follicular lymphoma subtypes (second most common NHL), as B cell NHLs are about eightfold more common than T cell lymphomas or Hodgkin lymphomas. Indeed, DLBCL and follicular NHL differ substantially as immunotherapeutic targets, with follicular NHL characterized by infiltration with CD8+ T cells, the level of which correlates with patient survival,[5] and gene expression signatures characteristic of either activated T cells or macrophages, that correlate with favorable or unfavorable prognosis, respectively.[6] This may account for the tendency of follicular lymphoma to undergo partial spontaneous regression in some cases. In contrast, DLBCL has a much higher growth rate, reduced surface expression of HLA and adhesion molecules, and less T cell infiltration, and has lower responsiveness to immunotherapeutic modalities such as allogeneic transplantation, antibodies, and cytokines.[7] B cell acute lymphoblastic leukemia (B-ALL) is a more immature and rapidly growing acute leukemia that shares some features with NHL, including expression of the B cell differentiation antigen CD19.

Interferon and Cytokine Therapies for Hematologic Malignancies

Interferon Alpha

There is now ample evidence that type I interferons (IFN-α and IFN-β) play a significant role in anticancer immunity.[8] Type I IFNs are promising anticancer agents owing to their direct antiproliferative and proapoptotic effects,[9–11] blockade of autocrine growth factor loops,[12] repression of c-myc oncogene expression,[13] downregulation of telomerase activity,[14] inhibition of angiogenesis,[15] and induction of tumor necrosis factor-related apoptosis-inducing ligand (TRAIL)-mediated lymphoma cell apoptosis.[16] Furthermore, the favorable immunologic effects of IFN-α/β for lymphoma treatment include activation of T, NK, and dendritic cell (DC) functions, as well as upregulation of class I major histocompatibility complex (MHC) and CD20 molecules on the tumor cell surface.[17–19]

IFN-α has shown efficacy and achieved U.S. Food and Drug Administration (FDA) approval in a number of hematologic malignancies, including follicular NHL, chronic myelogenous leukemia (CML), and hairy cell leukemia (the latter exquisitely sensitive, with response rate of 86%), and modest but measurable activity against multiple myeloma and CLL.[20–22] IFN-α also has a significant activity in the initial treatment of follicular NHL in combination with an anthracycline-containing chemotherapy. This approval is based on a randomized study of 249 patients treated with chemotherapy with or without IFN-α2a that showed a prolonged time to treatment failure (2.4 vs. 1.6 years, $P = .008$) and a clinically but not statistically significant improvement in overall survival (OS) favoring the combination arm.[23] A second study in follicular NHL used chemotherapy with or without IFN-α2b (5 million IU subcutaneously three times weekly for 18 months). The combination group had a significantly longer progression-free survival (PFS; 2.9 vs. 1.5 years, $P = 0.0001$) and OS (not reached vs. 5.5 years, $P = 0.004$).[24] Thus, prolonged IFN-α appears to improve survival in follicular NHL after chemotherapy. As a single agent, IFN-α also has documented activity in relapsed NHL.

In a single-arm study of the chemotherapy-refractory B cell NHL, high-dose IFN-α (50×10^6 IU/m² three times a week for at least 3 months) showed objective response rates (ORRs) of 54% (13 of 24 subjects) in low-grade (including follicular) NHL, 33% (two of six subjects) in intermediate-grade NHL (including DLBCL), and 14% (one of seven subjects) in high-grade NHL.[25] However, the potential of IFN therapy is hindered by dose-limiting toxicities that include flu-like symptoms, fatigue, nausea/anorexia, neuropsychiatric symptoms, injection site reactions, hematologic effects, and the agent's short serum half-life.[22]

One strategy to overcome the systemic toxicity of IFN as well as to efficiently deliver it to the tumor bed is through the use of antibody–IFN fusion proteins.[26,27] Our group has previously reported the ability of anti-CD20 antibody-IFN-α and IFN-β fusion proteins to induce apoptosis and promote in vivo eradication of CD20-expressing mouse and human B cell lymphomas.[26–28] In further preclinical studies, we found that relative to the standard anti-CD20 antibody rituximab (described in the following), anti-CD20-IFN-α demonstrates superior antiproliferative activity, enhanced complement and cell-mediated cytotoxicity, and improved in vivo survival in human NHL xenograft models.[29] Based on these results, the anti-CD20–IFN-α fusion protein IGN002 is being evaluated in a first-in-human, Phase 1 clinical trial (NCT02519270) for CD20+ B cell NHL.[30] If this approach using antibody-targeted IFN is successful, it may be possible to better exploit the potent antitumor effects of IFN against hematologic and other cancers. In preclinical solid tumor models, Yang et al. have also recently found that antibody–IFN-α fusion proteins targeting epidermal growth factor receptor (EGFR) or Neu could have antitumor efficacy.[31]

Interleukin-2

Behind melanoma and renal cell carcinoma (RCC), B cell NHL has the third highest clinical response rate to high-dose interleukin-2 (IL-2). Among eight trials in relapsed NHL, the ORR was 17%, with responses of 26% in follicular and 16% in diffuse histologies.[32] Although these response rates are not high enough to be clinically useful, they do point to the immune responsiveness of certain B cell lymphomas. An anti-CD20-IL-2 immunocytokine (DI-Leu16-IL-2) studied in a Phase 1 clinical trial combined with low-dose rituximab showed an ORR of 31% among all dosing cohorts in B cell NHL.[33]

Interleukin-12

IL-12 is a potent activator of IFN-γ production by T and NK cells. In animal studies, it has shown remarkable antitumor activity,[34] yet in clinical testing in a Phase 2 study of IL-12 and rituximab with follicular lymphoma, patients treated concurrently with rituximab and IL-12 showed a lower response rate than when treated sequentially.[35] One potential explanation is that IL-12 exposure to freshly isolated human CD4+ T cells actually leads to T cell exhaustion by induction of T cell immunoglobulin and mucin domain-containing 3 (TIM-3) through an IFN-γ-independent manner.[36]

Interleukin-21

IL-21 may be an attractive immunotherapeutic candidate in B cell NHL, as it has a number of regulatory effects on NK, B, and T cells.[37] Specifically, in xenograft DLBCL tumors, IL-21 leads to tumor regression via STAT3 activation and upregulation of c-myc, promoting a decrease in anti-apoptotic protein expression of bcl-2 and bcl-XL, thereby triggering cell death.[38] A Phase 1 clinical trial of IL-21 in NHL using weekly bolus recombinant human interleukin-21 (rIL-21) plus rituximab was evaluated using a 1-week lead-in with rituximab. B cell lymphoma subtypes included small lymphocytic lymphoma/chronic lymphocytic leukemia (SLL/CLL; $n = 11$), follicular lymphoma ($n = 9$), or marginal zone lymphoma ($n = 1$). The maximum tolerated dose for rIL-21 was 100 µg/kg among 19 evaluable patients, and eight had clinical responses (42%).[39]

Antibody Therapy for Lymphomas: CD20 and Other Surface Targets

Custom-Made Antibodies Targeting Lymphoma Idiotype

Although Kohler and Milstein's 1975 description of monoclonal antibody generation got scientists immediately thinking about using the technology to fight cancer, it took years to demonstrate the promise of antibody therapy in humans. The first target was not a shared antigen, but in fact the tumor-specific surface immunoglobulin expressed by B cell lymphomas.[40] The *idiotype* is defined as the collection of unique antigenic determinants present in the variable regions of the clonal immunoglobulin heavy and light chains expressed by B cells or B cell malignancies. Freda Stevenson et al. were the first to demonstrate that lymphoma idiotype could serve as a therapeutic target, using polyclonal antibodies to treat a guinea pig lymphoma.[41] Levy et al. moved this principle forward into humans, using lymphoma-derived idiotypic immunoglobulin (Ig) to vaccinate mice to generate mouse antihuman idiotype monoclonal antibodies. This tailor-made treatment was a spectacular success in the very first patient treated, who was suffering from widespread chemotherapy-refractory follicular lymphoma, showing for the first time the powerful antitumor effects that could be derived from monoclonal antibodies.[42] This led to the founding of IDEC, Inc., whose goal was to commercialize anti-idiotype antibody therapy for

lymphomas. Over the next 12 years, 45 patients were treated with these custom-made antibodies, and objective tumor regressions were seen in 66% of cases, with 8% complete response (CR), and some patients actually cured, remaining tumor-free without other lymphoma therapies for many years.[43] Today it is not widely appreciated how very effective this therapy was, since it was abandoned by IDEC after proving to be prohibitively complex and expensive. In its place, it was decided to focus on the shared B cell antigen CD20, because it was highly expressed on the surface of most B cell lymphomas but not on normal tissues, and was not appreciably shed or internalized on antibody binding.

Rituximab: A Broadly Effective Anti-CD20 Antibody for B Cell Lymphomas

The variable regions of the mouse antihuman CD20 monoclonal antibody 2B8 were engineered to have human IgG1 and κ constant region sequences, yielding the chimeric antibody C2B8, which would eventually come to be known as rituximab. In Phase 1 dose-escalation trials, C2B8/rituximab was found to be effective against B cell lymphomas, especially those of the follicular subtype.[44] In the pivotal study of rituximab, a response rate of 48% was observed in the chemotherapy-refractory indolent lymphoma patients (60% in follicular cases), with response lasting on average a year or more, and with negligible side effects.[45] These data led to FDA approval of rituximab in November 1997, making it the first antibody therapy approved for the treatment of cancer. Importantly, prolonged depletion of normal peripheral blood B cells was noted, but without immediate decline in serum immunoglobulin levels. Rituximab was quick to revolutionize the therapy of B cell lymphomas, with more than half of the patients with indolent forms of NHL responding to a single-agent therapy. Though more aggressive forms of NHL (such as DLBCL or mantle cell lymphoma) responded less frequently (approximately 20%–40%) and for shorter durations, the anti-CD20 antibody could easily be combined with chemotherapies, as it did not affect blood counts in most cases. Within a decade, improved OS was shown in common types of NHL using combinations of rituximab with chemotherapy in indolent/follicular lymphomas,[46,47] and in DLBCL when combined with standard CHOP chemotherapy (cyclophosphamide, adriamycin, vincristine, and prednisone).[48,49]

Mechanisms of Action for Anti-CD20 Antibodies

Meanwhile, laboratory efforts were unraveling the mechanisms of action behind the remarkable effectiveness of rituximab. Studies in B cell lymphoma xenografts in mice lacking activating or inhibitory Fc receptors suggested that antibody-dependent cellular cytotoxicity

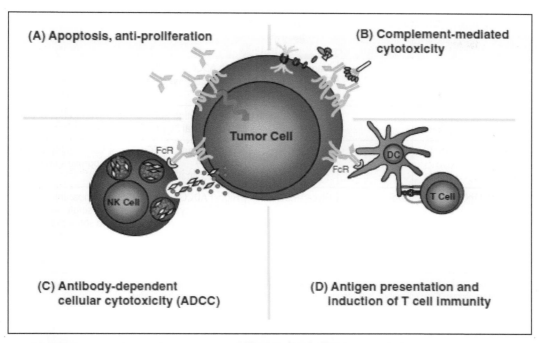

Figure 59.1 Potential mechanisms of action for anti-CD20 antibodies in lymphomas. (**A**) Direct growth inhibitory and proapoptotic effects can be demonstrated against some cell lines. (**B**) Complement-mediated cytotoxicity is elicited to varying degrees by different antibodies. (**C**) Antibody-dependent cellular cytotoxicity appears to be the dominant mechanism of action in vivo, mediated by Fc receptor-bearing NK cells and other phagocytes. (**D**) Antigen cross-presentation following uptake of antibody-coated cells into antigen-presenting dendritic cells, with subsequent stimulation of an adaptive T cell response is a proposed mechanism of action, but is likely inefficient.

DC, dendritic cell; NK, natural killer.

(ADCC) was a dominant in vivo mechanism of action for rituximab.[50] This hypothesis was corroborated not only by studies showing that rituximab could mediate potent ADCC in vitro against human lymphoma cells using peripheral blood-derived NK cells or monocytes, but also by studies of genetic polymorphisms in the Fcγ receptor IIIA gene (*FcγRIIIA*), which encodes CD16, the key receptor responsible for ADCC in human NK cells.[51,52] In subjects carrying *FcγRIIIA* alleles encoding receptors that bind more tightly to the Fc portion of the antibody, tumor responses were more frequent and longer lasting. Additional data have led to our modern view of the mechanism of action for anti-CD20 antibodies against lymphomas, in which ADCC plays the primary role, with direct growth-inhibitory/proapoptotic effects and complement-dependent cytotoxicity (CDC) playing lesser roles (Figure 59.1). This model has also provided a conceptual road map for how to make anti-CD20 antibodies more effective, by enhancing one or more of these effector mechanisms.[53]

Engineering Better Anti-CD20 Antibodies

Intensive efforts have been undertaken to reengineer antibodies with greater affinity binding to activating

Fc receptors, enhanced CDC, and improved proapoptotic effects against tumor cells on antigen binding at the tumor cell surface.[54] Ofatumumab is a fully human "second-generation" anti-CD20 monoclonal antibody having a different pattern of binding to the lymphoma cell surface, by way of the small loop of the CD20 molecule, in contrast to most other anti-CD20 antibodies that bind the large loop of the four-time membrane-spanning CD20 antigen. This antibody was found to have not only enhanced ADCC, but also markedly increased CDC, which unfortunately was found to be associated with more severe infusional toxicities. Efforts to generate antibodies not only with enhanced ADCC, but also with more potent direct cytotoxic effects via induction of apoptosis/programmed cell death, led to the development of the "third-generation" antibody GA-101 (now known as obinutuzumab). Obinutuzumab differs from other anti-CD20 antibodies in having an altered glycosylation structure low in fucose, which promotes higher-affinity interactions with activating receptors FcγRIIIA and IIA, promoting greater levels of ADCC. Obinutuzumab also differs in its CD20 binding characteristics by not recruiting lipid rafts, as seen with rituximab and ofatumumab ("type I" binding), but rather by inducing additional intracellular signaling events downstream from CD20

Table 59.1 Properties and Clinical Results of Approved Anti-CD20 Antibodies

ANTIBODY	FORMAT	GENERATION	MANUFACTURER	PROPERTIES	CLINICAL RESULTS
Rituximab (Rituxan)	Chimeric IgG1	1st	Biogen/IDEC, Genentech	High ADCC, high CDC, weak PCD ("type I")	First antibody approved to treat human cancer (1997); prolongs PFS and OS in all types of B cell NHL
Tositumomab (Bexxar)	Mouse IgG2a (approved for use as ^{131}I conjugate)	1st	GlaxoSmithKline	Low CDC, high PCD (prototypical "type II")	Potent efficacy against NHL, but impractical for routine clinical use
Ofatumumab (Arzerra)	Human IgG1	2nd	Genmab	High CDC and ADCC ("type I") Binds to small loop CD20	Comparable efficacy to rituximab; approvals now limited to CLL
Obinutuzumab (Gazyva)	Humanized IgG1	3rd	Glycart/Roche	Higher ADCC, high PCD, low CDC ("type II")	Comparable efficacy to rituximab as single agent; improved outcomes in some trials in combination with chemotherapy; CLL and FL, but not DLBCL Requires higher dosing

ADCC, antibody-dependent cellular cytotoxicity; CDC, complement-dependent cytotoxicity; CLL, chronic lymphocytic leukemia; DLBCL, diffuse large B cell lymphoma; FL, follicular lymphoma; Ig, immunoglobulin; NHL, non-Hodgkin lymphoma; OS, overall survival; PCD, programmed cell death induction; PFS, progression-free survival.

ligation that favor caspase-independent target cell death at the expense of less CDC ("type II" binding).[55,56] The characteristics of these approved anti-CD20 antibodies are summarized in Table 59.1.

Clinical Results With Newer Generation Anti-CD20 Antibodies of Atumumab and Obinutuzumab

Despite the tremendous efforts expended to reengineer anti-CD20 antibodies for greater efficacy, it has been difficult to show that these antibodies consistently improve outcomes in B cell lymphomas and CLL. Although ofatumumab has received regulatory approval for use in CLL for a 58% response rate in fludarabine-refractory disease,[57] and for superior outcomes compared with the oral alkylating agent chlorambucil in fludarabine-ineligible patients, it has never been shown to be superior to rituximab in the treatment of common B cell NHL.[58] Obinutuzumab, in contrast, has been extensively compared with rituximab, and has been found to have measurable advantages in some settings.[59] In Phase 1/2 testing of a single-agent obinutuzumab in indolent NHL, it was found that higher doses were required to achieve optimal antilymphoma activity.[60] Repeated dosing with 400 mg yielded only a 17% ORR (no CRs) and a 6-month median PFS, while dosing with 800 to 1,600 mg achieved an ORR of 55% (9% complete responders) and median 11.9-month PFS. These data showed that higher doses of obinutuzumab are required to achieve the same level of efficacy generally seen with rituximab dosed at the traditional 375 mg/m² dose. Obinutuzimab was then tested head-to-head in a prospective, randomized study comparing four weekly doses of obinutuzumab 1,000 mg/m² with rituximab

375 mg/m² (followed by maintenance doses every 2 months for 2 years) in relapsed, rituximab-sensitive indolent lymphoma, with the endpoints of ORR and PFS. Somewhat surprisingly, although patients with follicular lymphoma seemed to have a higher ORR with obinutuzumab compared with rituximab (44.6% vs. 26.7%; $P = 0.01$), there was no difference in PFS between the two arms, and thus the new glycoengineered antibody failed to show superiority over rituximab in this antibody-only setting.[61]

Subsequently, it has taken several very large randomized trials to sort out the relative clinical efficacy of obinutuzumab versus rituximab. The first study to show an advantage of rituximab was in previously untreated older adult patients with CLL who were too fragile to receive aggressive chemotherapy.[62] Subjects received mild oral alkylating agent chemotherapy with chlorambucil with either high-dose obinutuzumab (1,000 mg/m²) or standard-dose rituximab at 375 mg/m². Outcomes were superior in the obinutuzumab versus rituximab arms in terms of both response rates (78.4% vs. 65.1%) and PFS (26.7 vs. 15.2 months). This study has been criticized for using much higher doses of obinutuzumab than rituximab, since earlier data in CLL had shown that higher doses of rituximab (500–2,250 mg/m²) might also have greater efficacy.[63] Nonetheless, this randomized study did show a significant advantage to the newer generation antibody at the doses used, despite the remaining question of whether obinutuzumab is truly more potent than rituximab against CLL. A study in front-line treatment of follicular lymphoma recently showed a similar result. This large study of 1,202 patients compared obinutuzumab (1,000 mg/m²) plus chemotherapy with rituximab (375 mg/m²) plus chemotherapy, with maintenance doses of antibody given every 2 months for 2 years. A modest advantage of obinutuzumab was seen in terms of a 3-year PFS (80.0% vs. 73.3%), but there was no difference in the OS during the 4-year follow-up period.[64]

In contrast, obinutuzumab (Gazyva) combined with CHOP chemotherapy (G-CHOP) had no advantage over standard R-CHOP in a large randomized study of DLBCL, in terms of either PFS or OS.[65] Thus, while incremental efficacy advances have been made in the engineering of anti-CD20 antibodies for treating lymphoma, these have been relatively modest, and limited to specific disease settings and chemotherapy combinations. Can the efficacy of anti-CD20 antibodies be further improved? Perhaps, but after more than 20 years of research it has been difficult to show that any new anti-CD20 antibodies are significantly more potent than the original rituximab antibody. It may be that we have reached a plateau in the efficacy of these antibodies and that further advances will come from learning how best to combine these agents with other immunotherapeutic and targeted agents. It remains to be determined how much newer generation anti-CD20 antibodies improve outcomes in lymphoid malignancies when combined with such agents.

Antibodies Against Other Cell Surface Targets in Lymphomas

Monoclonal antibodies against a host of other B cell surface antigens have been studied since the original success of rituximab, including those targeting CD19, CD22, CD23, CD30, CD40, CD52, CD74, CD80, and others.[58] However, none has convincingly achieved or surpassed the clinical efficacy of anti-CD20 antibodies.[66]

Vaccines

The most advanced research efforts for vaccine therapies in hematologic malignancies have focused on tumor-specific idiotype vaccines for B cell lymphomas.[40] Despite early evidence of antilymphoma activity in single-center studies using patient-specific idiotype-KLH conjugate vaccines formulated with adjuvants including granulocyte-macrophage colony-stimulating factor (GM-CSF)[67] or DCs,[68] two of three large industry-sponsored Phase 3 randomized trials of Id-KLH vaccines in follicular lymphoma failed to show clinical benefits versus controls,[69,70] and the third showed only a modest benefit in PFS in the subset of patients with IgM+ tumors.[71] However, there is evidence that the chemical conjugation technique used in the manufacturing of these vaccines may have impaired the immunogenicity and efficacy of these vaccines.[72] The approach was thus abandoned due to the availability of newer immunotherapies, such as anti-CD20 antibodies.

Bispecific Antibodies for Lymphoid Malignancies: Bridging Tumor Cells to Effector Cells

Another approach to harness the immune system that is now showing promise in a variety of hematologic malignancies is the use of bispecific antibodies. Bispecific antibodies have antigen-binding domains of two different antibodies, one directed to a cell surface target and the other most often to CD3, in order to cross-link the CD3 complex on adjacent T cells, thereby leading to the killing of target cells.[66] However, challenges in bispecific-antibody constructs have included a short serum half-life, immunogenicity, and difficulty in large-scale production.[73]

Blinatumomab, the first FDA-approved bispecific antibody, is a first-in-class "bispecific T cell engager" (BiTE) made up of two single-chain variable fragments (scFvs), one targeting CD19 and another targeting CD3. Because the low molecular weight results in a 2-hour half-life, dosing is critical for clinical activity. Initial trials of blinatumomab in CLL and NHL, given as 2- to 4-hour infusions three times a week, consequently showed no objective responses.[74] Yet when given by continuous intravenous infusion in a trial of NHL patients, the increased drug exposure led to the elimination of target cells in the blood at very low doses (0.005 mg/m²/day).[75] Phase 1 clinical trial results of blinatumomab in relapsed/refractory NHL showed an ORR of 69%.[76]

In ALL, blinatumomab has achieved complete minimal residual disease (MRD) responses across multiple patient settings, including a second-line treatment and in heavy MRD burden. In the Phase 2 trial of blinotumomab in patients with persistent or relapsed MRD ALL patients, among 20 evaluable patients, 80% achieved MRD negativity within four cycles of treatment.[77] In a separate Phase 2 study among 189 relapsed/refractory ALL patients, 43% achieved CR or CR with partial haematological recovery of peripheral blood counts (CRh) after two cycles of blinatumumab. Among these patients, 40% were bridged to the only curative immunotherapeutic strategy yet known, allogeneic stem cell transplant.[78] Bispecific antibodies have therefore shown efficacy even in patients with negative prognostic features, but their roles in the treatment paradigm have yet to be determined.[79] Other platforms of bispecific antibodies include the dual-affinity retargeting antibodies (DARTs), tetravalent chimeric antibody construct (TandAb), and trispecific antibodies, which can potentially overcome the challenge of short serum half-life.[73] In a study of REGN1979, an anti-CD20 × anti-CD3 bispecific full-length antibody, in NHL and CLL patients, an ORR of 27% was seen at the two highest dose levels, with the added benefit of more convenient dosing (weekly) compared with continuous infusion.[80] Similarly, in refractory

Hodgkin lymphoma, the TandAb bispecific anti-CD30/CD16A antibody (AFM13) recruits NK cells via binding to CD16A on immune effector cells with a longer half-life of 19 hours. Among 13 patients treated at doses of greater than or equal to 1.5 mg/kg of AFM13, the ORR was 23%.[81]

Checkpoint Inhibitor Therapies for Lymphomas

Ipilimumab and Nivolumab

As checkpoint inhibitor antibodies were becoming available in the early 2000s, there were several reasons to believe that lymphomas might be responsive to these immunostimulatory agents. First, they can be infiltrated with T cells having a memory phenotype, the presence of which correlates with improved survival, suggesting the host's attempt at an antitumor immune response.[82] Second, as mentioned earlier, the common follicular subtype of NHL is prone to spontaneous waxing and waning felt to be immune-mediated.[83] Third, lymphomas can undergo regression in response to tumor-antigen vaccines.[68] Fourth, B cell lymphomas respond well to monoclonal antibodies targeting tumor idiotype or CD20.[40] Furthermore, as the first reports of therapeutic anticytotoxic T lymphocyte–associated protein 4 (CTLA-4) antibodies began to appear,[84] it was becoming known that populations of T cells infiltrating B cell NHL could have the phenotype of regulatory T cells (T_{reg} cells) and express CTLA-4.[85] These findings led us to test the new anti-CTLA-4 antibody ipilimumab in subjects with relapsed and refractory B cell NHL.[86] Eighteen patients were treated with four monthly doses of ipilimumab at 1 or 3 mg/kg, and treatment was well tolerated, with some manageable mild autoimmune side effects in a minority of subjects. Two tumor regressions were observed; one subject with follicular lymphoma had a partial response lasting 19 months, and a subject with DLBCL had a CR lasting more than 31 months (ongoing at greater than 7 years, S. Ansell, 2016, personal communication). Janik and colleagues also observed regression of follicular and mantle cell lymphoma in two of four patients who received ipilimumab when their tumors relapsed following idiotype vaccination.[87] While the number of responders was low in these studies, they demonstrated the proof-of-principle that lymphomas could respond to single-agent checkpoint inhibitor therapy.

With growing recognition of the importance of the PD-1/PD-L1 axis in mediating tumor immune evasion, investigators sought to explore the expression pattern of PD-1 ligands in hematologic malignancies. Early observations showed that myeloma cells could express low levels of PD-L1, which could be upregulated by exposure to inflammatory stimuli such as IFN-γ or Toll-like receptor (TLR) ligands.[88] More striking were the seminal observations of Yamamoto et al., who found that the malignant Reed-Sternberg cells of Hodgkin lymphoma expressed very high levels of PD-L1 that were functional in suppressing PD-1+ tumor-infiltrating T cells.[89] Shipp et al. then discovered that this exaggerated PD-L1 expression in Hodgkin lymphoma was explained by amplification of the 9p24.1 chromosomal locus, which contains not only PD-L1 and its homolog PD-L2, but also the *JAK2* gene, and that the locus copy number was correlated with the level of cell surface protein expression by immunohistochemistry.[90] PD-L1 expression was then also documented in many other cases of T cell[91] and B cell NHL.[92] In B cell NHL, PD-L1 expression on tumor cells was largely limited to a minor subset of the "activated B cell" DLBCL tumors, whereas expression on tumor-infiltrating macrophages could be found in most DLBCL cases. Importantly, PD-L1 expression was functional in suppressing the proliferation of autologous tumor-associated T cells, and this suppression could be reversed by blocking PD-1/PD-L1 interactions. Several other types of B cell NHL, including mantle cell, marginal zone, and small lymphocytic, did not have significant PD-L1 expression. The pattern of PD-L1 expression in follicular lymphoma was unique, with tumor cells in the malignant follicles largely devoid of PD-L1, but with macrophages scattered between the follicles expressing PD-L1, where they interacted with PD-1+ T cells.[92,93] Further studies confirmed that PD-L1 expression in B cell NHL was limited to selected additional less common subtypes, including primary mediastinal large B cell, T cell/histiocyte-rich, plasmablastic, Epstein–Barr virus (EBV)-associated, and human herpesvirus 8 (HHV8)-associated primary effusion lymphomas, where PD-L1 was highly expressed by malignant cells and tumor-infiltrating macrophages.[94] Together, these data provided strong rationale for testing PD-1 blockade in lymphoid malignancies.

In line with the earlier preclinical data, the first trial of PD-1 blockade (nivolumab) in hematologic malignancies (BMS CA209-039) included a total of 104 patients with B cell and T cell NHL, multiple myeloma, and Hodgkin lymphoma, who were refractory to numerous prior therapies.[95] Subjects were treated with the standard nivolumab regimen of 3 mg/kg every 2 weeks. Treatment was generally well tolerated, but 21% of subjects had significant (grade 3 or higher) toxicities. The pattern of autoimmune-like symptoms were similar to that observed in previous nivolumab trials in other cancers, and included rash, colitis, pneumonitis, hepatitis, and thyroid or kidney disorders, but only 14% required the discontinuation of treatment. Among the 31 subjects with B cell NHL, the most common histologic subtypes were represented. Objective tumor responses were seen in 4 of 11 DLBCL (36%) and 4 of 10 follicular (40%) patients, with durable responses more common in the latter. There were no responses seen in the B cell NHL with other histologies ($n = 10$, including mantle cell, primary mediastinal, small lymphocytic, and marginal zone lymphomas), though more than half had initial disease stabilization. Within the T cell NHL cohort ($n = 23$), only four subjects (17%) with mycosis fungoides or peripheral T cell lymphoma responded, but several of these responses were durable. Notably, none of the 27 multiple myeloma patients had an objective response during nivolumab therapy, though intriguingly, one patient did have normalization of serum paraprotein following radiation therapy to a solitary plasmacytoma, suggesting a possible abscopal effect.

However, the biggest story to arise from the Phase 1 experience of PD-1 blockade in hematologic cancers was the spectacular responsiveness of Hodgkin lymphoma.[96] In this cohort of 23 chemotherapy-refractory patients, 78% had received earlier autologous stem cell transplantation and brentuximab vedotin (anti-CD30-toxin conjugate). Remarkably, 100% of patients had some reduction of their tumors, with 87% meeting criteria for partial (70%) or CR (17%). Responses occurred rapidly, with many patients experiencing relief of tumor-related symptoms within days, and most achieving objective responses within 2 months. In correlative biomarker studies, it was found that the malignant Reed-Sternberg cells in 10 of 10 cases analyzed were positive for the 9p24.1 amplification, and for PD-L1 expression by immunohistochemistry. These data prompted a Phase 2 registration trial of nivolumab in Hodgkin lymphoma relapsing or progressing after both autologous stem cell transplantation and post-transplant brentuximab vedotin.[97] Thus, this population represented patients with the greatest unmet medical need, whose disease had resisted all standard therapies. In this study of 80 patients, the side effect profile was similar to the Phase 1 experience. The ORR was 72.5% (27.5% complete, 45% partial), and the median PFS was 10 months. More favorable outcome was correlated with the degree of 9p24.1 locus amplification and PD-L1 protein expression, with patients achieving CRs having the highest 9p24.1 copy number and PD-L1 staining. Based on these data, nivolumab was approved by the FDA in May 2016 for treatment of Hodgkin lymphoma recurring after autologous stem cell transplantation and brentuximab vedotin.

Given the earlier studies, additional trials of single-agent nivolumab in lymphomas include Phase 2 trials in relapsed and refractory DLBCL and follicular NHL. New checkpoint inhibitor combinations are also being explored in cohorts on the CA209-039 trial, including combined nivolumab plus ipilimumab, and nivolumab plus lirilumab (an NK cell-activating antibody against KIRs).

Pembrolizumab

The anti-PD-1 antibody pembrolizumab is a humanized IgG4 monoclonal antibody that has also undergone testing in lymphomas, and has achieved excellent results against Hodgkin lymphoma relapsing after brentuximab vedotin failure.[98] Thirty-one patients with relapsed, chemotherapy-refractory Hodgkin lymphoma were treated with pembrolizumab 10 mg/kg every 2 weeks until disease progression. A typical pattern of autoimmune side effects associated with PD-1 blockade was seen, but with just 14% of subjects having grade 3 or higher toxicities, including colitis, infusion reactions, pneumonitis, hepatitis, or thyroid or kidney dysfunction. The ORR was 65%, with 16% CR, and 48% PR, with a median PFS of approximately 1 year. Overall, the pattern of responses was very similar to the results achieved with nivolumab, as expected given the similar efficacy of these antibodies against other cancers. Additional studies of pembrolizumab are underway in B cell NHL and other hematologic malignancies.

Pidilizumab (CT-011)

Pidilizumab is a humanized IgG1 antibody reported to be a PD-1 antagonist. Based on preclinical studies in mice, it was first tested in a Phase 1 trial in patients with hematologic cancers (B cell NHL, Hodgkin lymphoma, CLL, and myeloma). Some clinical activity was seen, with one CR in follicular lymphoma, and stable disease in Hodgkin lymphoma and CLL.[99] It was next applied in 66 DLBCL patients following high-dose chemotherapy and autologous stem cell transplantation, with the goal of stimulating immunity to eliminate MRD.[100] Of the 35 patients with residual tumor after transplant, 34% went on to achieve CR, thus showing apparent clinical activity in this setting. Pidilizumab has also been combined with rituximab in a single-arm study of 32 patients with rituximab-sensitive follicular lymphoma.[101] Unlike studies with nivolumab and pembrolizumab, no grade 3 or higher autoimmune toxicities were seen. Although the observed ORR of 66% would not be unexpected with rituximab, a high CR rate of 52% was achieved, and T cell activation in the peripheral blood correlated with prolonged PFS. Although these trials do appear to show beneficial effects of the antibody in lymphomas, the pattern of tumor responses and lack of traditional PD-1 blockade-associated autoimmune toxicities has raised the question as to whether pidilizumab is actually a PD-1 antagonist. In this light, it is notable that the antibody, originally designated BAT, was generated by immunizing mice with membranes from Daudi B cell lymphoma cells,[102] yet Daudi lymphoma cells have been shown to be PD-1-negative.[92] Thus, the precise target of and mechanism of action for pidilizumab in lymphoma remain unclear.

Summary of Checkpoint Inhibitors in Hematologic Malignancies

As in all areas of oncology now, explorations into the use of checkpoint inhibitor antibodies have exploded in hematologic malignancies. More than 100 trials are underway using the PD-1 inhibitors nivolumab and pembrolizumab, the PD-L1 inhibitors durvalumab and atezolizumab, and other checkpoint inhibitors, in virtually all forms of blood cancer. They are being combined with a broad array of other agents, including other immunomodulatory antibodies targeting CTLA-4, LAG-3, or 4-1BB, antitumor antibodies (targeting CD20, CD38, and others), adoptive T cell therapies, immunomodulatory drugs (IMiDs), antibody-drug conjugates, kinase inhibitors, TLR agonists, DNA methylation inhibitors, indoleamine 2,3-dioxygenase (IDO) inhibitors, and tumor-antigen vaccines. With little human data available, they are even being combined with conventional cytotoxic chemotherapies, which may blunt the effector cells believed to be responsible for the action of checkpoint blockade. With tests of so many combinations underway, it will take years before optimal combinations become apparent, but patient outcomes are sure to improve following these diverse efforts.

Adoptive Cellular Therapy and Chimeric Antigen Receptor T Cells

Adoptive cell transfer entails treatment of patients with cell populations expanded ex vivo and reinfused to patients in order to traffic to tumor sites and mediate tumor cell killing. The rationale for adoptive T cell therapy is that naturally occurring tumor-infiltrating lymphocytes (TILs) are unable to exert their maximum in vivo potential because of the immunosuppressive influences within the tumor microenvironment. This leads to T cell expression of negative regulatory molecules, such as TIM-3, LAG-3, PD-1, and CTLA-4, that prevent optimal T cell function.[103,104] Expanding and activating T cells ex vivo may have the potential to preserve their tumor-killing capacity.

Transformative studies showed that adoptive transfer of TILs may afford durable immunity in malignant melanoma, leading to potential functional cures.[105] This seminal observation was followed by similarly critical findings utilizing genetically engineered TCR T cells in melanoma and synovial cell sarcoma,[106] and a number of independent observations using CAR-engineered T cells showing durability of clinical responses, in B cell malignancies, approaching or exceeding 10 years.[107] This prompted an unprecedented effort in research and development in this area; during an interval of only several years (2017–2021), research led to four breakthrough approvals for anti-CD19 T cell products covering diverse histologies such as relapsing/remitting DLBCL, pediatric B-ALL, and mantle cell lymphoma (Figure 59.1).[108–111] These products have a feature in common—they all target CD19; nevertheless, they are different in regards to the manufacturing process and CAR molecules design, potentially imparting differences in efficacy and safety profile.

In the text that follows, we are providing some additional specifics regarding research and development of such products for hematologic malignancies where several types of adoptive cell transfer therapy have been pioneered, including T cells recognizing viral antigens, minor histocompatibility antigens, or tumor-associated antigens in an MHC-restricted fashion, and, most recently, CAR T cells that recognize cell surface antigens in a non-MHC-restricted manner.[112]

Investigators at Baylor College of Medicine have carefully developed techniques for expanding EBV-specific cytotoxic T cells, using these cells to achieve remissions in EBV+ posttransplant lymphoproliferative disorders.[112] More recently, they have achieved impressive results in subjects with multiple-relapsed B cell NHL, with 62% responders, including 52% CRs.[113] In addition to using T cells expressing a native T cell receptor (TCR), tumor antigen-specific T cells can be generated by transfection of genes encoding a cloned TCR into host T cells. An example of this approach uses a NY-ESO-1 antigen-specific TCR to target multiple myeloma.[114] In a Phase 1/2 trial, 20 patients with advanced relapsed myeloma were treated. Clinical responses were seen in 16 of 20 patients (80%), with a median PFS of 19.1 months. However, disease recurrence was associated with a loss of T cell persistence or a loss of NY-ESO-1 expression.

Adoptive T cell therapy has grown rapidly owing to CAR T cell technology. CARs have an antigen-recognition moiety and a T cell activation domain that can be inserted into host T cells via retroviral or lentiviral transduction. This redirects the specificity of the T cell for a tumor-associated antigen. In the case of B cell malignancies, anti-CD19 CAR T cells are the most widely studied, with objective tumor responses and tolerable toxicities reported thus far.[103,115–117]

Chimeric Antigen Receptor Constructs and Treatment Procedures

The extracellular portion of the CAR is composed of the antigen-recognition domain, derived from the antigen-binding fragment (Fab) of monoclonal antibodies (mAbs), usually as a scFv fused to the transmembrane domain and the intracellular T cell signaling domain. The hinge region allows for flexibility and improved engagement of the CAR to its antigen. First-generation CARs linked the scFv to the intracellular signaling domain of the TCR, typically the CD3ζ chain. Initial studies using first-generation CAR were disappointing owing to lack of CAR T cell persistence.[118,119] Second-generation CARs were developed with the addition of a co-stimulatory domain (CD28, 4-1BB, DAP10, OX40, or ICOS), thereby amplifying the T cell response, inducing T cell proliferation and achieving CAR T cell persistence.[120–124] There are a number of second-generation CAR T cells under development with published results of efficacy in ALL, CLL, and

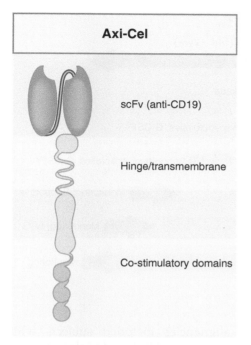

Figure 59.2 Typical structure of a CAR T cell construct using Axi-cel as an example.

NHL.[73] A typical structure of a CAR construct is depicted in Figure 59.2, exemplified through Axi-cel.[125] They correspond to the first wave of CAR T cell products that entered the standard of care in several B cell malignancies. Third-generation CARs use two co-stimulatory domains with the hope that this will direct even greater T cell potency.[126–128]

The history of research and development of anti-CD19 CAR T cells is widely described in several landmark reviews.[129–131] Various anti-CD19 CAR T cells have been constructed and tested in the clinical setting. At the U.S. National Cancer Institute (NCI), the anti-CD19 CAR construct consists of the variable region of the anti-CD19 mAb fused to the CD28 co-stimulatory molecule, plus the signaling domain of CD3ζ.[123,132] At the University of Pennsylvania, June et al. reported on the use of anti-CD19 CAR T cells in CLL patients using a CAR construct containing CD137 (4-1BB) and CD3ζ.[133] Lymphodepletion chemotherapy typically precedes CAR infusion and is thought to improve efficacy and persistence by (a) creating space for CAR T cells and reducing the competition for T cell homeostatic cytokines;[134] (b) removing competition of surface antigen-presenting cells (APCs);[135,136] and (c) removing the immunosuppressive effects of regulatory T cells (T_{reg} cells).[137]

Adverse Effects of Chimeric Antigen Receptor T Cell Therapy Including Cytokine Release Syndrome

Accumulating evidence, during the last decade or so, informed on CAR T cell treatment-related toxicities, particularly in the context of CD19 targeting in B cell malignancies. While six categories of adverse events (AEs) have been described mechanistically (Figure 59.3), much attention has been dedicated to the inflammatory ones occurring during the acute window post CAR T cell infusion, namely "cytokine release syndrome," or CRS, and neurotoxicity (ICANs).[138] Following infusion, CAR T cells rapidly proliferate in the host, and on contact with cells bearing the target antigen, they secrete large quantities of cytokines (including IL-6, TNF-α, and IFN-γ) that can result in CRS.[139,140] This AE can be severe in one-quarter to one-third of subjects, and even become life-threatening. This condition correlates with a number of factors related to CAR structure, tumor type and burden, and genetic polymorphisms.[141] Manifestations of CRS include fevers, malaise, myalgias, hypotension, and, in severe cases, hypoxemia, renal insufficiency, and multiorgan failure. A related but less common side effect is acute neurotoxicity, with delirium, aphasia, and motor disturbances, although this typically resolves completely within 1 to 3 weeks with supportive care. The severity of CRS appears to correlate with tumor burden, due to larger numbers of CD19+ tumor cells promoting higher-level cytokine secretion once the CAR is ligated after encountering its target antigen. CRS can be successfully managed in most cases using the anti-IL-6 receptor antagonist antibody tocilizumab, corticosteroids, and advanced supportive care. Fatalities in CAR T cell trials have highlighted the potential dangers of this therapy, noting increased rates of severe and fatal CRS and neurotoxicity with the use of higher cell doses, greater tumor burden in the host, and perhaps certain vector constructs. However, it is believed that with the lower doses of CAR T cells in current trials, safety and efficacy are appropriately balanced.

Correlative analysis in the context of clinical studies, complemented by interventional studies in the clinical and preclinical setting, established the mainstay of toxicities management based currently of IL-6R blockade for CRS and corticosteroids for ICANs. Continuous optimization of regimens based on these agents, coupled with earlier and measured introduction of corticosteroids, resulted in gradual decrease of grade 3+ inflammatory AEs toward single-digit percentages. Nevertheless, to maximize the footprint of this therapeutic modality, more progress is needed, so as to pre-empt acute toxicities in a majority of subjects and/or predict more accurately who can be reliably treated in an outpatient setting. To that aim, elucidation of pathogenesis of these two categories of toxicities is of paramount importance. The evidence to date suggests interaction of pretreatment and product-related factors in determining these toxicities, with differences between CRS and ICANs as reflected in Figure 59.4A and B. Excess CAR T cell activity, expansion, accompanied by myeloid cell mobilization, seems to be

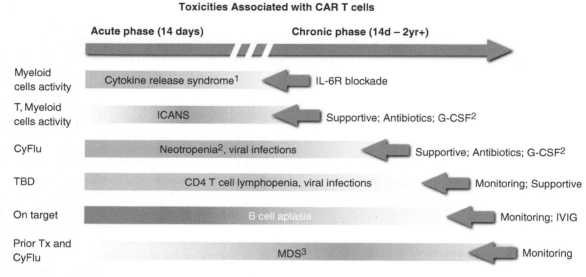

Figure 59.3 Categories of adverse events associated with CAR T cell intervention.

key to pathogenesis of ICANs, while systemic activation of the reticuloendothelial system mediated by IL-6/IL-6R axis is key in triggering CRS. Common to both categories of toxicities seems to be vascular endothelial damage, likely of an inflammatory nature. Strikingly, subjects with preexisting disease-related inflammation could be more prone to developing CAR T cell treatment-related AEs. The two major directions to optimize the CAR T cell treatment safety profile consist in prophylactic use of targeted agents[142] and optimization of product performance through CAR construct modification, signaling modulation, or changes in manufacturing, other product attributes.

Anti-CD19 Chimeric Antigen Receptor T Cells in Non-Hodgkin Lymphoma

CAR T cells have been studied in various hematologic malignancies, including NHL, ALL, and CLL, and those furthest in development are summarized in Table 59.2.[115,116,143–159] The first patient treated at the NCI using anti-CD19 CAR T cells had follicular lymphoma with progressive disease despite several lines of therapy. After a lymphocyte-depleting regimen of cyclophosphamide and fludarabine, this patient received anti-CD19 CAR T cells and had dramatic regression of his lymphoma. Also noted was eradication of B-lineage precursors and resultant hypogammaglobulinemia, but without infectious complications.[160]

In studies using the CD28 co-stimulatory domain, Kochenderfer et al. reported using the lymphodepleting agents fludarabine and cyclophosphamide followed by anti-CD19 CAR T cell infusion and a course of IL-2,[145] with tumor regressions noted in subjects with indolent NHL or CLL. A later study of 15 patients with advanced

B cell malignancies included subjects with aggressive NHL, including DLBCL, indolent NHL, and CLL. Four of seven evaluable patients with chemotherapy-refractory DLBCL achieved CR with durations ranging from 9 to 22 months, and two patients achieved PR. Substantial acute toxicities included hypotension (four of 15 patients), fever (12 of 15 patients), and neurotoxicity (six of 15 patients) including confusion, obtundation, or aphasia. Two patients received the IL-6 receptor antagonist tocilizumab and all toxicities were reversible within 3 weeks of CAR T cell infusion.[115] Additional results with a shorter 3-day lymphodepleting chemotherapy regimen continued to yield excellent responses in NHL; among 19 patients with various subtypes of DLBCL, there were eight CR (42%) and five PR (26%), while three patients with mantle cell or follicular lymphoma also attained CRs.[147]

Using CAR T constructs containing the 4-1BB co-stimulatory domain, Schuster et al. treated 38 patients (21 DLBCL, 14 follicular, and 3 mantle cell lymphoma), after a variety of lymphodepleting chemotherapy regimens.[149] Among 22 evaluable patients, the oRR was 54% in DLBCL (seven of 13), 100% in follicular lymphoma (seven of seven), and 50% in mantle cell lymphoma (one of two). CRS occurred in 16 patients, and its presence did not predict response. Investigators at the Fred Hutchison Cancer Research Center (FHCRC) and Juno Therapeutics have also used CAR constructs featuring the 4-1BB co-stimulatory domain.[144] This study included 32 subjects with various NHLs using a defined ratio of CD8+ and CD4+ CD19-specific CAR T cells after cyclophosphamide-based lymphodepleting chemotherapy with or without fludarabine. Importantly, response rates were higher in subjects receiving the cyclophosphamide/fludarabine

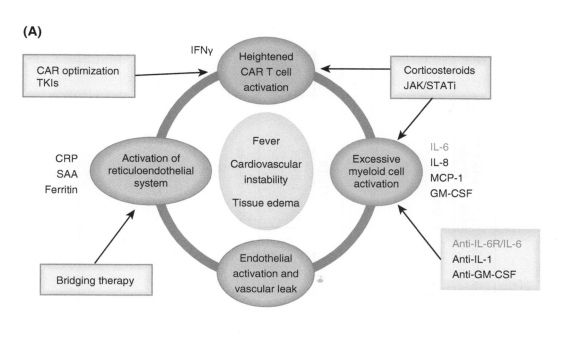

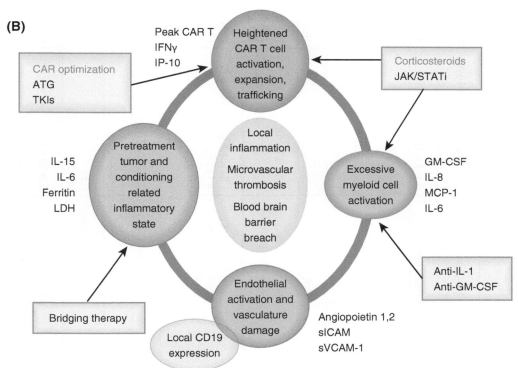

Figure 59.4 (A) Pathogenesis of CAR T related CRS; (B) pathogenesis of CAR T related neurotoxicity (ICANS).

combination (72% ORR, 50% CRs) than in those without fludarabine (50% ORR, 8% CRs).

Preliminary results have been reported for the ZUMA-1 trial of KTE-C19 (Kite Pharma), a CD19-specific CAR T cell product derived from the NCI CD28/CD3ζ vector.[143] This multicenter registration trial has enrolled

101 patients with chemotherapy-refractory DLBCL, 51 of whom were included in the interim analysis. Grade 3 or higher CRS and neurologic events were reported in 20% and 29% of subjects, respectively, and there was one death due to hemophagocytic lymphohistiocytosis. The ORR was an impressive 76%, which included 47% CRs

Table 59.2 Selected CAR T Cell Trial Results in Hematologic Cancers

INSTITUTION	ANTIGEN	CO-STIMULATORY DOMAIN	CONDITIONING REGIMEN	CAR T DOSE	DISEASE	N	ORR, CR%	REFERENCE
Non–Hodgkin lymphoma								
Kite Pharma (KTE-019)	CD19	CD28	Flu/Cy	2×10^6/kg	DLBCL	51	76%, 47% CR	143
FHCRC, Juno	CD19	CD28	Flu/Cy or Cy$^{+/-}$ E	2×10^5, 2×10^6, or 2×10^7/kg	NHL	20 Flu/Cy 12 Cy$^{+/-}$ E	72%, 50% CR in Flu/Cy 50%, 8% CR without Flu	144
NCI	CD19	CD28	Flu/Cy then IL-2	$0.3–3 \times 10^7$/kg	3 FL, 1 SMZL	4	100%, 0% CR	145
NCI	CD19	CD28	Flu/Cy	$1–5 \times 10^6$/kg	1 SMZL, 3 PMBCL, 4 DLBCL, 1 indolent lymphoma	9	89%, 56% CR	115
NCI	CD19	CD28	Flu/Cy	1×10^6/kg	8 DLBCL, 1 FL	9	66.7%, 11% CR	146
NCI	CD19	CD28	Flu/Cy		19 DLBCL	19	68%, 42% CR	147
MSKCC	CD19	CD28	BEAM conditioning and autologous SCT	$5–10 \times 10^6$/kg	2 FL (transformed), 3 DLBCL, 1 MZL	6	100%, 100% CR	148
UPenn	CD19	CD28	Bendamustine, Cy, Cy/Flu, modified EPOCH, XRT-Cy	5.84×10^6 (range: 3.08–8.87 $\times 10^6$)/kg	DLBCL 54% (7/13) FL 100% (7/7) MCL 50% (1/2)	22	68%, not reported	149
Chronic Lymphocytic Leukemia								
NCI	CD19	CD28	Flu/Cy then IL-2	$0.3–2.8 \times 10^7$/kg	CLL	4	75%, 25% CR	145
NCI	CD19	CD28	Flu/Cy	$1–5 \times 10^6$/kg	CLL	4	100%, 75% CR	115
UPenn	CD19	4-1BB	Physician discretion	$0.14–11 \times 10^8$ (median 1.6×10^8)	CLL	14	57%, 29% CR	116
UPenn	CD19	4-1BB	Unspecified	5 or 50×10^7	CLL	24	54%, 36% CR (high dose) 31%, 8% CR (low dose)	150
MSKCC	CD19	CD28	Pentostatin, Cy, rituximab	$3–30 \times 10^6$/kg	CLL	7	57%, 14% CR	151
FHCRC	CD19	CD28	Flu/Cy or Cy$^{+/-}$ E	2×10^5, 2×10^6, or 2×10^7/kg	CLL	6	67%, 50% CR	152

(continued)

Acute Lymphoblastic Leukemia								
UPenn	CD19	4-1BB	Unspecified	4.3×10^6/kg	ALL	53	94%, 94% CR	153
NCI	CD22	CD28	Flu/Cy	3×10^5/kg	ALL	5	20%, 20% CR	154
FHCRC	CD19	4-1BB	Flu/Cy or Cy $^{+/-}$ E	$2-200 \times 10^5$/kg	ALL	30	100%, 86% CR	155
Other Targets								
Baylor	CD30	CD28	None	2, 10, or 20×10^7/m^2	7 HL, 2 ALCL	8	25%, 13% CR	156
Zhejiang University	CD123	CD28	Cy	1.8×10^6/kg	AML	1	100%, 0% CR	157
NIH	BCMA	CD28	Flu/Cy	0.3, 1, 3, or 9×10^6/kg	Multiple myeloma	12	25%, 8.3% CR	158
Bluebird/Celgene	BCMA	4-1BB	Flu/Cy	5, 15, or 45×10^7	Multiple myeloma	9	67%, 22% CR	159

ALCL, anaplastic large cell lymphoma; ALL, acute lymphoblastic leukemia; AML, acute myeloid leukemia; B; BCMA, B cell maturation antigen; BEAM, carmustine, etoposide, cytarabine, and melphalan; CAR, chimeric antigen receptors; CLL, chronic lymphocytic leukemia; CR, complete response; DLBCL, diffuse large B cell lymphoma; EPOCH, etoposide, prednisone, vincristine, cyclophosphamide, hydroxydaunomycin; FHCRC, Fred Hutchison Cancer Research Center; FL, follicular lymphoma; Flu/Cy, fludarabine plus cyclophosphamide; IL, interleukin; MCL, mantle cell lymphoma; MSKCC, Memorial Sloan Kettering Cancer Center; NCI, National Cancer Institute; NIH, National Institutes of Health; ORR, objective response rates; SCT, stem cell transplantation; SMZL, splenic marginal zone lymphoma; XRT, X-ray therapy.

and 29% PRs, though follow-up is too short to assess the durability of these responses. This study clearly demonstrated that a potent CAR T cell product can be successfully manufactured and distributed to patient care centers with clinically meaningful results.

Alongside KTE-C19, two other CAR T cell products were approved for the treatment of relapsing/remitting DLBCL, as previously discussed. Notably, to date, the longest term follow-up in context of an NCI trial evaluating a product based on the KTE-C19 CAR construct showed a durable response rate in a subset of patients reaching a decade, thereby supporting the concept that this treatment modality could be curative.[161] Results with another product, based on a shorter follow-up, were consistent.[162]

Anti-CD19 Chimeric Antigen Receptor T Cells in Acute Lymphoblastic Leukemia

Several centers have now reported on CD19-specific CAR T cell therapies in both pediatric and adult B cell ALL, with CR rates as high as 70% to 92%.[163] Responses have been durable (more than 12 months) in up to half of patients, but CD19 antigen escape has been found associated with relapse in up to 20% of cases. A trial performed by the FHCRC/Juno group in adult B cell ALL highlighted the association between severe CRS and neurotoxicity with high cell dose and leukemia cell burden. Although 27 of 29 patients (95%) achieved bone marrow remission, two died—one from severe CRS, and another from late neurologic toxicity 122 days after T cell infusion. One of the two deaths was at a dose of 2×10^7 CAR T cells/kg, so this dose was deemed too toxic for further study. Furthermore, severe toxicity was mostly seen in patients with 20% or higher tumor infiltration in their bone marrow.[155]

Other Chimeric Antigen Receptor T Cell Target Antigens in Lymphomas

Although CD19 CAR T cells are the furthest along in clinical development, other tumor antigens are being targeted in lymphomas. A Phase 1 dose-escalation study of anti-CD30 CAR T cells in relapsed refractory EBV-negative CD30+ Hodgkin lymphoma and NHL has reported preliminary results.[156] Nine patients (seven with Hodgkin lymphoma and two with NHL) were treated with varying dose levels of CAR T cells without lymphodepleting chemotherapy. Six weeks after treatment, one patient had CR, one patient had very good PR, and four patients had stable disease (SD), while three patients progressed.

High response rates for CAR T cell therapies in NHL, ALL, and CLL suggest a promising future for this treatment platform. Despite these successes, the challenges of antigen escape and T cell persistence remain. Different targets are being explored to overcome these challenges, including anti-CD22,[164] anti-CD30,[156] and a

bispecific CD19/CD20 CARs.[165] Further refinements in vector design, cell dosage, and preparative regimens are eagerly awaited to improve the therapeutic index of this valuable technology.

Future Directions With Chimeric Antigen Receptor T Cell Therapy for Hematologic Malignancies

While the initial wave of CAR T cell products has been directed to diverse B cell cancer antigens, many product candidates are in various stages of development. Hence, CAR T cell intervention may witness label expansion to most if not all B cell histologies, including multiple myeloma, and also a shift to earlier line intervention as long as their curative potential will fare better compared to biologics and safety profile will improve. We can also envision next-generation dual or multitargeted CAR T cell products aimed to overcome mechanisms of resistance owing to individual target-related evasion. Other hematologic malignancies, most notably AML and Hodgkin lymphoma, are also targets of CAR T cell product candidates in development. Finally, the second major direction is represented by a transition to off-the-shelf cell products that may pose a formidable challenge to both custom-made CAR T cells and bispecific engagers owing to deployment of large numbers of "fit" immune cells derived from either healthy subjects or reprogrammed IPSCs. Product attributes are a major determinant of clinical performance of T cell intervention, and bispecific engagers or monoclonal antibodies may rely only on endogenous immune effector mechanisms. Long term, the success of off-the-shelf cell-based therapy, and cell therapy in general, as paradigm-shifting concepts will depend on their superior therapeutic index and scalability while keeping a competitive pricing.

MULTIPLE MYELOMA

Multiple myeloma is a clonal proliferation of malignant plasma cells that forms islands of tumor in the bone marrow (myelomas) that cause progressive destruction of bone and suppression of normal hematopoiesis. The tumor cells secrete large quantities of clonal immunoglobulins, which often leads to kidney failure. Measurement of these Igs in the serum correlates with tumor burden and can thus serve as a convenient measurement of disease activity. Though treatments including high-dose chemotherapy, proteasome inhibitors such as bortezomib, and IMiDs such as thalidomide and lenalidomide have improved the average survival to more than 5 years, the disease is still considered to be incurable.

Effects of Immunomodulatory Drugs in Myeloma

Until recently, myeloma was considered to be poorly responsive to immunotherapies due to a variety of immunosuppressive mechanisms within the tumor microenvironment (TME), including defective antigen presentation, T_{reg} cells, myeloid suppressor cells, macrophage production of immunosuppressive cytokines, and PD-L1 expression.[166] Newer-generation IMiDs, such as lenalidomide and pomalidomide, in addition to their direct suppressive effects on myeloma cells, have indirect mechanisms of action including disruption of supportive bone marrow, stroma-myeloma cell interactions, inhibition of angiogenesis, and multiple immunostimulatory properties.[167] These include enhanced CD4+ and CD8+ T cell activation and cytokine secretion, inhibition of T_{reg} cells, and inhibition of the proinflammatory cytokines TNF-α and IL-6. Based on this variety of mechanisms, lenalidomide has a single-agent activity in myeloma of 26% in relapsed/refractory disease,[168] and 47% in newly diagnosed patients.[169] Thus, the IMiDs can be an important building block in the design of immunotherapy regimens for myeloma.

Monoclonal Antibodies

Among monoclonal antibodies studied in myeloma (targeting signaling lymphocyte activation molecule F-7 [SLAMF-7], CD138, B cell maturation antigen [BCMA], CD56, and other antigens), the anti-CD38 antibody daratumumab deserves highlighting for the single-agent activity level that led to its regulatory approval in 2015. Daratumumab, a fully human IgG1, has potent CDC and ADCC activities against myeloma cells, even in the presence of bone marrow stromal cells.[170] In Phase 1/2 clinical trials, Lokhorst et al. demonstrated a response rate of 36% using daratumumab monotherapy in relapsed/refractory myeloma patients having had at least two earlier lines of therapy.[171] Furthermore, in a combined analysis of 148 patients from the GEN501 and SIRIUS studies, daratumumab monotherapy showed a response rate of 31%.[172] Subsequent trials have shown that daratumumab can significantly improve outcomes when added to standard myeloma therapies, such as proteasome inhibitors, IMiDs, and dexamethasone.

Immune Checkpoint Blockade

Although PD-L1 has been shown to be overexpressed in multiple myeloma tumor cells, no responses were seen in the Phase 1 clinical trial of the PD-1 antibody nivolumab in 27 myeloma patients.[95] However, when lenalidomide plus dexamethasone was added to the anti-PD-1 antibody pembrolizumab in combination with either lenalidomide/dexamethasone or pomalidomide/dexamethasone in refractory myeloma (including those previously treated with IMiDs), striking response rates of 76% and 50% were seen, respectively.[173,174] Thus, by mechanisms that are incompletely understood, IMiDs

and PD-1 blockade have apparently synergistic activity against myeloma.

Adoptive T Cell Therapies

As described previously, Rapoport et al. demonstrated that adoptive transfer of NY-ESO TCR-engineered T cells had clinical activity in HLA-A201+ patients whose myeloma cells expressed the cancer testis antigen NY-ESO-1/LAGE-1. Engineered T cells were able to traffic to tumor sites, had long-term engraftment, and had cytotoxic potential.[114]

Several surface antigens that have been selected for evaluation of CAR therapy in multiple myeloma have included BCMA, CD19, NKG2D, CD38, SLAMF-7, and kappa-light chain, with BCMA appearing to be the most promising target given its almost exclusive expression on late B cells and plasma cells.[175] A dose-escalation study of anti-BCMA CAR T cells was reported from the NCI using a CD28/CD3ζ construct.[158] In 12 patients treated at four dose levels, the best activity was seen at the two highest dose levels of 3 and 9×10^6 cells/kg, where among five patients there was one CR, two very good PRs, and two with stable disease. Therapy was well tolerated with mild to moderate CRS and cytopenias. In a more recent Phase 1 study using a 4-1BB/CD3ζ anti-BCMA construct (bb2121, Bluebird Bio), nine patients were treated at three dose levels of 5, 15, or 45×10^7 total CAR T cells. There were no dose-limiting toxicities or grade 3 or higher CRSs, and six of nine subjects had clinical responses (two CR, one very good PR, three PR).[159] Thus, the early experiences with anti-BCMA CAR T cells in myeloma appear quite promising and will likely lead to approvals in this space.[176]

ACUTE MYELOID LEUKEMIA

Finding effective immunotherapies against acute myeloid leukemia (AML) has represented a daunting challenge, given the disease's explosive growth rate and requirement for intensive chemotherapy that severely impairs host immune effector functions. However, several new approaches are beginning to show promise against this disease, which often carries a dismal prognosis. The first BiTE for AML therapy was the CD33/CD3 construct (AMG330).[177] CD33 is an attractive myeloid marker because it is expressed by greater than 90% of AMLs; also, treatment with epigenetic modifiers, such as azacitidine (an established AML therapy), has the potential to increase CD33 expression, thereby enhancing clinical efficacy with a CD33-targeted agent.[178] The use of CAR T cells targeting the CD123 myeloid antigen is also being explored, with clinical activity demonstrated in a single patient, offering positive proof of concept.[157]

CONCLUSION

It appears that in hematologic malignancies, there is a unique set of immunotherapeutic tools, each having substantial clinical activity. These include highly effective tumor targeting antibodies, checkpoint inhibitor antibodies, adoptive cellular therapies, cytokines, and small molecule immunomodulatory agents. Hence, many combinations will continue to be explored in the coming years, and are likely to lead to increased rates of cure for this large and diverse class of cancers. CAR T cell intervention—with four products approved to date in B cell lymphomas and leukemias, and several products in development for multiple myeloma, AML, Hodgkin lymphoma, and T cell lymphomas, carry substantial promise based on durable response rates suggestive of curative capability in a subset of patients. Future CAR T cell directions include expansion of applicability to broader histologies, outpatient and front-line setting, and utilization of off-the-shelf designer cells. Together with emergence of novel biologics including bispecific engagers and antibody drug conjugates, these advances carry the potential of radically changing the standard of care in hematological malignancies through therapeutic schemas applicable to earlier lines that lead to increased cure rates.

KEY REFERENCES

Only key references appear in the print edition. The full reference list appears in the digital product on Springer Publishing Connect: connect.springerpub.com/content/book/978-0-8261-3743-2/part/part04/chapter/ch59

45. McLaughlin P, Grillo-López AJ, Link BK, et al. Rituximab chimeric anti-CD20 monoclonal antibody therapy for relapsed indolent lymphoma: half of patients respond to a four-dose treatment program. *J Clin Oncol.* 1998;16(8):2825–2833. doi:10.1200/JCO.1998.16.8.2825

48. Coiffier B, Lepage E, Briere J, et al. CHOP chemotherapy plus rituximab compared with CHOP alone in elderly patients with diffuse large-B-cell lymphoma. *N Engl J Med.* 2002;346(4):235–242. doi:10.1056/NEJMoa011795

62. Goede V, Fischer K, Busch R, et al. Obinutuzumab plus chlorambucil in patients with CLL and coexisting conditions. *N Engl J Med.* 2014;370(12):1101–1110. doi:10.1056/NEJMoa1313984

71. Schuster SJ, Neelapu SS, Gause BL, et al. Vaccination with patient-specific tumor-derived antigen in first remission improves disease-free survival in follicular lymphoma. *J Clin Oncol.* 2011;29(20):2787–2794. doi:10.1200/JCO.2010.33.3005

75. Bargou R, Leo E, Zugmaier G, et al. Tumor regression in cancer patients by very low doses of a T cell-engaging antibody. *Science.* 2008;321(5891):974–977. doi:10.1126/science.1158545

107. Cappell KM, Sherry RM, Yang JC, et al. Long-term follow-up of anti-CD19 chimeric antigen receptor T-cell therapy. *J Clin Oncol.* 2020;38(32):3805–3815. doi:10.1200/JCO.20.01467

133. Porter DL, Levine BL, Kalos M, et al. Chimeric antigen receptor-modified T cells in chronic lymphoid leukemia. *N Engl J Med.* 2011;365(8):725–733. doi:10.1056/NEJMoa1103849

60

Brain Tumors

Hideho Okada and Noriyuki Kasahara

KEY POINTS

- Malignant brain tumors are classified into primary and secondary (metastatic) brain tumors. Despite recent advancements in conventional therapies, such as surgery, radiation therapy, and chemotherapy, prognosis for these tumors remain dismal.

- The "immunological privileged" status of the central nervous system (CNS) is not absolute and not only attributed solely to the blood–brain barrier (BBB) but also to immunosuppression and impaired antigen-presenting mechanisms.

- T cells are able to transmigrate the BBB, and immunotherapy trials should not exclude CNS lesions. Further understanding of CNS immunology will guide us to develop effective immunotherapy for brain tumors.

- Brain tumors produce a variety of immunosuppressive factors and recruit immunosuppressive cells, thereby escaping from the immune attack. The level of immunosuppression may be further enhanced by treatments, including the standard-of-care chemotherapy and radiation therapy.

- A variety of immunotherapy clinical trials are being conducted for both primary and secondary malignant brain tumors, including checkpoint blockade, vaccine, adoptive cell transfer, and oncolytic virus approaches.

- We should avoid significant autoimmunity in the brain. However, at present, one major challenge is paucity and heterogeneity of tumor-specific antigens. Further studies are warranted to discover and characterize target antigens for brain tumors.

- Proper response assessment criteria and management guidelines should be developed specifically for brain tumor patients receiving immunotherapy.

PRIMARY AND SECONDARY (METASTATIC) BRAIN TUMORS

Brain tumors can arise in the brain (a primary brain tumor) or other organs and metastasize into the brain (a secondary brain tumor).

Primary Brain Tumors

Primary brain tumors can arise from any tissue in the central nervous system (CNS) and occur in around 250,000 people a year globally. Primary brain tumors are classified into benign and malignant tumors. Benign tumors are usually demarcated from the surrounding brain tissue and thus are often totally resectable by surgery. On the other hand, malignant brain tumors invade the surrounding CNS tissue and are highly resistant to therapy. Gliomas, tumors arising from glial tissues, are the most common malignant primary brain tumors, accounting for 27% of all primary brain tumors and 80% of malignant tumors (Figure 60.1).[1,2] Gliomas are most commonly classified by the World Health Organization (WHO) grading system, which grades tumors from I (least advanced with best prognosis) to IV (most advanced with worst prognosis) with molecular parameters.[2] Glioblastoma multiforme (GBM; WHO grade IV) is the most common and most aggressive glial tumor, conferring a median survival of less than 15 months following the current standard of care using temozolomide chemotherapy combined with radiation therapy.[3] While the majority of WHO grade I gliomas are curable, WHO grade II gliomas have an extremely high risk of transforming into high-grade gliomas, and most grade II glioma patients eventually succumb to the disease.[4] Hence, gliomas, especially WHO grade II to IV gliomas, are considered malignant diseases, and novel and effective treatment options are needed.

Secondary (Metastatic) Brain Tumors

Secondary (metastatic) brain tumors are a common complication among patients with systemic cancer and more common than primary brain tumors. Lung and breast cancers, as well as melanoma, are responsible for up to three-quarters of metastatic brain lesions (Figure 60.2).[5–7] Clinically symptomatic metastases to the brain occur in

791

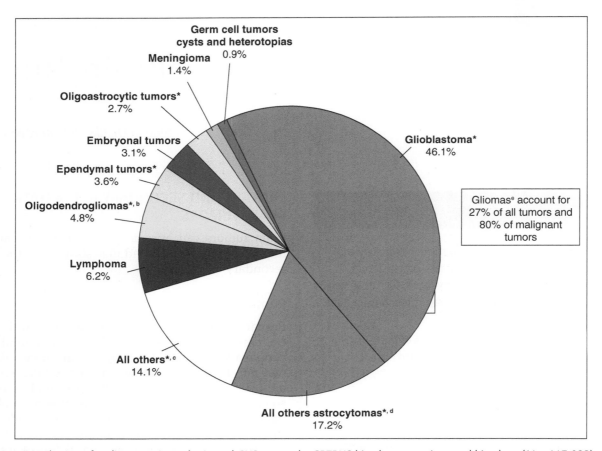

Figure 60.1 Distribution of malignant primary brain and CNS tumors by CBTRUS histology groupings and histology (*N* = 117,023).

†All or some of this histology is included in the CBTRUS definition of gliomas, including ICD-O-3 histology codes 9380–9384, 9391–9460 (Table 2b from Ostrom et al.). Percentages may not add up to 100% due to rounding.

‡Includes oligodendroglioma and anaplastic oligodendroglioma (Table 2b from Ostrom et al.).

§Includes glioma malignant, NOS, choroid plexus tumors, other neuroepithelial tumors, neuronal and mixed neuronal-glial tumors, tumors of the pineal region, nerve sheath tumors, other tumors of cranial and spinal nerves, mesenchymal tumors, primary melanocytic lesions, other neoplasms related to the meninges, other hematopoietic neoplasms, hemangioma, neoplasm, unspecified, and all others (Table 2b from Ostrom et al.).

**Includes pilocytic astrocytoma, diffuse astrocytoma, anaplastic astrocytoma, and unique astrocytoma variants (Table 2b from Ostrom et al.).

††Gliomas account for 27% of all tumors and 80% of malignant tumors.

CBTRUS, Central Brain Tumor Registry of the United States; ICD-O-3, International Classification of Disease Oncology; NPCR, National Program of Cancer Registry; SEER, Surveillance Epidemiology and End Result Program.

Source: Reproduced with permission from Ostrom QT, Gittleman H, Fulop J, et al. CBTRUS statistical report: primary brain and central nervous system tumors diagnosed in the United States in 2008–2012. *Neuro Oncol*. 2015;17:iv1–iv62. doi:10.1093/neuonc/nov189

15% to 20% of patients with metastatic breast cancer.[7,8] At autopsy, asymptomatic metastatic lesions are found in the brains of more than 30% of breast cancer patients.[5,8,9] Because of improvements in control of systemic disease and the consequent prolonged life span, the incidence of brain metastases is increasing in cancer patients. Recently, stereotactic radiosurgery (SRS) has emerged as a possible alternative to whole-brain radiotherapy and surgery.[10] Nevertheless, median overall survival for cerebral metastases remains less than 1 year.[11,12] Therefore, cerebral

metastases of cancers remain as major obstacles that must be overcome before cancers can be cured by any means.

IMMUNOLOGY OF THE BRAIN AND BRAIN TUMORS

Is the Brain Immunologically Privileged?

The concept of "immune privilege" in the CNS was shown as early as 1921, when Shirai observed that rat sarcoma

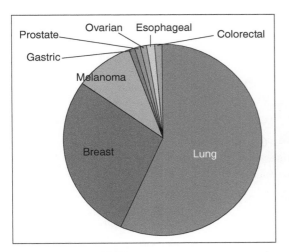

Figure 60.2 Breakdown of brain metastatic tumors according to originating cancer.

Source: Data from Bollig-Fischer A, Michelhaugh S, Ali-Fehmi R, Mittal S. The molecular genomics of metastatic brain tumours. *OA Mol Oncol*. 2013;1(1):759. https://www.ncbi.nlm.nih.gov/pmc/articles/PMC4229688

grew after being transplanted into the mouse brain parenchyma but not following subcutaneous or intramuscular implantation.[13] However, when recipient splenocytes were co-transplanted with the foreign tumor in the brain, it inhibited the tumor growth,[14] indicating that the xenograft tumor grew due to disconnection of the brain environment from the systemic immune system. Since then, extensive research on CNS immunology has not only confirmed the lack of immune response induction against bacterial or viral antigens inoculated into the CNS but also found that the "privileged" status is not absolute. More importantly, extensive studies have shown that the afferent arm of the cellular immune response is most impaired, while the

efferent arm is relatively intact (reviewed by Galea et al.; Figure 60.3).[15] While it has been controversial whether functional antigen-presenting cells (APCs) are able to migrate from brain parenchyma to lymph nodes, lymphatic drainage systems exist for the cerebral spinal fluid (CSF) space, including ones in the meninges of the dural venous sinuses in mice.[16,17] Further investigations are warranted to better delineate the afferent arm of the CNS immune system.

Immune Effector Mechanisms in the Brain— Does the Blood-Brain Barrier Shut the Immune Response?

Immune privilege in the CNS is often misattributed solely to the blood–brain barrier (BBB). Also, the presence of BBB has been often cited to dismiss the chance for exploiting the potential of immunotherapy for brain tumors. The BBB is formed by highly specialized endothelial cells in CNS microvessels, which inhibit uncontrolled transcellular passage of molecules by an extremely low pinocytotic activity and restrict the paracellular diffusion of hydrophilic molecules by an elaborate network of complex tight junctions between the endothelial cells (Figure 60.4).[18,19]

Although the access of circulating immune cells is tightly controlled by the BBB, T cells are able to traverse the BBB via chemokine axes and multistep adhesion processes.[20,21] In multiple sclerosis and in its animal model experimental autoimmune encephalomyelitis, inflammatory cells migrate across the endothelial BBB and gain access to the CNS via involvement of α4-integrins in mediating the initial contact to as well as firm adhesion with the endothelium.[18,19] In paraneoplastic cerebellar degeneration, patients with undiagnosed breast or ovarian cancer present with cerebellar signs. These are mediated by a

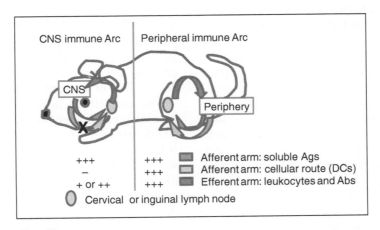

Figure 60.3 What is "immune privilege"?

Ab, antibody; Ag, antigen; CNS, central nervous system; DC, dendritic cell.

Source: Adapted with permission from Galea I, Bechmann I, Perry VH. What is immune privilege (not)? *Trends Immunol*. 2007;28(1):12–18. doi:10.1016/j.it.2006.11.004

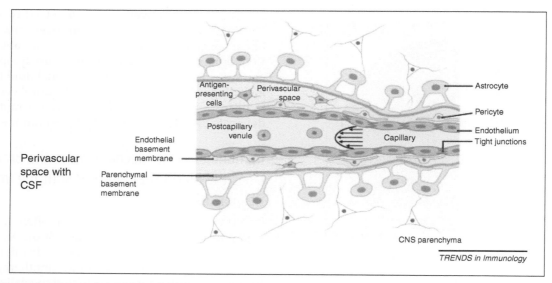

Figure 60.4 Neuroanatomy of the vascular BBB. Tight junctions link brain capillary endothelial cells together much more closely than what is observed in the systemic circulation. Much of the surface area of the CNS capillary system is also sheathed by the two layers of basement membranes of pericytes and the foot processes of astrocytes that comprise the parenchymal basement membrane.

BBB, blood–brain barrier; CNS, central nervous system; CSF; cerebrospinal fluid.

Source: Reproduced with permission from Engelhardt B, Ransohoff RM. Capture, crawl, cross: the T cell code to breach the blood-brain barriers. *Trends Immunol*. 2012;33(12):579–589. doi:10.1016/j.it.2012.07.004

specific T cell response reacting against an antigen, cdr2, which is expressed by breast/ovarian cancers and normal cerebellum.[22] Although cdr2 is expressed in normal cerebellum, the T cell response is activated only after the antigen is exposed to the systemic immune system through its expression in cancer tissues. This T cell response can then recognize and attack the targets located in the CNS. These findings suggest impaired antigen-presentation mechanisms for CNS antigens but provide us with rationale to develop effective peripheral immunization or systemic adoptive transfer strategies against CNS tumors.

Nonetheless, we have found that homing of effector cytotoxic T lymphocytes (CTLs) is weaker in brain tumors compared with cancer in other organs.[23] We subsequently found critical roles for the integrin receptor very late activation antigen (VLA)-4[24,25] and the chemokine CXCL10[26–28] in efficient homing of CTLs to the brain tumor environment. We subsequently found Toll-like receptor-3 agonist poly-ICLC as an immuno-adjuvant, which effectively induces expression of CXCL10 and VLA-4 in glioma and on vaccine-activated CTLs, respectively, thereby effectively promoting their migration to gliomas in the vaccine recipients.[25,29]

Glioma-Associated Immunosuppressive Leukocytes and Mechanisms

As is the case for other malignancies, brain tumors operate a variety of immune escape mechanisms. With the list of these factors constantly expanding, it seems almost unreasonable to expect a breakthrough by attacking just one or two of those pathways. However, major advances may be achieved by rational combination strategies targeting each of the critical pathways. In this section, we provide an updated review on immunosuppressive mechanisms that are most relevant to brain tumors, especially gliomas.

Glioma-Associated Immunosuppressive Leukocytes

Glioma-Associated Myeloid Cells

Among glioma-infiltrating hematopoietic cell populations, myeloid cells, including microglia and macrophages, are the most abundant[30] and constitute up to 30% to 70% of the tumor mass within gliomas.[31–33]

We and others have found that glioma-associated myeloid cells present key characteristics of myeloid-derived suppressor cells (MDSCs).[30,34] Cyclooxygenase (COX)-2 blockade can reverse the immunosuppressive role of MDSCs, thereby inhibiting the growth of glioma.[35] In regard to mechanisms underlying the induction of MDSCs in the glioma environment, glioma-derived granulocyte-macrophage colony-stimulating factor (GM-CSF) induces IL-4 receptor-α expression on glioma-infiltrating MDSCs, thereby inducing immunosuppressive phenotype, such as production of arginase-I, in the glioma microenvironment.[36] While the previously referenced study identified CD14-positive

MDSC subtype as the major MDSC population in the glioma environment, the CD15-positive population of MDSCs may also play important roles in glioma.[37] A variety of therapeutic approaches are being pursued based on solid understanding of these key mechanisms.[38]

Recent studies have underscored the importance of heterogeneous cell ontogeny of glioma-infiltrating myeloid cells. Single-cell-based analyses demonstrated that, in contrast to microglia, blood-derived myeloid cells aggregate in distinct compartments within GBM.[39] In this study, it was also noted that single myeloid cells can express both M1- and M2-markers, suggesting that the classical dichotomy of M1 versus M2 cells needs to be revised for glioma-infiltrating myeloid cells. Differences also exist in the activation profiles of different myeloid populations,[40,41] suggesting that myeloid cell responses in the context of targeted therapies are varied and their contributions to the tumor's adaptive resistance to treatment need to be considered.

Regulatory T Cells in the Brain Tumor

$CD4^+Foxp3^+$ T_{reg} cells in gliomas have been shown to express a variety of immunoregulatory molecules, such as CD25, CTLA-4, GITR (glucocorticoid-induced TNFR family-related gene), and CXCR4 at high levels.[42] Presence of T_{reg} cells correlates with a general paucity of CD4-positive T cells and impairment of T cell proliferation in peripheral blood specimens in GBM patients.[43] A recent study in a murine model demonstrated that the majority of tumor-infiltrating T_{reg} cells are thymus derived as opposed to induced T_{reg} cells.[44] GBM-derived CCL2 and other soluble factors can trigger the trafficking of T_{reg} cells to the tumor microenvironment.[45] Furthermore, macrophages and microglia within the glioma microenvironment produce CCL2, which recruit both $CCR4^+$ T_{reg} cells and $CCR2^+Ly-6C^+$ monocytic MDSCs.[46]

Multiple studies have examined the impact of depleting T_{reg} cells in bolstering antiglioma immunity. In murine models, systemic administration of anti-CD25 (IL-2Rα) mAb decreased the number of peripheral T_{reg} cells, inhibited their suppressive function, improved T cell effector responses, and improved the survival of mice-bearing gliomas.[47,48] However, in one study, while T_{reg} cell depletion alone failed to provide persistent immunological surveillance, the combination of T_{reg} cell depletion and DC vaccine established more potent immune rejection, as well as persistent antitumor immunity.[49] In human clinical trials of anti-CD25 mAb (Daclizumab) and EGFRvIII peptide vaccine, administration of Daclizumab depleted circulating T_{reg} cells after a single dose, which did not return to the baseline until 120 days post administration. There was a correlation between increased humoral response to epidermal growth factor receptor variant type III (EGFRvIII) and decreased T_{reg} cell populations.[50]

Glioma-Derived Molecular Factors Mediating Local and Systemic Immunosuppression

Gliomas suppress immune responses both locally and systemically. Gliomas secrete a variety of immunosuppressive factors, including TGF-β, prostaglandin E_2 (PGE_2), CCL2, vascular endothelial growth factor, and indoleamine 2,3 dioxygenase (IDO). Glioma cells also express immunosuppressive molecules on their cell surface, including Fas receptor (FasR)/Ligand (FasL), CD70, and lectin-like transcript 1.[51] In regard to recent findings on glioma-induced systemic immunosuppression, naïve T cells have been shown to accumulate in the bone marrow of glioma patients and mice, which appears to be the result of tumor-mediated loss of sphingosine-1-phosphate receptor 1 (S1P1).[52] In mouse models, blocking S1P1 internalization releases T cells and restores tumor-fighting capabilities, providing a possible avenue for therapeutic intervention. Furthermore, metabolites derived from glioma-specific mutation, such as production of 2-hydroxyglutarate in isocitrate dehydrogenase (IDH)-mutant gliomas,[53,54] mediate T cell exclusion, and suppression.

IMMUNOTHERAPEUTIC APPROACHES FOR BRAIN TUMORS—RECENT CLINICAL TRIALS

Adoptive Cell Transfer (ACT)

In a recently published comprehensive review on ACTs,[55,56] a variety of ex vivo propagated effector cells weren administered locally in the brain tumor site or systemically intravenously. In the past, ex vivo prepared cells with undefined, broad antigen-specificity were mainly used, such as lymphokine-activated killer (LAK) cells.[57] Also, expanded/activated γδ T cells from both healthy controls and selected patients have significant cytotoxicity against primary GBM explants.[58] γδ T cell therapy may be safe for brain tumor patients who undergo standard cytotoxic therapies.[59,60] While therapy with tumor-infiltrating lymphocytes (TILs) has shown reproducible and high objective response rates in metastatic melanoma,[61] in brain tumors only a few attempts have been made.[62-64] This may be because obtaining and expanding enough numbers of TILs require highly immunogenic, large, and accessible tumors.

Recently, antigen-targeted approaches have been developed, such as the use of chimeric antigen receptor (CAR). CARs have been generated for the glioma cell surface antigens, including IL-13Rα2,[65] EGFRvIII,[66-68] and HER2.[69]

IL-13Rα2 is overexpressed in approximately 75% of GBM and is linked to increased tumor invasiveness.[70] In a CAR T cell trial targeting IL-13Rα2 (NCT02208362), there was a dramatic response in one patient receiving intratumoral and intraventricular infusion of these CAR T cells.

The patient had no detectable lesions or spine metastases for 7.5 months following CAR treatment. However, four new lesions became detectable at 228 days after the first CAR T cell infusion. The emergence of new lesions was likely due to the outgrowth of cells not expressing surface IL-13Rα2.[71]

Another clinical trial (NCT02209376) employed a single intravenous infusion of autologous CAR T cells against EGFRvIII mutation in ten recurrent patients with EGFRvIII+ GBM.[67] The EGFRvIII mutation results in deletion of exons 2 through 7 and creates an immunogenic GBM-specific antigen.[72] The regimen did not result in cytokine release syndrome (CRS). All patients in this study demonstrated detectable transient expansion of CART-EGFRvIII cells in peripheral blood. In five of seven patients who underwent tumor resection post-CAR T cell infusion, trafficking of CAR T cells to tumor sites and reduction of EGFRvIII expression levels were noted. CAR T cell infiltration was associated with robust induction of inhibitory molecules, such as IDO1, PD-L1, and FoxP3, and infiltration by regulatory T cells.[68] The study also revealed a significant decrease of EGFRvIII-positive tumor cells. These results suggest immunoediting of the tumor and outgrowth of tumor cells without EGFRvIII expression.

HER2 is a receptor tyrosine kinase that is overexpressed in some GBM tumors and other cancer types, making it a possible CAR target. In a published trial (NCT01109095), investigators used virus-specific (CMV, Epstein-Barr, or adenovirus) T cells to express the CAR construct. This allows for enhanced immune activation by presentation of latent viral antigens. Although the trial was deemed safe, expansion of HER2-CAR T cells did not occur in the blood.[73]

These data imply that development of successful CAR T therapy for GBM will require further engineering and/or integration of strategies to improve CAR T homing and persistence in the GBM, overcome local immunosuppression, and address marked antigenic heterogeneity of GBM.

Checkpoint Blockade Approaches

Checkpoint inhibition approaches have been extensively evaluated in patients with GBM and metastatic brain tumors.

Checkpoint Blockade Approaches for Glioblastoma Multiforme

Among a variety of checkpoint blockade approaches, anti-PD-1 antibodies have been most extensively evaluated in GBM clinical trials. The Phase III CheckMate 143 (NCT02017717) study was one of the first large trials to evaluate the effectiveness of PD-1 blockade in GBM. The

trial compared bevacizumab (VEGF inhibitor) to either nivolumab monotherapy or nivolumab/ipilimumab (anti-CTLA-4 antibody) combination therapy in recurrent GBM patients.[74] As of 2017, nivolumab alone did not result in prolonged overall survival compared to bevacizumab; both arms of the trial resulted in a 42% 12-month overall survival. The trial resulted in significantly higher adverse effects in patients receiving the combination therapy. This arm of the trial (combination therapy) was discontinued and PD-1 monotherapy was continued.[74]

Standard GBM treatments, such as temozolomide (TMZ) and RT, further compound tumor-mediated immunosuppression by causing widespread lymphopenia, with a dramatic reduction in CD4+ T cells.[75] Two recent Phase III trials evaluated nivolumab in newly diagnosed GBM patients who also receive standard-of-care RT (NCT02617589; CheckMate 498) or RT+TMZ (NCT02667587; CheckMate 548). The former study failed to meet its primary endpoint of overall survival,[76] and the latter failed to meet improved progression-free survival (PFS) and, therefore, missed one of its primary endpoints; overall survival assessment is ongoing.[77]

A recent study evaluated molecular biomarkers associated with response to anti-PD-1 (pembrolizumab and nivolumab) therapy in recurrent GBM patients.[78] The authors profiled 66 patients via DNA, RNA, and imaging. Patients who responded to anti-PD-1 treatment had significant enrichment of MAPK pathway members, such as BRAF and PTPN11. Non-responders had an enrichment of phosphatase and tensin homolog (PTEN) mutations resulting in immunosuppressive gene signatures.[78]

In another study with neoadjuvant/pre-surgical administration of pembrolizumab, patients who received pre-surgical therapy and continued adjuvant therapy after surgery had improved overall survival than patients who received post-surgical pembrolizumab alone. Surgical specimens revealed that neoadjuvant anti-PD-1 therapy increased IFN-γ production by T cells and suppressed tumor cell cycles. Interestingly, pre/post-surgical tumor volume and dexamethasone administration were not identified as factors impacting patient outcome.[79]

Although some interesting biological impacts have been identified, checkpoint monotherapy is not likely to provide significant therapeutic benefits in patients with GBM. As such, there are a number of combination studies being evaluated in these patients (Table 60.1).

Checkpoint Blockade Approaches for Metastatic Brain Tumors

In 2013, 10% to 30% of all adult cancer patients developed brain metastases, which represents 170,000 newly diagnosed secondary brain malignancies in the United States.[80] Notably, up to 60% of metastatic melanoma

Table 60.1 Checkpoint Blockade Therapy Studies in Patients With Glioblastoma Multiforme and Other Malignant Glioma

TRIAL NO./PHASE	PATIENT GROUP	TREATMENT	CONTROL	PRIMARY OBJECTIVE	STATUS/ RESULTS/OS
NCT04323046; P1	Recurrent grade III glioma or GBM; $n = 45$; randomized	Ipilimumab, nivolumab, placebo	None	• Percentage change in cell cycle-related genetic signature after treatment • Safety	• Not yet recruiting
NCT04220892; Early P1	Grade III or GBM; $n = 22$; nonrandomized	Pembrolizumab vs. pemetrexed OR pembrolizumab vs. abemaciclib	None	• Tumor response rates	• Not yet recruiting
NCT03425292; P1	Newly diagnosed Grade III or GBM; $n = 90$; adult; nonrandomized	Nivolumab OR nivolumab plus ipilimumab OR nivolumab plus ipilimumab plus bevacizumab	Yes; standard radiation therapy with concurrent and adjuvant TMZ	• Rate of DLTs	• Recruiting
NCT 02017717; P3; Checkmate 143	Recurrent GBM; $n = 626$; randomized	Nivolumab Nivolumab + ipilimumab Bevacizumab		• Adverse events • % of G3 adverse events • Occurrence of laboratory abnormalities • OS	• Active
NCT02667587; P3 Checkmate 548	Newly diagnosed GBM; $n = 693$; adult; MGMT-methylated; randomized	Nivolumab, TMZ, RT Other: Nivolumab placebo + TMZ and RT	Nivolumab placebo	• PFS • OS (from date of randomization to death)	• Active
NCT02617589; P3; Checkmate 498	Newly diagnosed GBM; $n = 550$; adult; randomized	Nivolumab + RT	TMZ + RT	• OS (at 3 yrs)	• Active
NCT03173950; P2	Medulloblastoma, ependymoma, pineal region and choroid plexus tumors, meningioma; $n = 180$; adult; nonrandomized	Nivolumab	None	• OS • PFS	• Recruiting
NCT02794883; P2	Recurrent GBM; $n = 36$; adult; randomized	Durvalumab or tremelimumab alone vs. tremelimumab and durvalumab		• T cell (immunologic) changes in blood	• Active
NCT02336165; P2 MEDI4736	GBM; $n = 159$; nonrandomized	Durvalumab w/ or w/o RT, and w/ or w/o bevacizumab	None	• OS at 12 mos. • PFS at 6 mos.	• Active
NCT04013672; P2 SurVaxM	Recurrent GBM; $n = 51$; adult; nonrandomized	Pembrolizumab, SurVaxM, sargramostim, montanide ISA 51	None	• PFS (6 mos. since beginning of treatment	• Recruiting
NCT02337686; P2	Recurrent GBM; $n = 20$; adult	Pembrolizumab, then surgery	None	• PFS at 6 mos.	• Active
NCT04225039; P2	GBM; $n = 32$; adult; nonrandomized	GITR-agonist INCMGA00012, anti-PD-1 ab INCAGN01876, SRS, brain surgery		• Objective radiographic response	• Not yet recruiting

(continued)

Table 60.1 Checkpoint Blockade Therapy Studies in Patients With in GBM and Other Malignant Glioma (*continued*)

TRIAL NO./PHASE	PATIENT GROUP	TREATMENT	CONTROL	PRIMARY OBJECTIVE	STATUS/ RESULTS/OS
NCT03532295; P2	GBM; *n* = 55; adult; nonrandomized	INCMGA00012+RT+bevacizimab OR INCMGA00012+RT+bevacizumab +epacadostat	None	-OS at 9 mos.	- Not yet recruiting
NCT03174197; P1/P2	GBM, gliosarcoma; *n* = 60; adult; nonrandomized	Atezolizumab, TMZ, RT (as adjuvant or concurrent)	None	- DLTs - OS - Incidence of adverse events	- Recruiting
NCT03491683; P1/P2; REGN2810	GBM; *n* = 52; adult; MGMT methylation vs. nonmethylated; nonrandomized	INO-5401, INO-9012, cemiplimab, RT, TMZ	None	- Occurrence of adverse events	- Active
NCT02968940; P2	GBM; *n* = 4	Avelumab (anti-PD-L1 ab), hypofractionated radiation therapy (HFRT)	None	- Safety - PFS up to 6 months	- Active

Note: Search terms used:

Condition or disease: "GBM" OR "glioblastoma" OR "brain tumor" OR "DIPG" OR "DMG" OR "pediatric brain cancer" OR "glioma"

Other terms: "immunotherapy"

DLTs, dose-limiting toxicity; GBM, glioblastoma; MGMT, O6-Methylguanine-DNA Methyltransferase; OS, overall survival; PFS, progression-free survivial; RT, radiation therapy; TMZ, temozolomide.

patients develop metastases in the brain.[81] Brain metastases are also very common in patients with lung and breast cancer and occur in ~20% to 40% of patients across different cancer types.[81] In regard to the involvement of immunological mechanisms, the level of immune cell penetration has been found to be a favorable prognostic marker for melanoma brain metastasis.[82] Checkpoint blockade approaches have been actively investigated in these conditions, especially for melanoma brain metastases. There are excellent recent reviews in this regard.[83–87]

In a Phase 2 trial, ipilimumab showed activity in patients with advanced melanoma and brain metastases, in particular those who were asymptomatic and not receiving corticosteroids.[88] PD-1 monotherapy does appear less effective against brain metastases, with an intracranial response of 22% with pembrolizumab in melanoma patients with brain metastases not requiring steroids, compared with the 30% to 40% response rates usually seen in patients without brain metastases.[89] In regard to combination immunotherapy, in the CheckMate-204 study of nivolumab plus ipilimumab in patients with unirradiated brain metastases, intracranial and extracranial benefit was similar (57% vs. 56%).[90] However, complete responses were higher in the brain. Responses were also durable, with intracranial progression prevented for over 6 months in 64% of patients. However, with the exception of melanoma, immune checkpoint blockade has failed to achieve

significant brain control in patients with brain metastases of other solid tumors. It is also noteworthy that treatment of melanoma brain metastases with ipilimumab followed by nivolumab has led to subacute multifocal CNS demyelination[91] and a clinically unapparent but histologically prominent inflammation in the brain.[92]

Radiation therapy, such as SRS, is commonly used for treatment of brain metastasis. There have been a number of studies evaluating the efficacy of radiation in combination with checkpoint blockade, such as ipilimumab. If successful, these combinatorial strategies have the potential to result in enhanced rates of brain control, less brain exposure to radiation, and improved cognitive outcomes. In these combinations, the sequence of treatments may also be a critical factor. Patients treated with SRS during or before ipilimumab had higher rates of initial progression compared with those treated with SRS afterward.[93] This may, however, reflect induction of effective inflammatory response by the sequence of SRS followed by ipilimumab. It is also suggested that the combination of local radiation and checkpoint blockade therapy may elicit systemic antitumor immune response (the "abscopal effect").[94,95]

Challenges to determine the most effective regimen include retrospective comparison, different doses, and sequence of treatments, as well as patient eligibility criteria, such as the number of lesions. Nonetheless, recent meta-analysis studies may provide valuable information.

A report by Pin et al .performed a systematic review of 14 studies (11 on melanoma, three on lung cancers).[87] SRS plus immunotherapy showed better OS and regional control compared to SRS alone. Petrelli et al. searched 33 studies for a total of 1,520 patients, most of them with melanoma (87%).[86] Addition of immunotherapy to radiotherapy was associated with improved OS (HR = 0.54, 95% CI 0.44–0.67; p <.001). For patients with brain metastases from solid tumors, addition of concurrent immunotherapy to radiation increased survival and provided long-term control.[86] However, neurotoxic side effects also occurred more frequently.[83] More randomized controlled trials or prospective studies are warranted to generate proper evidence that can be used to change the standard of care for these patients.

Vaccination Strategies for Neuro-Oncology

Vaccine strategies have been extensively investigated in patients with malignant gliomas. As there are a number of recent, excellent reviews for more comprehensive explanation on this topic,[96–98] in this section, we will focus on selected, specific areas that are considered critical for the future directions. Table 60.2 summarizes currently ongoing vaccine trials in glioma patients.

Vaccinations With Glioma-Specific Antigens

As discussed earlier in this book, antigens expressed in tumor cells can be classified into two general categories: (a) tumor-associated antigens and (b) tumor-specific antigens. Most antigens that have been evaluated in glioma vaccines to date are nonmutated, glioma-associated antigens.[96–98] Concerns in directing vaccination strategies against glioma-associated antigens are central or peripheral tolerance against these self-proteins and the risk of autoimmunity directed at tissues with shared expression. While early phase studies of vaccination against these targets have shown safety, immunological activity, and some evidence of efficacy, further studies are warranted to determine whether a therapeutic window exists where vaccination against tumor-associated antigens can elicit sufficient immunity to mediate a clinical benefit without inducing intolerable autoimmunity. However, in recent immunotherapy trials using adoptive transfer of T cells, life-threatening and fatal events were caused by on-target[99–101] or off-target[102,103] cross-reactivity of T cells against normal cells, indicating the need for expanding the list of available tumor-specific antigens, such as mutation-derived antigens. While autologous glioma cell-based vaccines have been extensively developed as ways to target bulk antigens presented in patients' own tumors,[104,105] this chapter focuses on tumor-specific antigen-targeting approaches because this direction will become particularly important as we gain access to more robust immunotherapy modalities. Therefore, targeting of recurrent and immunogenic mutations, such as H3.3K27M in diffuse midline gliomas (DMGs)[106,107] and isocitrate dehydrogenase (IDH)1R132H in secondary GBMs and lower grade gliomas,[108] represents safe and potentially effective approaches.

EGFRvIII-Targeting Vaccines (Rindopepimut)

Rindopepimut is a 14 amino acid peptide from EGFRvIII encompassing the mutation site and conjugated to keyhole limpet hemocyanin (KLH) and is administrated subcutaneously along with GM-CSF.[109] In newly diagnosed GBM patients, a Phase 2 study demonstrated an impressive overall survival (OS) of 26 months in comparison with 15 months in historical controls receiving standard-of-care chemoradiation therapy.[110] Recurrence after treatment was associated with the outgrowth of EGFRvIII-negative tumor cells, suggesting a need for targeting multiple glioma-specific antigens. Unfortunately, the subsequent international Phase 3 randomized trial (ACT IV) failed to demonstrate survival benefit.

Vaccines Against the Isocitrate Dehydrogenase (IDH) Mutation-Derived Human Leucocyte Antigen (HLA)-DR Epitope

Mutations of the IDH metabolic enzymes IDH1 and IDH2 have been found to be early and frequent (70%–80%) genetic alterations in WHO grade II and III gliomas,[111] as well as secondary GBM which progress from lower grade gliomas.[112] All *IDH1* and *IDH2* mutations identified to date affect a single amino acid located within the isocitrate binding site [IDH1 (R132) or IDH2 (R140 and R172)] and confer a novel gain-of-function activity of converting α-ketoglutarate (2-OG) to the (R)-enantiomer of 2-hydroxyglutarate (R-2-HG). Reduced availability of α2-OG and increased production of 2-HG by mutant IDHs may coordinate genome-wide epigenetic changes and predisposing the cells toward malignant transformation.[111] The most common variant among these cancers is a single-base mutation at position 132 of *IDH1* replacing arginine (R) with histidine (H; IDH1R132H, approximately 90% of all *IDH* mutations).[113] These mutations occur very early in the progression of glioma development,[114] and can persist throughout multiple recurrences, chemotherapy, and resections.[115]

An HLA-class II-binding CD4[+] T cell epitope was recently found encompassing IDH1R132H (p123–142).[108] HLA-A2.DR1-transgenic mice-bearing IDH1R132H-transfected syngeneic sarcomas showed antitumor response upon immunization with the IDH1R132H (p123–142) peptide without toxicity beyond skin reactions. A Phase 1 vaccine trial targeting the IDH1R132H mutation has been recently conducted in IDH1R132H-mutated

Table 60.2 Vaccine Studies in Patients With Glioblastoma Multiforme and Other Malignant Gliomas

TRIAL NO./ PHASE	PATIENT GROUP	TREATMENT	CONTROL	PRIMARY OBJECTIVE	STATUS/RESULTS/OS
NCT01678352; P1	Grade II glioma; recurrent/post-chemotherapy; $n = 19$; adult; randomized	• Tumor lysate vaccine (BTIC: brain tumor-initiating cell) • Imiquimod	None	• DLT and safety • Induction of BTIC lysate-specific T cell response	• Completed • None reported
NCT01400672; P1	DIPG; $n = 8$; peds	• BiTumor lysate vaccine, imiquimod, radiation	None	• DLT and safety	Terminated (Treatment ineffective; extreme toxicity)
NCT03927222; P2	Newly diagnosed GBM, tumor resected, and MGMT unmethylated; $n = 48$; adult	• Human CMV pp65-LAMP mRNA-pulsed autologous DCs (dendritic cell) w/ GM-CSF • TMZ • Tetanus-diphtheria toxoid	None	• Median OS	• Recruiting
NCT02193347; P1 RESIST	Brain neoplasm, primary and recurrent w/ IDH1R132H expression in primary tumor; $n = 24$	• PEPIDH1M vaccine • Tetanus-diphtheria toxoid (Td) • TMZ		• Safety	• Active
NCT02549833; P1	WHO grade II glioma; $n = 30$	• GBM6-AD (tumor lysate vaccine) and poly-ICLC w/ resection		• Safety and feasibility • Measurement of vaccine-induced immune response	• Recruiting
NCT03334305; P1	Malignant, high-grade glioma; $n = 8$; peds. and adult; nonrandomized	• Dose-intensified TMZ with TTRNA-DC vaccines with GM-CSF and TTRNA-xALT plus Td vaccine with OR without autologous hematopoietic stem cells (HSCs)		• Evaluate safety of TTRNA-DCs and TTRNA-xALT	• Recruiting
NCT03396575; P1	DIPG; $n = 21$; peds. or young adult; nonrandomized	• TTRNA-DC vaccines with GM-CSF and TTRNA-xALT plus Td vaccine with autologous hematopoietic stem cells (HSCs) during cycles of dose-intensified TMZ OR with cyclophosphamide + fludarabine lymphodepletive conditioning	None	• Feasibility and safety of ACT therapy • Determine MTD for all treatment types	• Recruiting
NCT02149225; P1; GAPVAC-101	Newly diagnosed GBM; $n = 16$; adult	• APVAC1 vaccine plus Poly-ICLC and GM-CSF • APVAC2 vaccine plus Poly-ICLC and GM-CSF • Concurrent with TMZ	None	• Safety • Freq. of APVAC-specific CD8+ T cells	• Completed
NCT02122822; P1	Newly diagnosed GBM; $n = 20$; adult.	• Heat-shock protein gp96	None	• Blood analyses • Electrocardiogram • PFS (at 6 mos.)	• Completed
NCT01290692; P2 TVAX	Recurrent GBM; grade IV glioma; $n = 86$; adult	TVI-brain-1 following resection	None	• PFS	• Completed

(continued)

Table 60.2 Vaccine Studies in Patients With Glioblastoma Multiforme and Other Malignant Gliomas

TRIAL NO./ PHASE	PATIENT GROUP	TREATMENT	CONTROL	PRIMARY OBJECTIVE	STATUS/RESULTS/OS
NCT00643097; P2					• Completed
NCT01326104; P2	Medulloblastoma, neuroectodermal tumor; *n* = 17	TTRNA-xALT, TTRNA-DCs	None	• Safety • PFS, 12 mos.	• Active
NCT02960230; P2 PNOC	Newly diagnosed DIPG, DMG-HLA-A2+, and H3.3K27M-Mutant only; *n* = 49; peds. and young adult; nonrandomized	After radiation therapy, K27M peptide, plus poly-ICLC, w/ or w/o nivolumab	None	• Safety • OS at 12 months	• Recruiting; active
NCT03018288; P2	GBM; *n* = 14; adult; randomized	RT+pembrolizumab+TMZ w/ or w/o HSPPC-96; other: placebo	Vaccine placebo group	• Improvement of 1 year OS	• Suspended
NCT01280552; P2		ICT-107, dendritic cell vaccine; completed in ~2013			
NCT00045968; P3 DCVax-L	GBM, grade IV astrocytoma	Dendritic cell immunotherapy			
NCT01204684; P2	Anaplastic astrocytoma, anaplastic astro-oligodendroglioma, GBM; *n* = 60; adult	Autologous tumor lysate-pulsed DC vaccination, tumor lysate-pulsed DC vaccination+0.2% resiquimod, tumor-lysate-pulsed DC vaccination +adjuvant poly-ICLC	None	• Most effective combination of DC vaccine components	
NCT03382977; P1/P2	GBM; multiforme; *n* = 38; nonrandomized	VBI-1901 (includes granulocyte-macrophage colony-stimulating factor ("GM-CSF"), an adjuvant that mobilizes dendritic function and enhances Th1-type immunity)	None	• DLTs	-Recruiting
NCT02078648; P1/P2	GBM; *n* = 74	SL-701; poly-ICLC Bevacizumab	None	• Safety • OS (at 12 months) • Objective response rate	-Completed
NCT01480479; P3	GBM; *n* = 745; randomized	• Rindopepimut (CDX-110) with GM-CSF + TMZ	Active comparator: KLH plus TMZ	• OS	-Completed
NCT01920191; P1/2; IMA950	GBM; *n* = 19; adult	IMA 950 (multitumor-associated peptide vaccine) + Poly-ICLC		• Tolerability • Safety	-Completed

Note: Search terms used:

Condition or disease: "GBM" OR "glioblastoma" OR "brain tumor" OR "DIPG" OR "DMG" OR "pediatric brain cancer" OR "glioma"

Other terms: "immunotherapy"

ACT, adoptive cell transfer; APVAC, actively personalized vaccine; CSF, colony-stimulating factor; DC, dendritic cell; DIPG, diffuse intrinsic pontine glioma; DLT, dose-limiting toxicity; GBM, glioblastoma; GM-CSF, granulocyte-macrophage colony-stimulating factor; KLH, keyhole limpet hemocyanin; MTD, maximum tolerated dose; OS, overall survival; PFS, progression-free survival; TMZ, temozolomide; WHO, World Health Organization

gliomas (NCT02454634). While IDH mutations mediate T cell exclusion[54] and suppression,[53] coordinated approaches can be developed targeting the IDH1R132H as both a neoantigen and an inhibitory mechanism.

H3.3K27M-Neoantigen Vaccines in Diffuse Midline Gliomas

Within the majority of DMGs, a driver mutation in the histone H3 gene *H3F3A* confers a single amino acid mutation, K27M, in both histone 3 variant 1 (H3.1K27M) and variant 3 (H3.3K27M),[116] Studies conducted by our group[107] and others[106] led to the identification of the novel H3.3K27M p26–35 epitope (H3.3K27M$_{26-35}$). More than 70% of diffuse midline pontine gliomas (DIPGs) and the majority of DMGs harbor the H3.3K27M mutation, and the median survival of children with DIPG remains under 1 year. We recently completed a Phase 1 clinical trial (NCT02960230) evaluating the K3.3K27M-specific peptide vaccine with adjuvant Poly-ICLC in pediatric H3.3K27M-mutated gliomas. Our data demonstrated that expansion of non-exhausted H3.3K27M-reactive CD8[+] T cells was associated with improved survival while high levels of MDSC at baseline as well as use of corticosteroid were negatively associated with patients' survival (manuscript submitted).

Cytomegalovirus (CMV)-Derived Antigens for Glioma Immunotherapy?

A number of studies have demonstrated frequent detection of low-level expression of human CMV genes within malignant gliomas,[117,118] While it has been highly controversial whether CMVs are truly present in gliomas, early phase trials have been conducted targeting CMV, such as a DC vaccine in combination with the vaccine-site conditioning with tetanus-toxoid.[119] However, a recent Pan-Cancer Analysis of Whole Genomes (PCAWG) Consortium study reported that CMV was detected in none of 294 brain tumor cases, including 41 GBM and 107 low-grade gliomas.[120] As this study detected CMV in other cancer types, this almost irrefutably demonstrated the absence of CMV in gliomas.

Personalized Vaccines

Development of personalized vaccines targeting specific mutations in an individual patient's tumor is underway by multiple groups, taking advantage of novel genomic interrogation technologies.

The glioma-actively personalized vaccine (GAPVAC) 101 Phase 1 trial (NCT02149225) exploited both unmutated antigens (APVAC1) and neoantigens (APVAC2) as personalized vaccines.[121] APVAC2 vaccines were chosen from transcriptomes and immunopeptidomes of patient tumor samples. The study found that APVAC1 peptides were immunogenic and resulted in specific effector and memory T cells. Additionally, neoepitopes in APVAC2

elicited CD4[+] Th1 cell responses.[121] Another Phase 1/1b trial (NCT02287428) utilized a personalized neoantigen vaccine in conjunction with RT and pembrolizumab for newly diagnosed GBM patients. While patients who did not receive dexamethasone during vaccine priming had strong vaccine-specific immune responses, patients who received dexamethasone did not demonstrate a response.[122] While these personalized vaccine approaches may address interpatient heterogeneity and may induce truly tumor-specific (i.e., neoantigen-specific) immune responses, the magnitude of vaccine-specific T cell responses appears relatively low[121] compared to the levels that can be achieved by adoptive cell transfer approaches. Further, engineering and combination with potent immunoadjuvants may be necessary to improve the potency of vaccine approaches.

Immuno-Prevention of Recurrence and Transformation to High-Grade Glioma

The ultimate form of cancer vaccine may be represented by prophylactic vaccines. Although WHO grade II gliomas are classified as "low-grade," most grade II glioma patients eventually succumb to the disease due to inevitable progression and an extremely high risk of transforming into grade III or IV gliomas. Immunotherapeutic approaches, such as vaccines, may be particularly appropriate for patients with low-grade glioma because they are likely not to be as immunocompromised as patients with higher grade glioma. The slower growth rate of low-grade glioma should also allow sufficient time to administer multiple immunizations. We conducted two of the first Phase 1 vaccine trials using glioma-associated antigen peptides and poly-ICLC as the adjuvant in WHO grade II glioma patients with high-risk factor for recurrence (NCT00795457 and NCT00874861).[123] The regimen induced a robust T cell response against vaccine-targeted epitopes that are expressed at higher levels in high-grade glioma than in low-grade glioma, suggesting possible use as a prophylactic glioma vaccine against progression to higher grade glioma. Further refinements, such as selection of antigens, are warranted to improve the efficacy of the approach. We are currently conducting two vaccine studies in WHO grade II glioma patients with neoadjuvant designs to evaluate the effects of the vaccines in the tumor microenvironment (NCT02549833, NCT02924038).

ONCOLYTIC VIROIMMUNOTHERAPY FOR GLIOMA

Oncolytic viruses represent a novel class of biologic agents with a multimodal mechanism of action, which, in addition to direct cytolytic effects on cancer cells, include immunotherapeutic effects caused by release of danger signals, activation of innate inflammatory reactions, and induction of antitumor immunity. However, oncolytic virotherapy may run the risk of directing adaptive immune responses to viral antigens, eventually resulting in neutralization and clearance, and potentially detracting from antitumor immunity.[124–126] Furthermore, many viruses are able to suppress both innate and adaptive immunity through molecular mimicry and competitive inhibition, including viral proteins that act as immunomodulatory decoys and signaling pathway inhibitors[127–129] and may even actively induce recruitment of immunosuppressive cells into the tumor microenvironment.[130,131] Hence, current quandaries in the field include how to best manipulate immunological responses to minimize premature clearance by antiviral immunity and maximize induction of antitumor immunity. Nonetheless, this class of agents has considerable promise for both direct tumor mass reduction and for in situ tumor vaccination, and will likely show even more potency when combined with other immunotherapies such as checkpoint inhibition. Here, we will focus primarily on clinical development of oncolytic viruses for the treatment of gliomas, particularly focusing on immunological mechanisms of action contributing to therapeutic efficacy.

Adenovirus

One of the first oncolytic viruses to be commercially developed, ONYX-015, was previously evaluated in a Phase 1 dose-escalation trial involving 24 patients with recurrent malignant glioma, who received post-resection peritumoral injections at doses ranging from 10^7 to 10^{10} pfu; there were no significant adverse effects but also little evidence of therapeutic benefit in terms of median survival (6.2 months); however, 1/6 recipients at the 10^9 pfu dose and 2/6 at the 10^{10} pfu dose remained alive at 19 months of follow-up.[132] More recently, Delta-24-RGD (now designated DNX-2401 [*Tasadenoturev*]), a newer oncolytic adenovirus with a 24-bp deletion in the viral E1A gene, which prevents retinoblastoma protein (pRB) binding and an $\alpha v\beta 3 / \alpha v\beta 5$ integrin-binding RGD sequence inserted into the viral fiber,[133] has advanced to clinical trials for the treatment of recurrent GBM (NCT00805376, NCT01956734, NCT02197169). Preclinical studies have confirmed that this virus can elicit antitumor immunity,[134,135] and durable late-onset tumor regression suggesting immune-mediated responses have been observed in trial subjects. Phase 1 trial (NCT00805376) results showed that in patients who received a single intratumoral injection of DNX-2401 into biopsy-confirmed recurrent GBM ($n = 25$), 20% of patients survived >3 years from treatment, and three patients had a ≥ 95% reduction in enhancing tumor (12%) and >3 years of PFS.[136] Interim results from a Phase 2 dose-escalation study in combination with pembrolizumab (CAPTIVE/KEYNOTE-192 study, NCT02798406) demonstrated a favorable safety profile, and median overall survival of 12.3 months, with four of 48 subjects showing responses (5×10^{10} pfu dose, two subjects with >94% tumor regression), and three subjects alive >20 months.[137] Currently, DNX-2401 is also being evaluated in Phase 1 trials for diffuse intrinsic pontine glioma (DIPG; NCT03178032) and recurrent high-grade gliomas (NCT03896568), and a Phase 1 trial of DNX-2440, another version of Delta-24-RGD armed with OX40L,[138] has also recently been initiated for recurrent GBM.

Herpes Simplex Virus (HSV)

HSV-1716 and G207, oncolytic HSV with neurovirulence factor $\gamma_1 34.5$ and $\gamma_1 34.5/ICP6$ deletions, respectively,[139,140] were both safe and well-tolerated without evidence of encephalitis, and with signs of therapeutic benefit, especially when combined with radiation, which achieved partial responses or stable disease in six out of nine patients.[141,142] G207 is currently still under evaluation in pediatric brain tumor patients (NCT02457845, NCT03911388). A newer oncolytic HSV, G47Δ, in which a viral-encoded inhibitor of MHC class I expression is also deleted[143] has shown promising therapeutic results including durable tumor responses occurring several months after treatment, again suggesting that antitumor immunity had been induced.[144] Recently, patients with recurrent GBM received up to six repeated stereotactic intratumoral injections with 1×10^9 pfu G47Δ into different coordinates every 4 weeks in a Phase 2 trial in Japan, which reported a 1-year survival rate of 92.3% ($n = 13$).[145] Also, M032, a $\gamma_1 34.5$-deleted oncolytic HSV armed with human IL-12, has recently been developed for clinical application to gliomas (NCT02062827).[146] IL-12 is expected to mediate both immunostimulatory and antiangiogenic[147] effects, as recently suggested by clinical trial results after delivery of inducible IL-12 using a conventional adenovirus vector in high-grade gliomas.[148] Also, a clinical trial (NCT03657576) has recently been initiated for another $\gamma_1 34.5$-deleted oncolytic HSV with insertion of the *IRS1* gene from human cytomegalovirus (HCMV), which enables evasion from innate antiviral defense mechanisms triggered by double-stranded RNA-activated protein kinase (PKR).[149] Finally, another oncolytic HSV, rQNestin34.5, is also currently being evaluated in a clinical trial for recurrent high-grade glioma (NCT03152318); this virus is unique in retaining the neurovirulence gene $\gamma_1 34.5$ under transcriptional control of the nestin promoter.[150]

Reovirus

In a Phase 1 dose-escalation clinical trial evaluating Reolysin, an oncolytic reovirus, at doses of 10^7–10^9 $TCID_{50}$ delivered in a single stereotactic intratumoral injection in recurrent glioma patients, one out of 10 patients showed long-term survival.[151] In a subsequent study, Reolysin was infused slowly via convection-enhanced delivery at doses ranging from 10^8–10^{10} TCID$_{50}$ in patients with recurrent glioma; median survival was 4.7 months (range: 3.3–33 months), with two out of 15 patients surviving over 2 years, but this was not viral dose-dependent.[152] Currently, Reolysin is being evaluated in combination with sargramostim (GM-CSF) in pediatric patients with relapsed or treatment-refractory high-grade glioma (NCT02444546).

Poliovirus

In a Phase 1 trial for recurrent GBM (NCT01491893), oncolytic poliovirus PVSRIPO, derived from the Sabin vaccine strain and further attenuated by altering its translation-initiating Internal Ribosome Entry Site (IRES),[153] showed durable complete radiographic and clinical responses appearing several months after treatment in some patients, again suggesting that induction of antitumor immunity may be the primary mechanism of action. Poliovirus infection leads to innate inflammatory responses specifically through recognition by melanoma differentiation-associated protein 5MDA5.[154] However, increased toxicity occurred with virus dose-escalation, necessitating steroid treatment. Accordingly, a de-escalated dose level (5.0×10^7 TCID$_{50}$) was employed as the Phase 2 dose, still resulting in PVSRIPO-related adverse events of grade 3 or higher in 19% of the patients, but achieving an overall survival plateau of 21% that was sustained for at least 36 months.[155] PVSRIPO is currently under evaluation in a multicenter Phase 2 trial for adult GBM (NCT02986178), and a Phase 1b trial in children with recurrent high-grade glioma (NCT03043391).

Paramyxoviruses

Paramyxovirus infection results in the formation of host cell syncytia and triggers danger signals that elicit innate and adaptive immune responses, resulting in immunogenic cell death.[156,157] For the treatment of glioma, paramyxoviruses that have been clinically investigated as oncolytic agents are measles virus and Newcastle disease virus.

Measles

In a Phase 1 dose-escalation trial (NCT00390299), an attenuated Edmonston vaccine strain of measles virus genetically engineered to express carcinoembryonic antigen (MV-CEA) as a reporter gene was safe and well-tolerated in measles antibody-seropositive patients with recurrent GBM.[158,159] A recent study interrogated the impact of oncolytic measles virus on a panel of PDX lines

by RNA sequencing and gene set enrichment analysis.[160] A unique gene signature was identified that was predictive of response to measles virus, which suggests that it may be possible to select patients who would benefit from this therapy based on pretreatment gene signature analysis. Currently, an oncolytic measles virus expressing the sodium iodide symporter gene (MV-NIS) is being evaluated in a clinical trial for pediatric patients with recurrent medulloblastoma or atypical teratoid rhabdoid tumor (ATRT; NCT02962167).

Newcastle Disease Virus

Historically, tumor cells or oncolysates infected with Newcastle disease virus (NDV), an avian paramyxovirus, have long been investigated for use as cancer vaccines.[161,162] Csatary et al. reported durable remissions for over 5 to 9 years in four of 14 cases of GBM treated with MTH-68/H, an attenuated strain of NDV,[163] and significant regression of anaplastic astrocytoma in a pediatric patient when combined with the histone deacetylase inhibitor valproic acid, although remission lasted only 4 months before virus-resistant tumors emerged.[164] Similar results were observed in a clinical trial evaluating the oncolytic NDV-HUJ strain in GBM. While all patients eventually progressed, three out of 11 patients showed long-term survival ranging from 61 to 66 weeks, with one showing complete remission for some months.[165] More recently, a case series of 41 children with DIPG treated under compassionate use guidelines with individualized multimodal therapy combining NDV oncolytic virotherapy, hyperthermia, and autologous dendritic cell vaccines, reported median PFS of 8.4 months and median overall survival of 14.4 months, with 2-year overall survival of 10.7% and longer survival associated with Th1 responses, when this combinatorial therapy was in conjunction with first-line radiotherapy and chemotherapy; in contrast, median PFS and overall survival were 6.5 months and 9.1 months, respectively, when oncolytic virotherapy and immunotherapy were delayed until after disease progression.[166]

Parvovirus

Parvovirus H-1 PV has been shown to infect and kill human glioma cells, including glioma stem cells, in vitro.[167,168] Tumor lysates infected with H-1 PV were also shown to directly stimulate maturation of human APCs and cross-priming of human cytotoxic T cells,[169] an effect that could be potentiated by insertion of CpG motifs into the viral genome.[170] H-1 PV, now designated ParvOryx01, has recently been evaluated in a Phase 1/2a clinical trial in GBM patients (NCT01301430), using combined intratumoral and intravenous application,[171,172] and showed promising results in combination with bevacizumab.

Retrovirus

Retroviral replicating vectors (RRV) do not cause host cell lysis as a natural part of their infection cycle. Thus, RRV can maintain viral persistence in tumors through the combined characteristics of nonlytic replication, stable integration into the cancer cell genome, and reduced immunogenicity.[173] Toca 511 (*vocimagene amiretrorepvec*; now DB107) is an RRV encoding an optimized yeast cytosine deaminase (CD), which converts an antifungal prodrug, 5-fluorocytosine (5-FC), to the anticancer drug 5-fluorouracil (5-FU)[174] within infected tumors, leading to long-term survival benefit and development of durable antitumor immune responses.[175,176] Multicenter Phase 1 dose-escalation studies (NCT01156584, NCT01470794, NCT01985256) in recurrent high-grade glioma showed a highly favorable safety profile in over 128 patients to date with increased median PFS and OS compared to historical benchmarks.[177] Notably, 2-year survival rates (OS24) were 40% in higher dose cohorts, and post-treatment tumor specimens from some long-term survivors showed extensive necrosis and lymphocytic infiltrates, indicating radiographic pseudo-progression associated with induction of antitumor immunity.[177] An international randomized controlled Phase 2B/3 trial (NCT02414165) failed to meet its endpoints overall, but highly significant survival benefit was observed in pre-defined subgroups, including IDH mutant and grade III patients, as well as patients with two or more recurrences, which also correlated with those patients receiving more prodrug cycles.[178]

These results underscore the need to keep patients on immunotherapy trials for longer periods of time for effective antitumor immune responses to fully develop. Overall, the timeline for achieving partial response has been 1 to 2 years, and complete response may take about 3 years in the GBM patient population. Table 60.3 summarizes recent and current oncolytic virotherapy studies in patients with GBM and other malignant gliomas.

PERSPECTIVES OF IMMUNOTHERAPY IN BRAIN CANCERS

It has taken decades to revise the longstanding dogma that the CNS and tumors arising therein are "immunologically privileged." Well-designed preclinical and clinical studies, as reviewed in this chapter, have shown that brain tumors are susceptible to T cell-based immune responses to some degree. Nonetheless, the ultimate success of immunotherapy in brain tumor patients would require advancements in the following areas including, but not limited to, (a) strategies to address antigenic heterogeneity, (b) strategies to promote antigen-presentation and effector T cell trafficking, (c) strategies to overcome local and systemic immune suppression, and (d) proper

interpretation of imaging data for brain tumor patients receiving immunotherapy.

Address Antigenic Heterogeneity

Although the list of antigens that could be used for immunotherapy of brain tumors has expanded over the last decade,[97,98,179,180] there are not many shared and truly brain tumor-specific antigens, except for those derived from EGFRvIII,[66,67,110] H3.3K27M,[106,107] and mutant IDH1.[108] Due to marked heterogeneity of genetics and protein expression in solid cancers, targeting a single antigen may result in the evolution of variants that lack the target antigen.[110] These observations underscore the need for expanding the list of available tumor-specific antigens, such as mutation-derived antigens (i.e., neoantigens), for effective and safe immunotherapy.

Strategies to Promote Antigen-Presentation and Effector T Cell Trafficking

While brain tumors are heavily infiltrated by myeloid cells, the vast majority of them are suppressive for effector T cell functions but not effective APCs.[30] Efforts are being undertaken to modulate the function of these cells and promote their function as type 1 APCs.[181,182] In regard to improvement of T cell homing to brain tumors, to date, there have not been many immunotherapy regimens for brain tumors incorporating therapeutic agents that can facilitate T cell homing to the brain tumor site. Our regimens using poly-ICLC have been among the first to address this issue and are expected to enhance T cell homing to the glioma site.[25,28,123,183,184] Further refinements to this line of strategies are warranted to improve T cell homing.

Strategies to Overcome Local and Systemic Immune Suppression

As reviewed in earlier sections, brain tumors mediate a variety of immunosuppressive mechanisms. Furthermore, it is important to recognize that significant levels of systemic immunosuppression are likely caused by treatments for these patients. These include chemotherapy, such as temozolomide as standard-of-care,[75,185] and corticosteroids,[186] as well as radiation therapy.[75] Grossman et al. have suggested that lymphocyte counts alone are predictive of prognosis, with lower counts correlating with shorter survival in patients with GBM.[75] It is important to address how we can minimize the impact of treatment-induced immunosuppression by the time the patient receives immunotherapy, although for adoptive transfer of T cells, lymphopenic conditions induced by prior treatments may serve as a proper "conditioning," thereby promoting post-infusion expansion of T cells.

Table 60.3 Oncolytic Virotherapy Studies in Patients With Glioblastoma Multiforme and Other Malignant Gliomas

TRIAL NO./PHASE	PATIENTS	OV TREATMENT (STUDY TITLE)	CONTROL OR OTHER STUDY ARMS (ROUTE OF ADMINISTRATION)	PRIMARY OBJECTIVE	STATUS/RESULTS
NCT02031965 Phase 1	Recurrent childhood high-grade glioma; n = 2	Oncolytic HSV-1716 (Seprehvir) (Oncolytic HSV-1716 in Treating Younger Patients With Refractory or Recurrent High Grade Glioma That Can Be Removed By Surgery)	No control (intratumoral/peritumoral)	Safety DLT, MTD Radiographic responses	Terminated
2 Phase 1 studies (UK) 1 Phase 1/2 study (UK)	Primary or recurrent GBM or AA; 1st trial (Phase 1): n = 9 2nd trial (Phase 1): n = 12 Recurrent GBM; 3rd trial (Phase 1/2): n = 2	Oncolytic HSV-1716 (Seprehvir) (Phase 1 Trial of Single-Dose HSV-1716 in Patients With Primary or Recurrent Malignant Glioma) (Phase 1 Trial of Multiple-Dose HSV-1716 in Patients With Recurrent Glioblastoma)	No control 1st trial: HSV-1716 single injection 2nd trial: HSV-1716 single injection (expansion cohort) 3rd trial: HSV-1716 2 injections at 6-week intervals (intratumoral/peritumoral)	Safety Tolerability	Completed • 1 PR • 1st trial: four of nine subjects with 14–24 month survival • 2nd trial: three of 12 subjects with >15-month survival • 3rd trial: two doses of virus well tolerated
NCT00157703; Phase 1	Recurrent malignant glioma; n = 9	Oncolytic HSV G207 (G207 Followed by Radiation Therapy in Malignant Glioma)	No control (intratumoral)	Safety Tolerability AE	Completed • Well tolerated, no SAE • mOS 7.5 months • Six of nine patients w SD / PR
NCT00028158 (NGI-003); Phase 1b / 2	Recurrent GBM or GS (recurrent AA also included in Phase 1b); n = 21	Oncolytic HSV G207 (Safety and Effectiveness Study of G207, a Tumor-Killing Virus, in Patients With Recurrent Brain Cancer)	No control (intratumoral)	Safety Treatment response	Completed • No product-related SAE • Radiographic responses observed
NCT02457845; Phase 1	Pediatric progressive or recurrent supratentorial brain tumors (GBM, AA, PNET); n = 18	Oncolytic HSV G207 (HSV G207 Alone or With a Single Radiation Dose in Children With Progressive or Recurrent Supratentorial Brain Tumors)	No control G207 (intratumoral) + 5Gy radiation	Safety Tolerability AE ≥ Grade 3	Recruiting
NCT03911388; Phase 1	Pediatric recurrent or refractory cerebellar brain tumors (GBM, AA, PNET, etc.); n = 15	Oncolytic HSV G207 (HSV G207 in Children With Recurrent or Refractory Cerebellar Brain Tumors)	No control G207 (intratumoral) + 5Gy radiation	Safety Tolerability AE ≥ Grade 3	Recruiting
NCT02062827; Phase 1	Recurrent malignant glioma (recurrent or progressive GBM, GS, AA); n = 36	Oncolytic HSV M032 (NSC 733972) (Genetically Engineered HSV-1 Phase 1 Study for the Treatment of Recurrent Malignant Glioma)	No control (intratumoral)	Highest safe dose, MTD	Recruiting

(continued)

				Treatment-emergent AE Safety Tolerability	
NCT03657576; Phase 1	Recurrent GBM, GS, or AA; n = 24	Oncolytic HSV C134 (Trial of C134 in Patients With Recurrent GBM)	No control (intratumoral)		Recruiting
NCT03152318 Phase 1	Recurrent malignant glioma (recurrent or progressive GBM, AA, AO, etc.); n = 108	Oncolytic HSV rQNestin34.5v.2 (A Study of the Treatment of Recurrent Malignant Glioma With rQNestin34.5v.2)	Arm A: rQNestin (intratumoral) Arm B: rQNestin (intratumoral) + cyclophosphamide (intravenous)	MTD	Recruiting
UMIN000002661 Phase 1 / 2a	Recurrent GBM (n = 13 in Phase 2)	Oncolytic HSV G47Δ (now DS-1647)	No control (intratumoral, up to 6 injections)	MTD	Completed • OS12: 92.3%
NCT00805376 Phase 1	Recurrent malignant glioma (recurrent GBM, GS, AA, AO, etc.); n = 25	Oncolytic AdV DNX-2401 (DNX-2401 [Formerly Known as Delta-24-RGD-4C] for Recurrent Malignant Gliomas)	Arm A: DNX-2401 (intratumoral) Arm B: DNX-2401 + surgery	MTD	Completed • mOS 9.5 months • ORR 72% (18 of 25 subjects) • 3 CR, PFS ≥ 3 yr
NCT02798406 Phase 2	Recurrent GBM or GS; n = 49	Oncolytic AdV DNX-2401 + Pembrolizumab (Combination Adenovirus + Pembrolizumab to Trigger Immune Virus Effects [CAPTIVE/ KEYNOTE-192])	No control Three dose cohorts of DNX-2401 (intratumoral) + pembrolizumab (intravenous)	ORR	Active, not recruiting • mOS 12.3 months • Four of 48 subjects show responses • Two subjects with >94% regression • Three subjects alive >20 months
NCT02197169 Phase 1b	Recurrent GBM or GS; n = 37	Oncolytic AdV DNX-2401 (DNX-2401 With Interferon Gamma [IFN-γ] for Recurrent Glioblastoma or Gliosarcoma Brain Tumors [TARGET-I])	Arm 1: DNX-2401 (intratumoral) Arm 2: DNX-2401 (intratumoral) + interferon gamma (IFN-γ)	ORR	Completed
NCT03896568 Phase 1	Recurrent high-grade glioma (recurrent GBM, GS, AA with wild-type IDH1); n = 36	Oncolytic AdV-infected MSC (BM-hMSCs-DNX-2401) (Allogeneic Bone Marrow Human Mesenchymal Stem Cells Loaded With a Tumor Selective Oncolytic Adenovirus, DNX-2401, Administered Via Intra-Arterial Injection in Patients With Recurrent High-Grade Glioma)	Part 1: Oncolytic AdV DNX-2401 Part 2: Oncolytic AdV DNX-2401 + surgery (intra-arterial)	MTD, AE	Recruiting
NCT01956734 Phase 1	Recurrent GBM; n = 31	Oncolytic AdV DNX-2401 (Virus DNX-2401 and Temozolomide in Recurrent Glioblastoma)	No control DNX-2401 (intratumoral, peritumoral) + temozolomide	AE	Completed

(continued)

Table 60.3 Oncolytic Virotherapy Studies in Patients With Glioblastoma Multiforme and Other Malignant Gliomas (*continued*)

TRIAL NO./PHASE	PATIENTS	OV TREATMENT (STUDY TITLE)	CONTROL OR OTHER STUDY ARMS (ROUTE OF ADMINISTRATION)	PRIMARY OBJECTIVE	STATUS/RESULTS
NCT03178032 Phase 1	Newly diagnosed brainstem glioma (DIPG); n = 12	Oncolytic AdV DNX-2401 (Oncolytic Adenovirus, DNX-2401, for Naive Diffuse Intrinsic Pontine Gliomas)	No control (intratumoral, cerebellar peduncle)	Safety Tolerability Toxicity	Active, not recruiting
NCT03714334 Phase 1	Recurrent GBM; n = 24	Oncolytic AdV DNX-2440 (DNX-2440 Oncolytic Adenovirus for Recurrent Glioblastoma)	No control	Treatment-emergent AE	Recruiting
NCT01582516 Phase 1 / 2	Recurrent GBM; n = 20	Oncolytic AdV Delta24-RGD (Safety Study of Replication-Competent Adenovirus (Delta-24-rgd) in Patients With Recurrent Glioblastoma)	No control (intratumoral, convection-enhanced delivery)	Treatment-related SAE	Completed
NCT03072134 Phase 1	Newly diagnosed malignant glioma (GBM, AA, AO, etc.); n = 13	Oncolytic AdV-Infected NSC (NSC-CRAd-Survivin-pk7) (Neural Stem Cell-Based Virotherapy of Newly Diagnosed Malignant Glioma)	Arm 1: unresectable disease Arm 2: resectable disease (intratumoral)	Safety MTD	Completed
REO 003 Phase 1 / 2	Recurrent malignant glioma (GBM, AA, AO); n = 12	Oncolytic Reovirus (Reolysin) (Local Monotherapy of Reolysin for Patients With Recurrent Malignant Gliomas)	No control (intratumoral)	DLT, MTD	No SAEs related to treatment mOS 21 wks (range 6–234+), mPFS 4.3 wks (range 2.9–39) 1 SD, alive >54 mo
NCT00528684 Phase 1b	Recurrent malignant glioma (GBM, AA); n = 15	Oncolytic Reovirus (Reolysin)	No control (intratumoral, convection-enhanced delivery)	DLT, MTD	No DLT, MTD not reached mTTP 61 days (29–150), 2 SD w survival >2 yrs
ISRCTN 70443973 Phase 1b	Recurrent high-grade glioma or brain-metastatic cancer, any type; n = 6 (3 per cohort)	Oncolytic Reovirus (Reolysin) (REO13 Brain: A Clinical Study to Evaluate the Biological Effects of Preoperative Intravenous Administration of Wild-Type Reovirus (REOLYSIN®) in Patients Prior to Surgical Resection of Recurrent High-Grade Primary or Metastatic Brain Tumors)	No control Group A: recurrent high-grade glioma Group B: brain metastases, any tumor type. Cohort 1: Reolysin single dose Cohort 2: Reolysin three doses, days 1–3 Cohort 3: Reolysin 5 doses, days 1–5 (all intravenous)	Presence of reovirus in resected tumor specimens	Completed

(*continued*)

Trial	Population	Oncolytic Virus	Control/Delivery	Endpoint	Status/Results
ISRCTN 70044565 Phase 1/2	Newly diagnosed GBM; n = 24	Oncolytic Reovirus (Reolysin) (ReoGlio: Reolysin Plus GM-CSF in Combination With Standard-of-Care Chemotherapy and Radiotherapy for Patients With Glioblastoma Multiforme)	No control Reolysin (intravenous) GM-CSF (subcutaneous) TMZ (oral) Radiation	MTD	Active, not recruiting
NCT02444546 Phase 1	Pediatric recurrent or refractory cerebellar brain tumors (GBM, DIPG, AA, AO, medulloblastoma, PNET, AT/RT); n = 6	Oncolytic Reovirus (Reolysin) (Wild-Type Reovirus in Combination With Sargramostim in Treating Younger Patients With High-Grade Relapsed or Refractory Brain Tumors)	No control Reolysin (intravenous) GM-CSF (subcutaneous)	MTD, DLT	Active, not recruiting
NCT01491893 Phase 1	Recurrent GBM; n = 61	Oncolytic Poliovirus PVSRIPO (PVSRIPO for Recurrent Glioblastoma)	No control PVSRIPO (intratumoral, convection-enhanced delivery)	MTD, DLT Recommended Phase 2 dose	Active, not recruiting 1 DLT mOS 12.5 mo OS24: 21% (sustained at 36 mo) 2 CR, 6PR/SD
NCT03043391 Phase 1b	Pediatric recurrent high-grade glioma (GBM, GS, AA, AO, AT/RT, medulloblastoma, etc.); n = 12	Oncolytic Poliovirus PVSRIPO (Phase 1b Study PVSRIPO for Recurrent Malignant Glioma in Children)	No control PVSRIPO (intratumoral, convection-enhanced delivery)	Unacceptable toxicity	Active, recruiting
NCT02986178 Phase 2	Recurrent GBM; n = 122	Oncolytic Poliovirus PVSRIPO (PVSRIPO in Recurrent Malignant Glioma)	No control PVSRIPO (intratumoral, convection-enhanced delivery)	Objective radiographic response rate (iRANO)	Active, not recruiting
NCT00390299 Phase 1	Recurrent high-grade glioma (GBM, AA, AO); n = 23	Oncolytic Measles Virus MV-CEA (Viral Therapy in Treating Patients With Recurrent Glioblastoma Multiforme)	No control MV-CEA Arm A: peritumoral Arm B:	DLT, MTD Grade 3+ AE	Completed Arm A: SD in eight of nine subjects, mOS 11.8 mo, PFS6: 22% Arm B: SD in 12 of 13 subjects, mOS 11.4 mo, PFS6: 23%
NCT02962167 Phase 1	Pediatric recurrent medulloblastoma or AT/RT; n = 46	Oncolytic Measles Virus MV-NIS (Modified Measles Virus MV-NIS for Children and Young Adults With Recurrent Medulloblastoma or Recurrent AT/RT)	Local recurrence: MV-NIS (peritumoral) Disseminated: MV-NIS (intrathecal via lumbar puncture)	AE Recommended Phase 2 dose	Active, recruiting
(NCT01174537) Phase 1/2	Recurrent GBM; n = 11	Oncolytic Newcastle Disease Virus NDV-HUJ	No control NDV-HUJ (intravenous; intra-patient dose escalation	PFS	Completed OS: range 3–66 wks TTP: range 2–37 wks One CR, not durable Two possible pseudo-progression

(continued)

Table 60.3 Oncolytic Virotherapy Studies in Patients With Glioblastoma Multiforme and Other Malignant Gliomas (*continued*)

TRIAL NO./PHASE	PATIENTS	OV TREATMENT (STUDY TITLE)	CONTROL OR OTHER STUDY ARMS (ROUTE OF ADMINISTRATION)	PRIMARY OBJECTIVE	STATUS/RESULTS
NCT01301430 Phase 1/2	Recurrent GBM; n = 18	Oncolytic Parvovirus H-1 (ParvOryx) (Parvovirus H-1 in Patients With Progressive Primary or Recurrent Glioblastoma Multiforme)	No control ParvOryx (intratumoral, peritumoral, intravenous)	Safety, tolerability	Completed MTD not reached PFS 15.9 wks mOS 15.5 mo
NCT01156584 Phase 1	Recurrent high-grade glioma (GBM, AA, AO); n = 54	Retroviral Replicating Vector (Toca 511) + 5-Fluorocytosine Prodrug (Toca FC) (Study of a Retroviral Replicating Vector Combined With a Prodrug Administered to Patients With Recurrent Malignant Glioma)	No control Toca 511 (intratumoral) Toca FC (oral; tid for 6, 7, or 14 days every 4–6 wks)	MTD	Completed MTD not reached mOS 13.8 mo
NCT01470794 Phase 1	Recurrent high-grade glioma (GBM, AA, AO); n = 58	Retroviral Replicating Vector (Toca 511) + 5-Fluorocytosine Prodrug (Toca FC) (Study of a Retroviral Replicating Vector Combined With a Prodrug to Treat Patients Undergoing Surgery for a Recurrent Malignant Brain Tumor)	No control Toca 511 (peritumoral) Toca FC (oral; tid for 7 days every 4–8 wks)	DLT	Completed No DLT 6 CR, 10 SD mOS 14.4 mo, durable response rate 21.7%
NCT01985256 Phase 1	Recurrent high-grade glioma (GBM, AA, AO); n = 17	Retroviral Replicating Vector (Toca 511) + 5-Fluorocytosine Prodrug (Toca FC) (Study of a Retroviral Replicating Vector Given Intravenously to Patients Undergoing Surgery for Recurrent Brain Tumor)	No control Toca 511 (intravenous, peritumoral) Toca FC (oral; tid for 7 days every 4 wks)	MTD	Completed No DLT mOS 13.6 mo
NCT02414165 Phase 2/3	Recurrent high-grade glioma (GBM, AA); n = 403	Retroviral Replicating Vector (Toca 511) + 5-Fluorocytosine Prodrug (Toca FC) (Toca 5 Trial: Toca 511 & Toca FC Versus Standard of Care in Patients With Recurrent High-Grade Glioma)	Treatment arm: Toca 511 (peritumoral) Toca FC (oral; tid for 7 days every 6 wks) Control arm: physician's choice of TMZ (oral or intravenous), lomustine (oral), bevacizumab (intravenous)	OS	Terminated No DLT Overall mOS 11.1 mo (vs. controls 12.2 mo, N.S.) 2nd recurrence subgroup mOS 21.8 mo (vs. controls 11.1 mo, p = .016) AA, IDH mutant subgroups: median not reached (p = .009)

AA, anaplastic astrocytoma; AdV, adenovirus; AO, anaplastic oligodendroglioma; AS, adverse events; AT/RT, atypical teratoid/rhabdoid tumor; CR, complete response; DIPG, diffuse intrinsic pontine glioma; DLT, dose-limiting toxicity; GBM, glioblastoma multiforme; GS, gliosarcoma; HSV, herpes simplex virus; mOS, median overall survival; MTD, maximum tolerated dose; N.S., not significant; ORR, objective response rate; OS, overall survival; OS12, 1-year survival; PFS, progression-free survival; PFS6, PFS at 6 months; PNET, primitive neuroectodermal tumor; PR, partial response; SAE, severe adverse events; SD, stable disease; TMZ, temozolomide.

Proper Interpretation of Imaging Data for Brain Tumor Patients Receiving Immunotherapy

Immunotherapy clinical trials in brain tumor patients have revealed unique challenges associated with assessment of radiological changes reflecting delayed responses or therapy-induced inflammation.[187] Neuroimaging often reveals temporary worsening of abnormal findings and even appearance of new lesions. Clinical benefit, including long-term survival and tumor regression, can still occur following initial apparent progression. A multinational and multidisciplinary panel of neuro-oncology immunotherapy experts recently described immunotherapy response assessment for neuro-oncology (iRANO) criteria[188] that are based on guidance for determination of tumor progression outlined by the immune-related response criteria (irRC)[189] and the response assessment in neuro-oncology (RANO) working group.[190] The iRANO guidelines specifically address interpretation of initial progressive imaging findings in the context of neuro-oncology patients with a goal of decreasing the likelihood of premature discontinuation of potentially beneficial therapies while ensuring maximum patient safety. Prospective evaluation of the iRANO criteria in brain tumor immunotherapy trials for neuro-oncology patients will be required to improve their ultimate clinical utility.

CONCLUSION

Brain tumor immunotherapy research epitomizes translational research. As the brain is such a sensitive organ, we cannot afford significant autoimmune reactivity. Hence, we have to be particularly sensitive to the selection of target antigens and therapy strategies. Furthermore, the brain is located in the closed cranial space, making it particularly sensitive to treatment-induced inflammatory responses. This pertains to our needs to develop proper radiological response criteria. We have to integrate cutting-edge progresses in both cancer immunology and brain and CNS immunology. Multidisciplinary collaborations are the most essential method to move the field forward and provide patients with real hope for surviving the disease.

KEY REFERENCES

Only key references appear in the print edition. The full reference list appears in the digital product on Springer Publishing Connect: connect.springerpub.com/content/book/978-0-8261-3743-2/part/part04/chapter/ch60

39. Müller S, Kohanbash G, Liu SJ, et al. Single-cell profiling of human gliomas reveals macrophage ontogeny as a basis for regional differences in macrophage activation in the tumor microenvironment. *Genome Biol.* 2017;18(1):234. doi:10.1186/s13059-017-1362-4

68. O'Rourke DM, Nasrallah MP, Desai A, et al. A single dose of peripherally infused EGFRvIII-directed CAR T cells mediates antigen loss and induces adaptive resistance in patients with recurrent glioblastoma. *Sci Transl Med.* 2017;9(399):eaaa0984. doi:10.1126/scitranslmed.aaa0984

79. Cloughesy TF, Mochizuki AY, Orpilla JR, et al. Neoadjuvant anti-PD-1 immunotherapy promotes a survival benefit with intratumoral and systemic immune responses in recurrent glioblastoma. *Nat Med.* 2019;25(3):477–486. doi:10.1038/s41591-018-0337-7

90. Tawbi HA, Forsyth PA, Algazi A, et al. Combined nivolumab and ipilimumab in melanoma metastatic to the brain. *N Engl J Med.* 2018;379(8):722–730. doi:10.1056/NEJMoa1805453

121. Hilf N, Kuttruff-Coqui S, Frenzel K, et al. Actively personalized vaccination trial for newly diagnosed glioblastoma. *Nature.* 2019;565(7738):240–245. doi:10.1038/s41586-018-0810-y

136. Lang FF, Conrad C, Gomez-Manzano C, et al. Phase I study of DNX-2401 (Delta-24-RGD) oncolytic adenovirus: replication and immunotherapeutic effects in recurrent malignant glioma. *J Clin Oncol.* 2018;36(14):1419–1427. doi:10.1200/JCO.2017.75.8219

188. Okada H, Weller M, Huang R, et al. Immunotherapy response assessment in neuro-oncology: a report of the RANO working group. *Lancet Oncol.* 2015;16(15):e534–e542. doi:10.1016/S1470-2045(15)00088-1

Sarcomas

Seth M. Pollack

KEY POINTS

- Sarcomas are a family of rare cancers with incredible diversity. They are quite different from one another with respect to their tumor immune microenvironment and response to immunotherapy.

- While many sarcoma types do not respond well to programmed cell death 1 (PD-1) inhibitors, there are some subtypes including alveolar soft part sarcoma and undifferentiated pleopmorphic sarcoma that do appear to respond in some cases.

- Synovial sarcoma and myxoid round cell liposarcoma are translocation-related sarcomas that, despite having quiet immune microenvironments, may be good candidates for antigen-specific immunotherapy because of their consistent and homogenous expression of cancer testis antigens including NY-ESO-1.

INTRODUCTION TO SARCOMAS

Sarcomas are cancers of bone and soft tissue comprising approximately 1% of all new cancer diagnoses with an overall incidence averaging six new cases per 100,000/yr.[1] Together this group of mesenchymal malignancies accounts for over 20,000 new cases of cancer in the United States annually.[2] However, the approach to research and treatment of this group of diseases is complex as there are over 50 different sarcoma subtypes and some of them are quite rare; the individual subtypes frequently have completely unique biologic characteristics and clinical behavior.[3] Thus, while a busy oncologist in practice will generally see a handful of new sarcoma patients every year, that oncologist may never see patients with certain sarcoma subtypes in their entire career. Patients often will seek out care at large specialty referral centers as sarcoma specialists may be more experienced in treating patients with their specific subtype.[4,5]

Sarcoma classification is complex and even board-certified pathologists misclassify these tumors if they are not experienced with the nuances of bone and soft tissue pathology.[6] The first major dividing line in categorizing sarcomas separates the soft tissue sarcomas (STS) from the 12% of sarcomas originating from bone, an overwhelming majority of which are either osteosarcoma, chondrosarcoma, or Ewing sarcoma. Within STS subtypes, there are several additional critically important categories for classification purposes. Approximately 18% of sarcomas (1.5/100,000/yr) are gastrointestinal stromal tumors (GIST), a unique STS subtype driven by mutations of KIT and platelet-derived growth factor receptor A (PDGFRα) in most cases; treatment of these tumors has been transformed by tyrosine kinase inhibitors (TKIs).[7] Embryonal and alveolar rhabdomyosarcomas are pediatric STS subtypes that also have a unique paradigm of care and are often separated from the rest of STS for classification purposes.[2] The remaining 12,000 STS cases diagnosed in the United States annually (at least 4/100,000/yr) include over 50 different subtypes; the three most common subtypes—undifferentiated pleomorphic sarcoma (UPS), liposarcoma, and leiomyosarcoma (LMS)—together comprise a majority of the cases.[8]

The field of sarcoma has seen incredible success when investigators have focused on specific sarcoma subtypes. Ewing sarcoma, osteosarcoma, and the pediatric rhabdomyosarcoma subtypes each have a unique care paradigm combining locally targeted treatments with intensive cytotoxic chemotherapy that has completely transformed patient outcomes from very high mortaility (<20% survival at 5 years) to a situation where a majority of patients who present with localized disease are now likely cured.[9–11] Adjuvant imatinib has transformed the cure rate for patients with localized GIST and the development of multiple novel TKIs has made it so that now even patients with metastatic disease frequently live for more than 5 years.[7] Patients with perivascular epithelial cell tumors can have exquisite response to mammalian target of rapamycin (MTOR) inhibition[12] and patients with angiosarcoma can be surprisingly sensitive to weekly paclitaxel.[13] Tenosynovial giant cell tumor has an outstanding response to the CSF-1R inhibitor pexidartinib.[14] Epithelioid sarcoma may be sensitive to tazemetostat.[15] U.S. Food and Drug Administration (FDA) approvals have been grated to eribulin in liposarcoma and trabectedin in LMS and liposarcoma.[16,17]

However, these individual successes have only been transformative for a relatively small subset of patients and, for most, outcomes remain poor.[18] Surgery remains the mainstay of care for most STS patients and outcomes can be further improved through the use of adjuvant or neoadjuvant radiation and occasionally chemotherapy. However, even with properly administered multimodality therapy in the localized setting, patients with large, high-grade tumors have an over 50% chance of dying of their disease. Survival for patients with advanced disease remains less than 2 years for most sarcoma subtypes.[19–23] The traditional cytotoxic chemotherapy, doxorubicin, either alone or combined with the alkylating agent, ifosfamide, remains the standard front-line treatment.[24–26] Pazopanib is the only drug in the modern era to receive a broad FDA that includes all non-adipocytic STS subtypes.[27,28]

The use of immunotherapy in sarcoma has largely mirrored the successes and failures for therapeutics as a whole in this heterogenous family of cancers.[29,30] Broad investigations of the disease class as a whole have been disappointing and the field of immunotherapy in sarcoma has lagged behind other diseases.[31] However, it has become clear that individual sarcoma subtypes possess unique immunologic characteristics that make them uniquely suited for immunotherapeutic approaches, and in some instances may even be able to lead the rest of oncology. Alveolar soft-part sarcoma (ASPS) is a rare, translocation-driven cancer that strangely has an extremely high response rate to programmed cell death 1 (PD-1)-targeted therapies.[32] UPS is one of the most common genetically complex STS subtypes and also appears to respond to PD-1 inhibition.[33–35] Synovial sarcoma (SS) and myxoid/round cell liposarcoma (MRCL), by contrast, almost never respond to these agents but have remarkably high expression levels of cancer testis antigen immunotherapy targets.[36,37] Clinical trials that are not focused on specific sarcoma subtypes may not observe benefit, but when data are examined in more granular detail they may offer key insights into the strengths and weaknesses of various immunotherapies in individual contexts.[38] In this chapter, we will discuss the key clinical and immunologic factors shaping the development and application of immunotherapy for patients with sarcoma.

Coley's Toxin: The Original Immunotherapy

It is a sad irony that while sarcoma lags behind many cancers in the development of immunotherapy, it was actually one of the first malignancies ever targeted with immunotherapy. In the late 19th century Dr. William Coley, a sarcoma surgeon, noticed that osteosarcoma patients who survived postoperative infections might have improved long-term disease-free survival; this

effect was likely real in Coley's era though it is controversial whether this effect remains for patients with access to modern care.[39–42] This observation led Dr. Coley to hypothesize that intratumor injection of bacteria could provoke a life-saving immune response.[43] Given that sarcomas are frequently large and relatively superficial, they were well suited to percutaneous injection of "Coley's toxin," consisting of heat-inactivated *Streptococci*.[44] Despite anecdotal evidence of benefit in isolated patients, safety considerations, and difficulty demonstrating efficacy beyond individual case reports prevented Coley's toxin from becoming established as a part of standard care.[45]

Historic Perspective on Cytokine Therapies in Sarcoma

Perhaps because of the impressive, if isolated, successes of Coley's toxin, sarcomas were important malignancies for the clinical development of cytokine therapies in the 1980s and 1990s. Tumor necrosis factor-alpha became a key component of isolated limb perfusion, an important technique for sarcomas as well as melanoma,[46] where the vascular system of an extremity is connected to an oxygenated extracorporeal circuit, in such a way that a drug can be administered in the artery and removed from the vein and minimize systemic drug exposure. In practice, it is generally employed under mild hyperthermia conditions, in an effort to further increase the drug uptake in the extremity. Although isolated limb perfusion is quite effective at inducing tumor responses,[47] its use has been limited due to serious potential toxicities, particularly epidermolysis and deep tissue damage. However, it still plays an important role in limb tumors otherwise amenable only to amputation or as a substitute for mutilating surgery.

Interferon alpha (IFN-α) has been of great interest in osteosarcoma where early work has suggested potential benefit.[48] The EURAMOS-1 randomized clinical trial randomly allocated more than 700 patients with localized osteosarcoma following a good tumor response to standard neoadjuvant chemotherapy to receive four more cycles of chemotherapy with or without maintenance pegylated IFN-α2b for 18 months. The trial was negative, though some IFN proponents argued that there was a trend toward benefit in the IFN arm and a high attrition rate may have weakened the data set.[49] Case reports documenting potential clinical benefit to IFNs have been reported in selected STS histologies, most interestingly in hemangioendothelioma and ASPS.[50,51] Modern attempts to optimize systemic cytokine administration in novel formulation and in combination with potent, established immunotherapies for sarcoma are ongoing and discussed in the text that follows.

Mifamurtide

Mifamurtide (MTP: liposomal muramyl tripeptide phosphatidyl-ethanolamine) is a drug that activates macrophages, possibly through Toll-like receptor stimulation, derived from the cell wall of bacillus Calmette–Guérin (BCG) approved by European Medicines Agency (EMA) in 2009 for front-line treatment of osteosarcoma. Its role in sarcoma treatment is controversial as the evidence is based on a single trial with shortcomings; it is not currently approved in the United States. It was tested in a randomized clinical trial of the Children's Oncology Group in osteosarcoma patients treated with multi-agent chemotherapy.[52] MTP was thought to improve overall survival (OS) in one randomized clinical trial of localized osteosarcoma patients treated with multi-agent front-line chemotherapy.[53] Although the trial did observe an OS benefit, the trial had a factorial design, looking at both the efficacy of MTP and the addition of ifosfamide to standard chemotherapy with doxorubicin, cisplatin, and high-dose methotrexate. Although the trial was positive for MTP overall, it was negative for ifosfamide and additional analysis suggested that the benefit of MTP was in the negative ifosfamide-containing arm, which did not become standard of care. All this underlies the fact that the role of MTP in osteosarcoma remains controversial in the sarcoma community, with some practitioners still using it in Europe, though not in the United States.[54,55] Efforts to better define the proper role of MTP in the care of osteosarcoma patients are ongoing.[56]

THE SARCOMA TUMOR IMMUNE MICROENVIRONMENT

Sarcoma can be quite a frustrating field for immunotherapists who are looking for answers to some of the most basic immunotherapy-related questions about the sarcoma tumor microenvironment (TME): Are sarcomas highly mutated? Do sarcomas generally express programmed cell death ligand 1 (PD-L1)? Do they have infiltrating lymphocytes? Are they "hot" (inflammatory) or "cold" (non-inflammatory)? However, it bears repeating that sarcoma subtypes are different diseases with completely different underlying biologic features and clinical behaviors, so perhaps it should not be surprising there are no broad conclusions that summarize the TME.

Genetic Mutations and Microsatellite Instability

Mutational burden is a key factor determining responses to checkpoint inhibition.[57] It is a mistake to lump all sarcoma subtypes together and say the mutational burden is "low."[58,59] In fact, certain subtypes such as UPS, LMS, and de-differentiated liposarcoma (DDLPS) have above average numbers of genetic mutations. However, it is also true that some translocation-associated sarcomas will, in some instances, have no mutations other than the driving translocation.[60] Ideally, a nuanced approach is employed when discussing sarcoma biology, but when simplification is necessary it can be useful to classify sarcomas based on whether they are genetically "simple" or "complex" histologies, with genetically simple sarcomas having either few over/under expressed genes or a translocation that underlies them. The quarter of sarcomas classified as "simple-karyotype," characterized by chromosomal translocations (see Table 61.1), may be less inflammatory, but in some instances they may have other potential advantages for immunotherapy (see NY-ESO-1 targeting).[61]

Relatedly, microsatellite instability (MSI) can predict responses to CPI in a disease agnostic manner as mismatched repair genes can lead to large numbers of immunogenic mutations, particularly in malignancies, such as endometrial, gastric, and colorectal cancers.[62,63] MSI and mismatch repair deficiency are quite rare in sarcomas, likely in the 1% to 2% range, most commonly seen in unclassified sarcomas though it has been observed in cases of LMS.[64-66] However, there is one rare STS subtype which appears to frequently have inactivation of mismatch repair genes in a way that has proven to be critically important clinically. ASPS is a rare STS subtype (<1% of all STS) characterized by a nonreciprical t(X; 17) (p11.2;q25) translocation creating an ASPL-TFE3 fusion protein.[67] One of many downstream impacts of the fusion may be the silencing of hMSH2/hMSH1, resulting in mismatch repair deficiency.[68] This finding could, in part, explain why a translocation-related sarcoma is one of the most sensitive to PD-1 inhibitors.[32]

Programmed Cell Death Ligand 1 Expression, Major Histocompatibility Complex Expression, and Tumor-Infiltrating Lymphocytes

Similarly, some of the smaller series analyzing PD-1 and PD-L1 expression have at times had results that might initially appear to demonstrate conflicting results.[69-71] A registry of 2,539 patients with STS and bone sarcomas, evaluated with BD Pharmingen and R&D Systems antibody, found that 50% of them expressed PD-L1 by immunohistochemistry along with PD-1-positive tumor-infiltrating lymphocytes (TILs).[69] However, more granular analysis demonstrates that the sarcoma subsets differ widely with respect to their TME. UPS, a more mutated, genetically "complex" subtype, has significantly higher levels of PD-L1 expression as well as levels of T cell infiltration compared with other STS subtypes.[72] By T cell receptor (TCR) sequencing, these tumors have a higher clonality, which some propose as a metric for a more focused, possibly antigen-specific, response. These TIL are often organized together with tumor-associated macrophages (TAMs) and B cells into tertiary lymphoid structures which may play a critical role in patient survival as well as PD-1 inhibitor response.[73,74]

Table 61.1 Main Chromosomal Translocations in Sarcomas

HISTOLOGY	TRANSLOCATION	FUSION GENE
Alveolar rhabdomyosarcoma	t(2;13)(q35;q14)	PAX3-FOXO1A
	t(1;13)(p36;q14)	PAX7-FOXO1A
Ewing sarcoma	t(11;22)(q24;q12)	EWSR1-FLI1
	t(21;22)(q22;q12)	EWSR1-ERG
Desmoplastic small round cell tumor	t(11;22)(p13;q12)	EWSR1-WT1
Synovial sarcoma	t(X;18)(p11;q11)	SS18-SSX1
		SS18-SSX2
Myxoid liposarcoma	t(12;16)(q13;p11)	FUS-CHOP
Clear cell sarcoma	t(12;22)(q13;q12)	EWSR1-ATF1
Alveolar soft part sarcoma	t(X;17)(p11.2;q25)	TFE3-ASPL
Extraskeletal myxoid chondrosarcoma	t(9;22)(q22;q12)	EWSR1-NR4A3
Dermatofibrosarcoma protuberans	t(17;22)(q22;q13)	PDFGB-COL1A1
Inflammatory myofibroblastic tumor	t(1;2)(q22;p23)	TPM3-ALK
	t(2;19)(p23;p13)	TPM4-ALK
	t(2;17)(p23;q23)	CLTC-ALK
Low-grade fibromyxoid sarcoma	t(7;16)(q33;p11)	FUS-CREB3L2
	t(11;16)(p11;p11)	FUS-CREB3L1
Infantile fibrosarcoma	t(12;15)(p13;q26)	ETV6-NTRK3
Epithelioid hemangioendothelioma	t(1;3)(p36;q25)	WWTR1-CAMTA1
Solitary fibrous tumor	inv(12)(q13;q13)	NAB2/STAT6
Tenosynovial giant cell tumor	t(1;2)(p13;q37)	COL6A3-CSF1
Myoepithelial tumors of soft tissues	t(6;22)(p21;q12)	EWSR1-POU5F1
Endometrial stromal sarcoma	t(7;17)(p15;q21)	JAZF1/JJAZ1
	t(10;17)(q22;p13)	YWHAE/NUTM2

Some individual histologies (i.e., inflammatory myofibroblastic tumor, myxoinflammatory fibroblastic sarcoma, and follicular dendritic cell sarcoma) are by definition marked by an abundant chronic inflammatory infiltrate. Angiosarcoma, radiation-induced sarcomas, and myxofibrosarcomas have each been observed to have inflammatory infiltrates.[75–78] PD-L1 expression seems to be heterogeneous in osteosarcoma, with at least a subset of cases expressing high levels of PD-L1, correlating with the presence of TILs.[79]

Non-Inflammatory Microenvironments: Synovial Sarcoma and Myxoid/Round Cell Liposarcoma

In contrast, some of the less mutated, translocation-associated sarcomas SS and MRCL have a quiet TME with few T cells and low expression of PD-L1, though inflammatory infiltrates may accumulate outside the tumor margin.[80] By sequencing of the TCR, these tumors have a low T cell fraction, low clonality, and low expression of class I and II MHC molecules.[81] Some non-inflammatory translocation subtypes may evade immune recognition in part through expression of noncanonical MHC molecules despite T cell infiltration.[82] Despite strong non-inflammatory features, there has been hope that an endogenous immune response could be generated in SS and MRCL as they have consistent and strong expression of immunogenic self-antigens, particularly NY-ESO-1 as well as other cancer testis antigens.[36,37] It is important to recognize that while cancer testis antigens are expressed by many malignancies with patchy expression in a fraction of cases, SS and MRCL are in a different class with expression in over 80% of cases and most often homogenous expression throughout the tumor (see Figure 61.1).[83,84]

While the expression of numerous self-antigens has made SS and MRCL excellent candidates for targeted immunotherapy trials using adoptive cellular therapy and vaccines (see the text that follows), many investigators have speculated that they might also respond to non-antigen-specific immunotherapies only to be frustrated.[85] In an attempt to overcome this quiet TME, a

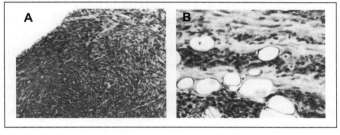

Figure 61.1 Classis strong, homogenous IHC staining of NY-ESO-1 in synovial sarcoma (A) and myxoid/round cell liposarcoma (B).

Phase 0 trial demonstrated that systemic weekly IFN-γ could alter the SS and MRCL TME through increased expression of MHC molecules and increased T cell infiltration, with a concomitant rise in PD-L1 expression.[86] These studies led to a trial of IFN-γ with adoptive cell therapy that proved toxic and a study through the Cancer Immunotherapy Trials Network IFN-γ and PD-1 inhibition with pembrolizumab (NCT03063632).[87]

Tumor-associated Macrophages, Regulatory T Cells, and Other Features of the TME

TAMs play a diverse set of consequential roles in the sarcoma TME, in addition to assisting in the organization of tertiary lymphoid structures as previously described.[88] TAM can be immune activating or inhibitory: M1 macrophages (HLA-DR^{high}) produce IL-12, can lyse tumor, and can be effective antigen-presenting cells (APCs). However, sarcoma tumors more commonly contain the immune inhibitory, M2 macrophages (CD163$^+$, CD206$^+$, CD115$^+$) that produce the inhibitory cytokines IL-10 and TGF-β. These cells have the potential to directly promote tumor growth, angiogenesis, and metastasis.[89] LMS tumors in particular have been noted to express gene signatures consistent with high levels of M2 TAM infiltration. High TAM numbers correlate with poor prognosis in LMS patients.[90] Gene expression profiles consistent with M2 phenotypic markers and increased expression of markers associated with M2 have been associated with worse outcomes independent of TAM presence.[91] Preclinical LMS models have demonstrated that elimination of TAM using an anti-CD47 antibody can result in tumor shrinkage and decreased number of metastasis.[92] While an extensive body of literature argues for the role of TAM in LMS immune evasion, TAM likely plays an important role in immunosuppression of many STS subtypes.[93]

Regulatory T cells (T$_{reg}$ cells) appear to be rare in most sarcoma subtypes; however, there may be some specific examples where they play an important role. In osteosarcoma, a high intratumoral CD8$^+$ T cell/Foxp3$^+$ (T$_{reg}$ cell) ratio assessed by standardized immunohistochemistry at the time of diagnosis was shown to correlate with a better prognosis.[94] T$_{reg}$ cells are likely quite important to the immunobiology of GIST through the actions of imatinib. GIST frequently has immune infiltrates and high density of T and natural killer (NK) cells correlate directly with progression-free survival (PFS).[95,96] Interestingly, imatinib has a complex interaction with the TME beyond inhibition of mutation KIT proteins through inhibition of T$_{reg}$ cells through decreased tumor production of indoleamine 2,3-dioxygenase (IDO)[97] while also shifting TAM from an M1- to an M2-like phenotype, though these converted macrophages ultimately revert again to the original M1-like cells.[98] High expression of PD-L1 in GIST correlates with a lower risk of both local and systemic progression, possibly because of an association between PD-L1 expression and immune cell infiltration.[99] A trial recently completed accrual at UCLA (NCT02880020) comparing single-agent nivolumab (anti-PD-1) alone or in combination with ipilimumab (anti-CTLA-4). A response observed in a refractory wild-type GIST may be further evidence that more exploration is warranted.[100]

IMMUNE CHECKPOINT INHIBITORS

Single-Agent Programmed Cell Death 1 Inhibition

Treatments targeting PD-1 and PD-L1 have transformed therapy for many solid tumors but adoption has been slow in sarcoma.[101] The first clinical trial testing the impact of a PD-1 inhibitor on sarcomas was the SARC28 trial of single-agent pembrolizumab. It demonstrated potential benefit for patients with UPS-inducing responses in 40% of that patient cohort, most of which were durable.[102] Dedifferentiated liposarcomas responded in two of 10 patients; however, an expanded cohort has raised questions regarding whether this is really a responsive tumor type.[103] Activity was poor for patients with SS and LMS, confirming a separate study using single-agent nivolimab to treat advanced uterine LMS saw little activity.[104] To be sure, a pooled analysis did demonstrate that LMS can respond, albeit infrequently;[105] a PTEN mutation may have led to treatment resistance in one particular case.[106]

The SARC28 trial also examined 40 patients with bone sarcomas. No responses were seen in Ewing sarcoma, one in osteosarcoma (5%), and one in chondrosarcoma (17%). At 1 year, PFS was consistent with a durable benefit in responding patients, reproducing the typical shape of curves seen within the initial studies of checkpoint inhibitors in other solid cancers (prolonged benefit in relatively few patients). Additional responses have been observed in chondrosarcoma, suggesting that this may be a subtype warranting further exploration.[107,108]

Given the paucity of options for metastatic sarcoma patients in the refractory setting, many centers are using these agents off label and observing clinical benefit though it is hard to discern subpopulations warranting additional study.[109] However, excellent responses in some patients, whether enrolled in a few prospective studies or through anecdotal reports, have been observed. Indeed, there are hints that patients with selected histologies might be more responsive than the average patient within heterogeneous and small clinical studies.[33,110] Angiosarcoma, for example, has been observed to respond in multiple series, and the activity of PD-1 inhibition is now being evaluated more formally in combination studies (NCT03512834).[111,112] Notable responses have been observed in epitheloid sarcoma[113] and GIST where additional evaluation is also pending (NCT02880020).[100,114]

Combination Therapies

CTLA-4 inhibition combined with anti-PD-1-targeted therapy improves survival for melanoma patients, albeit with more toxicity,[115] and this has been seen preclinically in some sarcoma models as well.[116,117] The Alliance trial combined nivolimab plus ipilimumab at a 1 mg/kg dose in refractory STS patients.[35] The combination was relatively well tolerated, and though a statistical comparison could not be made between the two trial arms, the response rate was 16% in the combination arm and 5% in the single-agent nivolimab arm. Further work exploring CTLA-4 targeting in combination with PD-1 blockage is ongoing (NCT03116529, NCT02834013).

Efforts to combine chemotherapy and checkpoint inhibition are ongoing. A Phase 1/2 trial of doxorubicin and pembrolizumab demonstrated the safety of the combination and found encouraging OS and PFS data, with responses that were durable as was disease stability, particularly for those patients with UPS and dedifferentiated liposarcoma.[34] Prior studies have demonstrated activity of low-dose cyclophosphamide in sarcoma patients.[118] Because this therapy is thought to decrease T_{reg} cell numbers, there was great hope that metronomic cyclophosphamide would synergize with pembrolizumab. However, a Phase 1/2 trial testing the combination saw little benefit, albeit with a small sample size for individual sarcoma subtypes.[119] Trabectedin is an FDA-approved chemotherapy used as part of the standard of care for LMS and liposarcoma, and is also frequently used in translocation-associated sarcomas.[120–122] Interestingly, trabectedin has been shown in multiple model systems to be highly potent in killing inhibitory macrophages, and this is likely an important mechanism of action in addition to its direct effect on tumor cells.[123,124] Trials combining trabectedin and checkpoint inhibitors (NCT03074318, NCT03138161) are ongoing. Gemcitabine may have a similar impact through its impact on the vasculature in addition to its direct antitumor activity (NCT03123276).

Small molecule "dirty" TKIs may act on numerous pathways, such as VEGF-R, that are highly relevant for success regarding checkpoint inhibition. The largest trial of a TKI in combination with a PD-1 inhibitor for sarcoma combined axitinib with pembrolizumab.[32] Because TKIs are such a critical part of the therapy regimen for ASPS patients, these patients were sought and accounted for 12 of the 36 patients despite their rarity among sarcoma patients. Partial responses were seen in six of the 11 ASPS patients evaluable for response; only two other partial responses were seen on the trial. Responses were durable and PFS at 6 months was 46.9%, which was viewed favorably for a refractory patient population. The results have made many sarcoma specialists incorporate this regimen as standard of care for ASPS patients. However, for other sarcoma patients, axitinib may make less sense as a TKI as it is not approved for sarcoma and lacks evidence of single-agent

activity. Pazopanib is an antiangiogenic TKI approved for advanced, refractory STSs with the exception of liposarcomas.[27,28] Activity of pazopanib and pembrolizumab has been observed in some case reports and series.[125,126] Sunitinib has been observed to facilitate TIL expansion by reducing the intratumoral content of myeloid-derived suppressor cells (MDSCs).[127,128] Work regarding further testing of a combination of nivolimab and sunitinib remains ongoing (NCT03277924) as do trials combining immune checkpoints and cabozantinib (NCT04551430).

ADOPTIVE CELLULAR THERAPY

Adoptive cell transfer (ACT) of genetically engineered and ex vivo selected endogenous T cells has induced durable complete responses (CR) in patients with otherwise incurable and fatal cancers.[129–131] One of the most important advances in ACT has been the development of chimeric antigen receptors (CAR) consisting of an extracellular antigen recognition domain coupled via transmembrane domains to the CD3ζ chain of the TCR, in addition to the CD28 and/or 41BB co-stimulatory receptor.[132] CARs have completely transformed the treatment of CD19+ lymphoid malignancies, particularly acute lymphoblastic leukemia leading to >90% CR rates in some settings.[133,134] Although CARs are extremely effective at recognizing and lysing cells expressing their target, the identification of promising targets is a huge challenge.

T cells that recognize their target through a TCR can be selected and cultured from the peripheral blood of patients but are more frequently engineered by inserting a T cell receptor (TCR) that may or may not have enhanced affinity.[135,136] Because TCRs recognize intracellular proteins displayed on the cell surface in the context of human leukocyte antigen (HLA), there are more established TCR targets; however, a given TCR will only work for patients with specific HLA types; HLA*0201 is one of the most common HLA types in the United States and in Europe.[137–139]

Cellular Therapy Targeting Cancer Testis Antigens in Synovial Sarcoma and Myxoid/Round Cell Liposarcoma

The consistent and robust expression of cancer testis antigens, including NY-ESO-1 and MAGE-A4, has allowed a wave of ACT trials that appear poised to change standard practice in the HLA*0201 expressing population of SS and MRCL patients. The original study piloted at the National Cancer Institute (NCI) in SS patients used a high affinity TCR that was altered to achieve even greater affinity.[140] Eighteen pretreated HLA-A0201 patients with a NYESO-1-positive SS were treated with TCR-engineered T cells, plus IL-2, after lymphodepleting chemotherapy (with cyclophosphamide and fludarabine).

Eleven of them (61%) demonstrated objective clinical response by the RECIST criteria, with 3- and 5-year estimated survival rates of 38% and 14%, respectively.[136,141]

Since this landmark study, a number of follow-up studies have each demonstrated similar results both in terms of response rate and potentially survival as well. Persistence has long been observed to be a critical factor in the success of ACT, and this is true for SS and MRCL as well.[142] Intensive lymphodepleting conditioning has long been known to improve T cell persistence possibly through inducing elevated levels of IL-7 and IL-15.[143] One study affirmed the critical importance of including lymphodepletion in the conditioning regimen as response rates seem to be less without it.[144] Ongoing trials are also targeting MAGE-A4, which is also a promising target and may have similar activity (NCT03132922).[145]

Additional trials targeting MAGE-A3, MAGE-A4, and MAGE-A10 are currently either in active enrolling clinical trials or follow-up analysis (NCT03139370, NCT02111850, and NCT02153905). CT antigen-specific T cells can also be purified and cultured from the blood of STS patients for use in treatment through stimulation with peptide-pulsed dendritic cells, sorting, and expansion; this has previously led to tumor regression in SS patients, and more trials are ongoing or in the analysis phase (NCT01477021, NCT02210104).[87,146] This method of T cell ACT-targeting multiple antigens (NY-ESO-1, MAGE family antigens, and PRAME) is being tested by Baylor (NCT02239861).

Other Adoptive Cell Therapies for Sarcoma

Historical attempts to treat sarcoma patients using lymphokine-activated killer cells[147–149] of ex vivo expanded TILs were essentially unsuccessful.[147] However, a new generation of TIL trials has emerged focusing on specific sarcoma subtypes and using modern approaches such as combination with checkpoint inhibitors (NCT04052334 and NCT03449108).[150]

A number of established CAR targets are now being targeted in the setting of sarcoma. Sarcomas may encode human epidermal growth factor receptor-2 (HER2) but lack of any amplification of the *HER2* gene, resulting in a low expression of HER2. Thus, an immunotherapy with HER2-specific CAR-modified T cells was tried in a Phase 1 and 2 study in osteosarcoma.[151] No responses were seen in this small study and there was no CAR T cell expansion (in the lack of any earlier lymphodepletion in this program); however, a truly impressive response to CAR T cells was seen in a rhabdomyosarcoma patient receiving HER2-targeted CAR T cells.[152] Targeting of the γ-subunit of the fetal acetylcholine receptor (fAChR) with CAR-engineered T lymphocytes has also been explored for the rhabdomyosarcoma patient; interestingly, this target can be induced with chemotherapy, specifically

on a rhabdomyosarcoma cell, suggesting potential synergy with CAR T cells.[153] A durable response to a CD56-targeted CAR has also been reported in rhabdomyosarcoma.[154] Among a variety of other targets that have been explored, VEGFR2 has been proposed as a target in Ewing sarcoma.[145] In chordoma, exploitation of the overexpression of chondroitin sulfate proteoglycan 4 (CSPG4), a melanoma-associated antigen, has been suggested as a target for T cell therapy.[155,156] CARs targeting the immune checkpoint B7-H3, EGFR, and GD-2 are currently being tested (NCT00902044, NCT02107963, NCT03618381, and NCT01953900).[157,158]

Other immune cells may also play a role in cellular therapy for sarcoma. Dendritic cell vaccines are being tested and these are discussed in the "Vaccination Strategies" section that follows. NK cells are being tested in the context of haploidentical allogeneic transplant (NCT02409576 and NCT02100891) as well as outside of the transplant setting (NCT02890758).[159,160] A recent report showed that MDSCs inhibited GD2-redirected T cells in a murine sarcoma model. Interestingly, all-trans-retinoic acid effectively blocked this inhibitory effect, restoring the antitumor efficacy against sarcoma xenografts, raising the possibility of possible therapeutic strategies for clinical investigation.[161]

VACCINATION STRATEGIES

Targeting NY-ESO-1 With Vaccination

Numerous prominent disappointments haunt the field of vaccination for sarcoma. However, clear isolated case reports of responding patients and clear immune monitoring data regarding an immune response suggest that the right vaccination, the right setting, and perhaps the right combination immunotherapy regimen could lead to success. The most recent disappointment in the field was the NY-ESO-1 vaccination LV305 by itself and as part of the CMB305 prime/boost vaccination regimen.[162] This unique vaccine was the first of a new class of agents leveraging an integration-deficient lentiviral vector selectively targeting CD209 on DCs via its envelope glycoprotein derived from Sindbis-virus,[163,164] inducing strong T cell responses in trials targeting NY-ESO-1 in SS and MRCL patients.[165,166] Presentation of an antigen expressed in the cytoplasm may induce a more potent CD8+ T cell response in comparison with the exogenously delivered peptides.[167] Phase 1/2 testing of this vaccine had impressive results with respect to 1 year OS (82%) with one notable patient developing a durable, near CR.[168,169] The combination of this vaccine with a Toll-like receptor 4 (TLR4) agonist and protein vaccine resulted in even further increased induction of antibody and CD4+ cell responses and with OS and PFS numbers that appeared better than historic controls.[170,171] However, this combination was most recently evaluated with a PD-L1 inhibitor (NCT02609984) without a clear positive outcome, and a proposed Phase 3 trial had difficulty with enrollment, leading to stoppage of the vaccine's development.[172] Another DC-targeted vaccine strategy uses a monoclonal antibody targeting CD-205 bound to the full-length NY-ESO-1 protein. This induced T cell responses in a pilot study for multiple tumor types including five sarcoma patients.[173]

Other Vaccine Approaches in Sarcoma

One exciting potential vaccine strategy currently in clinical trials uses autologous tumors engineered to express GM-CSF, with shRNA used to silence TGF-β, known as the "FANG" or "VIGIL" treatment. Isolated responses to this vaccination strategy have been previously observed and can be quite durable for some patients.[174,175] A randomized trial testing the vaccine with irinotecan and temozolomide chemotherapy is ongoing (NCT03495921).

A wide variety of other notable vaccine approaches have been tried in sarcoma-included whole tumor cells,[176] tumor lysates,[177] and irradiated cell lines.[178] One of the largest vaccine trials regarding sarcoma tested a trivalent peptide vaccine against widely expressed ganglioside antigens, which occurred in a placebo-controlled, multicenter trial, including 136 patients with a broad array of sarcoma subtypes who had no evidence of disease following metastasectomy.[179] Although more serological responses were seen following vaccination, there was no significant difference in PFS between the trial arms. A pilot study using peptides spanning the SYT-SSX fusion in SS patients resulted in one transient tumor response.[180,181]

Preliminary evidence of possible efficacy was reported in high-risk pediatric sarcoma patients of a tumor lysate and keyhole limpet hemocyanin-pulsed dendritic cell vaccine with or without recombinant interleukin-7 (IL-7) administered in the adjuvant setting following standard chemotherapy and autologous lymphocyte infusion.[182] Chordomas are marked in 95% of cases by overexpression of brachyury, a transcription factor related to the formation of the notochord, the remnants of which are thought to give rise to the tumor. Brachyury could well serve as an antigen,[183] and vaccination efforts are ongoing.[184] DC vaccines have been used to treat Ewing sarcoma and rhabdomyosarcoma using DC-pulsed tumor lysate or with peptides derived from the breakpoint regions of chromosomal translocations typical of these tumors, with potential evidence of immune response and better than expected survival.[182,185] One ongoing trial combines a DC vaccine with gemcitabine (NCT01803152).[186,187]

OTHER IMMUNOTHERAPY STRATEGIES

Oncolytic viral therapy has been limited in its application because it needs to be injected into tumors percutaneously.

However, because many sarcomas are large and superficial, they may be well suited to this therapy. Talimogene laherparepvec (T-VEC), an FDA-approved oncolytic virus for melanoma, may be well suited to STS as it is often superficial and injected at the bedside.[188] A trial of TVEC combined with pembrolizumab saw a response rate of 35% in a refractory patient population.[189] A trial combining T-VEC with nivolumab and trabectedin is also ongoing (NCT03886311). Oncolytic viral strategies are also being tested in other settings such as the University of Iowa, which is testing T-VEC in the neoadjuvant setting together with radiation (NCT02453191).

PLX3397 is a multitargeted TKI selective for the CSF1R kinase, c-Fms (CD115), and c-Kit.[190] A Phase 1 study combining PLX3397 and sirolimus is currently recruiting patients with unresectable sarcomas (NCT02584647). Humanized anti-CD47 monoclonal antibody (Hu5F9-G4) promoting macrophage phagocytosis has been tested in a Phase 1 trial for advanced solid tumors (NCT02216409).[191] Glucopyranosyl lipid A, a TLR4 agonist with similar impact on TAM that can recruit T cells to the TME, is being tested in combination with radiotherapy in order to increase tumor antigen release (NCT02180698)[192] Novel checkpoints with targets including B7-H3, OX40, GITR, and ICOS will surely be exciting to evaluate in sarcoma as the field continues to develop.[193-196] Compounds targeting inhibitory factor TGF-β must also be combined with these agents. New cytokine formulations, such as pegylated IL-2,[197] may work well in combination with many of these checkpoint strategies.

CONCLUSION

Immunotherapy in sarcoma has come a long way since the days of William Coley. Because sarcoma is such a complex group of diseases, it will undoubtably continue to be a major challenge to apply the lessons learned about immunotherapy from other cancers to sarcoma as a whole. However, breakthroughs will surely come as we examine the microenvironment of sarcoma subtype by subtype. The field of sarcoma research has much to offer the field of immunotherapy as there are so many unique diseases with individual biologic features that can be exploited by well-designed immunotherapeutic trials. Sarcomas can be large and superficial and thus are easy to biopsy and can be susceptible to therapies requiring percutaneous injection. Exploration of subtypes responsive to anti-PD-1 therapies, including ASPS and UPS may lead to unique insights regarding checkpoint inhibition. The uniquely high expression of cancer testis antigens in SS and MRCL allows these diseases to serve as models for the field as a whole. Through intensive study and focus, we are slowly starting to make progress in applying immunotherapy for sarcoma in a way that will help our sarcoma patients and improve the field of immunotherapy for cancer patients as a whole.

KEY REFERENCES

Only key references appear in the print edition. The full reference list appears in the digital product on Springer Publishing Connect: connect.springerpub.com/content/book/978-0-8261-3743-2/part/part04/chapter/ch61

32. Wilky BA, Trucco MM, Subhawong TK, et al. Axitinib plus pembrolizumab in patients with advanced sarcomas including alveolar soft-part sarcoma: a single-centre, single-arm, Phase 2 trial. *Lancet Oncol.* 2019;20(6):837–848. doi:10.1016/S1470-2045(19)30153-6

33. Tawbi HA, Burgess M, Bolejack V, et al. Pembrolizumab in advanced soft-tissue sarcoma and bone sarcoma (SARC028):
a multicentre, two-cohort, single-arm, open-label, Phase 2 trial. *Lancet Oncol.* 2017;18(11):1493–1501. doi:10.1016/S1470-2045(17)30624-1

35. D'Angelo SP. A multi-center Phase II study of nivolumab +/- ipilimumab for patients with metastatic sarcoma (Alliance A091401). *J Clin Oncol.* 2017;35:11007. doi:10.1200/JCO.2017.35.15_suppl.11007

72. Pollack SM, He Q, Yearley JH, et al. T-cell infiltration and clonality correlate with programmed cell death protein 1 and programmed death-ligand 1 expression in patients with soft tissue sarcomas. *Cancer.* 2017;123(17):3291–3304. doi:10.1002/cncr.30726

136. Robbins PF, Kassim SH, Tran TL, et al. A pilot trial using lymphocytes genetically engineered with an NY-ESO-1-reactive T-cell receptor: long-term follow-up and correlates with response. *Clin Cancer Res.* 2015;21(5):1019–1027. doi:10.1158/1078-0432.CCR-14-2708

62

Pediatric Cancers: Neuroblastoma

Maya Suzuki and Nai-Kong V. Cheung

KEY POINTS

- Pediatric embryonal tumors have few mutation-based neoantigens, are often downregulated in major histocompatibility complex (MHC), and are embedded in immunosuppressive tumor microenvironments (TMEs).

- The immune system in children is immature and tumor-specific immunity is not well developed.

- Immunoglobulin G (IgG)-driven natural killer (NK) and myeloid effector–based immunotherapy against disialoganglioside (GD2) have significantly improved the overall survival (OS) of patients with high-risk neuroblastoma.

- Compartmental radioimmunotherapy (cRIT) using ^{131}I-3F8 or ^{131}I-8H9 has changed the long-term outlook for neuroblastoma patients who relapse in the central nervous system (CNS).

- T cell–based therapies using chimeric antigen receptor (CAR) or bispecific antibodies could engage a potent effector immune cell population and are in clinical trials.

- Checkpoint blockade could potentially enhance immunotherapy during NK cell-based (e.g., inhibitory killer immunoglobulin-like receptor [KIRs]) or during T cell-based (B7-H1 or B7-H3) therapies.

- The vaccination effect following tumor-directed IgG (e.g., idiotype network) or T cell-engaging strategies (e.g., epitope spread) could potentially help maintain long-term remission.

- Vaccination strategies using whole tumors, tumor antigens, or anti-idiotypic antibodies in the presence of appropriate adjuvant (e.g., OPT-821 and oral beta-glucan) offer another opportunity to build long-term antitumor immunity.

- The clinical development of cytokines beyond interleukin-2 (IL-2; e.g., IL-7 or IL-15) holds promise for enhancing the antitumor effects of both antibody-based and cell-based therapies.

- With evidence-based targets and appropriate timing of the treatment strategies, immunotherapy, although most effective for eliminating minimal residual disease (MRD), has the potential to complement chemotherapy, radiation therapy, and small molecules in the curative approach to pediatric cancers beyond neuroblastoma.

INTRODUCTION

Immunotherapy is a proven modality against human cancers. Pediatric embryonal cancers and the immune system in children are unique. Childhood tumors have low mutational burden; hence, they have few mutation-based neoantigens, often downregulate their major histocompatibility complex (MHC) proteins, and are embedded in immunosuppressive tumor microenvironments (TMEs). In childhood, the immune system is immature and tumor-specific immunity is not well developed. Neuroblastoma is one of the few pediatric cancers where immunotherapeutic strategies have finally borne fruit. Monoclonal IgG antibody-driven natural killer (NK) and myeloid effector–mediated antitumor mechanisms against disialoganglioside GD2 have significantly improved the overall survival (OS) of patients with high-risk neuroblastoma. By summarizing the preclinical and clinical evolution of immunotherapies against neuroblastoma, including both passive and active immunotherapies, this chapter intends to bring clarity to their potentials and hurdles in order to formulate future directions for pediatric cancers in general.

PEDIATRIC CANCERS: NEUROBLASTOMA

Pediatric *embryonal* cancers and their tumor immune environment are unique. Although acute lymphoblastic leukemia is most common and curable among cancers in children, *metastatic* solid tumors are often fatal. The expression of MHC is often low or absent in pediatric solid tumors, including neuroblastoma, Ewing sarcoma, and alveolar rhabdomyosarcoma,[1] and is accompanied by overexpression of immune inhibitory molecules like programmed death-ligand 1 (PD-L1) and B7-H3.[2,3] In addition to the immunosuppressive TME, the *neoantigen* landscape based on mutation load is far more restricted among pediatric tumors (less than 10 mutations per tumor),[4,5] thereby limiting the potential actionable repertoire of immune targets. Furthermore, these cancers typically affect young children when the innate and adaptive immune systems are naïve, with little time to enrich tumor-specific adaptive immunity. Partly because of the limited repertoire of neoantigens, available targets for immunotherapy in children are seldom tumor specific and are often directed at differentiation antigens leading to autoimmune side effects—a consideration of particular relevance if cured patients are expected to live for decades. Unlike adult cancers, pediatric tumors are chemosensitive, and high chemotherapy doses and intensities are feasible in children, who generally have few comorbidities. Yet, relapse and death after achieving remission are common among patients whose disease is metastatic at diagnosis. Hence, treatment strategies to control or eliminate minimal residual disease (MRD) following induction have been a major focus since the 1990s. Not to be overlooked is the price for achieving this remission, which can be complicated by long-term crippling treatment-related toxicities in various organs. Hence, the reduction of upfront genotoxic therapy without compromising the chance of cure is an urgent and unmet need. Immunotherapy holds promise, not just for ablating MRD but also for complementing conventional therapies in the continuing effort to reduce late effects.

NEUROBLASTOMA

Neuroblastoma is the third most common cancer in childhood, following leukemia and brain tumor, with an incidence of 10.2 cases per million children younger than 15 years.[6] It is the most common solid cancer during the first year of life, accounting for more than 20% of malignancies.[7] Neuroblastoma is an embryonal tumor arising from neural-crest progenitor cells of the sympathetic nervous system, typically in the adrenal medulla or sympathetic ganglia. The clinical entity called *neuroblastoma* is not only heterogeneous in its seed (tumor) but also heterogeneous in its soil (immune system).[8] Despite widespread disease at diagnosis, neuroblastoma in infants (stage 4S) can regress without any treatment. Stage 4S neuroblastoma has more expression of class I MHC than neuroblastoma of other stages, which should make them susceptible to cytotoxic T cells.[9] Many have speculated that because 4S neuroblastomas develop in utero,[10] fetal circulating neuroblastoma cells may cross the placenta[11,12] to sensitize

the maternal immune system. However, only immunoglobulin M (IgM) antibodies have so far been reported among mothers,[13] an antibody class consistent with short immunological exposure during the gestational period. In adults, neuroblastoma characteristically has an indolent clinical behavior, and tumor-infiltrating lymphocytes (TILs) are more abundant than in neuroblastomas arising in adolescents or preadolescents,[14] suggesting an age-dependent immune response that could modulate the tempo of tumor progression. The relatively low frequency of somatic mutations in neuroblastomas in all age groups[4] has posed a major challenge for classic T cell–based immunotherapy and for targeted molecular therapy. Although the rationale for combining these targeted therapies is strong in adult cancers, which have a much larger mutational load, its application to pediatric cancers may be limited. A better understanding of the tumor biology and host immune system will be the key to the development of novel immunologic strategies. Here, we summarize the preclinical and clinical developments of immunotherapy for neuroblastoma and derive lessons learned that may explain immune resistance at different disease stages and in diverse age groups, from practice to principles potentially applicable to other malignancies in children.

PASSIVE IMMUNOTHERAPY

Table 62.1 summarizes clinical studies of passive immunotherapy in neuroblastoma using a variety of therapeutic approaches.

Anti-Disialoganglioside GD2 Monoclonal Antibody

Murine IgG3 Anti-GD2 Monoclonal Antibody 3F8

Disialoganglioside GD2 is overexpressed in a spectrum of embryonal cancers, including neuroblastoma, osteosarcoma, other sarcomas, and brain tumors,[37,38] and it is associated with tumor proliferation, invasion, and motility.[39] GD2 expression in normal tissues is restricted to the basal layer of skin, the central nervous system (CNS), and peripheral sensory nerves.[38] Because of its high expression on tumor cell surface and restricted expression in normal tissues, GD2 is an ideal target for cancer therapy. However, in young children, host immune response to carbohydrate antigens like GD2 is suboptimal. As polysaccharides are thymus independent (TI) type 2 antigens, generally not recognized by T lymphocytes, they (e.g., GD2) generally do not activate naïve B lymphocytes by themselves.[40,41] GD2 is a pentasaccharide anchored with ceramide tail embedded in the lipid bilayer; even with its clustering on the cell membrane, GD2 is not mitogenic for B lymphocytes. It is not surprising that anti-GD2 responses in young children are rarely detectable. The murine anti-GD2 IgG3 monoclonal antibody (mAb) 3F8 was developed and tested in the first-in-human Phase

Table 62.1 Clinical Trials of Passive Immunotherapy for Neuroblastoma (as of June 2020)

IMMUNOTHERAPY	TRIAL	PHASE	NCT	RESULT
Anti-GD2 mAb	Mouse 3F8 for metastatic NB in second complete remission	2	00002458	Not yet reported
	Mouse 3F8 + GM-CSF for first complete remission HR NB	2	01183429	5-year OS: 61%–80%[15]
	Mouse 3F8 + GM-CSF for primary refractory NB in bone marrow	2	01183897	Not yet reported
	Mouse 3F8 + GM-CSF for HR NB	2	00072358	2-year PFS: 48% in primary refractory NB patients[16]
	Mouse 3F8 + GM-CSF for first/second complete remission/refractory HR NB	N/A	02100930	58% no evidence of disease, 4.3% CR, 1.4% PR, 8.7% SD, 27.5%
	Mouse 3F8 + beta-glucan for metastatic NB	1	00037011	Not yet reported
	Mouse 3F8 + GM-CSF + beta-glucan for refractory NB	2	00089258	Not yet reported
	Chimeric 14.18 + GM-CSF + IL-2 for HR NB	1	00005576	Not yet reported
	Chimeric 14.18 + GM-CSF + IL-2 for HR NB	3	00026312	4-year OS: 74 ± 4% versus control 59 ± 5% side effects with IL-2[17]
	Dinutuximab (Chimeric 14.18) + lenalidomide for relapsed/refractory NB	1	01711554	1 CR, 3 PR out of 21 patients[18]
	Dinutuximab (Chimeric 14.18) + GM-CSF with irinotecan, temozolomide for relapsed/refractory NB	2	01767194	41.5% ORR, 1-year OS: 84.9 ± 4.9%, 1-year PFS 67.9 ± 6.4%[19]
	Dinutuximab beta (Chimeric 14.18/CHO) for primary relapsed/refractory NB	2	02743429	2-year OS: 64 ± 6%[20]
	Dinutuximab beta (Chimeric 14.18/CHO) ± IL-2 for HR NB	3	01704716	3-year EFS: 60% with IL-2 versus 56% without IL-2 3-year OS: 70% with IL-2 versus 69% without IL-2 Because of toxicity, only 62% completed dinutuximab beta with IL-2 versus 87% without IL-2[21]
	Chimeric 14.18/CHO + nivolumab	1	02914405	Not yet reported
	Humanized 3F8 for HR NB and GD2(+) tumors	1	01419834	MTD was not reached at 3 mg/kg/cycle. Pain was less than with m3F8[22]
	Humanized 3F8 + IL-2 for HR NB and GD2(+) tumors	1	01662804	Well tolerated at humanized 3F8 dosage 0.9 mg/kg (preliminary result)[23]
	Humanized 3F8 + GM-CSF for relapsed/refractory HR NB	1/2	01757626	75% CR in bone/bone marrow[24]
	Naxitamab (humanized 3F8) + GM-CSF for NB with refractory/incomplete response to salvage therapy in bone and/or bone marrow	2	03363373	67% CR, 8% PR[25]

(continued)

Table 62.1 Clinical Trials of Passive Immunotherapy for Neuroblastoma (as of June 2020) (*continued*)

IMMUNOTHERAPY	TRIAL	PHASE	NCT	RESULT
Anti-GD2 mAb	Naxitamab (humanized 3F8) + GM-CSF + irinotecan + temozolomide for chemoresistant HR NB	2	03189706	9 CR, 8 PR out of 46 patients after two cycles[26]
	Humanized 14.18K322A for NB, osteosarcoma, EWS, and melanoma	1	00743496	MTD and RP2D 60 mg/m^2. DLT including cough, asthenia, sensory neuropathy[27]
	The concomitant use of humanized 14.18K322A and induction chemotherapy for HR NB	2	01857934	80% PR/VGPR after two courses of induction chemotherapy (preliminary result)
Immunocytokine	Humanized 14.18-IL-2 fusion protein for relapsed/refractory NB and melanoma	1	00003750	MTD was 12 mg/m^2/day. DLT including hypotension, allergic reaction[28]
	Humanized 14.18-IL-2 fusion protein for relapsed/refractory NB	2	00082758	21.7% CR for MIBG or BM-only disease[29]
RIT	^{131}I-8H9 for CNS or LM cancers	1	00089245	62% alive (mean OS 82.6 months)[30]
	^{131}I-3F8 for CNS or LM cancers	2	00445965	
	^{131}I-omburtamab (^{131}I-8H9) for CNS or LM NB	2/3	03275402	Not yet reported
T cell-based immunotherapy	First-generation anti-GD2 CAR-modified T cells and EBV-specific CTL for NB	1	00085930	Three out of 11 patients achieved CR[31]
	Anti-GD2 CAR-modified T cells for relapsed/refractory NB	1/2	02919046	Not yet reported
	iC9-GD2-CAR-modified T cells for HR and/or relapsed/refractory NB	1/2	03373097	Not yet reported
	Second-generation anti-GD2 CAR-modified T cells for relapsed/refractory NB	1	02761915	One out of three patients treated with 1x10^8 cells had response in bone/BM[32]
	Third-generation anti-GD2 CAR-modified T cells for GD2(+) solid tumors	1	02107963	Not yet reported
	Third-generation iC9 -GD2 CAR-modified T cells for GD2(+) solid tumors	1	01822652	Not yet reported
	iC9-GD2-CAR-VZV-CTLs for refractory/metastatic GD2(+) sarcoma	1	01953900	Not yet reported
	Anti-GD2-Tri virus-CTLs for relapsed/refractory NB	1	01460901	Not yet reported
	Third-generation iC9-GD2 -CAR-IL-15 T cells for relapsed/refractory NB	1	03721068	Not yet reported
	Fourth-generation anti-GD2 CAR-modified T cells for relapsed/refractory NB	2	02765243	15% PR at 1-year observation point[33]
	Second/Third-generation anti-CD171 CAR-modified T cells for relapsed/refractory NB	1	02311621	Dose-limiting hyponatremia was observed in two patients. No objective response. (Preliminary result)

(*continued*)

Table 62.1 Clinical Trials of Passive Immunotherapy for Neuroblastoma (as of June 2020) (*continued*)

IMMUNOTHERAPY	TRIAL	PHASE	NCT	RESULT
T cell-based immunotherapy	C7R-GD2 CAR-modified T cells for relapsed/refractory NB and GD2(+) cancers	1	03635632	Not yet reported
	Second-generation anti-EGFR CAR-modified-T cells for relapsed/refractory solid tumors	1	03618381	Not yet reported
	Anti-GD2 BsAb-armed ATCs for NB and osteosarcoma	1/2	02173093	MTD was not reached. Out of seven NB patients, one achieved complete bone marrow response and one had minor response on MIBG scan. (Phase 1)[34]
	Humanized 3F8 bispecific antibody for relapsed/refractory NB, osteosarcoma, and other GD2(+) solid tumors	1	03860207	Not yet reported
NK cell-based immunotherapy	Autologous NK cells and rhIL-15	1	01875601	Not yet reported
	Allogeneic NK cells and anti-GD2 3F8 antibody for	1	00877110	29% CR/PR[35]
	Haploidentical NK cell and CD133+ autologous stem cell for HR solid tumors and lymphomas	1	02130869	Not yet reported
	Allogeneic NK cells and anti-GD2 humanized 3F8 antibody for HR NB	1	02650648	Not yet reported
	Haploidentical NK cells and anti-GD2 antibody (chimeric 14.18/CHO) for HR/relapsed NB	1/2	03242603	Not yet reported
	Autologous NK cells + anti-GD2 antibody (ch14.18) + lenalidomide for relapsed/refractory NB	1	02573896	Not yet reported
	Haploidentical NK cells and immunocytokine (humanized 14.18-IL-2) for relapsed/refractory NB	1	03209869	Not yet reported
	Autologous NK cells + irinotecan, temozolomide + dinutuximab for relapsed/refractory NB	1/2	04211675	Not yet recruiting
	Chemotherapy + humanized 14.18K322A + GM-CSF + IL-2 with allogenic NK cells for relapsed/refractory NB	1	01576692	61.5% response (pilot study)[36]
NKT cell-based immunotherapy	Second-generation anti-GD2 CAR-modified NKT cell for relapsed/refractory NB	1	03294954	Not yet reported
	Third-generation anti-GD2 CAR-modified NKT cells for relapsed/refractory NB	1	02439788	Not yet reported
	Anti-GD2-CAR-IL-15 NKT cells for relapsed/refractory NB	1	03294954	Not yet reported

ATC, activated T cell; BM, bone marrow; CAR, chimeric antigen receptor; CHO, Chinese hamster ovary cells; CNS, central nervous system; CR, complete response; CTL, cytotoxic T lymphocyte; CTR, constitutively active IL-7 cytokine receptor; DLT, dose limiting toxicity; EBV, Epstein–Barr virus; EFS, event-free survival; EWS, Ewing sarcoma; GM-CSF, granulocyte-macrophage colony-stimulating factor; HR, high risk; I, iodine; iC9, inducible caspase-9; IL, interleukin; LM, leptomeningeal; mAb, monoclonal antibody; MIBG, metaiodobenzylguanidine; MTD, maximum tolerated dose; N/A, not applicable; NB, neuroblastoma; NCT, National Clinical Trial number; NK cells, natural killer cells; NKT cells, natural killer T cells; ORR, overall response rate; OS, overall survival; PFS, progression-free survival; PR, partial response; rh, recombinant human; RIT, radioimmunotherapy; RP2D, recommended phase 2 dose; SD, stable disease; VGPR; very good partial response; VZV, varicella zoster virus.

1 study in patients with neuroblastoma in the mid-1980s.[42] Anti-GD2 mAbs engage Fc-dependent tumor lysis, including antibody-dependent cellular cytotoxicity (ADCC) mediated by NK cells and myeloid effector–mediated ADCC, antibody-dependent cell-mediated phagocytosis (ADCP), and complement-mediated cytotoxicity (CMC; Figure 62.1).[43] In addition, anti-GD2 mAbs can induce apoptosis and reduce motility of tumor cells by inhibiting focal adhesion kinase (FAK) phosphorylation and PI3K/Akt pathways, respectively.[44,45] By immunohistochemistry, the expression of GD2 in neuroblastoma is relatively homogeneous within a tumor and between tumors, and GD2 loss is rare but reported following anti-GD2 immunotherapy;[46,47] the wax and wane of GD2 expression could explain why anti-GD2 mAbs could fail.[47] In patients, iodine-131 (^{131}I)-labeled 3F8 (mouse IgG3) binds selectively to neuroblastoma with minimal nonspecific uptake in skin or CNS.[48] Major side effects (including pain, fever, hypertension, and urticaria) from

3F8 treatment are managed pharmacologically,[42] with no known long-term side effects during a 30-year follow-up. Phase 2 clinical trials using 3F8 in combination with granulocyte-macrophage colony-stimulating factor (GM-CSF) have shown long-term OS among patients with high-risk neuroblastoma (stage 4 diagnosed at 18 months or older age or stage 4 with tumor *MYCN* amplification) at 5 years of 61% to 80% compared to historical OS of less than 30% (Figure 62.2).[15] NK cells play key roles through ADCC and cytokine release when activated through FcγRIIIA (CD16A).[49] In retrospective analysis of large patient cohorts, outcome was strongly influenced by the level of expression of killer immunoglobulin-like receptor (KIR) 3DL1, a polymorphic receptor on NK cells that interacts with specific human leukocyte antigen (HLA)–B subtypes. The absence of interaction between KIR-3DL1 and HLA-B subtypes allows more robust ADCC, thereby improving both progression-free survival (PFS) and OS.[50] The potential importance of myeloid-ADCC (both

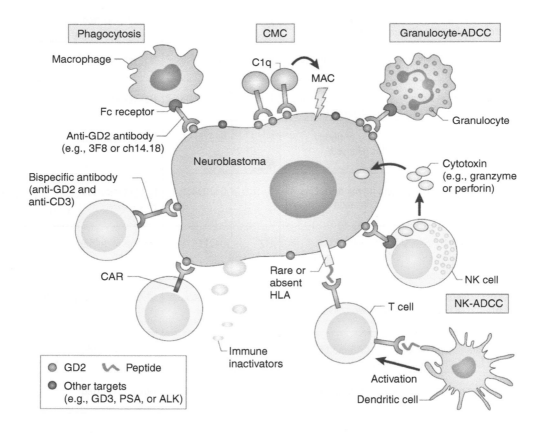

Figure 62.1 Immunotherapy in neuroblastoma. Anti-GD2 mAb can induce NK cell-mediated ADCC, granulocyte-mediated ADCC, phagocytosis, and CMC.

ADCC, antibody-dependent cellular cytotoxicity; ALK, anaplastic lymphoma kinase; CAR, chimeric antigen receptor; CMC, complement-mediated cytotoxicity; HLA, human leukocyte antigen; mAb, monoclonal antibody; NK, natural killer, PSA, polysialic acid.

Source: Adapted and modified with permission from Cheung NK, Dyer MA. Neuroblastoma: developmental biology, cancer genomics and immunotherapy. *Nat Rev Cancer*. 2013;13(6):397–411. doi:10.1038/nrc3526

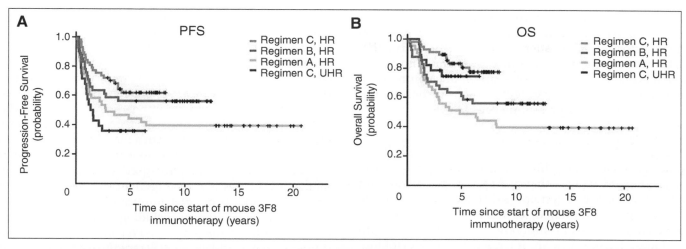

Figure 62.2 Survival for 169 patients with stage 4 neuroblastoma in first remission after consecutive anti-GD2 mAb immunotherapy regimens. (A) PFS: $p = .018$ (derived from log-rank test to compare PFS among these four groups). **(B)** OS: $p = .003$ (derived from log-rank test to compare OS among these four groups). Regimens: 3F8 alone (regimen A–HR; $n = 43$), 3F8 + intravenous GM-CSF + 13-*cis*-retinoic acid (regimen B–HR; $n = 41$), and 3F8 + subcutaneous GM-CSF + 13-*cis*-retinoic acid (regimen C–HR; $n = 57$ and regimen C–UHR; $n = 28$).

GM-CSF, granulocyte-macrophage colony-stimulating factor; HR, high risk; mAb, monoclonal antibody; OS, overall survival; PFS, progression-free survival; UHR, ultra-high risk.

Source: Adapted and modified with permission from Cheung NK, Cheung IY, Kushner BH, et al. Murine anti-GD2 monoclonal antibody 3F8 combined with granulocyte-macrophage colony-stimulating factor and 13-*cis*-retinoic acid in high-risk patients with stage 4 neuroblastoma in first remission. *J Clin Oncol.* 2012;30(26):3264–3270. doi:10.1200/JCO.2011.41.3807

neutrophil and macrophage-dependent) and its influence by FcγRIIA (CD32A) polymorphism on myeloid cells is also notable.[51] MRD negativity (measured by quantitative reverse transcriptase-polymerase chain reaction [qRT-PCR] of a four-marker panel) in bone marrow may provide an early response indicator predicting both PFS and OS—a powerful tool to evaluate treatment impact such as adjuvant immunotherapy after achieving remissions.[52] The ability to mount a human anti-mouse antibody (HAMA) response is consistently associated with a favorable OS (not compromised as one might expect),[53] though not PFS. The elicitation of the idiotype network by 3F8 (Ab1), whereby an anticarbohydrate GD2 antibody (Ab3′) response was induced in young children after four to five cycles of 3F8, appeared to be important for long-term maintenance of remission and survival[42,54] (see the section "Vaccines"). Even among neuroblastomas with poor outlook—namely, in patients with primary refractory disease or those in second remission or beyond—immunotherapy with 3F8+ GM-CSF has been followed by 25% to 40% cure rates.[55,56]

Chimeric and Humanized Anti-GD2 Monoclonal Antibody

Despite the favorable impact of the ability to make HAMA after mouse 3F8 on patient survival, an early or a persistent HAMA titer in patients could also neutralize the antibody and deny any benefit from repeat cycles of 3F8. In order to reduce HAMA, chimeric (murine x human) and humanized anti-GD2 mAbs have been developed. Chimeric 14.18, in combination with GM-CSF and interleukin (IL)-2, has been shown to significantly improve OS in patients with high-risk neuroblastoma in a Phase 3 Children's Oncology Group (COG) study,[17,57] forming the basis for U.S. Food and Drug Administration (FDA) approval of dinutuximab (chimeric 14.18) in 2015. However, significant toxicities from vascular leakage during IL-2 administration, along with its uncertain clinical benefit, have prompted subsequent treatment strategies without this cytokine.[58–61] Humanized anti-GD2 mAbs (e.g., hu3F8 and hu14.18) have also been developed and completed Phase 1 evaluations with or without cytokines (NCT00003750, NCT01419834, NCT01662804, NCT01757626, NCT00743496). As expected, the overall immunogenicity is substantially reduced by humanization of murine 3F8 even in the presence of GM-CSF, allowing a nearly threefold increase in maximum tolerated antibody dose, associated with a favorable clinical response. Whether the idiotype network continues to play a role in maintaining long-term remission when less immunogenic Ab1 antibodies are used will only be determinable after longer clinical follow-up.[62] Recently, anti-GD2 mAb and GM-CSF combined with irinotecan and temozolomide showed significant antitumor response in patients with relapsed or refractory NB, even with a history of failure after anti-GD2 mAbs.[19] How chemotherapy enhances immunotherapy is under investigation. It is possible that chemotherapy-induced tumor cell death releases tumor neoantigens to activate host immunity through antigen-presenting cells (APCs).

Immunocytokines and Antibody Drug Conjugates

Some cytokines, including IL-2, tumor necrosis factor (TNF), and IL-12, enhance ADCC when given with mAbs, but the risk of systemic side effects (e.g., capillary leak) is high.[58,59] Immunocytokines are IgG antibodies or single-chain Fv (scFv) antibody fragments fused with cytokines. These scFvs are intended to carry cytokines to tumor sites and activate immune cells (e.g., T cells, NK cells) locally around the tumor, although in the few studies where targeting has been studied, the immunocytokine might not home to the tumor site.[63] If immune stimulation is local, systemic side effects from cytokines should be reduced. Anti-GD2 mAb hu14.18-IL-2 fusion protein (hu14.18-IL-2) was administered intravenously to patients with relapsed/refractory neuroblastoma in a Phase 2 COG study. This study showed 21.7% complete remission in patients with disease only by metaiodobenzylguanidine (MIBG) scan or bone marrow test at the time of enrollment, whereas patients with bulky disease had no response.[29] Grade 3 and 4 acute vascular leak syndrome and hypotension were observed in 31.6% and 15.8% of the patients, respectively.[29] Hu14.18-IL-2 is also being tested after haploidentical NK cell infusions in patients with relapsed or refractory NB (NCT03209896).

To increase the potency of naked IgG antibodies, antibody drug conjugates (ADCs) have the potential to deliver cytotoxic agents selectively to tumors, although off-target toxicity is still unavoidable partly because of the unfavorable dwell time of these conjugates in blood.[64,65] Table 62.2 summarizes ADC clinical trials in pediatric cancers. Anti-GD2 mAb 14.G2a conjugated to calicheamicin analog, an antimicrobial chemotherapeutic agent that cleaves DNA, suppressed liver metastasis of murine neuroblastoma.[78] More recently, thienoindole, a DNA minor groove alkylating agent, when conjugated to an antianaplastic lymphoma kinase (ALK) mAb, also showed efficacy in preclinical models of neuroblastoma.[79,80] Further research on drug choice, conjugation method, off-target toxicities, and potential vaccination effects for pediatric application is needed.[81–83]

Radioimmunotherapy

Compartmental Radioimmunotherapy

Another class of payload deliverable by antibodies is the radioactive isotopes (see Table 62.3). Systemic administration of radiolabeled antibodies, though effective, has not been widely accepted.[102] One area with unique potential is compartmental radioimmunotherapy (cRIT). Primarily because the blood-brain barrier blocks entry of chemotherapy and antibodies, CNS or leptomeningeal (LM) relapse occurs in approximately 6% of neuroblastoma patients,[103] and occurs in nearly 20% of those who survived their systemic disease.[15] Once CNS/LM relapse occurs, prognosis is dismal, with a median survival of 4 to 14 months.[103,104] Historically, cure was unlikely even after combined craniotomy, cranial-spinal radiation, and chemotherapy. 8H9 is a mouse IgG1 mAb targeting B7-H3, an immunomodulatory glycoprotein expressed on a wide spectrum of solid tumors including neuroblastoma, sarcomas, and brain tumors.[105] By PET imaging, intrathecal (intra-Ommaya) [124]I-labeled 8H9 rapidly distributes within the cerebrospinal fluid (CSF) compartment, followed by a fast clearance except at the tumor sites (Figure 62.3).[106] Because of this selective tumor uptake and rapid exit from the CSF, radiation to the normal CNS is minimized. When cRIT using ^{131}I-labeled mAb [131]I-3F8 or [131]I-8H9 (10–60 mCi/injection) was used as an adjuvant to treat CNS recurrence, more than 40% of the patients became long-term survivors, with a median survival of at least 5.3 years after the CNS event (range: 1.3–10.8 years).[30,48,106] Because B7-H3 is not expressed at the protein level in the normal CNS,[107] no significant neurotoxicity has been reported other than mild chemical meningitis (headache, vomiting, fever) and hypothyroidism from radioactive iodine. Despite GD2 expression on neurons, neurotoxicity from intra-Ommya [131]I-3F8 was limited to transient chemical meningitis. Neither [131]I-3F8 nor [131]I-8H9 was associated with radionecrosis, and only occasional mild neurocognitive dysfunction in young infants was observed.[48] [131]I-8H9 (^{131}I-omburtamab) received breakthrough therapy designation by FDA in 2017. Phase 2/3 international clinical study of [131]I-8H9 (^{131}I-omburtamab) is currently ongoing (NCT03275402). This cRIT approach was recently applied to the convention-enhanced delivery (CED) of liquid radiation as an adjuvant therapy for diffuse intrinsic pontine glioma (DIPG), incurable dismal pediatric brain tumor with a median survival of less than 12 months. Here a positron-emitting isotope ([124]I) linked to 8H9 ([124]I-8H9) was injected directly into the epicenter of these brain tumors. This CED of [124]I-8H9 significantly improved the outcome of patients with DIPG with 12-month OS of 64.7%.[85] This cRIT is being applied to medulloblastoma, the most common brain cancer in childhood. The trial of ^{177}Lu-diethylenetriaminepentaacetic acid-8H9 (177Lu-DTPA-omburtamab) will be opened later in 2020 (NCT04167618).

Pretargeted Radioimmunotherapy

To overcome the hurdles of systemic radioimmunotherapy (RIT) using directly conjugated IgG,

Table 62.2 Clinical Trials of Antibody Drug Conjugates for Pediatric Cancers (as of June 2020).

ADC	TRIAL	PHASE	NCT	RESULT
SOLID TUMORS				
Lorvotuzumab mertansine	Anti-CD56/maytansinoid DM1 ADC for CD56 positive tumors	1		Out of 52 patients, one achieved CR, one had clinical remission[66]
	Anti-CD56/maytansinoid DM1 ADC for CD56 positive tumors	2	02452554	Five out of 47 patients had DLT (preliminary)[67]
Glembatumumab vedotin	Antiglycoprotein NMB/MMAE ADC for osteosarcoma	2	02487979	One out of 22 patients had PR[68]
Brentuximab vedotin	Anti-CD33/MMAE ADC for CD30 positive nonlymphomatous malignancies	2	01461538	Out of seven patients with germ cell tumors and sex cord stromal tumor, one CR, one PR[69]
ABT-414	Anti-EGFR/MMAF ADC for high-grade glioma	2	02342406	Not yet reported
HEMATOLOGIC MALIGNANCIES				
Gemtuzumab ozogamicin	Anti-CD33/calicheamicin ADC for AML	3	00372593	1-year EFS 38±14%, 1-year OS 53 ± 15%[70]
	Anti-CD33/calicheamicin ADC for APML	2	01409161	Not yet reported
SGN-CD19A	Anti-CD19/MMAF ADC for B cell lymphoma	2	01421667	Not yet reported
	Anti-CD19/MMAF ADC for leukemia and lymphoma	1	01786096	One out of eight patients with leukemia achieved CR[71]
Inotuzumab ozogamicin	Anti-CD22/calicheamicin ADC for B cell ALL	2		Three out of five patients achieved remission[72]
	Anti-CD22/calicheamicin ADC for B cell ALL	2	03913559	Not yet reported
Brentuximab vedotin	Anti-CD33/MMAE ADC for HL	1/2	01780662	58% CR[73]
	Anti-CD33/MMAE ADC for HL	2	01508312	Not yet reported
	Anti-CD33/MMAE ADC and rituximab for HL	Pilot	01900496	Not yet reported
	Anti-CD33/MMAE ADC for HL	2	00848926	5-year OS 41%[74]
	Anti-CD33/MMAE ADC for stage IIB, IIIB, IV HL	2	01920932	Not yet reported
	Anti-CD33/MMAE ADC for stage IIB, IIIB, IV HL	3	02166463	Not yet reported
	Anti-CD33/MMAE ADC for HL, ALCL	1/2	01492088	64% ORR[75]
	Anti-CD33/MMAE ADC for NHL	2	01421667	44% ORR for DLBCL
	Anti-CD33/MMAE ADC for ALCL	2	00866047	66% CR[76]
CAT-8015	Anti-CD22/pseudomonas endotoxin ADC for ALL, NHL	1	00659425	Three out of nine patients achieved CR[77]
JBH492	Anti-CCR7/ maytansinoid DM4 ADC for CLL, NHL	2	04240704	Not yet reported

ADC, antibody drug conjugate; ALCL, anaplastic large cell lymphoma; ALL, acute lymphoblastic leukemia; AML, acute myeloid leukemia; APML, acute promyelocytic leukemia; CCR, CC chemokine receptor; CLL, chronic lymphoblastic leukemia; CR, complete response; DLBCL, diffuse large B-cell lymphoma; DLT, dose limiting toxicity; EFS, event-free survival; HL, Hodgkin lymphoma; MMAE, monomethyl auristatin E; MMAF, monomethyl auristatin F; NCT, National Clinical Trial number; NHL, non-Hodgkin lymphoma; NMB, nonmetastatic melanoma protein B; ORR; overall response rate; OS, overall survival; PR, partial response.

Table 62.3 Clinical Trials of Radioimmunodetection and Radioimmunotherapy for Pediatric Cancers (as of June 2020)

RIT	TRIAL	PHASE	NCT	RESULT
SOLID TUMORS				
[131]I-3F8	[131]I-3F8 and bevacizumab for relapsed/refractory NB	1	00450827	Not yet reported
	Intrathecal [131]I-3F8 for CNS or LM cancers	2	00445965	62% alive (mean OS 82.6 months)[30]
[131]I-8H9	Intrathecal [131]I-8H9 for CNS or LM cancers	1	00089245	
	Intrathecal ^{131}I-omburtamab ([131]I-8H9) for CNS or LM NB	2/3	03275402	Not yet reported
	Intraperitoneal [131]I-8H9 for DSRCT and other peritoneal tumors	1	01099644	No DLT. Median PFS from RIT for CR1 was 17.9 months[84]
	[131]I-8H9 imaging study for CNS or LM cancers		00582608	Not yet reported
[124]I-8H9	CED [124]I-8H9 for DIPG	1	01502917	No DLT[85] 12-month OS 64.7%[86]
^{177}Lu-DTPA-omburtamab	^{177}Lu-DTPA-omburtamab(^{177}Lu-DTPA-8H9) for relapsed/refractory medulloblastoma	1/2	04167618	Not yet recruiting
[131]I-14G2a	^{131}I-anti-GD2 mAb for NB; melanoma; osteosarcoma; SCLC	1		Two out of 18 patients had PR[87]
[99m]Tc-ch14.18	^{99m}Tc-ch14.18 imaging study			Better sensitivity and specificity than ^{131}I-MIBG[88]
[131]I-chCE7	^{131}I-anti-L1CAM mAb imaging study for NB			Better sensitivity than ^{131}I-MIBG[89]
[111]In-R11D10	^{111}In-anti-myosin F(ab) fragments imaging study for RMS and leiomyosarcoma			Seven out of nine patients with RMS had uptake (one false positive)[90]
^{131}I-TP-1 F(ab)2 fragments	^{131}I-TP-1 F(ab)2 fragments imaging study for bone sarcoma			Three out of five patients had tumor detection[91]
^{99m}Tc-IMMU-30	^{99m}Tc-anti-AFP mAb imaging study for AFP secreting germ cell tumor			89% sensitivity; 58% specificity[92]
	^{99m}Tc-anti-AFP mAb imaging study for hepatoblastoma			Tumor detection comparable to MRI[93]
[131]I-81C6	Intrathecal ^{131}I-anti-tenascin mAb for recurrent glioma	1	00002753	One out of 31 patients PR; 13 out of 31 patients SD[94,95]
	Intrathecal ^{131}I-anti-tenascin mAb for primary or metastatic brain cancers	1/2	00002752	1-year OS 63% and 59% in patients with GBM/GS and AA/AO, respectively[96]
^{90}Y-MN-14	^{90}Y-anti-CEA mAb for thyroid cancer	1/2	00004048	Not yet reported
HEMATOLOGICAL MALIGNANCIES				
^{131}I-BC8	^{131}I-anti-CD45 mAb for AML	2	00002554	Not yet reported
	^{131}I-anti-CD45 mAb–based conditioning of HSCT for AML and MDS	2	00119366	Not yet reported

(continued)

Table 62.3 Clinical Trials of Radioimmunodetection and Radioimmunotherapy for Pediatric Cancers (as of June 2020) (*continued*)

RIT	TRIAL	PHASE	NCT	RESULT
HEMATOLOGICAL MALIGNANCIES				
90Y-ibritumomab tiuxetan	90Y-anti-CD20 mAb for relapsed/refractory NHL	1	00036855	No identified DLT. No CR or PR[97]
	90Y-anti-CD20 mAb–based conditioning of autologous HSCT for NHL	2	00336843	ORR 84.2%. No pediatric patients were included[98]
213Bi-HuM195	213Bi-anti-CD33 mAb for AML	1/2	00014495	Six out of 25 patients had response. No pediatric patients were enrolled[99]
90Y-anti-CD66 mAb	90Y-anti-CD66 mAb–based conditioning of HSCT for acute leukemia	2		DFS 46% at 2 years[100]
	90Y-anti-CD66 mAb–based conditioning of HSCT for acute leukemia	1	04082286	Not yet reported
131I-HD37	Intrathecal 131I-anti-CD19 mAb for CNS relapse of ALL	Pilot		Five out of six patients had response[101]
131I-WCMH15.14	Intrathecal 131I-anti-CD10 mAb for CNS relapse of ALL			

AA, anaplastic astrocytoma; AFP, alpha-fetoprotein; ALL, acute lymphoblastic leukemia; AML, acute myeloid leukemia; AO, anaplastic oligodendroglioma; Bi, bismuth; CED, convection-enhanced delivery; CNS, central nervous system; CR, complete response; DFS, disease-free survival; DIPG, diffuse pontine glioma; DLT, dose-limiting toxicity; DSRCT, desmoplastic small round cell tumors; GBM, glioblastoma multiforme; GS, gliosarcoma; HSCT, hematopoietic stem cell transplantation; I, iodine; LM, leptomeningeal; Lu, lutetium; mAb, monoclonal antibody; MDS, myelodysplastic syndrome; MIBG, metaiodobenzylguanidine; MRI, magnetic resonance imaging; NB, neuroblastoma; NCT, ; NHL, non-Hodgkin lymphoma; ORR, overall response rate; OS, overall survival; PFS, progression-free survival; PR, partial response; RIT, radioimmunotherapy; RMS, rhabdomyosarcoma; SCLC, small cell lung cancer; SD, stable disease; Y, yttrium.

multistep or pretargeted RIT (PRIT) strategies separate the tumor localization from the payload step and may reduce toxicity. Here, a bispecific antibody (one specificity for the tumor, the other for metal complex with 1,4,7,10-tetraazacyclododecane-1,4,7,10-tetraaceticacid [DOTA]) is first injected, and after 24 to 48 hours, the nonbinding surplus antibody is cleared from the blood before the administration of the small molecular size payload in the form of radiometal-Bn-DOTA. Because of the fast clearance of the Bn-DOTA payload, the therapeutic index of PRIT can be greatly improved (greater than 100:1), when compared with directly conjugated antibodies (less than 5:1). Because the metal-Bn-DOTA can be conjugated to drugs, toxins, or nanoparticles, this pretargeting strategy can achieve highly selective delivery with minimal bystander damage. A bispecific antibody built with hu3F8 (anti-GD2) and C825 (anti-177Lu-Bn-DOTA complex) was able to ablate rapidly growing neuroblastoma xenografts without histologic or clinical signs or symptoms of radiation damage.[108] The highly favorable therapeutic indices (the ratio of radiation dose received by the tumor versus that by normal organs) of 142 for blood and 23 for kidney[108] should provide an unprecedented selectivity to deliver radiation or drugs. This three-step PRIT approach has since been proven in preclinical models for other tumor antigens, including HER2 (breast cancer),[109] GPA33 (colorectal cancer),[110] CD20 (NHL), and CD38 (multiple myeloma).[111,112] A more advanced version, the two-step SADA (Self-Assembling Disassembly Antibody) system, has brought PRIT ever closer to clinical application by proving the curative potentials using both 177Lu and 225Ac (alpha emitter), without any myelo, renal, hepatic, or neurotoxicities.[113]

T Cell-Based Immunotherapy

Normally, the antigen-processing machinery (APM) converts protein antigens into peptides before transporting them in association with HLA to the cell surface, where they can be recognized by T cells.[114,115] Neuroblastoma cells escape T cell immunity by derailing the APM, whereby both HLA class I and class II expression are downregulated.[116] To engage T cells in immunotherapy of neuroblastoma, chimeric antigen receptor (CAR)-modified T cells and bispecific antibodies have been designed to bypass this requirement for HLA (Figure 62.4).[117] Here, tumor recognition is not through the classic peptide-MHC but instead through more common and abundant tumor-associated antigens (e.g., GD2) anchored on the cell surface without the requirement for or the restriction to specific HLA types. More importantly, polyclonal T cells can be exploited by both CAR and bispecific antibodies, thereby overcoming the limitation of low clonal frequency of classical antigen-specific T cells.[117] In infants and young children, because most T lymphocytes are naïve, memory T helper 1 (Th1), T

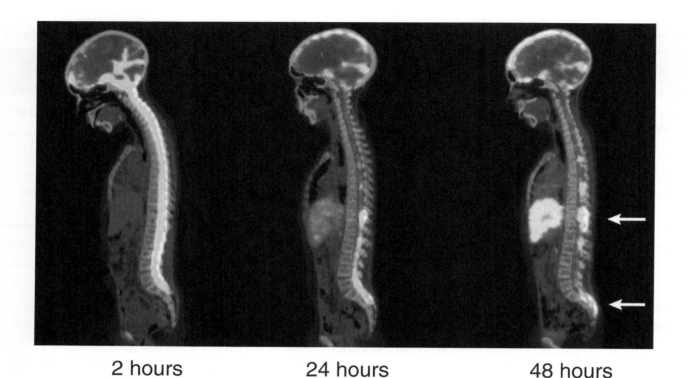

2 hours   **24 hours**   **48 hours**

Figure 62.3 Intrathecal RIT [124]I-labeled 8H9 antibody. PET images illustrate localization to LM tumor of the radioactivity. [124]I-labeled 8H9 antibody was completely filling the intrathecal space 2 hours after intrathecal injection via an Ommaya reservoir. It was progressively cleared at 24 and 48 hours, except at the tumor sites. At 48 hours, there is focal uptake at tumor sites evident in the thoracic and lumbar spine (arrows).

LM, leptomeningeal; PET, positron emission tomography; RIT, radioimmunotherapy.

Source: Adapted and modified with permission from Larson SM, Carrasquillo JA, Cheung NK, Press OW. Radioimmunotherapy of human tumours. *Nat Rev Cancer.* 2015;15(6):347–360. doi:10.1038/nrc3925

helper 2 (Th2), and T helper 17 (Th17) cells require a relatively long time to mature.[118,119] The absence of pre-existing adaptive immunity against their cancer among pediatric patients, thought to be required for a successful application of checkpoint blockade among adults,[120] is another compelling rationale to exploit CAR-modified T cells or bispecific antibodies in young patients where tumor-specific memory is not necessary.

Chimeric Antigen Receptor-Modified T Cells

Despite the clinical success in anti-CD19 CAR-modified T cells for lymphoblastic leukemia, CAR-modified T cells for solid tumors have generally not shown robust antitumor effects. Hurdles in the efficacy of CAR-modified T cells for solid tumors include T cell exhaustion,[121] tumor inaccessibility because of disorganized or abnormal tumor vasculature,[122] and the immunosuppressive TME because of regulatory T cells (T_{reg} cells), myeloid-derived suppressor cells (MDSCs), or tumor-associated M2 macrophages (TAMs).[123–125] Anti-GD2 CAR-modified T cells have achieved clinical responses against bone or bone marrow NB.[32,126] For soft tissue NB, however, antitumor

effects of CARs have not been observed. Many novel cell engineering approaches are being tested to (a) enhance CAR-modified T cell activation in two ongoing Phase 1 trials of third-generation anti-GD2 CAR-modified T cells (NCT02107963, NCT01953900), (b) prevent T cell exhaustion,[127] (c) stimulate T cell homing,[128,129] and (d) modify the immunosuppressive TME.[130]

Bispecific Antibodies

Anti-GD2 × anti-CD3 bispecific antibodies can engage GD2 on neuroblastoma while activating T cells through CD3 to initiate tumor-directed cytotoxicity. Unlike CAR-modified cellular therapy, bispecific antibodies are not patient restricted. As drugs, bispecific antibodies can be manufactured and distributed through the standard pharmaceutical network. Several structural platforms of anti-GD2 bispecific antibodies have been developed, including a highly immunogenic quadroma (rat × mouse) with enhanced Fc functions,[131] partial human tandem single chain (5F11-scBA) and its more potent dimeric form,[132,133] a fully human version with even higher potency (hu3F8-scBA),[133] as well as an

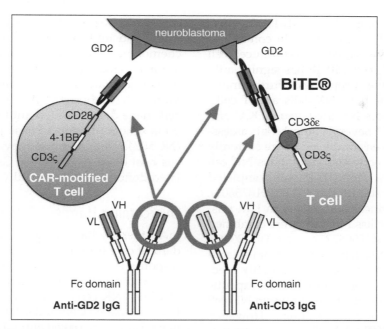

Figure 62.4 Anti-GD2 CAR-modified T cells (the third generation) recognize GD2 antigen on neuroblastoma cells via an anti-GD2 scFv-binding domain. Anti-GD2 x anti-CD3 BiTE® is composed of two scFvs joined in tandem, that is, anti-GD2 scFv and anti-CD3 scFv, recognizing GD2 on neuroblastoma cells and CD3 on T cells.

CAR, chimeric antigen receptor; IgG, immunoglobulin G; scFv, single-chain Fv.

Source: Adapted and modified with permission from Ref. (117). Suzuki M, Curran KJ, Cheung NK. Chimeric antigen receptors and bispecific antibodies to retarget T cells in pediatric oncology. *Pediatr Blood Cancer*. 2015;62(8):1326–1336. doi:10.1002/pbc.25513

aglycosylated IgG(L)-scFv format (hu3F8-BsAb) with a longer serum half-life.[134,135] In preclinical studies, hu3F8-BsAb drives circulating T cells into solid tumors to induce antitumor effects despite the expression of programmed death 1 (PD-1) and PD-L1 in the TME.[134,136] In addition, by removing Fc functions, cytokine release syndrome and pulmonary sequestration and destruction of T cells were substantially reduced. This hu3F8-BsAb is currently being tested in a clinical study for relapsed or refractory NB, osteosarcoma, and other GD2(+) solid tumors (NCT03860207). Bispecific antibodies have also been used to arm T cells from patients expanded ex vivo (EAT, *Ex vivo Armed T*), before reinfusion back to the patients with the addition of GM-CSF and IL-2 (NCT02173093).[137,138] Because gene engineering is not required, EATs armed with recombinant bispecific antibodies are easier to construct than CAR-modified T cells. In the absence of free unbound antibodies, nonspecific activation of T cells is also reduced.[139,140]

Natural Killer Cell-Based Immunotherapy

NK cells recognize tumors with downregulated HLA class I, which are known to silence NK function through KIRs.[141] NK cells also respond to activating receptors, whereupon perforin and granzyme B are injected into tumor cells through immune synapses. The intricate counterbalance of signaling from activating receptors (e.g., DNAX accessory molecule [DNAM-1] [CD226 and NKG2D]), and inhibitory receptors (e.g., KIRs and CD94-NKG2A) determines the cytotoxic output of the NK cell. When DNAM-1 binds to the poliovirus receptor (PVR) on neuroblastoma cells, the signal to kill is transmitted through adaptor proteins containing immune-tyrosine activation motifs.[142,143] Some neuroblastoma cells can escape NK cell surveillance by downregulating PVR.[49] B7-H3 expression on neuroblastoma is also associated with decreased NK cell cytotoxicity;[2] however, the exact lymphocyte receptor for B7-H3 is unknown. Among all the activating receptors, CD16 (FcγRIII) is by far the strongest; hence, the engagement of these receptors by IgG during the ADCC process is known to stimulate a very efficient antitumor effect, providing the rationale for the vast majority of antitumor mAbs in cancer therapy.[144] Among all the inhibitory receptors, KIRs, and especially 3DL1, have been shown to substantially influence the survival of neuroblastoma patients treated with anti-GD2 mAbs.[50]

Adoptive Natural Killer Cell Therapy

Despite the larger number of NK cells per body weight in young children versus adults, the cytotoxic potency of an individual NK cell is lower.[145] When these cells are stimulated with cytokines (e.g., IL-2 or IL-15) in vitro, their cytotoxic effects can be increased.[146] In contrast to IL-2, which causes capillary leak, activation-induced cell death, and induction of T_{reg} cells, IL-15 has significantly fewer of these undesirable properties. Furthermore, IL-15 expands and sustains both NK cells and T cells, matures APCs, and enhances NK-mediated ADCC and myeloid-mediated ADCC.[146] Several clinical trials assessing NK cell efficacy have been completed or are currently active: A Phase 1 study of activated autologous NK cell adoptive therapy with or without IL-15 was completed in children with advanced solid tumors (NCT01875601), and infusions of haploidentical NK cells with KIR mismatch (missing KIR/HLA class I ligand) were combined with anti-GD2 mAbs (NCT00877110, NCT02130869, NCT02650648). Although NK cells isolated from related or unrelated donor peripheral blood are commonly used, human NK cell lines have also been tested for therapeutic activity. NK-92 is an example of a cloned human NK cell line that is cytotoxic for many human tumors. However, while carrying inhibitory KIRs, NK-92 lacks the activating receptors, such as CD16, NKp44, and NKp46, found on fresh NK cells.[147,148] CD16-transfected NK-92 cell lines have been combined with antitumor monoclonal antibodies to enhance ADCC.[149–152]

Chimeric Antigen Receptor-Modified Natural Killer Cells and Bispecific Antibodies

Although NK cell cytotoxicity is not limited by low clonal frequency as in classic T cells, it is also not antigen specific and typically lacks long-term memory. In principle, modification with CAR or a bispecific antibody (one specificity for a tumor target and one specificity for NK cells) should endow NK cells with target-specific cytotoxicity. Anti-GD2 CAR has been used to enhance target-specific cytotoxicity of NK-92 cells or of fresh NK cells isolated from healthy donors. These anti-GD2 CAR-transfected NK cells, by virtue of their 2B4 cytoplasmic signaling through CD3ζ, have shown potent cytotoxicity against neuroblastoma cell lines in vitro.[153] Bispecific IgG antibodies (anti-GD2 × CD16) have also been shown to drive NK cells into GD2(+) tumors, where different polymorphic CD16 alleles can be activated equally.[154] This process is similar to that associated with the clinical strategy of retargeting NK cells to treat myelodysplastic syndromes (anti-CD16 × CD33 bispecific antibodies) or Hodgkin lymphoma (anti-CD16 × CD30 bispecific antibodies).[155,156]

Natural Killer T Cell-Based Immunotherapy

Natural killer T (NKT) cells, especially CD1d-restricted Vα24-invariant (type-I) NKT cells (iNKT cells), comprise a subset of lymphocytes that has high antitumor potential with properties that distinguish them from classic T cells and NK cells. The iNKT cells have been shown to traffic and infiltrate into neuroblastoma in response to chemokines released from tumor cells or tumor-infiltrating macrophages.[157] Furthermore, iNKT cells are a population appearing early during lymphoid development found in newborns.[158] Anti-GD2 CAR-modified iNKT cells have demonstrated antitumor effects in neuroblastoma xenografts, and a Phase 1 clinical trial was initiated (NCT02439788). Because they do not mediate graft-versus-host disease, allogeneic CAR iNKT cells from unrelated donors could potentially be clinically safe.[159]

Overcoming Hurdles of Passive Immunotherapy

mAb therapy has changed the prognosis and the standard of care for high-risk neuroblastoma. So far, the best response is seen in the marrow compartment, where NK cells and myeloid cells reside. The differential homing of CD16+ NK cells could account for organ specificity.[160] Indeed, isolated CNS and soft tissue relapses have become major hurdles to naked anti-GD2 IgG immunotherapies.[15] Another challenge for passive immunotherapy is how to maintain their antitumor effect with repeated treatment cycles or how to realize a vaccination effect (see the following section) for long-term protection. Antidrug antibodies (e.g., HAMA and human anti-chimeric antibody [HACA]) can neutralize both mouse and chimeric anti-GD2 mAb. Although there seems to be a strong association between the ability to mount a HAMA response and survival,[15] the immediate effect of HAMA or HACA during treatment is a decrease in the serum half-life and a reduction in drug exposure. The special class of pre-existing antitherapeutic antibodies (PATA) against the Fc of both human and mouse anti-GD2 antibody associated with better patient outcome was intriguing.[161] As the normal immune system is highly regulated to prevent autoimmunity or hyperinflammation, any manipulation to induce host immunity against self-antigens will likely encounter resistance. In adoptive cell therapy, the induction of T_{reg} cells, the interplay of inhibitory receptors (e.g., KIR or PD-1) and inhibitory ligands (e.g., HLA-C or PD-L1), and the maintenance of an immunosuppressive TME are natural reactions by the host and the tumor. Although the potential of passive immunotherapy is being tested with more sophistication, a better understanding of these complex regulatory immune networks and careful long-term patient follow-up should help design better passive immunotherapy while enhancing protective immunity with minimal autoimmune complications.

ACTIVE IMMUNOTHERAPY

Active immunotherapy clinical trials, including vaccines and immunomodulatory agents, for neuroblastoma are described in Table 62.4.

Table 62.4 Clinical Trials of Active Immunotherapy for Neuroblastoma (as of June 2020).

IMMUNOTHERAPY	TRIAL	PHASE	NCT	RESULT
Vaccines	Autologous NB cell vaccine secreting IL-2 for HR NB	1/2	00048386	Median EFS 13.7 ± 2.8 months[162]
	Allogeneic NB cell vaccine secreting IL-2/lymphotoxin for HR NB	1/2	01192555	Not yet reported
	Autologous NB cell vaccine secreting GM-CSF (GVAX) for relapsed/refractory NB	1	04239040	Not yet reported
	Allogeneic NB cell vaccine secreting IL-2/lymphotoxin for HR NB	1/2	00703222	Not yet reported
	KLH-conjugated GD2/GD3 vaccine with OPT-821 and oral β-glucan for HR NB	1/2	00911560	PFS 80±10% at 24 months in second remission[163,164]
	Autologous EBV-transformed B lymphoblastoid-tumor fusion cell vaccine with IL-2 for NB, EWS	1	00101309	Not yet reported
	Anti-idiotype antibody inducing anti-GD2 antibody (A1G4) with BCG			
	Anti-idiotype antibody inducing anti-N-glycolyl GM3 antibody (racotumomab) for HR NB	2	02998983	Not yet reported
	DNA vaccine encoding NB-associated antigen for relapsed NB	Pilot	04049864	Not yet reported
Immunomodulatory agents	Autologous tumor lysate/KLH-pulsed DC vaccines with IL-7 for relapsed/metastatic NB, EWS, RMS	1/2	00923351	5-year OS for EWS, RMS was 63%. No NB case was enrolled[165]
	Autologous NK cells with IL-15 for advanced solid tumors	1	01875601	Not yet reported

BCG, bacillus Calmette Guerin; DC, dendritic cell; EBV, Epstein-Barr virus; EFS, event-free survival; EWS, Ewing sarcoma; GM-CSF, granulocyte-macrophage colony-stimulating factor; HR, high risk; IL, interleukin; KLH, keyhole limpet hemacyanin; NB, neuroblastoma; NCT, ; NK cells, natural killer cells; OS, overall survival; PFS, progression-free survival; RMS, rhabdomyosarcoma.

Vaccines

The ability to mount HAMA response after mouse anti-GD2 mAb treatment has been consistently associated with a more favorable OS.[15] An idiotype network[166] accounting for long-term survival was hypothesized based on a pilot set of patients undergoing anti-GD2 antibody therapy.[167] Among the HAMA (Ab2), a subset of antibodies belonged to the anti-idiotypic type (Ab2β), which, in turn, could stimulate an anti-anti-idiotypic antibody response (Ab3), a subset of which belonged to Ab3' that interact with GD2. In a recent study in a larger cohort of patients after even longer follow-up, those with higher Ab3' or Ab2β at 12 to 18 months following anti-GD2 antibody therapy had a significantly better long-term outcome.[54] Although the idiotype network could be an indirect vaccine strategy, active immunization to build the patient's own immune defense against cancers is an idea as old as that against infections in humans. When autologous tumor cells are genetically modified to secrete IL-2, autologous tumor cell vaccines were proven safe when administered to neuroblastoma patients in remission.[162] These vaccines stimulated tumor-specific responses among both Th1 and Th2 T cells, associated with a median event-free survival (EFS) among treated patients of 13.7 +/- 2.8 months.[162] Gene-modified allogeneic neuroblastoma tumor cells secreting IL-2 or lymphotoxin have also been tested in a Phase 1/2 trial (NCT01192555, NCT00703222). Because MHC is downregulated on neuroblastoma cells, T cell immunity activated by these vaccines tends to be weak. To increase immunogenicity, dendritic cell vaccines targeting cancer testis (CT) antigens, such as MAGE-A1, MAGE-A3, and NY-ESO-1, have been tested in combination with decitabine, a potent inhibitor of DNA methylation that could upregulate expression of CT antigens.[168] Additionally, gangliosides conjugated to keyhole limpet hemacyanin

(KLH) are being tested on neuroblastoma-associated antigens GD2 and GD3.[169] When administered in combination with an immune adjuvant OPT-821 plus oral β-glucan,[170] OS was promising, with no major toxicities among a small cohort of patients with metastatic neuroblastoma in greater than or equal to second remission after heavy prior treatment.[163] β-glucan can stimulate phagocytosis, degranulation, and cytotoxicity of leukocytes by binding to a complement receptor CD11b (CR3).[171] This study has since been expanded to include a much larger patient cohort (NCT00911560).[164] Recently, DNA vaccine encoding NB antigens expressing on tumor biopsy materials by PCR or IHC (e.g., tyrosine hydroxylase, PHOX2B, surviving, MAGE-A1, MAGE-A3, or PRAME) and potato virus X coat protein in combination with oral Salmonella vaccine containing plasmid of the DNA vaccine is being tested in a clinical study (NCT04049864).

Immunomodulatory Agents

Cytokines and chemokines released from immune cells and stromal cells in the TME can strongly regulate the immune system in response to tumor growth and tumor metastasis. In children, these cytokine response patterns can differ from those in adults partly because of the immaturity of the immune system. For example, cord blood cells release higher levels of tumor necrosis factor α (TNF-α) and Th2 cytokines, including IL-6 and IL-10, than blood cells from adults, even though this ability rapidly decreases soon after birth. After birth, the capacity to produce cytokines mounts gradually, reaching adult levels after 4 years; however, interferon γ (IFN-γ), a Th1 cytokine, remains low until adolescence.[41] A patient's antitumor immunity can be enhanced by activating cytokines/chemokines (e.g., Th1) or by blocking receptors for inhibitory cytokines/chemokines on tumor cells. GM-CSF and IL-2 enhanced anti-GD2 mAb–mediated ADCC in patients with neuroblastoma, although the inflammatory side effects of IL-2, including capillary leak syndrome and hypersensitivity, have been difficult to manage.[17,57–59] IL-7 or IL-15 activates immune cells with less capillary leak than IL-2 and stimulates lymphocytes, including T cells, B cells, and NK cells.[172] Furthermore, in preclinical models, the combination of an anti-GD2 mAb, γδ T cells, and IL-7 could improve the survival of tumor-bearing mice.[173] IL-7 has also been combined with autologous tumor lysate/KLH-pulsed dendritic cell vaccines for treating relapsed or metastatic neuroblastoma, Ewing sarcoma, and rhabdomyosarcoma in a Phase 1/2 study (NCT00923351). Patients who received IL-7 had higher levels and CD4+ cells following the vaccine therapy than those who did not receive IL-7.[165] IL-15 is actively being tested in early phase trials using NK cell infusion therapies in children with solid tumors (NCT01875601). It is interesting to note that the complex of IL-15 receptor-α and IL-15 ligand can enhance anti-GD2 mAb–mediated ADCC better than IL-15 alone in vitro and in vivo.[174,175] Furthermore, a recent study demonstrated that IL-15 could play an important role in tumor immune surveillance by activating tissue-resident type 1-like innate lymphoid cells (ILCs) and type 1 innate-like T cells.[176] As the development of ILCs starts early during the fetal or neonatal period,[177] IL-15 may have the potential of enhancing innate cancer immunity in children.

Overcoming Hurdles of Active Immunotherapy

Active immunotherapy is a powerful strategy to initiate de novo immunity or to boost an existing immune response against cancer. The paucity of neoantigens, the immaturity of the immune system, and the damage from dose-intensive chemotherapy suffered by children with cancer combine to make this strategy more daunting for this age group. A critical assessment of tumor targets and the tumor immune environment, in addition to the establishment of monitoring and management algorithms for autoimmune side effects, will be necessary to enable us to forcibly tip the balance to achieve better tumor control.

FUTURE DIRECTIONS

To realize the true potential of immunotherapy in childhood cancer, the immunobiology of the seed and the soil need to be better understood. As the immunotherapeutic toolbox continues to expand, choosing the right strategies at the right timing during treatment course is critical for each cancer type.[178] With the convergence of genomic medicine, microbiome science, immune modulation by chemotherapy, and radiation therapy, vast opportunities exist for clinical applications in children.

Combination Therapy With Immune Checkpoint Inhibitors

The success of checkpoint inhibitors for T cells is accompanied by autoimmune side effects in adult cancers. For immune checkpoint inhibitors (ICIs) to produce meaningful tumor responses despite a paucity of neoantigens to drive de novo tumor-specific immunity in childhood cancer, autoimmune side effects are inevitable. When ipilimumab was administered to children with advanced solid tumors, including melanoma, sarcoma, and neuroblastoma in a Phase 1 study (NCT01445379), 27% developed grade 3 or 4 immune-related adverse events, among which gastrointestinal and hepatic toxicities were the most common. These frequencies were similar to those in adults, although they occurred sooner, even with the first administered dose. Unfortunately, no antitumor response was observed.[179] The combination of ICIs with

CAR–modified T cells or bispecific antibodies to overcome T cell exhaustion or the suppressive TEM is a logical extension, although toxicities will likely be severe. Strategies to reduce these autoimmune side effects in the young patient population represent a major unmet need. Anti-GD2 antibody therapy is a cogent example, where acceptance was slow despite the absence of late effects and the successful evolution of effective care plans to manage its acute toxicities. When used judiciously, immunotherapy has the potential to complement and/or reduce both dose and intensity of chemotherapy or myeloablative therapy (with stem cell transplantation).[180]

Timing of Immunotherapy—In Combination or in Sequence

Anti-GD2 antibodies are actively being combined with induction chemotherapy[181–183] or with salvage chemotherapy,[19,26,184] with initial evidence of an improvement in the quality of tumor response. Whether this combined chemo/immunotherapy will improve long-term survival will require longer follow-up. The vaccination effect of tumor-opsonizing antibodies, probably important for long-term tumor control, has been repeatedly shown in preclinical models.[185] However, proximity of chemotherapy to antibody treatment may derail the vaccination effects; hence, finding the right sequence and timing of modalities will be critical. T cells get exhausted by their tumor and repeat cycles of high-dose chemotherapy.[186] Understanding the age-dependent immune reconstitution after chemotherapy should guide the timing of immunotherapy. Autologous SCT, a standard consolidation therapy in high-risk neuroblastoma, and any high-dose chemotherapy will deplete most immune cells; however, NK cell recovery seems relatively intact in children.[187] Hence, anti-GD2 antibodies that mediate NK-mediated ADCC can be effective when applied at the end of induction therapy following lymphocyte recovery. B cell recovery, however, takes 6 months, and a normal isotype repertoire is not normalized even after 9 months. If the vaccination effect of anti-GD2 antibodies is to happen, it can be 6 to 12 months after the end of induction; thus, the continuation of anti-GD2 antibody therapy beyond the first 6 months could be beneficial. Although CD8+ T cells take 3 months to recover, the CD4+ T cell count remains low for 9 to 12 months, associated with a diminished response to phytohemagglutinin (PHA).[187] As active immunity requires CD4+ cells (e.g., to help B cells to mount antibody response), the 9 to 12 months wait may be necessary for a vaccine to be successful. Although CAR technology usually exploits CD8+ T cells and can be applied during the first 12 months following induction therapy, bispecific antibody technology may have the advantage of exploiting both CD8+ and CD4+ T cell populations, although the CD4+ T cell–mediated epitope spread or vaccination effects will likely have to wait until after the first year. The potential impact of the gut microbiome on the TME[188,189] and the effect of chemotherapy on the microbiome,[190] overlaying the changes of gut flora with age and with antibiotics during cancer treatment, add further complexity to the design of optimal immunotherapy approaches.[191,192]

Metastasis and Minimal Residual Disease

Although cytotoxic therapy with its unavoidable toxicities seems necessary to stop a galloping cancer such as neuroblastoma at diagnosis, its use at the time of MRD seems excessive if immunotherapy can offer an alternative. In randomized trials, megatherapy (e.g., autologous SCT) has not shown statistically significant impact on ultimate survival,[193,194] despite positive signals on surrogate endpoints such as PFS—a further reason for exploring alternatives. Tools have been developed for monitoring MRD of blood or bone marrow metastases, though few have been validated in large multicenter patient cohorts. The early detection of MRD could provide an early response signal, a measure of the quality of response, or even an actual measure of the amount of residual tumor, as demonstrated repeatedly in childhood acute lymphoblastic leukemia (ALL).[195] In one large study in neuroblastoma, four transcripts (e.g., CCND1, ISL1, PHOX2B, and B4GALNT1) in the bone marrow after two cycles of immunotherapy were highly predictive markers of treatment outcome.[52] Other studies using plasma cell–free DNA have shown promise, although their sensitivity and specificity must improve.[11] Armed with these MRD tools, various forms of immunotherapy can now be applied objectively to evaluate their efficacy when used as an adjuvant in rare pediatric cancers.

Integration Into Current and Future Modalities

So far, the timing of immunotherapy is tailored based on the kinetics of immune recovery following chemotherapy and the level of residual tumor, though evidence for synergism between chemotherapy and immunotherapy has recently emerged as potentially relevant. Some chemotherapeutic agents (e.g., low-dose cyclophosphamide or temozolomide) decrease T_{reg} cells,[196,197] and these immune-modulating chemotherapies may enhance the antitumor effects of T cell–based therapies, whether driven by CAR-modified T cells, by bispecific antibodies, or by vaccines. In fact, low-dose cyclophosphamide is commonly used for patient conditioning before injection of anti-CD19 CAR-modified T cells in ALL. Because temozolomide is routinely used for sarcoma and relapsed neuroblastoma, adding T cell–based immunotherapy to these chemotherapy courses could potentially boost the antitumor effect. Radiation is known to enhance the function of APCs, resulting in the activation of tumor-specific CD4[+] and CD8[+] T cells.[198] The best clinical example is the abscopal effect, where local radiation induces a distant antitumor effect after checkpoint blockade.[198] Total body irradiation, previously used during SCT, and as preconditioning for TIL therapy, could change the gut microbiota, elevating inflammatory cytokines to enhance CD8[+] T cell functions.[199] Going beyond cytotoxic therapies, targeted molecular therapy has also been exploited to modulate the immune system. PTEN-mTORC2 pathway is needed for maintaining T_{reg} cells,[200] so phosphatase and tensin (PTEN) inhibitors can modulate the immunosuppressive TME. The MEK pathway plays important roles in proliferation of both CD8[+] and helper CD4[+] T lymphocytes, and MEK inhibitors can potentially interfere with antitumor properties of T cells. Small molecule immunomodulators can also change TME and enhance immunotherapeutic effects. Indoleamine 2,3-dioxygenase (IDO) is an enzyme expressed in tumors, macrophages, and dendritic cells, and it suppresses immune cells. Indoximod, an IDO inhibitor, when combined with temozolomide was tested in pediatric tumors (NCT02502708). P2X7 receptor antagonist could inhibit MDSCs in the neuroblastoma microenvironment.[201] The advent of cytokines such as IL-7 or IL-15 (as IL-15Rα-IL-15) superagonists offers an alternative to IL-2 with fewer side effects, with potential to improve the survival and function of endogenous and transferred T cells and NK cells.[202,203] Given the many possible combinations, prioritization and careful toxicity monitoring are mandatory in order to rapidly eliminate false leads.

Target Discovery

Finally, efforts to circumvent the hurdles in T cell targeting against pediatric tumors (e.g., low frequency of somatic mutations and downregulation of MHC class I) have had varying degrees of success.[178] For instance, CAR engineering or bispecific antibodies have succeeded in steering T cells, NK cells, or iNKT cells toward non-HLA restricted cell surface antigens (e.g., GD2, B7-H3).

Various approaches using genomic testing have uncovered intriguing candidates for solid tumors in children, all waiting to be clinically validated.[204] Today, even internal proteins can be targeted once they get processed into peptides and presented on cell surface HLA,[205] although low expression of HLA in tumors, such as neuroblastoma, remains a challenge. Some surface antigens (e.g., ROR1 and ROR2) are too low in density for ADCC, but they are adequate for redirected T cell–mediated cytotoxicity. As mentioned earlier, another workaround is targeting immune checkpoints. ICIs (e.g., ipilimumab, nivolumab, pembrolizumab) have made major breakthroughs in the immunotherapy of several cancers in adults,[206] and many co-stimulatory or inhibitory receptors on T cells are being investigated as potential targets for cancer treatment.[207,208] Activating or inhibitory receptors/ligands on other immune cells, including NK cells and iNKT cells, are also promising targets, as was shown for the inhibitory KIR-3DL1.[50]

CONCLUSION

The immune system in children with cancer, although immature and damaged by chemotherapy, can recover. Advances in immunotherapy promise to improve the cure rate and to allow reduction in cytotoxic therapy, thereby minimizing long-term toxicities.

KEY REFERENCES

Only key references appear in the print edition. The full reference list appears in the digital product on Springer Publishing Connect: connect.springerpub.com/content/book/978-0-8261-3743-2/part/part04/chapter/ch62

15. Cheung NK, Cheung IY, Kushner BH, et al. Murine anti-GD2 monoclonal antibody 3F8 combined with granulocyte-macrophage colony-stimulating factor and 13-*cis*-retinoic acid in high-risk patients with stage 4 neuroblastoma in first remission. *J Clin Oncol.* 2012;30(26):3264–3270. doi:10.1200/JCO.2011.41.3807
43. Cheung NK, Dyer MA. Neuroblastoma: developmental biology, cancer genomics and immunotherapy. *Nat Rev Cancer.* 2013;13(6):397–411. doi:10.1038/nrc3526
106. Larson SM, Carrasquillo JA, Cheung NK, Press OW. Radioimmunotherapy of human tumours. *Nat Rev Cancer.* 2015;15(6):347–360. doi:10.1038/nrc3925

63

Immunotherapy in Combination With Radiation Therapy

Jean Philippe Nesseler, William H. McBride, and Dörthe Schaue

KEY POINTS

- Radiation therapy (RT) promotes the release of danger signals and tumor antigens while driving the antigen-presenting machinery.

- As a result, innate and adaptive immune systems can be activated locally and systemically.

- Local and systemic regulatory immune pathways are also induced, which can limit immune responses, especially out-of-field abscopal effects.

- Combining immune-modulating agents with RT can shift the immune balance toward effective tumor-immune eradication, which is further aided by radiation-induced reduction in tumor burden.

- Future challenges in the field of radiotherapy–immunotherapy combination include optimizing radiotherapy parameters, target sites, and therapeutic sequences; promoting de novo antitumor immunity; finding biomarkers for patients who could benefit most from this combination; and predicting treatment response.

INTRODUCTION

From its first use against cancer performed on July 4, 1896, by Victor Despeignes in France,[1] radiation therapy (RT) quickly became a crucial component of cancer care, together with surgery and chemotherapy, and most recently with immunotherapy as the fourth pillar of modern oncology. Today, over 50% of all cancer patients will receive RT at some point during their treatment.[2] It is used with curative intent for localized primary tumors and oligometastasis, as a palliative treatment to enhance the quality of life in patients with widespread metastatic disease, and, also, to the total body, as a conditioning strategy prior to transplantation. Recent technologic improvements, most notably intensity modulation, image-guidance, and stereotactic delivery, allow more precise dose delivery, minimizing acute and late side effects by sparing normal tissues and so widening the therapeutic window.

Historically, the therapeutic effect of ionizing radiation is attributed to direct DNA damage and indirect damage from free radical formation, which ultimately results in tumor cell death.[3] Until recently, the effects of radiation on the tumor microenvironment (TME), especially the inflammatory and immune components, remained underappreciated. The coming of age of immunotherapy renewed interest in the irradiated tumor-immune interface. Mounting evidence indicates that local RT can generate a state of systemic immunity that can have antitumor and antimetastatic effects.[4] The term "abscopal" refers to the regression of a non-irradiated tumoral lesion, which remains very rare in the clinic following RT alone.[5-7] In this chapter, we detail the immunomodulatory properties of RT (Figure 63.1), report preclinical and clinical results of combinations between RT and different immunotherapeutic agents, and discuss optimal strategies to develop this promising therapeutic duo.

THE IMMUNE SYSTEM CONTRIBUTES TO THE SUCCESS OF RADIATION THERAPY

In 1979, in an immunogenic chemically induced mouse fibrosarcoma model, Stone et al. found that the radiation dose necessary to control a tumor was 1.67 fold higher in immunodeficient compared with immunocompetent mice.[8] In most models, tumor regression requires CD8+ T cells, and Lee et al. showed they were involved in regression caused by a single fraction, ablative irradiation (20 Gy) delivered to mouse melanoma B16 tumors. Indeed, tumor control was not observed in nude or B6/Rag -/- (T cell-deficient) mice and was abolished by administration of anti-CD8 antibodies after RT.[9] Moreover, a clinical study found a correlation between a high number of tumor-infiltrating CD8+ T cells and survival after definitive chemoradiotherapy in head and neck cancer, supporting the hypothesis that immune system contributes to the efficacy of RT.[10]

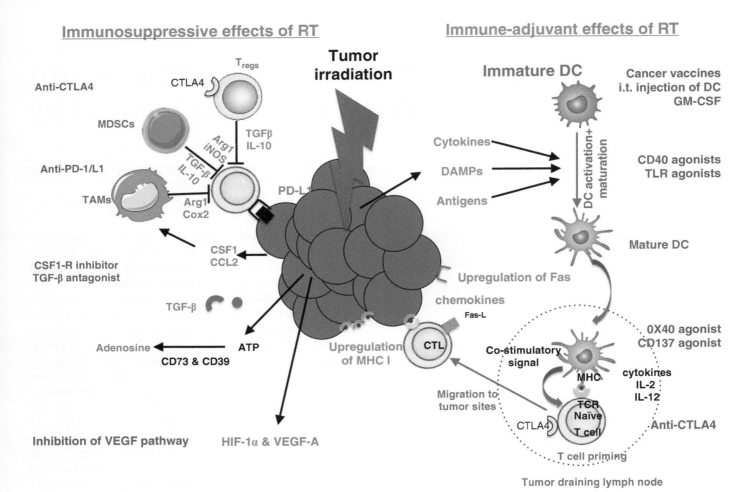

Figure 63.1 Opposing effects of radiation on the tumor-host interface. Radiation-induced tumor cell damage elicits the release of TAA, and the expression of DAMPs (calreticulin, HMGB1, ATP). These signals facilitate the production of proinflammatory cytokines and chemokines, the recruitment and maturation of DCs, the uptake of TAAs, and their migration to draining lymph nodes, where they present antigens to naïve T cells. Activated T cells proliferate and traffic to the tumor site. Overexpression of MHC class I by tumor cells after irradiation aids the presentation of TAA and their recognition by tumor-specific CD8+ T cells, which are then licensed to kill. Irradiation also induces Fas on tumor cells, which further sensitizes them to T cell-mediated killing. However, radiation also triggers several immunosuppressive pathways (highlighted in red). T_{regs} are overrepresented after irradiation, in part because of their relative radioresistance, and populations of MDSCs tend to expand post RT. Intratumoral CSF-1 and CCL2 levels increase, leading to a recruitment of monocytes, which differentiate into TAMs polarized toward the M2 phenotype. Irradiation induces upregulation of PD-L1 in the TME. ROS allows the dissociation of active TGF-β. ATP released during the immunogenic cell death is quickly catabolized into adenosine by ectonucleotidases CD39 and CD73. Irradiation upregulates HIF-1α and VEGF-A, two potent immunosuppressive forces. Different therapeutic strategies that integrate radiation and immunomodulatory agents (blue) are under investigation with the goal to shift the balance in favor of systemic tumor immune eradication. Cancer vaccines might be able to further boost the radiation in-situ vaccination effect. I.t. injection of autologous DCs can increase the DCs infiltration, further enhanced by immune-stimulatory pathways (CD40 agonists, TLR agonists, STING ligands, IFN-I) or T cells (OX40 agonists, CD137 agonists, IL-2, IL-12), in addition to immune checkpoint inhibitors (anti-CTLA-4, anti-PD-1, anti-PD-L1). Alternative immunosuppressive pathways that are promising in this context are TGF-β antagonists, as well as CSF-1R inhibitors that could limit M2 macrophage tumor infiltration.

DAMPs, damage-associated molecular patterns; DCs, dendritic cells; GM-CSF, granulocyte-macrophage colony-stimulating factor; IFN, interferon; IL, interleukin; MDSCs, myeloid-derived suppressor cells; MHC, major histocompatibility complex; RT, radiation therapy; TAA, tumor-associated antigens; TCR, T cell receptor; TLR, Toll-like receptors; T_{regs}, regulatory T cells; VEGF, vascular endothelial growth factor.

RADIATION SIGNALS DANGER AND ACTIVATES PROINFLAMMATORY PATHWAYS

Irradiated cells can release fragments of cellular materials that contain damage-associated molecular patterns (DAMP) capable of stimulating host cells, including innate immune and dendritic cells (DC; Figure 63.1). Some are recognized by surface Toll-like receptors (TLRs). Others, such as nucleic acid–sensing immune receptors TLR3 and TLR7-9, are expressed in endosomal compartments or in the cytoplasm (RIG-I-like receptors [RLRs], AIM2). DNA fragments formed by irradiation that escape digestion by extracellular and intracellular nucleases can have diverse fates, including forming micronuclei after cell division, or DNA-SCARS after radiation-induced cellular senescence, or persisting as cytoplasmic or extracellular fragments. It may also be transferred to other cells via gap junctions or endocytosis.

As a DAMP, extracellular DNA can be recognized by the receptor for advanced glycation end-products (RAGE), which promotes uptake into endosomes allowing activation of TLR9.[11] Cytosolic DNA can be recognized by cyclic GMP-AMP synthase (cGAS), producing cyclic GMP-AMP (cGAMP) that activates STING (stimulator of interferon genes). STING is an endoplasmic-reticulum-associated protein that can activate transcription of the type I interferon (IFN-1) gene via the STING/TBK/IRF3 signal transduction pathway.

The end result of DAMP signaling is production of proinflammatory cytokines and type 1 interferons, including activation of inflammasomes and IL-1b production.[12,13] Radiation can also activate the NF-κB pathway for proinflammatory cytokine/chemokine production. The DNA damage response (DDR) kinases ATM and DNA-PKcs that are activated by radiation-induced DNA double-stranded breaks (DSBs) may participate in NF-κB activation and inflammasome production. NF-κB is a transcription factor that translocates to the nucleus to induce gene expression of many proinflammatory cytokines, including TNF-α, interleukin-6 (IL-6), IL-1α, and IL-1β.[14,15]

These endproducts have been implicated both in causing further tissue damage and in the stimulation of tumor immunity. They participate in DC maturation and subsequent activation of antitumor T cells. For example, IFN-1 can activate and mature DC for antigen presentation, encouraging them to migrate to draining lymph nodes, where they efficiently cross-present tumor antigens to T cells, resulting in tumor-specific T cell responses.[16] STING expression in DCs was demonstrated to be essential for radiation-induced IFN-1 responses and initiation of a cascading innate and adaptative immune attack and tumor regression after RT.[17,18] It is interesting to note that the secretion of IFN-1 seems to be dependent on the radiation dose, where 8 Gy fractions induce a strong upregulation of IFN levels, while higher doses failed to achieve this effect, presumably due to three prime repair exonuclease 1 (TREX1) induction and hence degradation of cytosolic DNA before this pathway can be initiated.[19]

IMMUNE-ADJUVANT EFFECTS OF RADIATION THERAPY

Historically, RT has been considered foremost for its immunosuppressive effects because of the relatively high radiosensitivity of quiescent lymphocytes as they moved through the radiation field.[20–22] In fact, immune cells are not all created equal in radiation sensitivity. There is a wide spectrum ranging from very sensitive naïve T cells on one end to relatively resistant macrophages on the other, with cell activation and differentiation status adding further complexity. The effects of local RT on immune cells within the TME are therefore complex and will depend upon many tumor-related factors, such as hypoxia, vasculature, and immune balance (Figure 63.1). However, local RT can actually create a microenvironment to which T cells can traffick to cause tumor regression.[23]

T cells require three different signals in order to become activated and to mount an adaptive immune response. The T cell receptor (TCR) on T cells recognizes the antigenic peptides presented by DCs and tumor cells in the context of the major histocompatibility (MHC) class I or class II molecules and this is signal 1. Signal 2 is the costimulatory signal (B7.1 and B7.2 on mature antigen-presenting cells [APCs]) that binds to CD28 on T cells, being only required once to activate naïve T cells. Signal 3 is a supportive environment, including immunostimulatory cytokines like IL-2. The current school of thought is that RT might be able to support all three signaling axes (Figure 63.1).

Release of Tumor Antigens

The RT beam inflicts substantial damage on cancer cells, causing cell cycle arrest, senescence, and death, often by necrosis, which elicits the release of tumor antigens. The hope is that RT may at the same time broaden the tumor-antigen repertoire available for immune recognition. The available evidence for radiation-induced neoantigens is not very strong, but the antigenic profile presented by the MHC may change.[24,25] Moreover, irradiated tumor cells can alter their intracellular proteasome balance in favor of the more relevant immunoproteasomes and so modify the processing and presentation of cellular antigens compared with the standard proteasome.[26]

Immunogenic Cell Death

Some irradiated tumor cells can undergo an immunogenic death[27] and become a source of DAMPs. Translocation of calreticulin to the plasma membrane in dying cancer cells is a "eat-me" signal, which promotes uptake by phagocytic cells.[28–30] Release into the extracellular space of high-mobility group box-1 (HMGB1), a histone-chromatin binding protein, especially after radiation-induced necrotic death is another key hallmark of immunogenic cell death. HMGB1 interacts with Toll-like receptor 4 (TLR4) on DC that induces DC maturation through an NF-κB pathway.[31] The third key signal is the release of adenosine triphosphate (ATP), notably by autophagy-related stress. This is sensed by the purinergic receptor P2X7 on monocytes and DCs, which activates the inflammasome and causes the secretion of proinflammatory cytokines like IL-1β and IL-18.[32–34] What HMGB1, ATP, and other DAMPs have in common is their ability to induce DC maturation, that is, allowing them to present not only antigen to T cells but also the crucial co-stimulatory signal 2, without which T cell anergy would ensue rather than activation. This cross-talk tends to happen at the tumor-draining lymph node where DCs and T cells meet and form the immunological synapse.

Radiation Increases Intratumoral T Cell Infiltration

Irradiation can induce the secretion of chemokines that recruit CD8+ T cells to the tumor site. In a mouse breast cancer model, Matsumura et al. demonstrated that radiation induced chemokine C-X-C motif ligand 16 (CXCL16) in tumor cells and on blood vessels, peaking at 48 h after exposure. CXCL16 binds to C-X-C chemokine receptor type 6 (CXCR6) on activated CD8+ effector T cells to recruit them to the irradiated field.[35] Lugade et al. observed an upregulation of the adhesion molecule VCAM-1 on the tumor vasculature 24 h after irradiation of the B16 mouse melanoma, increasing the infiltration and retention of tumor Ag-reactive CD8+ T cells.[23] Radiation-induced reprogramming of tumor-associated macrophages (TAMs) can improve T cell trafficking to the tumor. TAMs in many tumors tend to express an M2 phenotype that promotes angiogenesis, tumor progression, invasion, and metastasis, and have immunosuppressive effects. In a mouse pancreatic cancer model, Klug et al. have found that low-dose irradiation (single 2 Gy dose) reprograms macrophage differentiation toward the iNOS(+)/M1 phenotype, which normalizes the tumor vasculature and facilitates T cell tumor infiltration[36] although many other radiation studies have pointed at an M2-type macrophage/MDSC bias or a myeloid-over-lymphoid bias post RT.[37–39]

Radiation Facilitates Recognition and Elimination of Tumor Cells by Effector CD8+ T Cells

RT increases the expression of MHC class I on DCs and cancer cells, likely due to the induction of interferons and proinflammatory cytokines. This facilitates tumor-antigen presentation and recognition by cytotoxic T cells.[24,40] Similarly, radiation can upregulate Fas family members on tumor cells, which can sensitize them to Ag-specific CTL killing via the Fas/Fas ligand pathway, as was shown in the murine MC38 adenocarcinoma model.[41]

Radiation Aids Recognition and Elimination of Tumor Cells by Natural Killer Cells

RT induces the expression of natural killer (NK) group 2 member D (NKG2D) ligands on the surface of cancer cells, which mediate tumor cell killing by NK cells.[42,43] As a backup immunosurveillance mechanism, cancer cells that have lost MHC class I expression can still be recognized and killed by NK cells, but NK cells can also lyse cancer cells in the presence of MHC expression if they express NKG2D ligands.[44] RT can also promote sensitivity to NK cells indirectly by downregulating Clr-b, a ligand for the inhibitory NK receptor NKR-P1B.[45]

ABSCOPAL EFFECT

The term "abscopal"—from "ab," away from, and "scopus," target—was proposed by Mole in 1953 to define radiation's effects at a distance.[5] In a series of experiments using BALB/c mice injected with 67NR mammary carcinoma cells or with A20 lymphoma cells, Demaria et al. demonstrated that radiation-induced abscopal responses could be immune mediated. This was based on the following observations: (a) the absence of abscopal regressions in T cell-deficient (nude) mice, (b) the need for the DC growth factor Flt3-L to be given with RT, (c) tumor-specificity, and (d) the systemic rise of tumor-specific cytotoxic T cells measurable in the spleen.[4] Together, this led to the argument that RT might act as an in-situ tumor vaccination approach.[46] In the clinical setting, genuine abscopal effects after RT alone, without additional systemic therapy, are extremely rare. Abuodeh et al. recently described that there have been only 21 reported cases of abscopal tumor regression of solid tumors in the literature over the past 45 years.[7] With the advent of immunoradiotherapy, the number of reported abscopal cases has grown, albeit while still remaining an exception rather than the norm.[47] This suggests that powerful immunosuppressive powers at play need to be overcome and/or that meaningful de novo immune responses fail to be evoked by RT.

IMMUNOSUPPRESSIVE EFFECTS OF RADIATION THERAPY

Radiation Therapy Enhances Regulatory T Cell Representation

Regulatory T cells (T_regs cells, or suppressor T cells) are a subset of CD4+ T cells that express the biomarkers CD25,

CTLA-4, CD39, CD73, and Foxp3, among many others.[48,49] They can be "hard-wired," naturally occurring CD4 T_{regs} cells that undergo thymic selection or they can be induced in the periphery, for example by chronic, low-dose antigen exposure in an immune suppressive environment that is driven by TGF-β.[50] T_{regs} cells limit inflammation, maintain peripheral tolerance to self-antigens, and prevent autoimmune diseases. This is best exemplified by the Scurfy mouse and the human equivalent immune dysregulation, polyendocrinopathy, enteropathy, X-linked (IPEX) syndrome that are both deficient in Foxp3 gene and that develop potentially lethal lymphoproliferative autoimmune disease. T_{regs} cells also play a key role in tumor immune evasion by accumulating in the TME, where they inhibit T effector cell function either directly through cell-to-cell contact or indirectly through secretion of immunosuppressive mediators, including TGF-β, IL-10, and adenosine, or by competing for T cell tropic factors such as IL-2.[51,52] Importantly, T_{regs} cells tend to increase in immune organs and tumors after local or whole-body radiation, in large part due to their radiation resistance relative to other lymphocyte subpopulations, resulting in their selection by survival.[53–55] Cross-talk with other immune cells may add to this. For instance, Price et al. showed that Langerhans cells (LCs) rapidly repaired DNA damage after exposure to radiation, migrated to the draining lymph nodes, and induced an increase in T_{reg} cell numbers.[56] RT might also enhance T_{regs} cells' immunosuppressive function by increasing expression of TGF-β, IL-10, or CTLA-4.[54]

RT Drives the Engagement of Myeloid Cell Lineages

While T cell biology tends to involve clear-cut lineages set early during development, myeloid cell biology has no such luxury. The lines between TAMs and myeloid-derived suppressor cells (MDSCs) are blurred in many ways. Plasticity is a hallmark of this lineage that makes definitions, investigations, and comparisons challenging.[57] Notwithstanding these obstacles, the literature is somewhat consistent in that tumor RT tends to drive expansion and/or recruitment of suppressive myeloid cells to the tumor site, most likely by stimulating bona fide inflammatory-wound-healing signaling cascades. What is more, rarely has a tumor that is heavily infiltrated with myeloid cells demonstrated effective antitumor immunity.

Through the expression of factors such as TGF-β, IL-10, and arginase, MDSCs accelerate tumor progression, angiogenesis, invasion, and metastasis, and suppress effector T cell function.[58–61] Xu et al. observed a systemic rise of MDSCs in spleen, lung, lymph nodes, and peripheral blood after irradiation of RM-9 prostate cancers implanted in C57BL6 mice, findings confirmed in patients with prostate cancer. Mechanistic investigations revealed the recruitment of the DNA damage-induced

kinase ABL1 into cell nuclei, where it bound the CSF-1 gene promoter and enhanced its transcription, leading to an increase in circulating MDSCs expressing the counterpart CFS-1R.[37] In that regard, STING, which plays a key role in promoting innate and adaptive immunity in response to RT, can also have negative effects. Several irradiated murine tumors kept recruiting myeloid cells along the CCR2/CCL2 axis in part via continued STING/type I IFN pathway engagement, which ultimately drove chronic, suppressive inflammation and extrinsic radiation resistance.[38]

Traditionally, macrophages are classified into classically activated M1 macrophages, phagocytic cells, and APCs secreting proinflammatory cytokines, essential for the recruitment of effector T cells and alternatively activated M2 macrophages, which are more immunosuppressive in nature, stimulating angiogenesis and tumor growth, and promoting invasion and metastasis.[62] Most tumors have M2-like TAMs that are associated with poor prognosis.[63] RT and the induced expression of CSF-1 in irradiated tumor cells recruit macrophages and cause their proliferation and polarization to an M2 phenotype.[37,64–66] Kalbasi et al. demonstrated that CCL2 is produced by pancreatic ductal adenocarcinoma cells after ablative RT, which recruits Ly6C+CCR2+ monocytes that differentiate into TAMs.[67] The influx of TAMs into irradiated murine tumors that ultimately polarize toward immunosuppression mediated by transcriptional regulation by NFκB p50 was also reported by Crittenden et al.[68] Similarly, Tsai et al. showed that TAMs in the irradiated TME express higher levels of arginase-I and cyclooxygenase 2, two immunosuppressive enzymes.[69] Activated tumor-specific T cells, however, drive an M1 phenotype and, therefore, TAM phenotype reflects the status of the immune system as a whole.[70]

Programmed Death-Ligand 1 Is Upregulated After Radiation Therapy

Programmed death-ligand 1 (PD-L1) is a transmembrane protein that is inducible in various cell types upon IFN-I or IFN-II stimulation.[71] PD-L1 binds to its receptor, programmed cell death protein 1 (PD-1), found on activated T cells to inhibit adaptive immunity.[72] Preclinical data have shown that PD-L1 is upregulated in the TME after RT, which was confirmed in esophageal squamous cell carcinoma patients receiving neoadjuvant RT but not following neoadjuvant chemotherapy without RT.[73–75]

Raditaion Therapy Activates Tumor-Growth Factor β (TGF-β)

TGF-β is a pleiotropic cytokine that is produced by many tumor types. It has major immunosuppressive effects: it inhibits cytotoxic T cell proliferation and function, contributes to the conversion of naïve CD4[+] T cells into T$_{regs}$ cells, inhibits the antigen-presenting function of DCs, and promotes the macrophages M2 phenotype and the neutrophil tumor-supportive N2 phenotype.[76–82] The role of TGF-β in radiation responses is infamous, and one likely to dictate the level of tumor immunity in radiation oncology patients. Radiation-induced reactive oxygen species cause a conformational change of the latency-associated peptide-TGF-β complex to release active TGF-β.[83,84]

Radiation Therapy Increases Adenosine in the Extracellular Space

Adenosine is a purine nucleoside. In tumors, accumulation of extracellular adenosine inhibits the activity of APCs and effector lymphocytes, induces proliferation of T$_{reg}$ cells, and promotes macrophages M2 phenotype through the expression of A2A adenosine receptor.[85–88] RT induces immunogenic tumor cell death with the release of ATP. In the TME, ATP is catabolized into adenosine by the action of ectonucleotidases CD73 and CD39 expressed not only on many tumor cell types but also on effector T cells, T$_{regs}$ cells, and MDSCs.[89–95] Hence, the conversion of ATP to adenosine can ultimately limit the ability of RT to induce antitumor immunity, attenuating both DC maturation and T cell activation.[96]

Radiation Therapy Upregulates Hypoxia-Inducible Factor-1α and Vascular Endothelial Growth Factor-A

Hypoxia-inducible factor-1α (HIF-1α) is a subunit of the heterodimeric transcription factor HIF-1, which is considered the master transcriptional regulator of cellular response to hypoxia, as well as being a central player in metabolism. In normal circumstances, the alpha subunits of HIF are hydroxylated at proline residues by prolyl hydroxylases allowing their recognition by VHL E3 ubiquitin ligase and proteasomal degradation. Since prolyl hydroxylases need oxygen as a cofactor, under hypoxic conditions, HIF-1α is stabilized. HIF-1α, when stabilized, associates with the beta subunit and acts by binding to HIF-response elements (HREs) in gene promoters and so upregulates gene transcription of many genes, in particular vascular endothelial growth factor-A (VEGF), which promotes angiogenesis. HIF-1α and VEGF-A have multiple, potent immunosuppressive effects. HIF-1 can also be stabilized under normoxic proinflammatory conditions through the NF-kB pathway.[97]

HIF-1α modulates TCR signal transduction[98,99] and upregulates PD-L1 expression on tumor cells and MDSCs, which inhibits T cell function.[100,101] HIF-1α also increases the number and suppressive properties of T$_{regs}$ cells;[102] promotes MDSCs differentiation and function;[103] induces chemokines BV8 and CXCL12, which

mobilize MDSCs from the bone marrow;[104] stimulates TGF-β expression;[105,106] suppresses NK cell cytotoxicity;[107] decreases MICA (NK cell ligand) levels on tumor cells;[108] and downregulates the surface expression of the activating NK cell receptors.[109]

VEGF-A, on the other hand, inhibits maturation of DCs,[110] suppresses the activation of T cells,[111] increases the expression of checkpoints on CD8[+] T cells (TIM-3, CTLA-4, PD-1, LAG-3),[112] induces Fas-L expression on tumor endothelial cells causing apoptosis of effector T cells,[113] and generates T$_{reg}$ cell proliferation[114] and accumulation of MDSCs.[115,116] Irradiated tumors have increased expression of HIF-1α, and, consequently VEGF-A, for tumor cell reoxygenation,[117–119] which could severely counteract immune activation by RT.

RADIOTHERAPY–IMMUNOTHERAPY COMBINATIONS

The potential of RT to convert a tumor into an in situ vaccine[46] has implications for both local and systemic tumor control. However, rarity of abscopal effects[7] suggests that RT as a single agent does not easily overcome endogenous immunosuppressive mechanisms, and/or it may not be as efficient in inducing de novo tumor immunity. The rationale for combining immunotherapies with RT is therefore mainly two-fold: to shift the balance in favor of systemic immune activation by "releasing the brakes," that is, removing immune suppressor mechanisms, and to "push the accelerator," that is, enhancing immune stimulation (Figure 63.1). Two clinical situations are of particular interest: (1) immunotherapy added to hypofractionated stereotactic body RT (SBRT) to treat oligometastatic disease in a curative setting and (2) irradiation of poorly immunogenic tumors to induce response to immunotherapy that wouldn't respond otherwise.

Stimulation of Innate Immunity

CD40 Agonists

CD40 is a member of the TNF-receptor superfamily. This protein, found on APCs, is required for DC activation and maturation. Several preclinical studies showed antitumoral synergy between agonist anti-CD40 monoclonal antibody (mAb) therapy and RT. In two syngeneic B cell lymphoma models, Honeychurch et al. saw that anti-CD40 mAb plus RT, although ineffective when each given alone, together were capable of providing long-term protection in a CD8[+] T cells-dependent manner.[120] Concomitant targeting of the co-stimulatory molecules CD40 and CD137 (the latter is a co-stimulatory receptor expressed on activated T cells) enhanced the antitumor effects of RT and promoted the rejection of subcutaneous BALB/c-derived 4T1.2 breast tumors, with CD8[+] T cells essential for curative responses.[121] Numerous clinical trials combining chemoradiation with CD40 agonists (NCT03165994) or with CD40 agonists and immune checkpoint blockade (NCT02304393, NCT03123783, NCT03214250, NCT02706353, NCT01103635) are underway.

Toll-Like Receptors Agonists

TLRs are pattern-recognition receptors that recognize pathogen-associated molecular patterns (PAMPs), in particular microbial products, in much the same way as they recognize DAMPs. The engagement of TLRs activates potent immune signaling pathways, triggers the release of key cytokines, and ultimately forms the bridge that ties innate to adaptive immunity. A variety of synthetic TLR agonists have been tested in combination with RT.

TLR9 Agonists

TLR9 recognizes unmethylated CpG oligonucleotide sequences (typical for bacterial DNA), resulting in production of IFN-I and upregulation of co-stimulatory molecules on DCs.[122,123] In a murine immunogenic fibrosarcoma tumor model, Mason et al. combined fractionated RT with subcutaneous peritumoral or intratumoral administrations of synthetic CpG oligodeoxynucleotides. The radiation dose for 50% tumor cure, that is, the TCD50, was lowered by a factor of 3.6.[124] Such impressive synergy in terms of local control was also observed in rats bearing glioma.[125] Furthermore, mice bearing ectopic Lewis lung adenocarcinoma, treated with a similar combination of an intratumoral TLR9 agonist plus 20 Gy single-fraction RT, inhibited tumor growth and the development of lung metastases, that is, translating into systemic effectiveness.[126] Clinically, Phase 1/2 studies combining intralesional CpG with low-dose local RT (2 Gy × 2) showed promise in heavily pretreated mycosis fungoides[127] and low-grade B -cell lymphoma, successfully inducing often durable systemic responses in about one-third of patients, and was well tolerated.[128] However, chronic TLR9 activation with RT can also drive chronic inflammation, upregulate indolamine 2,3-dioxygenase (IDO), generate immune suppression, including T_{regs} cells, and increase tumor recurrence.[129,130] Triple therapy combining RT, CpG, and IDO-blockade is one way to counteract this, as was evidenced by improved local and systemic antitumor effects in murine and canine models.[131]

TLR7 Agonists

Imiquimod, a synthetic TLR7 ligand, has been successfully tested in combination with RT. In a TSA breast carcinoma mouse model, topical administration of imiquimod plus RT significantly enhanced tumor control compared with either treatment alone. Regression of distant unirradiated tumors was also observed as long as they had also been treated with topical imiquimod. Mice that remained tumor-free after 90 days rejected a TSA rechallenge,

showing long-term immunologic memory. CD8$^+$ T cells were key to the success.[132] Dovedi et al. demonstrated that intravenous administration of a novel TLR7 agonist with RT in T and B cell lymphoma-bearing mice led to the expansion of tumor antigen-specific CD8$^+$ T cells, sustained clearance of tumors, and protection from subsequent tumor rechallenge, that is, the generation of a tumor-specific memory.[133] Similarly, systemic administration of a TLR7 agonist combined with local RT primed an antitumor CD8$^+$ T cell response leading to improved survival in mice bearing colorectal carcinoma or fibrosarcoma.[134] Early clinical trials of imiquimod and RT are ongoing.

TLR3 Agonists

The synthetic TLR3 ligand polyinosinic-polycytidylic acid, stabilized with polylysine and carboxymethylcellulose (poly-ICLC), has been tested intramuscularly in combination with RT in adults with glioblastoma in two-Phase 2 clinical studies, one after surgery[135] and one with definitive concurrent chemoradiotherapy.[136] Both studies suggested a survival advantage without additional significant toxicities.

Stimulator of Interferon Gene Agonists and IFN-I

In preclinical studies, STING agonists have demonstrated therapeutic synergy with RT. Distant disease control was achieved in a CD8$^+$ T cell-dependent manner.[137–139] A multicenter Phase 2 clinical trial evaluated adjuvant IFN-α-2b, cisplatin, and continuous infusion of 5-fluorouracil concurrently with external-beam RT in patients with resected (R0/R1) adenocarcinoma of the pancreatic head (50.4 Gy). A promising 18-month overall survival was observed albeit at a dismal all-cause grade ≥3 toxicity rate of 95% during therapy.[140] A similar level of toxicity (85% grade ≥3) was seen in a multicenter randomized Phase 3 clinical trial for patients with resected pancreatic adenocarcinoma. This time adjuvant chemoradiation plus IFN-α-2b was compared to fluorouracil and folinic acid but failed to demonstrate a survival advantage for the combinatorial treatment.[141] Similarly, RT given concomitantly with IFN-α-2b and 13-*cis*-retinoic acid (RA) did not demonstrate a survival advantage when compared to weekly cisplatin chemoradiation in a recent Phase 2, open-label, randomized trial for stage III cervical cancer patients despite being less toxic.[142]

Granulocyte-Macrophage Colony-Stimulating Factor and Flt3-Ligand

Driving APC proliferation has always been an appealing avenue for cancer immunotherapy, and Flt3 ligand or granulocyte-macrophage colony-stimulating factor (GM-CSF) are two ways to achieve that. In a preclinical study, Demaria et al. observed an abscopal effect with a combination of RT and Flt3-ligand.[4] In a proof-of-principle clinical trial, this abscopal response was detected in 26.8% of patients with extensively pretreated metastatic disease of varied histologies who received RT (35 Gy in 10 fractions) and concurrent GM-CSF.[143]

Release of T Cell Inhibitory Signals

Checkpoint Inhibitors

CTLA-4 Blockade

Many preclinical studies demonstrated that RT is synergistic with anti-CTLA-4 mAb.[144–147] In a poorly immunogenic, metastatic 4T1 mammary carcinoma mouse model, Demaria et al. showed that combination of RT and anti-CTLA-4 led to tumor-growth inhibition, inhibition of lung metastases formation, and a survival advantage. CD8[+], but not CD4[+], T cells were required for these therapeutic effects.[144] Similarly, fractionated RT plus CTLA-4 blockade enhanced tumor-growth delay in TSA mouse breast carcinoma and MCA38 mouse colon carcinoma compared to RT alone, and induced abscopal effects. The frequency of CD8[+] T cells showing tumor-specific IFN-γ production was proportional to the extent of inhibition of the distant tumor.[145] Clinical abscopal responses in individual patients who were on ipilimumab followed RT to a metastatic site in melanoma and non-small cell lung cancer (NSCLC).[148–151] Twenty-two melanoma patients with multiple metastatic sites, each of whom received hypofractionated irradiation to a single index lesion, followed by four cycles of ipilimumab as part of a Phase 1 clinical trial, generally tolerated the treatment well with no grade 4 toxicity. Evaluation of the unirradiated lesions indicated that 18% of patients had a partial response and 18% had stable disease.[146] A similar Phase 1 trial was done in patients with metastatic solid tumors refractory to standard therapies and with ≥1 metastatic lesion in liver or lung that received stereotactic ablative body radiotherapy (SABR) with ipilimumab every 3 weeks for a total of four doses. Again, the treatment was considered safe with no grade 4 toxicity, no grade >1 pneumonitis, and a rate of grade 3 at 34%, mostly self-limiting. Data on efficacy was encouraging with 10% of patients exhibiting out-of-field partial response and 23% with clinical benefit, that is a partial response or stable disease lasting ≥6 months.[152] Hiniker et al. conducted a prospective trial in 22 patients with stage IV melanoma treated with ipilimumab for four cycles and palliative RT to one or two disease sites initiated within 5 days of ipilimumab. Combination therapy was well tolerated without unexpected toxicities. Half the patients experienced clinical benefit from therapy, including three (27.3%) with ongoing systemic complete response at a median follow-up of 55 weeks.[153] A multicenter, double-blind, Phase 3 clinical trial randomized 799 patients with at least one bone metastasis from castration-resistant prostate cancer that had progressed after docetaxel treatment to receive bone-directed RT (8 Gy in one fraction), followed by either ipilimumab or placebo every 3 weeks for up to four doses. The trial nearly met statistical significance of overall survival benefit with ipilimumab ($p = 0.053$) but that was seen in a subset analysis of those patients with nonvisceral metastatic disease. Overall, there was a significant improvement in progression-free survival (PFS) at a level of toxicity that did not exceed what would have been expected from ipilimumab monotherapy.[154] An 18% objective response rate (ORR) and a 31% disease control rate to hypofractionated RT and CTLA-4 blockade have been recently reported in patients with metastatic NSCLC refractory to anti-CTLA-4 antibodies alone or in combination with chemotherapy. An increase in the frequency of T cell clones recognizing a mutated tumor antigen was noted.[155]

Programmed Cell Death 1/Programmed Death Ligand 1 Blockade

Many preclinical studies using a variety of tumor models have demonstrated the potential benefits from blocking the PD-1/PD-L1 axis when combined with RT. In an orthotopic murine glioblastoma model, improved survival and a change in the intratumoral balance in favor of cytotoxic T cells at the expense of T_{regs} cells was achieved, following stereotactic radiosurgery (SRS) plus PD-1 blockade compared to either modality alone.[156] Breast tumors also responded better to this therapeutic approach, both locally and systemically, through a T cell-dependent mechanism. Increased cytotoxic T cell proliferation and TNF-α production were seen that inadvertently limited the accumulation of MDSCs.[73]

In preclinical models, low doses of fractionated RT led to PD-L1 upregulation on tumor cells, but adding anti-PD-1 or anti-PD-L1 monoclonal antibodies (mAbs) concomitantly to RT generated meaningful CD8[+] T cell responses that improved local tumor control, long-term survival, and protection against tumor rechallenge.[157] Further, in a B16-F10 melanoma mouse model, resistance to the combination therapy of RT plus anti-CTLA-4 was partly due to upregulation of PD-L1 on tumor cells. This was associated with T cell exhaustion, and easily mitigated by PD-L1 blockade. The triple-combo of RT, anti-CTLA-4, and anti-PD-L1 appeared to promote tumor control and immunity through distinct mechanisms: while RT enhanced the diversity of the TCR repertoire of intratumoral T cells, anti-CTLA-4 predominantly inhibited T_{regs} cells, increasing the CD8[+] T cell-to-T_{reg} cell ratio (CD8/T_{reg}) with anti-PD-L1 reversing T cell exhaustion, counteracting a CD8[+]/T_{reg} ratio decline and further encouraging oligoclonal T cell expansion.[146]

Clinical data on this combination therapy is beginning to emerge. Brain metastases treated with SRS within 6 months of receiving nivolumab was well tolerated in a retrospective analysis of 26 patients, with one patient experiencing grade 2 headaches following RT, but no other treatment-related neurologic toxicities or scalp reactions were reported. Local control and overall survival appeared prolonged compared with standard treatment.[158] Pseudoprogression is another aspect of immunotherapy that may be enhanced when RT is added to the equation. Early clinical and radiologic progression was seen in two patients with metastatic brain malignancies who received SRS followed by pembrolizumab, or nivolumab with ipilimumab. Upon surgical resection and pathological examination, no tumor cells were detected but a marked inflammatory and immune reaction highlighted a potential pseudoprogression.[159] Another secondary analysis of the KEYNOTE-001 trial, a Phase 1 study assessing pembrolizumab in patients with advanced NSCLC, found that patients who received RT before the anti-PD-1 treatment experienced longer PFS and better OS than patients who did not have previous RT.[160] Blockade of the PD-1/PD-L1 axis in combination with RT has shown similar promise in prospective trials. In the PACIFIC trial, the anti-PD-L1 agent durvalumab used as consolidation after platinum-based chemoradiation in patients with stage 3 NSCLC demonstrated an improved OS compared to placebo. Interestingly, the patients who were randomized to receive durvalumab within a 14-day window after the completion of chemoradiation had better clinical outcomes.[161] In a multicenter, randomized Phase 2 study (PEMBRO-RT), patients with advanced NSCLC received pembrolizumab alone or in combination with SBRT (8 Gy × 3) that was administered to a single tumor site 1 week in advance. Better outcomes were observed in the combination treatment group, ironically especially in patients with PD-L1 negative tumors.[162] Many ongoing trials are assessing the value of integrating RT into PD-1/PD-L1 blockade and/or PD-1/PD-L1 blockade plus CTLA-4 blockade in varied histologies. The rationale behind this combination comes from the finding that these three therapies have nonredundant effects: T_{reg} cell depletion by anti-CTLA-4, possible TCR repertoire diversification and decreasing tumor burden by RT, and reversing T cell exhaustion by PD-1/PD-L1 inhibition.[141]

TGF-β Antagonists

A study on two breast cancer mouse models showed that priming of tumor-reactive CD8⁺ T cells after RT was enhanced by TGF-β blockade, leading to CD8⁺ T cell infiltration, and tumor-growth inhibition, locally and systemically. However, adaptive immune resistance along the PD-1 pathway ultimately limited the therapeutic efficacy, supporting the concept of targeting PD-1 alongside TGF-β in the context of RT.[163] In another preclinical study, TGF-β receptor antagonism sensitizes mouse rectal cancers to RT, which was dependent on CXCR3-mediated recruitment of CD8⁺ T cells.[164] Clinically, the

combination between RT and TGF-β inhibition has been studied in metastatic breast cancer patients who received the TGF-β blocking antibody fresolimumab at two different doses (1 or 10 mg/kg). Patients receiving the 10 mg/kg dose had a significantly higher median overall survival and an increase in CD8⁺ central memory T cells and a decrease of monocytic MDSCs in their circulation.[165]

Indoleamine 2,3 Dioxygenase (IDO) Inhibitors

IDO can be upregulated in the lymph node microenvironment by chronic TLR stimulation or by adaptive immune resistance fueled by IFN-γ from activated cytotoxic T lymphocytes, especially following CTLA-4 or PD-1/PD-L1 blockade.[166] IDO causes depletion of tryptophan, an essential T cell factor, as well as increasing kynerine, and suppressing T cell proliferation while promoting T_{regs} cells. A preclinical study showed that pharmacologic inhibition of IDO synergized with chemoradiation, prolonging survival of mice bearing intracranial glioblastoma tumors, which was associated with widespread complement component C3 deposition at the tumor site.[167]

Stimulation of Effector T Cells
Co-Stimulatory Antibodies
Agonistic Anti-OX40 Antibody

In murine models of lung cancer[168] and soft tissue sarcoma,[169] hypofractionated RT combined with anti-OX40 mAb led to prolonged survival compared to either single treatment. It was mainly CD8⁺ T cell-dependent with OX40⁺CD8⁺ T cells proliferation in tumor-draining lymph nodes. Mice bearing intracranial GL261 gliomas or MCA 205 fibrosarcomas that had been treated with a combination of local RT (5 Gy × 1), intrasplenic vaccination with DC/tumor fusion cells, and anti-OX40 mAb, showed durable survival in 50% to 80% of the mice.[170] The benefits of radiation followed by OX40 stimulation was also seen in anti-PD-1-resistant mouse lung tumors with local and systemic antitumor-growth delay and improved survival rates.[171] Two early clinical trials combining hypofractionated RT and anti-OX40 mAb have been conducted recently in patients with progressive metastatic prostate cancer (NCT01303705) and metastatic breast cancer (NCT0186290).

Agonistic Anti-CD137 Antibody

Combination of RT with CD137 activation showed promising results in intracranial models of murine high-grade glioma.[172,173]

IL-2 and IL-12

Treatment of MC38, a murine colon adenocarcinoma, with RT and IL-12 resulted in complete remission in 100%

of mice compared to only 12% with RT alone.[174] Similar results were observed in animals bearing large subcutaneous or orthotopic hepatocellular carcinoma, with dramatic local tumor regression, systemic effects against a distant tumor, and significantly prolonged survival.[175] In a pilot clinical study of SBRT (1, 2, or 3 doses of 20 Gy) followed by high-dose IL-2 in patients with metastatic melanoma or renal cell carcinoma, the response rate was significantly higher than expected from historical data, at least for those with melanoma. Responders had a greater frequency of circulating proliferating CD4+ T cells with an early activated effector memory phenotype.[176] To reduce side effects and improve the therapeutic index of cytokines, engineered immunocytokines have been developed. They are antibody-cytokine fusion proteins, with the potential to preferentially localize to the tumor site and to activate antitumor immunity. Various tumor-antigen targets (cell membrane antigens, extracellular matrix components) and antibody formats (intact IgG, antibody fragments) have been considered.[177] L19–IL-2, an immunocytokine that combines IL-2 with an antibody targeting altered tumor vasculature by binding to extradomain B (ED-B) of fibronectin,[178] has been evaluated in combination with RT. In a preclinical study of different cancer mouse models with different ED-B expression levels, data showed an increased CD8+ T cell-dependent therapeutic potential by combining single-dose local tumor RT with systemic administration of L19–IL-2.[179,180] NHS-IL-2 is a fusion of IL-2 and NHS-76, an antibody that binds to DNA-histone complexes and targets necrotic tumor cells,[181] Systemic administration of NHS–IL-2 plus local RT induced immune response activation and complete tumor-growth regressions in 80% to 100% of mice with lung carcinomas. A Phase 1b trial in metastatic NSCLC patients who achieved disease control with first-line palliative chemotherapy was conducted. RT (4 Gy × 5) of a single pulmonary nodule and NHS–IL-2 given i.v. in a dose-escalating design was well tolerated and two of 13 patients achieved long-term survival.[182]

Inhibition of Tumor-Associated Macrophage Recruitment and Polarization

As previously mentioned, colony-stimulating factor 1 (CSF-1) tends to increase in irradiated tumors, and targeting CSF-1/CSF-1R pathway promises to prevent the proliferation and differentiation of macrophages with an immunosuppressive phenotype as was seen in irradiated prostate tumors in mice given the CSF-1R small molecule inhibitor pexidartinib (PLX3397).[37] Similarly, GBM xenografts treated with RT plus concurrent PLX3397 prevented radiation-driven recruitment and differentiation of monocytes into immunosuppressive, pro-angiogenic TAMs, enhanced the tumor-growth delay, and extended survival.[183] PLX3397 is under investigation in association with

RT in two early clinical trials conducted in patients with intermediate- or high-risk prostate cancer (NCT02472275) and newly diagnosed glioblastoma (NCT01790503).

Inhibition of VEGF

Many preclinical studies have shown a synergistic effect of VEGF-targeting therapies, in combination with RT,[184–189] which is normally explained as a transient normalization of tumor vasculature, leading to improved tumor oxygenation and thus greater radiosensitivity.[190] Reversal of the immunosuppressive effects of VEGF-A is another possible explanation. Bevacizumab (Avastin), an anti-VEGF recombinant humanized mAb, is currently under clinical investigation in combination with RT for the treatment of glioblastoma. Sorafenib (Nexavar), a protein kinase targeting the VEGF receptor, is also being studied in RT patients with localized unresectable pancreatic cancer.

Intratumoral Injection of Autologous Dendritic Cells

RT and intratumoral (i.t.) injection of DC caused significant tumor-growth delay in a murine model of squamous cell carcinoma, which also inhibited the growth of untreated tumors in the same mouse.[191] Similarly, i.t. DC plus RT inhibited growth of D5 melanoma and MCA 205 sarcoma tumors in an additive or synergistic manner, respectively, with an increase in IFN-g-secreting T cells in the spleen.[192] A Phase 1 clinical study was conducted with i.t. injection of autologous, immature DCs plus single-fraction RT (8 Gy) in advanced/metastatic hepatoma patients. Treatment was safe and innate and tumor-specific immunity was induced with a partial or minor response in 50% of patients.[193] Another Phase 1 study evaluated neoadjuvant radiation with i.t. DC injections in 18 newly diagnosed high-risk soft tissue sarcoma patients, of whom 56% developed a tumor-specific immune response that often correlated with a clinical response.[194]

Cancer Vaccines

Therapeutic cancer vaccines may be classified into several major categories including (a) tumor cell vaccines, autologous or allogenic, typically irradiated; (b) protein/peptide-based cancer vaccines with tumor-associated antigens (TAAs); and (c) genetic vaccines, DNA plasmid TAA vaccines, RNA vaccines with mRNA from autologous tumor tissues, or viral-based vaccines.[195] They can be combined with immune adjuvants such as IL-2 or GM-CSF. Three preclinical studies in HPV-associated cervical cancer mouse models have clearly demonstrated that RT combined with HPV vaccination improved tumor-specific cytotoxic T cell responses.[196–198] A pancreatic mouse tumor model with limited CD8+ T cell infiltration and high PD-L1 expression revealed that local RT coupled with a tumor vaccine can drive T cell infiltration, but this was insufficient to translate into tumor-growth inhibition until an anti-PD-L1 antibody was added which enhanced TIL effector function and tumor regression with increased survival. This study is crucial as it highlights the possibility of shifting the balance toward T cell-inflamed tumor phenotype and tumor control.[199] A Phase 2 clinical trial in patients with clinically localized prostate cancer randomized 30 patients into a combination arm with recombinant vaccinia (rV) carrying a PSA gene, rV containing the co-stimulator B7.1, local GM-CFS, low-dose systemic IL-2, and standard RT, or RT alone. Seventeen of 19 patients in the combination arm completed all vaccinations and 13 of these 17 patients had increases in PSA-specific T cells of at least three-fold versus none in the RT-only arm.[200] Currently, clinical trials are underway in patients with castrate-refractory metastatic prostate cancer assessing RT to a metastatic site with sipuleucel-T, a therapeutic cancer vaccine consisting of autologous DCs loaded with the prostatic acid phosphatase (PAP) antigen, plus GM-CSF aiming to mature DCs.

Latest Immunotherapeutic Innovations

Chimeric antigen receptor (CAR) T cells and bispecific antibodies (bsAbs) are two recent engineered technologies. CAR is a modular fusion protein comprising extracellular target-binding domain, usually derived from the single-chain variable fragment (scFv) of antibodies, spacer domain, transmembrane domain, and intracellular signaling domain containing CD3zeta linked co-stimulatory molecules, such as CD28, CD137, and CD134. T cells are collected via apheresis from the patient, genetically modified with transfer of CAR coding sequence by retroviral vectors, then used for an autologous adoptive cell transfer. They are capable of specifically recognizing their target antigen through the scFv binding domain, resulting in T cell activation in a major histocompatibility complex (MHC)-independent manner.[201–206]

T cell-recruiting bsAbs consist of two scFvs, with one Fv directed at a tumor cell surface antigen and the second scFv binding the CD3epsilon subunit of the T cell receptor complex. They are able to recruit and activate T cells and bring together T cells and tumor cells for a specific lysis of tumor cells.[207] There is a rationale for combining RT with these therapeutics. However, a recent preclinical study reported that large melanomas treated with hypofractionated RT plus T cell-recruiting bsAbs relapsed faster than those treated with RT alone. Mechanistic investigations revealed that bsAbs mediated overstimulation of tumor-specific T cells and induced massive T cell apoptosis, calling for caution when considering CD3-engaging bsAbs for the treatment of solid tumors.[208]

OPTIMIZING RADIOTHERAPY-IMMUNOTHERAPY COMBINATIONS

Optimizing Radiation Therapy Parameters

Total Dose

A recent analysis of murine tumor models including breast, colon, lung, fibrosarcoma, pancreas, melanoma, and head and neck cancer provides evidence for a dose-response relationship between biologically effective dose (BED) of irradiation and the rate of occurrence of abscopal effects, suggesting a probability of abscopal effects of 50% for a BED of 60 Gy.[209]

Dose Per Fraction and Dose-Rate

A point worth noting here is the concept of BED, where the effective tumor cell-killing dose is not always the same as the numerically calculated dose, that is, 3 Gy × 5 is not necessarily equal to 5 Gy × 3 or 15 Gy. This is dependent on the a/b ratio of the tumor, that is, the ability to repair sublethal damage between fractions. Having said that, most murine tumors have relatively fast growth kinetics with very high a/b ratios and, therefore, show little response to fractions. In other words, in most of these preclinical tumor models, equating BED with the numerically calculated dose is probably acceptable. However, the fast proliferation rate makes it difficult to control tumors using low-dose daily fractions.

The optimal fractionation regimen that maximizes tumor immunity while keeping immunosuppressive effects to a minimum remains unknown. Hypofractionated RT appears to be the most promising in that regard. In mice bearing B16-OVA murine melanoma treated with up to 15 Gy given in various-size fractions of 3 Gy, 5 Gy, 7.5 Gy, or 15 Gy, fractionated treatment with medium-size radiation doses of 7.5 Gy/fraction gave the best tumor control and tumor immunity while maintaining low T_{reg} cell numbers.[210] Similarly, TSA mouse breast carcinomas and MCA38 mouse colon carcinomas responded best to anti-CTLA-4 mAbs, when combined with fractionated, local RT with 6 Gy × 5 or 8 Gy × 3, rather than 20 Gy single-dose RT, both in terms of local control and abscopal effect.[145] More recently, Vanpouille-Box et al. showed that radiation doses above 12 to 18 Gy likely activate the DNA exonuclease Trex1, and so degrade cytosolic DNA that would have otherwise activated cGAS-STING pathways for potent, immune-activating IFN-I responses.[211] This would support the idea of a "sweet spot" using the mid-range dose/fraction, although some preclinical studies found that single ablative doses can be just as effective, if not more so. For instance, B16-SIY mouse melanoma tumors irradiated with a single dose of 20 Gy responded much better in terms of immunity and growth control than following 5 Gy × 4.[9] Similarly, a single local dose of 15 Gy was superior to 3 Gy × 5 in the parent B16 mouse melanoma model for tumor-specific antigen presentation, priming of T cells, and T cell trafficking and tumor infiltration.[23] Other data indicate that conventionally fractionated RT could also effectively trigger an immune response. For instance, a retrospective study of 47 patients with metastatic melanoma treated with ipilimumab and palliative RT revealed that responses of index lesions outside the radiation field (i.e., abscopal responses) favorably associated with a radiation fraction size ≤ 3 Gy.[212]

Part of this discussion is the question of dose rate. When delivered at supra-high rates, as during FLASH RT, that is, >40 Gy/s compared to conventual dose rates of 0.01 to 0.2 Gy/s, there appears to be significantly less normal tissue injury for comparable tumor control.[213,214] The immunomodulatory impact of this novel radiation delivery method that is in early preclinical development remains to be explored.

Size of Treatment Field

Large treatment fields and/or large integral doses include more circulating blood, spleen, and bone marrow cells and tend to drive lymphopenia as lymphocytes are radiosensitive, whereas hypofractionation with less beam time tends to have the opposite effect.[215,216] Moreover, irradiation of tumor-draining lymph nodes could impact T cell priming and proliferation. So, highly conformal tumor irradiation techniques such as stereotactic RT are preferred to spare lymphocytic death and maximize immune responses. In contrast, intensity-modulated RT (IMRT), which results in a higher integral dose than 3D-conformal RT, might deplete more T cells. Proton therapy is promising in some settings, thanks to its advantageous ballistic properties. Because of their relatively large mass, protons have little lateral side scatter, resulting in only a small dose deposited in tissues bordering the tumor. The dose delivered is maximized in the Braag peak, that is, over the last few millimeters of the particle's range, with no exit dose beyond the tumor. This results in a lower integral dose. Proton therapy appears to induce an identical tumor immune response versus photons.[217] Brachytherapy may confer meaningful advantages over external-beam RT because of its powerful conformality. Finally, partial tumor volume irradiation could be sufficient to stimulate the immune system. Spatially fractionated GRID radiotherapy (SFGRT) has been designed for achieving tumor responses in bulky tumors too large to be treated safely with traditional RT. The radiobiologic mechanisms are postulated to involve radiation-induced bystander effects, microvascular alterations, and/or immunomodulation. A recent review summarized the early phase clinical trials in SFGRT and highlighted remarkable response rates at minimal toxicity although more biological data on the immunomodulatory impact of this radiation strategy are needed.[218]

Target Site

Thus far, most abscopal effects observed clinically were induced after RT to a visceral lesion. Looking at the systemic immune response in patients receiving SBRT to parenchymal (lung and liver) or nonparenchymal tumor sites (bone and brain), McGee et al. showed an increase in circulating activated memory CD4+ and CD8+ T cells only when RT was delivered to parenchymal sites.[219] However, targeting a deep site tended to increase the integral dose with an increased risk of lymphopenia. Irradiating multiple lesions within different tissue beds could circumvent the issue of tumor heterogeneity, broaden the repertoire of released TAAs, and activate immune signals from multiple TMEs.[220] A larger tumor presumably releases more antigens with greater diversity, but it likely also contains more hypoxic areas, which are radioresistant, and to be immunosuppressive. Irradiating a large tumor also increases integral dose and the risk of lymphopenia.

High-Linear Energy Transfer Radiation Therapy

Most studies assessing the combination between RT and immunotherapeutic agents have used photon irradiation. Carbon-ion therapy has an increased linear energy transfer (LET), that is, greater ionization density along the beam path and more clustered DNA lesions, defined as two or more lesions within one to two helical turns of DNA. These are harder to repair and so likely to cause more cell death. Carbon ions have a relative biological effectiveness (RBE) of 3 compared to photons, electrons, and protons.[221-223] This potent cell-killing capacity may have greater immunogenic potential. Moreover, carbon ions also have an advantage in terms of conformal dose distribution and a low integral dose. Thus, they might be superior for triggering an antitumor immune response and/or an abscopal effect. Preclinical studies have confirmed this. Even mice carrying a poorly immunogenic squamous cell carcinoma were able to develop tumor-specific, long-lasting antitumor immunity through CD8+ T lymphocytes following carbon-ion beam irradiation.[224] A single 6 Gy dose of carbon ions to a murine squamous cell carcinoma induced an intratumoral increase of ICAM-1 and activated DCs. When the treatment included the injection of α-galactosylceramide-pulsed DCs into the primary tumor in addition to carbon-ion RT, distant lung metastases formation was inhibited.[225] Fast neutron therapy is another high-LET irradiation with an RBE of 3. However, neutron therapy centers are few and far between owed to the challenging dose distribution. Their immunomodulating properties remain unknown.

Optimizing the Therapeutic Sequence

RT presumably releases TAAs and DAMPS, two immune-stimulatory factors in the cancer-immunity cycle.[226] With each additional therapy to be combined with RT, the scheduling of the different interventions should be adapted accordingly. For instance, therapies that promote cancer antigen presentation (CD40 agonists, TLR agonists, IFN-I, STING ligands, intratumoral injection of autologous DC) or priming and T cell activation (anti-CTLA-4 mAb, agonistic anti-OX40 mAb, agonistic anti-CD137 mAb) should be administered concomitantly to irradiation, whereas therapies that promote cytotoxic T cell activity (anti-PD-1/PD-L1, IDO inhibitors, IL-2) may be best administered after RT. A case in point is the preclinical study by Dewan et al., demonstrating that delaying administration of anti-CTLA-4 mAbs after conclusion of RT reduced the therapeutic effect of the combination therapy.[145] In fact, most clinical cases of abscopal responses occurred when anti-CTLA-4 was combined with RT concomitantly.[227,228]

Patient Selection

Personalized cancer therapy and the selection of patients who are most likely to benefit from RT-immunotherapy is crucial and remains one of the main challenges in the field.

Patient (Host) Criteria

Some patients' characteristics indicate immune depression and a decreased likelihood of immune response. Age is associated with impaired immunity.[229] Prior exposure to chemotherapy can induce myelodepression and lymphopenia, and should be taken into consideration. Similarly, multiple prior RT, especially with large fields and/or protracted fractionated regimens, likely induce lymphopenia. In fact, abscopal responses are more often seen in patients who have a lower baseline median neutrophil to lymphocyte ratio.[143] The gut flora can also affect the TME and the antitumor immune responses to therapy.[230] In preclinical models, efficacy of CTLA4[231] and PD-L1[232] blockade was shown to depend on gut microbiota. Similarly, in a mouse melanoma model, total body RT induced microbial translocation that increased DC activation via TLR4 signaling and tumor-specific CD8[+] T cell function, driving tumor regression.[233]

Tumor Criteria

Overall tumor burden might significantly impact the outcome of RT-immunotherapy. In a Phase 3 trial assessing ipilimumab versus placebo after RT in patients with metastatic castration-resistant prostate cancer that had progressed after docetaxel chemotherapy, an overall survival benefit for ipilimumab was only seen in a subset of patients without visceral metastases.[154] The TME is also immensely important. The number of tumor stroma-infiltrating lymphocytes was found to predict the response to irradiation. High densities of T cells (CD3[+])

and cytotoxic T cells (CD8[+]), as well as a low density of T_{reg} cells (CD25[+]Foxp3[+]), were associated with good clinical and pathological responses after chemoradiation in various cancer types such as rectum,[234,235] esophageal,[236] or NSCLC.[237] In many tumor types such as melanoma, NSCLC, HNSCC, or bladder, PD-L1 expression is associated with an increased rate of response to PD-1/PD-L1 blockade.[238–241] Tumor mutational burden, nonsynonymous mutations, in particular, can be important as well as it correlates with neoantigen load and local immunity.[242,243] A higher somatic mutational load was shown to be associated with the degree of clinical benefit in melanoma,[244] NSCLC,[245] and mismatch repair-deficient colorectal patients[246] receiving immune checkpoint inhibitors. It is likely that the genomic landscape of tumors also dictates radiation-induced immune responses.

Endpoints for Clinical Trials

Historically, assessing tumor response to a cytotoxic treatment is based on imaging results and RECIST (Response Evaluation Criteria in Solid Tumors). RECIST 1.1, updated in 2009, is the latest version.[247,248] RECIST takes into account size and number of tumor lesions. Partial response is a ≥30% decrease of sum of diameters of target lesions. Progressive disease is a ≥20% increase of sum of diameters of target lesions or appearance of ≥1 new lesion. RECIST may not provide a complete assessment of immunotherapeutic tumor response as antitumor response to immunotherapy may take longer compared to cytotoxic agents. Moreover, transient pseudoprogression often occurs due to vascular leakage and tumor infiltration. The irRC (Immune-Related Response Criteria) is a set of published rules that provide better assessment of the effect of immunotherapeutic agents.[249–251] New lesions identified at evaluation timepoints don't count anymore as "progressive disease" but are combined with index lesions as a measure of tumor burden. Immune-related progressive disease is defined by a new threshold of 25% increase in tumor burden from the lowest level recorded. Immune-related partial response is a 50% drop in tumor burden from baseline. Traditional endpoints to assess efficacy in clinical trials such as local control or PFS don't seem relevant. OS appears to be the most appropriate. Safety/toxicity of these new combinations between RT and immunotherapy must be carefully reported and graded. By unbalancing the immune system, immunotherapies generate immune toxicities, called immune-related adverse events (irAEs) that mainly involve the gut, skin, endocrine glands, liver, and lung but can potentially affect any tissue;[252] toxicities may be increased by RT. The inflammatory reaction at the irradiated site may also be increased by an immune stimulation, potentially amplifying acute and late toxicities. Finally, patient monitoring with the development of surrogate immune biomarkers would help to predict treatment responses long before radiologic evidence occurs. Examples are changes in peripheral CD8[+] T cells, CD8[+]/CD4[+] T cell ratio, neutrophil to lymphocyte ratio, and proportion of CD8[+] T cells expressing 4-1BB and PD-1.[152] Other peripheral biomarkers, such as circulating immune cells (T$_{regs}$ cells, MDSCs, macrophages, neutrophils) or soluble factors (CRP, IFNs, ILs, TNF-α, TGF-β), as well as post-therapeutic pathologic changes in the irradiated tumor, could be of value. Innovative radiomics approaches have also been proposed as non-invasive methods to predict clinical outcomes of patients treated with immunotherapy.[253]

CONCLUSION

Renaissance of cancer immunotherapy, therapeutic success of immune checkpoints blockade, and multiplication of immunotherapeutic modalities, associated with a better understanding of interactions between irradiated tumors and the immune system, lead to a potential paradigm shift in the use of RT. In addition to a direct cytotoxic effect, RT can be an adjuvant to immunotherapy, eliciting a stronger systemic antitumor response or even de novo antitumor immune responses. However, current evidence of the benefits of RT in this context is mainly based on results of preclinical studies and clinical case reports. Implementation in clinical practice requires the results of numerous ongoing prospective clinical trials. Moreover, high costs of most immunotherapies such as

the checkpoint inhibitors and financial constraints will force a more careful selection of patients, most likely to benefit from RT-immunotherapy and drive their optimal integration.

KEY REFERENCES

Only key references appear in the print edition. The full reference list appears in the digital product on Springer Publishing Connect: connect.springerpub.com/content/book/978-0-8261-3743-2/part/part04/chapter/ch63

4. Demaria S, Ng B, Devitt ML, et al. Ionizing radiation inhibition of distant untreated tumors (abscopal effect) is immune mediated. *Int J Radiat Oncol Biol Phys.* 2004;58(3):862–870. doi:10.1016/j.ijrobp.2003.09.012
5. Mole RH. Whole body irradiation; radiobiology or medicine? *Br J Radiol.* 1953;26(305):234–241. doi:10.1259/0007-1285-26-305-234
8. Stone HB, Peters LJ, Milas L. Effect of host immune capability on radiocurability and subsequent transplantability of a murine fibrosarcoma. *J Natl Cancer Inst.* 1979;63(5):1229–1235. doi:10.1093/jnci/63.5.1229
24. Reits EA, Hodge JW, Herberts CA, et al. Radiation modulates the peptide repertoire, enhances MHC class I expression, and induces successful antitumor immunotherapy. *J Exp Med.* 2006;203(5):1259–1271. doi:10.1084/jem.20052494
37. Xu J, Escamilla J, Mok S, et al. CSF1R signaling blockade stanches tumor-infiltrating myeloid cells and improves the efficacy of radiotherapy in prostate cancer. *Cancer Res.* 2013;73(9):2782–2794. doi:10.1158/0008-5472.CAN-12-3981
211. Vanpouille-Box C, Alard A, Aryankalayil MJ, et al. DNA exonuclease Trex1 regulates radiotherapy-induced tumour immunogenicity. *Nat Commun.* 2017;8:15618. doi:10.1038/ncomms15618

Regulatory Aspects of the Biological Therapy of Cancer

Raj K. Puri

Regulatory Considerations for Therapeutic Cancer Vaccines

Syed R. Husain, Karin M. Knudson, Laronna Colbert, Ramjay S. Vatsan, Thomas Finn, Jaikumar Duraiswamy, Ke Liu, and Raj Puri

KEY POINTS

- In this chapter, we summarize the chemistry, manufacturing, and control (CMC), as well as clinical information, relevant to cancer vaccine development.

- The U.S. Food and Drug Administration's (FDA's) general recommendation is to not retain unwanted foreign genetic materials in human therapeutic agents.

- We discuss general CMC considerations that apply to the manufacture and testing of synthetic peptide-based investigational products that may also be applicable to neoantigen-based peptide vaccines.

- As the selection of neoantigens is a fundamental part of the manufacturing process to produce the specific final product, details about the approach used should be included in the IND (21 CFR 312.23(a)(7)).

- CMC considerations for dendritic cell (DC) vaccines include the reagents used to purify peripheral blood mononuclear cells (PBMCs), generate immature DCs and mature them, the cell culturing process, the level of cellular characterization, the cell surface markers used to identify DCs, and the tests to evaluate the purity and potency of the DC product.

- Early clinical developmental protocols should specify in detail all the elements of the study that are critical to safety. Such elements may include all clinical safety assessments, toxicity monitoring, description of toxicity-based stopping rules, dose adjustment rules for individual patients and the overall trial, and adverse event recording and reporting.

- It is imperative that investigators fully detail anticipated toxicities and include a robust safety monitoring plan to appropriately characterize and document the safety profile of the investigational agent.

- In oncologic practice, investigational and approved treatments are generally discontinued when patients experience disease progression. Because of the time required for the host (patient) to elicit or amplify an immune response to a cancer vaccine (i.e., tumor-specific immune response), the vaccine may have a delayed effect in the study subjects.

- When the proposed mechanism of action involves a specific antigen or other therapeutic target, consideration also should be given to developing an assay or mechanism to measure the target antigen expression in tumor tissues of individual patients and using that information in subject selection or response monitoring.

INTRODUCTION

In the long catalogue of human ailments, cancer has occupied a prime space for millennia. However, we are at the dawn of a new, hopeful 21st century where it is conceivable to contemplate cures for what has been termed "the emperor of all maladies."[1] Over the last 50 years, the U.S. Food and Drug Administration (FDA) has approved over 200 new medications to treat cancer.[2] Of these 200 new medications, approximately 50% of the approvals are for targeted non-immune-based therapies for cancer, and about 10% to 20% correspond to new molecular entities representing cancer immunotherapy.[2,3] Cancer immunotherapy drugs are designed to target specific molecules expressed by the cancer cell (tumor targets or tumor-associated antigens [TAA]) or to enhance immune responses to cancer cells (e.g., checkpoint inhibitors [CHI]). Notable milestones include the approval of IFN-α2 (for the treatment of melanoma in 1995); approval of an anti-CD20 monoclonal antibody (rituximab, for the treatment of B cell non-Hodgkin lymphoma in 1997); and approval of IL-2 (for the treatment of stage IV melanoma in 1998).[4]

However, immunotherapies are not new. In 1891, William B. Coley, an American surgeon and cancer researcher, observed that injecting a mixture of live bacterial pathogens *Streptococcus pyogenes* and *Serratia marcescens* caused the remission of sarcoma. He later demonstrated that using heat-killed bacteria achieved remission of several types of malignancies, including sarcoma, lymphoma, and testicular carcinoma. However, due to a lack of knowledge of the immune mechanisms and risks associated with injecting virulent bacteria into cancer patients, the treatment termed "Coley toxins" was given up in favor of surgery[4] and chemotherapy. Attenuated bacterial therapy for cancer was revived when bacille Calmette-Guérin (BCG) was shown to prevent recurrence of nonmuscle invasive bladder cancer. Two different strains of BCG were approved by the FDA in 1990 (TheraCys, Sanofi Pasteur) and in 1998 (Tice, Merck). BCG is still used today, but the exact mechanism of BCG-based immunotherapy of cancer is not clearly understood.[5]

The successes of CHI in treating cancer and a greater understanding of the mode of action of CHI,[6,7] early promising results of tumor-infiltrating lymphocyte (TIL) therapies,[8] subsequent success of chimeric antigen receptor (CAR) T cell therapies,[9] and the identification of new TAAs revived interest in the development of cancer vaccines (please refer to the accompanying chapters on cell therapy [Chapter 65] and gene therapy [Chapter 66] for additional details on TIL- and CAR-based immunotherapies and how the FDA regulates these products). Cancer vaccines are primarily therapeutic vaccines designed to amplify cytotoxic T lymphocyte (CTL) responses to tumor cells through active immunization. Cancer vaccines utilize TAA as immunological targets on cancer cells. TAAs are made up of proteins and glycoproteins that were initially identified and characterized due to their value as diagnostic tumor markers.[10,11] TAAs are normal proteins or "self-antigens" that are: (a) expressed in higher abundance in tumor cells due to mutations (e.g., P53, a cell cycle regulatory protein); (b) embryonic proteins not normally expressed by adult cells but expressed in tumors due to gene regulation errors (e.g., CEA, an oncofetal protein); or (c) proteins typically restricted to immune-privileged sites in the human body but expressed in tumor cells due to errors in gene regulation (e.g., NY-ESO-1, a tumor-testis antigen). Antigens derived from infectious organisms, which have been conclusively identified as the causative agents of tumors (e.g., hepatitis B virus [HBV], human papillomavirus [HPV]), also serve as TAAs for diagnostic and therapeutic tumor markers.[10,11] To date, numerous TAAs associated with specific cancer types have been identified.

Active immunization of animal models with TAAs is effective in overcoming preexisting TAA-expressing tumor cells (therapeutic models) and preventing growth of implanted TAA-expressing tumors in a prophylactic setting.[12,13] However, TAAs are not always restricted to tumors. TAAs can be expressed in normal cells at a lower abundance than tumor cells or have shared epitopes with other proteins expressed by normal cells. Active immunization with such TAAs poses the risk of inducing autoimmune responses against self-antigens. Tumor-restricted TAAs have not been identified for all type of tumors, but during the ever-expanding search for unique TAAs, it was discovered that many tumors express patient-specific, tumor-specific mutated proteins known as neoantigens. Neoantigens differ from self-antigens in one or more antigenic epitopes, and they can serve as diagnostic targets for tumors and therapeutic targets for cancer vaccines.[14]

Thus, cancer vaccines can consist of an immunogenic target that is made up of TAAs, neoantigens, and/or one or more immunogenic epitope(s) derived from these antigens. Various vectors have been employed in delivering TAAs and neoantigens to the immune system, including viruses, bacteria, nucleic acid (DNA/mRNA), or a combination.[13,15] Cancer vaccines may also consist of proteins or peptides formulated with adjuvants to induce the desired immune response.

In this chapter, we summarize the chemistry, manufacturing, and control (CMC), and the clinical information, relevant to cancer vaccine development. In addition to the summarized CMC considerations generally applicable to all biologics, we provide specific considerations applicable to viral vectored cancer vaccines, protein and peptide cancer vaccines, and cellular cancer vaccines. We also provide an overview of the regulatory considerations for developing neoantigen-based cancer vaccines, which can utilize any of the vaccine delivery methods or may consist of a combination of these delivery methods in a prime-boost strategy.

CHEMISTRY, MANUFACTURING, AND CONTROL CONSIDERATIONS FOR CANCER VACCINES

Cancer vaccine manufacturing should meet all required GMP regulations set forth under 21 CFR 211 and be fully compliant with the biologic regulations (21 CFR 600s) at the time of a Biological License Application (BLA). The FDA has provided clarification on the extent of CGMP requirements for Phase 1 studies in "Guidance for Industry CGMP for Phase 1 Investigational Drugs."[16] Some cancer vaccines may also be classified as gene therapy products based on the FDA's definition of gene therapies.[17] To obtain more information on how gene therapy products are regulated, the reader is directed to the accompanying Chapter 66 and FDA guidances for gene therapy products, available at www.fda.gov/regulatory-information/search-fda-guidance-documents/guidance-human-somatic-cell-therapy-and-gene-therapy. CMC considerations for cancer vaccines that are administered as (a) a vectored vaccine, (b) a protein or peptide vaccine, or (c) a cell-based vaccine are discussed in the text that follows.

Vectored Recombinant Cancer Vaccines

Cancer vaccine vectors are vehicles consisting of, or derived from, biological material. They are designed to deliver a TAA to the immune system to initiate or enhance tumor antigen-specific immune responses.[18] Examples include plasmids or viruses and bacteria that are attenuated by either naturally occurring or engineered mutations or deletions. In this review, we use viral-vectored cancer vaccines as an example of vectored recombinant vaccines. We describe the FDA's expectations for characterization studies and lot release testing.

Recombinant viral vectors are naturally immunogenic and can be engineered to express tumor antigens and immunostimulatory molecules such as co-stimulatory ligands (i.e., CD80, CD86, 4-1BBL) and cytokines (i.e., IL-2, IL-12). Immunogenicity, tropism, safety profile, and transgene carrying capacity and expression are important considerations for virus selection and use.[19] Viral cancer vaccine vectors may include either viruses that replicate poorly in humans, such as modified vaccinia Ankara (MVA), canarypox, and fowlpox,[20,21] or viruses that are attenuated by targeted genetic deletions of virulence genes, such as thymidine kinase (TK)-deleted vaccinia virus (VV), ICP34.5-deleted herpes simplex virus (HSV), and E1, E3-deleted adenovirus.[22-25] A strategy used with considerable success in inducing immune responses to TAAs is the diversified prime/boost strategy. For example, priming with MVA expressing prostate specific antigen (PSA) followed by booster vaccinations with fowlpox expressing PSA induces immune responses against metastatic castration-resistant prostate cancer (mCRPC).[26,27]

GENERAL CHEMISTRY, MANUFACTURING, AND CONTROL CONSIDERATIONS FOR VIRAL VECTORED CANCER VACCINES

Viral cancer vaccine vectors that become a part of the drug product should be fully evaluated and lot release specifications with acceptance criteria should be set early during the product development phase of the clinical studies. The FDA normally recommends that IND sponsors discuss with the FDA before introducing any changes to the vector genome as changes to the vector may result in a new vector and may even require an investigational new drug (IND) application. All CMC requirements that apply to gene therapy vectors also apply to vectored cancer vaccines (see accompanying Chapter 66). All IND applications are required to comply with the 21 CFR 312 requirements for information to be included in the application. INDs should include the following information as elaborated in the FDA's CMC Guidance for Gene Therapy Products:[17] characterization of the vectors, cell substrate, cell banks, and viral banks; manufacturing per clinical phase-appropriate GMP requirements; and

release based on lot release tests with appropriate preset acceptance limits for appearance, safety (including tests for sterility, mycoplasma, endotoxin, adventitious viruses, other specific pathogens), process- and product-related contaminants, identity, potency, and stability.

As part of vector characterization, the FDA recommends that the vector derivations (e.g., generation of recombinant vectors; description of all intermediate plasmids and other intermediate viruses, if any; complete annotated sequence of the plasmids; and, in case the vectors are smaller than 40 kb, complete sequencing of the vectors) should be included in the IND.[17] In the case of a viral vector, such as poxviruses, the complete derivation history, plaque purifications, and genomic sequencing of the attenuating features should be part of the CMC information included in the IND.[17,28] The IND should also contain information on the reagents used in the manufacturing process. Information on the manufacturing facilities should also be in the IND, including quality assurance (QA) and quality control (QC) measures in place at the manufacturing facility to prevent cross contamination with other products manufactured in the same facility.

In general, the acceptance criteria for product characterization studies and lot release tests should be set based on manufacturing experience and available scientific knowledge about the product. For early product development, these acceptance criteria may be a set of broad limits that are based on data obtained during the production of preclinical materials and engineering manufacturing runs. However, when the manufacturing process used to produce the preclinical product is substantially different from that used to manufacture the clinical product, a comparability study (and in some instances a bridging preclinical study) may be necessary. An IND sponsor should understand the implication of manufacturing changes between preclinical studies and a proposed clinical study and discuss the changes with the FDA (e.g., during a pre-IND meeting).

The FDA recommends that a well-controlled, scalable manufacturing process be in place for the cancer vaccine vector prior to initiating a Phase 3 clinical study. It is essential for sponsors of INDs to develop knowledge of the product's critical quality attributes and to optimize the manufacturing process early in the product development cycle. This will enable early process optimization studies and help in setting meaningful acceptance criteria for lot release tests. The FDA recommends that prior to initiating a study designed to support licensure, the acceptance criteria for all lot release tests be fully defined and the test methods qualified as suitable for their intended purposes. All noncompendial test methods should also be validated prior to submitting a biologics license application (BLA). To help with setting in-process limits and process optimizations that are a part of process validation studies, please refer to the FDA's guidance on process validation[29] and ICH Q11.[30] In addition to developing and validating a manufacturing process, the sponsor should ensure that all the safety assays (assays used to evaluate sterility, endotoxin, and mycoplasma) are either compendial assays or are qualified as suitable for its intended purposes and evaluated to ensure that the assays are equal to or better than the compendial assays in terms of their sensitivity, specificity, and reproducibility. The FDA also recommends that sponsors retain samples from early phase studies and develop well-characterized, in-house standards or have sufficient stock of any qualified external standards. Qualified reference standards help in comparative evaluation of the product as well as in conducting any bridging studies required for product comparability during late stages of product development.

In addition to these general recommendations on product characterization, process validation studies, and lot release testing, there are specific issues that are relevant to vectored cancer vaccines. These issues are discussed in the text that follows.

SPECIFIC CHEMISTRY, MANUFACTURING, AND CONTROL CONSIDERATIONS FOR VIRAL VECTORED CANCER VACCINES

Residual Selection Markers

Selection markers such as neomycin gene or reporter genes such as beta-galactosidase and green fluorescence protein gene are often used in the derivation of recombinant vectored cancer vaccines. The FDA's general recommendation is to not retain unwanted foreign genetic materials in human therapeutic agents. A change in the selection marker may require a comparability study, a bridging preclinical or clinical study, and the IND sponsor should discuss with the FDA the role of a selection marker (if present).

Adventitious Viral Agent Assays

Adventitious viral agents (AVA) are a concern for all biologics, and vectors should be tested for the presence of AVA by an in vitro AVA assay[28,31] as well as for specific viral pathogens. The FDA recommends that all vectored cancer vaccines be tested for AVA. Depending on the type of cancer vaccine, these tests are typically performed on the production cell lines (master cell bank [MCB], working cell bank [WCB]), viral banks (master virus bank [MVB], working virus bank [WVB]), the final viral product at the bulk harvest stage, and as a one-time test on the end of production cells (EOPC).[17,28,31] The FDA also recommends that the MCB and the MVB also be tested by an in vivo AVA assay using animal models (e.g., inoculation of adult and suckling mice, inoculation of embryonated chicken eggs, antibody production tests).[28,31]

In addition to the in vitro and in vivo tests, AVA tests also include those for the detection of retroviruses (using reverse transcriptase assays and transmission electron microscopy analysis) and species-specific AVA (e.g., via species-specific antibody production tests or PCR).[17,28,31] Of note, use of human cell lines and reagents necessitate testing for human pathogens, including cytomegalovirus (CMV); human immunodeficiency virus (HIV)-1 and -2; human T-lymphotropic virus (HTLV)-1 and -2; human herpesvirus (HHV)-6, -7, and -8; JC virus; BK virus; Epstein-Barr virus (EBV); human parvovirus B19; HBV; HPV; and hepatitis C virus (HCV), as appropriate.[17]

The FDA normally recommends that the sponsors develop a testing plan and discuss the test methods with the FDA prior to implementation in their product manufacturing program. As with all other tests, the AVA tests should be qualified (evaluated for its ability to function as desired in the product matrix, and evaluated for the test's sensitivity, specificity, and accuracy) and any non-FDA approved or cleared test should be validated prior to submitting a BLA.

Replication Competence Assay

Candidate vectors for the development of cancer vaccines include replication-restricted viruses, such as MVA, and viruses that have deletions in their genome to prevent replication in humans, such as E1, E3-deleted adenovirus, ICP34.5-deleted HSV, or amplicon vectors. The manufacture of these vectors employs the use of complementing essential viral genes that are expressed in trans by either the production cell line or by the use of helper viruses.[25,28,31,32] These manufacturing strategies introduce the possibility of generating replication competent viruses (RCV) that may be co-purified during the manufacturing process and be present in the final drug product. Depending on the type of vectors that are used in the cancer vaccine, the FDA recommends that tests for RCVs be performed at different stages in the vector manufacturing process, such as the MVB and as part of the in-process or release testing of the drug substance (DS) or drug product (DP).[17] The FDA typically recommends that the acceptance criteria for the presence of RCV be less than 1 virus particle in the highest proposed dose. However, the acceptance limit and sensitivity of the test method are product dependent (e.g., for adenovirus, the FDA recommends a maximum of one replication-competent adenovirus in 3×10^{10} viral particles) and should be discussed with the FDA during a pre-IND meeting.[17]

Virulence Determination and Introducing Changes to the Viral Genome

Replication competent HSV and vesicular stomatitis virus (VSV) have known neurotropism.[19,32] In order to use these viruses as viral vectored cancer vaccines, assessment of their attenuating features and evaluation of neurovirulence is necessary. Viruses such as HSV also have the ability to become latent and to revive at a later date in response to environmental or other activation signals.[32] To ensure that the corrected intended virus is evaluated in preclinical studies, changes to the viral genome or inserted genetic elements should be done prior to initiating preclinical proof of concept and toxicity studies. Early discussion with the FDA through the Initial Targeted Engagement for Regulatory Advice on CBER Products (INTERACT, www.fda.gov/vaccines-blood-biologics/industry-biologics/interact-meetings) and pre-IND meeting process helps the sponsors in their product development (for additional guidance, please refer to the FDA's guidance on formal meetings).[33]

Dose

Viral vectored cancer vaccines may include incomplete, defective, or empty viral particles (product-related contaminants) that may get co-purified with the viral vector but may not contribute to the induction of immune responses to TAAs. The FDA typically recommends that an IND sponsor conducts characterization studies to fully understand the nature of the chosen viral vector, limitations of the purification process, and levels of product-related contaminants present in the final drug product. Based on the accumulated scientific knowledge and manufacturing experience gained from characterization and engineering manufacturing runs, an acceptance limit for the number of incomplete viral particles in the DP may be set early in product development. For example, the FDA recommends that the infectious to empty particle ratio for human adenovirus be less than 1:30.[34]* However, the acceptable limit for infectious to empty or defective particles will depend on the vector type and should be discussed with the FDA prior to initiation of a clinical study. An IND sponsor should discuss the dose-determining assays with the agency during the pre-IND meeting and during various developmental milestone meetings (e.g., EOP1, EOP2).

Purity

Product purity is defined as the relative freedom from extraneous matter in the finished product, whether or not it is harmful to the recipient or deleterious to the product (21 CFR 600.3(r)). Common process-related impurities for viral vaccine manufacture include residual cell substrate proteins, host cell derived nucleic acid sequences, and reagents used during manufacture,

such as cytokines, growth factors, serum, and solvents. Typical product-related impurities include defective or incomplete viral particles, empty capsid particles, degraded viral proteins, and aggregated viral proteins. The FDA recommends that sponsors develop in-process acceptance limits for product impurities by including in-process tests at appropriate process steps.[30,35] As a part of manufacturing process validations, the IND sponsor should determine the critical steps in the manufacturing process and include acceptance limits for the critical process parameters and action limits for noncritical process parameters.[30,36]

Potency

The word "potency" is defined as "the specific ability or capacity of the product, as indicated by appropriate laboratory tests or by adequately controlled clinical data obtained through the administration of the product in the manner intended, to effect a given result" (21 CFR 600.3(s)). A potency assay is required to assure product quality and should be a part of the lot release tests for a DP (21 CFR 610.10). A potency assay is also a part of the assays used to determine the drug product's stability. It is also used to evaluate product comparability after changes are introduced in the manufacturing process. A potency assay is typically an assay that measures the DP's biological function.[37] When a product has multiple biological functions, the FDA recommends that potency assays be developed to evaluate each one of the biological functions of the drug product. The FDA also recommends that the potency assay be quantitative, but a matrix of both quantitative and qualitative measures of potency may be used to measure the product's strength/activity.[37] A potency assay should ideally be developed early in the product development process and will typically represent a measure of one or more of the product's mechanism of action (e.g., quantitatively evaluate a transgene expression), and a biologically relevant assay should be developed to measure the activity of the DP prior to initiating studies to support licensure. Due to the complexities in developing a potency assay for a cancer vaccine, the FDA recommends that the sponsor develop orthogonal potency assays that measure different aspects of the product's function and discuss the potency assay(s) with the FDA during a milestone meeting (e.g., EOP1, EOP2).

Stability Studies

Stability studies are needed to establish the shelf life of the MCB, WCB, MVB, WVB, DS (if stored), and the final DP. DP stability testing must be performed during early stage development to demonstrate adequate stability for the duration of the clinical studies. The stability study

---

* Adenovirus Reference Material Working Group is a consortium of industry, government, and academic researchers to manufacture adenovirus reference standards and codify analytical methods under the auspices of the FDA.

should evaluate the drug product's stability while stored in the recommended storage temperature and storage container. The stability test parameters typically include the evaluation of the product's purity, quality, potency, and sterility. Alternatives to sterility testing as part of the stability protocol, such as replacing the sterility test with a container and closure system integrity testing, may be more useful than sterility testing in demonstrating the potential for product contamination over the product's shelf life or dating period.[38]

The FDA recommends conducting real-time stability studies during the IND phase of the product development and extending the investigational product's shelf life as additional stability data become available. The ICH guidance Q1A(R2) on stability recommends that product stability be evaluated every 3 months during the first year of storage, every 6 months during the second year of storage, and annually thereafter through the proposed storage period months.[39] For viral cancer vaccines that are expected to be stored for a short period of time (e.g., viral vectors expressing patient-specific neoantigens), the timing of stability testing may be determined based on the storage period. In the case of frozen cancer vaccines, stability testing should also evaluate stability of the DP for the acceptable duration it can be kept at the clinical site after thaw. Stability of the drug product in the delivery device should also be evaluated, and a thorough device compatibility study should be conducted to ensure that the delivery device does not affect the quality and quantity of the drug product.[39] Stability determining assays must be validated prior to submitting a BLA, and any change in DP formulation, container closures, or storage conditions will require additional stability testing.

Shedding Studies

The FDA recommends that the shedding of recombinant viral vectors be evaluated during clinical studies. Shedding studies are typically designed by taking into consideration the replication competence, immunogenicity, persistence and latency, and tropism of the viral vector. Stability of product attenuation and route of administration are also considerations for the shedding study design. For replication competent viral vectors, the FDA recommends that shedding studies be conducted during Phase 1 trials and may continue into Phase 2 and Phase 3 after a dose and regimen have been determined. Given their lower potential for release as an infectious virus, it is recommended that shedding studies for nonreplicating viral vectors be conducted during Phase 2 after a dose and treatment regimen have been determined. Shedding studies are typically not necessary for other modes of vaccine delivery such as plasmid DNA and mRNA-based cancer vaccines. For detailed FDA recommendations for the design of shedding studies, refer to the FDA guidance on shedding studies.[40]

Environmental Assessments

Vectored cancer vaccines that contain a TAA-specific transgene are not considered naturally occurring as discussed in the FDA's environmental assessment guidance,[41] and will not be eligible for categorical exclusion under 21 CFR 25.31(c), and will be subject to the requirement for an environmental assessment as required under 21 CFR 25.40. However, all biological INDs including cancer vaccines are eligible for a categorical exclusion under 21 CFR 25.31(e), and an IND sponsor should request a categorical exclusion at the time of IND submission. The FDA will normally grant the sponsor's request for categorical exclusion unless there are extraordinary circumstances (21 CFR 25.21) that exist to prevent the granting of a categorical exclusion. In the case of vectored cancer vaccines, a product (e.g., a replication competent virus) that has the potential to cause serious harm to the environment at the expected level of exposure due to use or disposal from use of the FDA-regulated article, can trigger the extraordinary circumstances clause. Serious harm to the environment includes the use of those organisms that can be toxic to the environment, or that can cause lasting effects on ecological community dynamics. Serious harm may also be due to disposal activities that adversely affect a species or the critical habitat of a species. An IND sponsor should discuss the issues related to the specific cancer vaccine vector with the FDA during the pre-IND or INTERACT meetings. For additional guidance on environmental assessment requirements, please refer to the FDA's guidance on this topic.[41]

Peptide Cancer Vaccines

Peptide cancer vaccines consist of minimal epitopes derived from one or more TAAs and are designed to induce CTL responses against tumors expressing the TAA(s). The peptide cancer vaccine may be specific to a single human leukocyte antigen (HLA) type or may be promiscuous epitopes that bind multiple HLA types and induce immune responses in a broader segment of the population.[42] Peptide vaccines may consist of multiple independent peptide epitopes mixed together, linked together in a linear multi-epitope sequence, or combined as hybrid peptide sequences consisting of CTL epitopes plus helper epitopes. The peptide epitopes may come from TAAs or may be derived from a patient's tumor as a neoantigen to make a personalized peptide vaccine. In this chapter, we will discuss the regulation of peptide vaccines using neoantigen-based cancer vaccines as an example.

SPECIFIC CHEMISTRY, MANUFACTURING, AND CONTROL CONSIDERATIONS FOR NEOANTIGEN-BASED PEPTIDE CANCER VACCINES

Tumor neoantigens arise from somatic mutations of the tumor and are therefore tumor-specific and are distinct from TAAs. Neoantigens are patient-specific, selected due to their unique expression in tumor cells, and expected to have lower risk of generating autoimmunity as compared to designer TAA that are modified to render them immunogenic. Early results from preclinical and clinical studies suggest that neoantigens play a critical role in eliciting tumor-specific T cell-mediated antitumor immune response, may play an important role in natural tumor regressions, and may be responsible for the induction of TILs.[42,43] Neoantigens arising from malignant clones of cancer cells are attractive targets, as they are expected to be perceived by the immune system as "non-self" due to their expression only in the tumors and their absence during the early immune education phase of T cells that determines "self" and "non-self" antigens in the thymus.[44] Higher neoantigen load may be associated with stronger T cell responses and consequently is expected to induce a better clinical outcome.[45]

Consistent with the complexity of the high polymorphism in HLA and high selectivity of peptide-HLA binding, correct epitope prediction and selection is vital for the success of personalized peptide cancer vaccines. The manufacturing process for a neoantigen-specific therapeutic cancer vaccine is complex and involves the identification of neoantigens, identification of CTL epitopes for the neoantigen, synthesis and assembly of one or more of the neoantigenic epitopes in a preferred sequence, and formulation of the vaccine with appropriate adjuvants. All these steps constitute the manufacturing process for a neoantigen peptide vaccine, and the FDA evaluates the manufacturer's ability to consistently produce a product with uniform quality attributes and compliance with the CMC requirements for an IND.

Identification of Neoantigens

Identifying all the mutated neoantigen sequences in tumor cells (termed "mutanome") typically involves the following steps: (a) sequencing genomic DNA isolated from the tumor cells (whole genome sequencing, WGS); (b) comparing the genomic DNA sequence with that obtained from normal cells from the same study subject; (c) identifying unique point mutations and/or insertion-deletions that are present within the open reading frames in the genome of the tumor cells; (d) comparing data obtained from step 3 with a cDNA library derived from mRNA isolated from the same set of tumor cells using WGS; and (e) confirming that the mutated

sequences are expressed in the tumors and ascertaining the relative abundance of the mutated transcripts.[46,47]

While there could be many different versions of this strategy for the identification of neoantigens, the principle for the identification of neoantigens remains the same: to identify unique patient-specific, tumor-specific mutations that are not present in the normal cells. In the text that follows, we discuss general CMC considerations that apply to the manufacture and testing of synthetic peptide-based investigational products that may also be applicable to neoantigen-based peptide vaccines. For additional discussion on the topics covered in this section, the reader should refer to the FDA's guidance for industry documents: "ANDAs for Certain Highly Purified Synthetic Peptide Drug Products That Refer to Listed Drugs of rDNA Origin" (Draft Guidance)(2017),[48] "Clinical Considerations for Therapeutic Cancer Vaccines" (2011),[49] "General Principles for the Development of Vaccines to Protect Against Global Infectious Diseases" (2011),[50] and "General Principles of Software Validation" (2002).[51] Since each set of circumstances are different, we recommend that IND sponsors planning a clinical study using a neoantigen-based cancer vaccine make full use of INTERACT and pre-IND meetings to discuss their manufacturing and testing strategies with the FDA prior to implementing them.

Process of Identifying Tumor-Specific Mutations

There are several unique challenges when the product is different for each individual study subject and, depending on the clonality of the tumor sample, each subject's tumor may exhibit a different set of neoantigens depending on the location of the tumor and the time point at which the tumor was isolated. The neoantigen manufacturing process begins with the isolation of tumor cells to identify neoantigens, and deviations in the manufacturing process may result in product differences. The entire manufacturing process from tumor isolation to neoantigen selection and manufacture should be standardized to yield a consistent product.

Epitope Prediction

Mutated sequences representing different patient-specific neoantigens are prioritized per the sponsor's requirements (e.g., abundance of the expressed mutated sequences, immunogenicity of the sequences, peptide length, presence of epitopes that could induce autoreactive immune responses, ability of the peptides to aggregate, presence of mutant epitope reactive T cells in the patients, etc.). Subsequently, epitopes within the mutated sequences that can bind the patient's HLA sequences are predicted based on an epitope prediction algorithm.[52,53] Epitope prediction algorithms are still evolving, and the predicted epitopes may differ depending on the algorithm. We discuss in the text that follows a few CMC considerations for epitope predictions. However, the sponsor should discuss their algorithm of choice with the FDA during INTERACT and pre-IND meetings to obtain the FDA's concurrence prior to implementing it in the manufacturing process.

Epitope Prediction, Selection, and Documentation

As the selection of neoantigens is a fundamental part of the manufacturing process to produce the specific final product, details about the approach used should be included in the IND (21 CFR 312.23(a)(7)). One complication is that identification of neoantigens, predicting major histocompatibility complex (MHC) binding, and relative immunogenicity is complex. Many of the algorithms and software used for these purposes is produced by third parties or in the public domain, and the end user has little control over changes made to these programs or how the predictions might change with software revisions.

Factors that contribute to peptide safety include: (a) control over and traceability of reagents and the synthesized peptide through GMP manufacturing; (b) levels of residual organic solvents used in peptide synthesis and cleavage; (c) purity of the peptide from truncated or altered sequences; (d) confirmation of peptide sequence; and (e) peptide stability with storage. Note that not all primary sequences are easy to synthesize—difficult sequences can lead to truncated or altered sequences, poor yield, and low purity. Neoantigen peptides can be highly hydrophobic, vary in length and charge, and some can have a strong tendency to aggregate, which could result in a more immunogenic form of the antigen.[54] Peptide-related impurities may create the potential for differences in immunogenicity or may otherwise affect the safety or effectiveness of a peptide.[48]

Lot Release Tests

Neoantigen-based peptide cancer vaccine DP broadly consists of the following vaccine components: the neoantigen peptide (may be one or more peptides), immunological adjuvant(s), and a vehicle or carrier. For early phase clinical studies, the manufacturing of the final formulated drug product, including control of individual components, should comply with the GMP requirements as outlined in the FDA's Phase 1 GMP guidance[16] and be fully GMP compliant for late-stage products as required under 21 CFR parts 210 and 211. Lot release testing requirements should comply with IND regulations (21 CFR 312.23) and biologics regulations (21 CFR 600). For a general description of FDA-recommended product characterization and lot release testing requirements applicable to neoantigen cancer vaccine drug substances and drug products, please refer to the FDA's

guidance documents.[17,48,55] A few specific issues that are relevant to neoantigen cancer vaccines that should be taken into consideration while designing product lot release tests include a need to establish product identity (to be established and verified based on the product's primary sequence), purity (the neoantigenic peptide product should be of the highest purity achievable and justified based on scientific knowledge and feasibility), potency (biological function of the product should be measured, or alternative methods justified),[37] and stability (stability period to be determined based on real-time stability measurements). As all these parameters are variable from product to product, all testing parameters and acceptance criteria should be discussed with the FDA during INTERACT, Pre-IND, or other meetings as appropriate.

Adjuvants

Adjuvants may be used in cancer vaccine formulations. These adjuvants are not generally licensed by themselves but are used in conjunction with vaccine antigens to augment or direct the specific immune response to an antigen. General requirements for inclusion of such adjuvants include submission of evidence that the proposed adjuvant does not adversely affect the safety or potency of a given vaccine formulation. Information supporting the value of adding the adjuvant should be provided, and may include evidence of enhanced immune response or antigen-sparing effects, and data supporting selection of the dose of the adjuvant. Examples of adjuvants that have been used in FDA-approved peptide/protein vaccines include Toll-like receptor (TLR) agonists, such as CpGs, Montanide™ ISA 51, QS21 and MPL, and AS02.[56]

Cellular Cancer Vaccines

Cellular cancer vaccines utilize the ability of antigen-presenting cells (APCs) such as DCs and macrophages to induce immune responses to tumors. The APCs may be from the same patient (autologous) or from a donor (allogenic). A typical APC used in a number of experimental cancer vaccine formulations is autologous or allogenic DCs. For an in-depth discussion on the FDA's regulatory requirements for cellular products, the reader is directed to the accompanying Chapter 65 and to the FDA guidance "Guidance for FDA Reviewers and Sponsors: Content and Review of Chemistry, Manufacturing, and Control (CMC) Information for Human Somatic Cell Therapy Investigational New Drug Applications (INDs)."[55] In this section, we have provided an overview of the regulatory considerations for cellular cancer vaccines using antigen-pulsed DC vaccines as an example of cellular cancer vaccines.

SPECIFIC CHEMISTRY, MANUFACTURING, AND CONTROL CONSIDERATIONS FOR DENDRITIC CELL CANCER VACCINES

CMC considerations for DC vaccines include the reagents used to purify peripheral blood mononuclear cells (PBMCs), generate immature DCs and mature them, the cell culturing process, the level of cellular characterization, the cell surface markers used to identify DCs, and the tests to evaluate the purity and potency of the DC product. Autologous DC used in cancer vaccines are produced from monocytes isolated from a cancer patient, and the number of circulating monocytes can vary greatly patient to patient. It may not always be possible to generate sufficient numbers of autologous DCs for every potential patient. Cell surface marker expression changes as monocytes become activated and mature into DC, and changes in cell surface marker expression is commonly used to monitor DC manufacturing. Cultured DC have the ability to stimulate specific T cell responses, though the level of stimulation may also vary by product lot. The source of cells to generate DCs can come from autologous or allogeneic donors. If allogeneic, then a donor eligibility determination must be made as described in 21 CFR 1271 Subpart C.

In order to direct a response to a specific tumor type, tumor-derived antigenic peptide epitopes generated from TAAs are typically used to pulse DCs. The antigenic epitope may be a dominant tumor epitope, a cocktail of known tumor epitopes, or neoantigenic epitopes. Overlapping peptides corresponding to an entire tumor protein have also been used.[42] CMC considerations for the selection of neoantigens were discussed previously in the peptide cancer vaccines section (refer to the previous section "Specific Chemistry, Manufacturing, and Control Considerations for Neoantigen-Based Peptide Cancer Vaccines"). For peptides used in conjunction with DC vaccines, specific consideration should be given to the selection of immunogenic epitopes, and the peptide design should be tailored for their ability to bind a specific HLA molecule present on the autologous DC.

Tumor lysates are unique in that they consist of cellular material and are not considered viable. However, lysates are often mixed with viable cells, such as DCs, to increase their ability to induce antitumor immune responses. In addition to characterizing the tumor lysate itself, testing of the final formulation (e.g., lysate admixed with DCs) would be necessary to assess safety of the final product. Tumor lysates can function as an immunotherapy product, or act as a source of antigen to induce or augment a tumor response in vivo or as a source of antigen for pulsing a DC product for the same purpose. An advantage of tumor lysates over purified peptides or recombinant proteins is that potentially all the relevant tumor antigens, both known and as yet unknown, are represented in the lysate and can be presented to the immune system to generate a response.

Because tumors can vary widely patient to patient, between tumors in the same patient, and even within different parts of the same solid tumor, tumor lysates can vary substantially lot-to-lot. They can vary in the amount and concentration of antigen, the number of antigens, the relative percentage of tumor antigens compared with total protein, and the types of tumor antigens present. The relative abundance or ratio of specific tumor antigens can also vary. It can be challenging to demonstrate manufacturing consistency for tumor lysate generation and to determine the performance of the manufacturing process. It can also be difficult to define minimum quality specifications. Different approaches can be taken to help characterize the product and evaluate consistency. One approach is to measure constitutively expressed proteins that would be expected in each preparation for comparison purposes. Another approach is to measure a specific tumor antigen that would be expected to be present in the particular tumor type of interest.

Tumor lysates can be from a number of sources: autologous tumors, tumors from a different person (allogenic tumors), or tumors from a cell line. When allogeneic tumors are used to generate tumor lysates, they should comply with donor eligibility requirements (21 CFR 1271). If a tumor cell bank is used as a source of tumor lysate, then as with all cell banks used in manufacturing, the history and properties should be described in the IND (21 CFR 312.23(a)(7)(i)) and the bank appropriately qualified.[31,55,57] Qualification should include in vitro and in vivo adventitious agent testing. Lysates should also be tested to be sure no viable tumor cells remain after processing. For additional considerations regarding cell therapy products, the reader is referred to the FDA's guidance on this topic.[55]

Preclinical Considerations

Tumor lysates are unique in that they consist of cellular material and are not considered viable CTs. However, these vaccines are often mixed with viable cells, such as DCs, to increase their antitumorigenic potential. In such cases, the considerations provided in the introduction still apply. In addition to characterizing the tumor lysate itself, testing of the final formulation (e.g., lysate admixed with DCs) would be necessary to assess safety of the final product. As with other products, consideration must be given as to the appropriate animal model to test the vaccine and whether it is most appropriate to test the human product or analogous product. Data to support that decision should be provided in the IND.

CLINICAL CONSIDERATIONS FOR CANCER VACCINES

Clinical Trial Design

An IND protocol for the study of cancer vaccine products should be adequately designed and include sufficient information to support the proposed study design. There are unique challenges in the design of cancer vaccine trials, which are informed by the type of product to be investigated. In this section we will set forth general principles that may serve to guide the design of therapeutic cancer vaccine trials.

Regardless of the type of vaccine product studied, the goal is to achieve disease control by enhancing the study subject's immune response through administration of the investigational agent either as monotherapy or in combination with other classes of agents.

Therapeutic cancer vaccines are intended to result in specific responses to tumor antigens and mediate their effect through in vivo induction or amplification of an antigen-specific host immune response. The mechanism of action for most cancer vaccines is thought to be mediated through induction of an antigen-specific T cell response or amplifying a preexisting antigen-specific T cell response, especially cytotoxic T cell responses. Cancer vaccines induce responses to tumor-specific antigens that are processed by the immune system through APCs. These APCs then present antigenic determinants in a HLA-restricted fashion to T cells, which in turn can attack tumor cells that express cognate antigenic determinants.

Certain subsets of T cells also provide help for B cell responses that produce antibodies, which in some cases could lead to tumor cell death. The course of antigen presentation and processing, activation of lymphocytes, and tumor cell killing are expected to require a substantial time *in vivo*. Thus, the development of a cancer vaccine can present different considerations for clinical trial design than development of a more traditional biological product or cytotoxic drug for the treatment of cancer.[49]

Early Phase Trial Objectives

Early developmental protocols should specify in detail all the elements of the study that are critical to safety. Such elements may include all clinical safety assessments, toxicity monitoring, description of toxicity-based stopping rules, dose adjustment rules for individual patients and the overall trial, and adverse event recording and reporting.

Study enrollment criteria should be written with consideration of the following: (a) background risks associated with the disease or condition studied, and (b) previous knowledge of toxicities of the investigational drug observed in animal studies or with human experience.

It is preferable that toxicity is assessed and graded according to a standardized grading scale relevant to the studied population and that adverse events are collected, recorded, and reported in a consistent manner.[58]

Dose Exploration

When feasible, preclinical in vitro and in vivo proof-of-concept (POC) studies are recommended to provide the rationale for the proposed clinical trial. These studies, in conjunction with appropriately designed preclinical studies characterizing biodistribution and the toxicology of the cancer vaccine, should guide the clinical doses and initial clinical dosing schedule. The dose levels used in the preclinical toxicology studies should be based on dose levels that showed biological activity in preclinical POC studies. The sponsor should submit justification, with supporting scientific data, for the extrapolation modality used to determine the proposed clinical starting dose, dose escalation scheme, and dosing schedule.[49]

Booster and Maintenance Therapy

Sponsors may wish to explore vaccination boosters and maintenance therapy to evaluate long-term immunogenicity and its correlation with clinical outcomes. The conduct of preclinical studies to evaluate such regimens is recommended, and subsequent clinical studies should be designed to support the safety and effectiveness of such regimens.[49]

Dose Escalation

In the early phase setting, dose exploration may be achieved by a dose-escalation study in which cohorts are enrolled in a "3 + 3" design, accelerated titration, or through use of a continuous reassessment model in order to determine the maximally tolerated dose. This dose may then be further explored in a Phase 2 study.

Irrespective of which dose-escalation approach is chosen, the study protocol should clearly define dose-limiting toxicities (DLTs), the subject "off-treatment" criteria, and the study stopping rules that will ensure subject safety. When no DLT is expected or achieved, optimization of other outcomes, such as immune response, can be useful to identify doses for subsequent studies.[58]

Toxicity Assessments

In the early phase trial setting, assessing early safety signals may allow for early implementation of additional safety measures throughout the study. Novel vaccine products may be studied in first-in-human studies, and for those products which lack an appropriate animal model there may not be sufficient preclinical data to guide the implementation of safety measures in early phase studies. Therefore, it is imperative that investigators fully detail anticipated toxicities and include a robust safety monitoring plan to appropriately characterize and document the safety profile of the investigational agent.

Additionally, since potential vaccine-related toxicities may be related to the presence of the target antigen in normal tissues, or to the presence of an unrelated protein in normal tissues that may contain a peptide sequence similar to a peptide in the vaccine, the presence of target antigen in normal human tissues should be determined.[49]

Feasibility Assessments

As some cancer vaccines may be manufactured from the study subject's own tumor specimen, attention must be given to the processes which will allow for production of sufficient amounts of the investigational product to be used throughout the study, particularly in protocols in which repeat dosing will be employed. The feasibility of manufacturing the product will influence the study design. Feasibility of manufacturing may be assessed by both a safety and efficacy measurement in the first-in-human study.[49]

Activity Assessments

As vaccines are intended to activate and enhance immune activity, assessments may include measurements of biologic activity such as cytokine levels. However, caution should be employed in drawing conclusions regarding clinical benefit from such measurements. The most reliable measurements of activity may be combined measurements of efficacy involving tumor measurement, laboratory evaluation of serum tumor markers or cytokine, and objective measurements of quality of life as well as survival.[49]

Phase 2-3 Trials

All of the previously described expectations for adequate safety elements also apply to Phase 2 to 3 trials. Detailed protocols describing both efficacy and safety endpoints should be submitted for Phase 2 to 3 trials. Objectives of a trial should be clearly stated, including description of the observations and measurements to be made to fulfill the objectives of the trial.

Clinical trial protocols should include a clear description of trial design and patient selection criteria as well as description of clinical procedures, laboratory tests, and all measures to be taken to monitor the effects of the drug.

Previous experience with the proposed primary endpoints should be discussed with relevant scientific references (including any available data regarding the measurement's validation as relevant to clinical outcomes, biomarkers, or patient-reported outcomes).[59]

Choosing a Study Population

In contrast to the clinical development plan pursued for chemotherapeutic agents in which initial clinical investigations may enroll subjects with advanced and metastatic disease with a variety of tumor types, there are inherent challenges in enrolling such a population in early phase studies investigating vaccine products. In designing trials to investigate the safety and efficacy of therapeutic cancer vaccines, consideration must be given to the fact that subjects with advanced and metastatic disease may have received numerous previous therapies (i.e. chemotherapy, radiation and immunotherapy). Therefore, the ability of such subjects to respond to a cancer vaccine may be limited. Differences in the clinical stage of the disease and prior treatments can affect the potential response to the cancer vaccine.

Additionally, studies in which vaccine products are derived from autologous patient material may yield uninterpretable results if heterogeneous patient populations are enrolled. This could potentially delay product development.

Evaluating the effectiveness of therapeutic cancer vaccine in the adjuvant setting in subjects with no evidence of disease may negatively impact the ability to accurately determine treatment benefit as such study subjects may need to be followed for considerable periods of time in order to achieve the desired number of events to reach a statistical threshold consistent with clinical benefit.[49]

Control Group and Blinding

To avoid the biases that can be introduced in the conduct of the trial and which confound the analyses of the trial results, cancer vaccine trials should have appropriate controls, either an active comparator or placebo. Studies involving a placebo should be carefully considered and planned. Withholding an available therapy with proven safety and efficacy may be unethical.

Blinding of subjects, investigators, and evaluators may be helpful to decrease the risk of bias in the study results. However, either cancer vaccines or coadministered immune stimulatory agents can cause reactions that make the subjects treated with the vaccine easily identifiable. To maintain blinding of treatment assignment, the study may need to provide separate personnel for each of the following: study agent administration, post-administration subject care, and endpoint assessment.[60]

Autologous Vaccine Trials

Design of studies using autologous vaccine products that are derived from the subjects' own tumors poses unique challenges and deserves special consideration. Manufacturing such vaccines may take up to several months. If complete remission or stable disease is an eligibility criterion, the time required for manufacture may mean that some trial subjects may become ineligible for vaccine administration because of disease recurrence or progression.

Additionally, the manufacture of autologous vaccine product may not be possible for every subject for a wide variety of reasons, including challenges with source material and/or the manufacturing process. Regardless of the cause, a sponsor's inability to treat randomized subjects with the vaccine may adversely affect the statistical power of the clinical study. Therefore, consideration should be given to optimization of the vaccine manufacturing process before the late phase clinical trials are initiated, to increase the proportion of the randomized subjects who can receive the vaccine.[49]

Study Design-Concomitant Therapies

The ultimate therapeutic effect of cancer vaccines may be diminished or enhanced by other cytotoxic or immunomodulatory treatments. Therefore, such cytotoxic or immunomodulatory effects of other treatments should be considered in the overall product development plan and specifically in the clinical trial design. Justification should be provided for the use of concomitant therapy (e.g., chemotherapy, biotherapy, radiotherapy, laser therapy), including the mode of action, dose and schedule of the concomitant therapy, and potential for negative or positive interactions of the concomitant therapy with the vaccine.

When standard therapies are available, consideration should be given to the timing and sequencing of these therapies, relative to the schedule of cancer vaccine administration, to optimize the evaluation of the safety and potential biological activities of the cancer vaccine. Preclinical exploration of the different options of timing and sequencing of cancer vaccine and standard therapy (such as cytotoxic chemotherapy) can help guide clinical development.[49,61]

Single-Arm Versus Randomized Phase 2 Trials in Early Development

Single-arm studies can be, and often are, used to demonstrate tumor shrinkage by cytotoxic agents; however, such evidence of therapeutic activity is more difficult to obtain in situations where the product is a cancer vaccine that may not be expected to cause tumor shrinkage. Therefore, due to their mechanism of action, single-arm studies of cancer vaccines may not provide reliable antitumor activity data to guide subsequent product development, although such studies may better characterize and estimate immunologic effects.

Randomized Phase 2 trials, due to their limited sample sizes, typically lack the statistical power for conclusive demonstration of the treatment effect of the investigational agent and provide a more limited patient experience for generalization of treatment effects to the general patient population. However, such randomized Phase 2 trials can provide more reliable data to guide the design of the later phase confirmatory trials (e.g., help to determine the appropriate sample size and estimate treatment effect) and take into account potential negative effects, including tolerance induction.[49,59]

General Monitoring Considerations

Immune monitoring is considered as mainly exploratory, especially in early phase clinical trials, with the major goals of establishing proof-of-principle for the proposed pharmacological effect and showing immunogenicity of the administered antigens. To this end, monitoring of the immune response can be useful as follows:

- To assess variations in immunocompetency that may affect the study results
- In early phase clinical trials, to optimize the dose and schedule, determine whether the vaccine induces the intended immune responses, assess immune tolerance, provide proof-of-concept, and aid the decision-making process concerning further product development and later clinical trial design
- In later phase clinical trials, to provide data regarding the types, magnitudes, and duration of response and the possible correlation with clinical efficacy parameters[49]

Disease Progression/Recurrence Immediately or Shortly After the Initial Administration of Cancer Vaccines

In oncologic practice, investigational and approved treatments are generally discontinued when patients experience disease progression. Because of the time required for the host (patient) to elicit or amplify an immune response to a cancer vaccine (i.e., tumor-specific immune response), the vaccine may have a delayed effect in the study subjects. In this situation, clinical progression may occur before the vaccine has had sufficient time to be effective. Therefore, clinical progression that is asymptomatic and/or is not likely to result in life-threatening complications with further progression (e.g., central nervous system [CNS] metastases or impending fractures from bony metastases) may not be sufficient reason for discontinuation of administration of a cancer vaccine.

One potential approach to this situation would be for the study protocol to clearly define the extent and location of clinical disease progression for which continued vaccination will be continued.

The following are potential clinical situations in which sponsors may wish to consider providing provisions in the protocol for continued vaccination despite evidence of disease progression:

- Subjects continue to meet all other study protocol eligibility criteria.
- No dose-limiting toxicity (DLT) has been observed, and all toxicities resolved to the baseline level, consistent with the study eligibility criteria.
- No deterioration of subject performance status was seen.
- No curative salvage therapy exists for the indication (e.g., resection of pulmonary metastases in osteosarcoma patients).
- Does not delay imminent intervention to prevent serious complications of disease progression (e.g., CNS metastases).
- Clinical evidence from early phase clinical trials suggests delayed effects.[49]

Delayed Vaccine Effect

As a consequence of their immunological mechanisms of action, cancer vaccines may require considerable time after administration to induce immunity. Therefore, tumors in subjects treated with cancer vaccines may show early progression followed by subsequent response. This potential phenomenon should be considered in the design of later phase clinical trials, particularly if nonclinical data or early phase clinical trials suggest that the phenomenon exists, and time-to-event endpoints are used. Due to delayed effect of the vaccine, the endpoint curves may show no effect for the initial portion of the study. If the vaccine is effective, evidence of the effect may occur later in the study. This delay in the effect may lead to an average effect that is smaller than expected and thus may require both an increase in sample size to compensate for the delay and a careful assessment of trial maturity for the primary analysis. In addition, possible violation of the proportional hazards assumption should be considered when selecting a statistical method for the primary analysis.[49]

Companion Diagnostics

When the proposed mechanism of action involves a specific antigen or other therapeutic target, consideration also should be given to developing an assay or mechanism to measure the target antigen expression in tumor tissues of individual patients and using that information in subject selection or response monitoring. These assays are generally regulated by the Center for Devices and Radiological Health (CDRH). Therefore, sponsors developing cancer vaccines who are considering including the use of an assay in the labeling of the cancer vaccine, or sponsors of such assays who are planning to develop the assay for use with a specific cancer vaccine, should request a meeting with both the relevant product review office (CBER) and the relevant device review division (CDRH). Discussions begun early in the development process, ideally before submission of an IND and/or investigational device exemption (IDE), may help ensure that product development provides data that establish the safety and effectiveness of the therapeutic product and assay pair. This is particularly important where use of the assay turns out to be necessary to the safe and effective use of the therapeutic product (referred to as companion diagnostics).[62]

An IND protocol for a study of tumor vaccine product should contain the following clinical components:

- rationale for use of product in chosen patient population;
- brief summary of previous human experience with the product;
- anticipated risks;
- hypothesis and objectives;
- inclusion and exclusion criteria;
- study design and detailed protocol;
- justification for starting dose;
- justification for dose regimen;
- safety and endpoint monitoring plans;
- definition of dose-limiting toxicity;
- definition of maximum tolerated dose;
- adverse event reporting plan;
- long-term follow-up plan;
- patient treatment discontinuation criteria;
- trial stopping criteria; and
- investigator's brochure (for multicenter trials).

EXPEDITED PROGRAMS FOR SERIOUS CONDITIONS

Fast Track Designation

Sponsors may request fast track designation when the IND is first submitted or at any time thereafter before receiving marketing approval of the BLA if nonclinical or clinical data demonstrate the potential to address an unmet medical need in patients with a serious condition. The IND and potential fast track designation may be discussed before an IND submission in a pre-IND meeting, but a decision on designation would await submission of the IND and an official request for fast track designation. If a product development program is granted fast track designation for one indication and has subsequently obtained data to support fast track designation for another indication, sponsors should submit a separate request.[63]

Breakthrough Therapy Designation

Sponsors may submit breakthrough therapy designation requests if there is preliminary clinical evidence indicating that the product may demonstrate substantial improvement over existing therapies on one or more clinically significant endpoints. Because the primary intent of breakthrough therapy designation is to provide intensive guidance to sponsors on efficient drug development support to support approval as efficiently as possible, the FDA anticipates that breakthrough therapy designation requests will rarely be made after the submission of an original BLA or a supplement. If a product development program is granted breakthrough therapy designation for one indication and has subsequently obtained preliminary clinical evidence to support breakthrough therapy designation for another indication, the sponsor should submit a separate request.[63]

Accelerated Approval

The accelerated approval pathway has been used primarily in settings in which the disease course is long, and an extended period of time would be required to measure the intended clinical benefit of a product. At the time a product is granted accelerated approval, the FDA has determined that an effect on the endpoint used to support approval—a surrogate endpoint or an intermediate clinical endpoint—is reasonably likely to predict clinical benefit. For drugs granted accelerated approval, postmarketing confirmatory trials have been required to verify the anticipated clinical benefit.[59,63]

Priority Review Designation

An application for a drug will receive priority review designation if it is for a drug that treats a serious condition and, if approved, would provide a significant improvement in safety or effectiveness over available therapies. Priority review has the benefit of a short review clock, and the FDA will take action on an application within 6 months (compared to 10 months under standard review) after a successful filing of a BLA.[63]

Rolling Biological License Application Review

Sponsors may request preliminary FDA agreement on the proposal for a rolling submission of completed sections of an application (e.g., the entire clinical section) at the pre-BLA meeting. If the FDA determines, after preliminary evaluation of the submitted clinical data, that the product may be effective, the FDA may consider reviewing completed portions of a marketing application before submitting the complete application.[63]

Regenerative Medicine Advanced Therapy

Regenerative medicine advanced therapies (RMATs) are defined in section 506(g)(8) of the FD&C Act as cell therapies, therapeutic tissue engineering products, human cell and tissue products, and combination products using any such therapies or products, except for those regulated solely under section 361 of the Public Health Service Act (PHS Act; 42 U.S.C. 264) and Title 21 of the Code of Federal Regulations Part 1271 (21 CFR Part 1271). The FDA interprets cell therapies, for purposes of section 506(g)(8) of the FD&C Act, to include both allogeneic and autologous cell therapies.

Based on the FDA's interpretation of section 506(g), human gene therapies, including genetically modified cells, that lead to a sustained effect on cells or tissues may meet the definition of a regenerative medicine therapy.

An investigational drug is eligible for RMAT designation if it meets these three criteria:

- It meets the definition of regenerative medicine therapy.
- It is intended to treat, modify, reverse, or cure a serious condition.
- Preliminary clinical evidence indicates that the regenerative medicine therapy has the potential to address unmet medical needs for such a condition.

Advantages of the RMAT designation include all the benefits of the fast track and breakthrough therapy designation programs, including early interactions with the FDA.[64]

CONCLUSION

Cancer vaccines are expected to be a long-term solution in the management of solid tumors and to prevent tumor metastasis. In the short run, cancer vaccines have been proposed as a means of preventing recurrence of cancer after surgical resections. Early preclinical and clinical studies in cancer vaccine-based immunotherapy[65-68] have demonstrated the potential of cancer vaccines in overcoming cancer. Global interest in this field has been fueled by the success of immunotherapies based on the use of CPIs (e.g., CTLA-4-specific or PD-1-specific monoclonal antibodies) and a possibility of developing combination therapies that combine CPI with cancer vaccines.[69] As with other products, consideration must be given as to the animal models used to test cancer vaccines and evaluate if it is the most appropriate model to evaluate the vaccine. The FDA recommends that the IND sponsors discuss their preclinical studies and pharmacology and toxicology data in an appropriate pre-IND or INTERACT meeting with the FDA. To help guide the sponsors, the FDA has published a guidance on the "Preclinical Assessment of Investigational Cellular and Gene Therapy

Products." This and other related guidance documents are available at the FDA's webpage (www.fda.gov/vaccines-blood-biologics/biologics-guidances/cellular-gene-therapy-guidances). Cancer vaccines are rapidly maturing, and the FDA is making significant efforts to provide timely regulatory advice to stakeholders based on the current science knowledge and regulatory requirements to help accelerate cancer vaccine development.

ACKNOWLEDGMENTS

We thank Drs. Andrew Byrnes, Chaohong Fan, Carolyn Laurencot, Steven Oh, and Tejashri Purohit-Sheth, of the Office of Tissues and Advanced Therapies (OTAT), CBER, FDA, for critical reading of the manuscript and for their comments and suggestions in drafting this chapter.

KEY REFERENCES

Only key references appear in the print edition. The full reference list appears in the digital product on Springer Publishing Connect: connect.springerpub.com/content/book/978-0-8261-3743-2/part/part05/chapter/ch64

8. Hinrichs CS, Rosenberg SA. Exploiting the curative potential of adoptive T-cell therapy for cancer. *Immunol Rev.* 2014;257(1):56–71. doi:10.1111/imr.12132

11. Vigneron N. Human tumor antigens and cancer immunotherapy. *Biomed Res Int.* 2015;2015:1–17. doi:10.1155/2015/948501

17. U.S. Food and Drug Administration. Chemistry, manufacturing, and control (CMC) information for human gene therapy investigational new drug applications (INDs): guidance for industry. https://www.fda.gov/regulatory-information/search-fda-guidance-documents/chemistry-manufacturing-and-control-cmc-information-human-gene-therapy-investigational-new-drug. Published January 2020.

19. Larocca C, Schlom J. Viral vector-based therapeutic cancer vaccines. *Cancer J.* 2011;17(5):359–371. doi:10.1097/PPO.0b013e3182325e63

30. U.S. Food and Drug Administration. Guidance for industry: Q11 development and manufacture of drug substances. https://www.fda.gov/media/80909/download. Published November 2012.

33. U.S. Food and Drug Administration. Formal meetings between the FDA and sponsors or applicants of PDUFA products guidance for industry. https://www.fda.gov/regulatory-information/search-fda-guidance-documents/formal-meetings-between-fda-and-sponsors-or-applicants-pdufa-products-guidance-industry. Published December 2017.

45. Yarchoan M, Johnson BA, Lutz ER, et al. Targeting neoantigens to augment antitumour immunity. *Nat Rev Cancer.* 2017;17(4):209–222. doi:10.1038/nrc.2016.154

52. Peters B, Nielsen M, Sette A. T cell epitope predictions. *Annu Rev Immunol.* 2020;38(1):123–145. doi:10.1146/annurev-immunol-082119-124838

A Regulatory Perspective on Cell Therapy for Cancer: Chemistry, Manufacturing and Control, Preclinical, and Clinical Considerations

Ke Liu, Jaikumar Duraiswamy, Thomas Finn, Brian Niland, Allen Wensky, and Raj Puri

KEY POINTS

- The U.S. Food and Drug Administration (FDA) reviews products based on an assessment of risk, and each product is reviewed on a case-by-case basis according to the associated risks with that product from intrinsic and extrinsic factors.

- Patient-specific autologous and allogeneic cell-based products present unique challenges in terms of manufacturing scale, the level of testing, stability, consistency/comparability, and logistics.

- The same CGMP regulations apply to cell therapy products as for other types of biologics, along with the additional expectations for donor screening and testing for infectious agents and tracking of donor material during manufacturing.

- The clinical assessment of cell therapy is similar in many ways to the clinical assessment of nonliving drugs.

- Safety and substantial evidence of effectiveness must be demonstrated through a rigorous program of nonclinical and clinical development. The totality of such data must show that the benefits expected from the cell therapy outweigh the risks.

- In addition to the many clinical considerations inherent in the design of any experimental agent in human beings, the additional complexity of the manufacture of cell products and their continued biological activity in the host add special concerns.

- Clinical development can often outpace product development, which can present issues for registration studies and biologics license applications.

INTRODUCTION

Regulation of Cell Therapies by the Food and Drug Administration

Cell therapies at the U.S. Food and Drug Administration (FDA) are reviewed within the Office of Tissues and Advanced Therapies (OTAT) in the Center for Biologics Evaluation and Research (CBER). Examples of cell therapies reviewed by OTAT include stem cells, cellular immunotherapies, and somatic cell therapies for treatment of metabolic disorders, neurological conditions, and cardiovascular diseases. Categories of cellular immunotherapies include both antigen-presenting cell (APC)-based therapies (monocytes, dendritic) and lymphocytes (CD4, CD8, regulatory T cells [T_{reg} cells], natural killer [NK]). Genetically modified versions of these same cell types would typically be classified as gene therapies (see Chapter 66 on gene therapy regulatory considerations in this section). Many of the same concerns and recommendations surrounding cell therapy manufacturing would also apply to gene therapy products. Clinical applications of such immunotherapy products have been most prominently investigated in the field of adoptive cellular immunotherapy of cancer.[1–3]

The majority of cellular products are regulated as biologics, but in some cases they are regulated as devices or combination products, under the authority of the Public Health Service Act (42 USC 262) and/or the Food, Drug and Cosmetic Act (21 USC) and the implementing regulations in Title 21 of the Code of Federal Regulations (21CFR).* It is important to understand that the regulation of cell therapies is accomplished with many of the same regulations and concerns about product manufacturing and testing as applied to other types of biologics (e.g., monoclonal antibodies). As biologics, the biologic regulations under 21 CFR part 600/610 apply. As a drug product, current good manufacturing practice (CGMP) facility and

---

* For a list of examples please see www.fda.gov/BiologicsBlood Vaccines/TissueTissueProducts/RegulationofTissues/ucm150485.htm

quality systems regulations (21 CFR part 210/211) apply. As human cells, tissues, and cellular and tissue-based products (HCT/Ps), 21 CFR part 1271 regulations that govern good tissue practices and the risk of transmission of communicable disease agents apply.* In situations where an HCT/P is classified as a medical device, medical device regulations found in 21 CFR part 820 apply.† Together these regulations help ensure product safety and quality, including safety and potency. The FDA's current thinking on these regulations can be found in numerous FDA and International Council for Harmonization (ICH) guidance documents. A list of relevant guidance documents can be found at CBER's and CDER's websites,‡ some of which are referenced in this chapter. Additional manufacturing advice is provided by the ICH, which publishes guidelines on product quality.[4] General concepts described in many ICH guidelines are consistent with the FDA guidance in general. The regulatory pathway most cell therapies fall under is as investigational new drugs (IND) for conducting clinical trials, and for licensure under a biologics license application (BLA). For cell therapies regulated as devices under the investigational device exemption (IDE) pathway, they are ultimately marketed either through the premarket approval (PMA) or humanitarian device exemption (HDE) regulatory pathways. This chapter will focus on the IND/BLA pathway, though many of the same preclinical, clinical, and manufacturing concerns apply to IDE/PMA products as well.

The type of manufacturing, preclinical, and clinical information that should be submitted in an IND is described in 21 CFR 312.23 and in the FDA guidance on somatic cell therapies.[5] Each IND must contain sufficient information to assure the identity, quality, purity, and potency of the investigational agent (21 CFR 312.23(a)(7)(i)). The required information may be provided by the sponsor either directly or by cross-reference to previously submitted information (21 CFR 312.23(b)). A standardized

way of organizing chemistry, manufacturing, and control (CMC) information in regulatory submissions is provided in the ICH M4 guideline describing the common technical document format.[6] The FDA now requires all BLAs, commercial IND submissions, and master files be submitted in the electronic common technical document (eCTD) format.[7] Excluded from the eCTD requirement are academic and noncommercial INDs (IND for a product that is not intended for commercial distribution; this exemption includes research and investigator-sponsored INDs). For academic and noncommercial INDs, the FDA will continue to accept submissions in alternative electronic formats.[8]

General Cell Therapy Product Manufacturing Considerations

The evaluation of product manufacturing is accomplished through the review of relevant CMC information. Although both protein-based and cell-based biologics are governed by many of the same regulations and have many of the same regulatory concerns, additional considerations apply to some types of cell therapies. For example, in the case of small molecule products and protein-based biologics, "personalized medicines" or "individualized medicine" can refer to biomarkers used to target-specific patient populations, to customized patient treatment schedules, or to products with unique specificities. For cell therapies, these terms can also refer to an allogeneic or autologous product manufactured at a lot size to treat a small number of patients, or a single patient "N-of-one." They can also be personalized to match properties of the source material with the target patient or patient population, such as the degree of HLA match. The degree of product specialization can also extend to a product designed to target a mutation specific to that one individual. It is therefore important when describing a product as a personalized medicine to understand the context in which it is being used.

Due to their smaller batch size, number of lots generated, and short manufacturing time windows and/or shelf life for many types of cell therapy products, some practical limitations can exist. For example, it may not be possible to perform the same level of rigorous in-process and final product testing on a product lot intended to treat a single patient, compared to a cell therapy product derived from a multitiered cell bank system that yields thousands of doses, or a well-characterized protein biologic.

Another consideration is that the precise mechanism of action can be more difficult to assess for some cell therapies. Although it is not a requirement that the mechanism of action be known, it is very important to have a good understanding of how the product likely functions so that appropriate critical quality attributes (CQA) and critical process parameters (CPP) can be established that

---

* Certain HCT/Ps are regulated solely under section 361 of the Public Health Service Act (42 USC 264). Those types of cellular products are minimally manipulated; intended for homologous use; not combined with other articles except for water, crystalloids, or a sterilizing, preserving, or storage agent; and either do not have a systemic effect dependent on cell metabolism or have such an effect but it is only for autologous use, for allogeneic use in a first -or second-degree relative, or for reproductive use (21CFR1271.10). Cellular products regulated solely under section 361 therefore generally include hematopoietic stem cells for autologous use or for use in a first- or second-degree relative, cells used in assisted reproduction techniques, and many tissue products used for their mechanical properties in surgical reconstruction.

† Please refer to www.fda.gov/medical-devices/how-study-and-market-your-device/investigational-device-exemption-ide

‡ CBER guidances can be found at www.fda.gov/vaccines-blood-biologics/guidance-compliance-regulatory-information-biologics/biologics-guidances, and CDER guidances can be found at www.fda.gov/regulatory-information/search-fda-guidance-documents

will help ensure product quality.[9] In-process and final product release specifications should be based on these defined CQA.[10,11] Specifications may change during the product development life cycle as additional manufacturing experience and product knowledge is gained and possible correlations with clinical outcomes are identified.[5] Some products may have more than one mechanism of action. In such cases, developers of cell therapies should decide what cellular properties are desirable for each proposed mechanism of action, and should rank their relative importance.

Logistics can also be of great importance for some types of products. Source material, product intermediates, and final products can have short dating periods (shelf lives). This can place important limitations on how source material is collected, stored, handled, and shipped.

Product intermediates can be very sensitive to manufacturing step holding times, the number of times cell lines are passaged, the length of time cells are kept in expansion phase, or the number of times cells are stimulated. Final products that are relatively unstable typically have short dating periods. These factors impact CPPs and can place restrictions on the manufacturing and shipping timelines, which may then impact clinical protocol design. For example, logistical factors can make multicenter trials more challenging. In some cases, this may necessitate cryopreserving source material, intermediates, or final products. Some cellular treatments may include administration of lymphodepleting or myeloablative conditioning to the patient prior to receiving the product. This can present a risk to the patient if the product cannot be manufactured or if testing cannot be completed before the product is released for administration. For such therapies it can be important to demonstrate the feasibility of the manufacturing process, including achieving the intended dose and the ability to meet the release testing criteria. Coordination of manufacturing and cell treatment schedules should align with donor or recipient conditioning, or specific stages of patient treatment.

General Cell Therapy Preclinical Considerations

In addition to considerations of autologous, allogeneic, or xenogeneic CT products, CT-derived products are also generally classified as stem cell-derived products or mature and functionally differentiated cell-derived products. Both types can vary greatly with respect to product origin, formulation, and genetic compatibility with the host (e.g., autologous, allogeneic, or xenogeneic). Therefore, it is important to thoroughly characterize and provide detailed information on these specific characteristics using both in vitro and in vivo studies when applicable. This includes characterization of: (a) the cellular phenotype(s); (b) the source of the cell(s); (c) the extent of ex vivo manipulation (e.g., selection, purification,

expansion, activation); (d) the fate of the cells post-administration (engraftment, migration, differentiation, tumorigenicity); (e) the host immune response to the administered cells; (f) administration site reactions; (g) potential inflammatory or adverse responses in target and nontarget tissues; and (h) unregulated proliferation of the cells within the host. Depending on the nature of the product and maturity of the product class, varying degrees of preclinical studies, which often include animal models of disease or injury, should be performed to address these issues. The level of preclinical studies that need to be conducted is decided on a case-by-case basis and is dependent on a number of factors. These factors include similarities and differences compared to other cellular products currently being studied in the clinic or licensed, and available data from the peer-reviewed scientific literature, "in-house" studies, or cross-referenced clinical trials. In considering the risk/benefit profile, the FDA also considers the cell source, manufacturing and final formulation, clinical indication to be studied (e.g., aesthetic treatments vs. late-stage cancer), the route of administration, dose, dosing regimen, and so on. For any application for cell therapies, the previously outlined issues should be addressed in the investigational regulatory application.

In most cases, the concerns for safety and bioactivity of a cell therapy product will need to be addressed in an animal model of disease or injury. Selection of the appropriate animal model for testing is important for properly assessing the activity and safety of the product. The comparability of the physiology and anatomy of the animal, susceptibility or permissiveness of the animal host to the cell therapy agent, immune tolerance, or the potential for rejection of the cell therapy product are all issues that need to be addressed. Careful consideration of the animal species and model to be used through the use of previous knowledge about the model, as well as pilot studies conducted with the intended CT product, are important before conducting definitive studies. The pilot studies should inform the design of definitive animal studies. Nonstandard test species are acceptable if adequate supporting data for their use is provided. This includes the previously mentioned factors as well as the similarities and differences to the indication to be studied.

General Cell Therapy Preclinical Considerations: Dose and Dosing Regimen

A justification for starting dose based on preclinical data and/or clinical experience should be provided in the IND. If animal or in vitro data are available, there might be sufficient information to determine if a specific starting dose has an acceptable level of risk. However, conventional allometric scaling methods for cell therapy products may be less precise than for small-molecule drugs. Therefore, it may be difficult to establish an initial starting dose based on the considerations used for small-molecule drugs.

Dosing of cellular therapies is not straightforward. Cell therapies may be a mixture of many different types of cells, and it may not be clear what cell type is responsible for the desired therapeutic outcome. Equally, if a toxicity occurs, it is not always clear if it is due to the final intended cell therapy cell type, due to other cell populations in the final formulation, or due to the host's reaction to the cell therapy. Practically, most trials of cellular immunotherapy of cancer describe the dose as the total number of cells delivered. In some situations, it is possible to base a dose on several different parameters, such as a desired number of CD34$^+$ cells not to exceed a total number of T cells in the infusion.[12]

Even when it is clear which cells mediate the biological effects, the linear relationship between dose and effect that characterizes cytotoxic therapies is much less apparent for cell therapies, where dose response curves are more often flat. Further complicating dose determinations is the fact that cells introduced into patients may divide, differentiate, and adapt. For this reason, it may be more important to consider the persistence of cells in the host. Because neither the therapeutic effects nor the toxicity may be necessarily related to administered dose, trial designs calling for a flat dose, rather than a dose based on the subject's weight or body surface area, may be more acceptable.

Specific criteria for dose escalation and de-escalation should be provided in the first-in-human cell therapy study. Clinical development of cell therapy products has often included dose escalation in half-log (approximately three-fold) increments. However, the dosing increments used for dose escalation should consider preclinical and any available clinical data regarding the risks and activity associated with changes in dose.

Additional information about dosing considerations and the design of early phase clinical trials may be found in the FDA "Guidance for Industry (June 2015): Considerations for the Design of Early-Phase Clinical Trials of Cellular and Gene Therapy Products."[13]

REGULATORY CHEMISTRY, MANUFACTURING, AND CONTROL CONSIDERATIONS FOR CELL THERAPY PRODUCTS

The FDA reviews product manufacturing in the context of safety risks to the subject or patient, as well as risks that might reduce product quality. Sources of risk include the manufacturing environment, starting materials, raw materials/reagents used during manufacturing, potential product-related impurities and process-related impurities and contaminants,[10] and container closures (such as vials).[5,14] These elements are discussed in greater detail in the text that follows.

Current Good Manufacturing Practices Manufacturing

CGMPs apply to both facilities that perform manufacturing and to the quality system that assures proper design, monitoring, and control of manufacturing processes.[15] This includes establishing strong quality management systems with an independent quality assurance (QA) unit to review and approve important procedures related to production, provide oversight, and perform trend analysis,[16] obtaining appropriate quality raw materials, establishing robust operating procedures, detecting and investigating product quality deviations, and maintaining reliable testing laboratories. Such a formal system of controls, if adequately put into practice, would help to prevent instances of contamination, mix-ups, deviations, failures, and errors.[9,14–17] The potential for product mix-ups or cross-contamination is of special importance for cell therapies where multiple lots may be manufactured at the same time in the same facility, and product lots are intended for specific patients.[5] For example, it is critical to ensure that autologous product lots are given back to the same patient. These risks can be mitigated using robust product tracking systems, including chain of identity and chain of custody, and appropriate product segregation strategies. The product label should contain the date of product manufacture, storage conditions, expiration date and time (if appropriate), product name, and two nonpersonal patient identifiers. Many manufacturers also include bar codes on in-process and final product labels.

The FDA understands that CGMP regulations in 21 CFR parts 210 and 211 may be difficult to fully adhere to for the manufacturer of many investigational drugs used for Phase 1 clinical trials. Therefore, for Phase 1 the FDA offers additional flexibility in how compliance with CGMP is achieved. The specific CGMP requirements in 21 CFR part 211 are not applicable to investigational products manufactured for use during Phase 1 clinical trials[18] and certain exploratory products (CFR 312.21(a)). Sponsors must still comply with the requirements of CGMP under section 501(a)(2)(B) of the FD&C Act, but sponsors may achieve this through other approaches than those specifically described in 21 CFR part 211. The FDA has issued a guidance document that describes some of the elements important to adherence to CGMP manufacturing and product testing during Phase 1.[18] For example, adherence to QC procedures during Phase 1 development occurs largely through: (a) having written procedures that are well defined, (b) the use of equipment that is adequately controlled, and (c) data from production, including testing, that are accurately and consistently recorded. Sponsors should carefully consider the risks from the production environment that might adversely affect the resulting quality of an investigational product, especially when the investigational product is produced in laboratory facilities that are not expressly or solely designed for drug or biologic production. For example, of particular importance is the susceptibility of a cellular product to contamination or cross contamination with other substances (e.g. chemicals, biological substances, adventitious agents) that may be present from previous or concurrent research or production activities.[19-23] To mitigate these risks, the FDA recommends that: (a) sponsors perform a formal evaluation of the production environment to identify potential hazards; and (b) take appropriate actions prior to and during production to minimize risks and safeguard the quality of the investigational product.[14]

Critical Quality Attributes and Critical Process Parameters and Their Relationship to Product Specifications

Quality must be designed into the product and reflected in the process through established CQA and CPP. A CQA is a physical, chemical, biological, or microbiological property or characteristic that is deemed important to help ensure product quality.[9] As such, each CQA should be within an appropriate limit, range, or distribution. A manufacturing process is typically established by examining CQA and processes will be needed to generate a final product consistent with those desired attributes. Critical process parameters are independent manufacturing process parameters most likely to affect the quality attributes of a product. CPPs are determined by sound scientific research and manufacturing experience. Product specifications are established based on identified CQA and CPP. A specification is a specific test method with a specific acceptance criterion. Specifications are chosen to confirm the quality of the drug substance (DS) and drug product (DP) rather than to establish full characterization, and should focus on those characteristics found to be useful in ensuring the safety and efficacy of the DS and DP.[10,11] Product specifications guide both in-process and final product parameters. A criterion could be a minimum lower limit, an upper limit, a range, or a qualitative parameter. It is important to understand that methods, assay criteria, and specifications often change during the product life cycle as improvements or refinements are made.[5] For example, consider an attribute for assuring the presence of a key cell population that according to the proposed mechanism of action is necessary for the intended therapeutic effect. Knowing that it is important to control this attribute, it should be considered a CQA. A specification could be set to assure that the final product contains at least 90% of this cell type, as determined by flow cytometry. The type of assay used for detection could change during the course of

product development as a more reliable, accurate, or sensitive method is established. Product knowledge is often limited in early stages of development. The FDA encourages manufacturers to test as comprehensively as is feasible and then refine testing later in development as the value of each test becomes more apparent.

Allogeneic Versus Autologous Cells—Donor Eligibility

Donor screening and testing are essential for ensuring that the cellular starting material is safe; however, this is a common deficiency in many cellular therapy IND applications. For allogeneic cellular products, prospective donors must meet the donor eligibility requirements as described in 21 CFR 1271 part C and in FDA guidance.[24-27] This is true for both patient-specific products involving the production of a single lot to treat one allogeneic subject, or for a cell line used as a master cell bank intended to manufacture product doses for many patients. A complete description of the testing and screening of the donors should be provided in IND submissions, and documentation of testing should be maintained in the study records (21 CFR 1271.50; 21 CFR 1271.55). Tracking should be able to trace the donor to the recipient and from the recipient to the donor (21 CFR 1271.290). Each prospective donor should be screened for high-risk behavior and tested for communicable disease agents as appropriate (21 CFR 610.40; 21 CFR 1271.85). The specific relevant communicable disease agents that donors of HCT/Ps must be tested for are listed in 21 CFR 1271.85 and FDA guidance. Additional expectations regarding the types of tests to be performed, the test or test kits that can be used, and the types of laboratories appropriate to conduct the tests are described in FDA guidance on donor eligibility.[24-28] Allogeneic donors must be tested, whereas for autologous donors screening and testing are optional (21 CFR 1271.90(a)). Some collection facilities prefer to test all donors as do some sponsors. If a complete donor eligibility determination is not performed, the product labels would need to include the statement "NOT EVALUATED FOR INFECTIOUS SUBSTANCES" per 21 CFR 1271.90 (b).[2] Autologous products must be labeled as "FOR AUTOLOGOUS USE ONLY" per 21 CFR 1271.90 (b).[1]

Testing of donors should be performed using FDA-licensed, -approved, or -cleared donor screening tests when they are available (21 CFR 1271.80(c)). An updated list of licensed, approved, or cleared tests can be found on the FDA website.[29] HCT/Ps' donors whose screening tests are reactive for HIV-1, HIV-2, HBV, or HCV should be excluded. Recent draft guidance documents with current proposed recommendations for screening and testing HCT/P donors for syphilis,[30] West Nile virus,[25] and Zika virus[31] are also available. Donors of leukocyte-rich

HCT/Ps should be tested for HTLV-I , HTLV-II, and CMV. Leukocyte-rich donors who are reactive for HTLV-I or HTLV-II should also be excluded. Additionally, note that if a donor tests positive for CMV, such a donor is not necessarily ineligible, but you must establish and maintain a standard operating procedure governing the release of an HCT/P from a donor whose specimen tests reactive for CMV (1271.85(b)(2)), and the test results indicated on the product lot label or accompany the product lot (21 CFR 1271.370).

Ancillary Materials

To mitigate safety risks that materials, reagents, or components that are in direct product contact might pose, and to help ensure consistent product manufacturing, the FDA recommends that a qualification program be established for all critical materials.[5,9,16] Upon receipt of an ancillary material, the certificate of analysis supplied by the vendor documenting all relevant test results should be reviewed. If vendor quality testing is insufficient, then additional testing by the product manufacturer should be performed. The qualification program should consist of appropriate safety tests, an analysis for purity, and a functional assay to ensure that these materials are performing as desired in the manufacturing process. These tests should be performed each time a new lot of material is qualified. An expiration date for each component should be established based on information provided by the supplier and/or stability studies conducted by the sponsor. For licensed products, an identity test is to be performed by either the component manufacturer or the sponsor (21 CFR 211.84(d)(2)). Only after the materials have been deemed adequate can they be released for use in the manufacturing process (21 CFR 211.84(a)).[15,16] If added reagents might interfere with final product function or present a safety concern, such as generate a possible allergic reaction, the manufacturing process should be designed to reduce their levels in the final product, and residual levels should be determined and appropriate limits should be established. For critical reagents or custom materials, we further recommend that sponsors consider identifying a second source supplier in the event of a material shortage or should a material performance issue arise.

Container Closures

Container closures are important because they have direct contact with the product and their performance can affect product quality. Careful selection and qualification of in-process and final product container closures should be made to be sure they are compatible with the product and are suitable for the intended purpose. Containers used to hold source material, product intermediates, or the final product for long periods should be carefully selected so that materials from the container do not leach into the product. They should also maintain their integrity during storage and shipment to maintain product sterility. For more information, please refer to the FDA guidance on container closure systems.[32,33]

Product Specifications

Specifications are one part of a total control strategy designed to ensure product quality and consistency.[10] The manufacturing process should be designed to ensure product quality if CQA and CPP are adhered to, with confirmation of adequate product quality assessed through product testing.[10,11] The level and type of testing performed on cellular product (DS and DP) is influenced partially by regulatory requirements and expectations, such as donor eligibility requirements, and partially by the manufacturer's established CQAs.[5] Some assays might serve more than one function. For example, viable cell number may be important both for determining cell dose and as a safety measure to minimize dead cells that might clump and lead to blocking of capillaries. Release criteria should be consistent with scientific and medical principles, and with the sponsor's manufacturing experience.

How some properties are categorized will vary by product and different types of products may involve different levels of testing for the same type of CQA. Potency or identity, for example, could involve a single measure for each, or multiple measures may be necessary in order to ensure adequate product quality. Appropriate measures of potency and identity in some cases may be best served using a matrix approach.[34] Note that these measures are not always mutually exclusive. For example, for a T cell therapy the number of $CD8^+$ cells could be part of both a potency specification matrix and an identity specification matrix. The level of testing intended to ensure adequate product quality should be justified. Any potential future labeling claims should also be considered, and an evaluation should be made as to whether sufficient data exist to support claims associated with specific product properties.

Specific Assays

Sterility (Bacterial and Fungal) Testing: Sterility testing must be performed on each lot of each biological product's final container material or other material, as appropriate (21 CFR 610.12), and be free of objectionable microorganisms (211.165). Previously, prescriptive methods to be used for sterility testing were specified in regulation. However, in 2012 the FDA amended the sterility testing requirements for biological products. These changes are intended to promote improvement and innovation in the development of sterility test methods by allowing manufacturers the flexibility needed for sterility testing of some novel products that may be introduced to the market, enhancing sterility testing of currently approved products, and encouraging manufacturers to utilize scientific and technological advances in sterility test methods as they become available.[35] Regardless of the manufacturer's choice in sterility test, the method used for testing should be appropriate for the type of product. The method should be described in detail in regulatory submissions and the assay will need to be initially qualified to demonstrate suitability and fully validated for licensure.

Rapid Microbial Methods: In cases where the product is released prior to complete sterility assay results being available, a rapid microbial method should be used to test the final product for release[5] in addition to a culture-based sterility test method. Results from the rapid test should be available prior to release. The most common rapid method is a Gram stain, though sponsors may choose other rapid methods. In such cases where full sterility results are not available at the time of release, an action plan should be included in the investigational plan to address the actions to be taken in the event sterility results indicate product contamination after the product is administered to the subject. This would include notifying the physician of the sterility failure and evaluating the root cause.[5] The event should be reported as an information amendment within 30 calendar days after initial receipt of the positive culture test result (21 CFR 312.31), along with any corrective actions taken. The investigator should evaluate the subject for any signs of infection that may be attributable to the product sterility failure. If the patient experiences any serious and unexpected adverse drug experience that could be attributed to the administration of the cellular product, this must be reported in an IND safety report no more than 15 calendar days after the sponsor receives initial receipt of the information (21 CFR 312.32).

Mycoplasma Testing: If the product manufacturer includes cell culture for more than 48 hours, the product should usually also be tested for mycoplasma contamination.[5,18] Sources of possible mycoplasma contamination include animal sera and cell lines, and these should be qualified to demonstrate they are free of mycoplasma contamination.

Purity Testing: Product purity can be defined as freedom from extraneous material, except that which is unavoidable in the manufacturing process (21 CFR 610.13). Testing for purity includes an assay for endotoxin and may also include assays for unintended cell populations (e.g., distinguished by phenotypes), residual proteins or peptides used to stimulate or pulse cells, and materials used during manufacture, such as cytokines, growth factors, antibodies, and sera. For any parenteral drug, except those administered intrathecally or by intraocular route, the FDA recommends that the upper limit of acceptance criterion for endotoxin be 5 EU/kg body weight/hour in accordance with USP <85>.[36,37] For intrathecally administered drugs, the FDA recommends an acceptance criterion upper limit of 0.2 EU/kg body weight/hour. The endotoxin limit for intraocular delivery should follow the specifications in USP <771> (not more than [NMT] 2.0 Endotoxin Unit [EU]/dose/eye or NMT 0.5 EU/mL).[38] Sponsors should describe in their IND submissions the endotoxin test method they will conduct, and the acceptance criterion for release.

Identity Testing: For licensed products, the identity of the final product must be verified by assays that will identify the product for proper labeling and will distinguish the product from other products being processed in the same facility (21 CFR 610.14). IND identity testing should adequately characterize the product for the cell population(s) that correspond to the active ingredient(s), as defined by the proposed mechanism of action, and for other cell types that may be present.[5]

Potency Testing: Potency is the specific ability or capacity of the product to effect a given result, as indicated by appropriate laboratory tests or by adequately controlled clinical data obtained through the administration of the product in the manner intended (21 CFR 600.3(s)). Ideally, a potency assay is a quantitative bioassay that measures biological function of the clinical mechanism of action. These may be by in vivo or in vitro tests (21 CFR 610.10). If direct measure of a biological function is not feasible, data must be provided to justify use of a test or combination of tests to ensure product potency. FDA guidance is available for potency testing of cell and gene therapy products.[34]

Process Development, Critical Process Parameters, and Process Changes

The product development life cycle encompasses early preclinical work through licensure and beyond. During the life cycle, it is expected that manufacturing changes will occur, either during the early stages as the process is fully being developed, later in development as the process is refined and optimized, and throughout the life cycle in response to either planned or unanticipated events, such as a material or reagent that is no longer available. Minor manufacturing changes can be reported in IND annual reports, but more substantial changes should be submitted as a manufacturing amendment. When there is a significant manufacturing change, a comparability study may be needed to assure that product quality has not been impacted.[39]

CPPs should be controlled and monitored to confirm that the quality attributes of the product are maintained or improved.[9] It is expected that the procedures used in manufacturing will be refined during early phase clinical studies, but the manufacturing process should be well established before late-phase studies are initiated, and changes to the process should be minimized once the late-phase studies are initiated. Because the clinical trial results could be confounded by manufacturing changes, changes in manufacturing procedures that affect clinical studies intended to support licensure may require a demonstration of product comparability. An objective product comparability study should include the use of appropriate prespecified statistical equivalence intervals along with an adequate justification for the equivalence interval(s) used. Validation of analytical methods, manufacturing and systems processes, and facilities must be completed by the time of submission of a BLA.[40,41] When manufacturers move into later development and prepare for licensure, additional considerations arise related to product manufacturing. Ideally, this involves a greater understanding and control of product manufacturing.[11,15]

Clinical Considerations for Cell Therapy Products

In many respects, clinical considerations for cell therapy products are similar to considerations for drugs, biologics, and devices not manufactured from human cells. Clinical development should proceed from a sound basis or preclinical theory and data, and should be carried out in a phased manner. Because of the complexity of the manufacture, logistics, administration, and monitoring of cell therapy products, there are certain considerations unique to this class of products.

As a dynamic "living drug," cell therapy products change over time as they adapt to their environment. As previously noted, this presents problems for manufacturing and characterizing the product. Once implanted, though, these same properties lead to clinical challenges. These include migration of cells from where they were implanted, the synthesis of membrane bound or excreted proteins not present during manufacturing, and the differentiation or dedifferentiation of cells along an unanticipated pathway.

Another complicating factor in cell therapy is the need for a cell donor to provide starting material. The ethical issues of asking an allogeneic donor to provide cells or tissues are well known from solid organ and bone marrow transplant literature.[42,43] The use of modified autologous cells may avoid some of these issues, but creates its own set of complications. Examples include the need for a potentially invasive procedure to obtain the cells in a subject who may already be immunologically or physiologically compromised by the disease to be treated, and possibility that a subject's clinical condition may change appreciably between procurement and administration of the cells, such that the risk-benefit of cell administration must be re-evaluated.

A discussion of concerns particularly relevant to cell and gene therapy, and of the impact of these concerns on trial design, can be found in the 2015 FDA guidance document, "Considerations for the Design of Early-Phase Clinical Trials of Cellular and Gene Therapy Products."[13]

Early Phase Trial Objectives

As in studies of conventional drugs and biologics products, an important objective in early phase clinical studies of cell therapies is to identify a safe dose and schedule. Because of the technical complexity of the manufacture of cells, simply demonstrating that it is feasible to manufacture and deliver a particular cellular product may also be an objective.

Trial Design

Due to the complexity of cell therapy products, the classic paradigm of performing large clinical trials, which enroll a diverse patient population to receive an off-the-shelf manufactured product, may be difficult. Smaller clinical trials offer a possible alternative for clinical trial design for cell therapy products, which may be highly active in a specifically defined patient population.[44] Knowing the cell therapy product's expected mechanism of action in a particular disease is essential to choose an appropriate study population, which might allow an early assessment of activity. It is important to enroll a study population whose responses to a new cell therapy will provide interpretable safety and activity data. Acute and chronic cell therapy toxicities are often different than cytotoxicities of other types of drugs. Dose-limiting toxicities may not occur during early phase trials, and a maximum tolerated dose may not be defined. However, possible serious late-occurring toxicities may occur, which require appropriate planning and monitoring during development. In addition, some cell therapy products may be locally administered and must have appropriate safety assessment for both localized and systemic toxicities.

General Monitoring Considerations

Toxicities may be graded using Common Terminology Criteria for Adverse Events (CTCAE).[45] In order to mitigate serious risks for cell therapy products, the definition of dose-limiting toxicity should usually include CTCAE grades 3 to 5 toxicities.

Specific monitoring considerations apply to cell therapy products, based on their biological nature. These include monitoring for transmission of infectious agents (and rarely, transmission of other donor diseases), graft-versus-host disease and other immune phenomena, monitoring of cells for migration from the target site and for persistence in the host, and the potential need for extended follow-up. A discussion of concerns particularly relevant to cell therapy, and of the impact of these concerns on trial design, can be found in the 2015 FDA guidance document, "Considerations for the Design of Early-Phase Clinical Trials of Cellular and Gene Therapy Products."[13]

As for all other drugs, biologics, and devices, rigorous safety monitoring and reporting to the FDA and other regulatory agencies is important for cell therapy products. Adverse events are reported as outlined in 21 CFR 312.32, including the reporting of suspected unexpected serious adverse reactions within 15 days and fatal events within 7 days. Additional information on standard monitoring requirements can be found in the 2012 FDA guidance, "Safety Reporting Requirements for INDs and BA/BE studies."[46] In addition to monitoring for routine adverse events, monitoring in the period immediately around the infusion or implantation of cellular products should include a plan to detect common reactions seen with cellular and biologic infusions, such as fevers, shortness of breath, hypotension, and allergic reactions. An additional concern common to cell therapy and other biologic products is monitoring for the transmission of infectious agents. This should be done as for more traditional blood products, relying primarily on donor screening to prevent such transmission. Such screening should be in accordance with 21 CFR 1271, subpart C. This topic is discussed in more detail in the "Allogeneic Versus Autologous Cells—Donor Eligibility" section in this chapter.

In addition to the general considerations that were previously discussed, special concerns apply to the safety monitoring of cell therapy products, deriving from their biological status as living drugs.

Immune cells used to treat cancer can cause complex reactions as they interact with the host immune system. The most often described such reaction is graft-versus-host disease (GvHD) occurring after bone marrow transplant, and more rarely after other infusions of hematopoietic cells. Other such complex reactions include autoimmunity due to the graft's immunocompetence or immunogenicity, graft failure, and cytokine release syndrome (CRS). Clinical monitoring for such immune-mediated complications is necessary in trials of cellular therapies. CRS has been most typically a problem after the treatment of subjects with high burdens of hematologic malignancy using certain genetically modified cell products, but can also occur after the infusion of cells that have not been genetically modified. A related concept, seen in both autologous and allogeneic transplant settings, is engraftment syndrome.

Endpoints for Cell Therapy Study

The primary endpoint for early phase clinical trials should focus on safety evaluation. One common secondary endpoint of early phase clinical trials for cell therapy product is to obtain preliminary data on clinical activity such as tumor response. In addition, exploratory endpoints should be considered for cell therapy studies and might include cell expression /

persistence, cell engraftment, or other aspects of the immune function.

For cell therapies whose mechanism of action depends on the host immune system. assessments of immune responses may provide mechanistically useful data, especially when they can be correlated to clinical outcomes.

Cell therapy trial endpoints must be carefully chosen and may include measures of clinical and/or biological activity of the cell product. Immunological endpoints may be considered, when applicable, to support or correlate with clinical outcomes.

Phase 3 trial endpoints can be challenging to choose, both in terms of specific selections and in terms of their assessments. Sponsors are encouraged to discuss the choice of Phase 3 endpoints with the FDA and refer to the FDA guidance document titled "Guidance for Industry: Clinical Trial Endpoints for the Approval of Cancer Drugs and Biologics."[47]

Later-Phase Clinical Trials

A Phase 2 trial can be a screening discriminator to determine if further progression to Phase 3 confirmatory trial is warranted. In addition, the clinical activity can be estimated in a well-conducted Phase 2 trial. Randomized Phase 2 trials typically lack the statistical power for conclusive demonstration of the treatment effect of the investigational cell therapy product.

Randomized Phase 2 trials may provide more reliable data about treatment effect size than single-arm trial data compared with historical controls. These Phase 2 data may be useful when planning the design of the subsequent Phase 3 trial. The quality and quantity of Phase 2 development should be sufficient to provide adequate data to make go or no-go decisions about proceeding to Phase 3 confirmatory trial.

Phase 3 trial usually provides primary evidence of efficacy and safety and may be used to support a marketing application. Sponsors may choose to submit a Phase 3 protocol to the FDA for special protocol assessment. SPA is a means by which the sponsor reaches an agreement with the FDA on the clinical design, endpoints, and statistical analysis plan prior to commencement of the Phase 3 trial. The FDA will document such an agreement in writing. To learn more about special protocol assessment agreements, please refer to the FDA's "Guidance for Industry—Special Protocol Assessment."[48]

Companion Diagnostics

When the proposed mechanism of action involves a specific antigen or other therapeutic target, consideration should be given to developing an assay or mechanism to measure the target antigen expression in tumor tissues of individual patients and using that information in patient selection or response monitoring. These assays may be considered as companion diagnostics and are generally regulated by the Center for Devices and Radiological Health (CDRH).[49]

Content of an Investigational New Drug Protocol

An IND for a cell therapy product should contain the following clinical components, as indicated in 21 CFR 312 part 23:

- rationale for use of product in chosen patient population;
- brief summary of previous human experience with the product;
- anticipated risks;
- hypothesis and objectives;
- inclusion and exclusion criteria;
- study design and detailed protocol;
- justification for starting dose;
- justification for dose regimen;
- safety and endpoint monitoring plans;
- definition of dose-limiting toxicity;
- definition of maximum tolerated dose;
- adverse event reporting plan;
- long-term follow-up plan;
- patient treatment discontinuation criteria;
- trial stopping criteria; and
- investigator's brochure.

Expedited Programs for Serious Conditions

Sponsors may request fast track designation when the IND is first submitted or at any time thereafter before receiving marketing approval of the BLA. The IND and potential fast track designation may be discussed before an IND submission in a pre-IND meeting, but a decision on designation would await submission of the IND. If a product development program is granted fast track designation for one indication and has subsequently obtained data to support fast track designation for another indication, sponsors should submit a separate request.

Sponsors may submit breakthrough therapy designation requests if there is preliminary clinical evidence indicating that the product may demonstrate substantial improvement over existing therapies on one or more clinically significant endpoints. Because the primary intent of breakthrough therapy designation is to develop evidence needed to support approval as efficiently as possible, the FDA anticipates that breakthrough therapy designation requests will rarely be made after the submission of an original BLA or a supplement. If a product development program is granted breakthrough therapy designation for one indication and has subsequently obtained preliminary clinical evidence to support breakthrough therapy designation for another indication, the sponsor should submit a separate request.

The accelerated approval pathway has been used primarily in settings in which the disease course is long and an extended period of time would be required to measure the intended clinical benefit of a product. At the time a product is granted accelerated approval, the FDA has determined that an effect on the endpoint used to support approval—a surrogate endpoint or an intermediate clinical endpoint—is reasonably likely to predict clinical benefit. For drugs granted accelerated approval, postmarketing confirmatory trials have been required to verify the anticipated effect.

An application for a drug will receive priority review designation if it is for a drug that treats a serious condition and, if approved, would provide a significant improvement in safety or effectiveness. Sponsors may request preliminary FDA agreement on the proposal for a rolling review at the pre-BLA meeting. If the FDA determines, after preliminary evaluation of the submitted clinical data, that a fast track product may be effective, the FDA may consider reviewing portions of a marketing application before submitting the complete application.

For further information regarding fast track designation, breakthrough therapy designation, and rolling review,* please see "Guidance for Industry: Expedited Programs for Serious Conditions—Drugs and Biologics."[50] For information on regenerative medicine advanced therapy designation (RMAT), please refer to the Chapter 64 on "Regulatory Considerations for Therapeutic Cancer Vaccines."

Expanded Access Uses

Expanded access is the use of an investigational drug outside of clinical trials to diagnose, monitor, or treat patients with serious diseases or conditions for which there are no comparable or satisfactory therapy options available.

Whenever possible, use of an investigational medical product by a patient as part of a clinical trial should be considered. However, when patient enrollment in a clinical trial is not possible, expanded access may be an option to gain access to an investigational medicinal product. The FDA is committed to increasing awareness about its expanded access process and the procedures for obtaining access to investigational drugs, biologics, and medical devices. Access to investigational treatments

---

* Rolling Review refers to a situation where a drug company can submit completed sections of its biologic license application (BLA) or new drug application (NDA) for review by the FDA, rather than waiting until the entire application is completed for submission. BLA or NDA review usually does not begin until the drug company has submitted the entire application to the FDA.

requires not only the FDA's review and authorization, but also the active involvement and cooperation of other parties, including drug companies and healthcare providers, in order to be successful. For more information about expanded access, sponsors can refer to the FDA guidance document entitled "Guidance for Industry-Expanded Access to Investigational Drugs for Treatment Use—Questions and Answers."[51]

Rare Disease Considerations

Many cell therapy products are developed for indications in rare diseases. A rare disease is defined in 21 USC 360 as either a disease that affects less than 200,000 people in the United States or a disease affecting more than 200,000 people for which a manufacturer is unlikely to be able to recover the cost of developing a drug to treat such disease through sales of such drug in the United States. Fundamental considerations in developing any drug for a rare disease include (a) the requirement for safety and substantial evidence of effectiveness is the same for rare and for common diseases and (b) the more that is known about a rare disease, the more straightforward it will be to demonstrate the evidence of safety and effectiveness. While it may be necessary to limit interventional trials in rare diseases to a small number of subjects specifically because few subjects are available, data from a small number of patients may provide evidence that an intervention is safe and effective if such a conclusion is backed by long-term and well-documented data on the natural history of the disease in question. To this end, it can often be beneficial to sponsors of therapies for rare diseases to have well-documented natural history data to bolster any claim that evidence from a small number of patients is sufficient to establish the safety and effectiveness of a product.

CHEMISTRY, MANUFACTURING, AND CONTROL, PRECLINICAL, AND CLINICAL REGULATORY CONSIDERATIONS FOR DIFFERENT CLASSES OF IMMUNOTHERAPIES

Examples are provided in the text that follows on some common cellular immunotherapy types of products that may illustrate some of the points raised previously in this chapter. Clinical trial design considerations are also provided. Please also refer to Chapter 64 on "Regulatory Considerations for Therapeutic Cancer Vaccines" for information on tumor lysates, peptides, and antigen-pulsed dendritic cells.

Ex Vivo Stimulated Cells

Chemistry, Manufacturing, and Control Considerations: Cells stimulated/activated ex vivo are typically autologous products or allogeneic cells targeted to treat a single donor.

Such patient-specific products often have high inherent lot-to-lot variability due to the nature of the source material. Such variability can make demonstrating manufacturing consistency more challenging and demonstrating product comparability after a manufacturing change more difficult. It is therefore important for such products to distinguish inherent variability due to source material from variability introduced as a consequence of the manufacturing process. Also, careful consideration should be given to assigning an appropriate range for source material properties. Some clinical treatments might involve the use of more than one lot per patient. It can be useful to evaluate the variation in lots derived from the same patient where it would be likely that the per-lot variation would be less, though these too can have significant variation due to cell collection differences and in some cases the clinical status of the patient. The lot variation can also profoundly affect acceptance criteria for final product release specifications. The variation may necessitate setting very wide acceptance criteria for release, but this can present challenges for assuring the manufacturing process is achieving the level of product quality as intended.

The stability of the source material, intermediates, and the final product should be established and an appropriate dating period (shelf life) be assigned for each. Process times and action limits should be established for process intermediates and critical processing steps. Logistics can be challenging for reasons outlined earlier.

Throughput is another consideration. While scaling is a concern for all biologics, in the case of ex vivo-stimulated cells and other types of autologous and patient-specific allogeneic products, scaling is more of a function of the number of lots generated at any one time (scale-out) than an increase in the number of doses produced from a single lot (scale-up). An increase in throughput creates its own challenges, and capacity studies may be needed to demonstrate the ability of the manufacturing process and facility(s) to produce the product consistently, while adhering to appropriate action limits and process step times, and avoid product lot mix-ups.

Clinical Considerations: An IND protocol for study of cell therapy products should be adequately designed with sufficient information to support the proposed study design.[44]

The use of ex vivo-stimulated cells introduces some unique features to the design of clinical trials of cell therapies, and these considerations differ depending on whether the cells are autologous, allogeneic but patient-specific, or nonpatient-specific ("off-the-shelf") allogeneic products.

In the case of autologous cell therapy, clinical trial analysis must account for all subjects from whom an attempt was made to collect cells. This would include subjects who did not actually receive the cellular product due to some intercurrent event such as a clinical complication.

Analysis only of subjects who have actually received a product can be performed as well, but such an approach would not be an intent-to-treat analysis, and would be likely to overestimate the true clinical benefit of an autologous cellular product. Similar considerations apply to allogeneic subject-specific products, but may not be relevant for subject-nonspecific off-the-shelf biologics.

The traditional standard dose-escalation schedule in the development of cancer therapeutics uses the so-called "3 + 3 design"; however, a maximum tolerated dose (MTD) is infrequently identified for a cellular immunotherapy. The dose–toxicity curve may be so flat that the highest dose that can be administered is limited by manufacturing or anatomic issues rather than toxicity. For additional considerations, please refer to Chapter 64.

Adjuvants may be used in cellular immunotherapy formulations. These adjuvants are not generally licensed by themselves but are used in conjunction with vaccine antigens to augment or direct the specific immune response to an antigen. General requirements for inclusion of such adjuvants include submission of evidence that the proposed adjuvant does not adversely affect the safety or potency of a given vaccine formulation. Information supporting the value of adding the adjuvant should be provided, and may include evidence of enhanced immune response or antigen-sparing effects, and data supporting selection of the dose of the adjuvant. In general, the use of adjuvants is not subject to the requirement that the contribution of each component be demonstrated. However, when products which may have independent clinical activity are used as adjuvants to enhance the effects of vaccine antigens, the study design and control group(s) should be discussed with the FDA. Study design requirements will be considered on a case- by-case basis.

Because cellular immunotherapy products may need time to elicit or amplify an immune response that could manifest as biological activity, a delayed effect can be expected in the subjects who received the vaccine. Shortly after the initial vaccine administration, subjects may experience disease progression prior to the onset of biological activities or effects from the vaccine (delayed effects). Clinical progression may not be a contraindication to continued administration of cellular immunotherapy products. One potential approach to this situation would be for the study protocol to clearly define situations in which vaccination therapy may be continued.

Natural Killer Cells

Recent interest in NK cells has intensified as a viable therapeutic platform along with T cell-based approaches. As solid tumors have a propensity to downregulate MHC-I, NK cells provide a failsafe mechanism in these circumstances where cytotoxic T lymphocytes (CTLs), which depend on MHC-I for tumor recognition and elimination,

are debilitated. Since early studies using autologous NK cells have failed to demonstrate significant clinical benefit, the current focus is on augmenting NK cell functions using adoptively transferred allogeneic NK cells.[52] As NK cells in cancer patients are highly dysfunctional and reduced in number, adoptive transfer of large numbers of allogeneic cytolytic NK cells offers the opportunity to induce relevant antitumor responses. The potential of allogeneic NK cells is being widely explored in cancer immunotherapy. Approaches are also being used to augment NK cell functions, including: Fc optimized mAbs (to mediate antibody-dependent cellular cytotoxicity [ADCC]), NK cell checkpoint inhibitors, bispecific Abs, genetic modification of NK cells using chimeric antigen receptors (CARs), iPSC-derived NK cells, and cytokine-induced NK cells. (Please see Chapter 66 for more information on CAR-modified cells.)

NK cells can be obtained from several sources. Human NK cells are generally categorized by their level of CD56 and CD16 expression into two subsets: $CD56^{dim}CD16^{bright}$ and $CD56^{bright} CD16^{dim}$ NK cells.[53] Other markers include CD2, CD57, CD94, CD127, CD161, and NKG2A. Most NK cells in the peripheral blood and spleen are $CD56^{dim} CD16^{bright}$ and are cytotoxic against a variety of tumor cells. Commonly used allogeneic NK cells are apheresis products collected from haploidentical and unrelated donor PBMC. Another source is umbilical cord blood (UCB), where NK cells are generated from $CD34^+$ progenitor cells that undergo expansion and differentiation using cytokines and growth factors and thereby mature into cytolytic NK cells. Apart from PBMC and UCB, NK cells have also been obtained from the clonal cell lines derived from immortalized lymphoma NK cells. Allogeneic NK cells can be haploidentical or partially MHC matched in origin. The major concern regarding source materials include risks of allogeneic residual T cell content and differing graft-versus-leukemia effects. Some of the criteria for selecting NK cell phenotype/activity include CMV-reactivity, HLA/KIR genotyping, and frequency of NK cells with activated phenotype. Although some viral infections increase NK cell activity, selecting donors with evidence of viral infection poses some risk.

NK cells can be selected for expansion using flow cytometry either by negative selection for $CD3^+$ T cells or positive selection for $CD56^{dim}CD16^{bright}$ and $CD56^{bright} CD16^{dim}$ population. Isolation of NK cells can also be accomplished using immunomagnetic selection using CD56 and CD16 antibodies and magnetic beads. Alternatively, negative selection with immunomagnetic beads can be used to enrich for NK cells by depleting specific populations of leukocytes. While T cell removal is usually efficient, selection of NK cells may result in variable yield because of the variable frequency within the source material.

Following selection, NK cell expansion is frequently performed using irradiated cell lines. Irradiation is performed to render immortalized or highly proliferative cell lines incapable of proliferation, which could present a safety risk if residual cells exist in the final product. Strategies to mitigate risk can include verifying the effectiveness of irradiation procedures,[5] or demonstrating the final product is free of residual cells from the cell bank. Cell banks used in product manufacturing should be qualified for safety, including adventitious agents.[19,20,38]

As previously described, lot release product testing typically includes measures of product safety, and other quality attributes, such as identity and potency. Considerations for final product release testing for safety could include residual allogeneic T cell content, especially for partially HLA-matched cellular products. For measuring potency, a matrix of multiple assays that measure different aspects of the product's activity may be helpful.[34] Such assays could include cytokine secretion, presence of degranulation markers, and/or measures of target cell killing. In some cases, a cell line of the same tumor type may exist that could be used as a cytolytic target.

Cytotoxic T Lymphocytes/Tumor-Infiltrating Lymphocytes

Chemistry, Manufacturing, and Control Considerations: Adoptive transfer of ex vivo-expanded antitumor-associated antigen (TAA) cytotoxic T lymphocytes (CTLs) and tumor-infiltrating lymphocytes (TIL) often involves several complex processing methods. For example, initial processing of TILs may include mechanical or enzymatic digestion steps to generate tumor-derived individual microcultures and may also use bulk lymphocytes. Information on chemically synthesized peptides for ex vivo pulsing and expansion of T lymphocytes should be included in the IND as important materials used in manufacturing (21 CFR 312.23(a)(7)(i). Useful information could include confirmation of peptide identity (e.g., amino acid sequencing confirmation, molecular weight by mass spec, isoelectric point, etc.) and the presence of impurities (e.g,. presence of truncated or altered sequences, residual solvents, etc.) in each peptide. Consistent with principles of CGMP, acceptance criteria should be established for the quality of materials used in manufacturing.[15,18] The safety of unintended peptide impurities present in the peptide reagents should be considered and justified.

Use of any cell selection device or separation device, including density gradients, magnetic beads, or fluorescence-activated cell sorting (FACS), should be described in detail along with descriptions of culture systems (flasks, bags, etc.), and an indication of whether the system is closed or open. Any in-process testing that would be performed during these procedures should also be described.[5] Sources of autologous or allogeneic APCs used during ex vivo stimulations and how they are processed should

also be described in detail.[5] If immortalized APCs are used, a potential safety concern would be uncontrolled growth after product administration of residual cells present in the final product. If APCs are irradiated, then the same concerns would apply as discussed previously for irradiated cells used in NK cell production.

Clinical Considerations: Initial trials of TILs or CTLs to treat solid tumors often includes in vivo administration of high dose IL-2.[54] The pharmacologic preparation of IL-2, aldesleukin, is an antineoplastic agent for a subset of patients with certain tumors, and presumably works by stimulating a host antitumor immune response. However, pharmacologic doses of IL-2 are quite toxic, so much so that the prescribing information advises that the agent only be administered in a setting where intensive care is readily available.[55] As has been described previously, an intervention requiring administration of aldesleukin may have potential toxicities of this FDA-approved agent in addition to toxicities attributable to the cell therapy itself. Trials of TIL therapy have also been conducted without aldesleuklin, and so the utility of adding this drug to TIL therapy remains an open question.

Lymphodepletion

Preclinical studies and clinical trials conducted in single institutions have shown that administration of chemotherapeutic agents may enhance the engraftment and persistence of infused CTL/TIL. The mechanism for such an effect is unclear, although it has been proposed that chemotherapy given prior to cell infusion may reduce or eradicate the suppressor T cells, thus creating space for infused cells to proliferate and persist.[56,57]

T Cell Subsets Versus Bulk Cultures

TILs have typically been given as bulk cultures containing a phenotypic heterogeneity of the T cell product. The alternative strategy is to select for a specific phenotype(s), such as CD8[+] killer cells, or for a specific mixture of phenotypes.[1] However, clinical considerations for trial design are similar for both T cell subsets and bulk culture.

Persistence of T Cells

The persistence of T cells after administration introduces clinical complications to the use of T cell therapy and the design of T cell trials. The optimal dose of T cells is unknown. As T cells survive and multiply in the host, it is unclear that a specific number of infused cells is correlated with the antitumor activity of T cell-based immunotherapies.

Adventitious immune activity of TILs is another concern. Graft-versus-host disease is a well-known complication of allogeneic hematopoietic cell therapy, the prototypical cellular therapy of malignancy. While this has not been a frequent problem in trials of autologous TILs, immunotoxicity is always of concern. For example, TIL treatment for patients with melanoma could lead to the development of vitiligo and uveitis deriving from the TILs attacking the normal melanocytes.[58] Therefore, the clinical protocol needs to describe approaches that will be used to detect and manage these immunotoxicities.

CONCLUSION

Chemistry, Manufacturing, and Control

CMC review of cell therapy products is based on an assessment of risk, and each product is reviewed on a case-by-case basis according to the associated risks with that product from both intrinsic and extrinsic factors. Examples of intrinsic factors include source material and cell banks. Examples of extrinsic factors include reagents, materials, excipients, container closures, and the manufacturing facility used during production. A good quality system should help mitigate these risks. Mitigation can be accomplished through thorough risk assessment, including an assessment of the ability to detect problems, find root cause, take appropriate corrective actions, and control change. Ancillary materials should be carefully selected and appropriately qualified. An independent QA unit should review and approve important procedures related to production, provide oversight, and perform trend analysis.

The high degree of lot-to-lot variation for some cell therapy products can make demonstration of manufacturing consistency more difficult, and demonstrating manufacturing comparability after a significant manufacturing change more challenging. It is therefore important to properly characterize process intermediates and the final products to aid in these assessments. Appropriate lot release specifications should be established as early as possible to help ensure adequate product quality, including safety and efficacy, particularly during late-phase studies.

Preclinical

As with any drug or biologics product, preclinical assessment of the safety of any cell therapy is based on a scientific risk-based approach. There are no requirements for using two species or nonhuman primates as a default testing paradigm. The in vitro and in vivo animal models selected should be based on the questions that are being addressed and include some of the factors outlined earlier in this chapter's introduction. For any novel cell therapy, additional considerations and tests may be necessary. Early communication with the appropriate regulatory agency is important to address these novel concerns.

Clinical

The clinical assessment of cell therapy is similar in many ways to the clinical assessment of nonliving drugs. Safety and substantial evidence of effectiveness must be demonstrated through a rigorous program of clinical development. The totality of such data must show that the benefits expected from the cell therapy outweigh the risks. In addition to the many clinical considerations inherent in the design of any experimental agent in human beings, the additional complexity of the manufacture of cell products and their continued biological activity in the host add special concerns, but do not change this fundamental drug-development paradigm.

ACKNOWLEDGMENTS

We would like to thank Carolyn Yong, Mohammad Heidaran, Ramjay Vatsan, Xiaobin Lu, Robert Sokolic, Laura Ricles, Graeme Price, Mercedes Serabian, Steven Oh, Kimberly Benton, Carrie Laurencot, and Wilson Bryan for their helpful comments, valuable discussions, and aid in editing this chapter.

KEY REFERENCES

Only key references appear in the print edition. The full reference list appears in the digital product on Springer Publishing Connect: connect.springerpub.com/content/book/978-0-8261-3743-2/part/part05/chapter/ch65

5. U.S. Food and Drug Administration. Guidance for industry: Content and review of chemistry, manufacturing, and control (CMC) information for human somatic cell therapy investigational new drug applications (INDs). Published April 2008. https://www.fda.gov/media/73624/download

10. International Council for Harmonization. Q6B Specifications: test procedures and acceptance criteria for biotechnological/biological products: guidance for Industry. Published August 1999. https://www.fda.gov/media/71510/download

13. U.S. Food and Drug Administration. Guidance for industry: Considerations for the design of early-phase clinical trials of cellular and gene therapy products. Published June 2015. https://www.fda.gov/media/106369/download

18. U.S. Food and Drug Administration. Guidance for industry: CGMP for Phase 1 investigational drugs. Published July 2008. https://www.fda.gov/media/70975/download

20. International Council for Harmonization. Q5D Quality of biotechnological/biological products: derivation and characterization of cell substrates used for production of biotechnological/biological products: guidance for Industry. Published September 1998. https://database.ich.org/sites/default/files/Q5D%20Guideline.pdf

34. U.S. Food and Drug Administration. Guidance for industry: Potency tests for cellular and gene therapy products. Published January 2011. https://www.fda.gov/media/79856/download

47. U.S. Food and Drug Administration. Guidance for industry: Clinical trial endpoints for the approval of cancer drugs and biologics. Published December 2018. https://www.fda.gov/media/97618/download

Gene Therapy-Based Immunotherapy Products for Human Clinical Trials: Chemistry, Manufacturing and Control, Preclinical, and Clinical Considerations: An FDA Perspective

Ramjay S. Vatsan, Y Nguyen, Allen Wensky, Chaohong Fan, Ke Liu, and Raj Puri

KEY POINTS

- This chapter discusses the information to be included in an investigational new drug application (IND) based on relevant Code of Federal Regulations (CFRs) and U.S. Food and Drug Administration (FDA) guidance documents, along with FDA's chemistry, manufacturing, and control (CMC), prelinical, and clinical review considerations related to human gene therapy (GT) products.

- GT vectors may differ greatly in their biology and manufacturing process, and may require additional CMC, preclinical, and clinical considerations. Three selected vector types are discussed here based on the current knowledge and state of the art in GT–related investigational agents for immunotherapy applications.

- Different meeting types are available to help sponsors, depending on the stage of product development and the issues to be considered. These include INitial Targeted Engagement for Regulatory Advice on CBER producTs (INTERACT) meetings, which provide early, nonbinding regulatory advice on issues such as a product's early preclinical program, and pre-IND meetings prior to submission of an IND. Pre-IND discussions can be helpful to obtain the FDA's guidance on the level of the product characterization and the types of preclinical studies required to initiate a human clinical trial.

- The FDA provides preclinical recommendations on a case-by-case basis, due to the differences in the GT vector types, vector tropisms, and the biological functions of transgenes.

- Once the IND is in effect, the FDA has a number of additional programs to facilitate and expedite the development and review of new drugs (including GT products) that are designed to address an unmet medical need for the treatment of a serious or life-threatening human condition.

INTRODUCTION

The U.S. Food and Drug Administration (FDA)'s primary objectives in the review of investigational new drug (IND) applications are to assure the safety and rights of subjects in all phases of an investigation, and in Phases 2 and 3, to help assure that the quality of the scientific information of the investigational product is adequate to permit an evaluation of its safety and effectiveness as stipulated in Title 21 of the Code of Federal Regulations part 312 section 22 (a) (i.e., 21 CFR 312.22(a)). Per 21 CFR 312.23(a)(7)(i), each IND must contain sufficient information to assure the identity, quality, purity, and potency of the investigational agent. All the required information may be provided either by the sponsor directly or by cross-reference to previously submitted information (21 CFR 312.23(b)). If the sponsor wishes to cross-reference information from another active file, a letter of authorization (LOA) must be obtained from the holder of the information, and the LOA must be included in the IND to give the FDA permission to review the cross-referenced file (21 CFR 312.23(b)). Also, the FDA now requires all biologics license applications (BLAs), commercial IND submissions, and master files to be submitted in the electronic common technical document (eCTD) format.

This requirement is meant to facilitate the ease of submission, archival, retrieval, and review of information, per congressional authorization under section 745A(a) of the FD&C Act. The requirement went into effect on May 5, 2017, for new drug applications (NDAs), abbreviated new drug applications (ANDAs), and BLAs, and on May 5, 2018, for commercial INDs and master files).[1] Excluded from the eCTD requirement are academic and noncommercial INDs (IND for a product that is not intended for commercial distribution; this exemption includes research and investigator-sponsored INDs), as well as submissions described in section 561 of the FD&C Act (e.g., expanded access INDs and protocols for individual patients, intermediate-sized patient populations, and for emergency use). The FDA will continue to accept submissions under section 561 in alternative formats (e.g., PDF files following the common technical document [CTD] organization).[2]

In this chapter, we have summarized the FDA's current recommendations for the information to be included in an IND for gene therapy (GT) products. The recommendations that are generally applicable to a broad range of human GT products are described first, and the later part of this chapter discusses additional recommendations for some of the more commonly used GT vectors and oncolytic viruses.

Human GT seeks to modify or manipulate the expression of a gene or to alter the biological properties of living cells for therapeutic use. The FDA generally considers human GT products to include all products that mediate their effects by transcription or translation of transferred genetic material, or by specifically altering host (human) genetic sequences. Some examples of GT products include nucleic acids (e.g., plasmids, in vitro transcribed RNA), genetically modified microorganisms (e.g., viruses, bacteria, fungi), engineered site-specific nucleases used for human genome editing, and ex vivo genetically modified human cells. GT products meet the definition of "biological product" in section 351(i) of the Public Health Service (PHS) Act (42 U.S.C. 262(i)) when such products are applicable to the prevention, treatment, or cure of a disease or condition of human beings.[3]

The considerations for chemistry, manufacturing, and control (CMC), preclinical evaluations, and clinical evaluations described in this chapter are based on current scientific knowledge and understanding of the GT products and the application of GT in treating human diseases and conditions.

The purpose of this book chapter is to give an overview of information contained in various previously published FDA guidance documents. The information included here is not complete. This chapter should not be considered an authoritative source of the regulatory information and the reader should consult the relevant guidance documents for the FDA's current recommendations related to GT products (available at the FDA website: www.fda. gov/vaccines-blood-biologics/biologics-guidances/cellular-gene-therapy-guidances).

CHEMISTRY, MANUFACTURING, AND CONTROL RECOMMENDATIONS FOR GENE THERAPY PRODUCTS

The overarching goal of GT product development is to establish a manufacturing process and quality control system that is able to produce a pure, safe, and potent product on a consistent basis. Due to the complexity of GT products, consistency in the manufacturing process can be challenging. The information an IND sponsor provides in the CMC section of an IND is critical for evaluating the adequacy of the manufacturing process and the control of product quality. The manufacturing process has to be controlled throughout the entire chain of the manufacturing steps from starting materials to finished final drug product. Ancillary materials used in the manufacturing should be verified through a review of the certificate of analysis supplied by the vendor documenting all relevant test results. If vendor quality testing is insufficient, then additional testing by the product manufacturer should be performed. In-process testing and monitoring should be strategically placed throughout the manufacturing process to ensure critical quality attributes (CQA) and critical process parameters (CPP) are within specified ranges. Justifications for specifications for drug substance and drug product lot release must be established during product development to ensure that the final product meets predefined quality (i.e., identity, safety, purity, and potency) requirements. To help sponsors and investigators better understand and prepare the CMC section of a GT IND, the FDA has developed various guidance documents (please see the reference list for this chapter). In the following sections, we will further elaborate and discuss some of the key considerations and recommendations in FDA and ICH guidance documents that are applicable to GT products.

Product Manufacturing—Reagents

Reagents are those materials that are used during the manufacturing process (e.g., for cellular growth, differentiation, selection, purification), but are not intended to be part of the final product. The quality of reagents can affect the safety, potency, and purity of the final product. Reagents used in manufacturing the product must be described in the IND (21 CFR 312.23(a)(7)(iv)(b)).

The FDA recommends that the manufacturing reagents be clinical grade reagents that are either FDA-approved or cleared, when available (for a current list of FDA-licensed products, please refer to the FDA's website: www.fda.gov/vaccines-blood-biologics/complete-list-licensed-products-and-establishments). If the reagent is not FDA-approved or cleared, it may be qualified for use in the manufacturing process by establishing a qualification program that includes safety testing as appropriate (e.g., sterility, endotoxin, mycoplasma, and adventitious agents), functional analysis, purity testing, and assays (e.g., residual solvent testing) to demonstrate absence of potentially harmful substances. Reagents derived from animal sources (e.g., fetal bovine serum, growth factors, protease, etc.) increase the risk of introducing adventitious agents. Certain cell selection and/or growth-promoting reagents (e.g., CD4, CD8, and CD28 antibodies) may also be derived from animal sources and should be evaluated for the presence of species-specific viruses. To reduce the risk of introducing zoonotic pathogens into products intended for human use, the FDA recommends the use of non-animal-derived reagents wherever possible (e.g., serum-free tissue culture media, recombinant protease, etc.).

An IND sponsor may include this qualification information either directly or through a cross-reference to information previously provided to the FDA by the manufacturer of the reagent. The extent of testing required to qualify a reagent will depend on how it is used in the manufacturing process. Often a Certificate of Analysis (COA) from the manufacturer will provide sufficient qualification information for early phase clinical studies.

Gene Therapy Vector Qualification

GT vectors are vehicles consisting of, or derived from, biological material that are designed to deliver genetic materials to modify or manipulate the expression of a gene or to alter the biological properties of living cells for therapeutic use.[3] Examples include plasmids, viruses, and bacteria that have been modified to transfer genetic material. Viral and bacterial GT vectors that directly deliver their payload (e.g., transgene) to specific target cells/tissues or cells may be a critical component of the final GT product. GT vectors may be naked genetic materials (DNA or RNA), viruses, or bacteria. When a GT vector is directly administered to a study subject, the vector in its final formulation for administration is considered a drug product (DP) and regulated as such. However, when a GT vector is used to modify a target cell ex vivo, the gene-modified cell becomes the final DP, and the GT vector becomes a critical component of the DP. Accordingly, the manufacturing process for a GT vector used for ex vivo gene modification should also be well controlled, and the release specifications for the GT vector should be established similar to those for directly administered GT products.[4] The following sections describe the general recommendations for the manufacture, characterization, and establishment of lot release specifications for GT vectors, including those used to modify cells ex vivo and those administered directly as DP.

A GT IND should contain sufficient detail regarding the vector to allow a rational, scientific evaluation of its characteristics, and to allow the verification of the submitted vector-related information.[4] The vector description should include the history and details regarding the derivation of the GT vector, an analysis of the genetic sequence of the vector with annotations for relevant restriction sites, and key vector elements such as regulatory elements and open reading frames (if the size of the vector is more than 40 kilobases, a genetic restriction map with annotated sequence of the inserted/modified region with a minimum of 0.5 Kb of the flanking sequences should be included). Information on the vector derivation should include any intermediate vector constructs, along with their sources, that are used to generate the final vector. The vector description should also include a detailed description and derivation of the gene insert (if any) and other regulatory elements, such as promoter, enhancer, splice donor/acceptance sites, and poly-adenylation signal. Frequently, the transgene in the vector is codon optimized.[5] If the gene is codon optimized, a detailed description of the codon optimization strategy/relevant information should be included in the IND. The genetic sequence of the entire vector (including the transgene and regulatory elements) should be fully analyzed and any significant discrepancies between the expected and the empirical sequences should be evaluated; this information should be included in the IND.

Viral Banks

To maintain control over safety and quality characteristics of viral vectors, a repository or a bank of the virus is generated. A viral bank typically consists of the primary bank or master viral bank (MVB).[6] A MVB is generally followed by the manufacture of one or more working viral banks (WVB), as needed. When a qualified WVB is generated, it serves as the source material for the manufacture of the vector or the final product. The MVB (and WVB, if applicable) should be generated using well-qualified cell substrates (e.g., MCB or WCB). To ensure the safety, purity, quality, and identity of the product, the viral banks should be qualified by appropriate testing, which should be documented in the IND.

The FDA evaluates the risk to human study participants through a review of the history and derivation of the viral banks, specifically the culture conditions and the reagents used during its production, and a review of the MVB's safety, purity, quality, and identity test results. The safety test results should include tests for sterility; mycoplasma; replication competent virus; in vivo and in vitro tests for unknown AVA (nonspecific tests for viruses); tests for the presence of specific pathogens, such as human viruses; and viruses specific to the animal-sourced reagents used in the growth and purification of the viral vector (examples of these animal-sourced reagents will include, for example, fetal bovine serum [FBS], porcine trypsin, or cell substrates derived from nonhuman primates, murine, or some other species).[4] Purity tests should include an evaluation of product-specific impurities (e.g., presence of incomplete/non-infectious viral particles) and process-specific impurities (e.g., residual reagents and cell substrate-derived impurities such as host cell DNA and host cell-derived proteins). Quality tests may include tests that evaluate the titer, vector particles, impurity profile, potency (e.g., transgene expression, assay for functional characteristics, etc.), and any other essential quality attributes of the virus. Identity tests should be tests that are specific to the vector used in the study and designed to uniquely identify the virus and to distinguish it from all other products that may be manufactured in the same facility. The stability of the viral banks should also be monitored to assure quality, potency, and sterility under their storage conditions (e.g., temperature, container closure, duration of storage, etc.). For detailed information, please refer to the FDA's "Guidance for Industry: Chemistry, Manufacturing, and Control (CMC) Information for Human Gene Therapy Investigational New Drug Applications (INDs)."[4]

Cell Substrate

The cell lines used to grow the viral vector should be fully characterized and described in the IND. A full cell substrate description will include the cell source and passage history (including a description of all animal-derived materials used in the cell culture). Documentation of all raw materials of human or animal origin used for the entire passage history should be retained and considered in developing a testing program for cell line qualification for vector manufacture. The FDA has defined the requirements for test methods used to evaluate manufacturing ingredients of animal origin used in production of biologics in 9 CFR 113.53 and 9 CFR 113.47 (Detection of extraneous viruses by the fluorescent antibody technique).

Cell Banks

The cells used for vector production should be banked. The derivation and history of the cell banks should be taken into consideration as discussed previously under MVB qualification when evaluating cell line suitability. The master cell bank (MCB) should be tested for the presence of unknown and known adventitious viral agents (AVA) (e.g., in vitro and in vivo AVA assays, tests for retroviral contamination using reverse transcriptase assays and TEM analysis, etc.) and species-specific viruses (e.g., rodent cell lines should be tested for the presence of rodent viruses). These viruses are usually detected by antibody production tests (e.g., murine antibody production [MAP], rat antibody production [RAP], or hamster antibody production [HAP]). When using human cell lines in the manufacture of a GT vector, the cell lines should be tested for human pathogens (i.e., CMV; HIV-1 and -2; HTLV-1 and -2; HBV; HCV; B19; human herpesvirus-6, -7, and -8 [HHV-6,-7, and -8]; JC virus; BK virus; Epstein–Barr virus [EBV]; and human papillomavirus [HPV]) and other human viral agents (e.g., Zika virus, West Nile virus), as appropriate. Species-specific viral agents may be tested using a PCR-based test system; however, each test should be qualified for its intended purpose with reference to sensitivity and specificity and fully validated prior to BLA. The FDA also takes into consideration the passage history of the MCB while evaluating suitability of the cell substrate.

End of Production Cells

Cell lines could become genetically unstable or acquire tumorigenic properties with increasing passage levels. It is therefore important that there be a passage level limit for the cells used in viral vector production and that cells be evaluated for tumorigenicity at or beyond this end of production (EOP) limit. The EOP passage limit should be determined by passaging the cells in a manner similar to that used in the production of the biological product. The genotypic and phenotypic stability of the cells should be demonstrated for the passages beyond the EOP cells used for full-scale manufacturing. Based on the findings from such studies, the passage level limit for the cells used in vector production should be established.

The FDA recommends that the EOP cells be qualified on a one-time basis to assess their genetic stability, tumorigenic potential, and for the presence of adventitious viruses. EOP cell qualification normally involves qualification of the cells at or beyond the expected EOP passage level.[7]

Product Manufacturing—Process Control to Produce a Final Drug Product

The manufacturing process for a GT product is typically complex and may be difficult to control due to variable and heterogenous starting materials (e.g., variability related to starting materials that may be patient specific) and the dynamic nature of a living system (e.g., cell substrate used for virus growth, or peripheral blood–derived mononuclear cells used to isolate and grow T cells). For a GT product manufactured by transducing cells using one or more GT vectors, terminal sterilization is not possible, so these types of products require a qualified aseptic manufacturing process that should be fully validated prior to commercial manufacturing. Furthermore, in these instances, the traditional concept of drug substance (DS) used in the pharmaceutical arena may not be obvious (e.g., an ex vivo vector transduced GT product is manufactured to the final drug product without a specific DS step). In such cases, to clarify the need for setting independent lot release specifications for the DS and DP, the IND sponsor should refer to the FDA's CMC guidance for GT.[4] The FDA encourages IND sponsors to discuss the lot release plan (i.e., release specifications for the DS and DP) with the FDA during the pre-IND meeting prior to submitting an IND.

The DP is a finished dosage form of the drug, and is typically manufactured from a DS. Active pharmaceutical ingredient (API) means any substance that is intended for incorporation into a finished drug product and is intended to furnish pharmacological activity or other direct effect in the diagnosis, cure, mitigation, treatment, or prevention of disease, or to affect the structure or any function of the body (21 CFR 207.1).

The FDA expects the API and DP manufacturers to apply current good manufacturing practices (CGMPs) to the manufacturing process beginning with the use of starting materials used to produce the API, and to validate all the critical process steps that impact the quality of the API, prior to submitting a BLA. Manufacturers should have controls over all the critical steps in the manufacture of the API. An IND sponsor should designate and document the point at which production of the API begins. CGMP requirements generally start applying to the product manufacture at the point of introduction of the API starting materials into the manufacturing process.[8]

Despite the previously mentioned challenges, the FDA expects the investigational drug product to be evaluated for identity, strength (potency), quality, and purity, and all this information should be described in the IND. Absence of this information may result in the IND being placed on "clinical hold" (21CFR312.23(a)(7)). DP is regulated under the authorization granted by the FD&C Act 501(a)(2)(B) and is expected to be qualified for human clinical evaluation when manufactured according to CGMPs as described in 21 CFR part 211. The 21 CFR part 211 regulations (CGMPs for finished pharmaceuticals) apply to GT products[9] that are in clinical evaluations through licensure. However, it may not be feasible or may be economically prohibitive to follow all the CGMP requirements in 21 CFR part 211 for investigational drugs used for Phase 1 clinical trials. Consistent with the FDA's CGMP for the 21st-century initiative,* the FDA has provided clarification on the extent of CGMP requirements for Phase 1 studies in "Guidance for Industry CGMP for Phase 1 Investigational Drugs."[9]

Setting In-Process Acceptance Criteria and Action Limits

The FDA recommends that the manufacturing process and the starting materials be well characterized, and acceptance criteria be established for critical intermediate process (in-process) steps.[10] In-process tests are typically performed at critical decision-making steps and at other steps where data from the tests serve to confirm consistency of the process during the production of either the DS or the DP. The results of in-process testing may be recorded as action limits or reported as acceptance criteria depending on the attribute tested and criticality of the in-process step. As an example, in a hypothetical GT vector production process, an in-process criterion such as cell viability or bio-burden tests may be classified as an acceptance criterion, while vector titer and clearance levels for process residuals may be action limits.

IND sponsors should establish acceptance criteria and/or action limits for the manufacturing process prior to initiating confirmatory clinical studies, and fully evaluate the operating ranges for these parameters during the process validation studies prior to submitting a BLA. For a detailed discussion on the FDA's recommendations for process validation studies, please refer to the FDA's guidance on this topic.[11]

An action limit may typically trigger an investigation followed by a corrective action and preventive action (CAPA); however, the action limit may or may not lead to lot failure. Internal action limits may be used by the manufacturer to assess the consistency of the process at less critical steps. All in-process control acceptance specifications (test methods and acceptance criteria) should be justified on the basis of manufacturing experience, a risk analysis associated with the process step, knowledge of the critical quality attributes of the product, and scientific reasoning—all these are typically part of the process validation studies.

Lot Release Testing

Lot release specifications are defined as a list of tests, references to analytical procedures, and appropriate acceptance criteria that are numerical limits, ranges, or other

---

* Pharmaceutical CGMPS for the 21st Century—A Risk-Based Approach: Second Progress Report and Implementation Plan. www.fda.gov/cder/gmp/21stcenturysummary.htm

criteria for the release of the product.[10] Lot release testing plans for DS and DP should include tests that adequately describe the physical, chemical, or biological characteristics of the DS and DP necessary to ensure that the DS and DP meet acceptable limits for identity, strength (potency), quality, and purity. Specifications establish the set of criteria to which a DS or DP should conform to be considered acceptable for its intended use. Specifications, along with the qualification of reagents and starting materials and adherence to CGMPs, ensure product quality.

Manufacturing experience for early stage product development may be limited and the inherent variability in some biological assessments may require careful considerations for setting acceptance criteria. For this reason, the FDA recommends that the final product be extensively characterized during the product development phases with reference to its physicochemical (and biological) properties, biological activity, immunochemical properties, purity, and impurities.[10] This early product characterization may be performed using lots made for preclinical studies or engineering manufacturing runs (pilot lots), using appropriate, qualified methods and techniques.

In the context of a GT product, a DS may be a bulk clarified harvest. The DS may be directly processed into a DP without an intermediate storage period. Release specifications for the DS (when applicable) should be set by taking into consideration the quality attributes that are uniquely associated with the DS.[12] In some instances, a process qualification study may be sufficient to document the removal of process-related residuals, and lot release testing for process-related impurities may not be required. The IND sponsor should clearly define the DS and DP of their product and discuss the testing plan with the FDA to obtain product-specific recommendations.

The FDA recommends that an acceptable range for DS and DP lot release limits be defined early in the product development cycle, and that these release limits be narrowed as the knowledge of the quality attributes and manufacturing experience grows during the course of the clinical trials. DS and DP lot release specifications are proposed and justified by the manufacturer, refined during product development, and set for commercial release of DS and DP lots. The test methods should be fully validated for testing the commercial product and would be a condition for product licensure.

Safety Assays

The FDA expects the following safety tests to be conducted on DP and at other manufacturing stages as appropriate. All safety assay methods need to be qualified with reference to their ability to perform as expected in the presence of the product matrix (excipients, buffers, and other cellular materials as appropriate), prior to Phase 1 studies and fully validated prior to BLA.

Endotoxin Assay

For any parenteral drug, except those administered intrathecally, the upper limit of acceptance criterion for endotoxin is set as 5 EU/kg body weight/hr. For intrathecally administered drugs, the upper limit of acceptance criterion is 0.2 EU/kg body weight/hour. These upper limits are set based on scientific data obtained from rabbit and human studies[13] and by calculated safety doses.[14]

Sterility Assay

Product sterility is defined as absence of viable microorganisms in the drug product as measured from the final container or other materials as appropriate (21CFR610.12). The FDA recommends that the sterility test be performed according to the USP<71> method (a 14-day growth-based sterility test) or an equivalent method such as a rapid microbial test method. Rapid microbial test methods must be qualified as suitable for the intended purpose with respect to sensitivity, specificity, and absence of interference from product matrix prior to use and fully validated prior to licensure. For DPs that have a short shelf life (e.g., patient-specific genetically modified chimeric antigen T cells) and that are administered immediately after manufacture, and where it may not be practical to wait for a 14-day sterility test result, an in-process sterility test on a sample taken 48 to 72 hours prior to final harvest, when combined with a rapid sterility test on the final DP and aseptic process qualification studies, may provide sufficient assurance of product sterility. The product may be released for administration to the study subject based on the in-process sterility test results, with an action plan in the event the full sterility test per USP <71> (or equally sensitive assay method) returns a positive sterility test result that is obtained after the product administration.

Mycoplasma Assay

For products made using living cells, a test for mycoplasma is required. Mycoplasma testing should be conducted on both cells and supernatant.[7] Due to the limited shelf life of some ex vivo genetically modified cellular products, it may not be feasible to perform culture-based mycoplasma assay for release testing. In those cases, a polymerase chain reaction (PCR)-based mycoplasma assay or another rapid detection assay may be used instead. However, the assay should be qualified as suitable for its intended purpose (assessed for equivalent or better performance for specificity and sensitivity, and free of interference from the product matrix) prior to use and fully validated prior to licensure.

Adventitious Viral Agent Assay

When cell lines are used, tests for AVA should be performed. The AVA assays are nonspecific tests for viral agents in the test sample. The assays typically involve an in vitro cell culture-based test method and an in vivo assay in suitable animal models.[4,7] In vitro viral testing should be performed on the MCB, WCB, MVB, WVB, and final vector product at the bulk harvest stage, and as a one-time test on the EOP cells. The in vivo assay should be performed at a minimum on MVB and MCB and at other stages in the DP manufacture as appropriate.[4]

Identity Assays

Identity assays are required to uniquely identify the drug product and distinguish it from all other products that may be manufactured in the same facility. When the final product is an ex vivo genetically modified cell product, the FDA recommends that both the vector and the final cell product be tested for identity. Such an identity test should include an assay to measure the presence of vector (e.g., transgene expression assay, restriction digest, or PCR) and an assay specific for the cellular component of the final product (e.g., cell surface markers).

Purity

Product purity is defined as relative freedom from extraneous material in the finished product, whether or not harmful to the recipient or deleterious to the product (21 CFR 610.3(r)). Purity testing includes assays for pyrogenicity/endotoxin, process-related impurities (process residuals) (e.g., host cell DNA and proteins or reagents/components used during vector manufacture, such as cytokines, growth factors, antibodies, and serum, and in the case of ex vivo modified cells, any unintended cellular populations or cell debris). For GT products that are ex vivo modified live cells, the FDA recommends that the final product should contain at least 70% viable cells (for additional information on the specific recommendations, refer to the FDA's guidance).[4]

Potency Assays

A potency assay is a measure of the biological function of the drug product. Potency assays may consist of a matrix of assays that measure different aspects of the product's activity.[15] The FDA recommends that potency assays be quantitative. A quantitative measure of transgene expression in vector-transduced cells may provide some assessment of product potency in early phase studies. Yet, for studies designed to collect efficacy data in support of licensure, a potency assay that measures the full extent of the biological activity of the product should be in place for product release. Potency assays are performed as part of GT vector and drug product lot release tests, are a key component of the comparability studies, and are a part of the stability assays. Biological potency assays tend to be highly variable due

to the variability introduced by the biological reagents (e.g., cell substrates), and require the use of well-characterized external or in-house standards and development of complementary assay procedures to ensure the assay's reproducibility and robustness. For these reasons, the FDA encourages sponsors to develop relevant potency assays early in the product development cycle in order to gain sufficient assay knowledge and understand the assay's limits. Like all other noncompendial assays, potency assays should also be validated prior to licensure.

Stability Studies

Stability studies are needed to establish the shelf life of a MVB, MCB, WVB, WCB, DS (if stored), and the DP. DP stability testing must be performed during early phases of the clinical trial to establish that the product is stable for the planned duration of the proposed clinical investigation (21 CFR 312.23(a)(7)(ii)). Data supporting a final formulation and dating period will be necessary for licensure. During the clinical evaluation period, the FDA recommends that there be a written stability protocol that describes the planned stability tests, along with test methods, acceptance criteria, and test periodicity. As the product development continues through the various clinical trial phases, any change in the formulation, container closure or cryopreservation conditions (in case of a frozen product), or storage conditions will require additional stability testing. The shelf life of the investigational product may be extended as more stability data become available.[16,17]

Some issues to be considered for stability evaluation are the need for external stability standards and controls that may be required to remake expired standards. GT products have traditionally had very few qualified external standards and the sponsors of INDs should take this into consideration when planning stability studies for viral stocks. One way to overcome this difficulty may be through extensive product knowledge. This product knowledge may be gained through a thorough product characterization study, knowledge of the product's critical quality attributes, understanding the mechanism of action (MOA) of the investigational product, and through the use of well-qualified and orthogonal analytical methods. Product knowledge will help in establishing in-house reference standards for evaluating product stability.

Product Comparability

During the product development process, manufacturing changes may be unavoidable due to process improvements, raw material changes, scale-ups, and so on. Manufacturing process changes can be managed by comparing the CQA, if known, between the pre- and post-change products. In order to show that the products are comparable, one must demonstrate that the product after change is highly similar and has no adverse impact on the product safety, potency, and quality.[18] Comparability tests should not be limited to lot release tests. Early and rigorous product characterization, along with tests conducted using archived retention samples and appropriate reference standards, will help evaluate manufacturing process change comparability studies. Product comparability studies are best performed by side-by-side studies using identical test methods and conditions. The test methods used in comparability studies must be qualified as suitable for their intended purposes.

Delivery Devices

Most GT products require some form of a delivery device to administer the product. In some instances, these devices may be complex, designed to deliver the GT product to a specific anatomical location, tissues, or target cells (e.g., intracranial delivery using MRI and stereotactic devices, in vivo electroporation devices, etc.). In order to ensure that the DP's quality attributes are not compromised during the delivery process and to ensure that the correct intended dose is delivered without loss due to adherence to the device (for example), device compatibility studies should be conducted. The FDA recommends that device compatibility studies include measures of both product quantity and product activity (e.g., for viral vectors, a measure of physical particles and infectivity, or potency to assess both adsorption and inactivation). The FDA recommends that the results of device compatibility studies be discussed with the FDA during INTERACT or Pre-IND meetings, to obtain guidance on the information to be included in the IND.

PRECLINICAL RECOMMENDATIONS FOR GENE THERAPY PRODUCTS

The preclinical program for a GT product is based on characterizing its benefit–risk profile to support administration to humans in a clinical trial. The requirement for the conduct of preclinical studies is specified in section 312.23(a)(8) of the Code of Federal Regulations. This section states that "[a]dequate information about the pharmacological and toxicological studies . . . on the basis of which the sponsor has concluded that it is reasonably safe to conduct the proposed clinical investigations. The kind, duration, and scope of animal and other tests required vary with the duration and nature of the proposed clinical investigations." The resulting data from in vitro and in vivo pharmacology and toxicology studies will inform regulatory and scientific decisions that are made regarding both early phase and late-phase clinical trial designs with an investigational GT product.

The key objectives of a preclinical program include: (a) establishing the putative mechanism(s) of action of the product; (b) identifying a biologically active and safe dose level and dose range; (c) selecting a reasonably safe starting dose level, dose-escalation scheme, and dosing regimen via the planned clinical route of product administration; (d) informing the human subject eligibility criteria, and (e) identifying key clinical monitoring aspects.

Safety concerns for GT products can be associated with: (a) vector persistence, (b) expressed transgene persistence, (c) viral replication, (d) biodistribution, (e) shedding and excretion, (f) insertional mutagenesis, (g) genomic integration, (h) germline transmission, and (i) immune responses to the vector or immune activation by the expressed product. Depending on the nature of the GT product, other concerns may arise. In cases where the GT product of interest, or a similar construct, has been well-studied in animals and/or in humans, data from peer-reviewed publications and completed preclinical and clinical studies may be leveraged to address the previously noted concerns. Nonetheless, all of these issues should be addressed, with supporting data, in an IND. Specific considerations for the safety assessment of GT product types are discussed in subsequent sections in this chapter.

Selection of appropriate animal species is important in order to facilitate translation of the resulting pharmacology/toxicology data to clinical studies. Factors such as susceptibility or permissiveness to infection, and immune tolerance or preexisting immunity to the GT product, should be considered. In addition, the safety and bioactivity profiles for a GT product can be studied in an animal model of disease or injury, if one exists. Comparability of various factors such as: physiology and anatomy, pathophysiology, route of administration, species specificity of the product, and species-specific immune responses should be considered. The conduct of pilot studies to ascertain the characteristics and biological relevancy of the animal species and model are important.

The pharmacology/toxicology considerations for a GT product will vary based on the investigational product, medical condition being treated, previously known and published information, and other factors. Thus, there is no "one size fits all" approach when designing the preclinical program. Stakeholders are recommended to consult the FDA guidance titled, "Preclinical Assessment of Investigational Cellular and Gene Therapy Products"[19] and the "Guidance for Industry: Gene Therapy Clinical Trials—Observing Subjects for Delayed Adverse Events."[20] In addition, investigators that are working toward submitting an IND for a GT product are encouraged to contact the FDA at a reasonably early stage in their product development program to discuss all aspects of their program, including the IND-enabling preclinical studies. This pre-IND meeting provides an opportunity for a targeted interaction with the regulators, in which specifics about product manufacturing, pharmacology/toxicology, and clinical trial design can be discussed.

CLINICAL CONSIDERATIONS FOR INVESTIGATIONAL GENE THERAPY PRODUCTS

Clinical Trial Design for Gene Therapy Products

An IND application protocol for study of GT products should contain sufficient information to support the proposed study design.[21] Due to the complexity of GT products, the classic paradigm of performing large clinical trials, which enroll a diverse patient population to receive an off-the-shelf manufactured product, may be difficult. Smaller clinical trials offer a possible alternative for clinical trial design for GT products, which may be highly active in a specifically defined patient population. Early phase trials should be designed to identify a safe, feasible dose and regimen to carry forward into a later-phase trial.

In general, the clinical protocol contained in an IND for a study of GT product should contain all of the information listed in Box 66.1.

BOX 66.1 CLINICAL COMPONENTS OF AN INVESTIGATIONAL NEW DRUG

- rationale for use of product in chosen patient population;
- brief summary of previous human experience with the product;
- anticipated risks;
- hypothesis and objectives;
- inclusion and exclusion criteria;
- study design and detailed protocol;
- justification for starting dose;
- justification for dose regimen;
- safety and endpoint monitoring plans;
- definition of dose-limiting toxicity;
- definition of maximum tolerated dose;
- adverse event reporting plan;
- long-term follow-up plan;
- patient treatment discontinuation criteria;
- trial stopping criteria; and
- investigator's brochure (for multicenter trials).

Early Phase Trial Objectives

The primary objective for early phase clinical trials, especially first-in-human trials, should focus on safety evaluation including an assessment of the nature and frequency of potential adverse events (AEs) and an estimation of their relationship to dose and schedule.

Some Phase 1 studies may include selected features of Phase 2 study design in order to gather preliminary evidence of clinical activity, the dose and schedule, sequencing, and feasibility of administration of combination therapies. In addition, the early phase trials for the complex GT products should consider investigating the clinical and biologic activity such as tumor responses, feasibility of administration, pharmacology, and pharmacokinetics, if applicable (e.g., in vivo transgene gene expression, immunologic changes after treatment, clearance and persistence of the GT product).

Additional information about design of early phase clinical trials may be found in the FDA "Considerations for the Design of Early-Phase Clinical Trials of Cellular and Gene Therapy Products: Guidelines for Industry."[21]

Study Population

Knowledge of the GT product's expected MOA in a particular disease is an important consideration in choosing an appropriate study population. It is important to enroll a study population whose responses to a new GT will provide interpretable safety and activity data. The treatment effect of some GT products depends on expression of transgenes (e.g., tumor-associated antigen [TAA]) that stimulate the immune system, which in turn destroys the cancer. These products are therefore expected to require a functional immune system of the host to manifest their treatment effect. In such a situation. it may not be informative to investigate these products in subjects with bulky or progressive metastatic disease who may have weakened immune function and ongoing immunosuppression from prior cancer treatment including cytotoxic chemotherapies. In contrast, some GT products (e.g., chimeric antigen receptor [CAR]-modified T cells) possess immediate, direct antitumor effect upon administration. Testing these products in subjects with bulky and metastatic cancers refractory to multiple prior treatment may be appropriate.

In trials of small molecule drugs intended for the treatment of non-oncologic diseases, normal volunteers are often the subjects of Phase 1 studies, whereas in therapies of drugs meant to treat oncologic diseases, the potential adverse outcomes of experimental chemotherapy are felt to be too high to ethically allow for healthy volunteers, and so subjects with cancer are asked to be participants of the trial. With respect to the study population for GT, similar considerations may apply. Because of the potential for acute, subacute, or latent toxicities, GT products are typically tested in subjects representing the population for whom these products are ultimately intended rather than in healthy volunteers. Furthermore, such trial participants with cancer typically have no other curative options. This consideration is particularly important for GTs whose mechanism of action involves their integration into the host genome, as they carry risks of potentially life-threatening genotoxicities.[22-26]

Children are generally considered to be vulnerable research subjects. As such, children are entitled to additional safeguards when they participate in clinical research. These safeguards are detailed in 21 CFR part 50, subpart D. In general, clinical research in children should present no more than minimal risk, should have the prospect of direct benefit to the child participants, or should likely yield generalizable knowledge about the child's clinical condition and such knowledge is of vital importance in understanding or ameliorating the indicated condition. In the last case, the research should entail no more than a minor increase over minimal risk. Research not falling into one of these categories may be approved with additional regulatory review and public discussion. Most GT products cannot be said to represent only a minimal risk, or only a minor increase over minimal risk, so trials of GT products in children should generally hold the prospect of direct clinical benefit. Evidence of the prospect of direct benefit may come from experience in adult subjects or in nonclinical studies.

Dose and Regimen

In early phase trials of GT products, there should be some dose and schedule exploration. For advanced cancer indications, significant treatment toxicities up to a predefined threshold are often expected and considered acceptable. However, substantial toxicities that will permit identification of a maximum tolerated dose may not occur in the expected or feasible therapeutic range of GT products. In this event, the intent of dose and schedule exploration may be to determine the optimal biologically active dose and regimen.

For some complex GTs, there may be substantial practical production limits on a quantity that can be produced or delivered. In this situation, the early phase trial objective may be to characterize the safety profile of the feasible dose and regimen.

Study Stopping Rules

Many early phase trials of GT products include study stopping rules. The purpose of these rules is to control the number of subjects put at risk, in the event that early experience uncovers important safety problems. Study stopping rules typically specify a number or frequency of events, such as serious AEs or deaths, that will result in temporary suspension of enrollment and dosing until the situation can be assessed. Based on the assessment, the clinical protocol might be revised to mitigate the risk to subjects. Such revisions could include changes in the enrollment criteria. Revisions might also include dose reduction, some other change in product preparation or administration, or changes in the monitoring plan. Well-designed stopping rules allow sponsors to assess and address risks identified as the trial proceeds, and to assure that risks to subjects remain reasonable.

Endpoints for Gene Therapy Studies

As discussed earlier, the primary endpoint for early phase clinical trials should focus on safety evaluation. One common secondary endpoint of early phase clinical trials for GT product is to obtain preliminary data on clinical activity such as tumor responses. In addition, exploratory endpoints should be considered for GT studies and might include gene expression/persistence, genetically modified–cell engraftment/persistence, or other aspects of the immune function.

For GTs whose mechanism of action depends on the host immune system, assessments of immune responses may provide mechanistically useful data, especially when they can be correlated with the clinical outcomes.

Phase 3 trial endpoints can be challenging to choose, both in terms of specific selections and in terms of their assessments. One is encouraged to discuss the choice of Phase 3 endpoints with the FDA and refer to the FDA guidance document titled "Guidance for Industry: Clinical Trial Endpoints for the Approval of Cancer Drugs and Biologics."[27]

Monitoring and Follow-Up

Acute and chronic GT toxicities are often different than those seen with cytotoxic agents in patients with cancer. Dose-limiting toxicities may not occur during early phase trials, and a maximum tolerated dose may not be defined. However, possible serious late-occurring toxicities may occur, which require appropriate planning and monitoring during development. In addition, some GT products may be locally administered (e.g., direct intratumoral injection) and thus necessitate appropriate safety assessment for both localized and systemic toxicities.

Since there may be prolonged biologic activity if there is integration of the therapeutic gene into the host genome, one should consider an appropriate duration of safety assessment. An additional complicating factor is that the GT vector itself may result in toxicities that require specific vigilant monitoring.

For an extended follow-up plan for subjects who have received GT products, please refer to the FDA guidance document titled "Long Term Follow-Up After Administration of Human Gene Therapy Products: Guidance for Industry."[3]

Duration of Follow-Up

A GT clinical trial that presents long-term risks to human subjects must include long-term follow-up (LTFU) observations in order to mitigate those risks.

If the GT product has a vector that is integrating, or if the vector has latency, the FDA normally recommends a 15-year LTFU to observe any delayed safety issues. Long-term safety monitoring can also be useful if the product involves a gene or vector component(s) that might predispose subjects to develop secondary malignancies. In other situations, a shorter period of observation may be more suitable. In assessing an appropriate observation period for delayed AEs, factors for consideration include pertinent preclinical and clinical experience with the GT product or similar experience with other products in the same vector class, route of administration, and clinical indication.

Long-Term Follow-Up Recommendations

A LTFU monitoring plan mainly monitors any delayed clinical events such as secondary tumors, new incidence or exacerbation of a preexisting neurologic disorder or other autoimmune disorder, or hematologic disorders.

One important part of LTFU is monitoring of the persistence of the infused GT product. This is typically done by following the specific and unique vector sequences in peripheral blood samples taken from the subject at various time points. Product persistence monitoring can inform the investigator of the status of the in vivo product levels and help to evaluate the product safety and efficacy as part of the product pharmacokinetics/pharmacodynamics profile. Under some circumstances, a lack of product persistence may serve as a basis to modify the LTFU monitoring plan. In the cases of gammaretroviral or lentiviral vector-transduced GT products, the LTFU monitoring plan should also include monitoring of RCR or RCL until negative results are obtained in consecutive testing.[3,28,29]

Phase 2 Trial

A Phase 2 trial can be a screening discriminator to determine if further progression to Phase 3 confirmatory trial is warranted. In addition, the clinical activity can be estimated in a well-conducted Phase 2 trial. Randomized Phase 2 trials typically lack the statistical power for conclusive demonstration of the treatment effect of the investigational GT product. However, randomized Phase 2 trials may provide more reliable data about treatment effect size than single-arm trial data with historical controls; thus, it is useful when planning the design of the subsequent Phase 3 trial. The quality and quantity of Phase 2 development should be sufficient to provide adequate data to make a go or no-go decision about proceeding to Phase 3 confirmatory trial.

Late-Phase Clinical Trials

Phase 3 trial usually provides primary evidence of efficacy and safety and may be used to support a marketing application. The sponsor may choose to submit a Phase 3 protocol to the FDA for special protocol assessment (SPA). SPA is a means by which the sponsor reaches an agreement with the FDA on the clinical design, endpoints, and statistical analysis plan prior to commencement of the Phase 3 trial. The FDA will document such an agreement in writing. To learn more about special protocol assessment agreements, one may refer to the FDA's "Guidance for Industry: Special Protocol Assessment."[30]

Expedited Programs for Serious Conditions

Expedited programs are intended to help ensure that therapies for serious conditions are approved and available to patients as soon as it can be concluded that the therapies' benefits justify their risks (21 CFR part 312 (E)). The FDA currently has multiple expedited programs: fast track designation (FTD), regenerative medicine advanced therapy (RMAT) designation, breakthrough therapy designation (BTD), accelerated approval (AA), and priority review.[31] Note that the expedited programs can be rescinded if they no longer meet the qualifying criteria.

Fast Track (FT)

A fast track designation can generally be requested when the IND is first submitted or at any time thereafter before receiving marketing approval of the BLA. The IND and potential fast track designation may be discussed before an IND submission in a pre-IND meeting, but a decision on designation would await submission of the IND. If a product development program is granted fast track designation for one indication and has subsequently obtained data to support fast track designation for another indication, a new designation request for the second indication will be required.

Fast track provides for frequent interactions with the FDA's review team, and such a product could be eligible for priority review if supported by clinical data at the time of BLA, NDA, or efficacy supplement submission. An IND with a fast track designation may also be eligible for a rolling BLA submission, where the FDA may accept portions (different complete modules) of a marketing application before the submission of a complete application.[31]

Breakthrough Therapy

A breakthrough designation can be requested if there is preliminary clinical evidence indicating that the product may demonstrate substantial improvement over existing therapies on one or more clinically significant endpoints. Because the primary intent of breakthrough therapy designation is to develop evidence needed to support approval as efficiently as possible, the FDA anticipates that breakthrough therapy designation requests will rarely be made after the submission of an original BLA or a supplement. If a product development program is granted breakthrough therapy designation for one indication and has subsequently obtained preliminary clinical evidence to support breakthrough therapy designation for another indication, the sponsor should submit a separate request. A breakthrough designation has all the benefits of the fast track designation and also includes provisions for intensive guidance on an efficient drug development program, beginning as early as Phase 1, along with an organizational commitment involving senior managers.

Regenerative Medicine Advanced Therapy: An investigational drug is eligible for RMAT designation if it meets the definition of regenerative medicine therapy; it is intended to treat, modify, reverse, or cure a serious condition; and preliminary clinical evidence indicates that the regenerative medicine therapy has the potential to address unmet medical needs for such a condition.[32] In general, regenerative medicine therapy includes cell therapies, therapeutic tissue engineering products, human cell and tissue products, and combination products using any such therapies or products. Based on the FDA's interpretation of section 506(g), human GTs, including genetically modified cells, that lead to a sustained effect on cells or tissues may meet the definition of a regenerative medicine therapy. Advantages of the RMAT designation include all the benefits of the fast track and breakthrough therapy designation programs, including early interactions with the FDA. Table 66.1 summarizes key similarities and differences between the breakthrough therapy designation and RMAT designation.

Accelerated Approval

Approval under an accelerated approval pathway is dependent on a determination that the product demonstrates an effect on the endpoint (a surrogate endpoint or an intermediate clinical endpoint) that is reasonably likely to predict clinical benefit. The accelerated approval pathway has been used primarily in settings in which the disease course is long and an extended period of time would be required to measure the intended clinical benefit of a product. For drugs granted accelerated approval, postmarketing confirmatory trials have been required to verify the anticipated effect.

Priority Review

If a drug treats a serious condition and, if approved, would provide a significant improvement in safety or effectiveness, a priority review may be granted. Priority review has the benefit of a short review clock, and the FDA will take action on an application within 6 months (compared to 10 months under standard review).

Expanded Access Uses

Expanded access is the use of an investigational drug outside of clinical trials to diagnose, monitor, or treat patients with serious diseases or conditions for which there are no comparable or satisfactory therapy options available. Whenever possible, use of an investigational medical product by a patient as part of a clinical trial should be considered. However, when patient enrollment in a clinical trial is not possible, expanded access may be an option to gain access to an investigational medicinal product.

The FDA is committed to increasing awareness about its expanded access process and the procedures for obtaining access to investigational drugs, biologics, and medical devices. Access to investigational treatments requires not only the FDA's review and authorization, but the active involvement and cooperation of other parties, including drug companies and healthcare providers, in order to be successful.[33]

Table 66.1 Comparison of Breakthrough Therapy and Regenerative Medicine Advanced Therapy

	BREAKTHROUGH THERAPY DESIGNATION	REGENERATIVE MEDICINE ADVANCED THERAPY DESIGNATION
Qualifying Criteria	A drug that is intended to treat a serious condition, AND preliminary clinical evidence indicates that the drug may demonstrate substantial improvement on a clinically significant endpoint(s) over available therapies.	A drug is a regenerative medicine therapy, AND the drug is intended to treat, modify, reverse, or cure a serious condition, AND preliminary clinical evidence indicates that the drug has the potential to address unmet medical needs for such disease or condition.
Features	• All fast track designation features, including actions to expedite development and review and rolling review • Intensive guidance on efficient drug development, beginning as early as Phase 1 • Organizational commitment involving senior managers	• All breakthrough therapy designation features, including early interactions to discuss any potential surrogate or intermediate endpoints • Statute addresses potential ways to support accelerated approval and satisfy post-approval requirements

Considerations for Rare Diseases

The FDA has an Orphan Drug Designation program that provides orphan status to drugs and biologics, which are defined as those intended for the safe and effective treatment, diagnosis, or prevention of rare diseases/disorders that affect fewer than 200,000 people in the United States, or that affect more than 200,000 persons but are not expected to recover the costs of developing and marketing a treatment drug.

Rare diseases represent several challenges in the design of clinical studies. As many rare diseases are of genetic etiology, such considerations are relevant to trials of GT products. With some rare diseases, the number of subjects available for research constrains the design of trials. In particular, the number of available subjects may not be sufficient to allow for a standard randomized controlled trial. In this setting, alternative designs can be considered. The use of historical, rather than concurrent, controls is often suggested. While historical controls are appropriate in certain limited circumstances, the interpretability of any historically controlled trial relies to a great extent on the comparability of the historical group and the subjects enrolled in the study. One way to maximize the possibility that a historical control group will be useful is to evaluate subjects in a uniform manner in a natural history study. Such studies should be considered very early in the development of GTs for rare diseases, typically well before any interventional study in humans is initiated. Additional information on the development of GTs for rare diseases can be found in the FDA draft guidance on rare diseases.[34]

Specific programs designed to aid in the assistance of drug development for rare diseases include designation of a product as an orphan product and, for products meant to treat children, the rare pediatric disease priority review voucher program.[35]

Companion Diagnostics

A companion diagnostic is a medical device, often an in vitro device, which provides information that is essential for the safe and effective use of a corresponding drug or biological product. Diagnostic tests make it possible to individualize, or *personalize,* medical therapy by identifying patients who are most likely to respond, or who are at varying degrees of risk for a particular side effect. These tests are generally reviewed by the Center for Devices and Radiological Health (CDRH). Such tests are generally developed in parallel with the biological product for which their use is intended. The label of the approved biological product will identify the approved patient population and specify use of an FDA-approved or -cleared IVD companion diagnostic device to determine specific required characteristics such as gene variants, protein expression profile, or other factors. The FDA will apply a risk-based approach to determine the regulatory pathway for IVD companion diagnostic devices, which are used in combination with a GT product. This means that the regulatory pathway will depend on the level of risk to patients, based on the intended use of the IVD companion diagnostic device and the controls necessary to provide a reasonable assurance of safety and effectiveness.[36]

CONSIDERATIONS FOR LATE-STAGE PRODUCT DEVELOPMENT

As the field of GT matures, and more GT products reach commercial stage, it is essential that sponsors of INDs pay attention to manufacturing process development and plans for process validation. Process validation includes the design of the manufacturing process, CGMP compliance, and the use of validated assay methods to ensure that the product manufactured during clinical stages and the commercial product are of consistent quality. The FDA recommends that IND sponsors gain sufficient product and process knowledge during product developmental stages. Key to this approach is a good understanding of the CQAs of the product and CPPs that will control for the variability of the process. Product knowledge can be gained by measuring the CQAs of the product using well-qualified orthogonal test methods at several steps during manufacturing (in process, drug substance, drug product, and during storage, i.e., stability). As product development continues, and changes are introduced into the manufacturing process, the product and process knowledge and availability of qualified test methods will be valuable in evaluating product comparability and setting in-process tests and acceptance limits to evaluate and control the manufacturing process. Given the various expedited product development pathways (covered earlier in this chapter), and/or limited manufacturing experience anticipated for GTs developed for rare diseases, the FDA recommends that the IND sponsor develop qualified assays and define the CQAs and CPPs earlier in an expedited product development plan than otherwise planned for standard product development. For additional guidance on these topics, please refer to the FDA's "Guidance for Industry Process Validation: General Principles and Practices."[11]

ADDITIONAL CONSIDERATIONS THAT ARE APPLICABLE TO SPECIFIC PRODUCT CLASSES USED IN IMMUNOTHERAPY APPLICATIONS

The FDA's general recommendations for information to be included in an IND with reference to a GT investigational agent were discussed in the preceding sections.

This section discusses the FDA's recommendations for three different vector classes that generally represent the current pipeline of GT-based immunotherapy applications being developed. In instances when there is insufficient experience in a product class, or when there are no specific recommendations that would apply to the entire product class, this section may not include specific recommendations, and the reader is advised to refer to the general recommendations given previously and approach the FDA for a presubmission meeting such as an INTERACT, or pre-IND meeting, to obtain additional guidance.[37]

Oncolytic Viruses

Oncolytic viruses (OVs) have been studied since the mid-20th century for the treatment of cancer.[38] A wide range of viruses have been harnessed as antineoplastic agents, including adenoviruses, herpesviruses, measles, and others.[39] An advantage of oncolytic virotherapy, as opposed to some other forms of immunotherapy, is the ability to kill cancerous cells directly due to active viral replication as a first act and follow this up with the induction of immune responses by the subject's own immune system to tumor antigens exposed by the lytic action of the oncolytic viruses.

The FDA approved the first-in-class oncolytic virus, Imlygic (talimogene laherparepvec; Amgen Inc). Imlygic is an HSV-based genetically modified oncolytic viral therapy indicated for the local treatment of unresectable cutaneous, subcutaneous, and nodal lesions in patients with melanoma recurrent after initial surgery. A number of other oncolytic viruses are in various stages of clinical evaluations (a simple search of the www.clinicaltrials.gov website with a key word of "oncolytic virus" lists 31 open studies and a total of 70 studies that are open and completed as of October 6, 2016). Oncolytic viruses are attenuated replication competent viruses that have a preferential cytolytic activity in tumor cells. The cytolytic activity is generally expected to be brought about by a tumor selective replication of the virus.

Chemistry, Manufacturing, and Control Considerations

In general, the CMC requirements for an oncolytic virus product are similar to that of other GT vectors. However, there are some special considerations for this class of products:

Characterization of Attenuating Factors

The attenuating mutations and deletions of an oncolytic virus should be fully characterized; as such, their genetic stability and their inability to revert to "wild type" (genotype and phenotype) should be fully evaluated. Of particular concern will be the potential for recombination of the attenuated oncolytic virus with a prevailing "wild type" strain of the same or related viruses. For this reason, the FDA routinely recommends that the attenuating genotype and phenotype be well characterized and there be multiple discontinuous attenuating deletions engineered into the virus to render the virus avirulent (and less likely to revert), while retaining its oncolytic abilities.

Assays for Adventitious Viral Agents in Oncolytic Virus Products

The FDA recommends that the oncolytic viruses be tested for the presence of AVA in the MVB and final DP.[4] Because the test article contains a replication competent virus as the active ingredient that may interfere in the in vivo and in vitro assays, it is essential to neutralize the oncolytic virus prior to evaluating for the presence of other AVA in the DP and in the MVB. The FDA recommends that every attempt be made to test for the presence of AVA in the neutralized DP and MVB. In case the neutralization of the oncolytic virus is not completely achievable, a parallel cell culture that uses mock infected cells and that are processed in parallel with the cells used to make the oncolytic virus may be an alternative, and the sponsor of an IND should consult with the FDA for additional guidance on the acceptability of their approach to AVA testing.

Potency Assay

All attempts should be made to develop potency measurements that reflect the relevant biological properties of the product,[15] which for oncolytic viruses include the ability to differentially infect normal and tumor cells.

Virus Shedding Studies

The possibility that the shed oncolytic product may be infectious raises safety concerns related to the risk of transmission to untreated individuals. To understand and evaluate this risk, shedding studies both in appropriate preclinical animal models (if applicable and depending on the biology and tropism of the oncolytic virus) and during clinical studies should be conducted in the target patient population(s) before licensure. For detailed recommendations for appropriate design of shedding studies, please refer to the FDA's guidance on the design and analysis of shedding studies.[40]

Preclinical Considerations

Preclinical programs for oncolytic viruses relate to concerns about viral infection and replication in normal cells along with increased viral spread and replication in nontarget tissue. The FDA's recommendations for preclinical evaluation of oncolytic viruses will depend on the individual study agent and should be discussed with the FDA prior to submitting an IND.

Clinical Considerations

As stated earlier, OVs can be administered locally (e.g., intratumorally) or systemically by intravenous infusion. Thus, clinical considerations vary according to the route of administration of OVs as outlined in the text that follows.

Intratumorally Administered Oncolytic Viruses

Efficacy Evaluation: Assessment of Systemic Effect From Oncolytic Viral Therapy as Part of Providing Primary Evidence of Effectiveness

One important consideration for intratumorally administered oncolytic viral therapy (OVT) is whether such a treatment would or would not have any systemic treatment effect. Most OVT trials use OVs injected intratumorally, and the primary endpoints of these trials are usually tumor response rates. Because of this route of administration, such a treatment would be expected to have a local treatment effect (i.e., tumor responses would be expected in the tumors that are injected with OVs). This mechanism of action is distinguished from that of systemically administered agents such as chemotherapy or biologic therapy. For a systemic therapy, tumor responses occur or are expected to occur not only in the target tumor lesion that can be visualized but also in subclinical micrometastases. Thus, the tumor response rate is typically considered in the context of a systemic therapy in solid tumors, and most commonly used as an accelerated approval endpoint, which is intended to predict a clinical benefit such as symptomatic relief or survival. In addition, most local therapies in oncology, such as palliative radiation therapy or bone-seeking radioisotopes, have used trials with a symptom endpoint (e.g., pain relief) rather than a tumor response endpoint. Therefore, it is challenging to interpret the tumor response rate when the OVs are injected into local tumor(s) in the setting of treated or untreated systemic diseases.

Thus, one important factor to consider in the efficacy evaluation for OVT is the evidence whether OVT has a systemic effect in mediating the regression of tumor lesions that are not locally administered with OVT. In the setting of metastatic diseases, such an abscopal effect would be contingent upon immune responses elicited by the treatment of injected lesions with OVT. One approach to address this issue is to monitor these immune responses. Knowledge of such responses could provide supporting evidence regarding whether or not an OVT could have a systemic effect. However, assays for such immune monitoring may not be available, or may not be standardized, which could pose important challenges for this approach.

Another, and perhaps more practical, approach to detect an abscopal effect is to meticulously measure and document the changes in size/volume of tumors that are not injected. If tumors are located in internal organs (e.g., lungs or liver) that are not injected, then measuring these lesions before and after OVT may be an optimal way to observe a systemic effect from a locally administered OVT. If tumors are not present in internal organs, or are not suitable for definitive measurement, then detailed measurement of non-injected cutaneous, nodal, or other accessible tumors could be crucial. The modalities for such measurement (e.g., clinical assessment, photographic documentation, and radiological assessment) need to be utilized consistently at each measurement to avoid assessment bias. Documenting such measurements in the case report forms (CRFs) could provide essential evidence of the presence or absence of an abscopal effect.

Still another consideration is whether progression-free survival (PFS), as assessed by a conventional approach (e.g., Response Evaluation Criteria in Solid Tumors [RECIST]), could serve as an interpretable primary endpoint in the efficacy assessment for the locally administered OVT. Following Imlygic administration,[41] some tumor lesions (either injected or non-injected) may initially show progression, but later regress after further treatment. Thus, it can be challenging to interpret PFS results based on the first progression by conventional criteria, since any difference in the observed PFS may not reflect an effect of OVT. Using immune-related Response Evaluation Criteria in Solid Tumors (irRECIST) could take such a scenario (i.e., initial progression followed by subsequent regression) into consideration.[42] However, the primary endpoint based on irRECIST has not yet been generally accepted to support regulatory approval.

For some locally administered OVTs, the most direct evidence of a systemic effect could be demonstration of an overall survival (OS) benefit. OS is a universally accepted direct measure of benefit, and is easily and precisely measured. However, trials using OS as the primary endpoint may involve a larger number of subjects, and interpretation of OS may be confounded by crossover therapy, sequential therapy, and noncancer deaths.[27]

Control Considerations

Intratumoral injection could result in tumor regression through a physical effect of the injection procedure (e.g., shearing effect from passing the needles), especially in the setting of multiple injections into a given accessible tumor. If a response is seen in the injected tumor(s), it could be difficult to discern whether the response reflects the effect of the OVT or the effect of the injection procedure. To confirm the effect of the OVT and address this concern regarding any effect from the intratumoral injection procedure, consideration should be given to a randomized trial design with a concurrent control that is also intratumorally injected. Such a concurrent control could be either a placebo or an active control, depending on the clinical situation (e.g., the availability of alternative available therapies).

Safety Evaluation

Almost all OVTs involve live viruses capable of replicating. One safety concern is that such viruses may be shed from the patients who receive such therapy, and then spread to individuals who are in close contact with the patients. Although OVs are often genetically modified to limit the ability of the OV to cause disease, shedding remains possible, particularly for systemically administered OVs

Therefore, early in the clinical development of OVTs, it is important to consider including plans to monitor for viral shedding into the clinical trial design. Such monitoring serves to safeguard the public health and inform the design of later-phase trials. Yet, it can be challenging to design a development and monitoring program that would fit all OVTs. Therefore, the monitoring approach, with its attendant sample collection, assay methods, and cut-off thresholds and their interpretation, should be tailored for the specific OVT. The FDA has published "Guidance for Industry—Design and Analysis of Shedding Studies for Virus or Bacteria-Based Gene Therapy and Oncolytic Products."[40] This guidance can help the sponsor to design the appropriate shedding studies.

Systemically Administered Oncolytic Viruses

Challenges for this route of administration include preexisting host immunity to and stability of the OVs in blood.[43] Additional factors to consider in the trial design include absorption/metabolism of OVs by the major organs such as liver and spleen that may limit the intended OV doses that can be delivered to the tumor sites. In addition, the systemic toxicities are expected to be relatively more frequent when compared to locally administered OVs. As previously discussed, viral shedding from systemically administered OVs need to be investigated early in the development.

Gammaretrovirus/Lentivirus Vectors

Gammaretroviruses and lentiviruses have been the most commonly used vectors to deliver GT since the 1990s. The predominant application of retroviruses in the immunotherapy of cancer has been in the creation of CAR-transduced T cells (CAR T cells) directed against CD19 to treat B cell malignancies.[44–53] Gammaretroviruses and lentiviruses, though, are distinct viruses for which distinct manufacturing processes are followed. However, for the sake of this review, gammaretroviruses and lentiviruses are discussed as a single group, and accordingly, the section that follows highlights considerations for the

development of these viral vectors for manufacturing GTs for cancer.

Chemistry, Manufacturing, and Control Considerations

Test for Replication Competent Retrovirus/Lentivirus

Replication competent retrovirus/lentivirus (RCR/RCL) represents a potential health risk due to the concerns of insertional mutagenesis and virus pathology. The FDA routinely recommends testing for the presence of RCR/RCL throughout the manufacturing process of an ex vivo transduced cell product (such as CAR T cells) at multiple points in production, including the MCB for vector producer cells, vector supernatant, end of production cells, and ex vivo modified cells.[28] A biological assay for RCR or RCL with sufficient detection sensitivity should be used with appropriate positive and negative controls and be evaluated for inhibitory effects due to the vector and the final DP matrix by using positive control samples. A biological test for RCR/RCL should include culturing the cells and supernatant in permissive cell lines.[28] Alternative methods for lot release RCR/RCL testing of ex vivo transduced cells in lieu of culture-based methods can be developed, but the sensitivity, specificity, and reproducibility of the assay should be evaluated to qualify the assay (as suitable for its intended purposes) before its use in product release testing. Current manufacturing experience indicates that a test sensitivity of less than one RCR/dose is achievable. Therefore, sufficient supernatant should be tested to ensure a 95% probability of detection when the RCR/RCL is present at a concentration of 1 RCR (or RCL)/dose. To detect RCR/RCL in the vector producer cells or ex vivo transduced cells, the FDA recommends that a minimum of 1% of the total number of cells or 10^8 cells (whichever is less) be tested by co-culture method using a permissive cell line. If there is accumulated manufacturing and clinical experience that demonstrates that the transduced cell product is consistently RCR-negative, this data can be used to support reduction or elimination of testing ex vivo genetically modified cells for RCR. For additional details on the current recommendations for RCR/RCL testing, please refer to the FDA's guidance on this topic.[28]

Control of Transduction Efficiency

The number of vector genomes integrated into the host genome of the transduced cells, reported as vector copy number (VCN), provides a measure of control of transduction efficiency and should be consistent between different batches of the product. The VCN for a product should be at an appropriate safe level to ensure that therapeutic levels of gene expression are achieved. The FDA generally recommends that the VCN number be kept to a minimum number and calculated as VCN/transduced cell. High levels of VCN in transduced cells may not be desirable as it may increase the potential for insertional mutagenesis.[54] The VCN required to induce a therapeutic benefit, along with justification based on scientific reasoning (e.g., based on the vector design, and built-in safety profile) and supporting safety data for the product (e.g., from developmental and preclinical studies), should be discussed with the FDA during the INTERACT or pre-IND meetings.

Autologous Chimeric Antigen Receptor T Cell Products

The retrovirus/lentivirus vector-transduced autologous CAR T cell manufacturing process should include procedures to ensure that the product is segregated from other products (i.e., in incubators, hoods, cryopreservation units [if applicable], etc.) to minimize the potential for mix-ups. To enable unambiguous identification of patient-specific products, the FDA recommends that the product label should contain sufficient and unique identifying information.[1]

Characterization of Chimeric Antigen Receptor T Cell Products

Cellular population subtypes (e.g., CD4+, CD8+, CD45+, CD62L+, etc.) of the CAR T cell products should be well characterized and the percentage of vector-transduced cells in the final CAR T cell product should be included in the certificate of analysis (COA) for the product (please refer to additional discussion on the characterization of cell populations in the accompanying cell therapy chapter [Chapter 65]).

Preclinical Considerations

Lentivirus- and retrovirus-based vectors pose a safety concern for their potential for insertional mutagenesis, resulting in oncogene activation. In addition, lentivirus- and retrovirus-based CAR T cell products and TCR T cell products (T cell receptor chimeric T cells) pose a risk of off-target toxicities and on-target off-site toxicities. These toxicities are primarily due to the binding specificities of the antigen-binding portion of these chimeric T cells, and its affinity to the ligand. Current efforts to generate off the shelf CAR T cells have increased the complexities of evaluating toxicological profiles of these genetically engineered T cell products and need to be evaluated on a case-by-case basis.

Clinical Considerations

The most active application for lentivirus- and retrovirus-based vectors in cancer GT in recent years has been in genetically modified T cells with re-directed specificity (CAR- or TCR-T cells). Thus, the following discussions focus on these lentivirus- or retrovirus-modified T cells.

General Safety Considerations

Insertional Mutagenesis/Oncogenesis

Retroviruses cause DNA double-strand breaks followed by integration into the host genome in order to express the therapeutic transgene(s) these viruses carry. This integration and the consequent genetic modification of the host genome raises the possibility of insertional oncogenesis, or genotoxicity. While this possibility had long been thought of as remote, cases of such genotoxicity have been reported in clinical trials of retroviral modification of CD34+ hematopoietic cells for the correction of primary immunodeficiencies.[22-26] While similar AEs have not been reported in trials of lymphocyte-directed GT for the treatment of cancer, the risk of insertional oncogenesis remains a clinical concern.

Both insertional oncogenesis and the generation of RCR may theoretically occur as either early or late toxicities. Management of these risks typically involves extended clinical follow-up.[28,29]

On-Target, Off-Tumor Effect and Off-Target, Off-Tumor Effect (Cross-Reactivity)

Retrovirally transduced lymphocytes may cause adverse effects by attacking noncancerous/normal tissues due to their expression of the targeted antigens (off-tumor effects, or cross-reactivity), or alloreactivity (mostly a concern in the less common setting of allogeneic engineered T cell therapy). When these effects occur, the clinical consequences can be life-threatening or even fatal.[55,56]

Therefore, when designing T cells with novel re-directed specificities, sponsors are expected to do their due diligence to ensure that the cross-activity of the novel T cells are minimized as much as possible. The approaches may include extensive sequence homology search, cell/tissue cross-reactivity studies, animal studies, and so on. The modified T cells may also attack the normal tissues or cells by virtue of the same antigen expressed in these cells as in the tumor cells, causing adverse reactions due to on-target, off-tumor effect. For example, anti-CD19 CAR T cells may cause prolonged B cell aplasia because CD19 is expressed on the normal B cells. In these situations, the sponsor needs to describe in detail in the clinical protocol plans or algorithms to manage these on-target, off-tumor effects.

Systemic Cytokine Toxicities and Cytokine-Release Syndrome

Increases in systemic cytokines have been reported in almost all patients who received CAR T cell treatment, suggesting robust interactions of CAR T cells with both tumor cells and host immune system. In some situations, the cytokine releases reach toxic levels, potentially life-threatening or fatal.[57,58] The toxicities include cytokine-release syndrome (CRS), hemophagocytic lymphohistiocytosis (HLH), macrophage activation syndrome (MAS), and a neurotoxicity named as immune effector cell-associated neurotoxicity syndrome (ICANS).[59] In order to achieve clinical efficacy while avoiding systemic cytokine toxicities in early phase trials with CAR T cells, initial dose and dose escalation schemes must be carefully established to reach optimal therapeutic windows.

Increases in CRS are characterized by increased serum levels, fever, hypotension, hypoxia, and organ dysfunctioning. The most commonly elevated cytokines are IL-6 and interferon-gamma. Anti-IL-6 receptor antibodies (e.g., toxicimab) and anti-IL-6 antibodies (e.g., siltuximab) have been reported to mitigate or reverse the CRS and so do corticosteroids, although the concern in using the latter is that they may lead to the apoptosis of CAR T cells, thus comprising their efficacy.[60] Sponsors should describe in their clinical protocols the grading system used for grading CRS toxicity, contributions of CRS to the DLT definitions, and algorithm of managing CRS including the timing of intervention and agents to be used.

Target Identification as Part of Screening for Eligibility

Some clinical studies of CAR- or TCR-T cells involve identification of a specific target antigen as part of the eligibility criteria. In this situation, the sponsor needs to consider developing an assay or mechanism to measure the target antigen expression in individual subjects. These assays may be considered as companion diagnostics that would be regulated by the Center for Devices and Radiological Health (CDRH). Sponsors are encouraged to engage early with CDRH[61] for the development of these assays.

Human Leukocyte Antigen Restriction

Some clinical trials for TCR-gene modified products may involve a specific antigen presented in the context of a given human leukocyte antigen (HLA). Presence of such an HLA allele by certain assays is required for eligibility. Such assays may be considered as companion diagnostics that would be regulated by the Center for Biologics Evaluation and Research (CBER), Office of Blood Research and Review (OBRR). Sponsors are encouraged to engage early with OBRR for the development of these assays.

Study Population

Because CAR T cell therapy can be associated with considerable, even life-threatening or fatal, toxicities, notably CRS and neurological toxicities, it is important to carefully consider these toxicities in the context of the potential benefit, disease stage, and the available therapies for the selected study population. In early phase trials, it may be appropriate to enroll subjects with severe or advanced disease who do not have adequate responses to available medical treatment, or have no acceptable alternative treatments.

Early phase trials in CAR T cell therapies may employ a tissue-agnostic approach so as to include subjects with different cancer types yet sharing common tumor antigen(s) targeted by the CAR T cells. However, this approach may present challenges to evaluating efficacy and toxicities due to differing toxicities and dose-response relationships with different tumors. Patient selection based on the presence of an antigen target may be acceptable for an early phase study, though the interpretation of later-phase efficacy data may be challenging in a population heterogeneous in their natural disease histories and clinical outcomes.

As the antitumor effect of CAR T cells depends on the binding of the CAR with the cognate antigen expressed on the surface of tumor cells, it is essential to develop a test that can accurately and reliably detect the antigen on the tumor cells. Such tests are generally considered as companion diagnostic devices,[37] and are described in the FDA guidances on using these tests for oncology trials.[62] and principles for codevelopment of an in vitro companion diagnostic device with a therapeutic product.[37]

If a CAR T cell therapy is developed for pediatric cancer, the clinical protocol should include additional safeguards for pediatric subjects. Usually, initial safety and tolerability data in adult patients are established first, before beginning studies in children, according to "Title 21 Part 50, Subpart D." Sponsors can refer to the FDA guidance as well.[21]

Selection of Starting Dose, Dose Escalation, and Repeating Dosing

To mitigate the potential risks associated with the administration of CAR T cell product, in particular CRS, CAR T cell dosing should consider several factors, including transduction efficiency, that can vary from lot to lot. There may be substantial variation in the percentage of CAR positively transduced T cells in the study product. This variation can lead to substantial differences in the active dose administered to different subjects. Other factors affecting transduction efficiency may include cell viability, the total number of cells administered to the subject, whether or not preconditioning lymphodepletion regimen will be used, and the individual subject's body mass index.

Justifications for a starting dose based on preclinical data and/or clinical experience should be provided in the IND. If animal or in vitro data are available, there might be sufficient information to determine if a specific starting dose has an acceptable level of risk. However, conventional allometric scaling methods for CAR T cell products may be less precise than for small-molecule drugs. Therefore, it may be difficult to establish an initial starting dose based on the considerations used for small-molecule drugs. Prior clinical experience with the CAR T cells, even with a different disease condition, may serve as an informative and valuable source to justify the selection of the starting dose in the proposed clinical protocol.

Specific criteria for dose escalation and de-escalation should be provided in the first-in-human CAR T cell study. The dosing increments used for dose escalation should consider preclinical and any available clinical data regarding risks and biological activities associated with changes in dose. Most CAR T cell toxicities are related to the rapid release of large amounts of cytokines, which may be correlated to the activation status of the CAR T cells and the level of tumor antigen load in vivo. Because tumor burden varies among subjects, a given dose that may be safe in one subject with a low tumor burden may cause considerable toxicities at the same dose in another subject with a higher tumor burden.

CAR T cells are considered a living medicine which can persist and have extended duration and activity in the study subjects. Therefore, administration strategies by repeating or splitting dosing may be unnecessary in CAR T cell therapy, and may even pose unacceptable life-threatening risks, particularly if combined with repeat or excessive lymphodepleting preconditioning treatment.

To mitigate potential life-threatening cytokine storms or other serious toxicities in CAR T cell trials, a staggered treatment can be used to limit the number of subjects to receive the study agents within and between dose escalation cohorts. The interval between study subjects within or across cohort(s) should be long enough to monitor acute and subacute AEs prior to treating additional subjects at the same dose or prior to increasing the dose in subsequent subjects. Time courses of the AEs observed in preclinical studies, prior clinical studies, and the expected duration of activity with the same or similar CAR T cell product may provide valuable information when developing overall study timeline and staggering strategy.

In addition, due to anticipated time for the manufacturing of the autologous CAR T cells, the study subject may develop disease progression and become ineligible for the treatment. Certain eligibility criteria may improve the likelihood for the study subject to maintain eligibility after the waiting period for the successful manufacturing of the CAR T cell product. On the other hand, there may also be a need for contingency plan(s) in case of a manufacturing failure. For example, a manufacturing failure or delay may prompt investigators to use "bridging therapy" in an attempt to ameliorate the underlying disease while waiting for the production of CAR T cells, or the clinical protocol may be designed such that the subjects will not receive any high-risk lymphodepleting preconditioning treatment until the CAR T cell product is available.

Adverse Event Monitoring

As previously discussed, cytokine-related toxicities in CAR T cell therapy, notably CRS and neuropsychiatric toxicities, are particularly concerning. The clinical protocol should include descriptions of a specific toxicity grading system to assess toxicities and provide algorithms for CRS management and dose escalation strategy. Toxicities may be graded using Common Terminology Criteria for Adverse Events (CTCAE).[63]

It is important to define dose-limiting toxicity (DLT) of CRS, including any grade 3 or 4 toxicities that may be exempted from DLT consideration as such toxicities are known to be associated with T cell therapies but are transient and manageable without significant clinical sequelae based on the available preclinical or clinical data. The following are potential examples of DLTs for CAR T cells: (a) any treatment-emergent grade 4 or 5 CRS; (b) any treatment-emergent grade 3 CRS that does not resolve to grade 2 within 7 days; (c) grade 3 or greater treatment-emergent autoimmune toxicity; (d) grade 3 and greater allergic reactions related to cell infusion; or (e) grade 3 and greater organ toxicity (cardiac, dermatologic, gastrointestinal, hepatic, pulmonary, renal/genitourinary, or neurologic) not preexisting or not due to the underlying malignancy and occurring within 30 days of cell infusion.

Furthermore, because transgenes carried by CAR T cells may not be endogenous to the recipient, the exogenous components administered may elicit immune responses with the potential to affect CAR T cell persistence or counteract the antitumor activity.

Finally, stopping rules can limit subject exposure to risks in the event that safety concerns arise. Such stopping rules serve as criteria to suspend the study for further evaluation and protocol revisions based on the observed incidence and severity of particular AEs. Examples of stopping rules for CAR T cell studies may include an increase in the number or frequency of expected or unexpected severe AEs (e.g., occurrence of DLTs in more than 33% of study subjects or two or more grade 4 CRS or any death associated with CAR T cell administration).

Monitoring Persistence of Engineered T Cells

CAR T cell products can persist in the subject or have an extended duration of activity. Attempts should be made to determine the duration of persistence of the CAR T cell product and its activity. Product persistence is assessed by testing for evidence of the presence of cells, vectors, or virus in biological fluids or tissues. Activity might be assessed through an evaluation of physiologic effects, such as gene expression or changes in biomarkers.

Additional studies are clearly needed to evaluate toxicities due to CAR T cells. All assays used to evaluate CAR T cells should be fully qualified through an evaluation of assay suitability (i.e., the assessment of the assay's specificity and sensitivity prior to use). The FDA recommends that a LTFU plan be developed and included as a part of the clinical protocol. For recommendations on the frequency and duration of long-term follow-up, please refer to the FDA's guidance on this topic.[3]

Microbial Vectors for Gene Therapy

Another growing area of vectors used in GT and immunotherapy applications are microbial vectors. Microbial vectors used for GT (MVGTs) include bacterial vectors such as Salmonella, Listeria, or *Escherichia coli* genetically modified to express human tumor antigens, cytokines, growth factors, enzymes, therapeutic proteins, or nucleotides. MVGTs may be generated by modifying chromosomal or episomal genes and by the insertion of foreign genetic material into the chromosome or naturally occurring episomes, or by introducing it into one or more plasmids. In addition, MVGTs may be modified to alter their growth characteristics that make MVGT replication restricted for use as oncolytic tumor therapies.[64] Live biotherapeutic products, such as gut microbiome used to potentiate or augment immunotherapies, are not discussed in this chapter and the reader is requested to refer to the FDA's guidance on this topic.[65]

Chemistry, Manufacturing, and Control Considerations for Microbial Vector Gene Therapy

The CMC requirements for MVGTs pose some unique challenges with reference to evaluation of purity, safety (e.g., sterility, endotoxin), and potency testing. The general requirements for MVGTs are consistent with other GT vectors in that the FDA recommends IND sponsors have a well-characterized microbial vector banking system and a qualified manufacturing process, tests for residual process and product-related impurities, and a lot release testing plan with predefined acceptance criteria. The unique aspects of MVGT product development are discussed in the text that follows, and the reader is advised to refer to the FDA's guidance on this topic for additional recommendations and considerations.[6]

Microbial Vector Gene Therapy Seed Stock and Banking System

The IND should include a detailed description of the history, source, and derivation of the MVGT. The characterization and testing of MVGT should adequately establish the safety, purity, identity, and stability of the cells. The MVGT stock should be derived from a single, well-isolated colony. Microbial purity, defined as freedom from microbes other than MVGT, should be evaluated using appropriate methods such as monoculture assays. Characterization of the MVGT should also include a description of the physical properties of the organism (e.g., shape and colony morphology), growth properties, growth conditions, and antibiotic sensitivity profile. The identity test should include the host genetic makeup such as chromosomal genetic marker(s) and distinguishing genomic restriction patterns and sequencing data (with annotation) for the genetically modified plasmids or chromosomally inserted foreign genes. For mutation(s) that result in attenuation of MVGT, descriptions of the size and stability of the attenuation should be included and confirmed by sequencing the relevant regions of the chromosome.

Manufacturing Process

A detailed description of all procedures used during the derivation, production, and purification of an MVGT product should be included in the IND. If the final product is an inactivated MVGT, the process should also describe the method and conditions of cell inactivation/killing along with related qualification data for the inactivation process and include this data in the IND to demonstrate that the bacteria is inactivated but maintains its desired characteristics.

Test for Microbial Purity

A live microbial product, by definition, is not sterile. As such, the live MVGT should be tested for freedom from specific human microbial pathogens and from other environmental microorganisms that may be present in the manufacturing facility. The FDA recommends the Centers for Disease Control and Prevention (CDC) list of invasive bacterial pathogens, and specific pathogens described in the United States Pharmacopeia (USP) <62>, as examples of common bacterial agents that should be assayed for to ensure freedom from other pathogens in the MVGT preparations. The FDA also recommends that the test volumes for microbial purity tests be consistent with that recommended by USP <61> (microbial examination of nonsterile products: microbial enumeration tests); however, an IND sponsor may justify alternative test methods that are equally or more sensitive and specific, based on scientific reasoning and supporting data. Microbial purity should be evaluated in the microbial seed stock, MCB and WCB, and the final DP.

Endotoxin in Microbial Vector Gene Therapy

Endotoxin is a bacterial pyrogen derived from the outer membrane of Gram-negative bacteria. The lipopolysaccharide (LPS) component of the outer membrane, when free from the bacteria, is highly toxic to humans and is the source of bacterial endotoxin. The FDA recommends that parenterally administered MVGT products be free from endotoxins and an acceptance criterion of <5 EU/kg/dose be set.

Other Product Tests

MVGTs should also be evaluated for other essential quality attributes including cell viability. The FDA recommends that live bacterial products be tested to establish minimum release criteria for viability and a live to dead bacterial cell ratio. Since dead microbial cells in a live MVGT may not contribute to the function of the product but may be a source of unwanted immune reactivity and toxicity, the FDA recommends that an acceptance criterion of greater than 60% live/viable cells be set. Lyophilized and/or frozen MVGT may contain a large proportion of dead cells and the IND sponsor should set the final drug product dose based on the number of viable cell count and live/dead cell ratio. The FDA evaluates the acceptance criterion for live/dead cell ratio for MVGT products on a case-by-case basis; the IND sponsors should set acceptance limits based on scientific reasoning and safety information from preclinical studies, and discuss these specifications with the FDA. MVGT viability should be tested at the MCB, WCB, DS, and DP stages. MVGT should also be tested for the presence of product aggregates, antibiotic sensitivity, and potency. The FDA recommends that the MVGT products be evaluated to ensure that antibiotic resistance was not introduced into the MVGT during the manufacturing process, and the MVGT continues to be sensitive to the first-line and second-line antibiotics that are routinely used to treat that class of microbes. Potency of MVGT should be evaluated as a part of the DP lot release tests. For early phase studies, the potency test may be an assay to quantify transgene expression.

Preclinical Considerations

The preclinical considerations for MVGT products are similar to the general considerations for CT and GT products. Additional preclinical guidance on the topic can be found in the "Guidance for Industry: Recommendations for Microbial Vectors Used for Gene Therapy."[6] Due to the wide range of MVGT products, indications, and unique routes of administration, early interaction with the FDA to discuss appropriate preclinical studies to establish the safety and activity of the MVGT is recommended.

Clinical Considerations

1. *General Considerations*

   MVGT products may pose substantial and unique safety concerns, especially infections (e.g., sepsis), among immune-compromised study subjects due to the infectious nature of MVGT products. Therefore, prophylactic and/or post-MVGT administration antibiotics may be indicated. Antibiotics sensitivity tests should be conducted to help select the first and second lines of antibiotics for prophylaxis and treatment of infections.

   Due to the hypothesized mechanism of action by MVGT product, the survival of MVGT product may rely on the concomitant administration of immunosuppressive drugs. However, the immunosuppressants may also substantially increase risks for infections in the study subjects. Therefore, the administration of immunosuppressive drugs should be carefully selected and justified with appropriate precautions in the proposed study (e.g., careful selections for dose levels and administrative route, monitoring, and management plan for potential infectious AEs). The proposed study protocol should include a detailed safety monitoring plan for detection, management, and reporting serious AEs.

2. *Prior Human Experience*

   If the specific investigational MVGT product or a relevant product has been administered to humans previously, the FDA recommends that the sponsor carefully assesses the relevance of prior product to the current product, and provides comprehensive assessment of the safety data from prior relevant data. Data collected from prior human experience may inform the safety of the proposed protocol and could obviate the need for conducting additional preclinical studies to determine starting dose and/or dose escalations for the current proposed study. In these situations, the FDA recommends that the sponsor contacts CBER to discuss dosing issues before conducting preclinical studies.

3. *Patient Population*

   The clinical development of MVGT products may involve initial testing in a wide spectrum of medical conditions, from relatively benign conditions to advanced stages of fatal diseases with limited treatment options or no available treatment. The general recommendation for early phase trials of MVGT product is to select a patient population that is relatively free of risk from the intrinsic or allergenic properties of the MVGT product. For instance, anaerobic bacterial spore-based MVGT products may produce spores that could proliferate in necrotic tissues. Therefore, FDA recommends the sponsor consider excluding patients with necrosis or risks to develop necrosis (e.g., patients with brain abscess, diverticulitis or recent radiation). For MVGT products with organ-specific tropism, we recommend that the sponsor consider excluding patients with underlying medical conditions in those organs in the initial trials of MVGT products.

4. *Starting Dose, Dose Escalation, and Dosing Schedule*

   The dose selection and dosing schedule in early phase clinical trials may substantially impact the risks associated with the MVGT product. Results from preclinical and early phase proof-of-concept clinical trials can help guide the initiation dose selection, dose-escalation scheme, and dosing schedule.

The FDA recommends that sponsors engage in discussions with the FDA early in product development to discuss what preclinical data are needed to support early phase trials.

The starting dose, dose-escalation scheme, and dosing schedule may also be supported by prior clinical experience. Sponsors should provide comprehensive assessment of clinical data and include justification for the proposed dosing scheme in the proposed trial. Sponsors should also consider including specific MVGT product-related risks when evaluating DLTs, MTD, recommended Phase 2 dose (RP2D), and study stopping rules. The following examples may serve as criteria for DLTs or study stopping rules: (1) symptomatic septicemia; (2) fever and positive blood culture for infections for locally injected MVGT product; and (3) prolonged fever and positive blood cultures for systemically administered MVGT products.

5. *Treatment Modifications*

In early phase clinical trials with safety as the primary endpoint, treatment discontinuation rules for individual participants and study stopping rules for the proposed study should be described in the trial protocol (e.g., an excessive incidence of abscess or increased severity of expected infections in a study with anaerobic MVGT products).

6. *Safety Monitoring*

A safety monitoring plan should consider the potential risks associated with the specific MVGT product and the transgene as identified in the preclinical and clinical experience, such as the potential of MVGT products to germinate and regerminate. Safety data, particularly the nature and timing of AEs, from prior human experience with related MVGT products may help determine an appropriate duration for long-term monitoring. Assessment of the relevance of the prior clinical experience with related MVGT products should include consideration of the dose level, route of administration, duration of exposure, and number of subjects exposed and evaluated. Examples of specific monitoring plans for MVGT products include blood cultures and imaging studies at the onset of nonspecific symptoms to mitigate risks for abscess formation due to anaerobic microbial products.

A safety monitoring plan for MVGT products should also include monitoring for shedding of MVGT products, and such monitoring should be continued until adequate successive measurements do not demonstrate the presence of the MVGT product. The choice of samples (e.g., bodily secretions and/or excretions) may depend on the specific MVGT product and the proposed route of administration. Please refer to the FDA's "Design and Analysis of Shedding Studies for Virus or Bacteria-Based Gene Therapy and Oncolytic Products" for additional information.[40]

CONCLUSION

Recent progress in GT has lent itself to the possibility of wider applications.

GT has the potential for a positive impact on not only cancer but also other diseases such as blood disorders; muscular dystrophy; pulmonary, hepatic, and cardiac disease; congenital retinopathies; neurodegenerative disorders; and other genetic and acquired diseases. A large number of GT products including vectors, modified virus and bacteria, gene-modified cells, and gene editing technologies are being tested in clinical trials. Recent advances in CAR T cell technology have generated tremendous interest due to the potential of a large clinical benefit in hematological malignancies. We are very encouraged by such advances and are highly committed to helping developers of GT products to advance the field to protect and enhance public health. The FDA offers developers of cancer immunotherapy products various mechanisms of interaction with FDA staff for their specific product development questions throughout the product life cycle. FDA staff are actively engaged in providing guidance to the GT sponsors through explicit guidance documents, discussions at conferences, and scientific publications.[66,67] Sponsors are encouraged to refer to various guidance documents and written resources; for example: CBER References for the Regulatory Process for the Office of Tissue and Advanced Therapies (OTAT)[68] and the OTAT Learn Webinar Series.[69]

ACKNOWLEDGMENTS

We thank Drs Thomas Finn, Yuxia Jia, Mercedes Serabian, Tajeshri Purohit-Sheth, Zenobia Taraporewala, Carolyn Laurencot, Steven Oh, and Iris Marklein of OTAT, CBER, FDA for critical reading of the manuscript and for their comments and suggestions in drafting this chapter.

KEY REFERENCES

Only key references appear in the print edition. The full reference list appears in the digital product on Springer Publishing Connect: connect.springerpub.com/content/book/978-0-8261-3743-2/part/part05/chapter/ch66

1. U.S. Department of Health and Human Services Food and Drug Administration. Drug master files: guidance for industry. Published October 2019. https://www.fda.gov/media/131861/download

4. U.S. Department of Health and Human Services Food and Drug Administration. Chemistry, manufacturing, and control (CMC) information for human gene therapy investigational new drug applications (INDs): guidance for industry. Published January 2020. https://www.fda.gov/media/113760/download

6. U.S. Department of Health and Human Services Food and Drug Administration. Recommendations for microbial vectors used for gene therapy: guidance for industry. Published September 2016. https://www.fda.gov

/files/vaccines,%20blood%20&%20biologics/pub-lished/Recommendations-for-Microbial-Vectors-Used-for-Gene-Therapy--Guidance-for-Industry.pdf

19. U.S. Department of Health and Human Services Food and Drug Administration. Guidance for industry: preclinical assessment of investigational cellular and gene therapy products. Published November 2013. https://www.fda.gov/media/87564/download

20. U.S. Department of Health and Human Services Food and Drug Administration. Guidance for industry: gene therapy clinical trials—observing subjects for delayed adverse events. Published November 2006. https://www.ngvbcc.org/pdf/gtclin.pdf;jsessionid=64AFB5DB8805374241D9FFBBD0137CCF

21. U.S. Department of Health and Human Services Food and Drug Administration. Considerations for the design of early-phase clinical trials of cellular and gene therapy products: guidance for industry. Published June 2015. https://www.fda.gov/media/106369/download

27. U.S. Department of Health and Human Services Food and Drug Administration. Guidance for industry: clinical trial endpoints for the approval of cancer drugs and biologics. Published December 2018. https://www.fda.gov/media/71195/download

29. U.S. Department of Health and Human Services Food and Drug Administration. Guidance for industry: supplemental guidance on testing for replication competent retrovirus in retroviral vector based gene therapy products and during follow-up of patients in clinical trials using retroviral vectors. Published October 18, 2000. https://www.govinfo.gov/content/pkg/FR-2000-10-18/pdf/00-26670.pdf

Combination Immunotherapies: Regulatory Considerations

Ke Liu, Marc Theoret, Allen Wensky, Thomas Finn, Ramjay S. Vatsan, and Raj Puri

KEY POINTS

- Combination immunotherapy for cancer has shown greater efficacy in some disease settings.

- Better understanding of the cancer immunity cycle and the rapidly increasing availability of agents in development that target different steps of the cycle provide fertile ground for combining immunotherapeutics.

- Unique regulatory challenges exist for combination immunotherapy with respect to trial designs such as identifying optimal dose, schedule, sequencing of different components combined, and contribution of each component to the efficacy and safety of the combination.

INTRODUCTION

Cancer immunotherapy has become the mainstay of cancer treatments. Of the U.S. Food and Drug Administration (FDA) approvals for cancer indications within the last 15 years (2006–2020), more than a third of these approvals are for a cancer immunotherapeutic either as monotherapy or in combination with other anticancer agents."[1] One of the recent advances in cancer immunotherapy is the realization that combining therapeutics that target different aspects or steps of the cancer immunity cycle holds great potential in improving efficacy. For example, combination of ipilimumab, an immune checkpoint inhibitor of cytotoxic T-lymphocyte-associated protein 4 (CTLA-4), with nivolumab, another checkpoint inhibitor of programmed cell death protein 1 (PD-1), represents the first approval of an immunotherapeutic combination. Compared to ipilimumab monotherapy, this combination had shown greater efficacy in increasing the objective response rate (ORR), prolonging response durations, improving progression-free survival (PFS) initially in patients with BRAF^{V600} wild-type, unresectable or metastatic melanoma,

and subsequently in patients with unresectable or metastatic melanoma irrespective of BRAF^{V600} mutation status, including an improvement in overall survival (OS).[2,3] Intensive efforts have also been devoted to investigate the combination of immunotherapy with other immunotherapeutic agents, chemotherapy, and radiation; and some trials have reported promising preliminary clinical activity of such combinations.[4]

This chapter will present a general description of regulatory review pathways for combination products followed by a discussion of some of the regulatory considerations for combination immunotherapy with a focus on clinical considerations.

COMBINATION THERAPY IS NOT SYNONYMOUS WITH COMBINATION PRODUCT

Combination immunotherapy holds great promise for definitive treatment of cancer. From a regulatory perspective, however, it is necessary to distinguish a combination product from combination therapy. FDA regulations strictly define a combination product as a product comprised of two or more regulated articles such as biologic-drug, biologic-device, drug-device, or biologic-drug-device that are specifically intended for use together in order to mediate the intended therapeutic effect for the labelled indication (21 CFR 3.2 [e]). An example of a combination product is PHOTOFRIN (porfimer sodium) for injection, a photosensitizing agent (a drug) activated by a laser device used in the photodynamic therapy (PDT) of tumors and of high-grade dysplasia (HGD) in Barrett's esophagus (BE). The two constituents become a therapeutic product only when used together. Without the specific laser device, the drug cannot cause the desired antitumor/antiproliferation effect.[5] A biologic or drug intended to be used together with a specific companion diagnostic device in order to have the intended therapeutic effect is, however, not considered a combination product. A combination therapy, on the other hand, involves two or more drugs or biologics developed independently or concurrently in order to be used in combination as part of the same clinical treatment regimen. Each component of a combination therapy may contribute to the effect but is not indispensable to the other medical product(s) used in the treatment regimen. Such combination therapies are not regulated as combination products.

COMBINATION IMMUNOTHERAPY FOR CANCER

As illustrated in the cancer immunity cycle described by Chen and Mellman,[6] cancer immunity contains multiple steps, starting with the release of cancer antigens in the tumor tissue and their presentation by antigen-presenting cells (APCs), priming and activation of T cells in the lymph nodes, then trafficking and infiltration of these activated T cells to the tumor where they recognize and kill tumor cells. Many agents can affect a given step and are being actively pursued in clinical trials or are already FDA-approved for cancer treatment. Thus, an understanding of the cancer immunity cycle, along with the rapidly increasing availability of agents that are approved or are in development which can affect each step of the cycle, provide a fertile ground for investigating combinations.

POTENTIAL OF THE COMBINATION OF CANCER IMMUNOTHERAPY

One recent advance in immunotherapy is the recognition of the potential power of combination therapies to improve efficacy. The FDA approved the first combination immunotherapy of ipilimumab and nivolumab for untreated melanoma in 2015, based on increased tumor response rate and duration, as well as prolonged PFS. The same combination has been approved for several other indications such as renal cell carcinoma (RCC), microsatellite instability-high (MSI-H) colorectal cancer, hepatocellular carcinoma, and non-small cell lung cancer (NSCLC) and mesothelioma.[7–9] Clinical trials have shown that combinations of different cancer immunotherapeutic agents also hold greater potential in improving activity in other disease settings.

However, many regulatory challenges exist for developing combination immunotherapies. We describe the following considerations to address some of these challenges.

PRECLINICAL CONSIDERATIONS FOR COMBINATION THERAPIES

Overall, the high-level regulatory considerations and expectations for preclinical testing are the same for combination products and therapies; however, combination therapies may require a wider or different set of preclinical assessments.

A thorough understanding of the individual components of the combination therapy, the final formulation of the combined components, proposed indication, and relevant guidances and standards, as well as early interaction with the FDA/regulatory agency are important for designing a thoughtful preclinical program with the highest probability of success. Early interaction with the FDA before submission of an investigational application (e.g., a pre-investigational new drugs [IND] interaction) is critical for these types of therapies.

CLINICAL CONSIDERATIONS

For the clinical development of combination immunotherapy, the FDA encourages the sponsor to communicate with the FDA as early as possible. When submitting an IND to investigate a combination therapeutic regimen, the IND sponsor may cross-reference existing INDs for the individual products to be used in the combination.

Similar to monotherapy studies, the overall clinical development for combination therapies focuses on safety and efficacy evaluations with some unique aspects described in the text that follows. The primary objective for initial clinical trials of a novel combination of products typically focuses on safety evaluation. One common secondary objective of early phase clinical trials for combination therapy is to obtain preliminary data that might indicate the clinical activity of the treatment regimen. In addition to assessing tumor responses, combination immunotherapy trials may also consider other exploratory endpoints such as immune responses. Assessments of immune responses may provide useful data to support the proposed mechanism of action, especially when they can be correlated to clinical outcomes.

In addition, the early phase clinical trials should consider investigating the dose/schedule, sequencing, and feasibility of administration of the combination therapy. The contribution of each component of the combination also may be evaluated early in the development program, for example, in small randomized trials utilizing clinically meaningful efficacy endpoint(s) that may be measured earlier than endpoints intended to demonstrate the ultimate clinical benefit. Late-phase trials focus on demonstrating the efficacy of the combination and, if not adequately demonstrated in the earlier development program, the contributions of each of its components should be evaluated, and the trial design will vary depending on the specifics of the combination.

To address issues related to the clinical development of combination therapies in general, the FDA has published "Guidance for Industry—Codevelopment of Two or More New Investigational Drugs for Use in Combination."[10] Although this guidance states that it is applicable to the therapeutic biological products that are regulated by the FDA's Center for Drug Evaluation and Research (CDER), the principles described in this guidance may provide useful information in designing early or late-phase trials that use other cancer immuno-therapeutics in combination, such as cellular and gene products.

Early Phase Studies

As stated earlier, the primary objective for early phase clinical trials mainly focuses on the safety evaluation, including an assessment of the nature and frequency of potential adverse reactions and an estimation of their relationship to dose/schedule. In addition to the safety evaluation, these early phase clinical trials also assess the biologic activity, feasibility of administration, and the effects of therapy sequencing and pharmacologic activity, if applicable.

Additional information about the design of early phase clinical trials for cellular and gene therapies applicable to cancer immunotherapy may be found in the FDA "Guidance for Industry—Considerations for the Design of Early-Phase Clinical Trials of Cellular and Gene Therapy Products."[11]

With respect to the exploration of the dose and/or schedule, as with combination chemotherapy, combination immunotherapy may require the use of a dose and schedule less intense than the dose and schedule of each individual component. Dose-escalation strategies may therefore not be straightforward. One option is to hold the dose of one component of a combination therapy constant, while escalating the other component.[12] A variation of this strategy is to escalate the dose of the first component once the maximum tolerated dose (MTD) of the second component is established.[13] Another option would be to increase the two components of a combination therapy in an alternating fashion.[14]

As opposed to cytotoxic chemotherapy, substantial toxicities that may permit identification of an MTD may not occur in the expected or feasible therapeutic range of combination immunotherapy. In this event, the intent of dose/schedule exploration may be to determine the optimal biologically active dose (OBD) and regimen rather than the MTD. Regardless of the dose-escalation options chosen, the IND sponsor would need to provide the rationale and justification, definitions of dose-limiting toxicities (DLTs), and the MTD or OBD in detail in the proposed clinical trial protocol. For some complex combination therapies, there may be substantial limitations on the quantity of the product that can be practically manufactured or delivered. In this situation, the early phase trial objective may be to characterize the safety profile of the feasible dose and regimen.

Combination immunotherapy trial protocols usually specify a scale for grading the severity of adverse events (AEs), and the latest version of the National Cancer Institute (NCI) Common Terminology Criteria for Adverse Events (CTCAE) is appropriate and often used in immunotherapy trials.[15] However, in situations where CTCAE may not be adequate for assessing some toxicities such as certain autoimmunity/immune reactions, trial protocols may consider specifying additional criteria for this purpose. In addition, plans/algorithms for certain potential immune toxicities need to be provided in the clinical protocols.

Early phase trials of combination therapy usually include study stopping rules. The purpose of these rules is to control the number of subjects put at risk if early experience uncovers important safety problems. Study stopping rules typically specify a number or frequency of events, such as serious AEs or deaths, that will result in temporary suspension of enrollment and dosing until the situation can be assessed. Based on the assessment, the clinical protocol might be revised to mitigate the risk to subjects. Such revisions could include changes in the enrollment criteria, dose reduction, some other change in product preparation or administration, or changes in the monitoring plan. Well-designed stopping rules allow sponsors to assess and address risks identified as the trial proceeds, and to assure that risks to subjects remain reasonable.

A Phase 2 trial can be used as a discriminator to determine if progression to a Phase 3 confirmatory trial is warranted. In addition, the clinical activity of the combination can be estimated in a well-conducted Phase 2 trial. Randomized Phase 2 trials typically lack the statistical power for conclusive demonstration of the treatment effect of the investigational combination therapy. However, randomized Phase 2 trials may provide more reliable data about treatment effect size than a single-arm trial with historical controls, and thus are useful when planning the design of the subsequent Phase 3 trial. Ultimately, the design and conduct of trial(s) in the Phase 2 portion of the development program would be tailored to the objectives and, typically, are sufficient to provide adequate data to decide whether to proceed to a Phase 3 confirmatory trial(s). In addition, randomized Phase 2 trials may provide for an earlier assessment of the contribution of each component of the combination therapy to the overall treatment effect.

One of the main objectives of the Phase 2 trial is to demonstrate the contribution of each individual new investigational product in the combination unless the contribution of components to the effect of the combination was sufficiently demonstrated earlier in the development program. To achieve such an objective, an important consideration in the Phase 2 trial design for the combination therapy is the number of trial arms needed to be included. The following several possible scenarios can be considered:

- Situations where each new investigational product alone has activity and they can be administered separately.

If preclinical information and/or Phase 1 studies suggest that each new investigational drug has activity, but the combination appears to have greater activity, and rapid development of resistance is not a concern, a four-arm, Phase 2 trial in the disease or condition of interest comparing the combination to each product alone and to placebo (in selected circumstances[16]) or standard of care (SOC; i.e., AB vs. A vs. B vs. SOC) may be used to demonstrate the contribution of the individual products to the combination and proof of concept.

An adaptive trial design with the same four treatment arms might also be used where appropriate, initially using the previously described treatment arms and terminating the single product arms early if it becomes clear that the single agents have much less activity than the combination. Such a design may demonstrate the contribution of each product to the activity of the combination without exposing the large number of patients typically required for Phase 3 trials to therapeutic products with inadequate activity. When determining whether to terminate monotherapy treatment arms early, it may be necessary to use endpoints that provide evidence of treatment effect more readily than endpoints that would be used in confirmatory Phase 3 trials to minimize the amount of time subjects may be exposed to a low activity product. For example, immune responses to treatment could be used to determine which arm may or may not be terminated early.

- Situations where the individual new investigational products in the combination cannot be administered separately or can be administered separately, but show no activity alone.

In such a situation, proof-of-concept evidence for the combination can come from a Phase 2 study design directly comparing the combination (AB) to SOC. Alternatively, if SOC is a known effective therapy (not solely palliative), an add-on design could be used comparing the combination plus SOC to placebo plus SOC.

- Situations when, administered separately, one new investigational product in the combination is active and one is inactive.

In this scenario, proof of concept and the contribution of each new investigational product could be demonstrated using a three-arm comparison of the active drug alone, the combination, and SOC (A vs. AB vs. SOC), or the combination and the individual drug added to SOC where SOC is a known effective therapy (AB + SOC vs. A + SOC vs. placebo + SOC).

Combination Therapy: Late-Phase Trials

Phase 3 confirmatory trials usually provide primary evidence of efficacy and safety for the combination studied and may be used to support a marketing application. The sponsor may choose to submit a Phase 3 trial protocol to the FDA for special protocol assessment (SPA). SPA is a means by which the sponsor reaches an agreement with the FDA on the clinical design, endpoints, and statistical analysis plan prior to commencement of the Phase 3 trial. The FDA will document such an agreement in writing. To learn more about special protocol assessment agreements, one may refer to the FDA's "Guidance for Industry—Special Protocol Assessment" at www.fda.gov/downloads/Drugs/GuidanceComplianceRegulatoryInformation/Guidances/UCM498793.pdf.[17]

Phase 3 trial endpoints can be challenging to choose in terms of the specific endpoints and how they are assessed. The sponsor is encouraged to discuss the choice of Phase 3 endpoints with the FDA and consult the FDA "Guidance for Industry—Clinical Trial Endpoints for the Approval of Cancer Drugs and Biologics," available at www.fda.gov/downloads/Drugs/GuidanceComplianceRegulatoryInformation/Guidances/ucm071590.pdf.[18] Novel endpoints such as immune-related response criteria (irRC) have been proposed and incorporated into cancer immunotherapy trials and as part of the management for patients who receive immunotherapy.[19,20] The FDA encourages sponsors to discuss the appropriateness and acceptability of these novel endpoints early in the clinical development.

In addition, as immunotherapeutic product classes used in combination are regulated across different FDA Review Divisions, Offices and Centers, sponsors are strongly encouraged to discuss their development plan with appropriate FDA Review Divisions/Offices early to most efficiently develop a combination therapy.

COMBINATION THERAPY: SAFETY CONSIDERATIONS

Acute and chronic toxicities from combination immunotherapy are often different than those seen with cytotoxic agents in patients with cancer. DLTs may not occur during early phase trials, and an MTD may not be defined. However, possible serious late-occurring toxicities may occur, which require appropriate planning and monitoring during development. In addition, some components of the combination therapy may be administered locally (e.g., intratumoral injection) and thus need appropriate safety assessment for both localized and systemic toxicities.

When toxicities occur in trial participants who receive combination immunotherapy, it is often difficult to ascribe observed toxicities (e.g., serious AEs) to a specific component of the combination due to multiple factors such as overlapping adverse effects of the combination therapy, the manifestations of the underlying disease, and untoward effects from other concomitant cancer treatment. Thus, it is important that the combination immunotherapy trials consider these factors in the definition of DLTs, study pausing/stopping rules, and safety reporting and management plans.

LONG-TERM FOLLOW-UP

Study subjects who receive a combination immunotherapy that utilizes genetic vectors may be at risk of developing delayed AEs months or even years after administration. Specific testing for replication competent retrovirus, replication competent lentivirus, adenovirus, and adeno-associated virus are recommended and discussed in the FDA's "Guidance for Industry—Testing of Retroviral Vector-Based Human Gene Therapy Products for Replication Competent Retrovirus During Product Manufacture and Patient Follow-Up."[21] Long-term follow-up after administration of human gene therapy products is discussed in the FDA's "Guidance for Industry—Long Term Follow-Up After Administration of Human Gene Therapy Products."[22] Depending on the vector type, its propensity to integrate, and other factors (for example, replication competence), a long-term follow-up observation plan may be required. If the combination therapy utilizes an integrating vector, or if the vector has latency, then the sponsor is typically expected to follow subjects for 15 years to identify any latent safety issues, such as insertional mutagenesis and secondary malignancies. Long-term safety monitoring can also be useful if the product involves a gene that might predispose subjects to develop secondary malignancies.

In other situations, a shorter period of observation may be suitable. In assessing an appropriate observation period for delayed AEs, factors for consideration include pertinent previous preclinical and clinical experience with the product or similar products, experience with other products in the same vector class, route of administration, and the clinical indication.

COMPANION DIAGNOSTICS

As with monotherapy, when the proposed mechanism of action of a combination immunotherapy involves a specific antigen or other therapeutic target, consideration includes developing an assay or mechanism to measure the target antigen expression in individual patients and using that information for patient selection or response monitoring. These assays may be considered as companion diagnostics if they provide information that is essential for the safe and effective use of the combination therapy. Companion diagnostics may be co-developed with the therapeutic biologic or drug product as investigational products and are typically regulated by the Center for Devices and Radiological Health (CDRH).[23]

CONCLUSION

Cancer immunotherapy has evolved tremendously in recent years. Many regulatory challenges exist, especially in the era of novel therapies and their combinations. Optimizing the approaches to determine efficacy and safety represents some of the major challenges for combination immunotherapy. Some of the challenges described in this chapter include identification of the contribution of each component, dose, schedule, and sequencing of the components combined and the toxicity evaluation. Early interaction with regulatory agencies and collaboration among stakeholders are important for future success of clinical development of new immunotherapy for cancer.

KEY REFERENCES

Only key references appear in the print edition. The full reference list appears in the digital product on Springer Publishing Connect: connect.springerpub.com/content/book/978-0-8261-3743-2/part/part05/chapter/ch67

4. Bashir B, Wilson MA. Novel immunotherapy combinations. *Curr Oncol Rep.* 2019;21(11):96. doi:10.1007/s11912-019-0851-x
6. Chen DS, Mellman I. Oncology meets immunology: the cancer-immunity cycle. *Immunity.* 2013;39(1):1–10. doi:10.1016/j.immuni.2013.07.012
10. U.S. Food and Drug Administration. *Guidance for Industry—Codevelopment of Two or More New Investigational Drugs for Use in Combination.* Published June 2013. https://www.fda.gov/regulatory-information/search-fda-guidance-documents/codevelopment-two-or-more-new-investigational-drugs-use-combination
16. U.S. Food and Drug Administration. *Guidance for Industry—Placebos and Blinding in Randomized Controlled Cancer Clinical Trials for Drug and Biological Products.* Published August 2019. https://www.fda.gov/media/130326/download.
17. U.S. Food and Drug Administration. *Guidance for Industry—Special Protocol Assessment Guidance for Industry.* Published April 2018. http://www.fda.gov/downloads/Drugs/GuidanceComplianceRegulatoryInformation/Guidances/UCM498793.pdf
18. U.S. Food and Drug Administration. *Guidance for Industry—Clinical Trial Endpoints for the Approval of Cancer Drugs and Biologics.* Published December 2018. https://www.fda.gov/media/71195/download

68

Regulatory Considerations for In Vitro Companion Diagnostic Devices

Shyam Kalavar, Pamela Gallagher, Reena Philip, and Wendy Rubinstein

KEY POINTS

- Some in vitro diagnostic devices (IVDs or tests) are used to identify cancer patients with specific biomarkers in order to "personalize" treatment.

- IVDs used in personalized medicine are often companion diagnostic devices that ideally should be developed along with the therapeutic product (drug) and tested/validated for safety and effectiveness in the same clinical trial that is used to assess the safety and efficacy of the drug.

- In the United States, clinical diagnostic tests are devices under the Federal Food, Drug, and Cosmetic Act (the FD&C Act) and are regulated by the U.S. Food and Drug Administration (FDA). In general, marketing applications for IVDs are reviewed by the FDA in order to ensure the safety and effectiveness of the device before being put to clinical use.

INTRODUCTION

Decades of research uncovering the biological mechanisms of cancer have not only been translated into a host of molecularly targeted therapies but have also led to the development of a multitude of in vitro diagnostic devices (IVDs or tests) performed on samples taken from the human body to measure or detect a specific analyte(s). In cancer medicine, IVDs are used to inform diagnosis, prognosis, monitoring of disease progression or recurrence, and cancer therapy selection. IVDs are also used in asymptomatic people to screen for the presence of cancer or to predict the risk of developing cancer in the future. Indeed, across all of medicine broadly, as well as in cancer medicine in particular, IVDs are an increasingly integral component of clinical care, influencing the majority of clinical decisions.

IN VITRO COMPANION DIAGNOSTIC DEVICES IN PRECISION MEDICINE

One of the most promising advances in the field of cancer medicine is the use of IVDs to determine whether or not a patient is likely to benefit from a particular therapy. This personalized, or precision, medicine approach has the potential to transform patient care into a more efficient and successful endeavor that delivers the right treatment to patients at the right time, and with better outcomes, fewer adverse reactions, and ideally at a lower cost. Getting the best possible treatment to a patient as soon as possible is particularly critical for many biomarker-targeted cancer therapies, and this relies on accurate and reliable IVDs. A particularly important group of IVDs identified as "companion diagnostic devices" play a critical role in informing treatment decisions, especially in the field of cancer medicine. A companion diagnostic device has been defined by the U.S. Food and Drug Administration (FDA) as an IVD that provides information that is essential for the safe and effective use of a corresponding therapeutic product.[1] Companion diagnostic devices have made important contributions to the field of precision medicine by enabling the identification of specific biomarkers in cancer patients that can be treated with targeted therapeutic products, thereby enabling "personalized" treatments.

One of the first examples of this "personalized" approach was the HER2 targeted therapy trastuzumab (Herceptin) and an accompanying IVD that measured levels of HER2/neu (HercepTest™), both approved by the FDA in 1998. Since the HER2 example, the number of companion diagnostic-therapeutic product pairs in oncology has steadily increased. As of August 31, 2020, 41 IVD companion diagnostic-therapeutic product pairs have been approved for cancer treatment (see Table 68.1).[2]

[1] Food and Drug Administration Staff. *In Vitro Companion Diagnostic Devices.* 2014. www.fda.gov/downloads/medicaldevices/deviceregulationandguidance/guidancedocuments/ucm262327.pdf

[2] List of cleared or approved companion diagnostic devices (in vitro and imaging tools). www.fda.gov/companiondiagnostics

Table 68.1 Approved In Vitro Diagnostic Companion Diagnostic Devices in Oncology

NUMBER	MEDICAL PRODUCTS
41	Approved IVD companion diagnostics in oncology
19	Approved IVD companion diagnostics for use with multiple cancer therapeutic products
7	Approved IVD companion diagnostics with multiple indications
4	Immunotherapy-companion diagnostic pair (e.g., pembrolizumab, atezolizumab, nivolumab, and ipilimumab)

IVD, in vitro diagnostic device.

Source: List of cleared or approved companion diagnostic devices (in vitro and imaging tools). U.S. Food & Drug Administration website. https://www.fda.gov/medical-devices/in-vitro-diagnostics/list-cleared-or-approved-companion-diagnostic-devices-in-vitro-and-imaging-tools. Updated May 28, 2021. Accessed August 31, 2020.

Table 68.2 Biomarkers Identified by Companion Diagnostic Devices by Methodology

MAJOR METHODOLOGY				
IHC TESTING	ISH TESTING	VARIANTS IDENTIFIED BY MOLECULAR TESTING		OTHER BIOMARKERS IDENTIFIED BY MOLECULAR TESTING
HER2/neu ALK c-KIT EGFR PD-L1	HER2/neu	*ALK* *BRAF* *BRCA1/* *BRCA2* *EGFR* *ERBB2* *FGFR2* *FGFR3* *FLT3*	*KRAS* *MET* *NRAS* *PDGFRB* *PIK3CA* *ROS1* 17p deletion	Homologous recombination deficiency (HRD) Homologous recombination repair (HRR) genes Tumor mutational burden (TMB)

EGFR, epidermal growth factor receptor; IHC, immunohistochemistry; ISH, in-situ hybridization; PD-L1, programmed death ligand 1.

Some companion diagnostics are paired with multiple therapeutic products (e.g., the EGFR PharmDx Kit is paired with two different targeted therapies). Some companion diagnostics are indicated for multiple therapeutic products across multiple tumor types (e.g., the FoundationOne®CDx [F1CDx] assay is approved for 22 targeted therapies across eight different tumor indications). Some therapeutic products have multiple options for corresponding companion diagnostics (e.g., trastuzumab [Herceptin], for which there are 10 different HER2 tests approved as companion diagnostics). Some companion diagnostics are approved for more than one specimen type, such as the cobas® EGFR Mutation Test v2, which is approved for use with non-small cell lung cancer (NSCLC) tissue and plasma, and the *therascreen* PIK3CA RGQ PCR Kit, which is approved for use with breast cancer tissue and plasma.

Many different types of IVDs may function as companion diagnostic devices. The assessment of specific biomarker status may be based on different testing methodologies such as protein-based testing (immunohistochemistry [IHC] assays), in-situ hybridization assays, and molecular diagnostics (polymerase chain reaction [PCR] and next-generation sequencing [NGS]-based testing). A list of biomarkers identified by companion diagnostic devices sorted by methodology is provided in Table 68.2.

In Vitro Diagnostics Used to Identify Biomarkers to Guide Therapy in Oncology but Not Considered as Companion Diagnostic Devices

Other tests used in clinical treatment decision-making may not be essential for the safe and effective use of the corresponding therapeutic product because the therapeutic product is approved in a population that can be identified without using a specific test. Although such tests do not meet the definition of a companion diagnostic, and therefore are not prerequisites to selecting the drug, they may provide useful information for individual patients and their health care providers. Such a test may, for example, identify a subgroup of the indicated population that exhibits a difference in therapeutic product response, and thus the test may inform the individual patient's benefit-risk profile.

One example of this type of test in the immunotherapy area is the PD-L1 IHC 28-8 pharmDx test, which measures levels of the PD-L1 protein in tumor tissue. In the clinical development of the PD-1 blocking immunotherapy nivolumab, subjects' lung cancer biopsies were tested to determine the levels of expression of PD-L1 protein, but the subjects were not enrolled or assigned to a treatment arm based on the test result.[3,4] A planned interim analysis of the pivotal trial (without analysis of the PD-L1 expression level) demonstrated a statistically significant improvement in overall survival for subjects randomized to nivolumab compared with docetaxel in the overall study population (patients with metastatic NSCLC who have disease progression on appropriate FDA-approved therapy). Since the responsive population could be identified without reference to the test result, the test was not essential for safe and effective

---

[3] Highlights of prescribing information—these highlights do not include all the information needed to use. www.accessdata.fda.gov/drugsatfda_docs/label/2015/125554s005lbl.pdf

[4] PD-L1 IHC 28-8 pharmDx. www.accessdata.fda.gov/cdrh_docs/pdf15/P150027c.pdf

---

BOX 68.1 EXAMPLES OF NONCOMPANION DIAGNOSTICS FOR PD-1/PD-L1 IMMUNOTHERAPIES

Stated Indications for Use (Excerpts)

PD-L1 IHC 28-8 pharmDx: PD-L1 expression as detected by PD-L1 IHC 28-8 pharmDx in nonsquamous NSCLC may be associated with enhanced survival from OPDIVO® (nivolumab).[5]

PD-L1 IHC 28-8 pharmDx: Positive PD-L1 status as determined by PD-L1 IHC 28-8 pharmDx in melanoma is correlated with the magnitude of the treatment effect on progression-free survival from OPDIVO®.[6]

Ventana PD-L1 (SP142) Assay: PD-L1 expression in ≥5% IC determined by VENTANA PD-L1 (SP142) Assay in urothelial carcinoma tissue is associated with increased objective response rate (ORR) in a nonrandomized study of TECENTRIQ™ (atezolizumab).[7]

[IC: tumor-infiltrating immune cells of any intensity]

Ventana PD-L1 (SP142) Assay: PD-L1 expression in ≥50% TC or ≥10% IC determined by VENTANA PD-L1 (SP142) Assay in NSCLC tissue may be associated with enhanced overall survival from TECENTRIQ.[8] (atezolizumab).

[TC: PD-L1 expressing tumor cells of any intensity; IC: tumor-infiltrating immune cells of any intensity]

IC, immune cell; IHC, immunohistochemistry; NSCLC, non-small cell lung cancer; PD-1, programmed cell death protein-1; PD-L1, programmed death ligand 1; TC, tumor cell.

---

use of the drug, and therefore, there was no requirement for a companion diagnostic. However, prespecified retrospective analyses of efficacy in subgroups according to PD-L1 expression level in tumor tissue showed subjects with higher levels of PD-L1 expression in tumors were associated with enhanced survival from nivolumab compared with docetaxel. This information, given the various options for therapy for NSCLC, may be useful for an individual patient's therapy decision-making. Information about the test was included in the Clinical Trials section of the immunotherapy's labeling. The test and the immunotherapy were approved at the same time in 2015. Since then, there have been several additional contemporaneous approvals for tests that inform the use of a specific immunotherapy (see Box 68.1).

FOOD AND DRUG ADMINISTRATION OVERSIGHT OF IN VITRO DIAGNOSTIC DEVICES

As additional cancer medicines, including new immunotherapies, are made available, it becomes even more important to understand the likely benefits and risks for an individual patient so as to select the therapy that is likely to be the most effective while minimizing adverse events (AEs). The need for accurate and reliable IVDs for this purpose is critical. In regulatory parlance, IVDs are devices that are regulated in the United States by the FDA under the Federal Food, Drug, and Cosmetic Act (the FD&C Act). As defined in the Code of Federal Regulations (CFR), in vitro diagnostic products are: "those reagents, instruments, and systems intended for use in diagnosis of disease or other conditions, including a determination of the state of health, in order to cure, mitigate, treat, or prevent disease or its sequelae. Such products are intended for use in the collection, preparation, and examination of specimens taken from the human body."[9]

In general terms, the FDA is charged with ensuring that devices, including IVDs in clinical use, are safe and effective for their conditions of use. The Office of In Vitro Diagnostics and Radiological Health (OIR–OHT7) in the Center for Devices and Radiological Health (CDRH) is the main component within the FDA that is responsible for oversight of IVDs.[10]

Some tests are indicated for over-the-counter (OTC) use, where a consumer performs the test directly (e.g., a home-use pregnancy test kit), and other tests are indicated to be performed at the point of care by health care providers, such as a rapid strep test. Most IVDs,

[5] PD-L1 IHC 28-8 pharmDx. www.accessdata.fda.gov/cdrh_docs/pdf15/P150027c.pdf
[6] bid.
[7] Ventana PD-L1 (SP142) Assay. www.accessdata.fda.gov/cdrh_docs/pdf16/P160002C.pdf
[8] bid.

[9] 21 CFR 809.3.
[10] Devices Regulated by the Center for Biologics Evaluation and Research. www.fda.gov/BiologicsBloodVaccines/DevelopmentApprovalProcess/510kProcess/ucm133429.htm

however, are for use in a clinical laboratory environment as they require specific instrumentation, complex procedures, and/or trained laboratorians to perform or interpret the test result. Such clinical laboratories require certification from the Clinical Laboratory Improvement Amendments (CLIA) program, which is overseen by the Centers for Medicare and Medicaid Services (CMS) to ensure quality laboratory testing.[11] The IVDs used in cancer diagnosis and treatment are typically only performed in CLIA-certified clinical laboratories.

Regulatory Requirements for In Vitro Diagnostic Devices[12]

FDA oversight of medical devices, including IVDs, is risk-based, meaning that the requirements applicable to a device type generally depend on what controls are necessary to adequately mitigate the risk of potential harms associated with use of the IVD. Typically, the potential harm of a given IVD is related to the effect of a false result and is therefore linked to how the test and the test's results will be used. Thus, there is greater potential harm, for example, when test results are relied on to make critical treatment decisions than when the test results are providing additional information about a condition.

Medical devices are classified into class I, II, and III, with the regulatory controls being applied increasing from the lowest risk devices classified into class I to the highest risk devices classified into class III. A device classification regulation informs the regulatory requirements applicable to a general device type.[13] One regulatory control is review of the IVD by the FDA prior to marketing. Class I IVDs are typically exempt from premarket review. Class II and class III IVDs generally require premarket review, which involves a premarket submission to the FDA.

A premarket submission to the FDA generally is either a premarket approval application (PMA) submission, de novo submission, or a 510(k) submission. When the FDA performs premarket review of devices submitted via a PMA submission or de novo submission, the FDA evaluates the scientific evidence supporting the IVD's analytical and clinical performance and its safety under its conditions of use. For example, in the context of the FDA's review of a PMA submission for a class III IVD, the FDA determines whether there is a reasonable assurance a test is safe (i.e., "that the probable benefits . . . outweigh

any probable risks"),[14] and whether there is a reasonable assurance a test is effective (i.e., "in a significant portion of the target population . . . the use of the device . . . will provide clinically significant results").[15] (See section "Food and Drug Administration Assessment of Device Performance" in the text that follows.) A 510(k) submission establishes that an IVD is substantially equivalent to a predicate device, which is an existing legally marketed device. Generally, submission for IVDs cleared through a 510(k) have included scientific evidence of the IVD's analytical performance and clinical performance to demonstrate that the IVD has similar technological characteristics to the predicate device or that any different technological characteristics do not raise different questions of safety and effectiveness than the predicate device.

Another regulatory control required for many IVDs is that they must be manufactured under a quality system and the manufacturer must comply with good manufacturing practices.[16] This is intended to ensure that a test is designed to meet the needs of the user(s) and is produced in a controlled manner over time. The FDA's regulatory controls also require a mechanism to identify and correct problems. For example, in the postmarket setting, a manufacturer is required to submit a report to the FDA upon learning that their IVD may have caused or contributed to a death or serious injury or has malfunctioned, and this device or a similar device that the manufacturer markets would be likely to cause or contribute to a death or serious injury if the malfunction were to recur.[17] Such medical device reporting allows the FDA to work with manufacturers to identify and correct problems in a timely manner, which helps to protect the public from faulty IVDs.

Food and Drug Administration Assessment of Device Performance

FDA premarket review generally includes the assessment of analytical and clinical performance based principally upon performance data included in a premarket submission. Analytical performance is the documented ability of the test to measure or detect the analyte that the test is purported to detect or measure (i.e., how reliable and accurate the test results are). Clinical performance is the established correlation between the test result and the specified clinical condition, predisposition, or outcome. Evidence to support clinical performance may

[11] Clinical laboratory improvement amendments. www.cms.gov/Regulations-and-Guidance/Legislation/CLIA

[12] Overview of IVD regulation. www.fda.gov/MedicalDevices/DeviceRegulationandGuidance/IVDRegulatoryAssistance/ucm123682.htm

[13] Classify your medical device. www.fda.gov/medical-devices/overview-device-regulation/classify-your-medical-device

[14] 21 CFR 860.7(d)(1).

[15] 21 CFR 860.7(e)(1).

[16] In vitro diagnostic (IVD) device studies frequently asked questions. www.fda.gov/regulatory-information/search-fda-guidance-documents/vitro-diagnostic-ivd-device-studies-frequently-asked-questions

[17] 21 CFR 803.50(a).

EXHIBIT 68.1 COMPANION DIAGNOSTIC CASE STUDY 1: PD-L1 BIOMARKER IN IMMUNOTHERAPY

Companion Diagnostic: PD-L1 IHC 22C3 pharmDx (Dako, North America, Inc.)

Stated Indications for Use (excerpt): PD-L1 IHC 22C3 pharmDx is indicated as an aid in identifying cervical cancer patients for treatment with KEYTRUDA® (pembrolizumab).[18]

Immunotherapy: PD-1-blocking antibody KEYTRUDA (pembrolizumab; Merck Sharp and Dohme Corp.)

Stated Indications and Usage (excerpt): Pembrolizumab is indicated for treatment of patients with recurrent or metastatic cervical cancer with disease progression on or after chemotherapy whose tumors express PD-L1 (combined positive score [CPS] ≥1) as determined by an FDA-approved test.[19]

[CPS is the number of PD-L1 staining cells (tumor cells, lymphocytes, macrophages) divided by the total number of viable tumor cells, multiplied by 100.]

Clinical Study: In a Phase 2 study, pembrolizumab efficacy was evaluated in 98 patients with recurrent or metastatic cervical cancer enrolled in a single cohort in a multicenter, nonrandomized, open-label, multicohort trial with PD-L1 expression CPS ≥ 1% as determined using the PD-L1 IHC 22C3 pharmDx Kit. The major outcome measure was overall response rate (percentage of patients who experienced complete and partial shrinkage of their tumors). Tumors shrank in 14.3% of patients treated with pembrolizumab and the effect lasted between 4.1 and 18.6 months (the median had not been reached at the time of reporting). Based on tumor response rate and durability of response, pembrolizumab was approved under the FDA's accelerated approval program.

The PD-L1 test was considered essential for identifying the population for which pembrolizumab had demonstrated efficacy and safety, and was approved as an IVD companion diagnostic device, contemporaneously with pembrolizumab, in June 2018.[20]

FDA, U.S. Food and Drug Administration; IHC, immunohistochemistry; PD-L1, programmed death ligand 1.

---

involve clinical studies or other valid scientific evidence that shows that the test results correlate with a biological truth (e.g., presence of a disease) or with a treatment outcome (e.g., a favorable response to therapeutic products). For companion diagnostics, clinical performance is usually demonstrated within drug trials.

The FDA examines the design and results of analytical validation studies included in the submission. For example, in the case of immunohistochemistry (IHC) assays, the following types of analytical validation studies have often been important to assess the analytical performance: biochemical characterization of the antibody; assay sensitivity; assay specificity; precision, including reader precision; interlaboratory reproducibility; assay robustness; impact of preanalytical variables; stability; and control cell line validation. For molecular assays, such as PCR- and NGS-based technologies, the following analytical validation studies are often conducted to evaluate the device analytical performance: analytical sensitivity, including limit of blank (LoB), limit of detection (LoD), and limit of quantitation (LoQ; for quantitative assays); analytical specificity, including cross-reactivity and interfering substances; analytical accuracy/concordance, relative to a reference method or validated comparator; precision, including intra-assay repeatability and inter-assay reproducibility; guard banding/

robustness; and stability (e.g., specimens, reagents, and controls). These studies have often been necessary to determine whether a test can accurately and reliably detect/measure the analyte.

The FDA also reviews the evidence submitted in support of the clinical validity of the IVD. In the case of the three approved PD-L1 IHC devices (22C3, 28-8, and SP142), the clinical trial results were examined to evaluate how well the test result correlated with the stated clinical outcome (e.g., overall response rate to the treatment). For each of these tests, a scoring algorithm is used to generate a clinical result, incorporating factors such as the inclusion of staining in tumor cells and/or immune cells and assessing the proportion of each cell type staining in order to assign a positive or negative status. Thus, the FDA review included examining the validation of the scoring algorithm (see Exhibit 68.1). Similarly, for the approved F1CDx NGS assay indicated for tumor

---

[18] PD-L1 IHC 22C3 pharmDx. 2015. www.accessdata.fda.gov/cdrh_docs/pdf15/P150013c.pdf

[19] Highlights of prescribing information—these highlights do not include all the information needed to use KEYTRUDA safely and effectively. www.accessdata.fda.gov/drugsatfda_docs/label/2019/125514s040lbl.pdf

[20] Summary of safety and effectiveness data—P150013/S009. www.accessdata.fda.gov/cdrh_docs/pdf15/P150013S009B.pdf

---

EXHIBIT 68.2 COMPANION DIAGNOSTIC CASE STUDY 2: TMB BIOMARKER IN IMMUNOTHERAPY

Companion Diagnostic: FoundationOne®CDx (F1CDx)

Stated Indications for Use (excerpt): F1CDx is indicated as a companion diagnostic for solid tumor patients with high tumor mutational burden (TMB) at the cut-off of 10 mutations per megabase (mut/Mb) who may benefit from treatment with KEYTRUDA® (pembrolizumab).[21]

Immunotherapy: PD-1-blocking antibody KEYTRUDA (pembrolizumab; Merck Sharp and Dohme Corp.)

Stated Indications for Use (excerpt): Pembrolizumab is indicated for the treatment of adult and pediatric patients with unresectable or metastatic solid tumors with tissue tumor mutational burden-high (TMB-H) [>10 mutations/megabase (mut/Mb)], as determined by an FDA-approved test, that have progressed following prior treatment and who have no satisfactory alternative treatment options.[22]

Clinical Study: In a Phase 2 multicenter, nonrandomized, open-label, multicohort study, the efficacy of pembrolizumab monotherapy was evaluated in 1,050 patients with multiple types of advanced (unresectable or metastatic) solid cancers that had progressed following prior treatment and who had no satisfactory alternative treatment options. TMB biomarker analysis with respect to the cut-point of 10 mutations per megabase (mut/Mb) was retrospectively analyzed by the F1CDx assay. The main efficacy outcome measures were objective response rate (ORR) and duration of response (DoR) in patients who had received at least one dose of pembrolizumab and assessed by blinded independent central review per Response Evaluation Criteria in Solid Tumors (RECIST) 1.1. All together, 102 patients had TMB-H solid tumors based on the cut-off of 10 mut/Mb, and the ORR for these patients was 29%. The median DoR was not reached, with 57% of patients having response durations ≥12 months and 50% of patients having response durations >24 months. Based on tumor response rate and durability of response, pembrolizumab was approved under the FDA's accelerated approval program.

The F1CDx assay was considered essential for the safe and effective use of pembrolizumab in patients with TMB-H (≥10 mut/Mb) solid tumors and was co-approved as an IVD companion diagnostic device with pembrolizumab in June 2020.[23]

FDA, U.S. Food and Drug Administration; IVD, in vitro diagnostic; PD-1, programmed cell death protein-1; TMB, tumor mutational burden.

---

mutational burden (TMB) biomarker detection (see Exhibit 68.2), the clinical trial results supported the safety and effectiveness of the device. TMB is measured by the F1CDx assay by counting the number of eligible mutations in the sequenced tumor DNA, and TMB is communicated as a score in mutations per megabase unit (mut/Mb). The clinical trial evaluated response rate in solid tumor patients with a TMB score ≥10 mut/Mb. FDA review included evaluating the clinical performance of the F1CDx assay for detecting TMB-High (TMB-H) patients with respect to the cut-off of 10 mut/Mb.

Regulation of Investigational Tests

When developing a new IVD for clinical use, or when developing a new use for an existing IVD, the test is typically considered investigational while the performance data are being generated. There are certain FDA regulations that apply to investigational tests, including the Investigational Device Exemption (IDE) regulation found in 21 CFR Part 812. The investigational regulations allow an investigational test to be used in human subjects to collect safety and effectiveness data in the absence of FDA marketing authorization for that test use subject to certain regulatory requirements. Regulatory requirements for an investigational device are determined by the risk posed to study subjects in the clinical studies. For investigational IVDs, the risk primarily derives from the consequences of a false result and the potential harm to study subjects.[24] The majority of IVD development involves investigations "exempt" from 21 CFR Part 812.[25] However, this is not always the case for investigational IVDs in the area of precision medicine, where investigational test results may be reported and used within the therapeutic product clinical trial.

---

[21] FoundationOne®CDx. www.accessdata.fda.gov/cdrh_docs/pdf17/P170019S016C.pdf

[22] Highlights of prescribing information—these highlights do not include all the information needed to use KEYTRUDA safely and effectively. www.accessdata.fda.gov/drugsatfda_docs/label/2021/125514s096lbl.pdf

[23] Next generation sequencing oncology panel, somatic or germline variant detection system. www.accessdata.fda.gov/cdrh_docs/pdf17/P170019S016B.pdf

[24] Note that invasive sampling procedures also may have the potential to introduce harm and therefore can contribute to risk of investigational devices.

[25] 21 CFR 812.2(c).

Some precision medicine trials have used the results from investigational tests to determine eligibility for enrollment of subjects into a clinical trial of an investigational therapeutic agent, or assignment to a particular trial arm, because, for example, there is prior evidence suggesting individuals with a particular marker status will respond better to the investigational agent. A false positive in this example scenario would result in the enrollment of a subject that does not have the marker of interest, and the potential harms to the subject include exposure to treatment side effects without any expectation of benefit and foregoing standard-of-care or other more effective treatments. Other precision medicine trial designs use the results from an investigational test to make sure that, in the randomization of enrolled subjects to the therapeutic treatment arms, there are an appropriate number of test-positive subjects in each arm. The test result in this example is not directing subjects to a particular treatment arm; therefore, a false result in such a trial likely is considered to pose little or no risk of harm to the subject.

For tests that present "significant risk" to study subjects for purposes of 21 CFR Part 812, an IDE submission must be approved by the FDA prior to initiating the clinical study. The FDA reviews the information submitted, including administrative and trial-related information, in assessing whether to disapprove a study under any of the criteria found at 21 CFR 812.30(b), including whether there is reason to believe that the risks to the subjects are not outweighed by the anticipated benefits to the subjects or whether informed consent is inadequate.

In Vitro Diagnostic Companion Diagnostics and Codevelopment

In 2014, the FDA issued a final guidance "In Vitro Companion Diagnostic Devices," defining IVD companion diagnostics as an IVD that provides information that is essential for the safe and effective use of a corresponding therapeutic product[26] and describes the applicable regulatory requirements. The guidance states the FDA's expectation for a companion diagnostic to be approved by the FDA contemporaneously with the approval of the corresponding therapeutic product, such that when a test is necessary for the safe and effective administration of a therapeutic product, a test with adequate performance is available clinically as soon as the therapeutic product is available.

The use of an IVD companion diagnostic device with a therapeutic product is specified in the instructions for use in the labeling of both the IVD and the corresponding therapeutic product, including the labeling of any generic equivalents of the therapeutic product.

Incorporating a test development program into the clinical development program of a therapeutic product is becoming more common in the era of precision medicine. This process is often referred to as codevelopment.[27] Although alignment of the two distinct development programs involves different considerations due to differences in business models and regulatory requirements for the therapeutic product and the IVD, there have been numerous successful codevelopment programs to date.

When it becomes clear that knowledge of the status of a particular biomarker may be important for administering a therapy, the therapeutic product developer often partners with a diagnostic test company that will develop a specific test to be used in the continued clinical studies and/or ultimately marketed for clinical use as the companion diagnostic. Codevelopment programs start at various points in the therapeutic product development process, depending on when the potential need for a diagnostic is identified and the IVD development program is initiated. In general, when a codevelopment program is established early, the therapeutic trial sponsor may be better able to incorporate the needs of the IVD developer (e.g., collection and banking of appropriate specimens for the IVD validation studies) and to design and implement studies that provide the evidence to support premarket applications for both products (e.g., obtaining outcome information about the test-negative population).

When a diagnostic test manufacturer partners with a therapeutic product developer with the goal of contemporaneous co-approval of an IVD and therapeutic, respectively, the device and therapeutic sponsors typically communicate expectations on the timing and execution of the clinical validation. When planning the clinical validation testing to support the performance of the IVD, the device and therapeutic developers align on the study inclusion and exclusion criteria so the primary efficacy population supporting the therapeutic regulatory approval is the same as the device validation population. Alignment on the study population in a codevelopment program ensures consistency in the therapeutic product and the IVD labeling. In addition, the IVD manufacturer typically completes the device analytical validation studies prior to conducting the clinical validation, such that the clinical validation is performed with a fully analytically validated device in its final configuration with the locked scoring algorithm and/or analysis pipeline for reporting results. Early alignment on the IVD validation studies needed to demonstrate

---

[26] Food and Drug Administration Staff. *In Vitro Companion Diagnostic Devices*. 2014. www.fda.gov/downloads/medicaldevices/deviceregulationandguidance/guidancedocuments/ucm262327.pdf

[27] Principles of codevelopment of an in vitro companion diagnostic device with a therapeutic product. www.fda.gov/ucm/groups/fdagov-public/@fdagov-meddev-gen/documents/document/ucm510824.pdf

the safety and effectiveness of the companion diagnostic may facilitate planning for contemporaneous marketing authorizations and thereby contribute to the success of codevelopment programs.

RESOURCES

1. U.S. Food and Drug Administration. *In Vitro Companion Diagnostic Devices*. Published August 2014. www.fda.gov/downloads/medicaldevices/deviceregulationandguidance/guidancedocuments/ucm262327.pdf

2. Bristol-Myers Squibb Company. Highlights of prescribing information—these highlights do not include all the information needed to use. Updated October 2015. http://www.accessdata.fda.gov/drugsatfda_docs/label/2015/125554s005lbl.pdf

3. PD-L1 IHC 28-8 pharmDx. http://www.accessdata.fda.gov/cdrh_docs/pdf15/P150027c.pdf

4. U.S. Food and Drug Administration. Devices Regulated by the Center for Biologics Evaluation and Research. https://www.fda.gov/BiologicsBloodVaccines/DevelopmentApprovalProcess/510kProcess/ucm133429.htm

5. U.S. Food and Drug Administration. Overview of IVD regulation. http://www.fda.gov/MedicalDevices/DeviceRegulationandGuidance/IVDRegulatoryAssistance/ucm123682.htm

6. U.S. Food and Drug Administration. In Vitro Diagnostic (IVD) device studies: frequently asked questions. Published June 2010. https://www.fda.gov/regulatory-information/search-fda-guidance-documents/vitro-diagnostic-ivd-device-studies-frequently-asked-questions

7. U.S. Food and Drug Administration. Principles for codevelopment of an in vitro companion diagnostic device with a therapeutic product. Published July 2016. https://www.fda.gov/ucm/groups/fdagov-public/@fdagov-meddev-gen/documents/document/ucm510824.pdf

Index

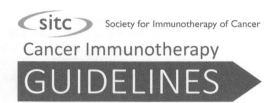

SITC Clinical Practice Guidelines Mobile App

The SITC Clinical Practice Guidelines (CPG) Mobile App is the first and only tool of its kind, offering direct, easy, portable access to SITC's clinical practice guidelines via phone or tablet. Highlighting key information from SITC's published guidelines, the SITC CPG App features evidence- and expert consensus-based recommendations on key aspects of immunotherapy treatment as well as interactive tools and companion educational resources. From biomarkers and therapy selection to quality of life and management of immune-related adverse events, busy clinicians will find the SITC CPG App as the go-to resource on when and how to use immunotherapy to help improve outcomes for patients with cancer.

Key Features

- Clean and simple navigation with a modern interface
- Interactive tools and tables at your fingertips
- Advanced search functionality for fast access to the content clinicians need
- Bookmarking and annotation capabilities throughout for future fast reference
- Timely updates when new practice-changing data or approvals become available
- Companion educational offerings to enhance understanding of guideline recommendations
- Free download with open-access content

sitcancer.org/CPG-app

   #SITCGuidelines

Explore the App

Download and explore the free SITC CPG App for iOS or Android.

Download on the App Store

GET IT ON Google Play

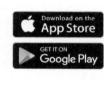

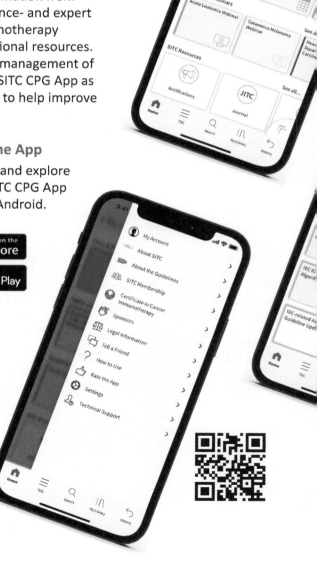